Oxford Textbook of Pathology

Volume 1
Principles of Pathology

Edited by

James O'D. McGee
Nuffield Department of Pathology
and Bacteriology
University of Oxford

Peter G. Isaacson
University College and Middlesex
School of Medicine
University College, London

Nicholas A. Wright
Royal Postgraduate Medical School
Hammersmith Hospital

Associate editors
Heather M. Dick
Department of Medical Microbiology
University of Dundee

Mary P. E. Slack
Nuffield Department of Pathology
and Bacteriology
University of Oxford

OXFORD   NEW YORK   TOKYO
Oxford University Press
1992

Oxford University Press, Walton Street, Oxford OX2 6DP

Oxford   New York   Toronto
Delhi   Bombay   Calcutta   Madras   Karachi
Petaling Jaya   Singapore   Hong Kong   Tokyo
Nairobi   Dar es Salaam   Cape Town
Melbourne   Auckland

and associated companies in
Berlin   Ibadan

Oxford is a trade mark of Oxford University Press

Published in the United States
by Oxford University Press, New York

A catalogue record for this book is available from the British Library

Library of Congress Cataloging-in-Publication Data
(Cataloging data is available)
ISBN 0–19–261976–4 (hbk. : set)
ISBN 0–19–261973–X (hbk. Vol. 1)
ISBN 0–19–261975–6 (hbk. Vol. 2a)   } Available as part of set only
ISBN 0–19–262273–0 (hbk. Vol. 2b)
ISBN 0–19–261972–1 (pbk. Vol. 1)
ISBN 0–19–261974–8 (pbk. Vol. 2)
ISBN 0–19–262274–9 (pbk. Vol. 2a)   } Available as part of Vol. 2 'set' only
ISBN 0–19–262275–7 (pbk. Vol. 2b)

Typeset by
Cotswold Typesetting Ltd, Gloucester
Printed in Great Britain by
William Collins Sons and Company Ltd, Glasgow

Preface

Pathology has been revolutionized over the past 20 years by an explosion of new knowledge generated by extensive scientific investigation of the cellular and molecular biology of human tissues. This has resulted from the introduction of a plethora of new molecular techniques, and the use of endoscopic and fine-needle tissue sampling which provide tissues previously only seen after surgical excision or at autopsy. What students of pathology need to know and learn today, therefore, is very different from the requirements two decades ago. The speed and magnitude of changes in pathology and in the pathologist's role are such that there is now a need to redefine the science of pathology and its future directions. It is in this context that we have embarked on this book. No textbook can ever take the place of careful study of original papers but we trust that this book will constitute an authoritative text for trainee and established pathologists as they get to grips with the new pathology.

The science of pathology does not lend itself easily to an encapsulating definition. The definitions proposed are either too narrow (the morphological basis of disease) or too broad (the study of disease) to be useful. It is clear, however, that pathology as we know it today grew from the gross morphological description of diseased organs, and following Virchow's discovery of the cellular basis of disease in the last century, pathology established itself as the core of medicine. As tissue preparative techniques and light microscopes improved, pathologists described natural and experimentally induced diseases in ever greater detail, culminating in the ultrastructural descriptions of the late 1950s and early 1960s. At about that time, Sir Roy Cameron summed up the direction of pathology as follows: 'The main endeavour has been to resolve the fundamental problems of pathology—injury, recovery, death—into simpler cellular, subcellular and eventually chemical components.' This we can now do with considerable accuracy. For some, this descriptive approach is sufficient; the problem is defined and the challenge is to treat the patient.

There is, however, a radically different view. In 1892, Victor Horsley wrote 'What is currently thought of as pathology is nothing of the sort—it is morbid anatomy. The pathologist should be a student of disordered function.' We strongly endorse this view. The advent of *in situ* phenotyping and genotyping of cells in the 1970s and 1980s respectively made it possible to ascribe synthetic function and dysfunction to intact cells. This, together with diagnostic morphology, has led to a new understanding of disease mechanisms and with it more accurate diagnosis and improved patient management. Over the past six years, new analytical nucleic acid techniques have emerged almost monthly. Some, such as the polymerase chain reaction, have had an immediate and profound impact on laboratory medicine, while others are being assimilated more cautiously. As practising clinicians, we foresee that these new and future methodologies will advance our knowledge of disease aetiopathogenesis and hence patient care. As medical scientists, we are excited by the future prospects because pathology laboratories will provide the largest repositories of fully documented DNA and RNA.

Volume 1 of the Oxford Textbook of Pathology examines the Principles of Pathology linking basic science and clinical observation to explain disease processes. Here, concepts of normal cell and chromosome/gene structure and function are described as a prelude to an account of the cellular, subcellular, and molecular mechanisms involved in genetic disorders, cell death, defence mechanisms, inflammation, pathophysiology of infection, neoplasia, and vascular disorders. Environmental and developmental pathology are also included. Emphasis is placed on the application of cell and molecular biology and the impact that these have had in unravelling the origins of disease. Because it is clear that we are far from a complete understanding of any single general principle, the text highlights our areas of ignorance and suggests ways of thinking and future experimental approaches. We believe it will provide a sound basis from which pathologists and basic scientists can approach the latest literature.

In Volume 2 (2a and 2b), we present the Pathology of Systems. Because of our conviction that the practice of clinical medicine should be multidisciplinary in its approach, we have shown the structural basis of disease in a clinical context. Each chapter starts with an overview of the normal structure and function of the system. The description of each disease is preceded by a précis of its clinical presentation and is followed by an analysis of aetiopathogenesis where this is known. In putting together Volume 2, we have been comprehensive in our approach without necessarily being encyclopaedic. The relevance of molecular pathology to specific disease processes is stressed. However, the main emphasis in this volume remains the cellular basis of disease and the role of pathology in clinical diagnosis. The book ends with a chapter on diagnostic and molecular investigative techniques which we hope will encourage pathologists to look deeper than the images conveyed by visible light through a microscope tube. By combining traditional methods of observation with the new molecular pathology, medical and non-medical scientists will each grow in their appreciation and understanding of disease processes. The future of pathology lies not only in the refinement of diagnosis and aetiology of disease but also in analysis of the mechanistic networks which regulate cellular responses to tissue and cell injury.

Our aim in this book has been to make a definitive statement. Thus we have elected to invite contributions from many leading experts. What may have been lost in continuity of style will, we hope, be compensated for by the high quality of the content. We have endeavoured to give the authors the opportunity to present their subjects comprehensively and encouraged the liberal use of colour diagrams and gross and microscopic photographs. This has resulted in a substantial book—rather more substantial than we originally envisaged—but one which we trust is pleasing to read in depth whilst being accessible for brief consultation. Our thanks are due to all contributors for their patience and for the care and enthusiasm with which they have approached their task. We believe that the finished product will expunge the memories of inevitable irritations along the way. To readers, we hope you enjoy the text and share in the excitement of discovery and the satisfaction of solving some of the problems we have outlined. We encourage readers to write to us with suggestions for improvement, or for changes of emphasis, which we will be glad to consider when planning future editions.

University of Oxford,   J.O'D.M.
University College, London, and   P.G.I.
Royal Postgraduate Medical School,   N.A.W.
    Hammersmith Hospital
November 1991

Acknowledgements

We would like to thank Mrs Penny Messer, Miss Lesley Watts, Mrs Sue Slaymark, Mrs Jean Garnet, and Miss Susan Chandler, whose organizational and administrative skills and eye for detail have kept this project flowing smoothly. We would also like to thank the many staff at Oxford University Press who have been involved in the production of this book. It has been a particular pleasure working with them as they have been professionally competent, encouraging, and effectively persistent over what sometimes seemed major problems.

Without the patience and encouragement of our wives and families, this book would not have seen the light of day. We express our gratitude to them for what they have had to endure during the gestation of this book.

The illustrations were drawn by Jane Fallows, Jane Templeman, and Focal Image Ltd.

List of chapters

Contents

11   Principles of developmental pathology   779

J. S. Wigglesworth

Contributors

M. Alison, Department of Histopathology, Royal Postgraduate Medical School, Hammersmith Hospital, Du Cane Road, London W12 0HS, UK

S. P. Allwork, British Heart Foundation Museum of Heart Diseases, Institute of Child Health, Guildford Street, London WC1N 1EH, UK

R. H. Anderson, National Heart and Lung Institute, Dove House Street, London SW3 6LY, UK

T. J. Anderson, University of Edinburgh, Department of Pathology, The Medical School, Teviot Place, Edinburgh EH8 9AG, UK

I. D. Ansell, Department of Pathology, City Hospital, Hucknall Road, Nottingham NG5 1PB, UK

P. P. Anthony, University of Exeter, Postgraduate Medical School, Area Department of Pathology, Church Lane, Heavitree, Exeter EX2 5DY, UK

J. P. Arbuthnott, Vice-Chancellor, University of Strathclyde, Glasgow, UK

J. K. Aronson, University of Oxford, Medical Research Council Clinical Pharmacology Unit, Department of Clinical Pharmacology, Radcliffe Infirmary, Woodstock Road, Oxford OX2 6HE, UK

N. A. Athanasou, Department of Histopathology, Nuffield Orthopaedic Centre, Headington, Oxford OX3 7LD, UK

F. Barker, Department of Histopathology, Royal Postgraduate Medical School, Hammersmith Hospital, Du Cane Road, London W12 0HS, UK

J. H. Baron, Department of Surgery, Royal Postgraduate Medical School, Hammersmith Hospital, Du Cane Road, London W12 0HS, UK

C. L. Berry, Department of Pathology, The London Hospital Medical College, The London Hospital, London E1 2AD, UK

M. Berry, Department of Anatomy, Guy's and St Thomas's Hospitals, London Bridge, London SE1 9RT, UK

E. Beutler, Department of Molecular and Experimental Medicine, The Scripps Research Institute, 10666 North Torrey Pines Road, La Jolla, CA 92037, USA

P. C. L. Beverley, Imperial Cancer Research Fund Human Tumour Immunology Group, The Courtauld Institute of Biochemistry, University College and Middlesex School of Medicine, 91 Riding House Street, London W10 8BT, UK

S. R. Bloom, Department of Medicine, Royal Postgraduate Medical School, Hammersmith Hospital, Du Cane Road, London W12 0HS, UK

L. G. Bobrow, Department of Histopathology, University College and Middlesex School of Medicine, University Street, London WC1E 6JJ, UK

A. R. Boobis, Department of Clinical Pharmacology, Royal Postgraduate Medical School, Hammersmith Hospital, Du Cane Road, London W12 0HS, UK

J. Bridger, Department of Histopathology, Royal Postgraduate Medical School, Hammersmith Hospital, Du Cane Road, London W12 0HS, UK

C. H. Buckley, Central Manchester Health Authority, Department of Pathology, St Mary's Hospital, Whitworth Park, Manchester M13 0JH, UK

J. Burns, University of Oxford, Nuffield Department of Pathology and Bacteriology, John Radcliffe Hospital, Headington, Oxford OX3 9DU, UK

K. A. Calman, Chief Medical Officer, Department of Health, Richmond House, 79 Whitehall, London SW1A 2NS, UK

S. Cameron, The Queen's University of Belfast, Department of Pathology, Grosvenor Road, Belfast B12 6BL, UK

R.L. Carter, Histopathology Department, Institute of Cancer Research, Royal Marsden Hospital, Sutton, Surrey SM2 5PX, UK

T.J. Chambers, Department of Histopathology, St George's Hospital Medical School, Cranmer Terrace, Tooting, London SW17 0RE, UK

I. Chanarin, Medical Research Council Clinical Research Centre, Watford Road, Harrow, Middlesex HA1 3UJ, UK

A. J. Chaplin, Department of Histopathology, John Radcliffe Hospital, Headington, Oxford OX3 9DU, UK

R. W. Chapman, Gastroenterology Unit, Level 2, John Radcliffe Hospital, Headington, Oxford OX3 9DU, UK

J. Cohen, Infectious Diseases Unit, Department of Bacteriology and Medicine, Royal Postgraduate Medical School, Hammersmith Hospital, London W12 0HS, UK

G. Cole, Department of Pathology, University of Wales College of Medicine, Heath Park, Cardiff CF4 4XN, UK

D. V. Coleman, Department of Cytopathology, St Mary's Hospital, London W2 1NY, UK

K. Cooper, University of Oxford, Nuffield Department of Pathology and Bacteriology, John Radcliffe Hospital, Headington, Oxford OX3 9DU, UK

T. Creagh, Department of Histopathology, Royal Postgraduate Medical School, Hammersmith Hospital, Du Cane Road, London W12 0HS, UK

J. Crocker, Department of Histopathology, East Birmingham Hospital, Bordesley Green East, Birmingham B9 5ST, UK

B. Crossley, 27422 La Cabra, Mission Viejo, CA 92691, USA

A. J. D'Ardenne, Histopathology Department, St Bartholomew's Hospital Medical College, West Smithfield, London EC1A 7BE, UK

D. S. Davies, Department of Clinical Pharmacology, Royal Postgraduate Medical School, Hammersmith Hospital, Du Cane Road, London W12 0HS, UK

M. J. Davies, St George's Hospital Medical School, Department of Cardiological Sciences, Cranmer Terrace, London SW17 0RE, UK

J. Denekamp, Cancer Research Campaign, Gray Laboratory, PO Box 100, Mount Vernon Hospital, Northwood, Middlesex HA6 2RN, UK

V. J. Desmet, Universitaire Ziekenhuizen Leuven, Dienst Pathologische Ontleedkunde II, Minderbroedersstraat 12, B-3000 Leuven, Belgium

T. M. Dexter, Paterson Institute for Cancer Research, Christie Hospital (NHS) Trust, Wilmslow Road, Manchester M20 9BX, UK

H. M. Dick, Department of Medical Microbiology, University of Dundee Medical School, Ninewells Hospital, Dundee DD1 9SY, UK

R. Doll, University of Oxford, Imperial Cancer Research Fund, Cancer Epidemiology and Clinical Trials Unit, Gibson Building, Radcliffe Infirmary, Oxford OX2 6HE, UK

M. S. Dunnill, Department of Histopathology, Level 1, John Radcliffe Hospital, Headington, Oxford OX3 9DU, UK

E. Duvall, University of Edinburgh, Department of Pathology, The Medical School, Teviot Place, Edinburgh EH8 9AG, UK

M. Eastwood, University of Edinburgh, Wolfson Gastrointestinal Laboratories, Western General Hospital, Edinburgh EH4 2XU, UK

H. A. Ellis, 16 Southland, Tynemouth, Tyne and Wear, UK

M. M. Esiri, University of Oxford, Department of Neuropathology, Radcliffe Infirmary, Woodstock Road, Oxford OX2 6HE, UK

D. J. Evans, Department of Histopathology, St Mary's Hospital Medical School, Paddington, London W2 1PG, UK

D. J. Fawthrop, Department of Clinical Pharmacology, Royal Postgraduate Medical School, Hammersmith Hospital, Du Cane Road, London W12 0HS, UK

M. Feldmann, The Charing Cross Sunley Research Centre, Lurgan Avenue, Hammersmith, London W6 8SW, UK

M. A. Ferguson-Smith, University of Cambridge, Department of Pathology, Tennis Court Road, Cambridge CB2 1QP, UK

J. D. Firth, Nuffield Department of Clinical Medicine, John Radcliffe Hospital, Headington, Oxford OX3 9DU, UK

A. M. Flanagan, Department of Pathology, St George's Hospital, Cranmer Terrace, Tooting, London SW17 0RE, UK

D. M. J. Flannery, University of Oxford, Nuffield Department of Pathology and Bacteriology, John Radcliffe Hospital, Headington, Oxford OX3 9DU, UK

K. A. Fleming, University of Oxford, Nuffield Department of Pathology and Bacteriology, John Radcliffe Hospital, Headington, Oxford OX3 9DU, UK

C. D. M. Fletcher, Cancer Research Campaign Soft Tissue Tumour Unit, United Medical and Dental Schools, Guy's and St Thomas's Hospitals, Department of Histopathology, St Thomas's Hospital, London SE1 7EH, UK

H. Fox, University of Manchester, Department of Pathology, Stopford Building, Oxford Road, Manchester M13 9PT, UK

A. P. Fraise, Microbiology Department, Selly Oak Hospital, Raddle Barn Road, Birmingham B29 6JD, UK

A. J. Franks, University of Leeds, Department of Public Health Medicine, 32 Hyde Terrace, Leeds LS2 9LN, UK

P. J. Gallagher, Department of Pathology, Southampton University Hospitals, Southampton SO9 4XY, UK

A. Gallimore, Department of Histopathology, Royal Postgraduate Medical School, Hammersmith Hospital, Du Cane Road, London W12 0NN, UK

K. C. Gatter, University of Oxford, Nuffield Department of Pathology and Bacteriology, John Radcliffe Hospital, Headington, Oxford OX3 9DU, UK

A. R. Gibbs, Department of Pathology, Llandough Hospital, Penarth, Glamorgan CF6 1XN, UK

J. M. Goldman, Medical Research Council Leukaemia Research Unit, Department of Haematology, Royal Postgraduate Medical School, Hammersmith Hospital, Du Cane Road, London W12 0HS, UK

S. Gordon, University of Oxford, Sir William Dunn School of Pathology, South Parks Road, Oxford OX1 3RE, UK

R. B. Goudie, University of Glasgow, Department of Pathology, Royal Infirmary, Castle Street, Glasgow G4 0SF, UK

C. F. Graham, University of Oxford, Cancer Research Campaign Growth Factors Group, Department of Zoology, South Parks Road, Oxford OX1 3PS, UK

D. G. Grahame-Smith, University of Oxford, Clinical Pharmacology Department, Radcliffe Infirmary, Oxford OX2 6HE, UK

G. A. Gresham, University of Cambridge, Department of Morbid Anatomy and Histopathology, The John Bonnet Clinical Laboratories, Addenbrooke's Hospital, Hills Road, Cambridge, CB2 2QQ, UK

D. Griffiths, Department of Pathology, University of Wales College of Medicine, Heath Park, Cardiff CF4 4XN, UK

M. Griffiths, University College and Middlesex School of Medicine, Department of Histopathology, Bland Sutton Institute, The Middlesex Hospital, London W1P 7PN, UK

P. D. Griffiths, Department of Virology, Royal Free Hospital, Hampstead, London NW3 2QG, UK

N. R. Grist, University of Glasgow, Communicable Diseases (Scotland) Unit, Ruchill Hospital, Glasgow G20 9NB, UK

B. A. Gusterson, Institute of Cancer Research, Royal Cancer Hospital, Department of Histopathology, The Haddow Laboratories, Clifton Avenue, Sutton, Surrey SM2 5PX, UK

T. J. Hamblin, Southampton University, Faculty of Medicine, Medicine 1, Level D, Centre Block, Southampton General Hospital, Tremona Road, Southampton, SO9 4XY, UK

D. G. Harnden, Paterson Institute for Cancer Research, Christie Hospital (NHS) Trust, Wilmslow Road, Manchester M20 9BX, UK

G. Hart, University of Oxford, Department of Cardiovascular Medicine, John Radcliffe Hospital, Headington, Oxford OX3 9DU, UK

D. A. Heath, University of Liverpool, Department of Pathology, Duncan Building, Royal Liverpool Hospital, PO Box 147, Liverpool L39 3BX, UK

C. S. Herrington, University of Oxford, Nuffield Department of Pathology and Bacteriology, John Radcliffe Hospital, Headington, Oxford OX3 9DU, UK

S. T. Holgate, Faculty of Medicine, Medicine 1, Level D, Centre Block, Southampton General Hospital, Tremona Road, Southampton SO9 4XY, UK

E. R. Horak, University of Oxford, Nuffield Department of Pathology and Bacteriology, John Radcliffe Hospital, Headington, Oxford OX3 9DU, UK

W. J. Hume, University of Leeds, Department of Dental Surgery, School of Dentistry, Clarendon Way, Leeds LS2 9JT, UK

S. E. Humphries, The Charing Cross Sunley Research Centre, 1 Lurgan Avenue, Hammersmith, London W6 8LW, UK

H. R. Ingham, Newcastle Regional Public Health Laboratory, Institute of Pathology, General Hospital, Westgate Road, Newcastle upon Tyne, Tyne and Wear NE4 6BE, UK

P. G. Isaacson, Department of Histopathology, University College and Middlesex School of Medicine, University Street, London WC1E 6JJ, UK

J. R. Jass, University of Auckland, Department of Pathology, School of Medicine, Private Bag, Auckland, New Zealand

H. M. H. Kamel, The Queen's University of Belfast, Department of Pathology, Grosvenor Road, Belfast BT12 6BL, UK

J. W. Keeling, Paediatric Pathology Department, Royal Hospital for Sick Children, 2 Rillbank Crescent, Edinburgh EH9 1LF, UK

P. M. A. Kelly, Department of Pathology, Mater Misericordiae Hospital, Eccles Street, Dublin 7, Ireland

T. Krausz, Department of Histopathology, Royal Postgraduate Medical School, Hammersmith Hospital, Du Cane Road, London W12 0HS, UK

P. J. Lachmann, University of Cambridge, Department of Pathology, Medical Research Council Centre, Hills Road, Cambridge CB2 2QH, UK

I. A. Lampert, Department of Histopathology, Ealing Hospital, General Wing, Uxbridge Road, Southall, Middlesex UB1 3HW, UK

P. L. Lantos, Department of Neuropathology, Institute of Psychiatry, de Crespigny Park, Denmark Hill, London SE5 8AF, UK

J. G. G. Ledingham, University of Oxford, Nuffield Department of Clinical Medicine, John Radcliffe Hospital, Headington, Oxford OX3 9DU, UK

F. D. Lee, University of Glasgow, Department of Pathology, The Royal Infirmary, Castle Street, Glasgow G4 0SF, UK

C. E. Lewis, University of Oxford, Nuffield Department of Pathology and Bacteriology, John Radcliffe Hospital, Headington, Oxford OX3 9DU, UK

P. D. Lewis, Department of Histopathology, Royal Postgraduate Medical School, Hammersmith Hospital, Du Cane Road, London W12 0HS, UK

G. B. M. Lindop, University of Glasgow, Department of Pathology, Western Infirmary, Glasgow G11 6NT, UK

J. Lorenzen, Universitat zu Koln, Abteilung Pathologie, Joseph-Stelzmann- Strasse 9, 5000 Koln 4, Germany

T. Lowhagen, Division of Clinical Cytology, World Health Organization Collaborating Centre, Department of Pathology, Karolinska Institute and Hospital, S 104 01, Stockholm, Sweden

D. R. Lucas, Department of Ophthalmology, Manchester Royal Eye Hospital, Oxford Road, Manchester M13 9WH, UK

S. Lucas, Department of Histopathology, University College and Middlesex School of Medicine, University Street, London WC1E 6JJ, UK

D. C. Linch, Department of Haematology, University College and Middlesex School of Medicine, University Street, London WC1E 6JJ, UK

I. C. M. MacLennan, The University of Birmingham, Department of Immunology, The Medical School, Vincent Drive, Birmingham B15 2JT, UK

I. A. Magnus, Institute of Dermatology, Guy's and St Thomas's Hospitals Medical Schools, London SE1 7EH, UK

D. Y. Mason, Leukaemia Research Fund, Immunodiagnostics Unit, University of Oxford, Nuffield Department of Pathology and Bacteriology, Haematology Section, John Radcliffe Hospital, Headington, Oxford OX3 9DU, UK

D. F. W. McCormick, The Queen's University of Belfast, Department of Pathology, Grosvenor Road, Belfast BT12 6BL, UK

J. O'D. McGee, University of Oxford, Nuffield Department of Pathology and Bacteriology, John Radcliffe Hospital, Headington, Oxford OX3 9DU, UK

P. H. McKee, Department of Histopathology, Guy's and St Thomas's Hospitals Medical Schools, St Thomas's Hospital, London SE1 7EH, UK

A. E. M. McLean, Department of Clinical Pharmacology, University College and Middlesex School of Medicine, 5 University Street, London WC1E 6JJ, UK

A. J. McMichael, University of Oxford, Nuffield Department of Medicine, John Radcliffe Hospital, Headington, Oxford OX3 9DU, UK

L. Michaels, Department of Histopathology, University College and Middlesex School of Medicine, London WC1E 6JJ, UK

A. Michalowski, Onkologiska Kliniken, Lasaretet 1 Lund,, 221-85 Lund, Sweden

N. A. Mitchison, Forschungslaboratorium, Robert Koch Institut, Haus 11, Nordufer 20, D-1000 Berlin 65, Germany

J. Monjardino, Department of Medicine, Queen Elizabeth the Queen Mother Wing, St Mary's Hospital Medical School, London W2 1PE, UK

W. J. Mooi, Netherlands Cancer Institute, Plesmanlaan 121, 1066 CX Amsterdam, The Netherlands

P. R. Morgan, Department of Oral Medicine and Pathology, Floor 28, Guy's Tower, Guy's Hospital, London SE1 9RT, UK

A. Morley, Department of Pathology, Royal Victoria Infirmary, Newcastle upon Tyne, Tyne and Wear NE1 4LP, UK

P. J. Morris, University of Oxford, Nuffield Department of Surgery, John Radcliffe Hospital, Headington, Oxford OX3 9DU, UK

A. M. Neville, Ludwig Institute for Cancer Research, Hedges House, 153/5 Regent Street, London W1R 7FD, UK

D. C. Old, University of Dundee, Department of Medical Microbiology, Ninewells Hospital, Dundee DD1 9SY, UK

E. G. J. Olsen, Department of Histopathology, Royal Brompton National Heart and Lung Hospital, Sydney Street, London SW3 6ND, UK

D. L. Page, Department of Pathology, Vanderbilt University Medical School, Nashville, TN 37232, USA

J. Parr, Department of Opthalmology, Manchester Royal Eye Hospital, Oxford Road, Manchester M13 9WH, UK

D. V. Parums, University of Oxford, Nuffield Department of Pathology and Bacteriology, John Radcliffe Hospital, Headington, Oxford OX3 9DU, UK

K. Paterson, Department of Haematology, University College and Middlesex School of Medicine, University Street, London WC1E 6JJ, UK

R. S. Patrick, University Department of Pathology, Royal Infirmary, Castle Street, Glasgow G4 0SF, UK

A. J. Pinching, Department of Immunology, St Mary's Hospital Medical School, London W2 1PG, UK

J. M. Polak, Histochemistry Department, Royal Postgraduate Medical School, Hammersmith Hospital, Du Cane Road, London W12 0NN, UK

A. Pomerance, Histopathology and Cytopathology, Harefield and Mount Vernon Pathology Laboratories, Mount Vernon Hospital, Northwood, Middlesex HA6 2RN, UK

J. S. Porterfield, University of Oxford, Sir William Dunn School of Pathology, South Parks Road, Oxford OX1 3RE, UK

B. Portmann, Institute of Liver Studies, King's College School of Medicine and Dentistry, Denmark Hill, London SE5 8RX, UK

C. S. Potten, Cancer Research Campaign, Department of Epithelial Biology, Paterson Institute for Cancer Research, Christie Hospital (NHS) Trust, Wilmslow Road, Manchester M20 9BX, UK

A. B. Price, Department of Histopathology, Northwick Park Hospital, Watford Road, Harrow, Middlesex HA1 3UJ, UK

L. Pusztai, University of Oxford, Nuffield Department of Pathology and Bacteriology, John Radcliffe Hospital, Headington, Oxford OX3 9DU, UK

P. Quirke, The University of Leeds, Department of Pathology, Leeds, Yorkshire LS2 9JT, UK

A. D. Ramsay, University of Southampton, Department of Pathology, Faculty of Medicine, Level E, South Lab/Path Block, Southampton General Hospital, Tremona Road, Southampton SO9 4XY, UK

J. G. Ratcliffe, Wolfson Research Laboratories, Department of Clinical Chemistry, Queen Elizabeth Medical Centre, Edgbaston, Birmingham B15 2TH, UK

P. J. Ratcliffe, University of Oxford, Nuffield Department of Clinical Medicine, John Radcliffe Hospital, Headington, Oxford OX3 9DU, UK

E. L. Rees, Department of Anatomy, Guy's and St Thomas's Hospitals, London Bridge, London SE1 9RT, UK

H. C. Rees, Department of Histopathology, St Bartholomew's Hospital, West Smithfield, London EC1A 7BE, UK

P. A. Revell, Department of Morbid Anatomy, The London Hospital Medical College, The London Hospital, London E1 1BB, UK

M. D. Richardson, Department of Medical Mycology, Anderson Building, 56 Dumbarton Road, Glasgow G11 6NU, UK

P. W. J. Rigby, Laboratory of Eukaryotic Molecular Genetics, Medical Research Council National Institute for Medical Research, The Ridgeway, Mill Hill, London NW7 1AA, UK

M. A. Ritter, Department of Immunology, Royal Postgraduate Medical School, Hammersmith Hospital, Du Cane Road, London W12 0HS, UK

C. R. Rizza, Oxford Haemophilia Centre, Churchill Hospital, Headington, Oxford OX3 7LJ, UK

J. W. Rode, Department of Anatomical Pathology, St Vincent's Hospital and University of Melbourne, 41 Victoria Parade, Fitzroy, Melbourne, Victoria 3065, Australia

J. Rosai, Department of Pathology, Sloan Kettering Institute of Cancer Studies, New York, NY, USA

R. Ross, University of Washington, Department of Pathology, School of Medicine, Seattle, WA 98195, USA

T. J. Ryan, Department of Dermatology, Slade Hospital, Oxford OX3 7JH, UK

V. Sams, Department of Histopathology, University College and Middlesex School of Medicine, University Street, London WC1E 6JJ, UK

P. J. Scheuer, University of London, Department of Histopathology, Royal Free Hospital School of Medicine, The Royal Free Hospital, Pond Street, London NW3 2QG, UK

J. B. Schofield, Department of Histopathology, Royal Postgraduate Medical School, Hammersmith Hospital, Du Cane Road, London W12 0HS, UK

A. W. Segal, Department of Medicine, University College and Middlesex School of Medicine, The Rayne Institute, University Street, London WC1E 6JJ, UK

J. B. Selkon, Oxford Regional Public Health Laboratory, Level 6/7, John Radcliffe Hospital, Headington, Oxford OX3 9DU, UK

N. A. Shepherd, Department of Histopathology, Gloucestershire Royal Hospital, Great Western Road, Gloucester GL1 3NN, UK

B. J. Shepstone, University of Oxford, Department of Radiology, John Radcliffe Hospital, Headington, Oxford, OX3 9DU, UK

P. R. Sisson, Newcastle Regional Public Health Laboratory, Institute of Pathology, General Hospital, Westgate Road, Newcastle upon Tyne, Tyne and Wear, NE4 6BE, UK

L. Skooge, Division of Clinical Cytology, World Health Organization Collaborating Centre, Department of Pathology, Karolinska Institute and Hospital, S 104 01 Stockholm, Sweden

J. M. W. Slack, University of Oxford, Imperial Cancer Research Fund Developmental Biology Unit, Department of Zoology, South Parks Road, Oxford OX1 3PS, UK

M. P. E. Slack, University of Oxford, Nuffield Department of Pathology and Bacteriology, Microbiology Section, Level 7, John Radcliffe Hospital, Headington, Oxford OX3 9DU, UK

P. M. Speight, Joint Department of Oral Pathology, The London Hospital Medical College and Institute of Dental Surgery, Eastman Dental Hospital, 256 Gray's Inn Road, London WC1X 8LD, UK

J. Spencer, Department of Histopathology, University College and Middlesex School of Medicine, University Street, London WC1E 6JJ, UK

C. J. F. Spry, St George's Hospital Medical School, Cardiovascular Immunology Research Group, Department of Immunology, Jenner Wing, Cranmer Terrace, London SW17 0RE, UK

M. W. Stanley, Hennipin County Medical Center, Department of Pathology and Laboratory Medicine, 701 Park Avenue South, MN 55415, USA

A. G. Stansfeld, Department of Pathology, St Batholomew's Hospital, West Smithfield, London EC1A 7BE, UK

J. E. Stickland, University of Oxford, Nuffield Department of Pathology and Bacteriology, John Radcliffe Hospital, Headington, Oxford OX3 9DU, UK

B. C. Sykes, University of Oxford, Nuffield Department of Pathology and Bacteriology, John Radcliffe Hospital, Headington, Oxford OX3 9DU, UK

P. J. Talmud, The Charing Cross Hospital, Sunley Research Centre, 1 Lurgan Avenue, Hammersmith, London W6 8LW, UK

D. Tarin, University of Oxford, Nuffield Department of Pathology and Bacteriology, John Radcliffe Hospital, Headington, Oxford OX3 9DU, UK

J. M. Theaker, Department of Pathology, Level E, Southampton General Hospital, Tremona Road, Southampton SO9 4XY, UK

H. C. Thomas, Department of Medicine, Queen Elizabeth the Queen Mother Wing, St Mary's Hospital Medical School, Praed Street, Paddington, London W2 1NY, UK

H. Thompson, Department of Histopathology, The General Hospital, Steelhouse Lane, Birmingham B4 6NH, UK

S. Tinkler, 53 Mount View Road, London N4, UK

P. G. Toner, The Queen's University of Belfast, Department of Pathology, Grosvenor Road, Belfast BT12 6BL, UK

J. Trowell, University of Oxford, Department of General Medicine, John Radcliffe Hospital, Headington, Oxford, OX3 9DU, UK

D. True, Department of Pathology, Yale University, Connecticut, USA

J. L. Turk, Department of Pathology, Royal College of Surgeons of England, Hunterian Institute, 35/43 Lincoln's Inn Field, London WC2A 3PN, UK

D. R. Turner, University of Nottingham, Department of Pathology, University Hospital, Queen's Medical Centre, Nottingham, NG7 2UH, UK

M. W. Turner, University of London, Molecular Immunology Unit, Institute of Child Health, 30 Guildford Street, London WC1N 1EH, UK

N. C. Turner, Department of Clinical Pharmacology, Royal Postgraduate Medical School, Hammersmith Hospital, Du Cane Road, London W12 0NN, UK

C.A. Wagenwoort, Erasmus University, PO Box 1738, 3000 Rotterdam, The Netherlands

J. C. Wagner, Medical Research Council External Staff, Team on Occupational Lung Diseases, Llandough Hospital, Penarth, Glamorgan CF6 1XW, UK

J. S. Wainscoat, Department of Haematology, Level 4, John Radcliffe Hospital, Headington, Oxford, OX3 9DU, UK

M. J. Waiport, Rheumatology Unit, Royal Postgraduate Medical School, Du Cane Road, London W12 0PP, UK

F. M. Watt, Imperial Cancer Research Fund Laboratories, PO Box 123, Lincoln's Inn Fields, London WC2A 3PX, UK

D. J. Weatherall, University of Oxford, Nuffield Department of Clinical Medicine, John Radcliffe Hospital, Headington, Oxford, OX3 9DU, UK

A. D. B. Webster, Clinical Research Centre, Division of Immunological Medicine, Watford Road, Harrow, Middlesex HA1 3UJ, UK

H. K. Weinbren, Royal Postgraduate Medical School, Hammersmith Hospital, Du Cane Road, London W12 0HS, UK

R. O. Weller, Department of Neuropathology, Level E, South Lab/Path Block, Southampton General Hospital, Tremona Road, Southampton SO9 4XY, UK

J. S. Wigglesworth, Department of Histopathology, Neonatal and Child Health, Royal Postgraduate Medical School, Hammersmith Hospital, Du Cane Road, London W12 0HS, UK

D. G. D. Wight, Department of Morbid Anatomy and Histopathology, The John Bonnet Clinical Laboratories, Addenbrooke's Hospital, Hills Road, Cambridge CB2 2QQ, UK

M. J. Wilkins, Department of Pathology, St Mary's Hospital Medical School, Paddington, London W2 1PG, UK

D. M. Williams, Department of Oral Pathology, Dental School, The London Hospital Medical College, Turner Street, London E1 2AD, UK

G. T. Williams, Department of Pathology, University of Wales College of Medicine, Heath Park, Cardiff CF4 4XN, UK

S. P. Wolff, Department of Clinical Pharmacology, University College and Middlesex School of Medicine, 5 University Street, London WC1E 6JJ, UK

C. G. Woods, Department of Histopathology, Nuffield Orthopaedic Centre, Headington, Oxford, UK

N. Woolf, Department of Histopathology, University College and Middlesex School of Medicine, The Bland-Sutton Institute, The Middlesex Hospital, London W1P 7PN, UK

D. H. Wright, The University of Southampton, Faculty of Medicine, South Lab/Path Block, Southampton General Hospital, Tremona Road, Southampton SO9 4XY, UK

N. A. Wright, Department of Histopathology, Royal Postgraduate Medical School, Hammersmith Hospital, Du Cane Road, London W12 0HS, UK

A. H. Wyllie, University of Edinburgh, Department of Pathology, The Medical School, Teviot Place, Edinburgh EH8 9AG, UK

E. P. H. Yap, University of Oxford, Nuffield Department of Pathology and Bacteriology, John Radcliffe Hospital, Headington, Oxford OX3 9DU, UK

1

Cell and matrix structure and function

1

Cell and matrix structure and function

1.1 Cellular organization and cellular interrelationships

Peter G. Toner and Derek F. W. McCormick

1.1.1 Cellular organization

The basic concepts of cellular organization are often illustrated with reference to some hypothetical 'typical' animal cell, in which some of the common properties of cells are displayed, while cellular diversity is conveniently overlooked. The cells that make up the tissues and organs of the human body are indeed diverse. Starting from the single totipotential cell of the zygote, the processes of differentiation produce over 200 morphologically distinct adult cell types, each identifiable by its unique combination of microscopic and ultrastructural features and each, in turn, possessing its own distinctive profile of metabolism and behaviour. This diversity translates from the steady state of normality to the various extremes of pathological response. Each cell type has its own limits of tolerance for environmental stress and its own pattern of reactions when these limits are exceeded. Each has a more or less consistent and distinctive range of pathological phenotypic variants associated with the somatic mutations of neoplasia. These we recognize as the various forms of cancer (see Section 9.3).

Nevertheless, despite the profound diversity of differentiated cells and of their neoplastic counterparts, these many cell types have more similarities than differences. The 'typical' cell does not exist, but all cell types are in fact built from quite a small range of structural subunits or organelles and have most of their basic metabolic pathways in common. Moreover, cells of different types subjected to a particular stimulus frequently follow common pathways of pathological response, irrespective of the nature of their specialization, implying the existence of common pathogenetic mechanisms, despite their anatomical and functional diversity.

The purpose of this section is to review briefly the basic structural and functional aspects of cellular organization, including the ultrastructural morphology of the nucleus and cytoplasm. The specific patterns of differentiation associated with various cell lineages will be described and the inter-relationships of cells with one another and with their surrounding tissue environment will be outlined.

1.1.2 Nucleus

The interphase nucleus typifies the paradox of wide structural diversity, derived from combinations of a limited number of common features. In many differentiated cell types, nuclear morphology is both distinctive and consistent when viewed in standard light and electron microscopic preparations. Thus the nuclei of the monocyte (Fig. 1.1), the plasma cell (Fig. 1.2), and the neutrophil (Fig. 1.3) can be distinguished easily by the pattern and texture of their chromatin, allied to the overall shape and size of the nucleus. Despite their biological equivalence, the structural contrast between the small, dense nucleus of the spermatozoon and the large, pale nucleus of the ovum could scarcely be more marked. The differences in this case can be rationalized as an efficient adaptation in the packaging of the nuclear material to assist the dynamics of the motile sperm cell. In other instances, nuclear contour, pattern, and texture may show equally striking, but often more puzzling, differences. These distinctive structural features seem, however, to be relatively minor variables in the expression of the fundamental molecular mechanisms which are common to every nucleated cell of the body.

Nuclear chromatin

The main substance of the nucleus consists of twisted masses of 30 nm fibres of nuclear chromatin, dispersed to variable degrees

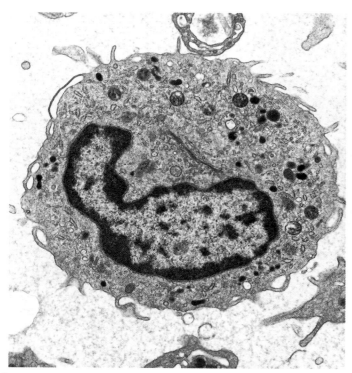

Fig. 1.1   Monocyte, showing indented nucleus of characteristic shape and chromatin distribution.

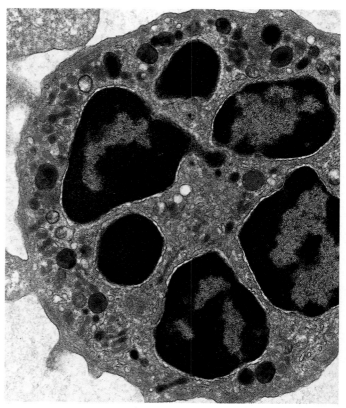

Fig. 1.3   Neutrophil polymorph, showing six nuclear segments with very dense peripheral heterochromatin and small central areas of pale euchromatin.

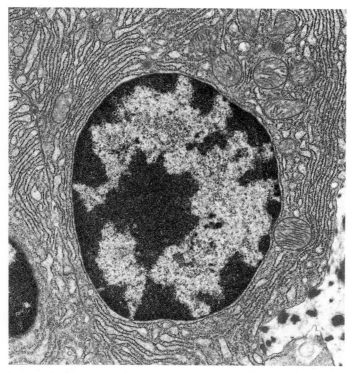

Fig. 1.2   Plasma cell, showing clear-cut demarcation of pale euchromatin and dense heterochromatin in the typical clock-face pattern.

in the surrounding nucleoplasm, or interchromatin space. Two patterns of chromatin aggregation are recognized: a dense form known as heterochromatin, consisting of clumped masses of chromatin granules; and a less densely aggregated paler pattern known as euchromatin. The individual chromatin fibres, consisting of strings of granules termed nucleosomes (see Sections 2.1, 2.3), are identical in different cell types: it is the relative proportions and the anatomical distribution of the euchromatin and heterochromatin areas which are mainly responsible for the various distinctive patterns referred to above.

Chromatin consists of nuclear DNA, closely bound to the nuclear histone proteins, which may control the coiling and packing of the nucleic acid. There are also close associations with non-histone proteins, which probably regulate nuclear functions in various ways. In functional terms, heterochromatin represents inactive areas of the genome, where the nucleic acid remains tightly coiled, whereas euchromatin contains its DNA in the extended form, implying an engagement in active transcription.

The chromatin pattern has certain consistent morphological features. A linear rim of heterochromatin granules is usually found lining the inner aspect of the nuclear envelope. In many cell types, large aggregates of heterochromatin are also seen towards the periphery of the nucleus, abutting against the nuclear envelope, but separated from one another by euchromatin

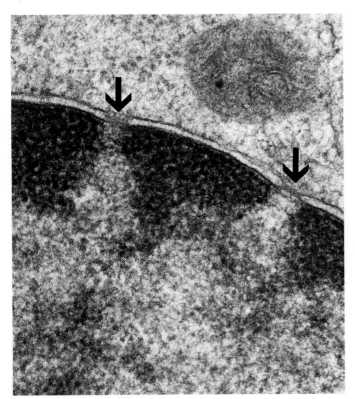

Fig. 1.4 Nuclear envelope, showing two nuclear pores (arrows), with euchromatin channels separating blocks of peripheral heterochromatin.

channels extending out to the nuclear pores (Fig. 1.4). Finally, there is often a heterochromatin mass consistently associated with the nucleolus. Despite the tremendous diversity of nuclear configuration and texture in specialized cells, these basic structural features are generally conserved.

Certain broad associations are recognized between nuclear morphology and function in normal cells. In general, cells which are relatively undifferentiated, or are engaged in active proliferation, tend to have a predominance of euchromatin, with an overall diffuse and ill-defined nuclear pattern. Most of the cells of the developing embryo, along with immature or proliferating cells in the adult, are in this category. The transformation, on antigenic stimulation, of the mature lymphocyte, with its small, dense nucleus, to a proliferating blast cell state, with a large, pale, euchromatic nucleus, provides a graphic example of this association of nuclear pattern with functional state. More highly differentiated cells, in which transcriptional activity and potential are progressively restricted, are likely to display more pronounced chromatin condensation, with accentuation or peripheral clumping of the heterochromatin masses. The classic example is the 'cartwheel' nucleus of the plasma cell (Fig. 1.2).

Nucleolus and other intranuclear structures

Nucleoli vary in number in different cell types, being more numerous and more prominent in highly active cells. The nuc-

leolus is not limited or defined by a membrane, but consists simply of a compact aggregate of dense and largely granular material suspended within the nuclear matrix and distinguished mainly by its texture. The nucleolus contains abundant RNA and is the site of manufacture of the component parts of the ribosomes.

On more detailed study, the nucleolus is seen to contain two main structural components, a granular portion and a fibrillar portion. A variable amount of nucleolus-associated chromatin is normally found surrounding or adjacent to the nucleolus. The overall configuration of the nucleolus is widely variable, from a sponge-like meshwork (Fig. 1.5) to a compact mass (Fig. 1.6). The pale fibrillary centres, also known as nucleolar organizing regions or nucleolar organizing DNA (if identifiable) are generally central or are interspersed with the denser fibrillar and granular components (Fig. 1.7).

Various other distinctive intranuclear structures are recognized, including 30 nm perichromatin and 15 nm interchromatin granules. These are small, dense aggregates, located near the margins or in the midst of heterochromatin masses. Their significance is unclear, but they should not be confused with virus particles or products. The same applies to nuclear bodies, which are rather larger intranuclear components (Fig. 1.6),

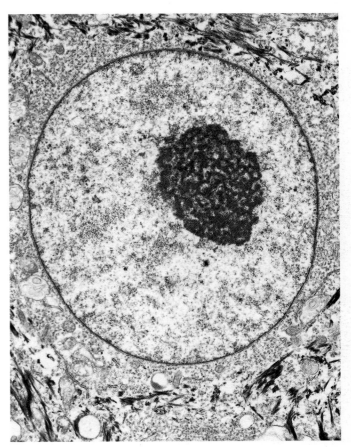

Fig. 1.5 Keratinocyte showing prominent nucleolus with a sponge-like configuration.

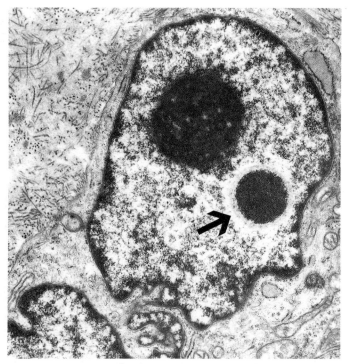

Fig. 1.6 Large dense nucleolus consisting of a granular core and a faint concentric filamentous ring. There is also an adjacent nuclear body (arrow).

sometimes multiple, consisting of variable combinations of granular, amorphous, fibrillar, and vesicular components. Nuclear bodies seem to reflect brisk metabolic activity; their specific functional associations have yet to be recognized. Numerous other heterogeneous inclusions have been described within the interphase nucleus, but their significance in most cases is not known. Finally, cell products (Fig.1.8), including secretory granules, and invaginations of cytoplasmic material (Fig. 1.9) may form inclusions or vacuoles within the nucleus in various circumstances.

Nuclear envelope

The nucleus is demarcated from the cytoplasm by a complex structural boundary known as the nuclear envelope. This consists of two membrane layers, an inner and an outer nuclear membrane, separated by an interspace termed the perinuclear cisterna (Fig. 1.4). The outer membrane is in contact with the cytoplasm, whereas the inner membrane defines the limit of the nuclear chromatin. A distinct component of the nuclear matrix, the nuclear fibrous lamina, can sometimes be detected at this boundary. The chromosomes of the interphase nucleus may have attachments to this region. The perinuclear cisterna is in structural and functional continuity with the cisternae of the granular endoplasmic reticulum in the cytoplasm. This is reflected by the attachment of ribosomes to the outer, or cytoplasmic, aspect of the outer nuclear membrane.

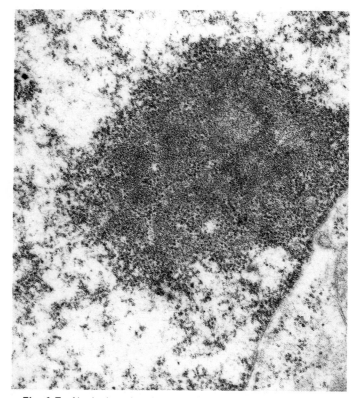

Fig. 1.7 Nucleolus, showing granular and fibrillar components.

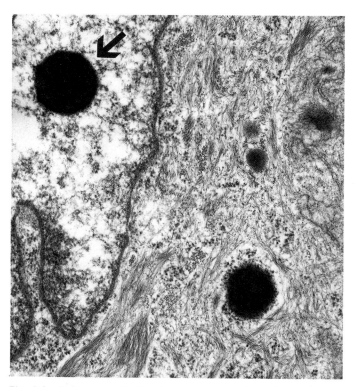

Fig. 1.8 Squamous cell, showing a cytoplasmic keratohyalin granule and surrounding cytokeratin filaments. The nucleus contains a similar granule (arrow).

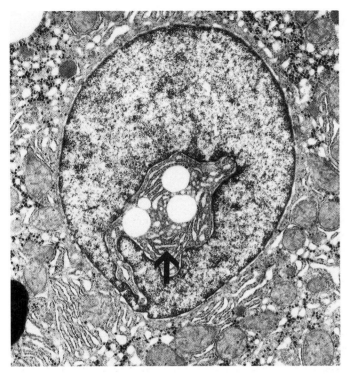

Fig. 1.9 Intranuclear pseudo-inclusion (arrow) consisting of a pocket of cytoplasmic material invaginated within the nucleus. It contains membranes of the endoplasmic reticulum and is surrounded by an intact nuclear envelope.

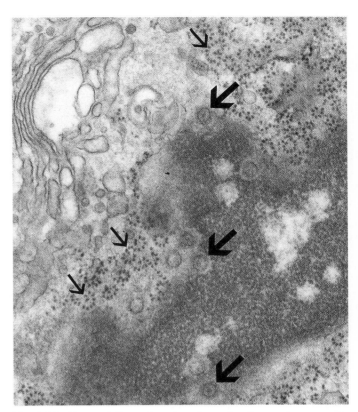

Fig. 1.10 Tangentially sectioned nucleus, showing nuclear pores in face view (large arrows). Note the spiral arrangement of nearby cytoplasmic polyribosomes (small arrows).

One of the most distinctive features of the nucleus is the presence of nuclear pore structures at intervals around the nuclear envelope (Fig. 1.4). These are circular discontinuities in the nuclear envelope, 80 nm diameter, bridged across by a tenuous diaphragm and embellished by a complex external collar structure which is composed of eight macromolecular subunits. Pores are often observed in tangential sections of the nuclear envelope (Fig. 1.10). They appear to represent channels for two-way nucleocytoplasmic exchange, through which, for example, the ribosomal subunits are transported out of the nucleus prior to their assembly in the cytoplasm and through which cytoplasmic molecules with a molecular weight of up to 60 000 Da can diffuse into the nucleus.

The nuclear envelope appears able at times to give rise to additional cisternal structures, which accumulate in parallel stacks in the cytoplasm as annulate lamellae. This name reflects the presence of nuclear pore structures, perforating the cisternae and often aligned in register to form striking parallel or concentric arrays. Annulate lamellae are seen most often in germ cells and their precursors, but may occur in many other situations, including various tumours (Figs 1.11, 1.12). They are of unknown function, but are thought to reflect increased nucleocytoplasmic exchange.

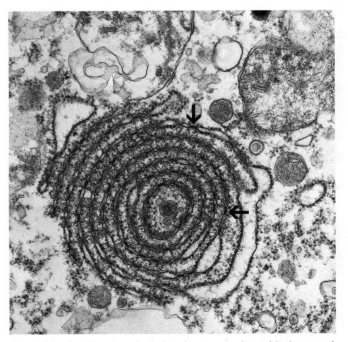

Fig. 1.11 Annulate lamellae, showing connection with the granular endoplasmic reticulum. The cisternae are perforated by structures similar to nuclear pores (arrows).

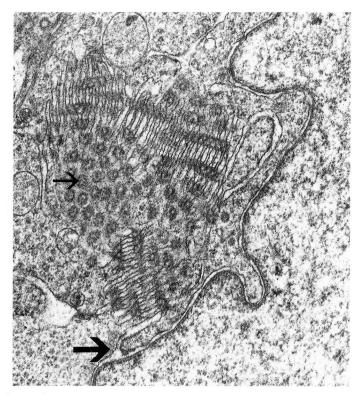

Fig. 1.12 Annulate lamellae in an ovarian tumour, showing some pore structures in face view (small arrows). The membranes connect with the nuclear envelope (large arrow). (Micrograph by courtesy of Mr A. Rennison.)

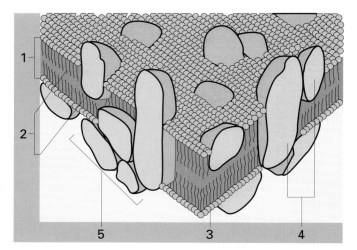

Fig. 1.13 Line diagram of membrane structure. 1, Phospholipid bilayer; 2, non-polar tails; 3, polar head groups; 4, membrane proteins; 5, cytoplasmic membrane-associated proteins.

from 7 to 11 nm thick, depending on the degree of specialization of the membrane (Fig. 1.14). Slight ultrastructural asymmetry is sometimes detectable. The presence of an external layer or cell coat, the glycocalyx, which is rich in carbohydrate, can be detected by special staining techniques (Fig. 1.15). The cell coat may be directly imaged in electron micrographs as a fuzzy layer

1.1.3 Cytoplasm

The cell surface

The contents of the cell are enclosed by a cell membrane, which forms the physical boundary between the cytoplasm and the extracellular tissue fluid. The cell membrane has numerous molecular, functional, and morphological specializations. Its basic framework consists of a lipid bilayer in which the polar ends of the phospholipid molecules are aligned on the outer and inner surfaces, the non-polar ends being opposed along the centre line of the membrane (Fig. 1.13). The associated membrane protein molecules may traverse the bilayer, forming a bridge across the entire thickness of the membrane, or may be anchored to the bilayer or to other proteins on either the inner or the outer aspect of the membrane. Transmembrane protein molecules can be individually visualized in freeze-fracture preparations as discrete intramembrane particles, the location and distribution of which can be correlated with known membrane specializations. Membrane functions include surface receptor mechanisms, molecular transport and ion pumping, cellular attachment, and intercellular communication.

High-resolution electron microscopy of cell membranes in tissues prepared by conventional fixation and sectioning techniques reveals a distinctive trilaminar or tramline structure,

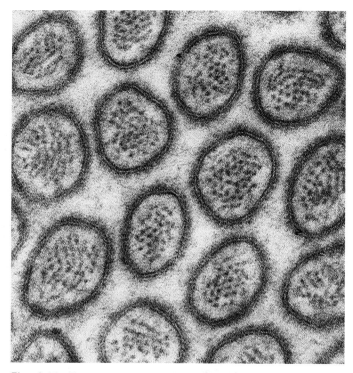

Fig. 1.14 Transverse section of intestinal microvilli, showing trilaminar membrane detail. The space between the microvilli contains the glycocalyx. The microvilli contain a central core of actin filaments. See Fig. 1.16 for a longitudinal section of villi.

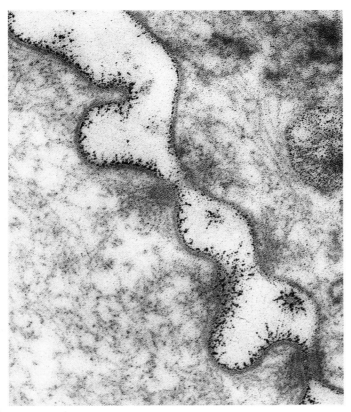

Fig. 1.15 Cell coat stained by the periodic acid silver proteinate technique, which reacts with carbohydrate residues at the cell surface.

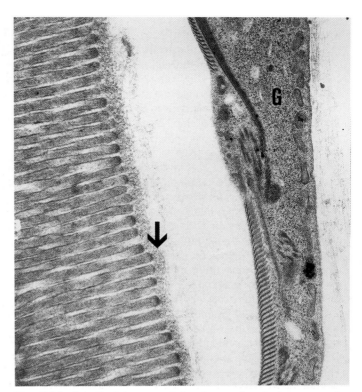

Fig. 1.16 Intestinal fuzzy coat forming a discrete layer over the intestinal microvilli (arrow). The adjacent structure is an intraluminal parasite, *Giardia lamblia* (G).

at the membrane surface in specialized cells, particularly at microvillous borders (Fig. 1.16), such as in the intestinal epithelium, although its visualization is inconsistent.

Membranes have fluid properties, allowing the lateral movement of many components by diffusion within the lipid bilayer. Both the lipid and the protein components are asymmetrically arranged, providing the outer and the inner faces of the membrane with quite different structural and functional properties, appropriate to their location. For example, the external surface of the outer face plays a role in cell-to-cell recognition and adhesion. The inner face provides attachment points for the components of the cytoskeleton, important not only mechanically, but perhaps also for the transmission of signals generated at surface receptors.

The membrane surfaces of individual cells display areas of distinctive specialization. Epithelial cells, for example, have prominent desmosomes (Fig. 1.17), attachment specializations that promote mechanical cohesion. These desmosomes are linked internally to the cytokeratin component of the cytoskeleton. In a columnar epithelium, the cell apices are linked by continuous bands or zones of occlusion and adhesion specialization, which firmly bind adjacent cells, prevent leakage between them, and have their own specific attachments to other cytoplasmic filaments. Surface specializations such as apical brush borders, consisting of parallel microvilli (Fig. 1.16), or labile

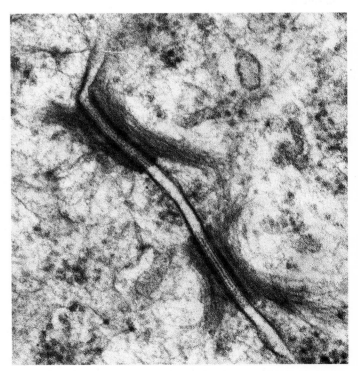

Fig. 1.17 Desmosomes, showing laminated structure and bundles of cytokeratin filaments inserted into the dense cytoplasmic plaque.

flaps (Fig. 1.18), folds, or basal infoldings, are all associated with specific functional properties such as absorption, locomotion, secretion, or molecular transport.

While much of the small molecular weight traffic across the cell membrane takes place through specific molecular transport mechanisms, there are also gross transmembrane movements, characterized as exocytosis and endocytosis. Exocytosis (Fig. 1.19) proceeds by fusion of the limiting membrane of an intracellular granule or vacuole with the inner aspect of the cell membrane, perhaps triggered by a localized increase in ionized calcium concentration. This is followed by discharge of the granule content to the exterior of the cell. This is one of the commonest mechanisms of secretion.

Endocytosis, which includes the processes of pinocytosis and phagocytosis, occurs on both a large and a small scale. This involves a localized invagination of the cell surface, followed by interiorization of the resulting vacuole or vesicle, with its content of extracellular fluid, macromolecules, or particulate material. Substances taken up in this way then enter the lysosomal system, where they are broken down.

Endocytosis is often mediated by surface receptors. This involves the formation of specialized coated vesicles, the cytoplasmic surfaces of which bear spiky projections indicating the presence of a membrane-associated protein called clathrin (Fig. 1.20). Surface receptors concentrated at these sites bind selectively to their target molecules in the extracellular fluid and the resultant complexes are incorporated into the cell by internalization of the coated vesicle, through this specialized form of

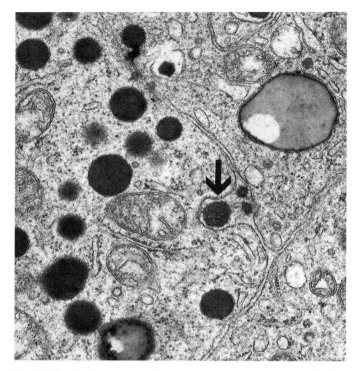

Fig. 1.19 Exocytosis, showing an endocrine secretory granule just released into the intercellular space (arrow), alongside remnants of two others.

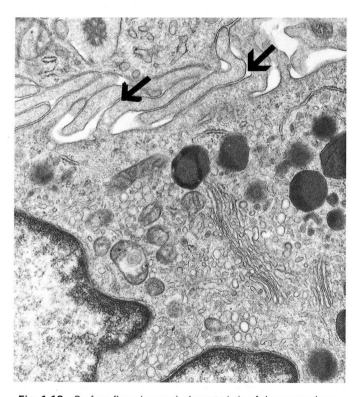

Fig. 1.18 Surface flaps (arrows) characteristic of the macrophage.

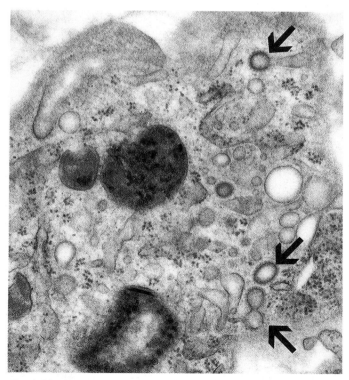

Fig. 1.20 Endocytosis, showing numerous vesicles at the surface of a macrophage. Some of these have the characteristic fuzzy or coated appearance associated with selective endocytosis (arrows).

endocytosis. The target molecules are finally detached from their receptors, which are then recycled to the cell surface. The uptake of low-density lipoproteins, bound to their specific receptor sites, is accomplished in fibroblasts by this mechanism. Phagocytosis of antibody-coated bacteria by polymorphs and macrophages is also triggered by specific surface receptors. The continuous dynamic interplay of exocytosis and endocytosis results in a constant recycling of cell membrane components. Delicate control mechanisms are postulated to regulate this process.

The membrane systems

The cytoplasm contains formed organelles and stored materials of various sorts, reflecting the distinctive differences between specialized cells. The cytoplasm is divided into two principal phases by its membrane systems, the cytoplasmic ground substance, or cytosol, and the cavities enclosed by the major membrane systems, which are identified as the endoplasmic reticulum and Golgi apparatus (Fig. 1.21). The barrier between these two phases consists of the membranes themselves, while the cavities, or cisternae, which they form are in functional continuity with each other and with the perinuclear cisterna. Encapsulated products, such as secretion granules, lysosomes, and microbodies, can be regarded as part of the cisternal phase, since they are formed by accumulation of material within a closed, membrane-limited sac, derived from either the endoplasmic reticulum or the Golgi apparatus.

The cisternae of the endoplasmic reticulum may be arranged in numerous distinctive configurations and, even when abundant, may appear to interconnect only infrequently. It must be recalled, however, that the images of the electron microscope are only snapshots, representing one moment in time, frozen by fixation. In life, time-lapse cinemicrography of cultured cells, using the phase-contrast microscope, clearly shows that the cytoplasm is a turbulent, dynamic system, in which continuity between component parts is constantly being broken and re-established. Thus, demonstrable interconnections may be infrequent, without calling into question the underlying functional continuity of the endoplasmic reticulum. Cisternae may be short, scanty, and widely separated; or elongated, numerous, and closely packed, depending on the functional profile and capacity of the cell.

The predominant form of endoplasmic reticulum, known as the granular endoplasmic reticulum, is distinguished by the presence of ribosomes attached to the outer, or cytoplasmic, surfaces of its cisternal membranes (Fig. 1.22). These 15 nm, dense particles are the site of cytoplasmic protein synthesis. The ribosomes are themselves highly complex structures, with two major subunits and some 50 separate components. The polypeptide chains that they synthesize are threaded through the

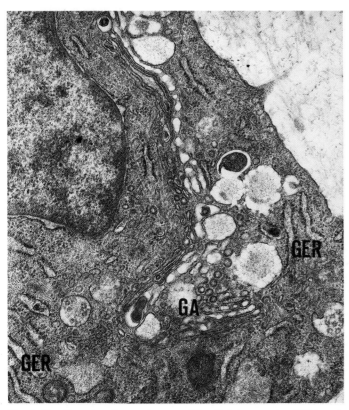

Fig. 1.21 Cytoplasmic membranes of the Golgi apparatus (GA) and granular endoplasmic reticulum (GER).

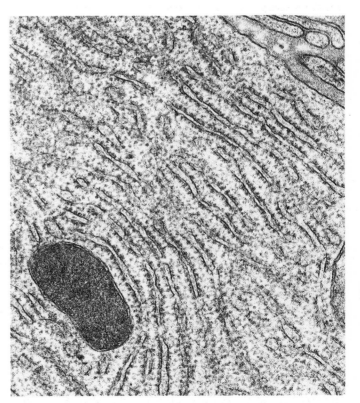

Fig. 1.22 Granular endoplasmic reticulum, showing parallel membrane-limited cisternae with attached ribosomes, separated by the cytoplasmic matrix.

membrane and accumulate within the cisternal lumen. The cisternae of the granular endoplasmic reticulum provide both a storage area and a transport pathway for newly synthesized proteins. These are next moved to the Golgi apparatus by a process of vesiculation of the endoplasmic reticulum membranes, to form transport vesicles which then fuse with the Golgi membranes.

The ribosome-rich granular endoplasmic reticulum is the major site of protein synthesis. This association is seen most clearly in active fibroblasts, zymogenic cells, and plasma cells (Fig. 1.2), where the granular endoplasmic reticulum is particularly abundant and elaborately organized, a feature of cells manufacturing proteins for export. Many ribosomes also lie free in the cytosol rather than attached to membranes, and these are concerned with the synthesis of protein for the internal use of the cell (Fig. 1.23). Both free and membrane-associated ribosomes are often grouped in small spirals or clusters (Fig. 1.10), termed polyribosomes, which are linked by a single molecule of messenger RNA.

The attached ribosomes are visible evidence of functional specialization in the endoplasmic reticulum, but similar cisternal membranes are also associated with other enzyme systems, which are not themselves ultrastructurally distinctive. In some cell types, there are abundant smooth-surfaced membrane cisternae (Fig. 1.24), identified as the agranular or smooth endoplasmic reticulum. Although not involved in protein synthesis,

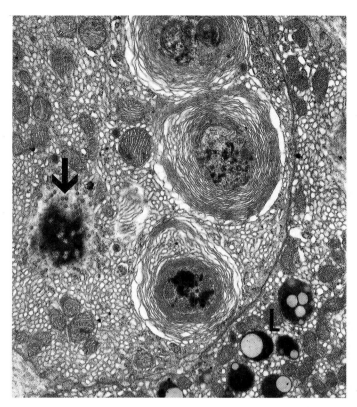

Fig. 1.24 Smooth endoplasmic reticulum in steroid-secreting interstitial cells of the testis, with prominent concentric arrays. Note the tangentially sectioned nucleus (arrow) and lipofuscin granules (L).

these membranes have many other metabolic functions in different cell types, including lipid metabolism and drug detoxification in the liver; steroid hormone synthesis in the adrenal cortex and testis; and the uptake and sequestration of ionized calcium in the muscle cell.

The Golgi apparatus consists of compact stacks of membrane-limited cisternae (Fig. 1.25), often focally dilated, along with numerous small vesicles, many of which are of the coated type associated with selective uptake (Fig. 1.26). Proteins are received by the Golgi system at its forming or input face, in transport vesicles derived from the adjacent cisternae of the granular endoplasmic reticulum. The full metabolic role of the Golgi apparatus is not entirely clear, but it is certainly involved in the modification of the carbohydrate components of glycoproteins and in the sorting and packaging of secretory products for subsequent discharge. Secretory granules form as condensing vacuoles at the maturing or output face, on the opposite surface of the apparatus from the intake of raw materials (Fig. 1.25). They then separate from the apparatus and accumulate at the secretory pole of the cell.

The Golgi apparatus is prominent in cells such as goblet cells, which secrete glycoproteins, but it is present in virtually all cells and has been shown, for example, to be involved in the synthesis of the carbohydrate-rich cell coat. In the gut, the Golgi apparatus takes part in the absorptive activities of the entero-

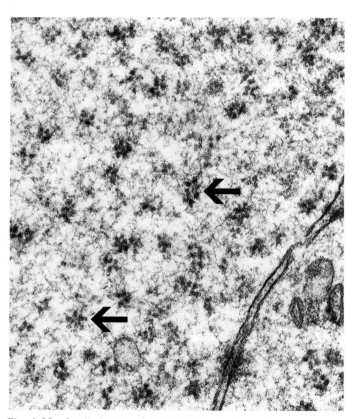

Fig. 1.23 Small clusters of ribosomes (arrows) are known as polyribosomes.

cyte, as shown by the accumulation of absorbed fat at this site, prior to its onward movement. The endoplasmic reticulum and Golgi apparatus may also play a role in membrane synthesis and in the membrane turnover of the entire cell.

Lysosomes and microbodies

These two organelles take the form of membrane-limited granules suspended within the cytosol, but derived from the endoplasmic reticulum and Golgi membrane systems described above. Lysosomes are discrete aggregates of acid hydrolytic enzymes, segregated from the cytosol by a limiting membrane. In their formation, lysosomes are similar to other encapsulated cell products, such as secretory granules. Their constituent enzyme proteins are synthesized by the granular endoplasmic reticulum and are sorted and segregated into discrete packages, or primary lysosomes, by the Golgi system, using a specific molecular recognition signal. A wide range of hydrolytic enzymes is involved, encompassing the full spectrum of cellular catabolic activities. The classic enzyme marker of the lysosome is acid phosphatase.

Lysosomes are the most distinctive feature of specialized phagocytic cells, such as neutrophil polymorphonuclear leucocytes and macrophages (Figs 1.3, 1.27), but in fact every cell possesses lysosomes. These are employed not only in the phagocytosis of external material, but in the internal recycling of cytoplasmic components in the course of normal intracellular

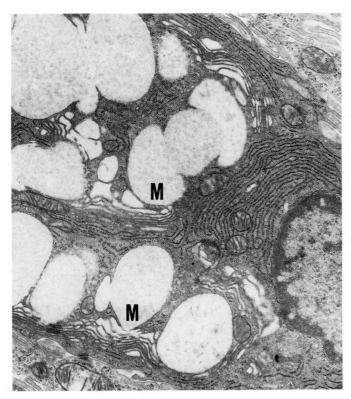

Fig. 1.25 Elaborate Golgi apparatus of intestinal goblet cell, in which foamy mucus granules (M) are forming.

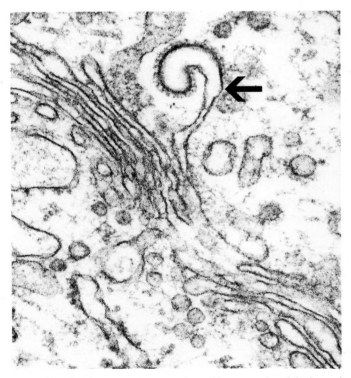

Fig. 1.26 Golgi apparatus connecting with a coated vesicle (arrow) associated with selective uptake.

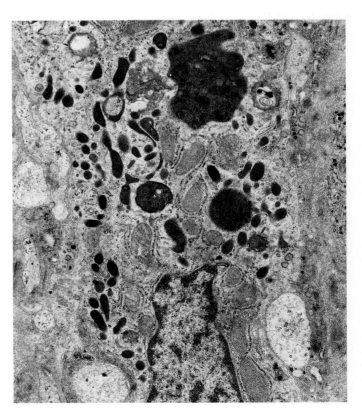

Fig. 1.27 Macrophage in liver, showing numerous lysosomes of different size and appearance.

maintenance and repair. Whatever the origin of the material for digestion, it becomes combined with the contents of a primary lysosome to form a secondary lysosome. These are morphologically heterogeneous inclusions, recognized typically as pleomorphic dense bodies, surrounded by a limiting membrane. Cytochemical methods can be used to demonstrate the presence of acid phosphatase and various other lysosomal enzymes. Following the digestion and resorption of the re-usable content of the secondary lysosome, the inert residue of digestion, generally rich in complex lipids, may persist as a dense residual body. These are recognized by light microscopy as brown lipofuscin granules.

Lysosomes play a central role in the metabolism of the cell and are intimately involved in many pathological processes, such as the response to cell injury and the inflammatory reaction. The process of ageing is reflected in an increase in the lipofuscin granule content of the permanent cells of the body, such as neurones and cardiac muscle cells, representing the accumulation of cellular 'wear and tear' over many years. The genetically determined absence of abnormality of one or other of the lysosomal enzymes results in the accumulation of its substrate within abnormal distended lysosomes, with consequent functional disturbances. These conditions, known as lysosomal storage diseases (see Section 2.5), typically have their onset in childhood and are relentlessly progressive. Each has its own distinctive pattern of organ and tissue involvement, determined by the particular metabolic pathway in question. For example, gangliosides are most abundant in the brain. Thus in gangliosidase deficiency, the substrate for the defective enzyme accumulates mostly in the lysosomes of neurones, leading to progressive neurological impairment and dementia.

Microbodies or peroxisomes are small, rather inconspicuous membrane-limited organelles which apparently form by budding off directly from the granular endoplasmic reticulum. They are best seen in liver (Fig. 1.28) and kidney tubule cells. Microbodies contain catalase and several oxidative enzymes. They are involved in the destruction of hydrogen peroxide, which is potentially lethal to the cell, as well as taking part in detoxification reactions, alcohol metabolism, and fatty acid breakdown. The presence of D-aminoacid oxidase is a curious finding.

Mitochondria

The mitochondria are discrete organelles composed of a double membrane envelope with a distinctive fine structure. Mitochondria are suspended in the cytosol and are generally either round or elongated (Fig. 1.29), but sometimes appear twisted and branching. The outer membrane is separated from the inner membrane by the narrow outer mitochondrial space. The inner membrane forms folds or internal shelves known as the mitochondrial cristae (Fig. 1.30). The inner mitochondrial space, bounded by the inner membrane, is also termed the mitochondrial matrix. The dense matrix granules which are sometimes observed here appear to be sites for calcium binding. The mitochondrial matrix also contains a small amount of DNA, in the form of a circular molecule similar to a bacterial chromosome,

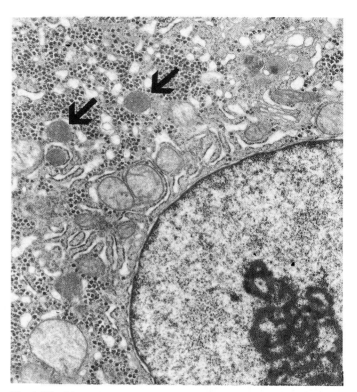

Fig. 1.28 Liver microbodies are small membrane-limited inclusions of moderate density (arrows). Mitochondria, endoplasmic reticulum, and glycogen are also present.

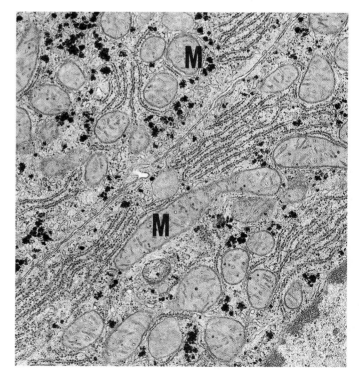

Fig. 1.29 Liver mitochondria (M) between cisternae of the endoplasmic reticulum. The internal cristae are not highly organized.

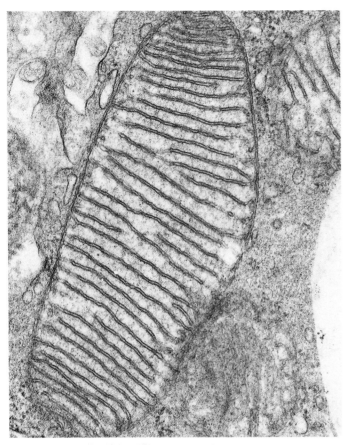

Fig. 1.30 Mitochondrion in brown fat, showing well-organized internal cristae.

a primitive eukaryotic cell and an oxidative bacterium. The presumption is that this proved a winning combination, providing the host cell with an efficient source of energy for the fullest possible exploitation of the eukaryotic genetic system.

The cytoskeleton

The cytosol is not simply a formless protein gel, as it has sometimes been portrayed, but has a well-defined framework of microtubules and filaments with a fundamental structural and functional role. The cytoskeleton has three major components, microtubules, actin filaments, and intermediate filaments, which are present in virtually all cells. These components form a complex network which extends to the furthest extremities of the cytoplasm and plays a vital role in determining the distinctive properties of each cell type. Increasingly, the cytoskeleton is seen not simply as a scaffolding mechanism for the maintenance of cell shape but as an active participant in cell function, providing a basis for locomotion, a mechanism for cytoplasmic translocation, and a link between surface receptors and cellular responses.

Cytoplasmic microtubules are 23 nm in diameter (Fig. 1.31) and of indeterminate length. They are formed by the self-assembly of macromolecular subunits of the cytoplasmic protein, tubulin. Microtubules are extremely labile structures, elongating rapidly in suitable circumstances by the addition of

providing a limited extranuclear genetic capability. Most of this DNA is derived from the ovum. Mitochondria also have their own ribosomes, which take part in protein synthesis. Most of the genes controlling the synthesis of the mitochondrial proteins, however, are located in the cell nucleus. These proteins are synthesized in the usual way on cytoplasmic ribosomes and are transported by selective mechanisms for incorporation into the mitochondrion.

Mitochondria are responsible for most of the oxidative metabolism of the cell and are the source of the ATP that drives virtually every aspect of cellular function. The total bulk of mitochondria in different cell types and the internal configuration of the mitochondrial membranes correlates with cellular differentiation and metabolism. Mitochondria are numerous and have complex, closely packed cristae in cells where the demands on oxidative metabolism are particularly high, such as the cardiac muscle cell and the acid-secreting gastric parietal cell. They have a semi-autonomous existence, increasing their numbers by growth and fission to keep pace with cell division.

On the basis of many genetic and metabolic similarities between mitochondria and bacterial cells, it is now generally accepted that the mitochondria arose early in the course of cellular evolution from an endosymbiotic relationship between

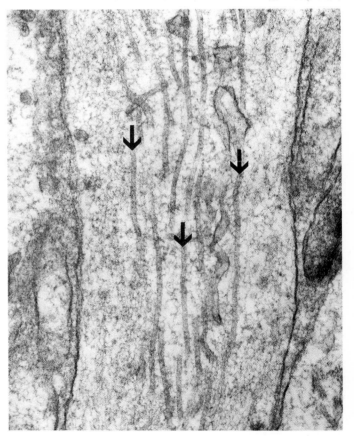

Fig. 1.31 Linear microtubules (arrows) in a nerve cell process.

tubulin molecules to their growing end, but capable of equally
rapid dissociation. Microtubule growth can be asymmetrical,
proceeding more rapidly at one end than the other, and a steady
state may be maintained in which assembly and dissociation
proceed simultaneously in dynamic equilibrium. Microtubules
are organized from specific cytoplasmic centres associated with
the centrioles, which are themselves composed of highly organized microtubular components and are often found close to the
nucleus and Golgi apparatus (Fig. 1.32). Centrioles form the
poles of the mitotic spindle and, in ciliated cells, divide to give
rise to the basal bodies from which the individual cilia originate
(Figs 1.33, 1.34).

The most dramatic appearance of microtubules in bulk is at
the time of formation of the mitotic spindle. During mitosis, the
movement of the individual chromosomes is controlled by
attached microtubule bundles (Fig. 1.35) which form part of the
spindle structure. A residue of the spindle persists for a time as
the mid-body, which joins the two daughter cells at a single
point until they finally separate (Fig. 1.36). Tubulin polymerization is blocked by the drug colchicine and by the antimitotic
agents vinblastine and vincristine, with resultant disruption of
the process of mitosis. These compounds are used therapeutically in cancer and experimentally (e.g. in preparing
chromosome metaphase spreads etc.).

Microtubules provide the central mechanism in ciliary movement, the main components of the axoneme being a ring of nine

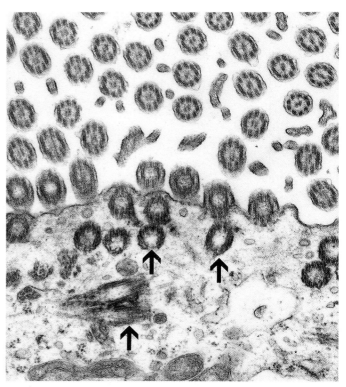

Fig. 1.33 The basal bodies of cilia (arrows) are derived from centrioles.

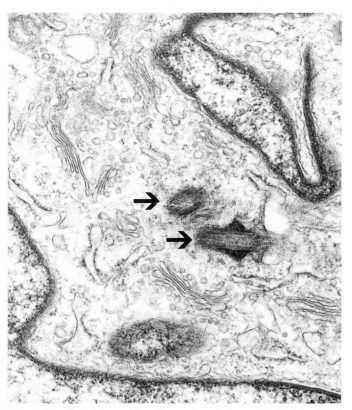

Fig. 1.32 Centrioles, obliquely sectioned (arrows), beside Golgi
apparatus and nucleus.

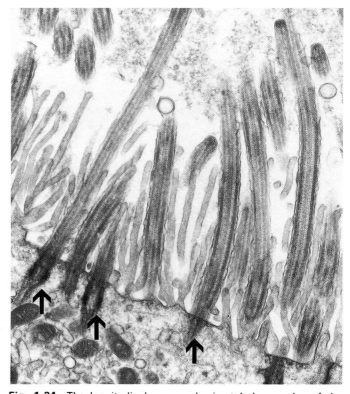

Fig. 1.34 The longitudinal axonemal microtubule complex of the
cilium originates from the underlying basal body (arrows).

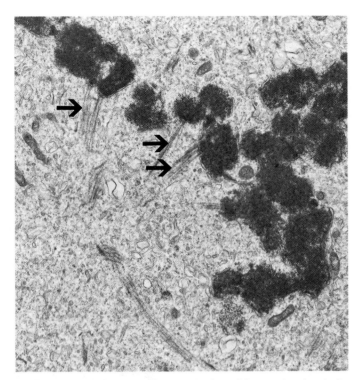

Fig. 1.35 Chromosomes during mitosis, with associated spindle microtubules (arrows).

highly organized microtubule doublets (Fig. 1.37), surrounding a further central pair of microtubules, all of which take origin from a basal body in the apical cytoplasm. Through the action of dynein (a special ATPase molecule), which is attached to the axonemal tubules, they are induced to slide in relation to one another in a regular, repetitive manner, resulting in the bending and recovery strokes of the characteristic ciliary beat. Absence of the dynein molecules, due to a genetic defect, results in immotile cilia. Although their structure is normal in every other aspect, the absence of the dynein arms can be detected by electron microscopy, which may be useful in the diagnosis of this rare condition (see Chapter 13).

Although other cytoplasmic microtubules are not organized in this complex pattern, they do appear to have an association with intracellular movements and translocations, of which the co-ordinated separation of the metaphase chromosomes is simply the most striking example. Microtubules are also associated with highly asymmetrical cell processes, being prominent in the extended cytoplasm of neurones and in renal glomerular podocytes. While here they may have a mechanical or structural role, there is also the likelihood that they are involved in transport mechanisms, carrying cytoplasmic components to parts distant from the main mass of the cell body.

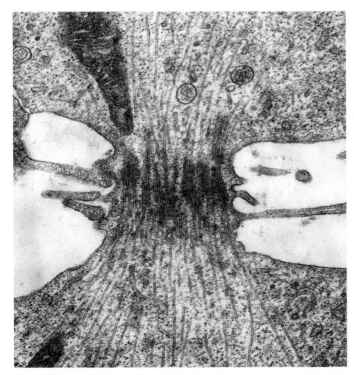

Fig. 1.36 At telophase, the mid-body is the only point at which the two daughter cells remain in contact before they finally separate. The mid-body is traversed by the residual microtubules of the mitotic spindle. (Micrograph by courtesy of Dr J. Kirk.)

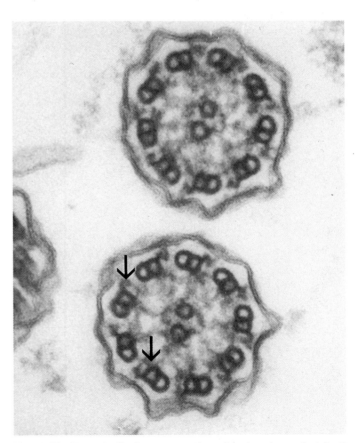

Fig. 1.37 Normal cilia in cross-section, showing the typical 9+2 tubular pattern, with recognizable dynein arms (arrows). See text for details.

Actin filaments, 7 nm in diameter, are present in all cells, although they are most abundant and organized in the different varieties of muscle cell (Fig. 1.38). Like microtubules, actin filaments are capable of rapid dissociation and reassembly from a cytoplasmic monomer pool, with which they coexist in a dynamic equilibrium. Actin filament bundles have an apparent mechanical stiffening role in certain situations, being present in the cores of microvilli (Fig. 1.14) and in the underlying terminal web to which they are connected and which links with the zonula adhaerens specialization close to the cell apex. The actin filaments associate here with myosin molecules, in a tension-generating role. In addition to these localized aggregates, actin filaments are distributed widely throughout the cytoplasm. Actin, indeed, is one of the most abundant of the cellular proteins. Small, ill-defined bundles of filaments, the so-called stress filaments, lie typically just beneath the surface of cells such as fibroblasts (Fig. 1.39), with mechanical attachments to the inner surface of the cell membrane.

The polymerization of actin molecules in the cytoplasm is blocked by cytochalasin B, which interferes in turn with various forms of cell movement, including locomotion and phagocytosis. This is taken to indicate the central role of actin in these functions. Actin filaments also play a role in mitosis, forming a

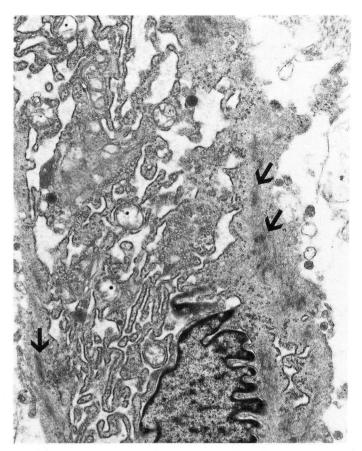

Fig. 1.39 Fibroblast, showing fine bundles of sub-surface actin filaments, sometimes termed stress filaments (arrows).

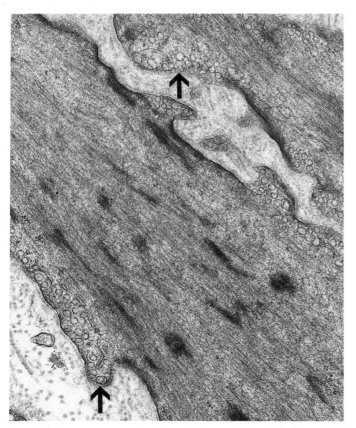

Fig. 1.38 Smooth muscle myofilaments and interspersed dense bodies. The small surface vesicles (arrows) are associated with endocytosis.

circular constricting band around the waist of the dividing cell, which causes the division of the cytoplasmic mass after the separation of the metaphase chromosomes. It is believed that in all of these situations associated with cell movement, the actin filaments are linked with myosin molecules. This exploits a molecular mechanism which is seen in its most highly evolved form in the striated muscle cell, but is, in fact, common to diverse forms of cell movement.

Intermediate filaments are so called because their diameter, 10 nm, lies between that of thin actin filaments and thick myosin filaments. They are mechanically strong, polymerizing from fibrous rather than globular protein subunits. Unlike microtubules and actin filaments, the intermediate filaments are stable and highly insoluble and they probably do not undergo rapid dissociation and reassembly. Intermediate filaments are predominantly associated with the mechanical functions of the cytoskeleton.

The major classes of intermediate filaments are cytokeratin, vimentin, desmin, neurofilaments, and glial filaments. Cytokeratin is the typical intermediate filament of epithelial cells, forming tonofilaments which attach to the desmosomes, providing mechanical cohesion and resistance to trauma (Figs 1.5, 1.8, 1.17). There is a large number of related cytokeratin molecules of different molecular weights and structures, present in different proportions in various cell types. A form of cellular differentiation particularly associated with cytokeratin accumulation is keratinization (Figs 1.8, 1.40) seen at its most extreme in horny layers such as thick skin and nails.

Vimentin is the typical intermediate filament of mesenchymal cells, such as fibroblasts and endothelium. Typically, these filaments are distributed diffusely in the cytoplasm, rather than in discrete bundles, as often seen in the case of cytokeratin. Desmin, a distinctive intermediate filament protein found in muscle cells, helps to align the sarcomeres in skeletal muscle. Neurofilaments are present in neurones, while glial fibrillary acidic protein forms the cytoplasmic intermediate filaments of the astrocytes. In all of these cases, it is likely that the differences in the intermediate filament content of different cell types relate closely to their various specialized functions, although it is not yet clear how. There are now reliable immunocytochemical staining methods for the detailed identification of intermediate filaments in histological sections. Although far from infallible, the intermediate filament phenotype is used as a guide to the differentiation of tumours of otherwise uncertain identity (see Section 9.4).

The functions of microtubules, actin filaments, and intermediate filaments are undoubtedly co-ordinated in many ways,

but the basic principles of cytoskeletal organization are still poorly understood. Even the precise anatomical interrelationship of the cytoskeletal components is controversial. After specialized tissue preparation, high-voltage electron micrographs of 1 μm thick sections of cells show delicate interconnections between the major cytoskeletal elements, as well as with the various formed organelles of the cytoplasm. This delicate mesh is known as the microtrabecular network. Its significance, its identity, and indeed its very existence as a meaningful biological 'system' in the living cell remain uncertain.

Other components of the cytosol

Stored material such as lipid, glycogen, and ferritin may accumulate within the cytosol. Lipid droplets lie free without a surrounding membrane, partitioned naturally by their physical nature from the hydrophilic cytoplasmic matrix. Glycogen exists in the form of dense particles, rather larger than ribobomes, sometimes lying singly (Fig. 1.41), but more often aggregated into clusters (Figs 1.28, 1.29). Ferritin is also a dense particulate substance, its discrete particles being smaller than ribosomes (Fig. 1.42). The ferritin molecule contains a dense iron core and is a major component of haemosiderin, the iron storage pigment of the body. These materials are normal

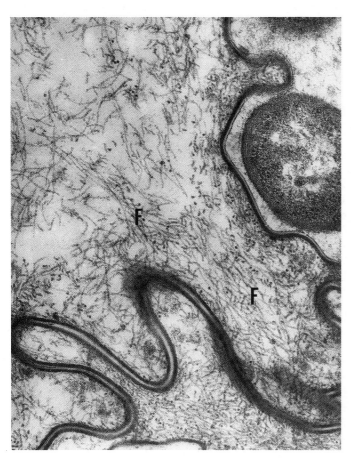

Fig. 1.40 Cytokeratin filaments (F) in a keratinized cell.

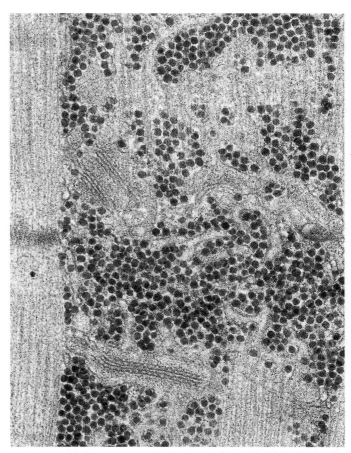

Fig. 1.41 Numerous solitary glycogen particles in the sarcoplasm of a skeletal muscle cell.

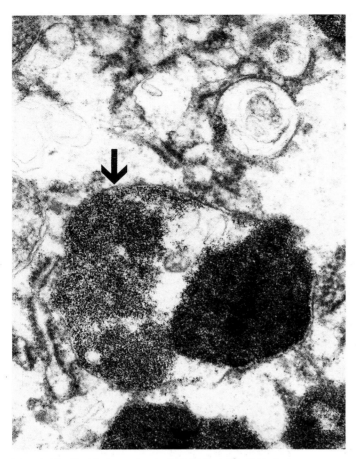

Fig. 1.42 Ferritin granules in a lysosome (arrow) in haemochromatosis ('iron overload' disease; see Chapter 17).

constituents of various cell types, but may accumulate abnormally in these and in other cells in various pathological conditions.

Cytoplasmic granules

In addition to the various organelles already described, many cells contain formed granules in their cytoplasm which relate to cellular function in various ways. These include secretory granules of different types, such as zymogen, mucin, and hormone products, as well as distinctive granular inclusions not directly associated with the secretory mechanism, such as the melanin granules of melanocytes, the Weibel–Palade granules of endothelial cells, and the Birbeck granules of Langerhans cells. Lysosomal granulation may have equally distinctive features. Granule morphology can often provide a key to cell identification, a commentary on cell function, and an insight into cell pathology.

Cells engaged in secretory activity often accumulate a store of formed secretory material, packaged into granules with distinctive morphological characteristics. Such granules are normally produced in the Golgi apparatus, using materials synthesized in the granular endoplasmic reticulum. Once detached from the Golgi apparatus, the secretory granule may undergo further maturation, often associated with a progressive condensation of its internal structure. In the case of exocrine cells, these secretion granules usually accumulate at the apical pole of the cell, from where they are released into a glandular lumen. Endocrine granules, on the other hand, are destined for release into the vascular system and tend to accumulate towards the basal pole, or around the periphery of the cell. Both exocrine and endocrine granules are released by a similar process of exocytosis (Fig. 1.19).

The balance between cellular synthesis and secretory discharge will generally determine the extent of accumulation of secretory granules within the cytoplasm, although a further regulatory mechanism termed crinophagocytosis may fine-tune the system. This describes the process by which undischarged and presumably ageing secretory granules are recycled through the lysosomal system. It is important to appreciate that a heavily granulated cell may not be particularly active in terms of synthesis or secretory discharge, whereas a cell with few stored granules may in fact be more active in both of these respects. The static evidence of the electron micrograph is insufficient to define such functional parameters with any accuracy.

The morphological features of specific secretory granules are often quite characteristic. The round homogeneous zymogen granules of the exocrine pancreas are very different from the endocrine granules of the islets of Langerhans (Fig. 1.43), and from the large foamy mucus granules of the goblet cell (Fig. 1.25), which in turn are structurally distinct from the much smaller mucin granules of the gastric surface cell. In the lung, the type 2 pneumocyte has distinctive laminated secretory granules (Fig. 1.44) associated with the production and release of surfactant. In the endocrine arena, the pancreatic islet cells and the various types of intestinal endocrine cell, to take only two examples, possess characteristic small, dense-cored granules, the precise features of which may make it possible to determine the cell type on morphological grounds alone. For example, the core of the β-cell granule of the islet often displays an internal paracrystalline structure (Fig. 1.45), whereas the α-cells have uniform, small, dense secretory granules. The human mast cell granule has a highly distinctive, complex laminated pattern, produced by close packing of whorled, scroll-like structures (Fig. 1.46).

Cytoplasmic granulation in secretory cells can easily be confused with granulation due to lysosomes. The phagocytic cells have their own distinctive morphological patterns. The primary lysosomes of the macrophage are small, dense granules, not unlike neuroendocrine granules, but these are usually mixed with larger, heterogeneous secondary lysosomes (Fig. 1.27). The granules of the neutrophil polymorph are of several structural types (Fig. 1.3), whereas those of the eosinophil polymorph are larger and typically contain an internal crystalline component (Fig. 1.47).

In most of the instances described above, the detailed ultrastructural appearances can be used as reliable markers of cellular identity. It must, however, be appreciated that granule

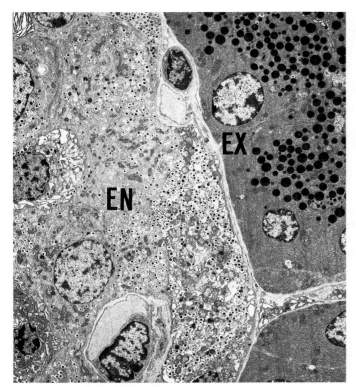

Fig. 1.43 Exocrine (EX) and endocrine (EN) pancreas, showing contrasting granule patterns; see also Fig. 1.45.

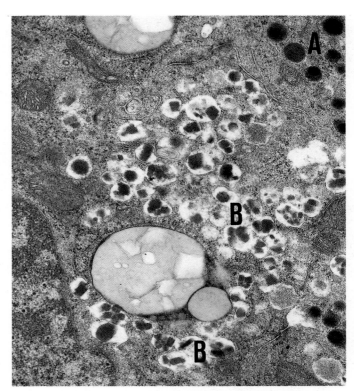

Fig. 1.45 β-cell granules (B), showing characteristic paracrystalline appearance, contrasting with adjacent round, dense α-cell granules (A).

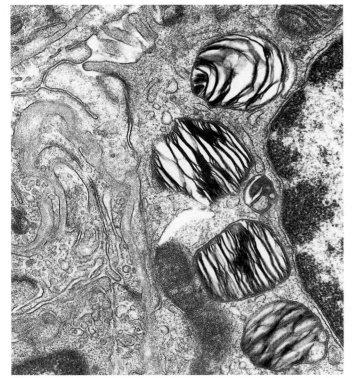

Fig. 1.44 Type 2 pulmonary alveolar cell, showing characteristic laminated secretory inclusions which contain surfactant.

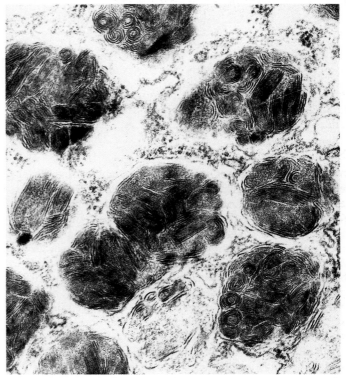

Fig. 1.46 Mast cell granules, showing characteristic whorled, scroll-like configurations.

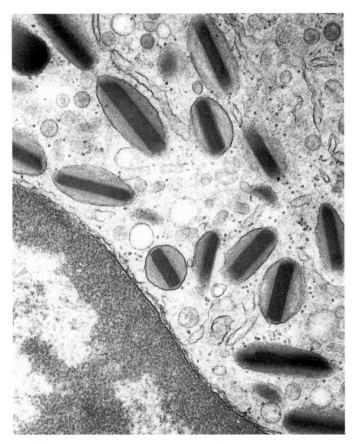

Fig. 1.47   Eosinophil granules, showing characteristic crystals.

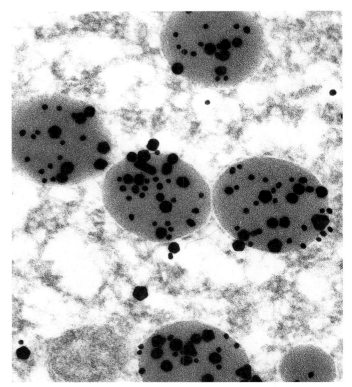

Fig. 1.48   Endocrine granules in a pituitary tumour, showing immuno-gold labelling with small and larger black gold particles. This confirms the presence of at least two distinct hormone products within each granule. (Micrograph by courtesy of Dr C. H. S. Cameron.)

morphology can give only limited guidance as to molecular composition or biological function. For example, it is often particularly difficult to distinguish between lysosomes and neuroendocrine secretory granules on morphological grounds alone. In tumours, disordered cellular function may lead to the production of atypical granules which correlate less well with cellular identity. Fortunately, there are now highly sensitive immunocytochemical techniques available for the ultrastructural localization of specific cellular products. For example, by the use of immunogold-labelling methods, specific hormones can be located in individual endocrine secretory granules and in some cells, double-labelling techniques can demonstrate the presence of two products within a single granule (Fig. 1.48).

Not all forms of secretion are associated with granule formation. Steroid hormones, for example, are not packaged in secretory granules, nor is collagen in fibroblasts, or immunoglobulins in plasma cells. Similarly, in the hepatocyte, the many synthetic and secretory activities of the cell are accomplished without the formation of secretory granules. Conversely, some cells have characteristic cytoplasmic inclusions which are not, themselves, destined for secretory release, but which reflect the metabolic functions of the cell. The cytoplasmic Reinke crystals of the Leydig cell (of the ovary and testis) are a striking example (Fig. 1.49).

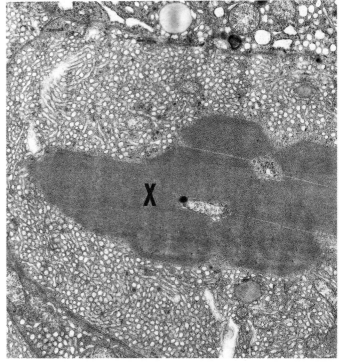

Fig. 1.49   Intracytoplasmic crystals of Reinke (X) in a Leydig cell tumour, with surrounding smooth endoplasmic reticulum.

Finally, it is worth mentioning three cell types which are not classified as secretory, but which are characterized by particularly distinctive cytoplasmic granules. These are the melanocyte, the vascular endothelial cell, and the Langerhans cell.

The melanocyte of the skin elaborates its characteristic pigment within granules known as melanosomes. The early immature form, or premelanosome, is a round or elliptical membrane-limited inclusion, which contains a distinctive internally structured matrix, composed of parallel longitudinal strands, each with a fine cross-periodicity (Fig. 1.50). It is within this framework that the biosynthesis of melanin is accomplished, leading to the accumulation of the amorphous, dense pigment of the mature melanin granule, which obscures the original fine structural detail of the granule matrix. Pigmented melanin granules such as these may be released from the cell and taken up through the process of endocytosis by neighbouring keratinocytes or macrophages. Melanin pigment taken up in this way is usually found in the form of larger heterogeneous inclusions, or secondary lysosomes, containing multiple discrete individual melanosomes. It is important to make the distinction between melanogenesis, which is the primary production of individual melanosomes, and secondary melanin uptake, or melanophagic activity. The recognition of melanin granules or premelanosomes (Figs 1.50, 1.51) is important in the diagnosis of certain poorly differentiated malignant tumours of melanocytes (see Chapter 28).

The Weibel–Palade body is a distinctive rod-shaped granule found in vascular endothelium (Fig. 1.52). It contains an internal longitudinal striation, translated in cross-section as a closely packed microtubulated pattern. The biological identity of this granule is uncertain, but it is no doubt related to endothelial cell function, perhaps representing part of the natural thrombolytic mechanism of vascular endothelium.

The Langerhans cell is a form of histiocyte, now identified as playing an important role in skin and mucosal antigen recognition and processing (see Chapter 4). Langerhans cells are normal intra-epithelial residents of skin and squamous mucosal surfaces, but are also found in the dermis, from where they migrate through lymphatics to regional lymph nodes. The Langerhans cell granule, or Birbeck granule, when imaged in three-dimensional reconstructions, appears as a complex membrane-limited disc, flattened and fused in one segment and dilated in another, resulting in a characteristic 'tennis racket' appearance in a typical cross-section (Fig. 1.53). These granules are found throughout the cytoplasm, but particularly

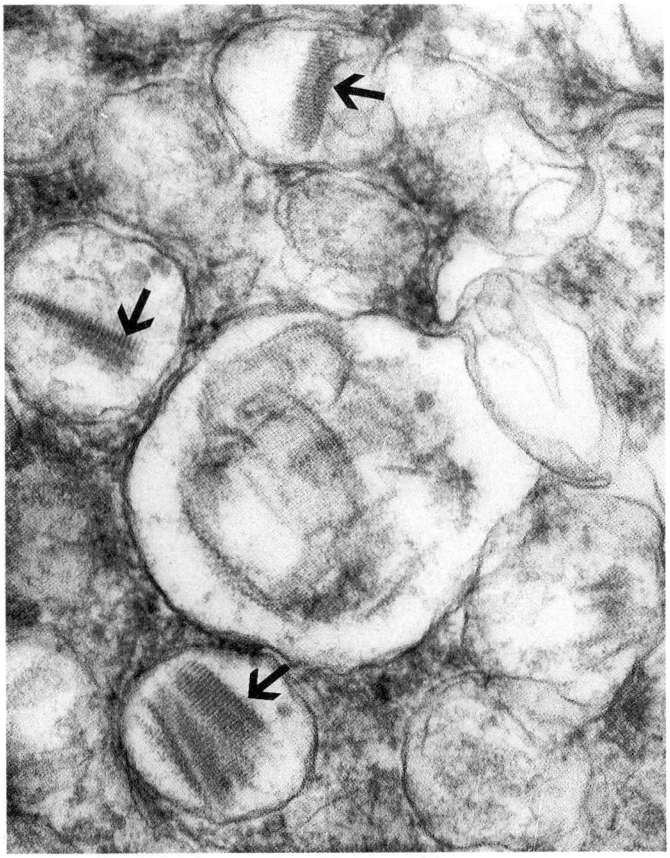

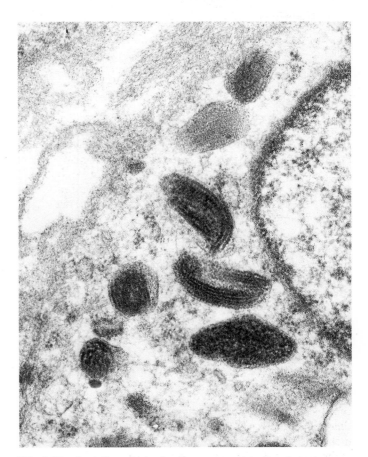

Fig. 1.50 Numerous premelanosomes in malignant melanoma, similar to those found in normal melanocytes. The internal periodicity is seen clearly (arrow).

Fig. 1.51 Partially melanized melanosomes in malignant melanoma, similar to those found in normal melanocytes.

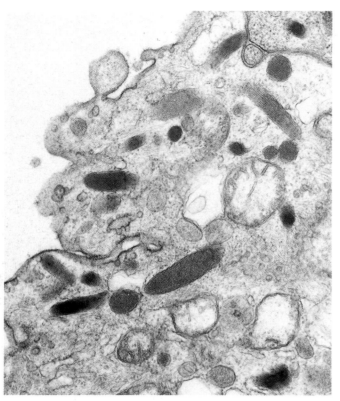

Fig. 1.52 Weibel–Palade endothelial granules.

around the Golgi apparatus. Similar structures appear to originate by the invagination and fusion of the cell membrane (Fig. 1.54), suggesting a specialized form of selective endocytosis. Generally, it is presumed that these images imply a sequence of granule formation at the cell surface, followed by internalization, in keeping with some role in antigen processing.

External and basal lamina

The histological concept of the basement membrane recognizes the existence of a specialized interface between certain cells and their surrounding connective tissue stroma. Typical examples are the basement membrane that underlies an epithelial sheet (Fig. 1.55), surrounds a gland, or envelopes a capillary vessel. A highly specialized adaptation of the same basic structure produces the filtration membrane of the renal glomerulus. The basement membrane can be delineated in histological preparations by various special stains, such as the periodic acid-Schiff (PAS) reaction and certain silver impregnation techniques.

Ultrastructural examination of the basement membrane region shows the consistent presence of a discrete, moderately dense layer (lamina densa), closely applied to the basal or external surface of the epithelial sheet, the gland, or the vascular tube. A similar external lamina invests various other cell types (Fig. 1.56), including Schwann cells, muscle cells, and fat cells.

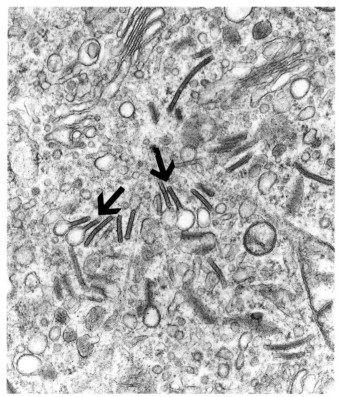

Fig. 1.53 Langerhans granules (arrows) in the Golgi region.

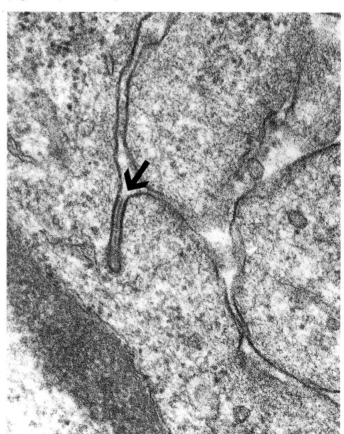

Fig. 1.54 Langerhans granule (arrow) at the cell surface.

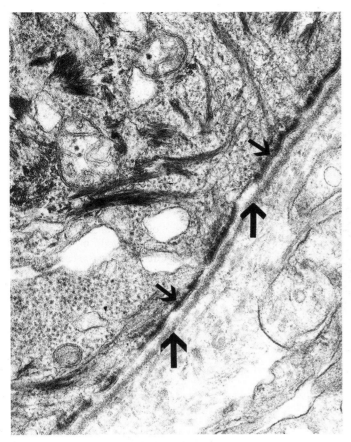

Fig. 1.55 Basal lamina at dermo-epidermal junction (large arrows), showing numerous hemidesmosomes (small arrows) and associated cytokeratin filament bundles.

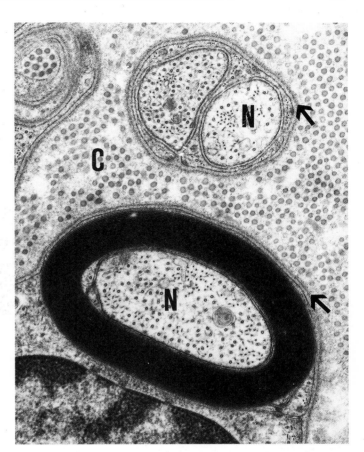

Fig. 1.56 Myelinated (lower nerve) and unmyelinated peripheral nerves, showing tightly fitting external laminae (arrows). Cross-sectioned collagen fibrils (C), neurotubules and neurofilaments (N) can be seen.

In the renal glomerulus, the filtration membrane arises through the fusion of an epithelial and an endothelial basal lamina to form a specialized combined structure, sandwiched between the podocytes of the glomerular epithelium and the capillary endothelial cells.

The lamina densa and its immediate macromolecular environment contain various defined constituents, such as laminin and type IV collagen. Although the role of the basal lamina is not yet fully established, it is clearly an interface of great biological significance, defining as it does the anatomical and functional boundaries within tissues and between cells of various types. It is clear from studies of the renal glomerular filtration membrane that the permeability characteristics of basement membranes are related closely to their physio-chemical properties (see Chapter 19).

1.1.4 Cell interrelationships

Interactions between cells have great biological significance in the multicellular organism and were, of course, a prerequisite of its evolution. From the earliest stages of embryonic development, the organization and compartmentalization of cells, and

the regulation of their activity, are dependent on cellular interactions such as endocrine and paracrine effects, which can take place either between spatially separated cells or between cells that are in close proximity. Interactions mediated by direct cell contact are involved in a wide range of general cellular physiological processes, in addition to their roles in morphogenesis and histogenesis. These include intercellular communications, movement, attachment, acquisition and maintenance of cell polarity, establishment of permeability barriers, growth control, and regulation of differentiation. Cell contact is also crucially involved in highly specialized cellular functions, such as lymphocyte homing, target recognition, and killing.

Mechanisms by which cell–cell contact is established and maintained involve molecular interactions at the surfaces of apposed cells. Some of these interactions occur at morphologically specialized areas of the cell membrane, such as desmosomes and gap junctions, whereas others take place in the absence of any morphological junctional organization. Several types of cell contact specialization are common to a wide range of cell types, whereas others are more restricted in their distribution. Since each type of junction is functionally distinct, it is not surprising that apposed cells often express more than one morphological class of adhesion mechanism.

Cell adhesion molecules

The cell adhesion molecules (CAMs) belong to a group of cell surface-associated glycoproteins which can promote cell–cell adhesion without necessarily being associated with morphological specialization. There is a growing number of confirmed and candidate CAMs which are believed to be involved in the processes of specific cell recognition and adhesion that take place during the organization of embryonic tissues, and organs in the cellular interactions of postnatal life. Those that appear in early embryonic development are known as primary CAMs, to distinguish them from the secondary CAMs which appear at later stages. CAMs can be subdivided into those that require Ca^{2+} for their activity and those that are Ca^{2+} independent.

Analysis of Ca^{2+}-dependent CAMs from different species and cell types indicates that they constitute a gene family of structurally and functionally related molecules. The human cell CAM 120/180, for example, is a homologue of chicken liver CAM (LCAM) and mouse uvomorulin. They are all integral membrane proteins with a long amino-terminal extracellular portion and a shorter carboxy-terminal cytoplasmic extension. The molecular mechanism of adhesion is not fully understood, but probably depends on homophilic interactions between apposed cells, with a CAM on one cell recognizing and adhering to an identical CAM on a neighbouring cell.

The neural adhesion molecule (NCAM) is a Ca^{2+}-independent CAM. It is a large, integral, membrane sialoglycoprotein and, as a primary CAM, it plays an important role in embryological development of the central nervous system. For example, it is involved in the guidance of developing optic nerve fibres. Its distribution over the cell surface may be localized rather than diffuse; in the optic nerve pathway it is concentrated at the end feet of neuro-epithelial cells. The form of NCAM may also differ between individual neural cell types, reflecting differences in glycosylation or in the structure of the protein itself. The binding mechanism is homophilic, depending on its ability to recognize and adhere to an identical molecule on the surface of an adjoining cell.

Also present in the central nervous system is NgCAM which mediates the adhesion of neurones to neurones and neurones to glia, properties that are of great importance in the architectural and functional organization of the nervous system. It is a secondary CAM which is present on the cell body of neurones. Its absence from glial cells indicates that its binding mechanism is heterophilic, the neuronal surface-associated NgCAM interacting with a different, and as yet unknown, molecule on the surface of glia.

Although CAM-mediated cell–cell interrelationships are of undoubted importance in cell physiology, the significance of interactions between the cell and the extracellular matrix must also be emphasized. Certain extracellular glycoproteins are known to have profound effects on cellular migration, morphology, and other phenotypic properties. Fibronectin is the best-characterized cell-substrate adhesion molecule. It is secreted by a number of cell types, including fibroblasts, and endothelial cells, and has several binding domains, one of which is recognized by a cell-surface receptor belonging to the integrin family. Other domains bind elements of the extracellular matrix such as heparin, collagen, and fibrin, suggesting that fibronectin plays a role in the structural organization of the extracellular matrix and its interactions with cells.

Another important molecule involved in linking cells and extracellular matrix is laminin, a glycoprotein with a distribution restricted to the basement membrane. Like fibronectin, it has a number of binding domains, including one that is recognized by the cell-surface laminin receptor and others that bind constituents of the extracellular matrix. The laminin receptor has been shown experimentally to be involved in cell adhesion and in the spread of malignant cells, but it seems likely that it may be implicated in other processes, such as cell migration, cytoskeletal organization, and mitogenesis. Cell matrix interactions are also discussed in Sections 1.4.3 and 1.4.4.

Cell interactions at morphologically specialized junctions

Cells demonstrate a wide variety of morphologically specialized junctional regions, some of which are cell type-specific whereas others have a more widespread cellular distribution. All of these junctions are, by definition, adhesive, but they have many additional physiological functions. They were first classified according to their ultrastructural appearances, but as information accumulates about their biochemical composition and functions these factors are also being taken into consideration. The major groups are tight junctions, adhaerens junctions, desmosomes, and gap junctions.

Tight junctions

The tight junction (or zonula occludens) is characteristic of epithelial cells. It acts as a selective barrier to luminal–serosal movement of materials and forms the most apical part of the junctional complex, a feature best seen in columnar epithelial cells. The junctional complex is a continuous circumferential zone of contact specialization occurring on the lateral aspect of the cell membrane, towards the apical or luminal margin (Fig. 1.57). In addition to the tight junctions, this area usually also displays adhaerens junctions and desmosomes. At the tight junctions, electron microscopy shows an apparent fusion of the outer leaflets of the cell membrane, with elimination of the extracellular space. Freeze-fracture studies demonstrate a continuous network of branching and anastomosing fibrils in the plane of the membrane, which appear to correspond to areas of membrane contact. There is fine filamentous material on the cytoplasmic surface of the tight junction, which suggests a possible interaction between the junction and elements of the cytoskeleton.

Transport across epithelia may take place through cells (the transcellular route), or between cells (the paracellular route). A prime function of an epithelial cell layer is to prevent the free passage of materials by the paracellular route. The tight junction represents the mechanism by which this is achieved.

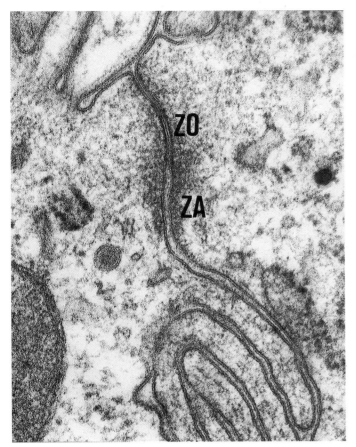

Fig. 1.57 Cell membrane at the apex of columnar epithelium, showing zonula occudens (ZO) and zonula adhaerens (ZA) specializations.

Tight junctions are impermeable to many molecules and the molecular size of excluded materials varies between different epithelia.

The permeability of tight junctions may fluctuate in response to physiological stimuli. In the mammary gland, for instance, the transepithelial paracellular movement of sucrose is increased during lactation. Recent research has indicated that absorption of some nutrients from the intestinal lumen may proceed by the paracellular route rather than by active transcellular passage. The mechanism suggested for this is that glucose or amino acids entering the cell by the Na^+-coupled active-transport system cause contraction in the actin–myosin cytoskeleton in the region of the junctional complex. This might increase paracellular permeability at the tight junction, resulting in the paracellular luminal–serosal movement of nutrients.

Epithelial cells have a marked morphological polarity, which is also represented in the chemical composition of the cell membrane. The protein and lipid components of the apical membrane differ from those of the lateral and basal membranes, the borderline between the two domains lying at the tight junction. Since proteins and lipids are normally free to diffuse within the plane of the membrane, it appears that the tight junction forms a barrier to molecular movement. This has been confirmed by

the finding of a loss of structural membrane polarity following disruption of tight junctions.

Little is known about the biochemical composition of the tight junction, but one protein is known to be specifically associated. This is a monomeric phosphoprotein ZO1 which is associated with the periphery of the junctional membrane. In addition, the presence of LCAM is essential for the formation of the tight junction and other components of the junctional complex.

Adhaerens junctions

Adhaerens junctions are formed with membranes of neighbouring cells or with extracellular substrates. They were originally known as belt desmosomes and classified within the desmosome group, because of morphological similarities. However, the two groups are now known to be sufficiently distinct, especially in their association with different classes of intracytoplasmic filaments, to merit separate classification. In polarized epithelia this junction is known as the zonula adhaerens (Fig. 1.57), since it forms a continuous belt around the cell. There is an intercellular gap of 15–20 nm. On the cytoplasmic face, actin filaments run along the membrane parallel to the junction. In other cell types in which they are found, such as myocytes (Fig. 1.58) and cultured fibroblasts, the adhaerens specialization has a patchy distribution and is called a fascia adhaerens.

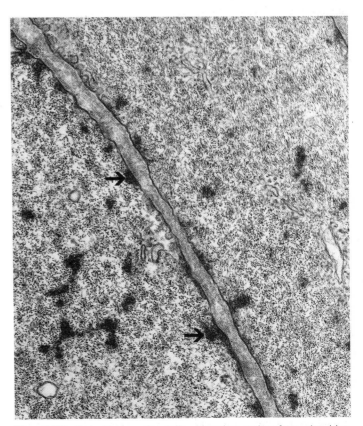

Fig. 1.58 Smooth muscle cells, showing subsurface densities (arrows) to which actin filaments attach.

Adhaerens junctions may also form between the cell and elements of the extracellular matrix. They may be found *in vivo* in association with intercellular connective tissue and basement membranes. The extracellular matrix has a profound influence on many aspects of cell morphology and of cellular behaviour, including locomotion, differentiation, and proliferation. It is likely that these effects are signalled through adhesive contact. Cultured cells possess similar structures which maintain contact with the growth substatum. These are known as focal adhesion plaques or focal contacts, and their study has led to considerable advances in the understanding of adhaerens junctions in general.

The adhaerens junction contains at least four distinct but interconnected molecular domains. The first of these is the surface to which the cell is attached. This may be the membrane of an adjoining cell, or the extracellular matrix, which must contain molecules that are specifically recognized by the attaching cell. Fibronectin, an extracellular matrix and cell-surface glycoprotein, is known to play this role. It is essential for the establishment of focal contact and for the induction of adhesion plaques, but it is removed from the junctional area at a later stage and so is clearly not essential for maintenance of the specialized junction.

The second is the plasma membrane domain. This consists of integral membrane proteins, which form links with the external domain and with the plaque inside the cell. In junctions between cells and the extracellular matrix, one of these proteins is an integrin, which acts as a fibronectin receptor. This integrin is absent from the junctional cleft in contacts between cells, and there is evidence that in this situation the Ca^{2+} LCAM may be involved. The membrane domain contains proteins that are restricted to that site, but it is unlike the tight junction membrane domain in that it does not act as a diffusion barrier to mobile membrane components.

The third domain of the adhaerens junction is the junctional plaque, which consists of a group of proteins interacting on one side with the integral membrane proteins and on the other with the cytoplasmic actin microfilaments. The best-characterized and most abundant plaque protein is vinculin, which acts as a marker for adhaerens junctions. It seems that the plaque consists largely of a multilayered structure of vinculin in association with other proteins. Vinculin has actin-binding properties and is probably responsible for inducing the assembly of actin filaments into the large bundles that are associated with the junction. In addition to being present as an anchored plaque protein, vinculin exists in a soluble, diffusible cytoplasmic form. In conditions encouraging cell contact, soluble vinculin would be converted into the plaque form and the reduction in cytoplasmic vinculin would lead to increased gene expression and replenishment of the cytoplasmic reserve. Another plaque-associated protein is talin, the presence of which is restricted to contacts between the cell and the extracellular matrix.

The cytoplasmic domain is the final component of the adhaerens junction. This consists of the actin microfilament system and its associated actin-binding proteins, which interact with the junctional plaque. The precise nature of this interaction is unknown but it is likely to reflect the known variability in morphological appearances. In the fascia adhaerens and in focal contacts, the filaments abut end-on with the plaques, whereas in the zonula adhaerens the filaments run parallel to the plaque. Whilst actin and its associated proteins are the major components of the cytoskeleton which interact with the plaque, there is evidence, at least in focal contacts, that intermediate filaments may also form linkages and play a part in the stabilization of the junction.

The presence of adhaerens junctions in a wide variety of cell types, including fibroblasts, epithelia, muscle, neurones, astrocytes, endothelia, and macrophages, suggests a fundamental role in cell physiology. The adhaerens junction probably has at least a purely mechanical role. The myotendinous junction, which shares structural and functional characteristics with focal adhesions, anchors cytoplasmic microfilaments and transmits their tension across the membrane to the extracellular matrix components of the tendon. In most normal cells, the ability to proliferate depends on attachment to a substratum, a property termed anchorage dependence. Proliferation stops when cells make sufficiently close contact with their neighbours, a phenomenon known as contact inhibition of growth. It seems likely that both of these processes are mediated by cell–substrate or cell–cell contacts of the adhaerens type. In this context it may be significant that the number of adhaerens junctions is reduced in malignant cells in which anchorage-independent growth occurs and which lose the ability to control growth by contact inhibition.

Desmosomes

The desmosome, or macula adhaerens, is structurally not unlike the zonula and fascia adhaerens, but has specific distinguishing features. Desmosomes are found principally in epithelia, where they link cells externally by spot-like adhesion and anchor intermediate filaments to the plasma membrane (see Fig. 1.17). This combination of properties gives tensile strength to the tissue as a whole, enabling it to resist mechanical forces. The desmosome is a highly organized focal attachment specialization, with an intercellular gap of 20–30 nm. The gap is bisected by a median density, representing a condensation of extracellular material at the site of the desmosome. On the cytoplasmic surface there is a dense plaque, to which cytoplasmic intermediate filaments of the cytokeratin class are attached.

The number and distribution of desmosomes differs from tissue to tissue. In epithelia that are naturally highly stressed, such as the epidermis, desmosomes are particularly numerous, large, and well-formed, whereas less mechanically stressed sites have much less prominent desmosomes. In simple epithelia, desmosomes are restricted to the lateral surfaces, whereas in the intermediate layers of stratified epithelia they are distributed over the entire surface of the cell, to provide all-round adhesion. At the base of a stratified squamous epithelium, such as the epidermis, hemidesmosomes (Fig. 1.55) provide equivalent mechanical linkages between the basal cell layer and the under-lying epithelial basal lamina. The hemidesmosome consists of the typical desmosomal membrane-associated plaque with attached cytokeratin filaments, associated with a patch of extra-cellular material equivalent to the median density which bisects the full desmosome. These structures ensure the firm attach-ment of the epidermis to its basement membrane.

As is the case with adhaerens junctions, desmosomes have membrane, plaque, and cytoskeletal domains, each of which is characterized by the presence of specific proteins. A number of glycoproteins have been localized to the membrane domain. At least some of these, the desmogleins, are involved in cellular adhesion, a property that resides in the glycosylated part of the molecule. Experimentally, it has been shown that desmosomes may form between cells isolated from different tissues and even from different species, suggesting a high degree of evolutionary conservation of adhesive protein structure.

In contrast with the membrane domain, the plaque contains non-glycosylated proteins known as desmoplakins. It seems likely that they play a part in the linkage between the plaque and the cytokeratin intermediate filaments, or tonofilaments, which results in their anchorage to the plasma membrane. Bundles of tonofilaments traverse the cell, forming loops which interconnect the desmosomes. It is not yet clear whether the filaments enter the plaque, or simply approach its surface tangentially before looping back into the cytoplasm.

Desmosomes first appear early in embryonic development, at the morula–blastocyst transition in the mouse, at a time that coincides with the first appearance of cytokeratin filaments. Their formation and stability is Ca^{2+}-dependent. Some of the desmogleins have calcium-binding properties and may be the site of action of Ca^{2+} in promoting desmosomal assembly.

The degree of permanance of desmosomal junctions may well vary from tissue to tissue. Areas of continuous cell rearrange-ment, such as the intestinal crypt, would require frequent breakdown and re-establishment of desmosomal contacts, whereas more permanent contacts would be expected in the upper layers of the epidermis. A curiosity of some desmosome-rich cells is the occurrence of occasional intracytoplasmic des-mosomes. These resemble the conventional structures, but they are disconnected from any continuous membrane surface and appear to lie isolated within the cytoplasm, sometimes showing a small remnant of the cell membrane from which they have become detached. Intracytoplasmic desmosomes probably arise by the engulfment and endocytosis of a conventional desmosome (Fig. 1.59). The quite frequent occurrence of this phenomenon in certain tumours is thought to reflect the greater instability of cellular contacts in the neoplastic state.

Desmosomes occur mostly in epithelia, but identical struc-tures have been observed in other tissues. They are present in the intercalated discs of the myocardium, where they differ from epithelial desmosomes only in as much as the intermediate fila-ments to which they are attached are desmin rather than cyto-keratin. Similar structures are found between the arachnoid cells covering the brain. In this instance, the attachments are with vimentin intermediate filaments.

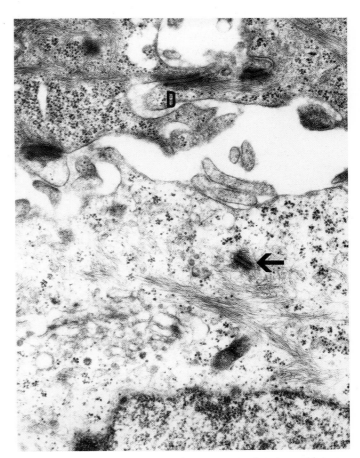

Fig. 1.59 Oesophageal squamous epithelium, showing desmosomes (D) linking adjacent cells. An intracytoplasmic desmosome (arrow) is associated with cytokeratin filaments.

Gap junctions

The gap junction is a specialized membrane complex which allows the exchange of ions and molecules between cells. In ultrastructural terms, the gap junction is a focal area of close membrane apposition, which falls short of complete fusion of the external leaflets of the contacting membranes (Fig. 1.60). Gap junctions are thus distinct from tight junctions. There is no obvious attachment of cytoplasmic cytoskeletal components to the inner aspect of the gap junction. Junctions such as these in smooth muscle were originally described as nexus specializa-tions. Gap junctions may occasionally become internalized by mechanisms analogous to the formation of intracytoplasmic desmosomes.

The unique molecular subunit of this junction is the con-nexon, a hollow cylinder of transmembrane proteins, six molecules of which surround the central 2 nm channel (Fig. 1.61). Each protein subunit is tilted at an angle to the axis of the connexon and a decrease in the angle of tilt results in closure of the channel at the cytoplasmic side. The gap junction channels tend to be grouped in particular areas of the mem-brane, into plaques ranging in size from a few connexons to

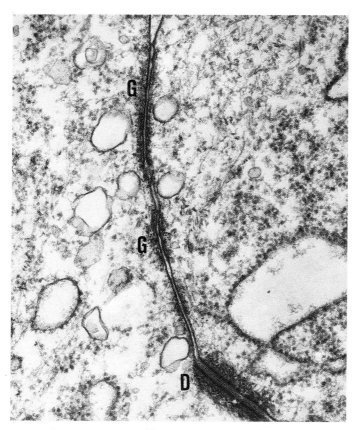

Fig. 1.60 Cell adhesion specializations between tumour cells, including a typical desmosome (D) and an area of linear and focal gap junction specialization (G).

many thousands. Connexons project about 1–2 nm into the extracellular space, where they abut directly on to connexons on the adjacent cell. Gap junctions are permeable to ions and molecules that are small enough to pass through the channel. In mammalian cells the exclusion limit is in the region of a molecular weight of 900, although the shape of the molecule is also important in determining permeability.

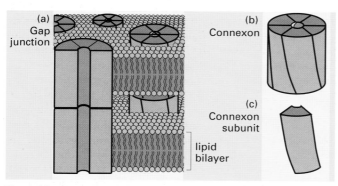

Fig. 1.61 The molecular structure of a gap junction. The gap junction traverses the cell membrane (a). The connexon (b) and its subunit (c) are the building blocks of these junctions. (Drawn after Bock and Clark 1987, with permission.)

A clear requirement of junctions involved in intercellular communications is rapid regulation. The normal state of gap junctions is the open position, but factors such as a falling pH and an increasing intracellular Ca^{2+} result in rapid closure. A consequence of this is the development of rapid isolation between normal cells and their damaged neighbours.

The formation of gap junctions is a cell-specific process, the incidence of junction formation being higher between similar cells than between unlike cells. This leads to the formation of 'communication compartments', characterized by the rapid exchange of molecules within a population of similar cells, but by very slow exchange with neighbouring heterologous cells. The mechanism of this specificity is unlikely to reside in the connexon proteins and is more likely to involve other cell-surface glycoproteins, which can recognize and adhere to homologous cells, thereby bringing them into close enough contact for gap junction formation. In tissue culture, the free exchange of small molecules across gap junctions can be demonstrated by introducing fluorescent dyes into individual cells and following the rapid diffusion of the marker throughout a whole sheet of coupled cells.

A result of widespread gap junction formation within a cell population is that changes occurring in one cell can be transmitted very rapidly to the rest of the group, and transmission between any two cells may, of course, be bidirectional. Action potentials can thus spread throughout a connected cell population more quickly and more widely than would be possible by chemical synaptic transmission. In tissues such as heart and smooth muscle, in which gap or nexus junctions are particularly frequent, they provide a very efficient mechanism for the spread of action potentials and thus for the propagation of waves of contraction. This, however, produces an 'all-or-none' effect, which would be inappropriate, for example, in skeletal muscle. In this tissue, gap junctions are lost during the later stages of differentiation.

The sharing of small molecules resulting from the presence of gap junctions may also be important in the response to hormonal signalling. Second messengers such as cyclic AMP and inositol phosphates, formed as a result of hormonal stimulation of one or a few cells, would rapidly spread throughout the connected group. This would result in the co-ordination and amplification of the tissue response to the hormonal signal.

Other morphological expressions of cell interaction

Even when cells form morphologically distinct contact specializations, the greater part of their contact surface remains structurally unspecialized. Cell membranes in mutual contact may display complex interlocking flaps and folds of cytoplasm, but a minimum intercellular gap of around 15 nm normally remains, as visualized by conventional ultrastructural techniques. This presumably corresponds to the layer of membrane-associated cell adhesion molecules, along with other components of the cell coat which are not positively imaged by electron microscopy.

The interrelationships of lymphocytes with other cell types

are of particular interest. Specific recognition signals facilitate the passage of lymphocytes to and fro across vessel walls, giving them access to the connective tissues. Lymphocytes also frequently traverse basement membranes to enter epithelial layers, such as the intestinal mucosa (Fig. 1.62), where they lie in apposition to the epithelial cells, but do not form specialized adhesions. Such relationships are presumably a normal part of immunological surveillance. Intra-epithelial lymphocytes are more numerous and apparently more active in various pathological conditions of the bowel.

In tissue culture and, on occasions, *in vivo* (Fig. 1.63), lymphocytes may push their way right inside large cells, such as tumour cells, so that they come to lie surrounded by the tumour cell cytoplasm, within a membrane-limited vacuole. The lymphocyte may move around inside the larger cell for substantial periods of time, without either cell coming to any apparent harm, since both cell membranes remain intact throughout the process. This phenomenon has been termed emperipolesis.

In the case of lymphocyte-mediated cytotoxic reactions, such as graft rejection, increased numbers of lymphocytes may be present, in keeping with an immune response (Fig. 1.64). It has been suggested that focal areas of close apposition of the cell membranes of the lymphocyte and the target cell provide morphological evidence of the mechanism of cell killing. Morpho-

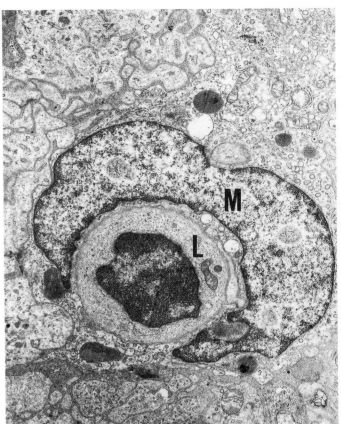

Fig. 1.63 Lymphocyte–macrophage interaction, showing a lymphocyte (L) lying embedded within the cytoplasm of the macrophage (M) and almost enveloped by its nucleus.

logy, however, has serious limitations in the study of phenomena such as these.

1.1.5 Subcellular phenotypes in pathological diagnosis

Much of the workload of the hospital pathologist involves the identification and classification of the various types of human tumour. Whatever the origins of the neoplastic process, the cancer cell can generally be pictured as a parody of some normally differentiated cell type. The neoplastic parody may come very close to the normal model, as in some benign tumours. Such tumours are described as well differentiated. In other cases, the parody may be so distant that routine histological examination shows no remaining recognizable markers of cellular identity. These tumours are known as poorly differentiated, undifferentiated, or anaplastic.

In general, however, when the diagnostic pathologist sets out to establish the identity of a tumour, it is the recognition of phenotypic similarities to related normal cells that will be the key to its classification. Thus gland-forming malignant tumours are termed adenocarcinomas, whereas keratinizing tumours

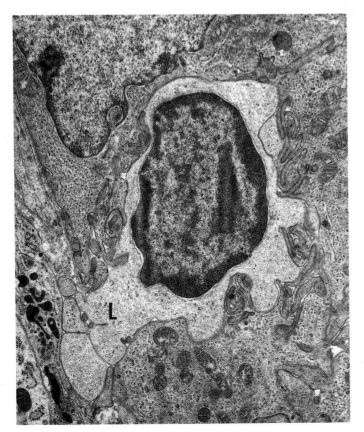

Fig. 1.62 Lymphocyte–enterocyte interaction, showing a lymphocyte (L) crossing the basement membrane.

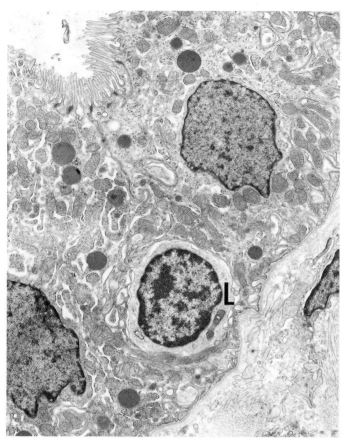

Fig. 1.64 Renal tubular epithelium in transplant rejection. A lymphocyte (L) lies between tubular epithelial cells, but these appear normal. (Micrograph by courtesy of Dr C. M. Hill.)

are identified as squamous cell carcinomas. Malignant tumours of connective and muscular tissues may be classified as sarcomas of smooth or striated muscle type, or of fibroblasts, fat cells or blood vessels. Pigment-forming tumours are known as melanomas. In brief, virtually every pattern of differentiated cell has a recognizable neoplastic counterpart.

Since the ultrastructure of the normal cell reflects its functional differentiation, the ultrastructure of the corresponding tumour cell can be expected to reflect whatever differentiated functions the malignant phenotype may retain. In tumours described by light microscopy as well differentiated, the ultrastructural phenotype usually corresponds closely to that of the normal cell. In light-microscopically undifferentiated tumours, however, only a minority of cases show no ultrastructural markers of identity.

In many of the problem cases which cannot be accurately classified by light microscopy, the ultrastructural phenotype may still be recognizable as a parody of some definable pattern of differentiation. In general, the evidence lies in some feature of cytoplasmic fine structure, or in characteristic associations between cells, or with stromal constituents. There are many examples. In poorly differentiated tumours, the persistence of

well-formed desmosomes or the formation of abortive but still recognizable glandular structures may point to an epithelial identity. In other instances, the presence of recognizable premelanosomes in a tumour which shows no histological evidence of pigmentation, or of neuro-endocrine secretory granules, may allow the confident identification of a malignant melanoma or of a neuro-endocrine carcinoma, whereas otherwise a non-specific diagnosis such as anaplastic malignant tumour might have been all that was available. In the classification of mesenchymal tumours, the recognition of fibroblastic features, of lysosomal accumulation, of myofilaments, or of lipid accumulation may be of importance in classification. Tumours of nerve sheath pattern are particularly distinguished by complex interlocking cytoplasmic processes, enveloped by external laminae.

It must be emphasized that there is no unique ultrastructural marker of neoplasia or of malignancy. This fundamental aspect of tumour classification still relies on traditional pathological criteria at the light-microscopic level. The contribution of electron microscopy to tumour classfication lies in its sensitive delineation of specific morphological patterns of differentiation, from which parallels can be drawn to normal cellular morphology. It follows that the pathologist who would use this technique in diagnosis must have an extensive experience of normal cellular ultrastructure, just as the histopathologist must have a mastery of the normal microscopic structure of human organs and tissues. Diagnostic morphological pathology is the practical application of anatomical knowledge to the diagnosis and classification of disease.

Similar parallels exist at the molecular level, between the normal and the neoplastic phenotype, in the form of specific molecular markers, detectable by biochemical or immunochemical methods. Various distinctive protein products expressed by cells during normal differentiation may continue to be produced by the neoplastic cell, thus providing a pointer towards tumour identity. Such tumour markers may be detectable not only in the tumour itself, but also in the patient's serum, thus providing a simple test for assessing recurrence after surgical treatment.

Diagnostic pathologists now have extensive panels of specific antibodies directed against various characteristic markers of phenotypic differentiation. The reactions of individual cells can be tested by the use of enzyme-labelling techniques, which produce a coloured reaction product in a histological section at the site of combination of labelled antibody with tissue antigen. On the assumption that the malignant phenotype retains certain features of corresponding normal gene expression, the reactions of tumour cells to such panels of antibodies can be taken as a basis for tumour classification (see Section 9.4).

Such 'functional' marker systems will often provide useful evidence of tumour identity quicker and more economically than electron microscopy. On the other hand, any individual immunodetectable marker reflects the function of only one or a handful of genes, which may be subject to unpredictable variations, whereas the patterns of ultrastructural differentiation detected by electron microscopy correspond to the expression and interaction of the much larger number of structural and organizational genes involved in the complex processes of morphogenesis. It can be argued that such polygenic characteristics may sometimes provide a more reliable indicator of cellular identity. It seems likely that our understanding of phenotypic variations in neoplasia will best be enhanced by the judicious use both of ultrastructural and of immunocytochemical technology.

Mechanisms involved in differentiation are discussed in the next section.

1.1.6 Further reading

Alberts, B., *et al.* (1989). *Molecular biology of the cell.* Garland Publishing, London.

Bock, G. and Clark, S. (eds) (1987). *Junctional complexes of epthelial cells,* CIBA Foundation Symposium 125. Wiley and Sons, Chichester.

Bruzzone, R. and Meda, P. (1988). The gap junction: a channel for multiple functions? *European Journal of Clinical Investigation* 18, 444–53.

Burridge, K., Fath, K., Kelly, T., Nuckolls, G., and Turner, C. (1988). Focal adhesions: transmembrane junctions between the extracellular matrix and the cytoskeleton. *Annual Review of Cell Biology* 4, 487–526.

Carr, K. E. and Toner, P. G. (1982). *Cell structure.* Churchill Livingstone, London.

Cereijido, M., Gonzales-Mariscal, L., and Contreras, R. G. (1988). Epithelial cell junctions. *American Review of Respiratory Disease* 138, S17–S21.

De Robertis, E. D. P. and De Robertis, E. M. F., Jr (1987). *Cell and molecular biology.* Lea and Febiger, Philadelphia.

Edelman, G. M. (1983). Cell adhesion molecules. *Science* 219, 450–7.

Edelman, G. M. (1986). Cell adhesion molecules in the regulation of animal form and tissue pattern. *Annual Review of Cell Biology* 2, 81–116.

Ellinger, A., Gruber, K., and Stockinger, L. (1987). Glycocalyceal bodies—a marker for different epithelial cell types in human airways. *Journal of Submicroscopic Cytology* 19, 311–16.

Fawcett, D. W. (1986). *A textbook of histology.* W. B. Saunders, Philadelphia.

Garrod, D. R. (1986). Desmosomes, cell adhesion molecules and the adhesive properties of cells in tissues. In *Prospects in cell biology* (ed. A. V. Grimstone, H. Harris, and R. T. Johnson), pp. 239–66. The Company of Biologists, Cambridge.

Gerace, L. (1986). Nuclear lamina and organization of nuclear architecture. *Trends in Biochemical Sciences* 11, 443.

Gerace, L. and Burke, B. (1988). Functional organisation of the nuclear envelope. *Annual Review of Cell Biology* 4, 335–74.

Ghadially, F. N. (1988). *Ultrastructural pathology of the cell and matrix.* Butterworths, London.

Glaumann, H. and Ballard, F. J. (eds) (1987). *Lysosomes—their role in protein breakdown.* Academic Press, London.

Heaysman, J. E., Middleton, C. A., and Watt, F. M. (eds) (1987). *Cell behaviour: shape, adhesion and motility,* The Second Abercrombie Conference. The Company of Biologists, Cambridge.

Jensen, C. G. and Smaill, B. H. (1986). Analysis of the spatial organization of microtubule-associated proteins. *Journal of Cell Biology* 103, 559–66.

Kemler, R., Ozawa, M., and Ringwald, M. (1989). Calcium-dependent cell adhesion molecules. *Current Opinions in Cell Biology* 1, 892–7.

Kessel, R. G. (1985). Annulate lamellae (porous cytomembranes): with particular emphasis on their possible role in differentiation of the female gamete. *Developmental Biology* 1, 179–84.

Lazarow, P. B. and Fujik, Y. (1985). Biogenesis of perioxisomes. *Annual Review of Cell Biology* 1, 489–504.

Mayne, R. and Burgeson, R. E. (eds) (1987). *Structure and function of collagen types.* Academic Press, London.

Nagle, R. (1988). Intermediate filaments: a review of basic biology. *American Journal of Surgical Pathology* 12 (51), 4.

Pitts, J. D. and Finbow, M. E. (1986). The gap junction. In *Prospects in cell biology* (ed. A. V. Grimstone, H. Harris, and R. T. Johnson), pp. 239–66. The Company of Biologists, Cambridge.

Scheer, U., Dabanvalle, M. C., Merkert, H., and Benevent, R. (1988). The nuclear envelope and the organisation of the pore complexes. *Cell Biology International Reports* 12, 660–89.

Stevenson, B. R. and Paul, D. L. (1989). The molecular constituents of intercellular junctions. *Current Opinions in Cell Biology* 1, 884–91.

Stevenson, B. R., Anderson, J. M., and Bullivant, S. (1988). The epithelial tight junction: structure, function and preliminary biochemical characterization. *Molecular and Cellular Biochemistry* 83, 129–45.

Tartakoff, A. M. (1982). Simplifying the complex Golgi. *Trends in Biochemical Sciences* 7, 174–86.

Tsanev, R. and Tsanev, J. (1986). Molecular organisation of chromatin as revealed by electron microscopy. In *Methods and achievements in experimental pathology,* Vol. 12 (ed. G. Jasmin and R. Simard), pp. 63–104. Karger, Basel.

Verheijen, R., Van Venrooij, W., and Ramaekers, F. (1988). The nuclear matrix: structure and composition. *Journal of Cell Science* 90, 11–36.

Weiss, L. (1988). The cell. In *Cell and tissue biology: a text book of histology* (ed. L. Weiss). Urban and Schwartzenberg, Baltimore.

Wheatley, D. N. (1982). *The centriole: a central enigma of cell biology.* Elsevier Biomedical Press, Amsterdam.

1.2 Cell differentiation

Fiona M. Watt

1.2.1 Introduction: what is differentiation?

The first section of this chapter has described the basic features common to all animal cells. This section deals with differences between cells. We shall consider the characteristics by which different cell types can be distinguished and how diversity of cell phenotype is established and maintained. The process by which different cell types arise to fulfil specialized functions within the body is known as differentiation.

1.2.2 Diversity of different cell types

How are different cell types distinguished from one another? They are found in different parts of the body, they differ in morphology, and there are qualitative and quantitative differences in the macromolecules they synthesize. Table 1.1 gives some examples of proteins with specific differentiated functions: these proteins are only expressed by certain types of cell; they are not essential for cell viability; and as such they may be defined as products of 'luxury' genes. In contrast, gene products with a

Table 1.1 Examples of 'luxury' gene products expressed by differentiated cells

Gene product	Function	Cell type
Haemoglobin	Transport of oxygen in the bloodstream	Erythrocytes
Involucrin	Precursor of the cornified envelope that provides the protective covering for skin	Keratinocytes
Insulin	Hormone regulating blood carbohydrate levels	Pancreatic β-cells
Crystallins	Transmission of light to the retina	Lens epithelial cells
Pepsinogen	Digestion of proteins in the stomach	Zymogenic cells

'housekeeping' function are present in virtually all cells, and without them the cells would die: the enzymes of the Krebs cycle are examples.

Other sections of this chapter (1.3 and 1.4) describe the properties and organization of a number of differentiated cell types in different tissues, e.g. liver. Here we shall consider general aspects of cellular diversity: cell morphology and the cytoskeleton; the extracellular matrix (ECM); and cell adhesiveness. The local cellular environment, consisting of the ECM and neighbouring cells, plays a central role in inducing and stabilizing the differentiated phenotype (see also Section 1.4).

Cell morphology

There is tremendous variation in the size of cells from different tissues: erythrocytes have a diameter of less than 5 μm, whereas skeletal muscle cells may be up to 0.5 m in length and individual neurones may extend axons over 1 m long. Most cells contain a single nucleus; however, mature mammalian erythrocytes are anucleate, and skeletal muscle cells and osteoclasts are multinucleate.

In addition to variation in size and nucleation, there are also wide differences in cell morphology, which are related to differentiated function. Thus erythrocytes are disc-shaped for ease of circulation in the blood; nerve cells have long processes for conducting nerve impulses; and cells in many epithelia are polarized, with apical surfaces specialized for absorption or secretion and a basal surface attached to a basement membrane.

The ultrastructure of cells also reflects their specialized functions. Thus the rough endoplasmic reticulum and Golgi are abundant in specialized secretory cells, such as those lining the gut, but are non-existent in erythrocytes. Lipid droplets are prominent features of the cytoplasm of adipocytes; synaptic vesicles are concentrated at nerve endings for release of neurotransmitters. Some cells have unusual cytoplasmic inclusions, such as melanosomes in melanocytes and keratohyalin granules in terminally differentiating epidermal keratinocytes (see also Section 1.1). Figure 1.65 illustrates the appearance of some of the specialized cell types found in the gut: even within a single tissue there can be considerable variation in ultrastructural appearance.

The cytoskeleton and cell motility

Most cells have a cytoskeleton consisting of three components: microtubules, actin filaments, and intermediate filaments (see Section 1.1). Although the basic structure and composition of each cytoskeletal element is conserved in all tissues, there are nevertheless differences in function, molecular composition, and spatial organization between differentiated cell types.

Microtubules

Microtubules are highly conserved structures assembled from heterodimers of α- and β-tubulin. They have two fundamental cellular functions: they form the mitotic spindle and they are the structures along which organelles are transported. Superimposed on this conservation, however, is some heterogeneity of function which is, in turn, reflected in variation in the biochemical composition and stability of microtubules.

Microtubule heterogeneity is observed at several levels. There are multigene families of α- and β-tubulins and there are tissue-specific differences in their expression. Another source of variation is in the degree of post-translational modification of tubulin: tyrosination, for example, is thought to affect microtubule stability. While tubulin isotype expression and post-translational modification vary to some extent between cell types, they may be more important as sources of microtubule diversity within individual cells. Differences between the microtubules of different cell types are more clearly observed with respect to microtubule-associated proteins (MAPs), a varied collection of proteins that bind to, or interact with, microtubules. Changes in MAP expression during embryonic development have been observed and these may influence microtubule distribution, stability, and function.

Microtubules grouped in the ordered arrays that constitute cilia and flagellae have a function in cell motility. Movement of sperm cells, for example, is dependent on flagellae. In tracheal epithelium, cilia move mucus-trapped particles from the lungs; and the ciliated epithelium of the fallopian tube moves oocytes from the ovary towards the uterus.

Microfilaments

Like the tubulins, the actins are highly conserved proteins that constitute a multigene family and have a variety of associated proteins in different differentiated cells. Actin microfilaments play an important role in cell shape and motility.

As with the tubulins, there is tissue-specific variation in actin isotypes. Non-muscle cells express β and γ cytoplasmic actins. There are two smooth-muscle actins: the γ form is the major actin in visceral tissue, and the α form is predominant in vascular smooth muscle. In addition there are two sarcomeric α-actins: one found in cardiac and the other in skeletal muscle.

A range of proteins interact with actin at the plasma membrane and along the length of microfilaments. Actin-binding proteins regulate actin assembly: there are proteins that sequester actin monomers; proteins that block the ends of actin filaments; and proteins that cross-link actin filaments. Some of these proteins are specifically expressed in different cell types:

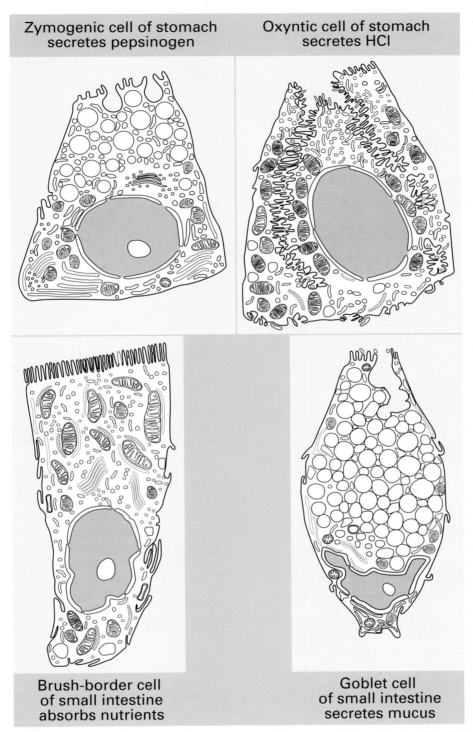

Fig. 1.65 Some of the specialized cell types found in the epithelial lining of the gut (After T. L. Lentz, *Cell Fine Structure*. Philadelphia: Saunders, 1971; redrawn after Alberts *et al.* 1983, with permission).

for example, spectrin connects actin oligomers into a two-dimensional network associated with the plasma membrane of erythrocytes, and the related protein, fodrin, is found in brain. Villin, originally purified from intestinal epithelial cells, cross-links actin filaments of microvilli into bundles.

Motile mechanisms based on actin and myosin are found in most eukaryotic cells. In muscle, actin molecules are mainly present in polymerized form, organized into stable structures, the sarcomeres, to allow contraction. In contrast, the non-muscle actins exist in dynamic equilibrium between monomer and polymer forms.

Intermediate filaments

Of the three classes of cytoskeletal elements, the intermediate filaments are those that show widest variation in molecular composition between types of differentiated cells, and their function is least well understood. Table 1.2 lists the different classes of intermediate filaments and their tissue distribution.

Proteins of the nuclear envelope, called lamins, have some sequence homology with intermediate filament proteins and, as such, may form an additional intermediate filament class. Of all the intermediate filaments, those assembled from keratins are the most heterogeneous. Fig. 1.66 shows that specific keratin polypeptides are associated with specific pathways of epithelial differentiation (the 'hard' keratins of nail and hair are not included).

Some cell types lack intermediate filaments, and microinjection of antibodies to intermediate filament proteins into cultured cells that do have them causes disruption of the filaments but no impairment of growth. These observations suggest that intermediate filaments do not fulfil a 'housekeeping' role in cells. There are situations, however, which implicate them in differ-

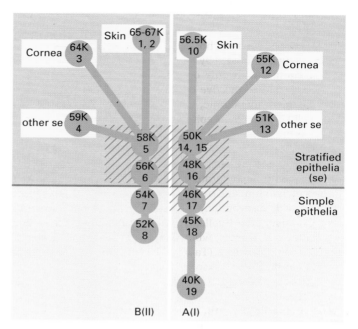

Fig. 1.66 A unifying model of keratin expression. Keratins of the acidic (A) (type I) and basic (B) (type II) subfamilies are arranged vertically according to their sizes. Keratins below the horizontal line are expressed mainly by simple epithelia and those above the line are expressed by stratified epithelia. The dashed box encloses the keratins commonly expressed by all stratified epithelia in neoplasms, hyperproliferative diseases, and in culture. The keratins are identified both by molecular weight in kilodaltons (K) and by the number assigned in the classification scheme of Moll *et al.* (1982). (Drawn after Cooper *et al.* 1985, with permission; copyright the United States and Canadian Academy of Pathology Inc., 1985.)

entiated functions. It is possible, for example, that keratin filaments in adjacent epithelial cells are functionally linked via desmosomal junctions, forming a supercellular skeleton (see Section 1.1.4). During myogenesis both the composition and distribution of intermediate filament proteins change, and desmin and vimentin become localized in the Z discs. Expression of lamins changes during early mouse embryo development, and this has been postulated to reflect changes in the structural organization of the nucleus. Finally, during adipocyte differentiation in culture the distribution of vimentin changes from an extended fibrillar array to a highly ordered monolayer of filaments surrounding lipid globules and ensheathed by endoplasmic reticulum.

Extracellular matrix

The extracellular matrix is generally defined as comprising the glycoproteins, proteoglycans, and glycosaminoglycans that are secreted by cells and assembled locally into an organized network. Detailed descriptions of the different extracellular matrix proteins are given in Section 1.4 of this chapter; here we will consider only those aspects of matrix expression that are associated with differentiation. Variation in ECM composition and location leads to differences in the physical properties of

Table 1.2 Different classes of intermediate filaments (after Osborn and Weber 1983, with permission; copyright the United States and Canadian Academy of Pathology Inc. 1983)

Type	Proteins	*In situ* examples
Epithelial	Cytokeratins, multiple polypeptides 40 000–68 000 Da	Keratinizing and non-keratinizing epithelia; these can be subdivided further
Neuronal	NF, 68 000, 160 000, and 200 000 Da	Most, but probably not all, neurones in central and peripheral nerves
Glial	GFA, 55 000 Da	Astrocytes, Bergmann glia (some GFA+, V+)
Muscle	Desmin, 53 000 Da	Sarcomeric muscle: smooth muscle, vascular smooth muscle; cells can be D+V+, D+V−, or D−V+
'Mesenchymal'	Vimentin, 57 000 Da	Fibroblasts, chondrocytes, macrophages, endothelial cells, etc.
No IF		Cells of the early embryo, certain neurones

Abbreviations: NF, neurofilaments; GFA, glial fibrillary acidic protein; V, vimentin; D, desmin; IF, intermediate filaments.

different tissues and in the interactions between different cell types.

Some cells, such as chondrocytes and dermal fibroblasts, are completely surrounded by ECM. Others, such as epithelial cells, make contact with only one surface. Cells may be separated from adjacent connective tissue by a specialized matrix called the basement membrane, which may make contact with only one cell surface, as in epithelia, or may completely surround cells, as in muscle or nerve (see Section 1.1.4).

All ECMs generally include one or more types of collagen (Table 1.3) and proteoglycan (Table 1.4). Other molecules that are frequently incorporated into the ECM include fibronectin, tenascin, laminin, and hyaluronic acid. Some ECM components have a wide distribution, whereas others are more restricted. For example, type I collagen is found in skin, tendon, bone, placenta, and arteries, whereas type X collagen is localized to hypertrophic cartilage (Table 1.3). Laminin and entactin are found specifically in basement membranes.

Different combinations of ECM molecules affect the physical properties of a tissue. In cartilage, for example, type II collagen provides tensile strength, while proteoglycans aggregated with hyaluronic acid give compressive resilience. In bone, type I col-

Table 1.3 Some vertebrate collagens: types and tissue distribution (reproduced [with modifications] from Cheah 1985, with permission; copyright 1985 the Biochemical Society, London)

Collagen type	Constituent α-chains	Major tissue distribution
I	α1(I)	Skin, tendon, bone, placenta, arteries
	α2(I)	
I trimer	α1(I)	Skin, tendon, liver, dentine, cultured skin, fibroblasts, tumours
II	α1(II)	Cartilage, vitreous humour, chondrosarcoma, intervertebral disc
III	α1(III)	Skin, lung, arteries, uterus, chorioamnion, liver, stroma and connective tissue of organs
IV	α1(IV) α2(IV)	Basement membranes
V	α1(V) α2(V) α3(V)	Placenta, skin, chorioamnion, pericellular/stromal in most connective tissue, rhabdomyosarcoma
VI	α1(VI) α2(VI) α3(VI)	Blood vessels, uterus, ligament, skin, lung, kidney
VII	α1(VII)	Chorioamniotic membranes, skin, oesophagus
VIII	α1(VIII)	Culture medium from endothelial, astrocytoma, and other cells from normal and malignant tissues
IX	α1(IX) α2(IX) α3(IX)	Cartilage, vitreous humour, intervertebral disc
X	α1(X)	Cartilage
XI	α1(XI) α2(XI) α3(XI)	Cartilage, vitreous humour, intervertebral disc

Table 1.4 Range of proteoglycans in different cell types (reproduced with modifications and permission from Hassell *et al.* 1986, *Annual Review of Biochemistry*, vol. 55, copyright Annual Reviews Inc., 1986)

PG source	GAG type*	Protein core preparation†
Mast cell	Hep,CS	10
L-2 cell	CS	25
Hepatocyte	HS	35
PG-I‡	CS,DS	45
PG-II§	CS,DS	43, 47
Cornea	KS	53
Epithelial	CS,HS hybrid	53
Epiphysis¶	CS,DS	68
Skin fibroblast	HS	90‖
Granulosa cell	DS,HS	240
Melanoma	CS	250
Smooth muscle cell	CS	320
Cartilage	CS,KS hybrid	400
Granulosa cell	DS	400
EHS,L-2	HS	400
Skin fibroblast	CS	500

* Abbreviations used: PG, proteoglycan; GAG, glycosaminoglycan; Hep, heparin; HS, heparan sulphate; CS, chondroitin sulphate; DS, dermatan sulphate; KS, keratan sulphate.
† Molecular mass in kDa.
‡ Cartilage, bone.
§ Skin, bone, tendon, cartilage, cornea.
¶ Chick growth cartilage, also sternum.
‖ Exists as a 180 kDa disulphide-bonded dimer.

lagen confers tensile strength, but this is combined with rigidity through the deposition of calcium phosphate in the ECM. Tenascin can act as an 'anti-fibronectin', inhibiting cell attachment and spreading on fibronectin-coated substrates.

Cell adhesion

Through adhesion to one another and to the extracellular matrix, cells remain together in the defined spatial arrays that characterize most tissues. Four different types of adhesive mechanism can be distinguished: both cell–cell and cell–matrix adhesion can be junctional or non-junctional. Junctions are defined as regions of plasma membrane specialization. Figure 1.67 illustrates the multiple adhesion mechanisms found in epithelial cells.

Intercellular junctions can be divided into three categories (see Section 1.1). Desmosomes and adhaerens junctions are junctions that hold cells together; tight junctions not only hold cells together, but also provide a seal that prevents passage of extracellular molecules. The third category of junction is involved in intercellular communication and consists of gap junctions and chemical synapses. Gap junctions and adhaerens junctions have a widespread tissue distribtion, tight junctions and desmosomes are found primarily (though not exclusively) in epithelia, and synapses are found in nervous tissue.

Hemidesmosomes and adhaerens junctions mediate cell–matrix adhesion. Like desmosomes, hemidesmosomes are found almost exclusively in epithelia and have keratin filaments associated with them. Adhaerens junctions with the ECM are, like intercellular adhaerens junctions, of more widespread distribu-

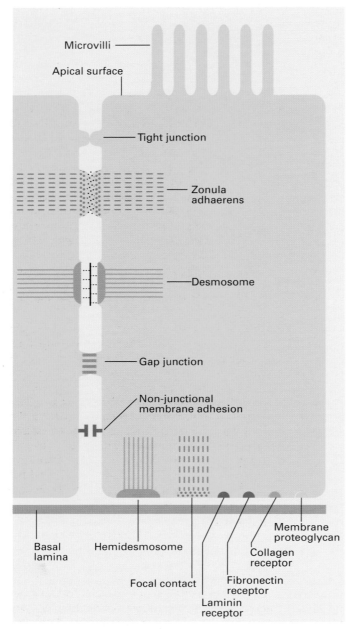

Fig. 1.67 Multiple adhesion mechanisms of epithelial cells. The diagram shows a probable maximum number of mechanisms, not all of which are present in all epithelial cells. Note that focal contacts are a form of adhaerens junction. (Drawn after Garrod 1986, with permission from the Company of Biologists Ltd.)

tion and are linked to microfilaments. Ultrastructurally hemidesmosomes resemble half desmosomes, but they differ in molecular composition. Cell–cell and cell–matrix adhaerens junctions both contain vinculin, but only cell–matrix junctions contain talin.

Non-junctional cell–cell adhesion molecules have generally been identified by the ability of antibodies raised against them to disrupt cell–cell adhesion in culture. The molecules are known collectively as CAMs (cell adhesion molecules). Different CAMs are expressed in different tissues and there are precise changes in their patterns of expression during embryonic development, suggesting a role in morphogenesis. Examples of CAMs and their sites of expression are: E-cadherin in epithelia; N-CAM and N-cadherin in nerve; and Ng-CAM mediating neural–glial cell adhesion.

The fourth type of adhesive mechanism involves plasma membrane receptors for extracellular matrix molecules. One family of such receptors are the integrins, which mediate binding to a variety of ECM components, including fibronectin, laminin, and vitronectin. In some cases, the integrin-binding site is a region of the matrix molecule that includes the sequence Arg–Gly–Asp. Mammalian integrins consist of one α- and one β-subunit, non-covalently linked and spanning the plasma membrane. The cytoplasmic domain of the integrin complex interacts with the cytoskeleton. Members of the integrin family include glycoprotein IIb/IIIa on platelets, the VLA antigens on T-lymphocytes, and Mac-1 antigen on macrophages and granulocytes.

In conclusion, variation in the adhesive properties of different cell types can occur at a number of different levels. Different cells may express different types or combinations of adhesive mechanisms; the number and distribution of junctional and non-junctional molecules can vary, as can their composition. Finally, the distinction between junctional and non-junctional molecules is not always absolute, since, for example, uvomorulin is found in tight junctions and integrins are associated with cell–substrate adhaerens junctions.

1.2.3   Differentiative mechanisms

Through embryonic development, a single fertilized egg gives rise to a multicellular organism that consists of at least 200 different cell types, arranged in precise spatial patterns that correspond to tissues. The transition from egg to mature organism involves a combination of cell division (to increase total cell number) and differentiation (to generate new cell types). In the adult, some cells (such as nerve cells) never divide, whereas others are renewed through proliferation. Renewal can occur by simple duplication (for example, of hepatocytes), in which both daughter cells must 'remember' and express the differentiated characteristics of the parent cell. Alternatively, regeneration may depend on division of a distinct subpopulation of cells, called stem cells (see Section 1.3), which may have different characteristics from their progeny (for example, in the haemopoietic system). It is therefore possible to distinguish three distinct aspects of differentiation: differentiation during embryonic development, maintenance of the differentiated state during division of cells in the adult, and differentiation of the progeny of stem cells.

At all levels, differentiation involves the switching on or off of specific genes in specific cells. For example, epidermal keratinocytes express keratins, but not haemoglobin, and red blood cells contain haemoglobin, but no keratins. One question, then, is whether genes that are not expressed in a given differentiated cell are still present in the nucleus, or whether they have been lost. It appears that, with a few exceptions, differentiation does not involve loss of genes. One piece of evidence for this comes from an experiment in which the nucleus of a keratinocyte taken from the skin of an adult frog was transplanted into an enucleated frog egg. In a small proportion of cases, the egg underwent normal development to form a tadpole (Fig. 1.68). Thus, although the cell that donated the nucleus was fully differentiated and expressing only those products, such as keratins, which were characteristic of its differentiated state, it nevertheless contained all the genes expressed in all the other differentiated cell types of the tadpole.

Differentiation, therefore, does not involve loss of genes but, rather, regulated expression of particular genes. Sequences of DNA, called promoters and enhancers, located near to individual genes, are required for regulated expression of those genes. Specific proteins bind to these sequences and promote or repress transcription (see Chapter 2.3). There is some evidence that the strategies for control of transcriptional initiation may differ between luxury and housekeeping genes. A crucial question, then, is how the regulatory mechanisms at the level of individual genes are co-ordinated during acquisition and maintenance of the differentiated state.

Differentiation during embryonic and fetal development

The details of embryonic development vary greatly between species. There are, however, certain steps that are common to all

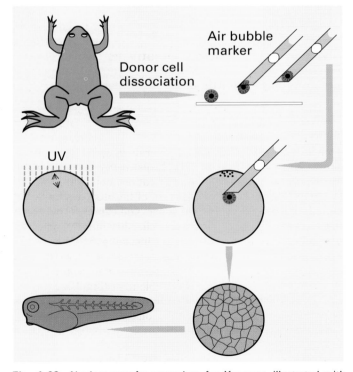

Fig. 1.68 Nuclear transfer procedure for *Xenopus*, illustrated with transfers from adult foot skin cells. (Drawn after Gurdon 1986, with permission from the Company of Biologists Ltd.)

vertebrate embryos which mark important stages in the differentiation process (see Chapter 9). In all species the fertilized egg undergoes a series of cleavage divisions to form a ball of cells, called the blastula. In lower vertebrates, such as amphibia, all the cells of the blastula contribute to the embryo, but in mammals many give rise to extra-embryonic material, such as the placenta. As a result of a programmed series of cell movements the blastula invaginates or involutes in a process called gastrulation. Through gastrulation the three 'germ layers' of the body, namely, ectoderm, mesoderm, and endoderm, are established. The ectodermal cells are on the outside of the embryo and form predominantly skin and nervous tissue; the brain and spinal cord form during neurulation when dorsal ectodermal cells roll into a tube. Mesodermal cells occupy a layer just inside the ectoderm and form muscle, cartilage, and connective tissue. Endodermal cells constitute the innermost cell layer and give rise to the gut and associated organs. Differentiation in the embryo thus occurs in steps, with a progressive restriction in cell potency: whereas a fertilized egg has the potential to give rise to all the different cell types of the body, a neural tube cell can only yield progeny that will differentiate into cells of the nervous system.

In the embryo, there is evidence that cells become committed to undergo a particular pathway of differentiation some time before they express the differentiated characteristics of that cell type. Cells that have made this decision, or commitment, are said to be determined; they may undergo division prior to differentiation, but all their progeny will share the same differentiated fate. The experiment that establishes whether a particular cell or group of cells is determined is to transplant them from their normal position in the embryo to a different site. If the cells were determined prior to transplantation they will form the differentiated cell types characteristic of their original position; if not, then they will make cell types characteristic of their new position in the embryo.

What are the mechanisms that result in determination and differentiation during embryonic development? These will be discussed below.

Cytoplasmic determinants

One way in which a pattern of differentiated cell types can be set up in the embryo is through localized distribution of cytoplasmic determinants. Regulatory molecules are distributed throughout the cytoplasm of the fertilized egg in such a way that cells derived from a part of the egg containing, for example, a muscle cell determinant would form muscle, while other cells might inherit a nerve cell determinant, and so on. A requirement of this developmental strategy is that the egg must be a remarkably complex structure, which, in effect, is a miniature of the resulting embryo. In fact, ascidian embryos, which develop into a tadpole-like larva, use cytoplasmic determinants as a major mechanism for specifying cell differentiation; the identity of the cytoplasmic determinants is, however, unknown.

In vertebrate embryos, cytoplasmic determinants rarely act to specify cell types directly. However, cytoplasmic inhomogeneities are correlated with the future embryonic axes. In amphibia, for example, there are maternal mRNAs that are restricted either to the animal hemisphere of the egg or the vegetal hemisphere; one of these is related to transforming growth factor-β (TGF-β). The polarity thus established in the egg can be amplified by later interactions between different cell types, as described below.

Inductive interactions

There are a number of situations during vertebrate embryonic development when the differentiation of one population of cells (the responding tissue) is controlled by interaction with an adjacent population of cells (the inducing tissue). This process is known as induction.

The nature of the inducing signals in development is largely unknown. However, there are some clues as to the mechanism of one important inductive interaction in amphibian development: the induction of mesoderm from ectoderm. An inducing protein secreted by *Xenopus* cells in culture has been identified recently as activin, and may turn out to be the natural inducer in embryos. In addition, fibroblast growth factor and a variety of other heparin-binding growth factors can induce animal pole ectoderm to form mesoderm and TGF-β potentiates the effect of fibroblast growth factor. The observation that a maternal mRNA which is localized to the vegetal hemisphere of *Xenopus* eggs encodes a protein related to TGF-β raises the possibility that mesoderm formation is specified by the products of maternal mRNAs that are localized in the egg.

Glial progenitor cells

One situation in which the mechanisms controlling differentiation in mammals have been studied in some detail is in the developing rat optic nerve. Oligodendrocytes and type 2 astrocytes develop from a common progenitor, the bipotential oligodendrocyte–type-2 astrocyte (O–2A). The differentiation of progenitor cells has been studied in culture, where the pathway taken can be determined by the composition of the culture medium: in the presence of 10 per cent fetal calf serum O–2A cells differentiate into type 2 astrocytes, whereas in $\leqslant 0.5$ per cent fetal calf serum the cells differentiate into oligodendrocytes.

O–2A cells can proliferate in culture in 0.5 per cent fetal calf serum if grown on a feeder layer of type 1 astrocytes. There is good evidence that the time when a progenitor cell differentiates is determined by counting the number of divisions it undergoes. After a certain number, the cells become unresponsive to growth factors produced by the type 1 astrocytes; the cells stop dividing and differentiate into oligodendrocytes. The divisions prior to differentiation are symmetrical, in that daughter cells tend to share the same fate (division or differentiation); this is in contrast to differentiation of stem cell progeny, in which there is potential for both self-renewal and differentiation.

In contrast to oligodendrocyte differentiation, differentiation of type 2 astrocytes requires an inducing signal. In culture this is provided by a component of fetal calf serum; *in vivo* an inducing protein that appears late in the developing rat optic nerve has been identified. Interestingly, the choice of differentiation pathway taken by O–2A cells in culture is initially reversible

and only becomes fixed after 1–2 days in the presence or absence of fetal calf serum. Such initial reversibility preceding irreversible differentiation has also been observed in a melanoma cell line in culture.

Maintenance of the differentiated state

When differentiated cells divide in the adult, their daughters usually have the same characteristics as their parents. Thus, cells 'remember' their differentiated phenotype. Many of the insights into the nature of this cell memory have come from experiments with cultured cells: it is now possible to grow cells from many body tissues in culture.

Environmental modulation

Although most cells remain differentiated in culture (i.e. remain recognizably one cell type or another), there is quite frequently some loss of differentiated function. For example, when mammary epithelial cells are placed in culture, production of milk-specific proteins, such as caseins, declines; furthermore, epidermal keratinocytes often fail to express all the keratins normally found in intact epidermis; and hepatocytes in culture generally stop synthesizing albumin. In each of these examples, differentiated gene expression can be restored by appropriate modification of the culture environment. Casein expression is stimulated when mammary epithelial cells assume a cuboidal morphology on floating collagen gels; reduction in the vitamin A content of the culture medium induces expression of the 67 kDa keratin (no. 1, see Fig. 1.66) by epidermal keratinocytes; and co-cultivation with non-parenchymal liver epithelial cells leads to a marked increase in albumin synthesis by hepatocytes. Thus by analysing the factors, such as nutrients, substratum, and cell–cell interactions, which regulate gene expression in culture, it is possible to gain some understanding of the factors that stabilize the differentiated state *in vivo*.

Transdifferentiation and dedifferentiation

One situation in which the differentiated state is not stable is the process of transdifferentiation, when one cell type is transformed into a different one. There are examples of epithelial and mesenchymal transformation during normal embryonic development, but in culture it is possible to induce transformation into mesenchyme of epithelial cells which never form mesenchyme *in vivo*. Thus, a number of adult and embryonic epithelia will give rise to mesenchymal cells if the epithelial sheet is suspended in a collagen gel (Fig. 1.69). Transdifferentiation involves changes both in morphology and gene expression: for example, lens epithelial cells switch off expression of crystallins, type IV collagen, and laminin, and express type I collagen *de novo*.

Studies of the mechanism of transdifferentiation provide some clues as to the signals that normally stabilize the differentiated phenotype. In the example of lens epithelium described above, exposure of the apical cell surface, which does not normally contact the extracellular matrix, to collagen appears to be important. In another example, retinal pigment epithelial cells

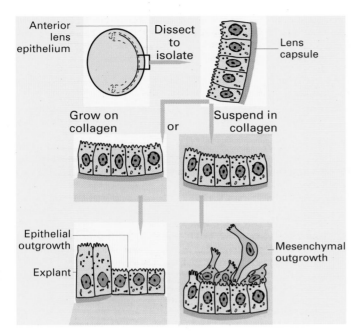

Fig. 1.69 Transdifferentiation of lens epithelial cells in culture. Following dissection of pure lens epithelial explants with the associated basal lamina (lens capsule) explants are placed either on the surface of (left) or suspended within (right) type I collagen gels. On the left, a monolayer of epithelial cells spreads out over the gel surface and lays down a new basal lamina. On the right, the explants form multiple cell layers (Greenburg and Hay 1982): the apical cell surface acquires motility and the cells elongate, forming bipolar mesenchyme-like cells that break free of the explant and migrate within the gel. (Drawn after Greenburg and Hay 1986, with permission.)

form neurones if cultured on a substrate of laminin. Furthermore, dissociation of retinal glia cells causes them to acquire the lens cell phenotype: it appears that the glial phenotype is normally stabilized by cell contacts and disruption predisposes the cells to phenotype transformation. These experiments point to the importance of the position and composition of the extracellular matrix, and of cell–cell interactions, in stabilizing the differentiated phenotype of cells.

In addition to cell memory and transdifferentiation, cell culture studies have identified potentially a third phenomenon: dedifferentiation. During prolonged cultivation of chondrocytes from cartilage, the cells lose their polygonal or rounded shape, and stop synthesizing type II collagen and cartilage-specific proteoglycans; instead they assume a fibroblastic morphology and express type I collagen and low molecular weight, non-aggregating proteoglycans. This loss of differentiated phenotype has been termed dedifferentiation. Under some culture conditions, in which chondrocytes are forced to resume a rounded morphology, the cells may re-express type II collagen. At present the significance of dedifferentiation of chondrocytes in culture is not clear. It could represent dedifferentiation to a more primitive progenitor developmental state; transdifferentiation to the differentiated phenotype of a fibroblast; or it could simply reflect reversible environmental modulation of the chondrocyte phe-

notype, as noted earlier for hepatocytes and keratinocytes. Chondrocytes provide a further demonstration that the differentiated phenotype may be labile and may depend on appropriate environmental signals for its maintenance. An understanding of this process *in vitro* may shed light on the failure of chondrocytes *in situ* in cartilage to repair the ECM in degenerative arthritic diseases.

Differentiation of stem cell progeny

The term 'stem cell' is confusing because, although it is widely used, it is defined differently in different contexts. A general definition, and the one used here, is that it is a cell which has the capacity for unlimited divisions and whose daughters have a choice: they can either remain stem cells or undergo terminal differentiation. Stem cell progeny that are committed to a differentiation pathway may undergo several more rounds of division, but eventually give rise to cells that cannot divide further and are thus terminally differentiated.

Stem cells are found in tissues in which there is a recurring need for newly differentiated cells and the differentiated cells themselves cannot divide. Examples of tissues that are constantly turning over and which contain stem cells are the lining of the small intestine, the epidermis, and the haemopoietic system. Section 1.3 will describe these stem cells and the concept of cell lineage in more detail. Here we will only consider some common features of stem cells and the signals that regulate self-renewal versus differentiation.

Stem cells are identified by their proliferative and differentiative potential. Haemopoietic stem cells were first identified by injecting bone marrow cells from one mouse into another mouse that had been lethally irradiated: some of the cells lodged in the host spleen and after several days nodules developed, each derived from a single cell and yet consisting of a mixture of different haemopoietic cells. Such assays of clonogenicity have now been extended to other tissues. In addition to the ability to regenerate tissue, stem cells are often identified by cell kinetic parameters: they tend to have a longer cell cycle time than their progeny.

Stem cells also differ from their progeny in phenotype and location. In the epidermis there is only one pathway of terminal differentiation, the end-point of which is the formation of cornified squames in the outer epidermal layers. In contrast, the differentiated progeny of a haemopoietic stem cell may be any of a number of cell types, including erythrocytes, neutrophils, and megakaryocytes. The epidermal stem cell compartment is in the basal layer of the epidermis; haemopoietic stem cells are thought to occupy specific niches in bone marrow; and the stem cells of the lining of the small intestine are found at the base of the intestinal crypts.

What factors control the initiation of differentiation among stem cell progeny? It is important that there be a balance between proliferation and differentiation, such that the total number of differentiated cells is sufficient for the body's requirements. In both the epidermis and the haemopoietic system there is evidence that interaction with the stroma is required for maintaining stem cells: both cell–ECM and cell–cell contacts are important. Also of importance are growth factors; these are best characterized in the haemopoietic system, where factors acting at different points in the differentiation pathways have been identified. In addition to factors that regulate proliferation, factors that promote differentiation along specific haemopoietic lineages have been identified.

1.2.4 Conclusions

In this section we have considered the nature of the differentiated phenotype and the mechanisms by which cells differentiate in the embryo and the adult. A common theme that emerges is the importance of environmental cues, from the extracellular matrix and interactions with other cells, that both direct the process of differentiation and maintain the differentiated phenotype.

1.2.5 Further reading

Alberts, B., Bray, D., Lewis, J., Raff, M., Roberts, K. and Watson, J. D. (1983 and 1989). *Molecular biology of the cell*. Garland Publishing, New York.

Bennett, D. C. (1983). Differentiation in mouse melanoma cells: initial reversibility and an on-off schochastic model. *Cell* **34**, 445–53.

Bennett, V. (1985). The membrane skeleton of human erythrocytes and its implications for more complex cells. *Annual Review of Biochemistry* **54**, 273–304.

Benya, P. D. and Shaffer, J. D. (1982). Dedifferentiated chondrocytes reexpress the differentiated collagen phenotype when cultured in agarose gels. *Cell* **30**, 215–24.

Burridge, K., Molony, L., and Kelly, T. (1987). Adhesion plaques: sites of transmembrane interaction between the extracellular matrix and the actin cytoskeleton. *Journal of Cell Science* (Suppl.) **8**, 211–29.

Cheah, K. S. E. (1985). Collagen genes and inherited connective tissue disease. *Biochemical Journal* **229**, 287–303.

Cleveland, D. W. (1987). The multitubulin hypothesis revisited: what have we learned? *Journal of Cell Biology* **104**, 381–3.

Cooper, D., Schermer, A., and Sun, T.-T. (1985). Classification of human epithelia and their neoplasms using monoclonal antibodies to keratins: strategies, applications, and limitations. *Laboratory Investigation* **52**, 243–56.

Dexter, T. M., Whetton, A. D., Spooncer, E., Heyworth, C., and Simmons, P. (1985). The role of stromal cells and growth factors in haemopoiesis and modulation of their effects by the *src* oncogene. *Journal of Cell Science* **3**, 83–95.

Edelman, G. M. (1986). Cell adhesion molecules in the regulation of animal form and tissue pattern. *Annual Review of Cell Biology* **2**, 81–116.

Franke, W. W. (1987). Nuclear lamins and cytoplasmic intermediate filament proteins: a growing multigene family. *Cell* **48**, 3–4.

Franke, W. W., Hergt, M., and Grund, C. (1987). Rearrangement of the vimentin cytoskeleton during adipose conversion: formation of an intermediate filament cage around lipid globules. *Cell* **49**, 131–41.

Fraslin, J.-M., Kneip, B., Vaulont, S., Glaise, D., Munnich, A., and Gugen-Guillouzo, C. (1985). Dependence of hepatocyte-specific gene expression on cell–cell interactions in primary culture. *EMBO Journal* **4**, 2487–91.

Freshney, R. I. (1983). *Culture of animal cells. A manual of basic technique*. A. R. Liss, New York.

Fuchs, E. and Green, H. (1981). Regulation of terminal differentiation of cultured human keratinocytes by vitamin A. *Cell* **25**, 617–25.

Garrod, D. R. (1986) Desmosomes, cell adhesion molecules and the adhesive properties of cells in tissues. *Journal of Cell Science* (Suppl.) **4**, 221–37.

Geiger, B., Volk, T., and Volberg, T. (1985). Molecular heterogeneity of adherens junctions. *Journal of Cell Biology* **101**, 1523–31.

Greenburg, G. and Hay, E. D. (1982). Epithelia suspended in collagen gels can lose polarity and express characteristics of migrating mesenchymal cells. *Journal of Cell Biology* **95**, 333–9.

Greenburg, G. and Hay, E. D. (1986). Cytodifferentiation and tissue phenotype change during transformation of embryonic lens epithelium to mesenchyme-like cells *in vitro*. *Developmental Biology* **115**, 363–79.

Gumbiner, B. and Simons, K. (1987). *The role of uvomorulin in the formation of epithelial occluding junctions*, Ciba Foundation Symposium No. 125, pp. 168–86. J. Wiley and Sons, Chichester.

Gundersen, G. G., Kalnoski, M. H., and Bulinski, J. C. (1984). Distinct populations of microtubules: tyrosinated and non-tyrosinated alpha tubulin are distributed differently in vivo. *Cell* **38**, 779–89.

Gurdon, J. B. (1986). Nuclear transplantation in eggs and oocytes. *Journal of Cell Science* (Suppl.) **4**, 287–318.

Gurdon, J. B. (1987). Embryonic induction—molecular prospects. *Development* **99**, 285–306.

Hassell, J. R., Kimura, J. H., and Hascall, V. C. (1986). Proteoglycan core protein families. *Annual Review of Biochemistry* **55**, 539–67.

Hay, E. D. (1981). *Cell biology of extracellular matrix*. Plenum Press, New York.

Hughes, S. M. and Raff, M. C. (1987). An inducer protein may control the timing of fate switching in a bipotential glial progenitor cell in rat optic nerve. *Development* **101**, 157–67.

Hynes, R. O. (1987). Integrins: a family of cell surface receptors. *Cell* **48**, 549–54.

Jeffery, W. R. (1985). Specification of cell fate by cytoplasmic determinants in ascidian embryos. *Cell* **41**, 11–12.

Jones, J. C. R., Yokoo, K. M., and Goldman, R. D. (1986). Is the hemidesmosome a half desmosome? An immunological comparison of mammalian desmosomes and hemidesmosomes. *Cell Motility and the Cytoskeleton* **6**, 560–69.

Kimelman, D. and Kirschner, M. (1987). Synergistic induction of mesoderm by FGF and TGF-β and the identification of an mRNA coding for FGF in the early *Xenopus* embryo. *Cell* **51**, 869–77.

Lackie, J. M. (1986). *Cell movement and cell behaviour*. Allen and Unwin, London.

Lazarides, E., Granger, B. L., Gard, D. L., O'Connor, C. M., Breckler, J., Price, M., *et al.* (1982). Desmin and vimentin-containing intermediate filaments and their role in the assembly of the Z disk in muscle cells. *Cold Spring Harbor Symposium on Quantitative Biology* **36**, 351–78.

Lee, E. Y.-H. P., Lee, W.-H., Kaetzel, C. S., Parry, G., and Bissell, M. J. (1985). Interaction of mouse mammary epithelial cells with collagen substrata: Regulation of casein gene expression and secretion. *Proceedings of the National Academy of Sciences, USA* **82**, 1419–23.

Mackie, E. J., Thesleff, I., and Chiquet-Ehrismann, R. (1987). Tenascin is associated with chondrogenic and osteogenic differentiation *in vivo* and promotes chondrogenesis *in vitro*. *Journal of Cell Biology* **105**, 2569–79.

Maniatis, T., Goodbourn, S., and Fischer, J. A. (1987). Regulation of inducible and tissue-specific gene expression. *Science* **236**, 1237–45.

Melton, D. W. (1987). Strategies and mechanisms for the control of transcriptional initiation of mammalian protein-coding genes. *Journal of Cell Science* **88**, 267–70.

Moll, R., Franke, W. W., Schiller, D. L., Geiger, B., and Krepler, R.

(1982). The catalog of human cytokeratins: patterns of expression in normal epithelia, tumors and cultured cells. *Cell* **31**, 11–24.

Moscona, A. A., Brown, M., Degenstein, L., Fox, L., and Soh, B. M. (1983). Transformation of retinal glia cells into lens phenotype: Expression of MP26, a lens plasma membrane antigen. *Proceedings of the National Academy of Sciences, USA* **80**, 7239–43.

Nose, A., Nagafuchi, A., and Takeichi, M. (1987). Isolation of placental cadherin cDNA: identification of a novel gene family of cell–cell adhesion molecules. *EMBO Journal* **6**, 3655–61.

Olmsted, J. B. (1986). Microtubule-associated proteins. *Annual Review of Cell Biology* **2**, 421–57.

Osborn, M. and Weber, K. (1983). Tumor diagnosis by intermediate filament typing: a novel tool for surgical pathology. *Laboratory Investigation* **48**, 372–94.

Pollack, R. (1981). *Readings in mammalian cells culture* (2nd edn). Cold Spring Harbor Laboratory.

Potten, C. S. (1983). *Stem cells: their identification and characterisation.* Churchill Livingstone.

Raff, M. C., Miller, R. H., and Noble, M. (1983). A glial progenitor cell that develops *in vitro* into an astrocyte or an oligodendrocyte depending on culture medium. *Nature* **303**, 390–6.

Raff, M. C., Williams, B. P., and Miller, R. H. (1984). The *in vitro* differentiation of a bipotential glial progenitor cell. *EMBO Journal* **3**, 1857–64.

Rebagliati, M. R., Weeks, D. L., Harvey, R. P., and Melton, D. A. (1985). Identification and cloning of localized maternal RNAs from Xenopus eggs. *Cell* **42**, 769–77.

Reh, T. A., Nagy, T., and Gretton, H. (1987). Retinal pigmented epithelial cells induced to transdifferentiate to neurons by laminin. *Nature* **330**, 68–71.

Revel, J. P., Yancey, S. B., Nicholson, B., and Hoh, J. (1987). *Sequence diversity of gap junction proteins,* Ciba Foundation Symposium No. 125, pp. 108–27. J. Wiley and Sons, Chichester.

Rheinwald, J. G. and Green, H. (1975). Serial cultivation of strains of human epidermal keratinocytes: the formation of keratinizing colonies from single cells. *Cell* **6**, 331–44.

Roberts, R. A., Spooncer, E., Parkinson, E. K., Lord, B. I., Allen, T. D., and Dexter, T. M. (1987). Metabolically inactive 3T3 cells can substitute for marrow stromal cells to promote the proliferation and development of multipotent haemopoietic stem cells. *Journal of Cellular Physiology* **132**, 203–14.

Sachs, L. (1987). The molecular control of blood cell development. *Science* **238**, 1374–9.

Sengel, P. (1976). *Morphogenesis of skin.* Cambridge University Press, Cambridge.

Slack, J. M. W. (1983). *From egg to embryo.* Cambridge University Press, Cambridge.

Slack, J. M. W., Darlington, B. G., Heath, J. K., and Godsave, S. F. (1987). Mesoderm induction in early *Xenopus* embryos by heparin-binding growth factors. *Nature* **326**, 197–200.

Smith, J. C. (1987). A mesoderm-inducing factor is produced by a *Xenopus* cell line. *Development* **99**, 3–14.

Stewart, C. and Burke, B. (1987). Teratocarinom stem cells and early mouse embryos contain only a single major lamin polypeptide closely resembling lamin B. *Cell* **51**, 383–92.

Stossel, T. P., *et al.* (1985). Nonmuscle actin-binding proteins. *Annual Review of Cell Biology* **1**, 353–402.

Takeichi, M. (1987). Cadherins: a molecular family essential for selective cell–cell adhesion and animal morphogenesis. *Trends in Genetics* **3**, 213–17.

Temple, S. and Raff, M. C. (1986). Clonal analysis of oligodendrocyte development in culture: evidence for a developmental clock that counts cell divisions. *Cell* **44**, 773–9.

Vandekerckhove, J. and Weber, K. (1978). At least six different actins are expressed in a higher mammal: an analysis based on the amino acid sequence of the amino-terminal tryptic peptide. *Journal of Molecular Biology* **126**, 783–802.

von der Mark, K. (1986). Differentiation, modulation and dedifferentiation of chondrocytes. *Rheumatology* **10**, 272–315.

Watt. F. M. (1986). The extracellular matrix and cell shape. *Trends in Biochemical Sciences* **11**, 482–5.

Weeks, D. L. and Melton, D. A. (1987). A maternal mRNA localised to the vegetal hemisphere in *Xenopus* eggs codes for a growth factor related to TGF-β. *Cell* **51**, 861–7.

1.3 Cell lineages

C. S. Potten

1.3.1 General considerations

The tissues of the adult mammalian body can be broadly classified into three types.

1. *Essentially non-replacing.* There is little or no cell replacement, or capacity for regeneration, for example, the female germ line and the central nervous tissue.

2. *Conditionally renewing.* Under normal circumstances, there is little or no cell replacement but there is a considerable capacity for regenerative proliferation of the tissue if it is damaged; for example, liver, kidney, and various glandular epithelia (merocrine or apocrine glands where the cell secretes its product through its membrane or where part of the cytoplasm is secreted but the body of the cell remains).

3. *Steady-state renewal.* These are tissues in which there is a steady appreciable level of cell loss and a steady level of counterbalancing cell replacement: for example, the surface epithelia (internal and external); some glandular epithelia (holocrine glands where the entire cell disintegrates to release its secretory product); the bone marrow; and the male germ line in the testis.

Within all of these tissues the individual cells can also be categorized. There will be functional cells (all tissues) which are mature, differentiated cells (see Section 1.2) performing the function for which the tissue was evolved and these cells eventually become senescent and die. There may also be potentially proliferative cells (conditional renewal tissues and possibly some renewing tissues where they might be referred to also as reserve proliferative cells) which are not sequentially passing through the series of biochemical events that prepare the cell for division, the cell cycle (Fig. 1.70). These are in a dormant, quiescent state sometimes referred to as G_0. It remains unclear whether mature functional cells may also ever be potentially proliferative. Finally, there may be actively proliferative cells mainly in the steady-state renewal tissues; these are in active cell-cycle progression.

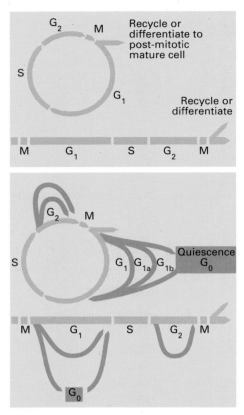

Fig. 1.70 The cell cycle. A sequence of biochemical or morphological events in the life of a cell can be mapped on a time scale which represents the cell cycle. In principle, many transition points can be mapped; only a simplified map is shown here. The onset and completion of mitosis (M) and the onset and completion of DNA synthesis (S) are the most frequently used transition points; the periods between these phases are known as gaps (G_1 and G_2). The time map can be represented as a cycle, implying that the cells at the beginning and end are identical; this is particularly relevant to stem cells. Alternatively, the time map can be regarded as a linear map where the cells at one end may differ slightly from the cells at the other end; this is possibly relevant to dividing transit cells where at each division the cells are closer to their terminal division, i.e. they are more mature or differentiated. Not all cells may progress through the cycle at the same rate. Most of the variability is observed in G_1 or, to a lesser extent, in G_2. Thus there is a considerable variability in the length of G_1, G_{1a}, G_{1b}, etc. Yet other cells may leave G_1 phase, cease progression altogether, and enter a quiescent phase commonly referred to as G_0.

At least from a theoretical point of view, the cells of a tissue may be further categorized as illustrated in Fig. 1.71. In the essentially non-replacing tissues the functional cells simply decline in number with time, i.e. they represent a decaying population. In the steady-state renewal systems there may, in theory, be up to three classes of cells.

1. *Simple transit cells*. These are mature functional cells that become senescent and die and require constant replacement;
2. *Dividing transit cells*. These are maturing cells that retain some limited capacity for cell division before becoming

simple transit cells, but similarly require constant replacement; and

3. *Stem cell compartment*. This is an immature proliferative compartment that maintains its numbers.

The stem cells do not require an input, but do provide an output of cells which can thus feed into any of the other cell compartments. It is not entirely clear how the stem cell numbers are maintained. It is possible that the stem cells always divide to produce two daughters, both of which can function as stem cells—a symmetric form of cell division—in which case, under steady-state conditions, mechanisms must be present that effectively remove half of all the stem cells produced. This may be achieved by the stochastic interaction of differentiation-inducing factors with the stem cells. This process is often assumed to exist but direct evidence is largely lacking. Alternatively, the spatial architecture of the tissues, that is cell position, may determine which of each pair of stem cell daughters remains as the stem cell. This may be more likely in tissues where there is a high degree of tissue polarity and spatial organization. In either case the net result is a situation that approximates to, or may even in some cases actually be, an asymmetric division. This arrangement is often implicitly assumed when diagrams are drawn of stem cell populations.

Thus for a steady-state renewal tissue there may be stem cells feeding directly into a simple transit population or feeding into a dividing transit population which itself feeds a simple transit compartment. Although the former was for many years assumed to occur for most surface epithelia (in the absence of hard supporting data), it is now becoming evident that wherever large numbers of cells are to be continually replaced the latter, hierarchical scheme is applicable.

The situation in conditional renewal systems remains unresolved. Several possibilities exist. They may, in fact, be simply steady-state renewal systems, complete with a similar hierarchy, that have cells which, although passing through the cell cycle extremely slowly, can be easily stimulated. They may represent a tissue that was hierarchical during development but within which all the cells simply stopped cycling and entered quiescence. This is referred to as a 'frozen' hierarchy, which can be reactivated by wounding. They could also be derived from an embryonic hierarchy where only the stem cells enter quiescence and the dividing transit cells continue into the simple transit state, in which case regeneration is achieved entirely by a re-activation of the stem cells. Finally, all the cells could be either in a closed or decaying compartment, or a slow simple transit compartment, but on appropriate stimulation they might be capable of reverting to a proliferative state. This would require some complex readjustments to the proliferation/differentiation genome, for which there is little or no evidence at present.

Definitions

Before proceeding further it is perhaps worthwhile defining more precisely a few of the terms that have already been used, since this may avoid confusion and prevent misconceptions.

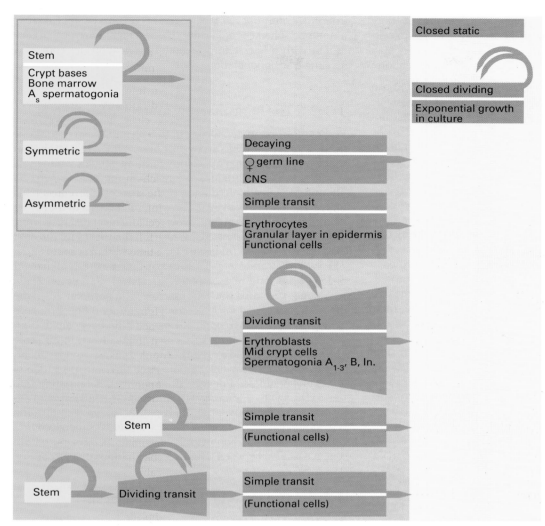

Fig. 1.71 The possible proliferative cell population types in tissues. Transit cell types are part of a 'pipe-line' system and require a constant input and provide a constant output. There may be some divisions within some transit populations. The input is provided by the output from the stem cell compartment. It is now fairly widely accepted that a hierarchical scheme, comprising stem, dividing transit, and simple transit cells, is common to all steady-state renewal tissues; see Fig. 1.74 for spermatogonia. (Drawn after Gilbert and Lajtha 1965, with permission.)

The terms differentiation (see also Section 1.2) and maturation are sometime used rather loosely and interchangeably.

Differentiation is a qualitative and relative term used to describe a change in the characteristics of a cell or population of cells. It represents a change in the pattern of gene expression, i.e. a reprogramming of the genome or a change in the balance of activated and repressed genes. It may be the consequence of changes either in the internal programming of the cell or of the external stimuli that affect the cell. It may be detected by a change in function, or appearance, or by the detection of novel biosynthetic products within the cell, or on its surface. Thus, the initial change in differentiation clearly involves a change in the activation and repression pattern of the genes, and the earliest detection of the change will depend on the sensitivity of

the technique being used. A cell will have a particular differentiation status relative to other cells.

Maturation, in contrast, can be thought of as a quantitative term describing the quantity or time changes initiated by differentiation. It thus represents an increase in quantity, or further metabolism, of novel cellular constituents with time.

Differentiation events begin early in embryogenesis and may continue throughout the life of a cell. Differentiation thus represents a spectrum of relative changes that are related to the life history of the cell, or cells, being considered. All cells in an adult tissue, including stem cells, are differentiated relative to embryonic cells. Transit populations in an adult tissue can be regarded as differentiated relative to the tissue stem cells, and maturing cells may continue to undergo differentiation events until they die. Stem cells may be capable of undergoing a variety of different initial differentiation steps. Or may give rise to cells that undergo a range of differentiation events; that is they may possess a multi- or pluri-potentiality in terms of differentiation.

Stem cells in an adult tissue can be defined as cells with an extensive self-maintenance capability (without detectable changes in the properties of the cell). They are the cells ultimately responsible for all cell replacement in the tissue for the life-span of the animal, in spite of physiological or accidental cell loss (Potten and Loeffler 1990). They may be capable of producing a range of differentiated cell lines and, because of this large division potential, are likely to be the most efficient tissue regenerators. These are commonly measured in practice by colony-forming assays. Hence colony- or clone-forming cells (*clonogenic cells*) and stem cells can be regarded as cell populations that overlap. However, largely because of technical limitations, they may not overlap precisely; i.e. they are not identical to each other, although it seems reasonable to assume that all stem cells are clonogenic cells. But it is probably not valid to assume that all clonogenic cells are stem cells. The question of whether there is a limit, or what the limit is, for stem cell division capacity remains unclear, but the division capacity of stem cells in adult mammalian tissues during one life-span is extensive (more than 200 cell cycles in mouse and probably more than 1000 in man). There are even indications from transplantation experiments that mouse bone marrow stem cells may be capable of the divisions involved in the cell replacement required for up to five life-spans. There are indications that the cell cycle duration of stem cells is slower than that of other proliferative cells, or that they spend appreciable periods of time in G_0.

Transit cells are relatively short-lived cells produced by a stem cell compartment. They may, or may not, possess a limited division potential. They are not self-maintaining, being totally dependent for their replacement on the stem cells. The facts that they have a limited, as opposed to extensive ('unlimited') division potential and may display features of differentiation as they mature suggest that they should be regarded as differentiated cells relative to the stem cells.

They usually mature and differentiate further as they pass through their life span and hence may possess an 'age structure'. Their division capacity, in practice, would seem to be limited in tissues to about 12 cell cycles at most, and in many cases considerably fewer.

The division of transit cells as they mature increases, or amplifies, the cell output from the stem cell compartment and hence these divisions are sometimes referred to as *amplifying cell divisions*. Three transit divisions amplify eightfold and 10 divisions 1024-fold. Since transit cells are derived from stem cells and may undergo amplifying cell divisions before maturing to a point beyond which divisions no longer occur, i.e. the cells become *post-mitotic maturing cells*, the family of cells derived from each stem cell represents a *lineage* or family tree and the tissue can be regarded as having an *hierarchical* organization.

Details of the proliferative organization in conditional renewal systems remain unclear, but in situations where extensive continual cell replacement is required it appears that a common scheme is applicable, based on a hierarchical organization with a few stem cells and amplification divisions in a dividing transit population.

1.3.2   The bone marrow and haematopoiesis

Perhaps the best understood system is haemopoiesis in the bone marrow where the hierarchy has been extensively studied in the mouse using *in vivo* colony-forming studies and, more recently, *in vitro* techniques. A key article appeared in 1961 by Till and McCullogh, describing how stem cells in mouse bone marrow can be assayed by the presence of colonies in the spleen after transplantation of bone marrow into irradiated recipients. This was shortly followed by the development, in the first instances, of short-term *in vitro* techniques (Pluznick and Sachs 1965; Bradley and Metcalf 1966) and then by the development of long-term culture techniques (Dexter *et al.* 1977). These techniques permitted the bone marrow cellular hierarchy in the mouse to be defined fairly precisely (Fig. 1.72). The stem cells here make up only a fraction of 1 per cent (probably about 0.25 per cent) of the bone marrow cells. They consist, in all probability, of both a non-cycling and a cycling compartment. About 5–10 per cent differentiate each day and enter one of several differentiated lineages, the majority differentiating into the erythrocytic or granulocytic lineages. The full range of differentiation options is large (high pluripotency). The dividing transit population, for the erythrocytes, can be subdivided into committed and morphologically definable precursors, within which a total of between 8 and 13 cell divisions may occur.

1.3.3   The testis and spermatogenesis

The tubules of the testis, in which spermatogenesis occurs, provide another example where there is clear evidence of a hierarchical organization. Here there is dispute about some fine details (Clermont and Bustos-Oberegan 1968; Hackins 1971; Oakberg 1971) but the most generally accepted scheme describing the testicular cell lineage is shown in Fig. 1.73. In this system, in contrast to others, the stem cell population can be identified with some degree of certainty in rodents by its morphology and position. The unique feature of cell division in spermatogenesis is that cytokinesis is incomplete, resulting in the retention of small cytoplasmic bridges between all cells in the lineage. Although this does not result in the formation of true syncytia (in the sense that a mass of cytoplasm may contain many nuclei) it does mean that large families of cells retain an intimate communications link that may, in principle, run through a chain of up to about a 1000–2000 late type-B spermatogonia. This linkage between cells probably accounts for the fact that all the nuclei are synchronized in relation to the cell cycle and mitosis, and it is possible that they are all influenced by the death of one nucleus, which may result in the death of all the nuclei in the chain. There are between nine and 11 mitotic divisions before meiosis of the spermatocytes and a significant

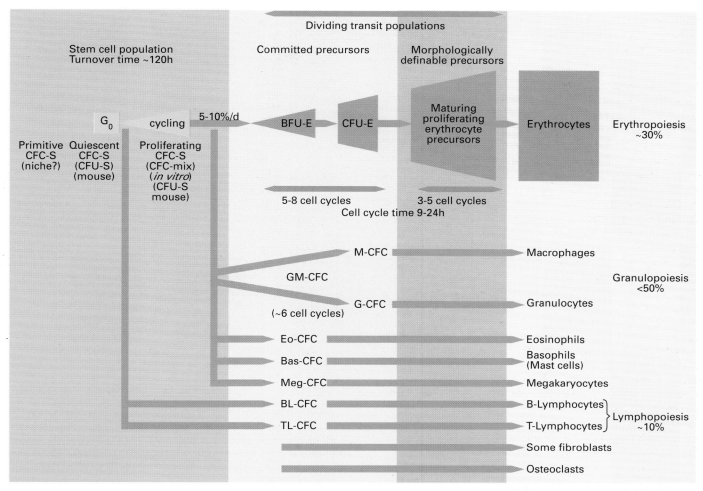

Fig. 1.72 Haematopoietic cell lineages. Haematologists have, over the years, developed a rather complex system of acronyms or abbreviations. CFC = colony-forming cells; S designates spleen. CFC-S is thus a cell that possesses the potential to form a colony in the spleen and CFU-S is a colony-forming unit (cell) that actually does make a colony in the spleen. The CFC-mix and the committed precursors are assayed using *in vitro* techniques (sometimes indicated by −c). BFU-E is an *in vitro* erythroid colony-forming cell that produces a cluster or burst of colonies, which is a more diffuse type of colony. Mix = a CFC with the ability to form mixed colonies. M, macrophage; G, granulocyte; Eo, eosinophil; Bas, basophil; Meg, megakaryocyte; BL, B-lymphocyte; TL, T-lymphocyte. (Drawn after Lord and Testa 1988, with permission.)

amount of spontaneous cell death within the lineage (particularly at the A_2 and A_3 levels), which means that the actual amplification factor is less than the theoretical factor of 2000–8000.

For many years it has been assumed, in the absence of any hard supportive data, that for all tissues other than bone marrow and testis proliferation was achieved via a stem cell compartment alone, which produces a simple transit functional population of cells. However, recent studies have tended to indicate that, at least in surface epithelia, an hierarchical scheme also operates. A feature of surface epithelia is their clear polarization into proliferative and functional zones. As a consequence, the proliferative organization cannot be considered without taking into account the architecture of the tissue.

1.3.4 The epidermis and keratopoiesis

Mouse epidermis has been most extensively studied and hence is best understood. The interfollicular epidermis on the back of the mouse is relatively thin. It has few keratinizing strata, is flat and not undulating with rete ridges or pegs (as in man). Here the cells in the 10–15 strata are organized characteristically into columns of cells. These can be viewed in appropriate 1 μm resin sections, electron micrographs, or specially swollen thicker sections. They can also be easily deduced from the regular hexagonal packing pattern seen when the surface is viewed either in the light microscope after suitable silver staining techniques or in the scanning electron microscope. The epidermis can be easily separated from the dermis and these epidermal sheets can

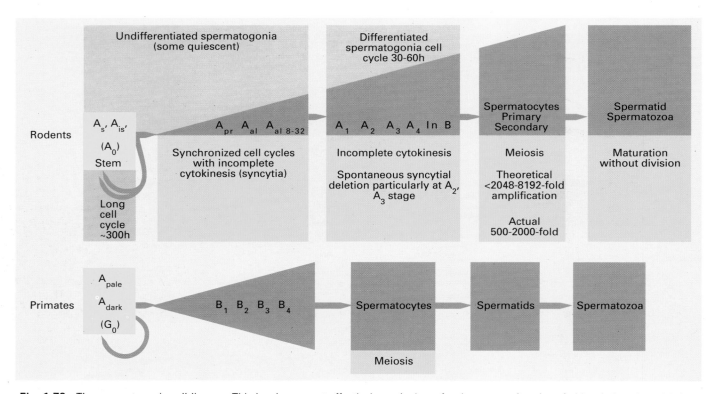

Fig. 1.73 The spermatogenic cell lineage. This has been most effectively worked out for the mouse. A series of abbreviations has also been adopted here, which can be summarized as follows. A_s is a stem or single spermatogonia, sometimes also called A_{is} (isolated) or A_0 (undifferentiated) spermatogonia. When these divide they produce either other A_s or a pair of linked type-A spermatogonia, A_{pr} (paired). On further division, the A_{pr} produce linked or aligned spermatogonia, A_{al}, $A_{al\,8-32}$ (see text). After 3–5 divisions the spermatogonia become differentiated type A_1 and with each successive division A_2, A_3, A_4, indeterminate (In), and B spermatogonia are produced. The latter mature into spermatocytes, where the two meiotic divisions occur. The spermatocytes then mature to form spermatids and then spermatozoa without further divisions. Most of the mitotic activity results in incomplete cytokinesis. Throughout the lineage, but particularly at the A_2 and A_3 stages, significant levels of cell death can occur. A different nomenclature is used for primates. (Drawn after de Rooij 1983, with permission.)

then be viewed by optical sectioning techniques to look at each level (stratum) in turn. When this is done it can be seen that the cells on the basal layer, which are responsible for the maintenance of the superficial column of cells, are arranged in a particular pattern. The superficial column of cells does, in fact, represent the historical record of the proliferative activity of this group of basal cells. The epidermis should therefore be regarded as being composed of a series of discrete units of proliferation, which have been termed epidermal proliferative units, EPU (Potten 1974). The structural organization of the EPU is illustrated in Fig. 1.74. Such an organization is seen in rodent epidermis but also in some sites in humans.

Clearly, the stem cell population must be located in the basal layer and in the past many have assumed that essentially all basal cells are equally important in functioning as stem cells, since essentially all basal cells appear to be in active progression through the cell cycle. However, the evidence now suggests that only a small fraction of the basal cells function as stem or clonogenic cells. In fact, clonal regeneration studies suggest that slightly fewer than 10 per cent of the basal cells are clonogenic cells (5–12 per cent, depending somewhat on how the

calculations are performed). There is now considerable evidence for cell population heterogeneity in the basal layer of mice and an accumulating amount of similar data for humans (Clausen and Potten 1990). Some of this heterogeneity is clearly related to a hierarchy amongst the proliferating cells. Clonal regeneration studies; detailed simultaneous analysis of several cell kinetic experiments; consideration of several ionizing radiation, ultraviolet light, and cytotoxic drug experiments; and a detailed analysis of the spatial patterns of clusters of cells labelled in DNA synthesis all suggest a hierarchy with three amplifying divisions in the dividing transit population (see Fig. 1.74). It is possible that some of these divisions produce daughters that become mature post-mitotic cells prematurely in terms of the cell lineage: the fine details of the hierarchy thus remain to be fully elucidated.

There have also been studies on stratified epithelia where the basal layer undulates; for example the filiform papillae of the tongue have a corresponding dermal papilla over which the epithelium is folded. The proliferative organization here is very similar to that shown in Fig. 1.74, with proliferative units and a subpopulation of stem cells. The difference is that the stem cells

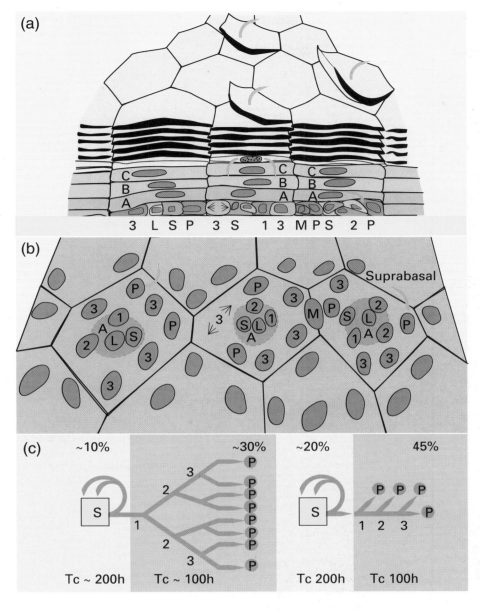

Fig. 1.74 Tissue and proliferative units in the epidermis. Murine interfollicular epidermis is structurally arranged with columns of cells and proliferative units as shown here. 10^7 cells/day are produced from the mouse epidermis.

(a) The top panel is a cross section through skin. The surface consists of hexagonally tesselated cornified cells. Such a pattern implies a columnar packing of the underlying cells. A, B, C indicate different strata in the epidermis. L, Langerhans cells; S, stem cell; P. postmitotic cell preparing for differentiated function; M, melanocyte.

(b) The centre panel is an *en face* view of a sheet of epidermis separated at the dermal–epidermal junction. The nuclei of the basal cells in this sheet, viewed through stratum A (indicated by a blue circle), are shown with a possible distribution according to the cell lineage model shown in the bottom left panel (c).

(c) In this panel, the lineage that most adequately explains all aspects of cell replacement and clonal regeneration is illustrated on the left. An alternative possible lineage based on an analysis of the clustering pattern of DNA synthesizing cells labelled with a radioactive precursor (and studied at various times thereafter) is illustrated on the right. Tc, cell cycle duration. (Drawn after Potten 1974, 1976, 1981, 1983; Potten *et al.* 1982, with permission.)

are inevitably located at the lowest epithelial position. The precise number of stem cells remains somewhat unclear, but it seems likely that the lineage cannot contain more than 2–3 transit cell divisions. The presence of an undulating basal layer with pegs or ridges extending into the dermis is common. It has been suggested that wherever such a structure exists the stem cell population will be found at the deepest part of the epithelium and that this will inevitably mean that there is some movement (or displacement) of cells along the basal lamina towards the top of the dermal peg.

In humans it has been suggested that the cells at such deep epidermal positions are morphologically less differentiated than those at the top of the dermal peg or ridge (Lavker and Sun 1983).

1.3.5 The intestine

The mucosa lining the small intestine of the mouse is probably the most extensively studied tissue from the point of view of its cell replacement. Cell proliferation is restricted here to small flask-shaped bags of cells that are probably derived during development from a single cell, representing clones. These bags of cells, the crypts, are tucked inconspicuously at the base of the large, functional, finger-like projections into the lumen of the gut, the villi. Within the crypts, cells rapidly (twice a day) pass through the cell cycle, and the progeny of the division activity of the 150 proliferative cells per crypt move, or are displaced, at a rate of 1–2 cell positions per hour from the crypt on to the villus. Thus they have a total life expectancy of about 3 days before

Mouse 2x10^8 cells shed/small intestine/day

Man ~10^{11} cells shed/small intestine/day

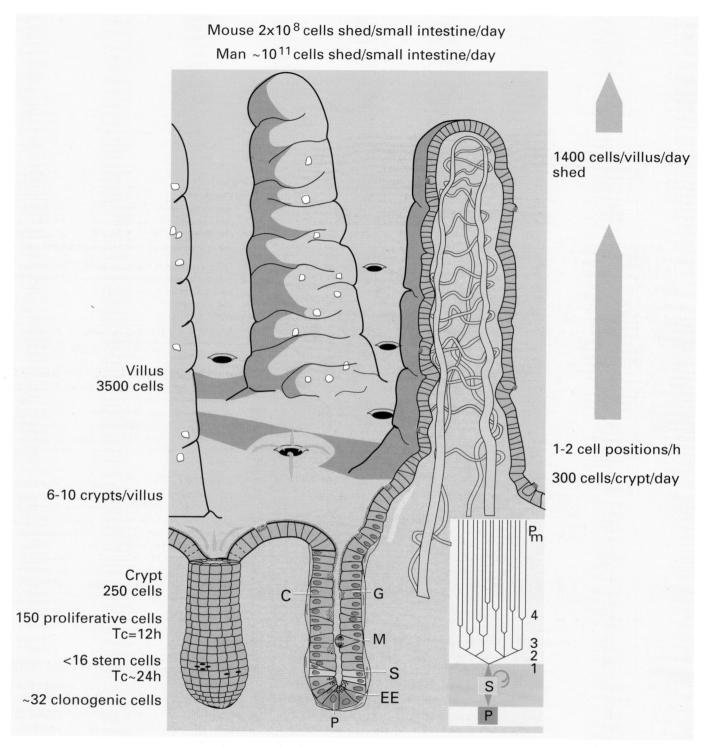

1400 cells/villus/day
shed

Villus
3500 cells

6-10 crypts/villus

1-2 cell positions/h

300 cells/crypt/day

Crypt
250 cells

150 proliferative cells
Tc=12h

<16 stem cells
Tc~24h

~32 clonogenic cells

Fig. 1.75 Tissue and proliferative organization in the small intestine. The proliferative units, the crypts, contain about 250 cells (about 16 in circumference), amongst which are at least three distinct differentiated cell lineages: Paneth cells (P), mucus-secreting goblet cells (G), and the predominant columnar epithelial cells (C); there is also a small population of entero-endocrine cells (EE). About 150 cells are proliferating. The majority divide twice a day, thus producing about 300 cells/day/crypt. These emigrate on to the villus at a velocity of 1–2 cell positions/h as postmitotic cells (Pm). The stem cells (S) are located at the base of the crypt and probably do not consist of more than about 16 cells/crypt. M, mitotic cell; Tc, cell cycle duration. (Drawn after Cheng and Leblond 1974; Leblond and Cheng 1976; Bjerknes and Cheng 1981; Potten and Hendry 1983; Potten and Loeffler 1987; Potten *et al.* 1987, with permission.)

being extruded from the villus into the gut lumen, where they are digested and the cellular constituents effectively salvaged. With a system such as this, it is particularly relevant to ask where the cells are upon which the whole system depends, i.e. the stem cells. It is fairly clear that these must be located at the origin of the movement. All other cells will inevitably be displaced when the cells below them divide. The very base of the crypt contains some mature functional cells, the Paneth cells. Situated above the Paneth cells, at about the fourth cell position from the base, are cells that could represent the origin of all other cells. There are about 16–18 cells in an annulus around the crypt at this position. There are also some cells interspersed between the Paneth cells that may also represent part, or even all, of the stem cell compartment. Clonal regeneration studies are feasible in this system and these studies suggest that only about 32 cells per crypt are clonogenic. This could mean two circumferential rings of cells or one ring plus the cells interspersed between the Paneth cells. Thus, in this system it would appear that the crypts contain relatively few functional stem cells. A current model for the proliferative operation of the crypt proposes between 4 and 16 functional stem cells, probably about twice as many potential stem cells (clonogenic cells), and about 120 rapidly dividing transit cells: in other words a lineage with four to six transit cell generations (Fig. 1.75). There are at least three distinct differentiated cell types in the mucosa—the Paneth, goblet, and columnar cells—all of which

are believed to originate from a common stem cell population, which therefore has at least a tripotentiality in terms if differentiation.

1.3.6 Concluding remarks

It is evident that in all cases of cell renewal tissues studied in detail, cell replacement is achieved via an hierarchical organization with dividing transit and stem cells. The picture can be summarized as in Fig. 1.76.

The precise number of transit divisions is, in some cases, uncertain and is in all probability an element of the scheme that can be modulated according to the requirements of the tissue from time to time. Figure 1.76 illustrates the level of 'amplification' achieved for each division in the dividing transit population, and the inverse relationship between the number of transit divisions and the proportion of stem cells. With the hierarchical scheme illustrated, a range of levels of control on cell output is possible. Output can be controlled by 'determinant' factors:

1. the number of transit divisions;

2. the rate of cell cycle progression of transit cells; and

3. the rate of cell cycle progression of the stem cells.

These may not necessarily be the same as factors that determine the rate of entry to and exit from G_0 for the stem cells. However,

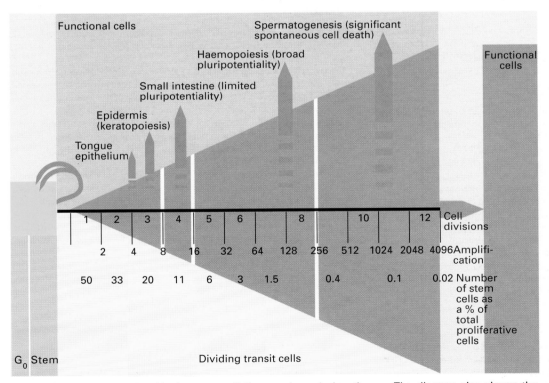

Fig. 1.76 The interrelationship between cell lineages in replacing tissues. The diagram also shows the relationship between the number of cell divisions in the dividing transit population; the degree of amplication that results from these divisions; and the progressive dilution of the stem cell population as the amplification increases.

both cycle progression rate and G_0 residence time would determine the input rate of cells to the dividing transit population.

A fourth determinant factor is the probability of differentiation, or its inverse the probability of self-maintenance of the stem cell compartment. If the probability of self-maintenance is raised above 0.5, the stem cell compartment will expand àt the expense of the dividing transit, and hence functional, cell compartments.

Some aspects of these hierarchically dependent control systems are currently becoming evident, particularly for the haematopoietic cell lineage.

1.3.7   Further reading

General

Gilbert, C. W. and Lajtha, L. G. (1965). The importance of cell population kinetics in determining response to irradiation of normal and malignant tissue. In *Cellular radiation biology*, p. 474–96. Williams and Wilkins, Baltimore.

Howard, A. and Pele, S. R. (1953). Synthesis of desoxyribonucleic acid in normal and irradiated cells and its relation to chromosome breakage. *Heredity* 6, 261–73.

Lajtha, L. G. (1979). Haemopoietic stem cells: concepts and definitions (rapporteur's summary). *Blood Cells* 5, 447–55.

Lajtha, L. A. (1979). Stem cell concepts. *Differentiation* 14, 23–34.

Potten, C. S. and Lajtha, L. G. (1982). Stem cells versus stem lines. *Annals of the New York Academy of Sciences* 397, 49.

Potten, C. S. and Loeffler, M. (1990). Stem cells: attributes, cycles, spirals, pitfalls and uncertainties. Lessons for and from the crypt. *Development* 110, 1001–20.

Potten, C. S., Schofield, R., and Lajtha, L. G. (1979). A comparison of cell replacement in bone marrow, testis and three regions of surface epithelium. *Biochimica et Biophysica Acta* 560, 281–99.

Bone marrow

Bradley, T. R. and Metcalf, D. (1966). The growth of mouse bone marrow cells *in vitro*. *Australian Journal of Experimental Biology and Medical Science* 44, 287–300.

Dexter, T. D., Allen, T. D., and Lajtha, L. G. (1977). Conditions controlling the proliferation of haemopoietic stem cells *in vitro*. *Journal of Cellular Physiology* 91, 335–45.

Lord, B. I. and Testa, N. G. (1988). The haemopoietic system: structure and regulation. In *Bone marrow damage* (ed. N. G. Testa and R. P. Gale), pp. 1–26. Marcel Dekker, New York.

Pluznik, D. H. and Sachs, L. (1965). The cloning of normal 'mast' cells in tissue culture. *Journal of Cellular and Comparative Physiology* 66, 319–24.

Till, J. E. and McCulloch, E. A. (1961). A direct measurement of the radiation sensitivity of normal mouse bone marrow cells. *Radiation Research* 14, 213–22.

Testis

Clermont, Y. and Bustos-Obregon, E. (1968). Re-examination of spermatogonial renewal in the rat by means of seminiferous tubules mounted *in toto*. *American Journal of Anatomy* 122, 237–48.

de Rooij, D. G. (1983). Proliferation and differentiation of undifferentiated spermatogonia in the mammalian testis. In *Stem cells: their identification and characterisation* (ed. C. S. Potten), pp. 89–117. Churchill Livingstone, Edinburgh.

Huckins, C. (1971). The spermatogonial stem cell population in adult rats.·I. Their morphology, proliferation and maturation. *Anatomical Record* 169, 533–58.

Oakberg, E. F. (1971). Spermatogonial stem cell renewal in the mouse. *Anatomical Record* 169, 515–32.

Epidermis

Clausen, O. P. F. and Potten, C. S. (1990). Heterogeneity of keratinocytes in the epidermal basal cell layer. *Journal of Cutaneous Pathology* 17, 129–43.

Lavker, R. M. and Sun, T. T. (1983). Epidermal stem cells. *Journal of Investigative Dermatology* 81, 121–7.

Potten, C. S. (1974). The epidermal proliferative unit: the possible role of the central basal cell. *Cell and Tissue Kinetics* 7, 77–88.

Potten, C. S. (1976). Identification of clonogenic cells in the epidermis and the structural arrangement of the epidermal proliferative unit (EPU). In *Stem cells of renewing cell population* (ed. A. B. Cairnie, P. K. Lala, and D. G. Osmond), pp. 91–102. Academic Press, New York.

Potten, C. S. (1981). Cell replacement in epidermis (keratopoiesis) via discrete units of proliferation. *International Review of Cytology* 69, 271–318.

Potten, C. S. (1983). Stem cells in epidermis from the back of the mouse. In *Stem cells: their identification and characterisation* (ed. C. S. Potten), pp. 200–32. Churchill Livingstone, Edinburgh.

Potten, C. S., Wichmann, H. E., Loeffler, M., Dobek, K., and Major, D. (1982). Evidence for discrete cell kinetic subpopulations in mouse epidermis based on mathematical analysis. *Cell and Tissue Kinetics* 15, 305–29.

Intestine

Bjerknes, M. and Cheng, H. (1981). The stem cell zone in the small intestinal epithelia I, II & III. *American Journal of Anatomy* 160, 51–91.

Cheng, H. and Leblond, C. P. (1974). Origin, differentiation and renewal of the four main epithelial cell types in the mouse small intestine. V. Unitarian theory of the origin of the four epithelial cell types. *American Journal of Anatomy* 141, 537–63.

Leblond, C. P. and Cheng, H. (1976). Identification of stem cells in the small intestine of the mouse. In *Stem cells of renewing cell populations* (ed. A. B. Cairnie, P. K. Lala, and D. G. Osmond), pp. 7–31. Academic Press, New York.

Potten, C. S. and Hendry, J. H. (1983). Stem cells in murine small intestine. In *Stem cells: their identification and characterisation* (ed. C. S. Potten), pp. 155–99. Churchill Livingstone, Edinburgh.

Potten, C. S., and Loeffler, M. (1987). A comprehensive model of the crypts of the small intestine of the mouse provides insight into the mechanisms of cell migration and the proliferative hierarchy. *Journal of Theoretical Biology* 127, 381–91.

Potten, C. S., Hendry, J. H., and Moore, J. V. (1987). Estimates of the number of clonogenic cells in crypts or murine small intestine. *Virchows Archiv B* 53, 227–34.

1.4   Extracellular matrix

Introduction

In the preceding sections of this chapter, cell structure, function, differentiation, and lineage have been considered in isolation. All tissues, however, are composed not only of cells but also of extracellular matrix (ECM). In fact, mammalian tissue and organs could not exist in the organized way that they do but for the evolution of the matrix components that hold the specialized tissue cells together. The extracellular space is occupied by water, plasma proteins, and other plasma constituents; these and the cells embedded therein are held together by extracellular matrix proteins and proteoglycans. The matrix components are synthesized mainly by cells in the immediate locality, and the extracellular matrix varies in molecular, microscopic, and gross structure and function from one tissue to another (see Section 1.4.4). In diseases where connective tissue production and deposition are prominent, the normal molecular constitution of ECM changes dramatically. For examples, see atherosclerosis (Chapter 12) and cirrhosis (Chapter 17).

Here we will consider the two major connective tissue proteins, viz. collagen and elastin. These proteins form a fibrous meshwork which confers structural/physical and functional properties on individual tissues and organs. The space between the fibrous meshwork is filled up by 'ground substance' (Section 1.4.3) and plasma derivatives. Matrix specialization will be discussed in Section 1.4.4. It is important to realize that collagen and other extracellular proteins not only serve as structural supporting skeletons for organs but may also have a profound influence on morphogenesis and the stability of organ differentiation (see Section 1.2.3).

1.4.1 Collagen

Bryan Sykes

Introduction

Until the mid-nineteenth century the prevailing view was that all tissues were made up entirely of fibres of one sort or another. When the new achromatic objectives made it possible to see cells clearly for the first time, interest rapidly shifted towards cellular explanations of biological and pathological processes. From then until very recently the 'cell theory' achieved a dominance so complete that it largely eclipsed all interest in extracellular events. A few unconnected events have re-awakened this interest so that it has now become a very active area for study and research.

The first of these events arose from the interest of textile chemists in the structures of natural and synthetic fibres. By applying the newly developed science of X-ray diffraction to biological fibrils, Astbury and Schmitt opened the door to the solution of the molecular structure of collagen and muscle.

The second was the observation that rats fed on a diet of sweet peas (*Lathyrus odoratus*) developed abnormalities like scoliosis and aortic rupture, reminiscent of those seen in the Marfan syndrome, a dominantly inherited disorder of man. This discovery was made during experiments designed to isolate the toxin responsible for the neurological symptoms of lathyrism which developed when livestock, and people, were forced on to a diet rich in the seeds of this hardy genus when regular crops had failed. It emerged that a simple chemical, β-aminopropionitrile (BAPN), was responsible for the disruptive effect on the mechanical strength of the tissues. The subsequent work into the mechanism of this effect provided the way into all modern studies of collagen and elastin because it was now possible to isolate the sub-units of these otherwise totally insoluble fibres which could then enjoy a conventional biochemical characterization.

The third unconnected event was the description by Klemperer of the conspicuous visible effects on the extracellular matrix of diseases like scleroderma and systemic lupus erythematosus. This marked the re-emergence of the concept of intercellular tissue as a functional biological system, though Klemperer's term 'collagen-disease' coined for these conditions has since been degraded by its popularity as an inappropriate non-specific diagnosis.

In the last three decades the major effort has been towards a complete chemical description of the extracellular matrix. This process has yielded an abundance of detailed information about the individual components. Nevertheless, the field still lacks a synthesis which will fit these components into an overall functional scheme though their influence on, for instance, differentiation and tumour development, is being recognized (Section 1.2).

Morphology

Histochemistry distinguishes three fibre systems in the extracellular matrix: collagen, elastin, and reticulin. Birefringence under polarized light or reaction with van Gieson's picrofuchsin stain reveals the collagen fibres. These have a rich variety of form in different tissues which can, with a bit of imagination, be correlated with the engineering demands made on each one. In tendon, for instance, the fibres are thick and run parallel to the direction of applied stress. This is collagen at its most impressive. With a tensile strength of 18,000 lbs per square inch, comparable to that of cast-iron, yet able to withstand rounds of tension and relaxation without fatigue, it is a remarkable material. The fibres in skin are arranged in a criss-cross pattern which resists stretching in any lateral direction (Fig. 1.77). Cornea has a special arrangement of laminated sheets of parallel fibres with, as in plywood, the orientation changing in each layer. It is a tribute to the versatility of the protein that the same basic molecule has such an extensive repertoire.

The fine branching filaments of the reticulin system which are picked out by silver stains are also made up predominantly of collagen, although a slightly different version of the basic molecule. This is not the case with the elastic fibre system revealed by orcein. Once thought to be degenerate collagen fibres, we now know that these fibres are composed of the rubbery protein elastin assembled round a scaffold of an acidic microfibrillar glycoprotein.

The consistency and ubiquity of collagen is even more

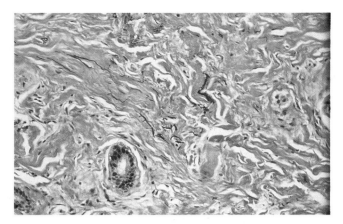

Fig. 1.77 Collagen fibres in skin. The collagen fibres stained red (with van Gieson's stain) are thick bundles between skin appendages such as the sweat duct shown in the lower half. The collagen fibres around the sweat duct are much thinner.

evident on electron microscopy. This reveals another level of order, the fibril, with its unmistakable cross-banding pattern (Fig. 1.78). Though fibril diameters vary, the banding interval does not. This is because it is a direct function of the molecular length and a direct result of the way in which these molecules pack to form the fibril.

Several types of cell are capable of synthesizing collagen but the major production sites are the mesenchymal cells within each tissue. Their production schedule is very dependent on the local environment and it can change substantially and unpredictably when the cells are grown *in vitro*. This has hampered efforts to identify subsets of fibroblasts, osteoblasts, chondroblasts, and others of the series. They appear to retain the potential to synthesize different collagens and, by changing their immediate culture environment, cells can be persuaded to go through several switching cycles from one collagen to another.

Molecular structure

Collagen occurs in the tissues as beautifully ordered, almost crystalline molecular arrays—the fibrils. Within the fibrils, each collagen molecule is a continuous 1.5×300 nm three-stranded helix. Each strand of the helix is 1014 residues long and each of these chains, save for a few residues at either end reserved for crosslinking purposes, is a 338-fold tandem repeat of the tri-

peptide Gly-X-Y. Positions X and Y can be occupied by any amino acid without damaging the helix but the glycine positioning at every third is absolutely crucial. This is known because single base changes in glycine codons which substitute other amino acids are so disruptive that they lead to a lethal form of the heritable bone disease osteogenesis imperfecta. The reason is that only glycine, lacking a side-chain, is small enough to pack into the centre of the tightly-wound helix. As it is, X and Y positions are often occupied by the imino acids proline (at X) and its hydroxylated derivative hydroxyproline (at Y). These residues give each strand a coarse-pitched (0.95 nm) left-handed twist which positions the glycines in such a way that they can pack precisely along the central axis of the three-stranded right-handed superhelix (Fig. 1.79). The wound-up helix is mechanically strong but thermally rather unstable and begins to unwind, or literally melt, at $42°C$. Hydrogen bonds between the adjacent chains counteract this tendency. Additional hydrogen bonds are created by hydroxylated Y position prolines and this serves to increase the melting temperature. In this context, the collagen of fish species, like the cod, which inhabit very cold seas and operate at a lower body temperature, contains very much less hydroxyproline than warm-blooded mammals. Fig. 1.80 illustrates diagrammatically the molecular and supramolecular structure of collagen.

Biosynthesis

Hydroxylation of proline is one of several steps between translation of collagen mRNA and self-assembly of the finished fibril. The first cellular product is actually an elaborate precursor, procollagen, with globular domains at both ends (Fig. 1.81). In common with other secreted polypeptides, the procollagen subunits each have a short-lived signal sequence at the amino terminus to get them into the cisternae of the rough endoplasmic reticulum. Once there, several things happen at once. Membrane bound enzymes modify the unwound strands hydroxylating not only Y position prolines but also lysines. The resulting hydroxylysines can then be glycosylated by addition of, first, galactose and, secondly, glucose.

These modifications can only take place while the strands are unwound. The folding process is initiated by aggregation of three propeptides at the carboxy-terminus. Interchain disulphide bond formation signals the winding process to begin and it continues from right to left. Finally, the short minor helix in the N-propeptide forms to complete the process.

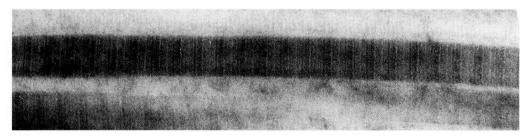

Fig. 1.78 Electron micrograph of a collagen fibre. It is composed of collagen fibrils which have a cross-striated appearance due to the 'quarter stagger' arrangement of the collagen molecules composing the fibril.

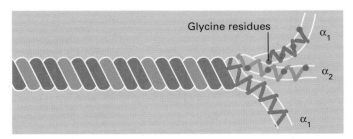

Glycine residues

α_1

α_2

α_1

Fig. 1.79 Different levels of structure within the collagen helix. The left-handed α-chain helices place the glycine residues in such a way that when the right-handed super helix folds they are arranged along the central axis. Any disturbance of this arrangement by, for instance, the substitution of another amino acid for glycine, prevents the helix from folding at that point.

Procollagen then leaves the cell via the Golgi apparatus and, soon after, loses the C-propeptide. The N-propeptide stays on while molecules jockey for position in the growing fibril and it is then removed after aggregation. Some of the propeptide finds its way into the blood where measurement of the concentration has been used as an index of active collagen synthesis in diseases such as scleroderma, liver cirrhosis, and pulmonary fibrosis.

The distribution of charges and hydrophobic residues along the collagen molecules obliges them to aggregate in a very precise way. Rather than simply lining up side by side, the ends of adjacent molecules are staggered by exactly 67 nm (Fig. 1.82). This arrangement, which is repeated throughout the fibril, has two consequences. The first is to create, along the fibril, zones of overlap between molecules in *adjacent* rows alternating with gap zones between molecules in the *same* row. Electron-dense stains can penetrate the gap zones but not the overlap zones and this results in the well-known appearance of negatively stained fibrils—alternating light and dark striations with a periodicity of, naturally, 67 nm.

The second and more important consequence of this stagger is to create a network of molecules that can be effectively interlocked. This interlocking is achieved by covalent cross-links formed between lysine (or its hydroxylated derivative hydroxylysine) residues in the short non-helical segments (telopeptides) at each end of the helix and lysine/hydroxylysine residues in the helical region of the staggered adjacent molecule.

First, the side-chain ε-amino group of teleopeptide lysine residues are removed by the enzyme lysyl oxidase, creating an

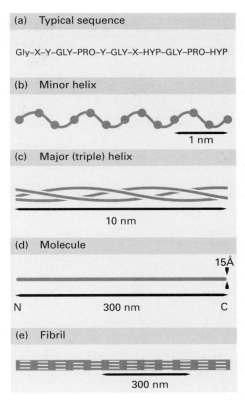

(a) **Typical sequence**

Gly–X–Y–GLY–PRO–Y–GLY–X–HYP–GLY–PRO–HYP

(b) **Minor helix**

1 nm

(c) **Major (triple) helix**

10 nm

(d) **Molecule**

15Å

N   300 nm   C

(e) **Fibril**

300 nm

Fig. 1.80 The molecular and supramolecular structure of collagen (see text for details).

active aldehyde group. Then, a series of chemical condensation and rearrangement steps between the precisely opposed reactive groups follow, not all of which are completely understood, resulting in stable cross-links joining together either two or three chains. As with many other steps in the sequence of post-translational modification there is a lot of scope for variation. Some tissues, for instance adult skin, cornea, sclera, prefer to construct cross-links by starting with lysine while others like bone, cartilage, ligament, and most tendons use hydroxylysine aldehydes. The reasons for these alternatives in cross-link construction and the effects of one pathway compared to another are a mystery. Nevertheless, the overall purpose is quite clear: to transmit the mechanical properties of the helix to the fibril as a whole. The overall scheme of biosynthesis is illustrated in Fig. 1.83.

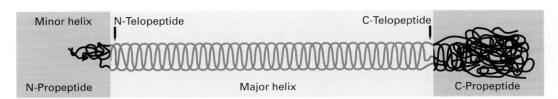

Minor helix   N-Telopeptide   C-Telopeptide

N-Propeptide   Major helix   C-Propeptide

Fig. 1.81 A procollagen molecule. The black arrows show the points where the molecule is cleaved to remove the propeptides. Only the major helix and the short, non-helical, telopeptides at either end remain in the collagen fibril.

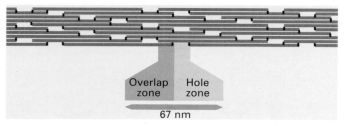

Fig. 1.82 The overlapping arrangement of collagen molecules in a fibril generates zones of hole and overlap. Negative stains penetrate the hole zones but are excluded from the overlaps. This leads to the appearance of regular striations across the fibril so characteristic of collagen under the electron microscope.

Collagen breakdown

During growth and remodelling there is an evident need for a mechanism for removing collagen fibres. This process is accomplished by a series of enzymatic digestions initiated by a specific collagenase. This enzyme makes a single clip across all three chains of the helix between residues Gly 772 and Ala 773, that is, about three-quarters of the way along starting from the N-terminus. The two fragments are further broken down by cathepsins operating at acidic pH within the intracellular lysosomes. These enzymes are also capable of initiating extracellular collagen breakdown without collagenase when, as happens with the osteoclast, the cell creates an acidic extracellular microenvironment on the resorptive surface of the bone. The amino acids resulting from complete proteolytic digestion are neutralized with the exception of hydroxyproline. This amino acid is excreted into the urine where the concentration has been used to assess collagen turnover in resorptive disorders like Paget's disease of bone.

Different types of collagen

Fibrillar collagens

The structures and events described above have all sprung from detailed study of tendon—the most collagen-rich of all tissues and the one which, in its strength and resilience, epitomises the collagen fibril at work. In 1969, during investigations of cartilage collagen, it became obvious that its subunit structure was different to that in tendon. In tendon, there are two different chains contributing to the helix. Each molecule comprises two α_1-chains and one α_2-chain. The subscripts refer to the order of elution from chromatographic columns used in their separation. They are the products of different structural genes and have a different amino-acid sequence. Cartilage collagen, on the other hand, contains only a single α-chain but one that is different again from the tendon α-chains. The discovery of tissue-specific collagen species required the formulation of a classification, intially Type I (the original) and Type II (the cartilage molecule). These days collagen I and collagen II are the preferred labels for these molecules. Two other collagens have been discovered which have a very similar molecular structure and which are capable of forming fibres either alone

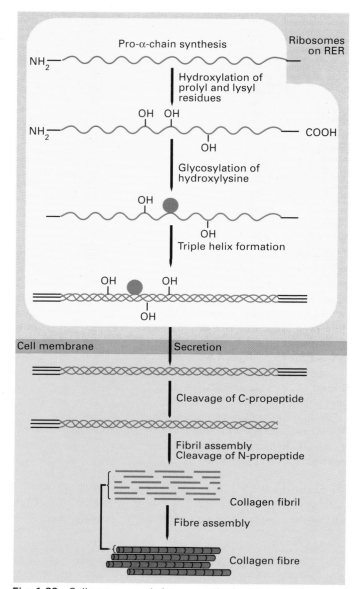

Fig. 1.83 Collagen pro-α-chains are synthesized in the rough endoplasmic reticulum (RER) and hydroxylated and glycosylated in the RER or Golgi apparatus. Triple-helical aggregates are secreted and the N- and C-termini are cleaved so that each trimer can assemble into fibrils (see Fig. 1.78 and text). These fibrils then further aggregate to form fibres (see Fig. 1.77).

or in combination with other collagens. Collagen III occurs in distensible tissues like skin, gut, and blood-vessel walls and is found at high concentrations in foetal tissue and during wound healing. Collagen V is found in small amounts in many tissues, particularly placenta. For obvious reasons, these four are collectively known as the fibrillar collagens. This is to distinguish them from the non-fibrillar collagens whose inclusion into the overall list has interrupted the arithmetical numbering sequence. Though the differential tissue distribution of the fibrillar collagens is well known, what it is about one collagen rather than another that makes it appropriate for a particular tissue is still a mystery (see Table 1.3, Section 1.2).

Non-fibrillar collagens

Just as 'collagen-disease' has lost its original meaning through indiscriminate and careless usage, so too has 'collagen'. These are several other extracellular molecules which are known to contain regions of Gly-X-Y triple helix. Sometimes this has come to light during sequencing, either amino acid or nucleotide, of proteins with known functions.

Examples of these are the complement component C1q, the asymmetric form of acetylcholinesterase, a mannose-binding protein synthesized in the liver and a pulmonary surfactant apo-protein. Otherwise, proteins have been deliberately traced either by the intrinsic property of the triple-helix to resist proteolytic digestion or by characteristics of the nucleotide sequence that encodes it. If the discovery is the result of a search via this second route, then the new molecule becomes known as a collagen and, probably wrongly, tends to assume its engineering function along with title. The distinction between the two groups of molecule is more administrative than anything—collagens being molecules discovered in collagen laboratories.

Of the non-fibrillar collagens, collagen IV is the best understood. It appears to form an open network in basement membranes. It has two subunits (α1 and α2) and the helix has several discontinuities in the Gly-X-Y repeat. At the C-terminus, a large globular domain is linked through disulphide bonds to the same domain of another molecule, while at the N-terminus several molecules are cross-linked together. Fluorescent antibodies to collagen IV are an excellent tool for outlining the basement membrane in tissue sections.

Gene structure

The organization of collagen genes (Fig. 1.84) is remarkable and certainly emphasizes the close relationship between the fibrillar collagens. The helical domain is encoded by forty-two exons with a very limited number of different sizes. The most common size is 54bp and the others are simple recombinational derivatives 108 (i.e. 54 × 2), 99 (108–9), 45 (54–9), and 162 (54 × 3). Each encodes a complete set of Gly-X-Y triplets. At either end of this domain, junction exons encode helix, telopeptide, and part of the propeptide sequences. Other than that, the propeptide exons have a much more conventional organization. Except for one very minor difference (the fusion of two 54bp exons), the organization of the genes encoding the subunits of all fibrillar collagens are, as far as is known at this time, identical.

The simplest explanation for the similarities between the different genes is that they were at one time duplicated from a common ancestor which itself evolved from a 54bp precursor. Estimates of divergence, calculated from non-critical amino acid substitutions between the different collagens, place the duplication from the common ancestor about 500–1000 million years ago. Exon evolution since then has evidently been severely constrained, probably by the strict discipline imposed by fibril formation. It is indeed a tribute to the original collagen molecule that the basic material used to build structures as diverse as Wharton's jelly, vitreous humour, intervertebral disc, gut wall, cartilage, and bone, is encoded by fossil genes unwilling or unable to improve upon a design first used to construct the creatures drifting in a Palaeozoic sea.

1.4.2 Elastic fibres

James O'D. McGee

Elastic fibres are present to a greater or lesser degree in all tissues and organs. They form a fibrillar meshwork (Fig. 1.85) in

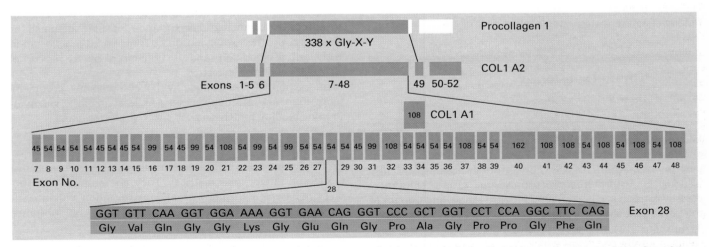

Fig. 1.84 The organization of a fibrillar collagen gene showing the exons coding for the major helix all of them simply related to 54bp. One of these, exon 28, is expanded. All helix exons have a full glycine codon at their 3′-ends. The sequence shown is from the human COL1A2 gene which codes for the α2 chain of collagen 1 but the arrangement of exons is almost exactly the same in all mammalian fibrillar collagen genes except for the condensation of exons 33 and 34 in COL1A1—the gene encoding the α1 chain of collagen 1.

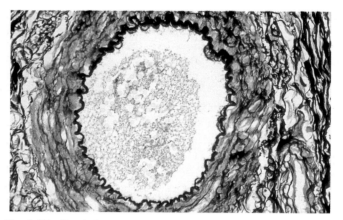

Fig. 1.85 Elastic fibres in and around a blood vessel. The elastic fibres (black) are arranged as an internal elastic lamina on the inside part of the vessel wall. Other elastic fibres extend from the vessel into the adjacent connective tissue (green). Elastic recoil is provided for the blood vessel and the adjacent connective tissue.

connective tissues such as skin, or lamellae in large arteries like the aorta They confer the necessary functional elasticity in organs, such as lung and blood vessels which return to their 'resting' size after inspiration and cardiac systole, respectively. An easily observed example of elastic recoil is that skin squeezed between two fingers immediately returns to a flat surface when finger compression stops. Elastic fibres consist of at least two components: elastin and microfibrillary proteins. Fibrillin is one component of the electron microscopically visible microfibrillar proteins. Elastin is a large, highly insoluble, hydrophobic molecule containing about 830 amino acids. Like collagen, it is rich in proline and glycine but, unlike collagen, few of the prolines are hydroxylated. This protein is highly cross-linked through lysine residues, analogous to the cross-links in collagen. Elastin is secreted into the extracellular matrix locally by cells, such as smooth muscle cells in the aorta. It achieves its elasticity through its random coil structure and the cross-linking of adjacent elastin molecules.

1.4.3 'Ground substance'

A. Jane d'Ardenne

Microscopic examination of connective tissues reveals collagen and elastic fibres (see Sections 1.4.1, 1.4.2) embedded in an amorphous matrix. This was called 'ground substance' by early histologists. A substantial proportion of the 'ground substance' is easily extracted, e.g. with physiological saline, and belongs to the extravascular pool of plasma proteins. In addition, however, it contains hyaluronate, proteoglycans, and other non-collagenous glycoproteins, which are essential for the organization of the tissue. These molecules have varying and important interactions with cells, fibrillar and basement membrane collagens, and elastin.

Hyaluronic acid

Hyaluronic acid is a major constituent of 'ground substance'.

Structure

Hyaluronic acid is a linear polysaccharide built from repeating disaccharide units of D-glucuronic acid and N-acetyl-D-glucosamine. It is not covalently linked to protein, unlike related substances present in proteoglycans (see below). At physiological pH its carboxyl groups are completely dissociated, and hence it is called hyaluronate.

Site

The highest concentrations of hyaluronate are found in mesenchymal tissues, but most cells synthesize it in culture. It is found bound to cell membranes, aggregated with other macromolecules, or free. Every tissue fluid contains hyaluronic acid, although in varying amounts. High concentrations are found in synovial fluid and in cartilage, where it is bound to proteoglycan. Human serum contains small quantities of hyaluronate derived from lymph. Increased serum levels are found in conditions associated with increased production, such as rheumatoid arthritis, or with impaired degradation by the liver.

Function

In body fluids, the presence of hyaluronate confers important physical properties, notably visco-elasticity. Hyaluronate also undergoes important interactions with cells. It may provide a protective coat for some, such as those of the synovium, and prevent attack from infective agents. There is also evidence that it can affect immunological responses. This may occur in a concentration-dependent manner. In high concentrations, it inhibits macrophage response to cytokines and phagocytosis; in low concentrations it enhances phagocytosis. It can also interact directly with lymphocytes.

Hyaluronic acid probably plays an important role in embryogenesis and differentiation. In areas where there is morphogenetic movement, extracellular matrices are rich in hyaluronate. Following differentiation, it may diminish or disappear. Synthesis of hyaluronate is increased in association with cell proliferation and is influenced by a variety of hormones and growth factors.

Interaction of hyaluronate with cells probably occurs by more than one mechanism, but, at least in part, via hyaluronate binding proteins on cell surfaces, or 'receptors'.

Proteoglycans

Proteoglycans are important components of most connective tissue and intercellular matrices. They are found on cell surfaces, in basement membranes, and in association with interstitial collagen and elastin, as well as free in the ground substance (see Table 1.4, Section 1.2.2).

Structure

A proteoglycan molecule consists of a central core protein to which one or more glycosaminoglycan (GAG) chains are covalently bound. Glycosaminoglycans consist of linear polymers of repeating disaccharides bearing anionic groups. Chondroitin sulphate, dermatan sulphate, keratan sulphate, heparan sulphate, and hyaluronic acid are all different types of GAG. Sulphate groups are found on all GAGs except hyaluronic acid, and all sulphated GAGs are linked to protein. Proteoglycans vary considerably in size, depending on the nature of the core protein and the number and class of GAG attached. They may be classified according to their site, size, nature of GAG side-chains or nature of the core proteins. In the following account they will be considered according to the site in which they are found.

Interstitial proteoglycans

These may be defined as proteoglycans which are situated in between, or associated with, interstitial collagen fibres. They have chondroitin sulphate, dermatan sulphate, or keratan sulphate side-chains, and may be large or small.

The largest, most complex proteoglycan is that found in cartilage, and it was the first to be discovered. It has a core protein of nearly 400 000 Da to which about 100 keratan sulphate GAG chains and 80 chondroitin sulphate GAG chains are bound, giving a 'bottlebrush' appearance on electron microscopy. In addition, there are linked oligosaccharides. Four of these proteoglycan monomers are associated with a single central molecule of hyaluronic acid via a globular domain at the N-terminal end of the core protein (Fig. 1.86). Other large 'aggregating' proteoglycans (i.e. those that interact with hyaluronic acid) are found in aorta, sclera, and tendon. Cartilage also contains large non-aggregating proteoglycans.

Very much smaller interstitial proteoglycans, with core proteins of less than 50 000 Da, have been isolated. These carry only one or two GAG side-chains (Fig. 1.86).

Basement membrane proteoglycans

Basement membrane proteoglycans are of two main types: those with heparan sulphate side-chains and those with chondroitin sulphate side-chains. Evidence for the presence of GAG in basement membranes first came from studies in embryonic tissues. Subsequently, polyanionic sites in glomerular basement membranes were observed by ruthenium red staining which disappeared on treatment with heparitinase or heparinase. Proteoglycans containing four chains of heparan sulphate per core protein have been isolated from glomerular basement membrane and Engelbreth–Holm–Swarm (EHS) sarcoma matrix (Fig. 1.86). Basement membranes in different sites may have a different proteoglycan content, reflecting their different functions.

Cell-surface proteoglycans

Heparan sulphate proteoglycan is present on the surface of nearly all mammalian cells. It is attached via a protein core which is inserted into the plasma membrane. The core proteins are of varying size depending on their cell of origin. For example, heparan sulphate proteoglycan isolated from hepatocytes has a core protein of 35 000 Da to which four heparan

sulphate chains are attached (Fig. 1.86). Heparan sulphate proteoglycan from ovarian granulosa cells has a core protein of 50 000 Da substituted with 8–14 heparan sulphate side-chains. Heparan sulphate proteoglycans from epithelial cells may also carry chondroitin sulphate chains.

Intracellular proteoglycans

Although this section is primarily concerned with extracellular molecules, it should be noted that proteoglycans may also have important functions within cells. For example, heparin proteoglycans are present in the granules of connective tissue mast cells, and chondroitin sulphate proteoglycans in granules of mucosal mast cells and natural killer cells.

Function of proteoglycans

'Space-filling' Large interstitial proteoglycans have been referred to as 'space-fillers'. They occur free in interstitial fluid

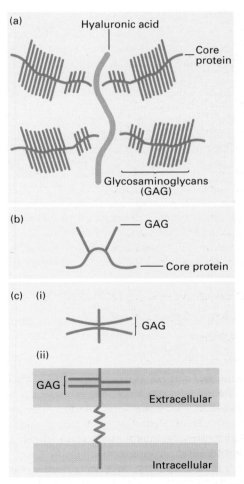

Fig. 1.86 Diagrammatic representations of some proteoglycans (not to scale). (a) Cartilage proteoglycan, large interstitial aggregating; (b) small interstitial proteoglycan; (c) basement membrane proteoglycan (i) and cell-surface proteoglycan (ii).

on which they confer visco-elastic properties. This is attributable to the polyanionic character of these high molecular weight polymers. In solution they have an extended structure. In hyaline cartilage swelling of proteoglycan is limited by the network of collagen fibrils. Here they are present in high concentrations with a consequent reduction in molecular volume and increase in charge density. This provides resistance to compressive loads and allows a return to normal shape when the load is removed.

Interaction with interstitial collagens Small interstitial proteoglycans interact with interstitial collagen fibrils, on which there are different binding sites for different types of proteoglycan. The type and amount of proteoglycan bound is dependent on the tissue, reflecting different functional requirements in different sites. In cornea, dermatan sulphate proteoglycans and keratan sulphate proteoglycans are arrayed regularly along collagen and preserve the regular fibrillar spacing necessary for transparency. A genetic defect in synthesis of keratan sulphate proteoglycans produces the human disorder of macular corneal dystrophy, characterized by corneal opacity.

Small interstitial dermatan sulphate proteoglycans may play a role in the regulation of collagen fibril assembly, since they inhibit fibrillogenesis of collagen types I and II. In bone, the keratan sulphate and dermatan sulphate binding sites on type I collagen are not occupied, but there is a chondroitin-sulphate-rich proteoglycan orientated mainly in parallel with the collagen fibrils. Since the dermatan sulphate binding sites on collagen are occupied in soft connective tissues and empty in bone, and since they correspond to the postulated site of nucleation of calcification, it has been suggested that dermatan sulphate proteoglycan may play a role in inhibition of calcification in soft tissues.

Basement membrane permeability Proteoglycans in basement membranes bind to other basement membrane molecules, including laminin, fibronectin, and type IV collagen. They are important for the permeability properties of basement membranes, since their anionic charge hinders the passage of other anionic molecules across the membrane. This may be of particular importance in the renal glomerulus, where the net anionic charge of the glomerular basement membrane normally helps to prevent the passage of plasma proteins through it. In the diseased glomerulus, loss of proteoglycan may contribute to the occurrence of proteinuria.

Cell–cell and cell–matrix interactions Cell-surface proteoglycan can interact directly with both extracellular and intracellular molecules. The intracellular moiety of the core protein interacts with actin. The extracellular portion bearing glycosaminoglycans can interact with other similar molecules and with extracellular proteins such as fibronectin.

Heparan sulphate has the capacity to self-associate with heparan sulphate of similar structure in a specific manner. Since cell-surface heparan sulphate varies with cell type, this may play a role in cell–cell recognition and in interaction with heparan sulphate proteoglycans in basement membranes. Sur-

face heparan sulphate proteoglycans are lost in dividing cells and in rapidly growing tumour cells.

Interaction of fibronectin with cells may occur partly via heparan sulphate proteoglycan as well as via fibronectin-specific cell-surface receptors (see below). Heparan sulphate promotes adhesion of fibroblasts to fibronectin matrices. Other proteoglycans may have an inhibitory effect on cell adhesion. Dermatan sulphate proteoglycans from cartilage inhibit attachment and spreading of fibroblasts on type I collagen and fibronectin. These observations suggest a regulatory role for proteoglycans in cell–matrix interactions as well as in cell–cell interactions.

Endothelial proteoglycan Proteoglycan on endothelial cells binds antithrombin III and thrombin and is important for the non-thrombogenic properties of endothelial surfaces. Endothelial proteoglycan may also promote lipid metabolism by binding lipoprotein lipase.

It is evident that proteoglycans are a very complex and varied class of macromolecule with many different functions. They play an essential role in tissue organization and in cellular interactions. Further studies will undoubtedly reveal more about the mechanisms by which they exert their effects and define more precisely their functional significance.

Fibronectins

Fibronectins are non-collagenous glycoproteins which, like proteoglycans, are widely distributed throughout the body. They exist in varying molecular forms derived from a single gene, and are collectively referred to as fibronectin. A soluble form produced by the liver is present in plasma and extracellular body fluids; an insoluble form is found on the surface of cells growing in culture and in extracellular matrices. Cells synthesizing fibronectin in culture include: fibroblasts, endothelial cells, epithelial cells, macrophages, and Schwann cells.

In human plasma, fibronectin is present at a concentration of around 300 μg/ml (range 150–800 μg/ml). It varies with the sex and age of the individual. Tissue fibronectin is present in association with basement membranes, on some cell surfaces, and in association with some interstitial collagen fibres, principally those that have a loose reticular arrangement. These fibres have the property of argyrophilia and have been collectively termed 'reticulin' fibres. They probably consist of a complex mixture of macromolecules and are not all identical in composition.

Properties

Interest in fibronectin was stimulated by its properties in tissue culture. If fibronectin is added to some lines, it promotes cell attachment to the substratum and subsequent cell spreading. Plasma and cell-surface fibronectin are equally active in this respect. Binding of cells to a fibronectin substratum complex is dependent on divalent cations and the expenditure of metabolic energy. The name 'fibronectin' is derived from the Latin '*fibra*', meaning fibre, and '*nectere*', to bind.

Several observations have indicated a relationship between

cell-surface fibronectin, the cytoskeleton, and cell morphology. Fibronectin made by cells in culture polymerizes into long fibrils a few nanometres in diameter, which remain in contact with the cell membrane. Immunofluorescence studies have demonstrated a relationship beween extracellular fibrillar fibronectin and intracellular actin filaments. Loss of cell-surface fibronectin may occur in association with loss of microfilament bundles, e.g. during mitosis or after treatment of cells with cytochalasin B. Transformation of cells with oncogenic viruses may also cause loss of cell-surface fibronectin and disorganization of intracellular actin. Addition of fibronectin to the medium may reverse these changes and restore cell morphology, but not growth control, to normal.

In addition to promoting cell adhesion, fibronectin can promote cell migration. This may be achieved not only by a direct interaction with the cytoskeleton, but also by chemotaxis. *In vitro*, fibronectin is chemotactic for fibroblasts and for neural crest cells.

Molecular structure

Some of the properties of fibronectin can be explained by knowledge of its molecular structure. All fibronectins are composed of subunits of molecular weight 210 000–250 000. Soluble plasma fibronectin is a disulphide-bonded dimer of two such subunits; cell-surface fibronectin is found as disulphide-bonded dimers and multimers. The amino-acid sequences of the molecule have been determined both directly and indirectly using recombinant DNA techniques. The amino-acid composition of fibronectin consists of three types of short amino-acid sequence repeated many times. The repeats are similar but not identical. Plasma fibronectin differs from cell-surface fibronectin in lacking a type III protein repeat. This is achieved by alternative splicing of the fibronectin gene's RNA transcript.

Fibronectin binds to a variety of molecules, including fibrin, glycosaminoglycans, DNA, and actin, as well as to cell surfaces. Proteolytic digestion of fibronectin with different enzymes has demonstrated several protease-resistant domains, each with different binding properties. These stable domains are globular and linked by more extended, protease-sensitive, polypeptide chains. The distribution of the amino-acid repeats varies in each part of the molecule and each has a corresponding functional significance. Type I repeats are present in the fibrin-binding domains at each end of the molecule, types I and II in the collagen-binding domain, and type III repeats are found in the central part of the molecule, including the cell- and heparin-binding domains (Fig. 1.87).

The property of cell adhesion is related to possession of a tripeptide (RGD) with the amino-acid sequence arginine, glycine, aspartate. Synthetic peptides with this sequence can promote cell adhesion to Sepharose beads or inhibit cell adhesion to fibronectin-coated substrata. This tripeptide is common to several proteins capable of cell attachment. In the fibronectin molecule it is present in one of the type III repeats in the cell-binding domain. It is absent from other type III repeats. However, cell surface receptors for fibronectin which are not dependent on the RGD sequence have also been characterized.

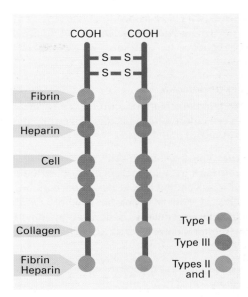

Fig. 1.87 Diagram of a fibronectin dimer indicating the different binding sites and the location of different types of amino-acid repeat (see text for details).

Cell-surface receptors for fibronectin have been identified by using the cell-binding domain of fibronectin to isolate proteins from cell lysates. Another approach has been to immunoprecipitate cell-surface proteins with antibodies that inhibit cells from binding to fibronectin. With these methods a family of glycoproteins has been isolated. Each receptor consists of two non-covalently linked α- and β-subunits, each with a molecular mass of around 140 000 Da. It is now recognized that the fibronectin receptors belong to a larger family of extracellular matrix receptors known as *integrins* (Table 1.5). A variety of different α

Table 1.5 Integrins (adapted from Ruoslahti 1991)

Alpha chain	Beta chain	Ligand
α1	β1	Collagen I, Collagen IV, Laminin
α2	β1	Collagen I, Collagen IV, Laminin
α3	β1	Collagen I, Laminin, Fibronectin
α4	β1	Fibronectin (non-RGD dependent)
α5	β1	Fibronectin (RGD dependent)
α6	β1	Laminin
αX	β2	?
αm	β2	Factor X, Fibrinogen, C3bi
αL	β2	ICAM-1, ICAM-2
αv	β1	Fibronectin (RGD-dependent)
αv	β3	Fibronectin, Vitronectin, von Willebrand factor
αv	β5	Vitronectin
αv	β6	?
αIIb	β3	Fibrinogen, von Willebrand's factor, Vitronectin, Fibronectin (RGD dependent)
α4	βp	Peyers Patch addressin
α6	β4	Laminin

and β chains exist. These associate in varying combinations giving rise to varying ligand specificities. Some are dependent on the RGD sequence for adhesion, whereas others are RGD independent.

Functions of fibronectin

The probable functions of fibronectin can be surmised from its properties in cell culture, its molecular structure, and its tissue distribution in health and disease.

Normal tissues The distribution of fibronectin in normal tissues suggests a role both in cell attachment to substrata and in the formation of extracellular fibres. The latter contain collagens and proteoglycans, both of which have affinity for fibronectin. The multiple binding properties of fibronectin allow mediation of cell–matrix interactions as well as participation in fibrillogenesis.

Embryogenesis Fibronectin appears early in development and has been demonstrated in pre-implantation mouse embryos. As in maturity, it is conspicuous in limiting membranes between epithelium and mesenchyme, and in loose connective tissue. Like hyaluronate, it is prominent in areas associated with morphogenetic movement and is probably important in cell migration. It is also prominent in undifferentiated mesenchymal tissue, but may disappear on differentiation. There are analogous observations in cell culture. For example, fibrillar fibronectin on the surface of myoblasts is lost when they fuse to form myotubes. All these findings suggest an important role for fibronectin in embryogenesis.

Haemostasis A role for plasma fibronectin in haemostasis is indicated by its interactions with fibrin and its presence in platelets. In the presence of activated factor XIII it is bound covalently to fibrin and to itself. The serum concentration of fibronectin is 20–50 per cent less than the plasma concentration, and it can be calculated that it constitutes 4.4 per cent of the mass of a clot. In platelets, fibronectin is found in association with α-granules and in varying quantities on the platelet surface. It is involved in platelet aggregation and possibly in platelet adhesion to subendothelial collagen. Platelets interact with fibronectin, fibrinogen, and von Willebrand's factor via a surface integrin receptor known as the platelet glycoprotein IIb–IIIa complex.

Macrophage function Fibronectin promotes phagocytosis of particles by macrophages in culture and may augment their response to cytokines. *In vivo*, diminished levels of fibronectin in plasma result in impaired plasma clearance of particulate debris. Decreased levels of plasma fibronectin are found after major trauma, burns, or major surgery. Administration of cryoprecipitate to such patients restores plasma fibronectin and results in clinical improvement.

Inflammation and repair Stromal fibronectin is diffusely increased in sites of active inflammation and during tissue repair. In healing wounds it appears early, together with invading fibroblasts. Interstitial collagen appears later, at 2–7 days,

at which time fibronectin diminishes. Fibronectin in sites of wound healing is probably initially derived from plasma but may subsequently be produced locally, e.g. by fibroblasts or endothelial cells.

The functional significance of fibronectin in sites of injury is probably multiple. A fundamental role in tissue repair is indicated by its ability to promote phagocytosis and by its interactions with clotting factors, platelets, and fibroblasts. Covalently linked fibrin and fibronectin form a temporary scaffold on which wound healing can occur. Fibronectin acts as a chemoattractant for fibroblasts and enables them to adhere to the fibrin substratum.

Neoplasia The role of fibronectin in neoplasia is poorly understood. It is diffusely increased in the stroma of the majority of malignant tumours and is sometimes, though not invariably, lost from the surfaces of neoplastic cells. It may be lost along with other basement membrane constituents at the margins of invasive carcinomas. The significance of these changes remains hypothetical.

Other 'nectins'

Other 'nectins' have been isolated which have adhesive properties similar to fibronectin but which are molecularly distinct. 'Chondronectin' is secreted by chondrocytes and promotes their adhesion to collagen type II. 'Vitronectin', like fibronectin, is found in human plasma and serum and in connective tissues. Its tissue distribution is similar but not identical to that of fibronectin.

Laminin

Laminin is one of the largest known proteins, with a molecular weight of about 1 000 000 Da. It was originally isolated from cultured tumours producing excess basement membrane material, specifically murine EHS (Engelbreth–Holm–Swarm) tumour and teratocarcinoma. Unlike fibronectin, it is found exclusively in basement membranes and is present in all sites where an organized basal lamina can be demonstrated by electron microscopy. It can, therefore, be demonstrated in basement membranes of epithelia, endothelia, and striated muscle fibres, and pericellularly around smooth muscle cells, Schwann cells, and adipocytes.

Properties of laminin

Native laminin binds to cell surfaces, type IV collagen, heparan sulphate, and to itself. It promotes binding of epithelial cell lines to type IV collagen and may also have a chemotactic effect for epithelial cells. Like fibronectin, interaction of cells with laminin may affect their morphology and differentiation via an interaction with the cytoskeleton.

Molecular structure

Laminin contains two types of polypeptide chain, an A-chain with a molecular weight of approximately 400 000 Da and two B-chains with molecular weights of about 230 000 (BI) and 220 000 (B2). Ultrastructural studies have shown that the con-

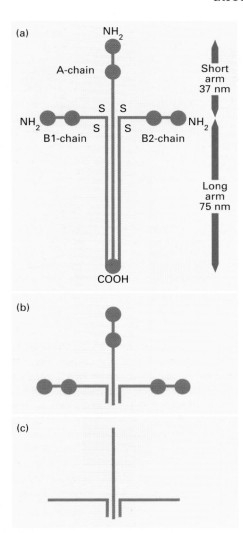

Fig. 1.88 Model of a laminin molecule. (a) Native laminin, which binds to cell surfaces, type IV collagen, and heparan sulphate. (b) the α3 fragment which binds to cell surfaces and type IV collagen. (c) The C1 or P1 fragment which binds only to cell surfaces.

figuration of the laminin molecule is an asymmetric cross with one long arm (75 nm) and three identical short arms (37 nm). The arms all have globular end-regions corresponding to different functional domains with different binding properties. Like fibronectin, the functional significance of different domains on the laminin molecule has been determined by restricted proteolytic digestion with different enzymes (Fig. 1.88). Removal of the long arm of laminin by digestion with α-thrombin abolishes heparan sulphate binding, but binding to type IV collagen and cell surfaces are retained. Digestion with pepsin gives the 'P1' fragment. This binds to cell surfaces but not to type IV collagen or other laminin molecules.

A cell-binding site has been further localized to a nonapeptide in the B1-chain. This peptide does not contain the cell-binding sequence arginine–glycine–aspartate present in fibronectin and many other adhesion molecules and it appears to recognize a cell surface receptor for laminin which does not belong to the integrin family. However, several laminin-binding integrins also exist (Table 1.5).

Function of laminin

The ubiquitous presence of laminin in basal lamina suggests that it has an important role in the organization of this structure. In this location it can promote cell attachment and differentiation. Like fibronectin, it is found in basement membranes in early embryos and is probably important in morphogenesis.

Neoplasia Immunohistological studies of human tumours have demonstrated a trend towards loss of laminin and other basement membrane constituents around invasive neoplastic cells. This may be due to decreased synthesis or increased breakdown of these proteins. Whether loss of basement membrane integrity is essential for the development of invasive malignancy is debatable. It is possible that loss of basement membrane proteins around malignant tumours reflects loss of differentiation of the neoplastic cells rather than their literally 'breaking through' a basement membrane barrier (see Chapter 9).

Experimental studies on transplantable murine tumours have placed a different emphasis on the role of laminin in neoplasia. It was found that the ability of some tumours to metastasize is related to their ability to secrete or bind to laminin. This might be due to its promotion of vascular invasion by binding of tumour cells to vascular basement membranes. Synthetic peptides with sequences akin to that of the cell-binding site on the laminin molecule have the ability to inhibit lung metastases in experimental models. It is suggested that this is due to competitive binding of the peptides with laminin receptors on tumour cells, thereby preventing their attachment to basement membranes. Synthetic peptides related to the fibronectin cell-binding sequence have a similar inhibitory effect. The precise significance of these observations in relation to human neoplasia has yet to be determined.

Nidogen and entactin

Nidogen is another major basement membrane constituent, which was originally isolated from the EHS tumour. It has a molecular weight of 150 000 Da and exists in a 1 : 1 molar ratio to laminin in many basement membranes. A basement membrane glycoprotein of similar molecular weight is entactin. This was isolated from cultured teratocarcinoma cells. Entactin and nidogen have many similar properties, including complex formation with laminin, and it is possible that they are related, if not identical, proteins. Both appear to be confined to basement membranes.

1.4.4 Matrix specialization

James O'D. McGee

The main components of extracellular matrices are collagen, 'ground substance' molecules, elastin, and fibronectin (see

Sections 1.4.1–1.4.3). It is obvious, however, that the extra-cellular matrices of skin and aorta are not only structurally dissimilar but functionally different. These differences result partially from the selective quantitative switching on of different matrix genes in both of these organs. In skin, for example, the main collagen type is collagen I, while in arteries it is collagen type III. Mechanisms other than selective gene switch on in indigenous cells must be invoked to provide a molecular explanation for the complex morphological forms of matrix found in these two organs in disease. These mechanisms, which are poorly understood, are outwith the scope of this section. However, it is worth emphasizing the morphology of matrix specializations since these are often lost as a result of disease processes. Skin, blood vessel, kidney, and liver matrices will be used as illustrative examples.

Skin extracellular matrix

The epidermis lies on a meshwork of collagen and elastic fibres. The epidermis is separated from this matrix by a specialized basement membrane which lies at the interface between the epithelium and connective tissue (Fig. 1.89). The basement membrane consists of laminin, fibronectin, and collagen type IV (and others). This basement membrane directly influences epidermal differentiation and limits cellular movement from the epidermis into the dermis and vice versa. Basement membranes under other epithelia, like the small bowel, allow selective cells to emigrate through them into the epithelium. In small bowel, lymphocytes normally enter and exit the epithelium.

The connective tissue of the dermis is organized into two distinct layers: the papillary dermis, composed of thin collagen fibres arranged in a loose meshwork; and a subpapillary dermis, in which the collagen fibres are thicker (Figs 1.89, 1.90). Within the dermis there are further morphological specializations of matrix around blood-vessels and hair shafts. When skin is cut and healing ensues, this specialized matrix organization is lost. The wound space is generally filled with a thicker diameter collagen fibre meshwork arranged roughly parallel to the epidermal surface.

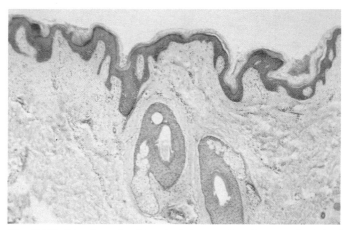

Fig. 1.90 Dermis and epidermis demonstrating the organization of connective tissue within the dermis. There is a loose layer of fine collagen fibres immediately under the epidermis. The collagen fibres in the deep dermis are much thicker except around hair shafts (centre).

Arteries

In large arteries, collagen confers tensile strength and elastic fibres the ability to recoil after cardiac systole. These fibres, particularly elastic fibres, are arranged in two lamina concentrically around the circumference of arteries (Fig. 1.91). This type of matrix organization is lost in atherosclerosis, which is the single largest cause of death in Western countries. In atherosclerosis, the regular arrangement of elastic fibres is destroyed or fragmented and collagen is deposited in the vessel wall in much larger amounts than normal. The loss of recoil locally in the aorta results in dilatation of the vessel (aneurysm formation) and sometimes rupture with massive blood loss (see Chapter 12).

Kidney

The renal glomerular basement membrane consists of a tri-laminar structure as visualized by electron microscopy. There

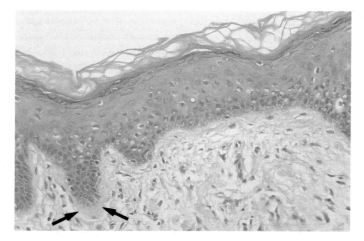

Fig. 1.89 The epidermis is separated from the papillary dermis (containing fine collagen fibres) by basement membrane (arrows).

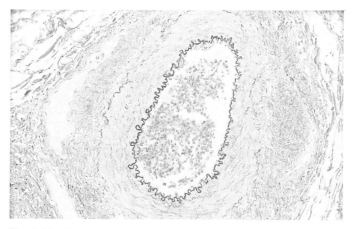

Fig. 1.91 Cross-section of normal artery. There are continuous internal and discontinuous external elastic laminae (black). Collagen is bright pink.

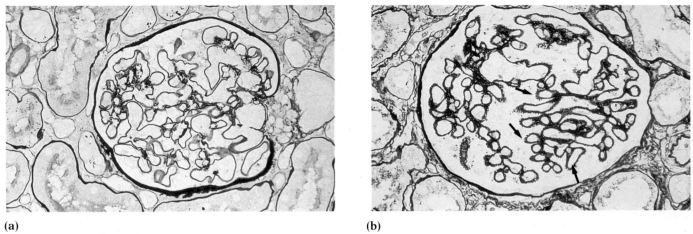

(a) **(b)**

Fig. 1.92 (a) Normal renal glomerulus. The capillary loops are outlined in black by silver impregnation of basement membrane components. (b) Renal glomerulus in immune complex nephritis. The capillary loops are generally much thicker than in (a); spikes of basement membrane (arrows) are also formed between the submicroscopic immune complexes. The basement membranes around renal tubules in (a) and (b) are normal. (Courtesy of N. J. Atkins.)

are two outer electron lucent layers (lamina rara) and an electron dense middle layer (lamina densa). These layers are products of the endothelial and epithelial cells that lie on each side of this basement membrane. The latter is composed of a mat of collagen type IV (non-fibrillar collagen), fibronectin, laminin, and proteoglycans. The glomerular basement membrane has selective molecular filtration function (see Chapter 19). In a variety of kidney diseases, the basement membrane of the glomerulus is grossly thickened by the presence of extra basement membrane components and immune complexes (Fig. 1.92a, b). Contrary to what might be expected, glomerular filtration function is less selective rather than more selective in spite of the

increase in basement membrane thickness. This leads to protein loss in the urine, which can in turn lead to generalized water retention and oedema (see Chapters 7 and 19).

Liver

The overall architecture of liver is discussed later (Chapter 17). For the present purpose only, the structure of liver sinusoids will be described. The hepatocytes are arranged in single-cell-thick plates which are in intimate contact with blood flowing through sinusoids on each side of these plates (Fig. 1.93). Plasma has free access to the surface of hepatocytes, and hepatocyte products (albumin, fibrogen, etc.) are secreted into the plasma; at

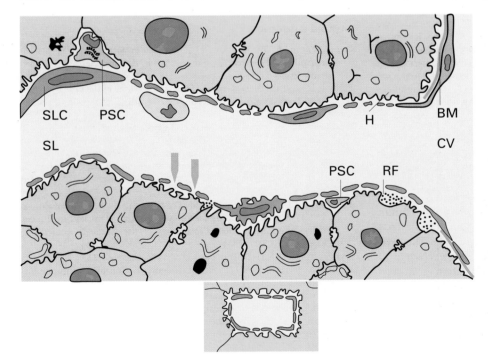

Fig. 1.93 Diagrammatic representation of a normal liver sinusoid. The sinusoidal lumen (SL) carries blood to the central vein (CV). The plasma in the sinusoidal lumen has free access to the surface of hepatocytes through gaps in the sinusoidal lining cells (SLC) indicated by arrows. Physiologically, there is very little connective tissue in the space (of Disse) which separates the sinusoidal lining cells from the surface of hepatocytes; the small amount of collagen fibrils, sometimes called reticulin fibres (RF), is indicated in the space of Disse. There is a true basement (BM) underneath the lining of the central vein but this is absent in the space of Disse. There is a specialized cell along sinusoids called perisinusoidal cells (PSC) which probably has a connective tissue formative and vitamin A storage function. The insert shows a hepatic sinusoid in cross-section.

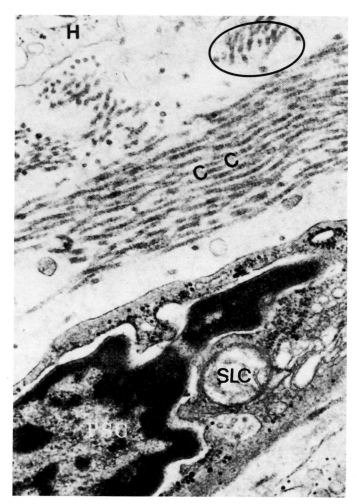

Fig. 1.94 Electron micrograph of hepatic sinusoid in end stage liver disease (cirrhosis) due to alcohol. The space of Disse is almost completely filled by collagen fibrils (C). This imposes at least a physical barrier to molecular interchange between the sinusoidal lumen (lower right corner), sinusoidal lining cell (SLC), and the adjacent hepatocyte (H). The amount of collagen along a normal sinusoid (at this magnification) is roughly that contained within the circle (top right corner).

the same time the villous surface of the hepatocyte actively removes bilirubin, fats, etc. from the plasma. At the interface between hepatocytes and the sinusoidal lining cells, there are very few recognizable collagen fibres and there is no visible basement membrane. In a variety of liver diseases, however, the space between the hepatocyte surface and the sinusoidal lining cells becomes filled with collagen fibres and sometimes a true basement membrane forms in this space (Fig. 1.94). The consequences are interference in the bilateral free exchange of molecules. When the normal matrix specialization of liver is totally lost in end-stage liver disease, the patient may go into liver failure and develop portal venous hypertension.

These few examples serve to emphasize the consequences of disruption in matrix specialization which can be induced by

physical agents (e.g. wound healing), immune-associated disorders (e.g. glomerulonephritis), and environmental agents such as viruses and alcohol (e.g. end-stage liver disease).

1.4.5   Further reading

General

Alberts, B., Bray, D., Lewis, J., Raff, M., Roberts, K., and Watson, J. D. (1989). The extracellular matrix. In *Molecular biology of the cell* (2nd edn.), pp. 802–23. Garland Publishing, New York.

Collagen molecular structure

Bornstein, P. and Sage, H. (1980). Structurally distinct collagen types. *Annual Review of Biochemistry* **49**, 957–1003.

Collagen biosynthesis

Fessler, J. H., Doege, K. J., Duncan, K. G., and Fessler, L. I. (1985). Biosynthesis of collagen. *Journal of Cellular Biochemistry* **28**, 31–7.

Collagen breakdown

Murphy, G. and Reynolds, J. J. (1985). Current views of collagen degradation. *Bioassays* **2**, 55–60.

Collagen gene structure

Sykes, B. C. (1987). Collagen gene structure. In *Oxford Surveys on Eucaryotic Genes* (ed. N. Maclean) **4**, 1–33. Oxford University Press.

Vuorio, E. and de Crombrugghe, B. (1990). The family of collagen genes. *Annual Review of Biochemistry* **59**, 837–72.

Inherited collagen diseases

Prockop, D. J. and Kivirikko, K. I. (1984). Heritable diseases of collagen. *New England Journal of Medicine* **311**, 376–86.

Ground substance

Cunningham, L. W. (ed.) (1987). *Methods in enzymology*, Vol. 145, *Structural and contractile proteins. Part E. Extracellular matrix.* Academic Press, London.

Evered, D. and Whelan, J. (eds) (1986). *Functions of the proteoglycans*, Ciba Foundation Symposium 124. John Wiley and Sons, Chichester.

Fitzgerald, L. A., Poncz, M., Steiner, B., Roll, S. C., Bennett, J. S., and Phillips, D. R. (1987). Comparison of cDNA derived protein sequences of the human fibronectin and vitronectin receptor subunits and platelet glycoprotein IIb. *Biochemistry* **26**, 8158–65.

Hay, E. D. (ed.) (1981). *Cell biology of the extracellular matrix.* Plenum Press, New York.

Hayman, E. G., Pierschbacher, M. D., Ohgren, Y., and Ruoslahti, E. (1983). Serum spreading factor (vitronectin) is present at the cell surface and in tissues. *Proceedings of the National Academy of Sciences USA* **80**, 4003–7.

Hynes, R. O. (1986). Fibronectins. *Scientific American* **254**, 32–41.

Iwamato, Y., *et al.* (1987). YIGSR, a synthetic laminin pentapeptide, inhibits experimental metastasis formation. *Science* **238**, 1132–4.

Poole, A. R. (1986). Proteoglycans in health and disease: structures and functions. *Biochemical Journal* **236**, 1–14.

Ruoslahti, E. (1988). Fibronectin and its receptors. *Annual Review of Biochemistry* **57**, 375–413.

Ruoslahti, E. (1991). Integrins. *Journal of Clinical Investigation* **87**, 1–5.

2

Chromosome organization, gene structure and function

2

Chromosome organization, gene structure and function

2.1 Chromosome structure

M. A. Ferguson-Smith

2.1.1 A résumé of basic genetics

Chromosomes are the vehicles of inheritance. They carry the genetic information during somatic cell division from parent cell to daughter cell, and through gametogenesis and fertilization from one generation to the next. Normal human somatic cells have 23 pairs of chromosomes, one member of each pair contributed by each parental gamete. Mendel first realized that inherited characteristics are determined by pairs of elements (genes) which separate from one another during the formation of the gametes. As there are 23 pairs of chromosomes (each member of a pair separating from one another during gametogenesis) there are 23 groups of genes. Each group of genes is linked together in its chromosome to form a genetic linkage group. Each gene has a specific position in the linkage group and on the chromosome, and this position is the gene locus. As there are two chromosomes of each sort (homologous chromosomes) there are two similar genes at each locus, one on the maternal homologue and the other on the paternal homologue. Genes at the same locus are sometimes referred to as allelomorphic pairs, or alleles. Alleles are thus alternative forms of the *same* gene, and for most gene loci there are many alternatives. When the two alleles at the same locus are identical, the individual is said to be *homozygous* at that locus; if the two alleles are different, e.g. by mutation, the individual is *hetero-*

zygous at that locus. It is sometimes helpful to refer to genes at different loci as being *non-alleles*.

Simple genetic traits or diseases may be determined by gene mutation and may affect several members of one family. The pattern of inheritance of single gene defects depends on whether the gene locus is on an X-chromosome or on a non-sex chromosome (autosome) and whether the condition is expressed by a single dose or a double dose of the mutant allele. Dominant inheritance occurs when the disease or trait is expressed by a single dose of the mutant allele. The affected individual is heterozygous and will transmit the mutant allele (and the condition) to half the offspring. If the condition is only apparent when both alleles at the locus are mutant, inheritance is recessive. The unaffected parents of an individual with a recessive condition, must both be heterozygous for the mutant allele (which is thus hidden) and the risk of recurrence in the same family is 1 in 4. Sometimes both alleles at a genetic locus are expressed (e.g. AB blood group); this is referred to as co-dominant inheritance. The essential difference between the inheritance of an X-linked and an autosomal mutation is that in X-linked inheritance, the mutant allele is not transmitted from father to son; a normal male always receives his X-chromosome from his mother.

Chromosomes consist essentially of protein and nucleic acid, and the genetic information is stored in deoxyribonucleic acid (DNA). DNA consists of two nucleotide chains which are coiled clockwise around one another to form a double helix. The two chains are linked together by pairs of nitrogenous bases, adenine:thymine (A–T) and guanine:cytosine (G–C). The order of base pairs constitutes the genetic code, each triplet of bases (codon) determining the type of amino acid incorporated into a particular polypeptide—which is the product of that gene. In molecular terms, a gene can be defined as the sequence of bases in DNA that codes for one polypeptide. The coding sequence of an average gene constitutes about 10 000 base pairs.

Although it is estimated that each cell nucleus contains at least 6000 million base pairs, the number of functional genes may be no more than 50 000, i.e. only a fraction of the total DNA. Much of the remainder is repetitive DNA, which may be moderately repetitive with several hundred copies, or highly repetitive with many thousands of copies. The moderately repetitive DNA includes some functional genes, including the genes for ribosomal ribonucleic acid (RNA), but the highly repetitive DNA is generally not transcribed into protein.

The DNA in each chromosome can be regarded as one extremely long molecule, some segments of which are DNA sequences which represent individual genes. The linear arrangement of genes on the chromosome, and the knowledge that each gene is located at a fixed position in the chromosome, implies that gene loci have a particular order along the chromosome. Gene mapping is the process of determining the order of gene loci in chromosomes and the relative distances between them. There are a number of methods for constructing such maps; some methods depend on family studies and others on physical methods. As will be apparent below, human gene maps are fundamental to the study of medical genetics and especially to the study of the molecular pathology of genetic disease.

Clearly Mendel's great contribution was the realization that inherited characteristics were determined by pairs of genes which segregate into different gametes (Mendel's first law). The behaviour of chromosomes follow the same pattern, although this was appreciated much later. Mendel also concluded from his experiments that non-alleles assort to gametes independently of one another (his second law); chromosomes do the same, maternal and paternal homologues segregating randomly during first meiosis.

Genes that are close together on the same chromosome tend to be transmitted together. This is the basis of genetic linkage and is the exception to Mendel's second law of independent assortment. However, it has been found that gene loci that are further apart on the same chromosome need not be transmitted together. This is due to the phenomenon of meiotic recombination, which is the physical exchange of DNA between homologues during meiosis. This achieves new combinations of parental genes in the gametes and is an important factor in maintaining genetic variation between individuals. As there are only a comparatively small number of such exchanges during each meiotic division, 1–6 exchanges for each chromosome pair (depending on size), there is plenty of opportunity for linkage. In male meiosis the average number of exchanges (or crossovers) is about 52, and there are rather more in female meioses.

Different gene loci on the same chromosome are said to be linked to one another if the proportion of offspring in which they are separated, i.e. the recombination frequency, is less than 50 per cent. Fifty per cent recombination is equivalent to independent assortment. The recombination frequency between two loci is therefore a measure of how far they are apart on the same chromosome. It is usual to express the genetic distance between two loci in terms of centimorgans, where one centimorgan is equivalent to a recombination frequency of 1 per cent. The genetic distance can be determined most easily in pedigrees where one parent is heterogygous at both loci and the other parent homozygous at both loci. The distance in centimorgans is determined from the proportion of offspring that do not show the same combination of loci as in the heterozygous parent. For closely linked loci, a large amount of family data may be required to establish genetic distances with accuracy. Analysis of this information is greatly aided by computer programs and, in recent years, linkage maps of parts of each chromosome have been assembled showing approximate genetic distances between many gene loci.

When it comes to defining genetic distance in terms of base pairs of DNA, difficulties are encountered because recombination occurs more frequently in some regions of the chromosomes (particularly the ends of the arms) than others. Also, recombination is more frequent in female meiosis than male meiosis. However, on average, the genetic distance of one centimorgan is roughly equivalent to 1000 kilobase pairs (one megabase).

Chromosomes have been seen with the light microscope for over 100 years and gross chromosome aberrations have been detectable for 30 years. However, it is still imperfectly understood how the DNA molecule is packaged with its associated protein into each chromosome. Electron microscope studies have shown that the smallest fibre that can be identified measures about 10 nm in diameter (Fig. 2.1). This appears to be composed of repeating units, called nucleosomes, each consisting of eight histone molecules around which the DNA molecule is coiled one and three-quarter times. The part of the DNA molecule between nucleosomes is associated with a linker molecule of histone. The linked nucleosomes are in turn coiled into a fibre of 36 nm diameter. This is the chromatin fibre that is most readily resolved by examining chromosomes under the electron microscope. It seems that each chromatid has a central scaffold of acidic protein to which the chromatin fibre is attached at regular intervals, and possibly by regions of repetitive DNA, so that loops of chromatin fibre (Laemli loops—each containing about 200 000 base pairs) radiate out at right angles to the central scaffold, rather like a bottle-brush. The structure is coiled once more and compacted into a chromatid, which is now visible under the light microscope during cell division. This method of packaging allows the replication and transcription of the DNA molecule in its extended form in the interphase nucleus and also the condensation of the chromosome into a compact structure to ensure its ready passage through cell division.

This brief résumé of basic genetics is designed to allow the reader to visualize the structure of the chromosome, so that pathological changes of the gene and chromosome may be more easily understood. It may also serve to define most of the common terms used in genetics which so often confuse the uninitiated. A more extensive description of the principles of medical

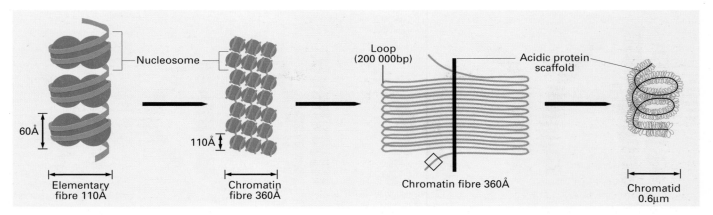

Fig. 2.1 Diagrammatic representation of a possible arrangement of DNA and protein in the nucleosome, chromatin fibre, and chromatid. (Drawn after Connor and Ferguson-Smith 1991, with permission.) 1 Å = 0.1 nm.

genetics is out of place here and the reader is referred to Connor and Ferguson-Smith (1991) for a fuller account.

2.1.2 Chromosome abnormalities

Pathological changes of the genetic material involve duplication, deletion, or rearrangement of DNA. The extent of the change varies from the gain or loss of a single nucleotide (a point mutation) to gain or loss of a whole chromosome. It is customary to refer to those changes which are large enough to be detectable by the light microscope as chromosome abnormalities, but it must be stressed that structural chromosome abnormalities differ from molecular mutations involving individual genes only in terms of scale. An understanding of the types of structural chromosome aberrations and their origins is thus useful in understanding the aetiology of gene mutations. This is fortunate because chromosome abnormalities are comparatively easy to study in patients and families, requiring only a culture of dividing cells and a good quality light microscope.

As cytogenetic techniques improve, the lower limits of resolution of chromosome abnormalities decrease. Currently, it is unusual to detect under the microscope a duplication or deletion that involves less than 4 million base pairs (0.13 per cent of the amount of DNA in the gamete—the haploid genome). This degree of resolution has been achieved by the introduction of chromosome-banding techniques which can resolve the chromosome complement into more than 800 bands, allowing each individual chromosome to be unambiguously identified (Fig. 2.2).

The procedure of chromosome analysis is comparatively simple. A heparinized blood sample is taken from the patient and 0.5 ml of whole blood is added to 5 ml of culture medium containing phytohaemagglutinin. The latter stimulates the T-lymphocytes to transform and divide. After 48–72 h incubation, cell division is arrested at metaphase by colchicine (which interferes with the production of spindle fibres) and a hypotonic solution is added to swell the cells and separate the individual chromosomes before fixation. The fixed cell suspension is dropped on to microscope slides and dried in air; this spreads the chromosomes out in one optical plane. The chromosome preparations are stained by an appropriate banding method and examined under the × 100 oil-immersion lens of a microscope. Similar preparations can be made from cultures of any living tissue, including skin, bone marrow, malignant tumour, and placental tissue.

The analysis of chromosomes under the microscope (karyotype analysis) is labour intensive and several automated systems are now available which find metaphases and arrange the chromosomes according to a standard karyotype. These systems require considerable interaction with a trained cytogeneticist but may be of value for preparations in which metaphases are scanty or in cases where large numbers of cells have to be analysed, as in assessing radiation damage or in carrier detection for the fragile-X syndrome of mental retardation (see below). The equipment is highly expensive and, as yet, not widely available.

Flow karyotyping is an alternative approach to automating classical karyotype analysis. This procedure exploits the ability of flow cytometry to measure the DNA content of individual chromosomes as they pass in a fluid stream at a speed of up to 2000 per second through the laser beam of a fluorescence-activated cell sorter. The suspension of chromosomes if first stained by a fluorescent dye (e.g. ethidium bromide), and the fluorescence generated by the laser beam in each chromosome is collected in a photomultiplier and stored in a computer. After several minutes, sufficient individual measurements have been collected to generate a histogram or flow karyotype (Fig. 2.3) which groups the chromosome measurements according to increasing DNA content. Many chromosomes form separate peaks, and the median of each peak provides an accurate and reproducible measure of the relative DNA content of a particular pair of chromosomes, which is useful in detecting chromosomal deletions and duplications. The area under each peak represents the relative number of chromosomes in each peak, and this has application in the diagnosis of numerical aberrations such as trisomic Down syndrome.

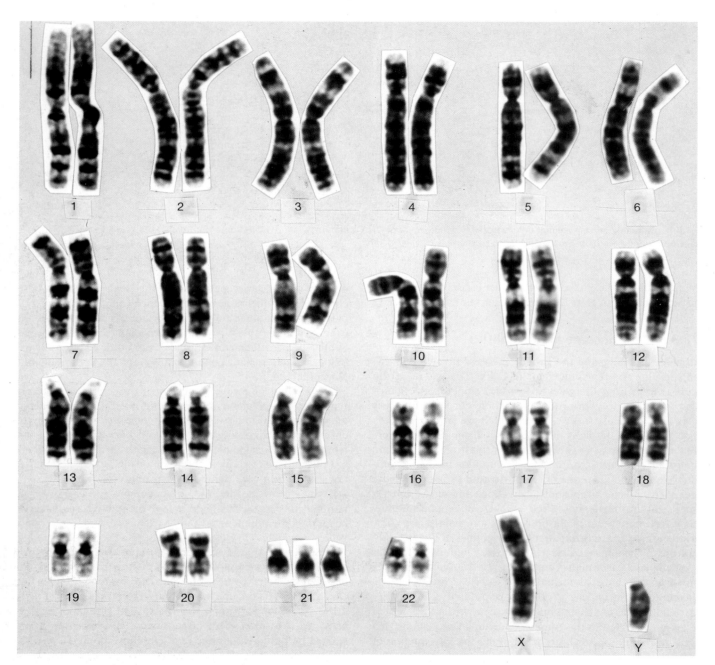

Fig. 2.2 The chromosome complement (karyotype) of a male patient with trisomic Down syndrome. The chromosomes have been arranged in pairs according to their Giemsa-banding appearance, and ordered roughly according to size (although chromosome 20 is larger than 19, and 22 larger than 21). The X and Y sex chromosomes are shown separately (lower right). Note the additional chromosome 21 responsible for Down syndrome.

As shown in Fig. 2.3, the flow karyotypes from normal males and females are easily distinguished by the area under the X-chromosome peak, which in the female karyotype is twice the size of the male peak. Normal chromosome variation can be distinguished from the changes associated with chromosome aberrations by family studies. Further resolution is possible using bivariate flow karyotyping, in which the chromosomes are stained by two dyes: Hoechst 33258 distinguishing A–T-rich chromosomes, and Chromomycin A3 for distinguishing G–C-rich chromosomes. The chromosomes pass sequentially through two lasers which produce a bivariate karyotype in which the chromosomes are grouped according to size and

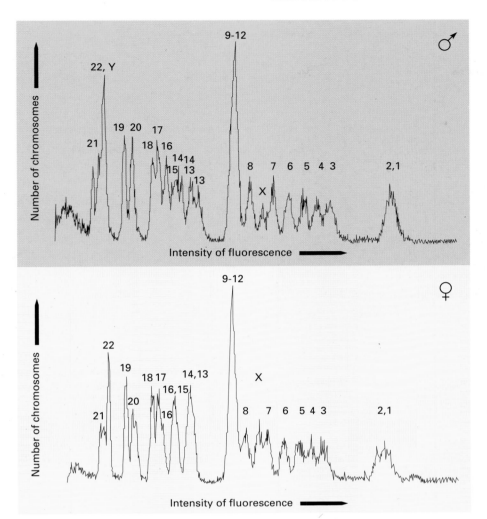

Fig. 2.3 Univariate flow karyotypes prepared from chromosome suspensions from normal male and female cell cultures. The peaks correspond to individual chromosome pairs or groups of chromosomes as indicated. The area under each peak represents the relative number of chromosomes in that peak, and the median of each peak provides an accurate and reproducible measure of the relative DNA content of a particular pair of chromosomes. (Drawn after Ferguson-Smith 1988, with permission.)

base-pair ratio (Fig. 2.4). Using this technique, individual homologues can often be distinguished from one another and chromosome rearrangements are readily detected.

An additional advantage of the fluorescence-activated cell sorter is that it can sort chromosomes according to DNA content and base-pair ratio so that sufficient chromosomes of one type can be collected for the construction of chromosome-specific DNA libraries. Chromosomes sorted directly on to nitrocellulose filters can be used in human gene mapping studies to localize cloned DNA sequences of genes to specific chromosomes (see Section 2.2). Unfortunately, as with all automated chromosome analysis, the application of flow karyotyping is presently limited due to the expense of the equipment, and most chromosome analysis is undertaken by conventional microscopy.

Like all mutations, chromosome aberrations can arise either in the germ line or in somatic cells. If in the germ line, they will usually affect all cells in the body (constitutional abnormalities) and may be transmitted to offspring. Somatic chromosome abnormalities are not transmissible; they occur commonly in neoplastic conditions.

Constitutional chromosome abnormalities occur in at least 7.5 per cent of recognized conceptions. Most miscarry spontaneously and so the frequency among live births is 0.6 per cent. Thus 60 per cent of early miscarriages have a chromosome abnormality, as do 5 per cent of late miscarriages and 5 per cent of still births.

Chromosome abnormalities are classified into numerical abnormalities (where the somatic cells contain an abnormal number of normal chromosomes) and structural abnormalities (where the somatic cells contain one or more abnormal chromosomes). Aetiological factors are different in these two groups; the former are essentially errors of cell division, while the latter involve breakage and reunion of DNA.

2.1.3 Numerical chromosome abnormalities

Normal human somatic cells contain 46 chromosomes (the diploid number). Mature sperm and eggs have 23 chromosomes (the haploid number), i.e. one member of each chromosome pair. The diploid number is thus reconstituted at fertilization. Cells with a chromosome number that is an exact multiple

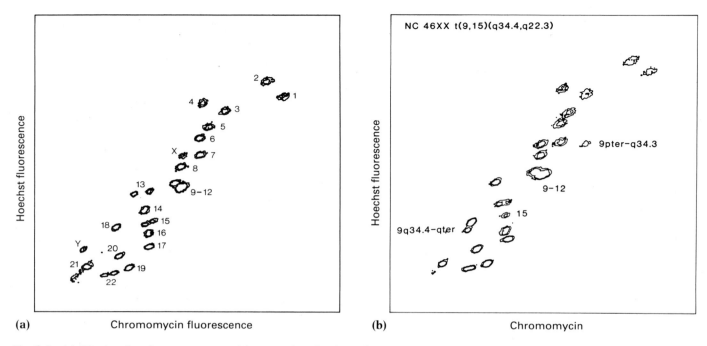

Fig. 2.4 (a) Bivariate flow karyotype prepared from a male cell culture. Chromosomes are distinguished not only by size but by base-pair ratio. A–T-rich chromosomes sort above and G–C-rich chromosomes below the diagonal. Note that the individual homologues of chromosomes 13, 15, and 22 can be distinguished from one another. (b) Bivariate flow karyotype from a female carrier of a 9;15 reciprocal translocation. Note the larger X area compared to (a) and the absence of the Y. Chromosome 15 is represented by one homologue and the two derivatives of the 9;15 translocation occupy novel positions.

of the haploid number and exceeds the diploid number are polyploid.

Triploidy

This is the most important form of polyploidy. There is a complete additional set of chromosomes resulting most commonly from fertilization by two sperm (dispermy) or from failure of one of the maturation divisions of the egg (digyny). It occurs in about 2 per cent of all conceptions but most of these miscarry and only a few survive to term. The affected fetus is dismature, has a disproportionately small trunk to head size, multiple congenital malformations, including syndactyly, and often a large placenta with hydatidiform changes. The latter is an example of genomic imprinting as it occurs when there is a double chromosomal contribution from the father but not when the extra chromosome set comes from the mother. (This is reminiscent of the hydatidiform mole, an abnormal conception in which the embryo is never formed and the chorionic villi contain no vasculature and become greatly swollen. Chromosome analysis reveals a 46XX karyotype but the chromosomes are derived solely from the father. It is likely that the female pronucleus of the fertilized egg degenerates and the mole develops from diploidization of the male pronucleus).

Tetraploidy

This is common in many tissues, including regenerating liver, where tetraploid cells arise by endomitotic reduplication, i.e.

the chromosomes divide twice and the cell divides only once. Failure to complete the first zygotic division occasionally results in a tetraploid embryo, which invariably aborts in the first trimester.

Aneuploidy

Somatic cells which contain an irregular number of normal chromosomes are termed aneuploid. Aneuploidy arises from failure of paired chromosomes to separate from one another during first meiosis, or from sister chromatids to separate from one another during second meiosis or during somatic mitosis. Both thus pass into one daughter cell while the other daughter cell receives neither. Failure of separation of chromosomes is usually referred to as non-disjunction. Failure of homologous chromosomes to pair in first meiosis is termed non-conjunction. Delayed movement of a chromosome at anaphase may result in it being incorporated into the wrong daughter cell or excluded from either. All these mechanisms may lead to an embryo having one or more chromosomes missing or extra. If the abnormal event occurred in a somatic cell division after fertilization, cell lines with different chromosome complements may be maintained in the embryo and/or extra-embryonic fetal membranes; this is referred to as chromosomal mosaicism.

Very little is known about the causes, as opposed to the mechanisms, of aneuploidy. Meiotic non-disjunction occurs with increased frequency with increasing maternal age and possibly with maternal hypothyroidism. However, it is not known how either of these factors operate.

Down syndrome Trisomy 21 (Fig. 2.2) was the first human chromosomal syndrome to be recognized (in 1959 by Lejeune and colleagues). It is also the most frequent chromosomal aberration, occurring in 1 in 700 live births. It is much more common at conception, but over 66 per cent of affected embryos are lost by miscarriage or still birth. The incidence increases with maternal age (Table 2.1) and extensive data on maternal-age-specific rates have been obtained from amniocentesis data. These show that the incidence at the 16th week of pregnancy is approximately 1 in 200 at a maternal age of 36 years, rising to 1 in 100 at 39 years and 1 in 50 at 42 years. The incidence is approximately 30 per cent lower at the time of birth due to fetal loss between 16 weeks and delivery. In line with the maternal age effect, it can be shown by chromosomal and DNA marker studies that in 80 per cent of cases of trisomy 21 the extra chromosome is contributed by the mother. At least 1 per cent of cases have chromosomal mosaicism with normal cells and trisomy 21 cells; in these cases the clinical features may be less severe. In approximately 5 per cent of cases, Down syndrome is due to an unbalanced translocation (see Fig. 2.7b) in which there is duplication of the long arm of chromosome 21; in 40 per cent of such cases the translocation is familial.

Down syndrome accounts for about 30 per cent of all moderate and severe mental handicap in children of school age; the IQ is usually less than 50. Affected children have a characteristic face with oblique palpebral fissues, mid-face hypoplasia with small nose, large tongue, and open mouth. The skull is brachycephalic and the ears are small and low-set. The fifth finger is short and incurved, and there may be a transverse palmar crease. Congenital heart disease, especially endocardial cushion defects, occur in 40 per cent and the incidence of duodenal atresia, short neck, speckled irides, epilepsy, leukaemia, and hypothyroidism are all increased. Presenile dementia with the characteristic neuropathological features of Alzheimer disease

is common. Affected females rarely reproduce and, when this occurs, less than one half of offspring are similarly affected.

Young parents of children with trisomy 21 have a risk of recurrence of trisomy 21 or other form of aneuploidy of about 1.5 per cent. Although this is a low risk, many couples will seek the reassurance of prenatal diagnosis in subsequent pregnancies. When the mother is over 35 years of age the maternal-age-specific rate should be used for determining the risk of recurrence (but see Section 2.1.7 for prenatal screening).

Other autosomal trisomies Trisomy 18 (Edwards syndrome) and trisomy 13 (Patau syndrome) occur in 1 in 3000 and 1 in 5000 live births, respectively. In both the incidence increases with maternal age.

Infants with trisomy 18 have low birth weight and multiple malformations of the heart, kidneys, and brain. Characteristic dysmorphic features include short sternum, clenched hands with overlapping index and fifth fingers, rocker-bottom feet, and single palmar creases. Anterior abdominal wall defects and spina bifida are common. There is micrognathia, a prominent occiput, and low-set ears with pointed helices. There is a preponderance of females and most die shortly after birth or within the first few months of life.

The trisomy 13 syndrome is characterized by microcephaly, microphthalmia, cleft lip and palate, post-axial polydactyly, small low-set ears, scalp defects, and single palmar creases. Holoprosencephaly and arhinencephaly are frequently associated, and occasionally cyclopia occurs. Congenital heart disease is almost invariable and most infants do not survive more than a few weeks.

While most other chromosomes can be involved in trisomic conceptions, these are always inviable and most are anembryonic. The rare exceptions are chromosomal mosaics where the trisomic cell line appears to be supported by the presence of a normal cell line. Thus adult patients with mosaic trisomy 8 are described with a characteristic dysmorphic syndrome, although non-mosaic trisomy 8 is inviable.

The XXY Klinefelter syndrome This is well known as an important cause of male infertility. Rather more than 1 in 1000 male births are affected and the risk increases with maternal age. The extra X-chromosome is maternal in 60 per cent and paternal in 40 per cent. The condition occurs in 1 per cent of males in institutions for the mentally handicapped, and in 10 per cent of infertile males. In the adult the testes are small (about 2 cm in length), plasma gonadotrophins are elevated, and there may be signs of androgen insufficiency, including poor growth of facial and body hair and lack of libido. Gynaecomastia (hyperplasia of breast ducts and periductal fibrosis) is present in 40 per cent of cases and there is skeletal disproportion from childhood. Patients are above average height, and 20 per cent are mildly mentally retarded with IQs 10–15 points below that of unaffected siblings.

The triple-X syndrome This is the equivalent syndrome in women, with a frequency among female live births of 1 in 1000. The incidence increases with maternal age. There are no characteristic clinical features and patients are slightly below

Table 2.1 Maternal-age-specific incidence for Down syndrome

Maternal age (years)	Frequency of Down syndrome at amniocentesis	Frequency of Down syndrome at birth
20		1 in 1500
25		1 in 1350
30		1 in 909
35	1 in 263	1 in 384
36	1 in 204	1 in 307
37	1 in 159	1 in 242
38	1 in 123	1 in 189
39	1 in 96	1 in 146
40	1 in 75	1 in 112
41	1 in 58	1 in 85
42	1 in 46	1 in 65
43	1 in 36	1 in 49
44	1 in 28	1 in 37
45	1 in 22	1 in 28

average height and tend to have lower IQs than their normal sisters. Most affected females are fertile and offspring are normal. Similarly, males with the *XYY syndrome* are usually fertile and asymptomatic. The incidence among male live births is 1 in 1000 and among mentally deficient adult males is about 3 in 1000. A rather higher incidence of 2 per cent has been found among males in penal institutes for the mentally subnormal, reflecting perhaps the association of mild mental handicap, aggression, and personality disturbance. In general, IQ tends to be 10–15 points less than normal siblings. Patients tend to be 4–5 cm taller than average. The condition usually arises from paternal non-disjunction of the Y-chromosome in the second meiotic division and there is no effect of parental age.

Turner syndrome Monosomy of the X in 45,X Turner syndrome appears to have a more profound effect. At least 98 per cent of affected conceptions abort and many of these are anembryonic. The incidence at birth is 1 in 5000 female live births. Stillborn embryos often have massive cystic hygroma of the neck associated with hydrops fetalis. At birth, this has resolved almost completely and there remains only redundant skin folds at the neck and some peripheral lymphoedema. Short stature and webbing of the neck are common presenting features in childhood. In the fetal ovaries the follicular cells fail to support the maturing ova and by early adolescence most of the ova have degenerated and the gonads atrophy into streaks of ovarian tissue. There is thus failure of secondary sexual development and most patients present with primary amenorrhoea and short stature (adult height 140–145 cm). Other clinical features may include broad chest, widely spaced inverted nipples, webbed neck, low hair-line, hypoplasia of the distal phalanges and nails, short IVth metacarpals, and multiple pigmented naevi. Coarctation of the aorta and atrial septal defect may be present, and 25 per cent of patients have unexplained systemic hypertension. Occasionally ovarian dysgenesis is incomplete and menstruation may occur irregularly over several months. Unlike some of the other sex-chromosome abnormalities, intelligence is normal. Oestrogen therapy allows the development of secondary sexual characteristics but does not influence the infertility or ultimate stature. The non-disjunctional error in monosomy X arises most often during male meiosis, or post-fertilization, as 75 per cent of patients have the maternal X-chromosome. Many cases show evidence of sex-chromosome mosaicism, with a variable proportion of somatic cells showing either a normal male or female karyotype. Turner syndrome may result from structural abnormalities of the X-chromosome, the most common being isochromosomes of the long arm of the X and deletions involving the short arm. In general, deletions of the short arm of the X are associated with the classical features of the syndrome, while deletions of the long arm alone produce streak ovaries without the short stature and associated dysmorphic features.

2.1.4 Structural chromosome abnormalities

Structural chromosome abnormalities occur as a result of breakage and abnormal reunion of DNA. This can be reproduced experimentally by treating cells with mutagenic agents, including radiation. However, most spontaneous structural rearrangements in both somatic cells and germ cells probably arise by errors of recombination. Normally, meiotic recombination is preceded by the synapsis of homologous chromosomes, and this is thought to involve the recognition by one homologue of complementary sequences in the other homologue. The precision with which homologous regions undergo synapsis is readily observed in the prophase of meiosis, particularly in individuals heterozygous for chromosomal translocations or inversions. Mismatching can occur sometimes during this process, particularly where there are multiple tandem repeats of DNA sequences. The most obvious examples of repeated sequences occur at the heteromorphic regions of normal chromosomes, notably the blocks of heterochromatin adjacent to the centromeres of chromosomes 1, 9, and 16 and chromosomal satellites on chromosomes 13, 14, 15, 21, and 22. These regions show great variation in DNA content between individuals (see Fig. 2.4a for example) and, as they are composed of multiple repeats of satellite DNA, it is likely that the variation is due to unequal crossing-over during meiosis. Examples of unequal recombination at specific gene loci include the X-linked colour vision locus, the α-globin locus and the locus for 21-hydroxylase. At each of these loci there are normally two copies of the gene adjacent to one another; the occurrence of individuals with either one or three copies of the gene, or individuals with a hybrid gene produced by unequal recombination within rather than outside the gene, suggest that mismatching during synapsis followed by recombination is the cause of the rearrangement. Similarly, synapsis between homologous regions on non-homologous chromosomes may lead to accidental recombination between non-homologous chromosomes, so causing translocations. It may be significant that the most common translocations in human populations occur between the short arms of satellited chromosomes which contain only repetitive DNA; these regions can be observed during first meiosis to take part frequently in non-homologous pairing.

Recombination also occurs between homologous chromosomes in somatic cells. Examples of pairing and chromatid exchange are occasionally seen during routine chromosome analysis, but the main evidence comes from studies of DNA markers in neoplasia. For example, Cavanee *et al.* (1983) demonstrated in a number of retinoblastoma tumours that the tumour cells were homozygous at several gene loci on chromosome 13, although the patients' normal cells were clearly heterozygous. Homozygosity at the retinoblastoma gene locus with loss of a tumour suppressor gene was shown to be an essential part of the malignant process. In some tumours, homozygosity was achieved by loss of one chromosome 13 and duplication of the other chromosome 13. In other tumours only part of one chromosome 13 was lost, and this could be shown by appropriate DNA markers to have occurred by recombination between the two homologues.

Chromosome analysis of cell cultures exposed to X-rays and other mutagens reveals that when a chromosome breaks two unstable (sticky) ends are produced. Repair mechanisms usually ensure that the two ends are rejoined. However, if more than one break has occurred, rejoining of the correct ends is not assured and (if the mutagen acts before the nucleus undergoes DNA synthesis) abnormal chromosomes composed of parts of different chromosomes result. Various combinations can occur, including acentric fragments, ring chromosomes, dicentric, and multicentric chromosomes. Chromatid aberrations, in which chromatids rather than whole chromosomes are seen to be involved in exchanges, are produced when breaks are induced during or after DNA synthesis. These studies show that somatic cells are capable of DNA repair and also that ends of chromosomes are unstable unless they possess an organized telomere. Constitutional terminal deletions which are associated with a number of chromosomal syndromes (e.g. the cat-cry syndrome associated with loss of the distal short arm of chromosome 5) must occur in such a way as to retain a functional telomere; most are generated by reciprocal translocations or interstitial deletions.

The main categories of structural aberration are translocations, deletions, duplications, isochromosomes, and inversions.

Translocations

A translocation is the transfer of DNA between chromosomes. It may result from accidental recombination between non-homologous chromosomes during meiosis or from the action of a mutagen. When the transfer occurs in the germ line and involves no loss of DNA, the phenotype is unchanged, and the individual is said to have a balanced translocation. The medical significance is for future generations, because a balanced translocation carrier is at risk of producing chromosomally unbalanced gametes. Translocations can be either reciprocal, centric fusion (Robertsonian), or insertional.

Reciprocal translocation

The break points are at the ends of two non-homologous chromosomes and the DNA distal to these breakpoints is exchanged (Fig. 2.5). When these chromosomes pair during the prophase of first meiosis, a cross-shaped quadrivalent is formed involving the two translocation chromosomes and their two normal partners. The homologous segments of the four chromosomes undergo recombination in the normal way, and chiasmata (exchanges) can be observed when the quadrivalent opens out into a ring of four during first meiotic interphase. At the anaphase of first meiosis these four chromosomes must segregate to the two pregametic cells (secondary spermatocytes or oocytes) (Fig. 2.6). Twelve possible combinations of these four chromosomes can enter one gamete: all four chromosomes, none of the four chromosomes, four combinations of three chromosomes (3 : 1 segregation), and six combinations of two chromosomes (2 : 2 segregation). If one considers 2 : 2 segregation, only one possibility leads to a normal gamete and one to a gamete with the balanced translocation. The other four possibilities result in various imbalances, which could lead to affected conceptions which miscarry or, if liveborn, to offspring with mental retardation and multiple malformations. The smaller the imbalance the greater the chance that the conception will be viable. The risk of abnormality in the offspring of translocation carriers is thus highly variable and depends not only on the extent of the imbalance but also on the gene loci involved. For translocations involving the smaller chromosomes, viable unbalanced offspring may result from 3 : 1 segregation.

Centric fusion translocation

This occurs when the breakpoints are at or near the centromere

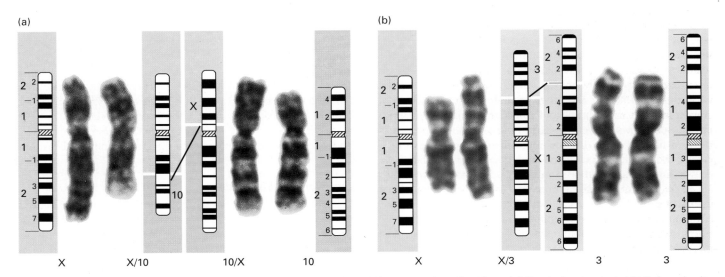

(a)   (b)

X   X/10   10/X   10   X   X/3   3   3

Fig. 2.5 Partial karyotypes showing balanced and unbalanced reciprocal X-autosome translocations. (a) Breaks have occurred in the proximal short arm of chromosome 10 and in the middle of the long arm of the X with reciprocal exchange of fragments; the translocation is balanced as both fragments are present. (b) In this case the breakpoints are in 3p21 and Xp22.1 and only the X-chromosome derivative of the translocation is present. The translocation is unbalanced because there is duplication of the distal part of 3p and deletion of the distal part of X.

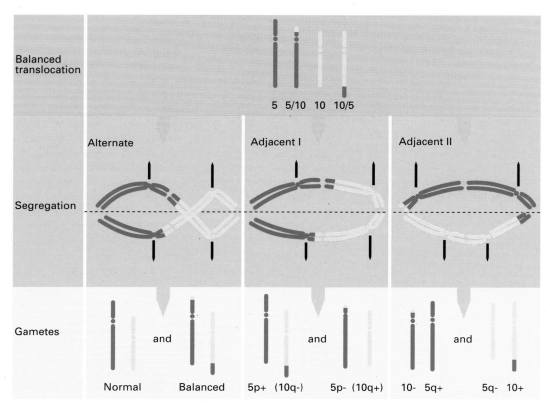

Balanced translocation

5 5/10 10 10/5

Segregation

Alternate   Adjacent I   Adjacent II

Gametes

and   and   and

Normal   Balanced   5p+ (10q-)   5p- (10q+)   10- 5q+   5q- 10+

Fig. 2.6 2:2 segregation in a reciprocal translocation between 5p and 10q. During first meiosis alternate segregation of the four chromosomes in the ring leads to normal and balanced translocation gametes. Adjacent segregation leads to four types of unbalanced gametes. In two of these (the products of adjacent II segregation) the gametic inbalance is so gross that embryos resulting from them are likely to be inviable. Grossly malformed and handicapped offspring are known to have resulted from both products of adjacent I segregation. In this case 50 per cent of conceptions are therefore at risk of fetal abnormality. (Reproduced with permission from Connor and Ferguson-Smith 1991.)

of two acrocentric (satellited) chromosomes. In most cases the breakpoints are in the short arms, which contain highly repetitive DNA, and the translocation arises from end-to-end pairing followed by accidental recombination during first meiosis. The resulting translocation is expected to have two centromeres close together, and these can usually be demonstrated by G-banding techniques. The other product of the translocation, containing the short arms and ribosomal RNA loci of both chromosomes, would be expected to have no centromere, and thus would be easily lost during subsequent cell divisions. Again, this prediction is fulfilled, and individuals with balanced centric fusion translocations have only 45 chromosomes. They show no phenotypic effect from loss of the ribosomal RNA genes, presumably because sufficient copies are present on the remaining eight satellited chromosomes.

Centric fusion of satellited chromosomes is the single most frequent type of translocation in humans, occurring in 1 in 500 live births. The chromosomes most commonly involved are 13 and 14, and this is followed by 14 and 21 (Fig. 2.7). Offspring with translocation trisomy 13 and translocation trisomy 21 respectively may result from unbalanced segregation during meiosis. When the chromosomes pair during meiosis a trivalent

is formed, so that six possible combinations from 2:1 segregation are possible. Only one is normal, one is balanced, and four are unbalanced. As trisomy 14 is inviable (and likewise monosomy 13, 14, and 21) the outcome in these two translocations is either normal, balanced or trisomy 13 (in 13;14 carriers) and trisomy 21 (in 14;21 carriers). In practice, the risk of translocation trisomy in 13;14 carriers is about 1 per cent. In 14;21 carriers the risk is 15 per cent when the mother is the carrier and about 1 per cent when the father is the carrier. This parental difference implies gametic selection in the father.

Insertional translocations

These appear to be less common than reciprocal or centric fusion translocations. They may occur within a chromosome or between two chromosomes. Three breakpoints are involved; two lead to an interstitial deletion of a chromosome fragment which is then inserted into the gap formed by the third breakpoint. The balanced carrier is healthy, but segregation of the two translocation chromosomes during meiosis may lead to unbalanced offspring with either a duplication or a deletion of the DNA involved in the insertion.

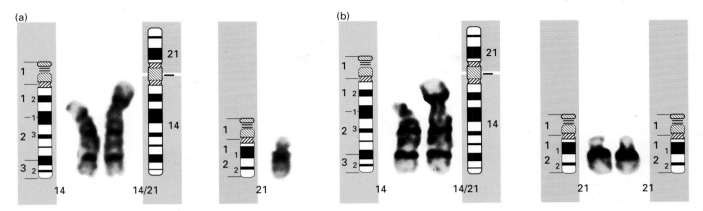

Fig. 2.7 Partial karyotypes showing balanced and unbalanced centric fusion (Robertsonian) translocations. (a) Only one normal chromosome 14 and one normal 21 are present; the centric fusion translocation t(14;21) chromosome has the long arms of both chromosomes 21 and 14. The translocation carrier therefore has 45 chromosomes and is clinically normal because the loss of the short arms of chromosomes 14 and 21 is unimportant. (b) 2:1 segregation in a t(14;21) carrier may produce a gamete with the 14/21 translocation chromosome and one normal chromosome 21. At fertilization with a normal egg or sperm, the resulting zygote will have an additional copy of the long arm of chromosome 21 and will develop Down syndrome.

Deletions

These arise as above from a parental translocation or from loss of DNA between two breakpoints (interstitial deletion) (Fig. 2.8). Both small and large deletions may result from unequal crossovers during meiosis. They may occur at one or other breakpoint of a reciprocal translocation at the time of origin, and this sometimes causes concern when a *de novo* apparently balanced translocation is discovered at prenatal diagnosis. Ring chromosomes may be associated with significant terminal deletions of DNA. They arise when breaks occur at both ends of a chromosome with reunion of the proximal ends and loss of the distal telomeric fragments. They are seldom inherited (unless very small) and are a common feature in irradiated cells. Sister chromatid exchanges within ring chromosomes not infrequently generate double-sized rings and this

may contribute to some of the phenotypic abnormality associated with constitutional ring chromosomes (Fig. 2.9).

Duplication

This refers to the presence of an additional copy of a particular sequence of DNA. Like deletions, they may originate by unequal crossing-over, or result from other chromosomal rearrangements, including translocation, inversion, or isochromosome formation. Duplications are more common than deletions and are generally less harmful. Small tandem duplications have probably played a useful role in evolution.

Isochromosome

This is an abnormal chromosome in which there is duplication of one arm and loss of the other; it is usually metacentric as

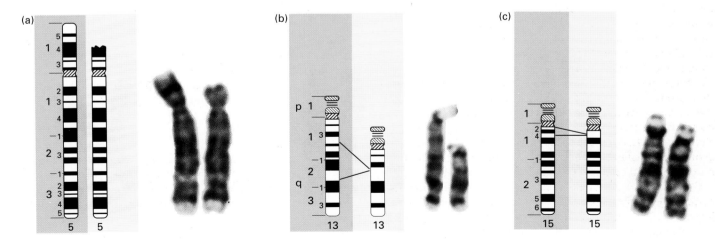

Fig. 2.8 Chromosomal deletions. (a) 'Terminal' deletion of the short arm of chromosome 5 in the cat-cry syndrome; this can result from a *de novo* unbalanced reciprocal translocation in parental meiosis. (b) Large interstitial deletion of the long arm of chromosome 13; this can predispose to retinoblastoma. (c) Small interstitial deletion of proximal end of chromosome 15 associated with the Prader–Willi syndrome.

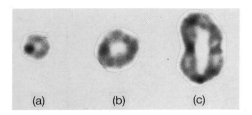

Fig. 2.9 Ring X-chromosomes. (a) This ring has a single centromere. (b) Dicentric and (c) quadracentric rings are generated from a mono-centric ring in somatic cells by sister-chromatid exchange.

each arm contains identical gene loci. It may arise from transverse instead of longitudinal division of the centromere, or from an isochromatid break and fusion above the centromere (in which case it is dicentric, one centromere usually becoming non-functional). The commonest isochromosome is an isochromosome for the long arm of the X-chromosome, which is sometimes found in the Turner syndrome (associated with monosomy for Xp) and rarely, in Klinefelter syndrome (XiXqY). Isochromosomes for the long and short arms of the Y-chromosome are associated with infertility and a variety of male, female, and intersex phenotypes (Fig. 2.10). Isochromosomes for autosomes are rare with the exception of short-arm isochromosomes of chromosomes 9 and 12, which both cause characteristic dysmorphic syndromes, and isochromosome 21, which causes Down syndrome.

Inversions

These arise from two breaks within the same chromosome and inversion through 180° of the segment between the breaks (Fig. 2.11). If the breaks occur on either side of the centromere the inversion is pericentric. If the breaks occur on the same side the inversion is paracentric, and the implications for offspring are different. Inversions simply change the order of gene loci on a chromosome and this has no phenotypic effect. However,

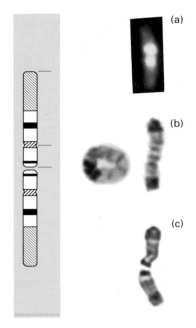

Fig. 2.10 Dicentric isochromosome for the long arm of the Y-chromosome. In dicentrics one centromere is frequently non-functional. (a) *In situ* hybridization with Y-specific DNA probe (GMGY10) which maps to Yp. (b) C-banding showing heterochromatin at distal ends of the long arms. Note the ring dicentric isochromosome Yq. (c) G-banded preparation showing non-functional lower centromere.

inversions interfere with the pairing of homologous chromosomes during meiosis, and crossing-over tends to be suppressed within the inverted segments. For pairing to occur, one homologue must form a loop in the inverted region, otherwise the chromosome arms distal to the inversion fail to pair. If a crossover occurs within a paracentric inversion, the recombinant chromosomes will be a dicentric chromosome and an acentric fragment. Both are unstable and tend not to be found in

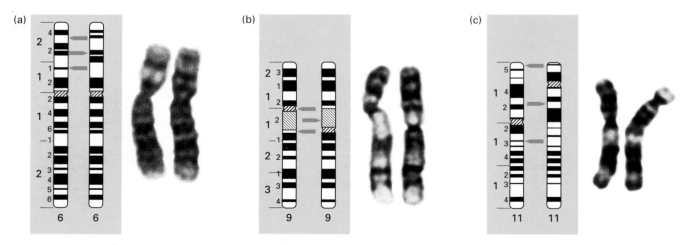

Fig. 2.11 Paracentric and pericentric inversions (see text). (a) Paracentric inversion of the short arm of chromosome 6. (b) Pericentric inversion of chromosome 9. This is the commonest inversion. It is found in about 1 per cent of the population and has no clinical significance. (c) Large pericentric inversion of chromosome 11.

offspring. Crossing-over within a pericentric inversion, on the other hand, results in recombinant chromosomes with duplication-deletion of the chromosome distal to the breakpoints of the inversion. The closer the breakpoints are to the ends of the chromosome, the greater the chance there is of fetal viability and hence the production of disabled offspring.

2.1.5 Microdeletion syndromes

The gradual transition between mutations visible with the light microscope and mutations detectable only by molecular methods is well illustrated by the microdeletion syndromes. These are complex phenotypes resulting from the loss of several closely linked genes which lie within the deleted chromosome segment. The deletion may be apparent by routine chromosome analysis or by flow cytogenetics, or may be undetectable by either. Most are sporadic, with the exception of several X-linked examples which may be transmitted through carrier females. The main characteristics are multiple dysmorphic features, malformation, mental deficiency, and sometimes the simultaneous presence of two or more characteristic single-gene defects. In fact the association of a Mendelian disorder with a detectable deletion may be the first evidence for mapping the gene locus for that disorder. The microdeletion syndromes are most usefully classified according to the chromosomal location of the deletion, as outlined below.

Microdeletion 8q23.3–24.1

The clinical features make up the Langer–Giedion syndrome and comprise multiple cone-shaped epiphyses; cartilagenous exostoses; microcephaly and mental deficiency; early balding; facial dysmorphism, including bulbous nose, large ears, upturned nares, and thin lips. The gene locus for the autosomal dominant disorder of multiple exostoses may be located within this deletion.

Microdeletion 11p13

This is probably the best known of the microdeletion syndromes and is referred to as the Wilms tumour–aniridia–genitourinary abnormalities–retardation syndrome (WAGRS) (Fig. 2.12). The features are nephroblastoma (Wilms tumour), aniridia, male genital hypoplasia, gonadoblastoma, mental retardation, and facial dysmorphism. The aniridia is often associated with corneal clouding, cataract, glaucoma, and optic atrophy. The gene for the enzyme catalase maps to 11p13 and is almost always deleted in patients with WAGRS.

Microdeletion 13q14

A small proportion of patients with retinoblastoma have a detectable deletion at 13q14. This can be associated also with deletion of the gene for the enzyme esterase D and a syndrome of mental retardation and facial dysmorphism (Fig. 2.8b).

Microdeletion 15q11–12

Approximately two-thirds of patients with the Prader–Willi syn-

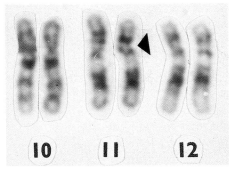

Fig. 2.12 11p13 deletion in the Wilms tumour–aniridia syndrome (WAGRS). (Reproduced with permission from Connor and Ferguson-Smith 1991.)

drome have detectable deletions of 15q11–12 (Fig. 2.8c). The clinical features are hypotonia and difficulty with feeding at birth, followed by hyperphagia and excessive obesity in childhood and adolescence. There is hypoplasia of the external genitalia in boys; small hands and feet and short stature; psychomotor retardation; seizures; life expectancy is reduced to 25–30 years. About 10 per cent of cases have unbalanced chromosomal translocations.

An apparently identical microdeletion of 15q11–12 is also present in a proportion of patients with the Angelman (happy puppet) syndrome. These children have severe mental retardation, seizures, no speech, paroxysms of laughter, microcephaly, prognathism, and ocular abnormalities. There appear to be few clinical features in common with the Prader–Willi syndrome and the difference between the two syndromes has been found to be associated with the parental origin of the deleted chromosome. DNA marker studies have shown that the deletion is paternal in the Prader–Willi syndrome and maternal in the Angelman syndrome. It is postulated that genomic imprinting (possibly mediated through differential methylation) occurs during gametogenesis, so that the structural loci active in the paternal homologue are different from those active in the maternal homologue.

Microdeletion 17p13.3

A small terminal deletion of the short arm of chromosome 17 has been observed in a large proportion of patients with the Miller–Dieker syndrome of lissencephaly. Affected children have severe mental retardation, seizures, microcephaly, narrow forehead, congenital heart disease, and growth retardation. Many have unbalanced chromosome translocations involving 17p.

Microdeletion 22q11

This particular microdeletion is associated with the Di George syndrome, which is due to abnormal development of the third and fourth pharyngeal pouches. There is hypoplasia or agenesis of the thymus and parathyroid glands, atresia of the external auditory canal, mental retardation, congenital heart disease (ventricular septal defect), and facial dysmorphism. Tetany and susceptibility to infections are characteristic.

Microdeletion Xp21

Boys with microdeletions involving this part of the short arm of the X-chromosome have been shown to have the following combinations of disorders:

1. Duchenne muscular dystrophy (DMD) and mental retardation (MR);

2. DMD, MR, chronic granulomatous disease, MacLeod syndrome, and retinitis pigmentosa;

3. DMD, MR, adrenal hypoplasia, and glycerol kinase deficiency;

4. MR and adrenal hypoplasia.

Each of the constituent disorders are known to be inherited as X-linked traits whose gene loci map to Xp21. Patients with microdeletions involving various combinations of these loci have provided the evidence required to determine the order of these loci along the X-chromosome.

Microdeletion Xp22.3

The distal end of the short arm of the X-chromosome appears to be particularly prone to microdeletion. The gene for steroid sulphatase (STS) maps in this region. STS deficiency causes X-linked ichthyosis, and approximately 80 per cent of patients with this condition have a deletion, some detectable by flow cytometry. More extensive deletions in the same region lead to the inclusion of other X-linked loci, including Kalmann syndrome (anosomia and hypogonadotrophic hypogonadism), chondrodysplasia punctata, and Rud syndrome (ichthyosis, hypogonadism, and neurological defects).

Microdeletion Xq21.1

This microdeletion of the long arm has been described in families with choroideraemia and mental retardation, with and without deafness.

2.1.6   The fragile-X syndrome of mental retardation

This condition deserves special mention because it is such a common cause of severe mental retardation in males and moderate mental handicap in females. Approximately 1 in 1000–2000 male births are affected by X-linked mental retardation, and in over half of these a fragile site on the X-chromosome at Xq27.3 can be induced in 4–60 per cent of cells by culture in folate-deficient medium (Fig. 2.13). The main clinical features in affected males are mental retardation and enlarged testes (30–50 mm); less constant features include a long face, large ears, prognathism, and epilepsy. Mental retardation of some degree is present in 20–30 per cent of heterozygous females, who may also show a small percentage of cells with a fragile site on one X. One-half of obligate carriers have apparently normal chromosomes and this makes carrier detection difficult. Affected carriers probably account for about 7 per cent of mild and 1 per cent of moderate to severe mental

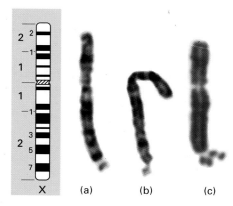

Fig. 2.13   The fragile-X chromosome of X-linked mental retardation. In some cells (a) the fragile-X site is seen as a Giemsa-negative gap at Xp27.3, in others (b) there is a chromatid break, or (c) a triradial resulting from a chromid break followed by non-disjunction of the fragment in the previous cell division.

retardation in females. In general, the pattern of inheritance is as for other X-linked traits, but many families are known in which a predisposition to the condition has been transmitted by apparently normal males to all their daughters, and to about half their grandsons who have the typical disorder. Carrier detection and prenatal diagnosis by DNA linkage analysis has been hampered until recently by the high frequency of recombination in the Xq27 region of the X-chromosome and the shortage of suitable DNA markers. An abnormal pattern of cytosine methylation is found close to the fragile site (Vincent *et al.* 1991). DNA studies have now revealed a breakpoint cluster region within a gene (FMR-1) which exhibits variable increase in length in affected males and females. Normal transmitting males and their daughters can be identified by an enlargement in DNA which is distinctly smaller than that found in affected individuals (Oberle *et al.* 1991); this smaller variation can be regarded as a premutation which is changed to the full mutation during female gametogenesis.

2.1.7   Prenatal screening for chromosome abnormalities

In view of the seriously disabling nature of the autosomal trisomies (including Down syndrome), the 1.5 per cent risk of recurrence in young mothers, and the increasing risk with advancing maternal age in older mothers, many couples at risk have chosen the option of prenatal diagnosis and selective termination in planning their families. For Down syndrome (trisomy 21) this has led to the avoidance of between 10 and 20 per cent of affected births, depending on the utilization rate in different regions. Clearly some more efficient means of identifying affected pregnancies would be helpful. Ultrasound scanning has led to the detection of the small proportion of cases associated with severe developmental malformations, such as duodenal atresia and non-immune hydrops fetalis. However, the most promising approach stems from the observation that affected pregnancies tend to be associated with a low maternal serum α-fetoprotein level in the second trimester. Unconjugated oestriol levels are also low in the maternal blood and, more recently, it has been found that maternal chorionic gonadotrophin levels are elevated in affected pregnancies.

It is estimated that by using a combination of maternal age and the levels of maternal serum AFP, oestriols, and chorionic gonadotrophin, it should be possible to identify about 60 per cent of pregnancies associated with trisomy 21. However, approximately 4–5 per cent of all pregnant mothers would have to be submitted to amniocentesis to achieve this reduction in affected births. A number of trials are currently in progress to determine the best way to conduct this form of prenatal screening.

2.1.8 Acknowledgements

The following people are thanked for the preparations of figures: Lionel Willatt (Figs. 2.2, 2.5, 2.7–2.11, 2.13) and Dr Nigel Carter (Fig. 2.4).

2.1.9 Further reading

Cavanee, W. L., et al. (1983). Expression of recessive alleles by chromosomal mechanisms in retinoblastoma. Nature 305, 779–84.

Connor, J. M. and Ferguson-Smith, M. A. (1991). Essential medical genetics (3rd edn). Blackwell Scientific Publications, Oxford.

Cuckle, H., Wald, N. J., and Thompson, S. G. (1987). Estimating a woman's risk of having a pregnancy associated with Down's syndrome using her age and maternal serum alpha-fetoprotein level. British Journal of Obstetrics and Gynaecology 94, 387–402.

Ferguson-Smith, M. A. (1988). Progress in the molecular cytogenics of man. Philosophical Transactions of the Royal Society of London 319, 239–48.

Ferguson-Smith, M. A. and Yates, J. R. W. (1984). Maternal age specific rates for chromosome aberrations and factors influencing them: report of a collaborative European study on 52 965 amniocenteses. Prenatal Diagnosis 4, 5–44.

Oberlé, I., et al. (1991). Instability of a 550-base pair DNA segment and abnormal methylation in fragile X syndrome. Science 252, 1097–102.

Schinzel, A. (1984). Catalogue of unbalanced chromosome aberrations in man. De Gruyter, Berlin.

Vincent, A., Heity, D., Petit, C., Kretz, C., Oberlé, I., and Mandel, J.-L. (1991). Abnormal pattern detected in fragile-X patients by pulsed field gel electrophoresis. Nature 349, 624–6.

Weatherall, D. J. (1991). The new genetics and clinical practice (3rd edn). Oxford University Press.

2.2 Inheritance of genetic information

M. A. Ferguson-Smith

2.2.1 Pedigree patterns for single gene defects

It is customary to collect information on families with genetic disease by identifying the affected family members, determining their relationships with one another and constructing a pedigree. The symbols used in drawing a pedigree follow conventions used internationally. Males are represented by squares, females by circles, miscarriages by a dot; husbands and wives are connected by a horizontal line, children are suspended on vertical lines from horizontal bars which represent individual sibships; generations are connected by vertical lines between sibships and parents, and are numbered using Roman numerals; individuals in each generation are given Arabic numbers, so that every family member has a unique number, e.g. I.1, I.2, etc., signifying his/her place within one generation.

As indicated in Section 2.1, the pattern of inheritance of a single gene defect (or trait) depends on whether the gene locus is on an X-chromosome or an autosome, and if the disease is manifest by a single or double dose of an abnormal allele at that locus. Thus an autosomal dominant disease is one that is expressed by a single dose of a mutant allele whose locus is on an autosome, e.g. Huntington chorea which results from a mutant allele at a locus on the short arm of chromosome 4. For true dominant diseases like Huntington chorea, the phenotype is similar in individuals either heterozygous or homozygous for the mutant allele. In other dominant disorders, such as achondroplasia, the disability is greater in the homozygote. Codominance occurs in heterozygotes where both alleles are evident in the phenotype, e.g. an individual who types AB at the ABO blood group locus.

An autosomal recessive disease, on the other hand, is only expressed in individuals homozygous for the mutant allele, e.g. cystic fibrosis which is due to a double dose of a mutation on the long arm of chromosome 7. Heterozygotes, with only one dose of the mutant allele, do not express the disease and the mutant is said to be recessive (or hidden) in the carrier. It should be noted that it is the phenotype that is either recessive or dominant and not the disease gene.

A person heterozygous for a dominant disease transmits the mutant allele on average to half his offspring. Each child has a 1 in 2 chance of being affected. Inheritance is therefore vertical, from one generation to the next. Only a person with a new mutation will not have an affected parent. Sometimes the mutant gene for a dominant disease may not be apparent in the heterozygote. This is referred to as non-penetrance. The degree of penetrance is the proportion of heterozygotes that express the disease. It is often related to the variability in expression of the gene, which is a characteristic of dominant disorders.

An individual with a recessive disease, such as cystic fibrosis, is homozygous for the mutant gene. He must have received one copy of the mutant gene from each parent. If both parents are unaffected, they are likely to be heterozygous for the mutant allele. As each parent has a 1 in 2 chance of passing the mutant allele to a child, on average 1 in 4 children will be homozygous affected, 1 in 4 will be homozygous normal and 1 in 2 will be heterozygous carriers like the parents. Affected individuals will tend to be confined to particular sibships, so that the pedigree pattern appears to be horizontal rather than vertical, and the condition is unlikely to appear in the next generation. For rare recessive diseases, the first clue as to the nature of the disease may be the observation of consanguinity in the parents. The same mutation has been transmitted to both parents from a common ancestor.

When the mutant gene is carried by the X-chromosome it will be transmitted from an affected father to all his daughters and to none of his sons (who receive the Y-chromosome). If the disorder is dominant, i.e. expressed in a single dose, all the daughters of an affected father will be affected, and half the daughters and half the sons of an affected mother will be affected. If the disorder is recessive, i.e. expressed in females only in double dose, half the sons of a carrier mother will be affected and half the daughters will be carriers. All X-linked mutant alleles are expressed in the hemizygous male.

The Y-chromosome carries important determinants for primary sex differentiation, for skeletal growth, for spermatogenesis, and possibly for other functions, but so far no Y-linked disease has been described. The pairing, or pseudoautosomal, segment of the Y is homologous to the pairing segment of the X, and gene loci in this region undergo recombination during meiosis like other homologous chromosomes. Occasionally accidental recombination occurs between the X and Y within the differential (non-pairing) regions, and this can result in the transfer of male determinants from the Y to the X. This is the usual cause of apparent sex reversal in XX males with a variant of Klinefelter syndrome (Fig. 2.14). X–Y interchange may also cause gonadal dysgenesis in XY females.

2.2.2   Gene mapping and reverse genetics

Some 130 different gene loci are known to be carried on the X-chromosome, largely because they show the characteristics of X-linked inheritance. The colour blindness locus was the first to be formally assigned, and this was published in 1911. However, it was not until 1968 that the first autosomal locus was assigned; this was the Duffy blood-group locus which maps to chromosome 1. In recent years there has been an explosion of activity in assigning gene loci to their respective chromosomes, and at the time of writing almost 2000 gene loci have been assigned to specific regions of chromosomes. This is a substantial proportion of the 5000 gene loci listed in McKusick's 1990 encyclopaedic catalogue of Mendelian traits, but a small proportion in relation to the total number of gene loci in our species, which has been estimated to be at least 50 000.

The mapping of the human genome should not be regarded as an academic exercise. It has important practical application in the diagnosis and carrier detection of genetic disease through linkage of genetic-marker loci to disease loci (see below). It also has fundamental importance in human biology, as it may be the means of identifying the gene product and determining the function of disease genes. This approach is sometimes referred to as 'reverse' genetics, in contrast to the classical approach which progresses from identification of a gene product through a number of stages, including amino acid sequencing and isolation of the specific messenger RNA to cloning the gene and finally finding its position in the human genome. Reverse genetics is used when the product of a gene is unknown. The disease

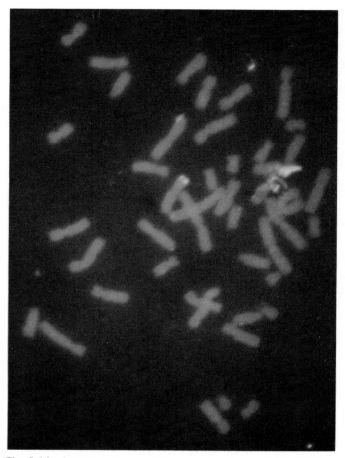

Fig. 2.14 A metaphase spread from a male patient with 46,XX Klinefelter syndrome (an XX male). The chromosomes have been hybridized with a biotinylated Yp-specific DNA probe (GMGY10) labelled with peroxidase. The Y-specific probe is annealed to the distal end of the short arm of one X-chromosome, demonstrating that Y-specific sequences, including the primary male determinants, have been transferred to one of the X-chromosomes by accidental recombination during paternal meiosis. (Reflectance contrast microscopy.)

locus is first mapped by family linkage studies; the gene is then identified by molecular methods and cloned; its product is synthesized by expression vectors and used to raise antibodies to assist in isolating the complete protein. This protein can then be characterized and its function determined. The products of a number of important genes are being analysed in this way, and examples include the Duchenne muscular dystrophy gene, the X-linked chronic granulomatosis disease gene, the retinoblastoma gene, and the gene for cystic fibrosis.

The main methods used for constructing the human gene map are given below.

Somatic cell hybridization

Human cells and rodent cells can be fused to form interspecific hybrid cell lines. These hybrids have the interesting property of losing human chromosomes preferentially. Selective systems can be used to retain human chromosomes of interest. This allows the correlation of loss of human gene products in the hybrid with loss of specific human chromosomes. Similarly, retention of the ability to produce human proteins can be correlated with the presence of specific human chromosomes. Large numbers of different hybrid cell lines can be tested so that significant correlations are readily obtained. The method has been highly productive.

Family linkage studies

The simultaneous transmission of several gene loci through three generations and in most members of a large family suggests that the loci are carried together on the same segment of the same chromosome. The recombination frequency is a measure of the distance any two loci are apart on the chromosome (see Section 2.1.1). Chromosome heteromorphisms or translocation breakpoints can be used as markers in linkage studies so that the locus in question can be assigned to part of a specific chromosome. The most useful markers are loci at which several different alleles can be distinguished. Before the days of recombinant DNA technology, useful markers included the blood groups, serum protein types, and red cell enzyme polymorphisms. These have now been replaced as markers by restriction fragment length polymorphisms (RFLPs). These are variations at the level of the DNA molecule recognized by site-specific restriction endonucleases. Point mutations can abolish restriction enzyme cleavage sites or generate new ones, and as variation at these sites is very common and comparatively easy to detect by the Southern blotting technique, DNA probes that recognize RFLPs are extremely valuable as genetic markers for linkage studies.

In situ hybridization

Cloned DNA sequences from genes of interest can be used to identify the complementary sequences within the chromosome complement. The DNA probe is usually radiolabelled and made single-stranded by heating and rapid cooling. It is then applied to a standard air-dried chromosome preparation that has been similarly denatured. The probe anneals to its complementary sequence on the chromosome, and the site of hybridization is revealed by autoradiography. This technique is the simplest and most widely used method for assigning DNA sequences to chromosomes, but probes that contain widely dispersed repeated sequences cannot easily be used. Biotin-labelling procedures are now replacing radiolabelling and autoradiography (Fig. 2.14). *In situ* hybridization with biotinylated chromosome-specific probes are increasingly used for the rapid diagnosis of chromosome aberrations by chromosome 'painting' (Fig. 2.15).

Gene dosage methods

Chromosomal deletions and duplications can sometimes give information on the mapping of gene loci. Normally both alleles at a given locus are expressed equally in somatic cells. If the gene product is an enzyme, the heterozygous carrier of a mutation that causes enzyme deficiency in the homozygote will have 50 per cent activity in his cells. The same effect is produced if an allele is involved in a chromosomal deletion. When a locus is involved in a duplication, three copies of the gene will be present and this is reflected in the enzyme activity, which may be 150 per cent of normal. The gene for acid phosphatase was assigned to chromosome 2 by such a deletion and confirmed by

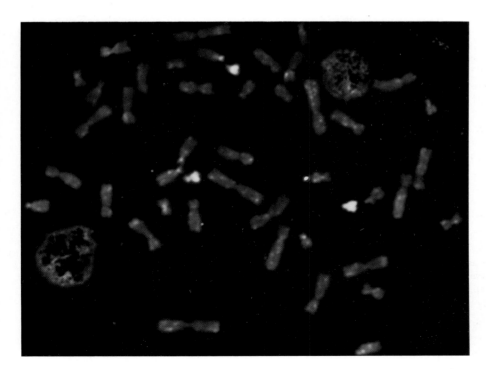

Fig. 2.15 Chromosome 'painting' by *in situ* hybridization. Multiple chromosome 21 specific biotinylated probes have been hybridized to this trisomy 21 cell; the result is that the three chromosomes 21 are identified by the hybridization signal—in this case peroxidase-labelled biotin detected by reflectance contrast microscopy.

a similar duplication. Other examples include the ABO:adenylate kinase:nail-patella linkage group, which was assigned to chromosome 9q34 by gene dosage studies of red cell adenylate kinase.

Other methods

The chromosome complement can be sorted into groups of different size by the technique of flow cytometry (Fig. 2.4). An unassigned cloned DNA sequence can then be mapped by hybridizing the labelled probe to Southern blots or dot blots of sorted chromosomes. Regional localization is then achieved by sorting chromosomes from individuals carrying translocations involving the chromosome of interest (Fig. 2.16).

A quite different approach exploits the remarkable conservation of linkage groups in mammalian species. Genes that have been mapped experimentally in mice may be assigned to the equivalent chromosome in man simply by knowing the linkage relationships in the mouse. Thus, as the β-galactosidase locus maps to chromosome 3 in man and chromosome 9 in the mouse, its linkage to the locus for transferrin in the mouse assigns the transferrin locus correctly to chromosome 3 in man.

As a result of these various strategies for mapping genes in man, the point has been reached where each chromosome is marked by a series of gene loci, none of which is less than 25 centimorgans from its nearest neighbour. Some regions are more closely mapped, with mapping points between 5 and 10 centimorgans apart. This represents a major achievement because it means that any unmapped gene locus could theoretically be assigned to its correct place on the map by linkage studies. Within the next 5–10 years it is expected that the resolution of the genetic map will be increased to between 1 and 2 centimorgans. As indicated in Section 2.1.1, this genetic distance is roughly equivalent to between 2 and 5 million base pairs, and this is currently at the upper limit for resolving the DNA molecule by physical and molecular methods (see below).

In addition to these achievements in expanding the human genetic map, considerable progress is being made with methods which aim eventually to sequence the entire human genome. When one considers that the haploid genome consists of 3000 million base pairs, the task is formidable and would require major improvements in existing technology if it is to be achieved in the foreseeable future. Development towards this goal of a complete physical map, depends on the construction of an ordered series of cloned DNA sequences which span each chromosome from end to end. Depending on the type of cloning vector used, the size of the cloned DNA sequence varies from 20 kilobases to several megabases (using yeast artificial chromosomes). Overlapping clones can be recognized by 'fingerprinting' techniques and computer analysis, so that a contiguous series of ordered clones ('contigs') can be assembled and

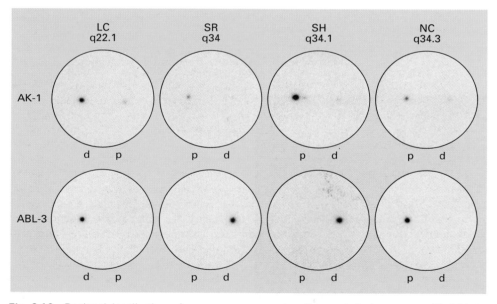

Fig. 2.16 Regional localization of gene sequences using flow-sorted chromosome 'dot' blots. Bivariate flow cytometry has been used to sort both derivatives of four different reciprocal translocations involving chromosome 9 (see Fig. 2.4b). In each case, 10 000 chromosomes have been sorted directly on to nitrocellulose filters; each filter contains the derivative with that part of chromosome 9 proximal (p) or distal (d) to the translocation breakpoint. The four filters were probed successively with ^{35}P-labelled sequences from the adenylate kinase-1 locus and the Abelson oncogene locus, respectively. Hybridization detected by autoradiography shows that the AK-1 locus maps proximal to the chromosome 9 translocation breakpoints in NC, SR, and SH, but distal to the breakpoint in LC. ABL-3 maps distal to the chromosome 9 breakpoints in LC, SR and SH, but proximal to the breakpoint in NC. AK-1 is therefore proximal to ABL-3 on chromosome 9.

assigned to their position on the physical map. The physical map can then be related to the genetic map by standard techniques, such as *in situ* hybridization and genetic linkage analysis. A complete, ordered set of DNA clones would be an ideal resource, e.g. for identifying disease genes and determining their function, and also for studying the molecular pathology of genetic disorders. Preliminary work on species with considerably smaller genomes, such as *Escherichia coli*, *Saccharomyces cerevisiae*, *Drosophila melanogaster*, and *Caenorrhabditis elegans*, attest to the feasibility of this approach.

2.2.3 DNA methods for diagnosis and carrier detection of genetic disease

The classical approach to the diagnosis of genetic disease depends on the knowledge of the gene product, which may be either altered or deficient in the affected patient. In sickle-cell disease, for example, the gene mutation results in an amino-acid substitution in the β-globin chain, which can be detected by starch gel electrophoresis. Carriers of the sickle-cell trait show both normal and sickle-cell haemoglobin on electrophoresis. Advances in recombinant DNA technology have led to a new approach, namely the direct analysis of the gene itself. This in turn has led to a knowledge of the molecular pathology of a number of single gene defects, including the haemoglobinopathies, enabling improved carrier detection and prenatal diagnosis using DNA probes and Southern analysis. The same approach has been helpful in the investigation of chromosomal and multifactorial disease, including cancer and congenital malformations.

As indicated above, the basis of DNA diagnosis lies in the recognition of restriction fragment length polymorphisms (RFLPs). Cloned sequences of parts of genes, or intervening sequences, are used as probes in Southern blots to detect RFLPs, which are of two main types. One type is known as a cleavage-site polymorphism. These usually consist of single base changes which occur every 200–500 base pairs and are usually asymptomatic unless they occur in a critical part of the coding sequence (exon). If the base change occurs in a restriction endonuclease cleavage site, it may abolish the cleavage site and result in a larger DNA restriction fragment apparent on Southern blotting. The base change may also create a new cleavage site and thus result in a smaller restriction fragment.

The second type of polymorphisms are variable-length polymorphisms. These occur in regions of the genome that contain tandem repeats of the same core sequence (which is usually not transcribed). A DNA probe containing the core sequence will recognize different lengths of DNA depending on the number of repeats present at that site on the chromosome. Probes that recognize this type of repeat are often referred to as VNTR probes (variable number of tandem repeats). Due to the phenomenon of unequal crossing-over, these regions are highly polymorphic and many different 'alleles' can often be distinguished. VNTR probes can be chromosome specific, or may recognize repeated sequences on many chromosomes. The

latter are sometimes called minisatellite probes and are now widely used for DNA fingerprinting in paternity suits and in forensic pathology, because the pattern of fragments on Southern blots is unique for each individual.

DNA probes for use in diagnosis should be chromosome specific and be able to recognize polymorphisms that occur frequently in the population. Intragenic probes are those which contain sequences from within the gene. Any polymorphism recognized by an intragenic probe will effectively mark the gene itself and, provided that the gene is not exceptionally large, will not be constrained by the possibility of recombination. Intragenic probes can therefore usually be used safely in tracking a particular gene through the family for the purposes of diagnosis or carrier detection.

Sometimes it happens that the gene of interest has not been cloned and so there are no intragenic probes available, or that the RFLPs recognized by the probe are not informative in a given family. Recourse is then made to probes that recognize polymorphisms outside the gene itself, but sufficiently closely linked to reduce the possibility of recombination to an acceptable level. To be useful for diagnostic purposes, the recombination rate between a disease locus and its marker locus should be less than 2–3 per cent. Much greater reliability is achieved when the disease locus is flanked by two closely linked markers. Recombination between either marker and the disease locus can be readily recognized and the only hazard is the occurrence of double recombination, the probability of which is the product of the two recombination frequencies.

Diagnosis by the polymerase chain reaction

Once a disease gene, or part of it, has been cloned and sequenced, and the mutation has been identified in the genetic code by DNA sequencing, it is possible to undertake direct diagnosis by molecular methods. A synthetic oligonucleotide comprising 17–19 base pairs is synthesized which is complementary to the stretch of DNA containing the mutation. Another synthetic oligonucleotide is constructed of the same region but with the normal DNA sequence rather than the mutated sequence. These are used as probes to determine whether or not an individual's DNA contains the mutation. This can be very readily accomplished by amplifying the corresponding sequence of DNA from the patient using the polymerase chain reaction technique. Only a small amount of DNA is required from the patient, either from a small blood sample or from buccal cells from the inside of the cheek. The polymerase chain reaction requires appropriate DNA primers for the sequence in question, a supply of DNA polymerase which is stable at high temperature, and a system of heating and cooling to allow repeated cycles of denaturation followed by DNA replication. As the reaction proceeds, multiple copies of the DNA sequence are produced. Dot blots of the DNA from the reaction are transferred on to nylon membranes and hybridized with the two ^{32}P-radiolabelled oligonucleotide probes. Under stringent hybridization conditions, the probe that recognizes the normal sequence will not hybridize to the dot blot containing only the mutant sequence, neither

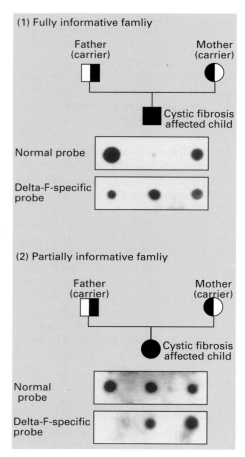

Fig. 2.17 Dot blot analysis of the cystic fibrosis delta F-508 mutation. Dot blots from amplified DNA from the CF locus in the affected child and both parents have been probed with an oligonucleotide probe from the normal allele and from the mutant allele, respectively. In (1) the affected child is homozygous for the mutant gene and both parents are heterozygous. In (2) the affected child and her mother are heterozygous, indicating that the mutant allele inherited from the father is not detected by the delta-F probe.

will the probe that recognizes the mutant sequence hybridize with the dot blot containing only the normal sequence. Homozygous affected, homozygous normal, and heterozygotes for the mutant allele are all readily detected by the two oligonucleotide probes (Fig. 2.17). An added advantage is that with the polymerase chain reaction a diagnosis can be made within 48 h. This is, of course, provided that the DNA sequence is known and that suitable DNA primers are available for the gene in question.

An example of the diagnosis of genetic disease by DNA analysis is given in Fig. 2.17.

2.2.4 Acknowledgements

The following people are thanked for the preparation of figures: Lionel Willatt (Fig. 2.15), Dr Sultan Habeebu (Fig. 2.14), Dr Nigel Carter (Fig. 2.16), and Dr David Barton (Fig. 2.17).

2.2.5 Bibliography

McKusick, V. A. (1990). *Mendelian inheritance in man: catalogues of autosomal dominant, autosomal recessive, and X-linked phenotypes.* Johns Hopkins University Press, Baltimore.

2.3 Eukaryotic gene structure and expression

Peter W. J. Rigby

2.3.1 Introduction

Our knowledge of the structure and function of eukaryotic genes has been revolutionized during the 19 years which have elapsed since the first segment of eukaryotic DNA was cloned in *Escherichia coli*. The advent of recombinant DNA techniques allowed the isolation of any segment of DNA from any organism, in pure form and in large quantities. The subsequent development of rapid methods for determining the sequence of DNA has led to an outpouring of structural information, culminating in current discussions on the sequencing of the entire human genome (see Section 30.7). Another vitally important step forward was the advent of effective protocols for the reintroduction of DNA into cultured mammalian cells, thus allowing studies of the mechanisms of gene expression and of the functions of the encoded protein. Such DNA-mediated gene transfer procedures culminated in transgenic mouse technology, by which genes can be stably introduced into the germ line of the mouse and the expression and function of a gene can be manipulated within the context of the whole organism. All of these studies of expression and function depend upon the ability to manipulate DNA molecules at will; it is now a straightforward matter to remove, insert, or change sequences within a cloned DNA molecule, and long stretches of DNA can be chemically synthesized. This technical facility underlies the approach of reverse, or surrogate, genetics in which the investigator introduces the mutation and then searches for a phenotype.

The details of these immensely powerful methodologies are beyond the scope of this chapter but they are well explained in several textbooks (Glover 1984; Kingsman and Kingsman 1988; Old and Primrose 1989).

I shall summarize here our current picture of the organization of the eukaryotic genome and of the structure and expression of the genes, concentrating on those aspects of higher eukaryotic molecular biology which are relevant for an understanding of human pathology.

2.3.2 The organization of eukaryotic genomes

The DNA sequences within a eukaryotic genome are classically divided into three broad classes, based on their behaviour in renaturation kinetic experiments. 'Unique' sequences, which are present once, or a few times, per haploid genome and include most protein-coding genes; middle repetitive sequences, which include gene families and individual genes present in tens to hundreds of copies, e.g. ribosomal RNA (rRNA) genes and histone genes; and highly repetitive sequences, which are often considered to be primarily structural but which do include certain transcribed elements.

Highly repetitive sequences are found dispersed throughout the genome, although some are clustered in certain areas, for example at the centromeres of chromosomes, and most of the Y-chromosome is comprised of such elements. These sequences are divided into a number of families, the members of which are clearly related in evolutionary terms, and many of them appear to belong to a class of elements found in all organisms, called retrotransposons. Sequences of this type can move within the genome via a process in which RNA transcribed from them is copied into DNA by reverse transcriptase and the resulting DNA copy integrates into the genome at a location remote from that of the original copy (reviewed by Finnegan 1989). Such transposition can, when the new copy inserts into a gene, be mutagenic, and it is also clear that the fact that these elements are present in the genome in multiple copies can lead to inappropriate recombination events, which can disrupt gene structure with pathological consequences (Lehrman *et al.* 1985; Nicholls *et al.* 1987). In the majority of cases the RNAs transcribed from such elements are of unknown function, and many believe that

some of these elements have no biological function and that they are merely parasitic on the rest of the genome.

Middle repetitive sequences can be divided into two broad classes. The first is exemplified by the genes encoding the large rRNAs. All of these genes encode the same sequence and thus there must be special correction mechanisms that eliminate the sequence divergence which would normally accumulate. The second class includes multigene families, the members of which have divergent sequences which give rise to products of different but related function; examples of this include the histone genes, the genes encoding the class I antigens of the major histocompatibility complex (MHC), and the multiple genes which encode a particular species of transfer RNA (tRNA). In some cases, of which the large rRNA genes are again the best example, the multiple genes within the family are located together, sometimes in a long tandem array, whereas in others, for example the genes encoding actin, the individual members of the family are dispersed throughout the genome.

'Unique' genes include the majority of protein-coding genes, and their location in the genome does not normally reflect functional relationships. In most cases genes which are co-ordinately regulated are not next to each other and there is no evidence for operons as found in bacteria. This may well be a reflection of the fact that any eukaryotic gene has to respond to a wide variety of regulatory signals. Thus, while genes A, B, C, D, and E might all be induced in response to the binding of a

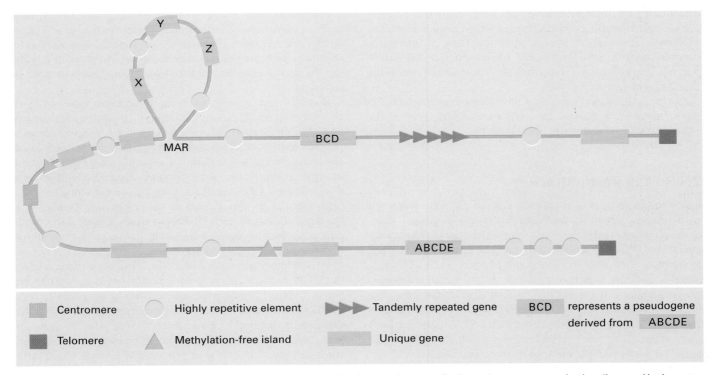

Fig. 2.18 A highly schematized view of a human chromosome, showing the main features of eukaryotic genome organization discussed in the text. The unique genes labelled X, Y, and Z are located within a single chromatin domain and may well thus be co-ordinately controlled. Middle repetitive gene family is organized in this case as a tandem array. Methylation-free islands are immediately upstream of housekeeping genes. MAR = matrix attachment region.

particular hormone to its surface receptor, genes A and E will respond to stimuli provided by viral infection, genes B and D to an environmental cue during embryonic development, and genes C and E to mitogenic stimulation. This necessity to respond to regulation by multiple stimuli requires that each gene be isolated and also leads to the complex organization of regulatory sequences discussed in Section 2.3.8. However, there are cases in which genes which are of related function and which are co-ordinately regulated are found in the same chromosomal locus, the classic example being the globin genes (Section 2.4). The unique sequences also include a large number of pseudogenes. These are defective genes which cannot give rise to a functional gene product and which are generally produced via reverse transcription of mRNA and subsequent integration in a fashion analogous to retrotransposons.

The genome can also be divided up according to the prevalence of the major base modification found in eukaryotic DNA, namely the methylation of cytosine residues. Large segments of DNA are heavily methylated, and in such regions the dinucleotide CpG is under-represented, probably because methylcytosine readily undergoes mutation. In other regions there is almost no methylation and the representation of CpG is that which would be expected on the basis of random base composition. Such unmethylated regions, called HTF islands, are often found at the 5′ ends of genes (Bird 1987).

The genome also contains a number of sequences that play a role in chromosome structure and function. These include centromeres and telomeres, and the sites at which DNA is attached to the nuclear matrix or scaffold. This is a proteinaceous structure, the precise nature of which is somewhat controversial. However, it is clear that the DNA of interphase chromosomes is highly organized by sub-nuclear structures, and it is likely that such structures play an essential role in the regulation of gene expression.

Figure 2.18 shows a highly schematized representation of the structure of a human chromosome containing all of the features discussed above (see also Fig. 2.1).

2.3.3   Chromatin structure

Inside the nucleus of a eukaryotic cell the DNA is complexed with protein, primarily histones. These nucleoprotein complexes show several levels of structure which lead to the packing of 1.8 m of DNA into a nucleus that can be as small as 0.06 μm in diameter. Dimers of the four major histones, H2A, H2B, H3, and H4, assemble to form an octamer around which is wrapped two superhelical turns of DNA to form the nucleosome core particle, in which the packing ratio is 6 (see Section 2.1 and Fig. 2.1). Histone H1 binds to the linker DNA between each nucleosome. This basic structural unit, which appears like beads on a string in the electron microscope, forms the 10 nm fibre which is then helically coiled to give the 30 nm fibre, in which the packing ratio is 40. This is itself further coiled into the interphase chromosome in which the packing ratio is 1000. In mitotic chromosomes the DNA is packed even more tightly and

thus the level of chromosome condensation must alter every cell cycle.

If detergents or polyanions are used to strip most of the protein from an interphase chromosome and the residual structure is observed in the electron microscope, it is apparent that the DNA is organized into a series of loops, the base of each loop being attached to a proteinaceous scaffold. It is also the case that if similarly deproteinized DNA is digested with restriction endonucleases then a small fraction of the DNA remains attached to the insoluble protein. This DNA, which has in some cases been characterized in detail, is called matrix attachment sites. The precise relationship between the biochemically characterized matrix and the morphologically characterized scaffold is unclear.

These multiple levels of structure mean that even within an interphase nucleus the DNA is extremely tightly packed and surrounded by protein, and is thus relatively inaccessible to the enzymes responsible for both replication and transcription. The controlled decondensation of particular chromatin domains is clearly a part of the mechanisms that impose selective gene expression. Transcriptionally active chromatin is much more sensitive to nuclease digestion than inactive chromatin, reflecting the unpacking that must occur to allow access of the transcriptional machinery. Particular sequences, both within and adjacent to active genes, become hypersensitive to digestion and are generally thought to represent the binding sites for regulatory proteins. Indeed, in some cases such hypersensitive sites can be helpful in identifying important control sequences.

Chromatin also contains many other proteins, generally called non-histone chromosomal proteins, the functions of which are not well understood, as well as a multitude of enzymes; for example, topoisomerases are involved in modifying the precise structure of the DNA during processes such as replication.

Histones are subject to several different types of posttranslational modification, including methylation, acetylation, and phosphorylation. There has been much speculation as to the role of such modifications in regulating the accessibility of chromatin to the transcriptional apparatus, and thus in regulating gene expression, but a clear causal connection has yet to be established. However, it has been known for a long time that histone H1 is phosphorylated as cells enter mitosis, leading to the suggestion that such phosphorylation is part of the mechanism of chromosome condensation. It has now been shown that the mitosis-regulated H1 kinase is the product of the cell cycle regulatory gene called cdc2 $^+$ in *Schizosaccharomyces pombe* or *CDC28* in *Saccharomyces cerevisiae* (reviewed by Moreno and Nurse 1990). The powerful genetic systems available for these yeasts have allowed unequivocal demonstration of the fact that this gene is required for progression through the cell cycle and that there is a functionally equivalent human gene which will work in yeast. Thus at least one type of histone modification appears to play a role in an important cellular process.

The fact that the DNA within the nucleus is wrapped around the outside of the histone octamer and that the 10 nm fibres are themselves helically coiled and arranged into loops indicates that the DNA is under considerable torsional stress. This stress leads to distortions in the classical double-helical structure of DNA. For example, studies of the accessibility of nucleosomal DNA to nuclease cleavage show that the strand farthest from the histone core can be readily distinguished from its partner, and the X-ray structure of the nucleosomal core particle shows that the DNA molecule kinks quite abruptly as it wraps around the histones. Other studies have shown that the precise structure of DNA, even in the absence of histone, varies considerably according to its sequence. The shape of a DNA molecule is thus not constant along its length and it can be perturbed by interaction with protein. These facts have profound consequences for the specific recognition of DNA by proteins that underlies much of the control of gene expression (Travers 1989).

2.3.4 Mechanisms of gene expression

The transfer of information from a chromosomal sequence to a functional polypeptide involves a large number of steps, each of which is a potential control point and each of which represents a potential failure point in a genetic disease. The first step is the decondensation of a chromosomal domain, which allows the access of *trans*-acting protein factors to their cognate binding sites; the combinatorial action of these factors then imposes the tissue-, cell type-, or developmental-specific pattern of transcription. The pre-mRNA molecule which is synthesized is then post-transcriptionally processed in a number of ways. Its 5′ end is capped, its 3′ end is generated by an endonucleolytic cleavage, the polyA tail is added, and the introns are removed by splicing. Either during or following these processing steps the RNA molecule is engaged by the transport machinery which ultimately delivers it to the cytoplasm. The information in the mRNA molecule is then decoded by the translational apparatus, which comprises ribosomes, tRNAs, and associated protein factors and enzymes, resulting in the synthesis of a polypeptide chain. This chain may then be processed (e.g. by specific proteolysis), modified (e.g. by glycosylation or phosphorylation), transported to a particular subcellular location or organelle, and then assembled into a supramolecular structure. These post-translational processing steps are often linked in a highly ordered pathway. This overall scheme is given in Fig. 2.19.

2.3.5 Eukaryotic gene structure

The only genes transcribed by RNA polymerase I are those that encode the precursor to the large rRNAs. They are organized in large tandem arrays, located on several different chromosomes, in which the transcribed sequences are separated by large non-transcribed spacers (see Fig. 2.20). In mammals these genes do not contain introns. The non-transcribed spacer contains the transcriptional control sequences which comprise a quite well-defined minimal promoter immediately upstream of the initiation site, together with a series of elements that have enhancer-like properties. Polymerase I transcription terminates at particular sequences and it appears that there is coupling between termination at the end of one gene and initiation at the beginning of the next. At least one of the components of the

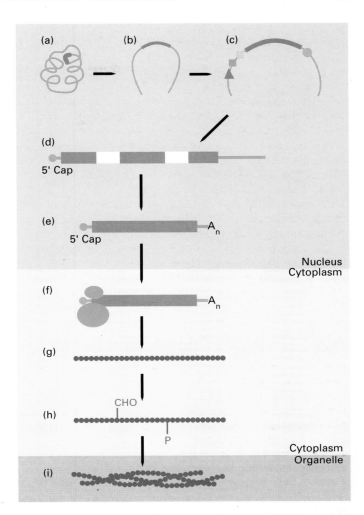

Fig. 2.19 Overall scheme for eukaryotic protein-coding gene expression (see also Fig. 2.23). (a) The purple segment represents an inactive gene located within highly condensed chromatin; (b) the chromatin domain is decondensed, rendering the gene accessible to *trans*-acting factors; (c) transcription factors ($\triangle$, $\square$, $\bigcirc$) bind to *cis*-acting control sequences adjacent to the gene and activate transcription by RNA polymerase II; (d) the immediate product of transcription is a 5′-capped pre-m RNA which still contains intron sequences and which extends, at its 3′ end, well beyond the last nucleotide that will appear in the mature mRNA; (e) the 3′ end is created by endonucleolytic cleavage and polyadenylation (A_n) and the introns are removed by splicing. The mRNA is then transported to the cytoplasm; (f) ribosomes recognize the 5′ end of the mRNA and initiate translation; (g) the initial product of translation is a pre-protein; (h) the mature protein is generated from the pre-protein by proteolytic processing and post-translational modification (CHO, carbohydrate; P, phosphate); (i) the protein is transported across a membrane into an organelle and assembled into a supramolecular structure.

polymerase I transcription machinery is highly species-specific; thus an extract of mouse cells will transcribe only mouse genes and not human ones, whereas a human cell extract has the opposite properties. This is a striking observation when contrasted with the fact that the polymerase II machinery has been

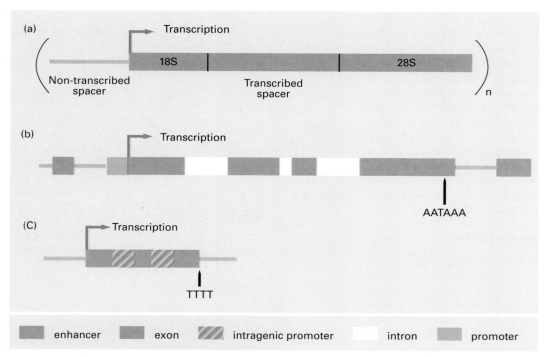

Fig. 2.20 General structure of eukaryotic genes. (a) Gene encoding the precursor to the large rRNAs, transcribed by RNA polymerase I. These genes are organized in long, tandem, head-to-tail arrays. (b) Protein-coding gene transcribed by RNA polymerase II. AATAAA is the signal for polyadenylation and 3'-end processing. (c) Gene transcribed by RNA polymerase III. TTTT is the termination signal. Such genes can be organized in tandem arrays but often are not.

so strongly conserved throughout evolution that yeast factors will work well on human genes and vice versa.

Protein-coding genes transcribed by RNA polymerase II can vary enormously in size. Some, most notably those encoding the core histones synthesized during each S-phase, are extremely compact and contain no introns. At the other extreme are genes that contain large numbers of small exons separated by many, in some cases very large, introns; such genes, for example that encoding dystrophin, which is mutated in Duchenne muscular dystrophy, can be spread over 2000 kb of DNA. The positions of introns within a gene are often conserved over very long periods of evolutionary time, suggesting that such positioning is of functional significance. Perhaps the location of introns crucially affects the tertiary structure of the pre-mRNA, which is assumed to be important for proper splicing. Introns are often located at points within the gene which demarcate functional domains within the encoded protein, and this observation has been interpreted in terms of the mobility of individual exons during evolution, thus allowing a given functional domain, for example a nucleotide-binding site, to be incorporated within many different genes. The location of introns between functional domains is not, however, an absolute rule; there are, for example, multiple introns within that segment of a myosin gene which encodes the single helical domain involved in the formation of myosin rods.

At, and immediately upstream of, the start site of transcription are elements, generally called the minimal promoter,

required for correct, albeit often very inefficient, initiation of transcription. Efficient, and properly controlled, transcription depends on two other classes of element, and all three types of element operate by binding, in a sequence-specific fashion, proteins which are generally called transcription factors. Upstream promoter elements are located within a few hundred bases of the start site and generally act in a manner that depends upon both their position and their orientation. Enhancer elements can be located far upstream of the gene, within it, or far downstream, and function in a position- and orientation-independent fashion. Enhancers are, in many cases, crucial for the imposition of correct cell type-specific transcription. Locus control regions (LCRs), originally discovered in the human β-globin locus, can be over 50 kb from the gene that they affect, and appear to be involved in the primary activation of a chromosomal domain.

The majority of genes transcribed by RNA polymerase III have a quite different structure in which the sequences required for transcription are located within the gene. However, these sequences appear to operate in the same way as those that control polymerase II transcription, i.e. by binding proteins which are required for accurate and efficient initiation by the polymerase. In some cases, exemplified by genes encoding small nuclear (sn) RNAs, the transcriptional control elements are positioned upstream of the coding sequence. Polymerase III transcription terminates precisely, in response to a well-defined signal. Some genes transcribed by polymerase III contain a single intron, but the mechanism of splicing is quite distinct from that which operates on pre-mRNAs transcribed by polymerase II.

2.3.6   Regulation of gene expression

The decision as to whether or not to express a eukaryotic gene product can be taken in many ways. The most dramatic of these is to create the gene only in those cells in which it is to be expressed, and this mechanism is involved in the regulation of the expression of the genes encoding immunoglobulin and T-cell antigen-receptor molecules. In both of these cases the functional gene is assembled from a number of segments in a series of rearrangement events that occur only in cells committed to express the gene in question (Lewis and Gellert 1989). It should be emphasized that rearrangement does not guarantee expression, the gene is still subject to many of the regulatory mechanisms discussed below, but expression clearly cannot occur in the absence of rearrangement. The joining of the gene segments is mediated by an enzyme; defects in the enzyme prevent effective rearrangement and cause the severe combined immunodeficiency in *scid* mice (Lieber *et al.* 1988). In some lower eukaryotes functional genes are created by a mechanistically distinct form of rearrangement best exemplified by the genes encoding the variant surface glycoprotein of trypanosomes. These parasites evade the host immune response by changing the structure of their surface coat, and this is achieved by having multiple genes which can only be expressed when they are moved into a functional expression site by a duplicative transposition event (Clayton 1988). This mechanism has not been found to operate in higher eukaryotes but it would not be surprising if it remains to be discovered.

Most genes exist in intact form in all cells of the organism and in such cases the primary decision is whether or not to transcribe the DNA sequence into an mRNA molecule. The first step in this process is a decondensation of the chromatin structure, which allows regulatory proteins to interact with their cognate binding sites in order to regulate the efficiency with which RNA polymerase can initiate transcription. Once RNA synthesis has begun, the polymerase moves through the gene unless it encounters sites at which it pauses; regulation of such pausing may be used to control the level of mRNA synthesis. It is not uncommon for a single gene to contain multiple polyadenylation signals and for these signals to be differentially utilized. It is thus possible to synthesize from a single gene mRNAs with different 3′ untranslated sequences, and it is highly likely that such differences affect the functioning of the mRNA, most likely by altering its processing or its stability. The pre-mRNA molecule is then heavily processed and modified, most notably by the removal of intron sequences by splicing. There are a large number of genes the transcripts of which can undergo alternative splicing, thus enabling the generation of multiple protein species from a single gene. Alternative splicing can be cell-type specific, thus enabling one gene to make different proteins in different cells. The mature mRNA molecule is then transported to the cytoplasm where it acts as a template for protein synthesis. Transport is a poorly understood process but it is fairly clear that it is controlled during the synthesis of the mRNAs encoded by human retroviruses and it would be surprising if such control mechanisms were not used by cellular genes. The output of an individual cytoplasmic mRNA molecule can be controlled in a number of ways. Firstly, its stability can be varied, and such changes in half-life are known to be important in such diverse processes as embryonic development and inflammatory responses. Secondly, the efficiency with which ribosomes bind to the mRNA and initiate translation can be altered dramatically. Once a protein molecule has been synthesized its function can be varied by altering its post-translational modification and by controlling its transport to particular subcellular locations or organelles. Finally, the assembly of individual polypeptide chains into macromolecular assemblies can be modulated. Failures in any one of these extremely complicated regulatory processes are likely to lead to pathological consequences.

2.3.7   Mechanisms of transcription

Higher eukaryotic cells contain three RNA polymerases, called I (or A), II (or B), and III (or C). RNA polymerase I is found only in nucleoli and is involved only in the transcription of the genes encoding the precursor of the large ribosomal RNAs. RNA polymerase II is found in the nucleoplasm and is responsible for the transcription of protein-coding genes into messenger RNA and of some genes encoding snRNAs. RNA polymerase III is found in both the nuclear and cytoplasmic fractions in a conventional subcellular fractionation but the enzyme in the cytoplasm is presumed to result from nuclear leakage during the fractionation. This polymerase is responsible for the transcription of genes encoding small, stable RNAs, e.g. tRNA, 5.8S ribosomal RNA, and some snRNAs. The activities of the three polymerases can be distinguished by their differential sensitivities to the fungal toxin α-amanatin.

All three polymerases have been purified to homogeneity from a variety of organisms and their subunit structures have been determined. Each enzyme contains multiple subunits, some of which are found in more than one enzyme. However, because it has not yet proved possible to dissociate the subunits and then reconstitute enzymatic activity, it is not clear that all of the polypeptides found in 'pure' polymerase are required for activity, nor is there direct evidence as to the functional roles of the majority of the subunits. The genes encoding some of the subunits of all three polymerases have now been cloned, and the DNA sequences of the genes encoding the largest subunits reveal a remarkable conservation with those encoding the relatively well-characterized subunits of the single RNA polymerase of *E. coli*. The largest subunit of polymerase II contains at its carboxyl terminus a variable number of heptapeptide repeats which have been shown to be required for function; these repeats are not present in the bacterial enzyme and it is conjectured that they are involved in interactions between the polymerase itself and accessory factors (Corden 1990).

While each of the purified polymerases will synthesize RNA, they do so in a non-specific fashion i.e. they are incapable of efficiently recognizing the signals in the DNA that mark the beginnings of genes. For RNA polymerase II such recognition requires the activities of a number of general transcription factors and ATP. The first factor to recognize the DNA is TFIID (the protein which recognizes the TATA box in promoters that contain this element), and this is followed by TFIIA and TFIIB. Polymerase itself then binds, followed by the factor TFIIE (Buratowski *et al.* 1989). Following the assembly of this initiation complex, elongation begins; several factors involved in the elongation process have been identified but their precise roles are not known. Elongation does not occur at a uniform rate across the gene; the polymerase can pause at defined sequences within genes, and such pausing sites have been called attenuators. The use of this term should not be taken to imply a mechanistic similarity with bacterial attenuators, which do cause pausing but which are regulated by a coupling between transcription and translation. There is no evidence for such coupling in eukaryotic cells, in which transcription and translation occur in distinct subcellular compartments.

RNA polymerase II transcribes through the whole gene, including all exons and introns, until it reaches a hexanucleotide signal, the consensus for which is AATAAA. This sequence is an essential part of the mechanism by which the vast majority of eukaryotic mRNAs are polyadenylated at their 3′ ends. It must be stressed that the creation of the 3′ end of an mRNA does not, at least in the cases of those higher eukaryotic genes which have been analysed in detail, involve a termination event such as occurs in bacterial transcription and in transcription by RNA polymerase III. The polymerase appears to continue transcription well past the last nucleotide that appears in the mature mRNA. There is then an endonucleolytic cleavage event, positioned, at least in part, by the AATAAA signal followed by the addition of the polyadenylic acid (polyA) tail. Cleavage and polyadenylation are concerted events performed by ribonucleoprotein particles, which appear to be similar to the better-characterized spliceosomes (see below), and a number of the proteins involved have now been identified. RNA polymerase III does terminate in response to a clearly defined signal, TTTT, in a fashion that appears to be analogous to the termination of bacterial transcription. The termination of polymerase I transcription is complex; rRNA genes are organized in long tandem arrays (see above) and the termination of the transcription of one gene is intimately connected with the initiation of transcription of the next gene.

Once polyadenylation has occurred, the synthesis of the pre-mRNA molecule is complete and there then follows a complicated series of post-transcriptional processing events which culminate in the transport of the mature mRNA to the cytoplasm. The first step in this process is splicing, in which the intron sequences are removed and the exons are ligated together. Splicing is mediated by ribonucleoprotein particles, called spliceosomes, which contain a number of snRNAs, each of which is complexed with several proteins. The reaction is ATP dependent and of exquisite specificity. It is clear that splicing must be extremely precise because otherwise exons would be missed out or introns would not be removed. Moreover, each individual mRNA molecule must be sequestered from all others during this process otherwise *trans*-splicing would occur, i.e. sequences from one transcription unit would become joined to sequences from another; uncontrolled *trans*-splicing would lead to the production of nonsense mRNAs. *In vitro* splicing systems derived from human cells will *trans*-splice but there is no evidence that this reaction is of physiological significance. However, it should be noted than in lower eukaryotes, e.g. the trypanosome *Trypanosoma brucei* and the nematode worm *Caenorhabditis elegans*, such *trans*-splicing is of great importance, and it would not be surprising to find it employed in the expression strategies of some human genes.

Recently it has become apparent that not all of the nucleotides found in mature mRNA molecules are encoded in the DNA template. This phenomenon was first discovered in certain *T. brucei* mitochondrial genes, the DNA of which carries a mutation which, if directly transcribed, would cause a frameshift. Either during or after transcription non-templated nucleotides are inserted into the mRNA in order to correct the frameshift. This process was subsequently shown to occur in other trypanosome genes (reviewed by Stuart 1991). The human gene encoding apolipoprotein B is transcribed into a 14 kb mRNA, which in liver is translated to give rise to a 512 kDa protein whereas in intestine the protein product is 242 kDa. This occurs because in intestine a C in the middle of the mRNA is modified to a U or a U-like base, thus introducing a stop codon which terminates translation after only the N-terminal half of the protein has been synthesized (Chen *et al.* 1987; Powell *et al.* 1987). Non-templated insertions of bases have also been shown to be a part of the expression strategies of a number of viruses, including that causing measles (Thomas *et al.* 1988; Cattaneo *et al.* 1989).

2.3.8 Regulation of transcription

The methodologies of reverse genetics have been applied widely in order to define the *cis*-acting DNA sequences that control the initiation of transcription. Two broad classes of sequence element have thus been defined. Promoters are elements located close to the site of transcriptional initiation which act in a position- and orientation-dependent fashion to allow initiation and to fix the correct start point. Enhancers are elements that can be located far upstream of the gene, within it, or at its 3′ end, and which act in a position- and orientation-independent fashion to increase the level of transcription from a linked promoter. The name silencer has been given to elements that have the other properties of enhancers but which act negatively, i.e. they repress transcription. These definitions are functional and to some extent arbitrary. As is discussed below, both enhancers and promoters are comprised of modules, each of which acts by binding a particular protein or proteins (reviewed by Johnson and McKnight 1989 and Mitchell and Tjian 1989), and an individual module can act as a promoter element in one context but as an enhancer element in another.

Promoters can be divided into two broad classes. Those which contain an element known as the TATA box (which serves to fix the site of initiation), and which generally also contain binding sites for a number of other *trans*-acting factors; such promoters are often associated with genes that encode terminal differentiation products. The second class is composed of GC-rich sequences which often exist in methylation-free islands; such promoters are often associated with genes that encode housekeeping products, i.e. proteins required for the basic functions of every cell, e.g. metabolic enzymes and structural components. Transcription driven by GC-rich promoters often initiates at multiple sites and appears to require fewer upstream factors. It is not clear how the initiation sites are fixed for transcription units of this type. Figure 2.21 shows idealized representations of the control sequences of two genes, one of each class. Let us first consider the gene that encodes a tissue-specific, terminal differentiation product, for example globin (expressed only in erythroid cells) or immunoglobulin (expressed only in B-lymphocytes). In each case the promoter contains the TATA element which directs the binding of TFIID. The binding of TFIID is necessary in order to assemble a pre-initiation complex, and this binding will be modulated accord-ing to whether or not the adjacent binding sites are occupied by the other requisite factors, e.g. Sp1, CAAT-box factor, etc. These factors, acting in concert, then determine the efficiency with which RNA polymerase II can engage the template. The promoter itself may or may not have autonomous activity but its efficiency is regulated by the enhancer, which can be upstream or located in an intron or at the 3′ end of the transcription unit. The enhancer is itself composed of multiple protein-binding sites, each of which may interact with more than one polypeptide, and it is clear that it is the combinatorial action of these proteins that mediates enhancer function. The fact that enhancers can act in a position-independent fashion raises the question of how the proteins bound to them influence the rate of initiation. It seems likely that the chromatin must assume complex structures in order to facilitate such interactions, as is indicated schematically in Fig. 2.21.

A simplistic view of this scenario would lead to the conclusion that the restriction of immunoglobulin gene expression to B-lymphocytes is accomplished by restricting the expression of the requisite *trans*-acting factors to B-cells. However, this view rapidly degenerates into an infinite regression; if the transcription factor is only expressed in B-cells, then what restricts the

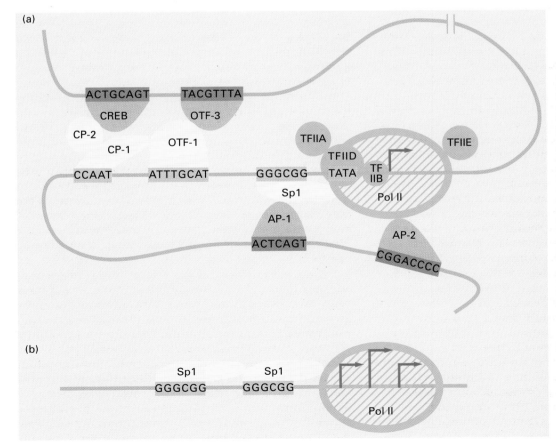

Fig. 2.21 Idealized representations of the transcriptional control region of protein-coding genes. (a) TATA-box containing gene. The initiation complex, assembled over the start site, contains polymerase II and the general transcription factors TFIIA, TFIIB, TFIID, and TFIIE, together with other general factors which are not shown. Upstream promoter elements bind factors (Sp1, OTF-1, CP1/CP2) which interact with each other and/or with the general transcription machinery to modulate the efficiency of initiation by the polymerase. In some cases, e.g. CP1/CP2, these factors are heterodimeric complexes in which only one subunit binds directly to DNA. Enhancer elements bind factors (AP-1, AP-2, OTF-3, CREB) which interact either with the factors bound to promoter elements or directly with the general machinery. More than one factor can bind to a given motif, e.g. OTF-1 and OTF-3 both bind to ATTTGCAT. It is not necessarily the case that all factors are bound to the DNA at any one time. The interactions shown are representative and should not be taken to indicate the mechanisms of action of particular factors. (b) Gene with GC-rich promoter. The mechanism by which the initiation site is fixed is unknown as is the involvement, or otherwise, of the general transcription factors.

expression of the factor itself? The simplest way out of this dilemma is to suppose that the activity of the factor is regulated post-translationally, and there is evidence in support of this view. For example, the factor NF-κB, which is required for efficient immunoglobulin gene expression, is not detectable in pre-B cells which do not express their rearranged immunoglobulin genes; if such pre-B cells are induced to differentiate into B-cells by treatment with bacterial lipopolysaccharide, NF-κB activity is induced, even in the presence of cycloheximide, a potent inhibitor of *de novo* protein biosynthesis. In pre-B cells, and in other cells that do not contain detectable NF-κB activity, the protein is present but it is located in the cytoplasm, where it cannot function, because it is bound to another protein, the inhibitor of κB(I-κB). The induction of differentiation leads to the breakdown of this complex and the NF-κB then translocates into the nucleus where it can act (Baeuerle and Baltimore 1988).

The binding of hormones to their surface receptors leads to many changes within the cell, including the activation of the transcription of particular genes. The signal initially provided by ligand binding is transduced via second messenger systems, one of which involves the activation of adenylate cyclase and thus an increase in intracellular cAMP, which in turn activates a cAMP-dependent protein kinase. Genes that respond to cAMP contain within their control sequences an element, the cAMP response element (CRE), to which binds a transcription factor called CREB. The ability of CREB to activate transcription depends on its phosphorylation state (Gonzalez and Montminy 1989) and one expects that many other transcription factors that regulate genes which respond to extracellular signals will be similarly regulated. It seems likely that much regulation of transcription factor activity is achieved by such mechanisms. However, there are clearly cases in which at least the first step of the regression operates. The expression of growth hormone and prolactin is restricted to certain pituitary cells; transcription of these genes depends upon the activity of a factor, variously called PIT-1 or GHF-1. The gene encoding this factor has been cloned and *in situ* hybridization and immunocytochemical analyses show that the expression of the factor is restricted to the appropriate pituitary cells. In this case, therefore, the question is: what regulates the expression of the regulatory factor?

Defects in such *trans*-acting factors can cause disease. The best example is provided by a factor called RF-X which binds to sequences essential for the proper transcription of human class II MHC genes. Patients suffering from class II deficient combined immunodeficiency have been shown to lack this factor (Reith *et al.* 1988); they are thus unable to express their class II MHC genes, the products of which are required for the proper functioning of the immune response.

While most of the regulation of transcription occurs at the initiation step, it is clear that the sites as which the polymerase pauses can also play a regulatory role. The best-characterized pausing site occurs within the first intron of the *c-myc* proto-oncogene (Bentley and Groudine 1988) and regulation at this site is involved in the response of the gene to haematopoietic cell differentiation.

2.3.9   Mechanisms of RNA processing

The primary transcript, i.e. that RNA molecule produced directly by RNA polymerase-mediated transcription of the gene, is, in eukaryotic cells, subject to an extensive series of post-transcriptional processing events, many of which represent potential points for the control of gene expression (reviewed by Krainer and Maniatis 1988). Defects in several of these processing reactions have been shown to underlie particular pathological conditions.

The first modification of the structure of mRNA molecules occurs shortly after RNA polymerase II has initiated transcription, and leads to the attachment to the 5′ end of the nascent transcript of an additional base which is not encoded in the DNA. This guanosine residue is joined to the terminal base via a 5′-5′ phosphodiester bond and is subsequently methylated to generate the structure 7meG5′ppp5′XpY; the first and second transcribed bases (X and Y) may be subject to methylations on their ribose rings. This complex terminal structure is called the cap and is essential for the initiation of translation (see below). The polymerase then continues transcription through the gene until it has passed the 3′ end of those sequences that will be represented in the mature mRNA. It is not clear whether polymerase II transcription terminates in the conventional sense of the word. However, the vast majority of polymerase II transcription units contain, some 30 bases upstream of what will be the end of the mRNA, the sequence AATAAA, which directs, in conjunction with other less well-defined signals (reviewed by Proudfoot 1991), an endonucleolytic processing event which cleaves the primary transcript to generate its 3′ end. To this end a polyadenylic acid tail, of several hundred nucleotides, is added by the enzyme polyA-polymerase.

This capped and polyadenylated transcript is now engaged by the splicing machinery. While polyadenylation normally precedes splicing temporally, it is not essential for it to occur. An individual transcription unit can contain many introns; collagen genes, for example, contain over 50. While there may be preferred orders for intron removal, there does not appear to be any required order, and even preferred orders are not obviously related to either the size of the intron or its location within the transcription unit. However, it is clear that splicing is an amazingly precise process; errors at the nucleotide level in the joining of exons, or the missing out of a single intron, would generate non-functional proteins.

The mechanics of splicing are now quite well understood, primarily due to the availability of cell-free *in vitro* systems which will effectively process artificial precursor molecules generated by the *in vitro* transcription of cloned genes or segments thereof (Lamond *et al.* 1990; Ruby and Abelson 1991). The analysis of wild-type and mutant genes in such systems has confirmed the importance of the consensus sequences which demark the beginnings and ends of introns, and also allowed the elucidation of the mechanism of splicing. The first step in the reaction is an endonucleolytic cleavage at the 5′ end of the intron which is guided by base pairing between the U1 snRNP and the consensus sequence at the 5′ boundary (Fig. 2.22). The

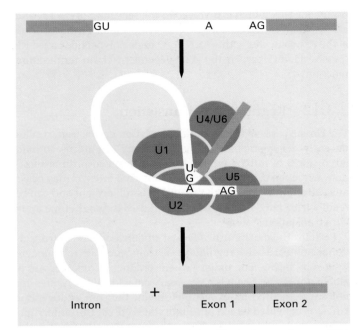

Fig. 2.22 RNA splicing. A highly simplified picture of pre-mRNA splicing. The snRNPs, together with other proteins, make up the spliceosome. The snRNAs within them recognize consensus sequences at intron/exon junctions and within the intron by base pairing.

5′-most base of the intron, which is always a G, then attacks an A residue situated within a less well-conserved consensus sequence at the branch-point, to generate a lariat structure. The branch point appears to be demarcated via an interaction with the U2 snRNP. The previously released first exon now attacks the 5′ end of the second exon, in a reaction that generates a properly spliced RNA together with an isolated lariat, which appears to be rapidly degraded. Other snRNPs are known to be involved in the assembly and operation of the complex splicing machine called the spliceosome, which can be thought of as an analogue of the ribosome.

The complexity of the splicing process means that many types of failure are possible. If an intron is not removed, the ribosomes will translate the intronic sequences, and in so doing will eventually encounter a chain termination codon and prematurely cease synthesis of a protein which has an improper sequence. Similarly, the inappropriate utilization of cryptic splice sites, or the missing out of an exon, will lead to the production of a nonfunctional protein. Many mutations that affect splicing in these ways have been characterized in human globin genes and underlie various forms of thalassaemia (see Section 2.4). If *trans*-splicing occurs in mammalian cells, the consequences are likely to be catastrophic; such mutants have not been discovered, presumably either because they are lethal or because the splicing machinery has multiple fail-safe mechanisms built into it.

Other splicing mechanisms operate on the products of transcription by RNA polymerase I and III in lower eukaryotes, and on certain mRNAs transcribed by the mitochondrial RNA polymerase of fungi. While these mechanisms have not thus far

been shown to have equivalents in mammals, that which operates in the splicing of the rRNA precursor of the protozoan *Tetrahymena thermophila* is of considerable theoretical importance as the classic case of self-splicing RNA, i.e. the RNA molecule itself acts as the catalyst for the excision reaction in the absence of any protein cofactor.

The capped, polyadenylated, and fully spliced mRNA molecule is then transported to the cytoplasm by mechanisms that remain poorly defined. Once in the cytoplasm the mRNA acts as a translational template until it is degraded, the signals that target the degradation machinery often being located in the 3′ end of the mRNA.

2.3.10 Regulation of RNA processing

The polyadenylation, splicing, transport, and stability of an mRNA molecule can all be regulated as a means of controlling the overall output of polypeptide from a particular gene. It is quite common for a transcription unit to contain multiple polyadenylation signals at its 3′ end, and such signals can be differentially utilized in different cell types. The usage of such alternative signals leads to the generation of mRNA molecules with 3′ untranslated regions of different lengths, which may act to control the stability or transport of the mRNA. Infection with herpes simplex virus type 1 induces an activity that alters the pattern of polyadenylation-site usage (McLauchlan *et al.* 1989), and one expects other examples of the regulation of this processing step.

Splicing can be controlled in a number of ways, the most potent of which is tissue-specific control of alternative splicing, by which a single gene can give rise to different protein products in different cell types. An instructive example of this phenomenon is provided by the calcitonin/calcitonin-gene-related-protein (CGRP) gene which is spliced in one way in the C-cells of the thyroid to give rise to calcitonin and in another way in neurones to give rise to CGRP (Amara *et al.* 1982; Crenshaw *et al.* 1987).

mRNA transport is also controlled, most notably during the life cycle of the viruses human T-cell lymphotrophic virus (HTLV-I) and human immunodeficiency virus (HIV). The products of viral genes, *rex* in the case of HTLV-I and *rev* in the case of HIV, regulate the appearance of mature mRNA in the cytoplasm of infected cells (Siomi *et al.* 1988; Malim *et al.* 1989).

Once the mRNA arrives in the cytoplasm, the number of protein molecules to which it can give rise via translation is a function of its stability. The levels of many mRNAs that encode proteins involved in growth regulation or in inflammatory responses are regulated at the level of stability, and in these cases the *cis*-acting target sequence appears to be an AU-rich sequence in the 3′ untranslated region. A particularly interesting case of the regulation of mRNA stability is provided by the transferrin receptor, the protein responsible for transporting Fe^{2+}-transferrin into the cell and thus satisfying its requirement for iron. Under conditions of iron deprivation the receptor mRNA is stabilized, thus increasing iron transport into the cell. This regulation of stability is mediated by a protein which binds to sequences in the 3' untranslated region, and which also binds to the 5' untranslated region of ferritin mRNA, where it regulates the translation of another protein involved in iron metabolism (Casey *et al.* 1988; Mullner *et al.* 1989).

2.3.11   Mechanisms of translation

All eukaryotic cellular mRNAs carry at their 5' end the modification called the cap (see above), and experiments in which the cap is chemically removed or in which mRNAs lacking the cap are synthesized *in vitro* show that in *in vitro* systems the cap is absolutely required for the initiation of translation. However, some viral mRNAs, for example poliovirus mRNAs, do not have a cap but, rather, have a covalently linked, virus-coded protein at the 5' end of the mRNA. This exception is exploited by the virus as part of the mechanism by which it suppresses the translation of host cell mRNAs and subverts all of the translational machinery of the cell to its own ends.

Mammalian 80S monoribosomes comprise two subunits of 60S and 40S, and the initial steps of protein synthesis involve the binding of initiation factors eIF3 and eIF4C to a 40S subunit, followed by the binding of an eIF2/GTP/Met-tRNA$_i^{met}$ ternary complex to generate the 43S pre-initiation complex. Meanwhile, the mRNA has interacted with the cap-binding protein (CBP) and three other initiation factors, eIF4A, eIF4B, and eIF4F, in an ATP-dependent reaction, to generate a complex to which the 43S pre-initiation complex binds, such that it is positioned over the 5' end of the mRNA. In a second step requiring ATP hydrolysis the small subunit positions itself over the initiating AUG codon and eIF5 then acts to dissociate those factors that were involved in assembling the 43S complex; following this the 60S subunit binds and elongation begins. When eIF2 dissociates it does so in a complex with GDP, which is recycled to the eIF2/GTP complex needed for the next cycle of initiation under the influence of eIF2B.

A major question raised by the above mechanism is how the small ribosomal subunit identifies the correct AUG codon at which to initiate translation. It appears that this is done by a process of scanning, by which the ribosome begins at the cap and moves down the mRNA looking for the first AUG codon that is in a favourable sequence context (see Kozak 1989). A survey of a very large number of mRNA sequences has led to the identification of the consensus sequence GCCGCC$_G^A$CC$\underline{A}$UGG as being that most favourable for initiation. Thus ribosomes will ignore an upstream AUG which is in an unfavourable sequence context and continue to scan until they encounter the correct one. Mutations in this consensus sequence can have pathological consequences; for example, there is a thalassaemia in which the crucial purine at position -3 (the A of the AUG is taken as $+1$) is mutated giving the sequence CCCC$\underline{AUG}$ rather than CACC$\underline{AUG}$. This single base change drastically impairs the efficiency with which α-globin mRNA is translated (Morle *et al.* 1985).

The polypeptide chain is elongated in a process that requires the factors eEF1α, which is the equivalent of the prokaryotic EF-Tu and binds the incoming aminoacyl-tRNA to the ribosome; eEF1$\beta\gamma$, which is involved in the recycling of eEF1α, and eEF2, which is involved in the energy-dependent translocation of the ribosome along the mRNA. A single polypeptide called RF (release factor) acts in the ATP-dependent chain-termination reaction.

2.3.12   Regulation of translation

The classic cases of translational regulation derive from studies on early development. The eggs of many organisms contain large stores of mRNA which are not translated until fertilization, while the translation of other maternal mRNAs may cease at fertilization even though the mRNA is still present and can be readily translated if it is extracted and used to programme an *in vitro* translation system.

Perhaps the mechanistically best-understood case of translational control is the regulation of translation in reticulocyte lysates by haem. The major protein product of reticulocytes is globin, for which haem is a necessary cofactor. If the lysates are not supplemented by exogenous haem, then an endogenous kinase is activated which phosphorylates eIF2α, thus interrupting the cycle which normally regenerates the eIF2/GTP/tRNA$^\bullet$ ternary complex and so inhibiting polypeptide chain initiation. eIF2 phosphorylation by a distinct kinase is also involved in cellular responses to interferon.

The overall levels of translational activity within a cell are regulated by external stimuli. Thus, treatment of quiescent cells with growth factors leads to the activation of a kinase that phosphorylates one of the proteins, S6, of the small ribosomal subunit, thus increasing the proportion of ribosomes that are assembled into polysomes. The response of cells to heat shock involves the selective translation of the mRNAs that encode the proteins which protect the cell against hypothermia.

2.3.13   Protein processing and trafficking

Relatively few proteins function in the form of the primary translation product. Most are modified in one, several, or many ways (e.g. phosphorylation, glycosylation, or fatty acylation), and such modifications have, in many cases, been shown to be essential for particular aspects of function. The modifications are often targeted by particular motifs within the sequence of the polypeptide. The primary translation product may also be proteolytically processed, the classic example being preproinsulin. Finally, the protein must be delivered to its correct location within, or outside, the cell. Such trafficking is mediated by signals which generally comprise a short, 4–20, amino-acid sequence within the protein. These signals target a protein for secretion, transport to the nucleus, or localization within a cytoplasmic organelle, for example the mitochondrion or the lysosome, and in many cases are cleaved off the protein during transport. Once properly localized, proteins may be assembled into complex structures, such as ribosomes, secretory granules, or the cytoskeleton.

All of these processes are tightly controlled and some types of post-translational modification are reversible. As was discussed above, the activity of some transcription factors is regulated by phosphorylation, and the synthesis and degradation of glycogen is controlled by complex interrelationships between the activities of protein kinases and protein phosphatases. Key steps in one of the most fundamental cellular processes, mitosis, are regulated by phosphorylation (see above) and recent work has identified phosphatases encoded by genes which are essential for this process. Processing can be cell-type specific, for example the primary translation product of the proopiomelanocortin gene is proteolytically cleaved to give rise to different peptide hormones in different lobes of the pituitary. Some types of post-translational modification also play a role in protein localization; the product of the *ras* oncogene must be fatty acylated in order to be properly located on the cytoplasmic face of the plasma membrane. If fatty acylation is prevented, the protein cannot exert its oncogenic function.

Failures in these mechanisms can lead to disease, an excellent example being provided by I-cell disease. Patients suffering from this condition lack a post-translational modification enzyme which phosphorylates mannose residues. Mannose-6-phosphate is a trafficking signal; proteins carrying this modification being recognized by a specific receptor and thus transported to lysosomes. The defect in phosphorylation means that degradative enzymes are secreted rather than being packaged into lysosomes and toxic intracellular wastes thus accumulate (see Section 2.5).

2.3.14   Further reading

Alberts, B., Bray, D., Lewis, J., Raff, M., Roberts, K., and Watson, J. D. (1989). *Molecular biology of the cell* (2nd edn). Garland, New York.

Darnell, J., Lodish, H., and Baltimore, D. (1986). *Molecular cell biology.* Scientific American Books, New York.

Lewin, B. (1990). *Genes IV*. Oxford University Press/Cell Press, Oxford and Cambridge, Mass.

Watson, J. D., Hopkins, N. H., Roberts, J. W., Steitz, J. A., and Weiner, A. M. (1987). *Molecular biology of the gene*, Vols 1 and 2. Benjamin/Cummings, Menlo Park, California.

2.3.15   Bibliography

Amara, S. G., Jonas, V., Rosenfeld, M. G., Ong, E. S., and Evans, R. M. (1982). Alternative RNA processing in calcitonin gene expression generates mRNAs encoding different polypeptide products. *Nature* **298**, 240–4.

Baeuerle, P. A. and Baltimore, D. (1988). IκB: A specific inhibitor of the NF-κB transcription factor. *Science* **242**, 540–6.

Bentley, D. L. and Groudine, M. (1988). Sequence requirements for premature termination of transcription in the human c-*myc* gene. *Cell* **53**, 245–56.

Bird, A. P. (1987). CpG islands as gene markers in the vertebrate nucleus. *Trends in Genetics* **3**, 342–7.

Buratowski, S., Hahn, S., Guarente, L., and Sharp, P. A. (1989). Five intermediate complexes in transcription initiation by RNA polymerase II. *Cell* **56**, 549–61.

Casey, J. L., *et al.* (1988). Iron-responsive elements: regulatory RNA sequences that control mRNA levels and translation. *Science* **240**, 924–8.

Cattaneo, R., Kaelin, K., Baczko, K., and Billeter, M. A. (1989). Measles virus editing provides an additional cysteine-rich protein. *Cell* **56**, 759–64.

Chen, S.-H., *et al.* (1987). Apolipoprotein B-48 is the product of a'messenger RNA with an organ-specific in-frame translational stop codon. *Science* **328**, 363–6.

Clayton, C. E. (1988). The molecular biology of the Kinetoplastidae. In *Genetic Engineering*, Vol. 7 (ed. P. W. J. Rigby), pp. 2–56. Academic Press, London.

Corden, J. L. (1990). Tails of RNA polymerase II. *Trends in Biochemical Science* **15**, 383–7.

Crenshaw III, E. B., Russo, A. F., Swanson, L. W., and Rosenfeld, M. G. (1987). Neuron-specific alternative RNA processing in transgenic mice expressing a metallothionein-calcitonin fusion gene. *Cell* **49**, 389–98.

Finnegan, D. J. (1989). Eukaryotic transposable elements and genome evolution. *Trends in Genetics* **5**, 103–7.

Glover, D. M. (1984). *Gene cloning: the mechanics of DNA manipulation.* Chapman and Hall, London.

Gonzalez, G. A. and Montminy, M. R. (1989). Cyclic AMP stimulates somatostatin gene transcription by phosphorylation of CREB at serine 133. *Cell* **59**, 675–80.

Johnson, P. F. and McKnight, S. L. (1989). Eukaryotic transcriptional regulatory proteins. *Annual Review of Biochemistry* **58**, 799–839.

Kingsman, S. M. and Kingsman, A. J. (1988). *Genetic engineering.* Blackwell Scientific, Oxford.

Kozak, M. (1989). The scanning model for translation: an update. *Journal of Cell Biology* **108**, 229–41.

Krainer, A. R. and Maniatis, T. (1988). RNA splicing. In *Frontiers in molecular biology: transcription and splicing* (ed. D. Hames and D. Glover), pp. 131–206. IRL Press, Oxford.

Lamond, A. I., Barabino, S. M. L., and Blencowe (1990). The mammalian pre-mRNA splicing apparatus. In *Nucleic acids and molecular biology 4* (eds F. Eckstein and D. M. J. Lilley), pp. 243–57. Springer-Verlag, Berlin.

Lehrman, M. A., Schneider, W. J., Sudhof, T. C., Brown, M. S., Goldstein, J. L., and Russell, W. W. (1985). Mutations in LDL receptor: Alu–Alu recombination deletes exons encoding transmembrane and cytoplasmic domains. *Science* **227**, 140–6.

Lewis, S. and Gellert, M. (1989). The mechanism of antigen receptor gene assembly. *Cell* **59**, 585–8.

Lieber, M. R., *et al.* (1988). The defect in murine severe combined immune deficiency: joining of signal sequences but not coding segments in V(D) J recombination. *Cell* **55**, 7–16.

McLauchlan, J., Simpson, S., and Clements, J. B. (1989). Herpes simplex virus induces a processing factor which stimulates polyA site usage. *Cell* **59**, 1093–1105.

Malim, M. H., Hauber, J., Le, S.-Y., Maizel, J. V., and Cullen, B. R. (1989). The HIV-1 *rev trans*-activator acts through a structured target sequence to activate nuclear export of unspliced viral mRNA. *Nature* **338**, 254–7.

Mitchell, P. J. and Tjian, R. (1989). Transcriptional regulation in mammalian cells by sequence-specific DNA binding proteins. *Science* **245**, 371–8.

Moreno, S. and Nurse, P. (1990). Substrates for p34^{cdc2}. In vivo veritas? *Cell* **61**, 549–51.

Morle, F., Lopez, B., Henni, T., and Godet, J. (1985). α-Thalassaemia associated with the deletion of two nucleotides at positions −2 and −3 preceding the AUG codon. *EMBO Journal* **4**, 1245–50.

Mullner, E. W., Neupert, B., and Kuhn, L. C. (1989). A specific mRNA binding factor regulates the iron-dependent stability of cytoplasmic transferrin receptor mRNA. *Cell* **58**, 373–82.

Nicholls, R. D., Fischel-Ghodsian, N., and Higgs, D. R. (1987). Recombination at the human α-globin gene cluster: sequence features and topological constraint. *Cell* **49**, 309–78.

Old, R. W. and Primrose, S. B. (1989). *Principles of gene manipulation* (4th edn). Blackwell Scientific, Oxford.

Powell, L. M., Wallis, S. C., Pease, R. J., Edwards, Y. H., Knott, T. J., and Scott, A. J. (1987). A novel form of tissue-specific RNA processing produces apolipoprotein-B48 in intestine. *Cell* **50**, 831–40.

Proudfoot, N. (1991). Poly(A) signals. *Cell* **64**, 671–4.

Reith, W., *et al.* (1988). Congenital immunodeficiency with a regulatory defect in MHC class II gene expression lacks a specific HLA-DR promoter binding protein, RF-X. *Cell* **53**, 897–906.

Ruby, S. W. and Abelson, J. (1991). Pre-mRNA splicing in yeast. *Trends in Genetics* **7**, 79–85.

Siomi, H., Shida, H., Nam, S. H., Nosaka, T., Maki, M., and Hatanaka, M. (1988). Sequence requirements for nucleolar localization of human T cell leukaemia virus type 1 pX protein, which regulates viral RNA processing. *Cell* **55**, 197–209.

Stuart, K. (1991). RNA editing in mitochondrial mRNA of trypanosomatids. *Trends in Biochemical Science* **16**, 68–72.

Thomas, S. M., Lamb, R. A., and Paterson, R. G. (1988). Two mRNAs that differ by two nontemplated nucleotides encode the amino coterminal proteins P and V of the paramyxovirus SV5. *Cell* **54**, 891–902.

Travers, A. A. (1989). DNA conformation and protein binding. *Annual Review of Biochemistry* **58**, 427–52.

2.4 Molecular pathology of single gene disorders

D. J. Weatherall

2.4.1 Introduction

Over the past few years enormous progress has been made in the application of recombinant DNA technology to the study of genetic diseases. Considering that it is little over 10 years since the first human genes were cloned and sequenced, a remarkable amount has been learnt about the molecular pathology of single gene disorders. Indeed, we probably have a fairly good idea about the total repertoire of the different types of mutation that can underlie these conditions.

In the 1990 edition of Victor McKusick's *Mendelian inheritance in man*, he lists 2656 proven mutant phenotypes and an additional 2281 probables. Of the definite phenotypes, 1864 are classified as autosomal dominant, 631 as autosomal recessive, and 161 as X-linked; the proportional distribution in the probable group is similar. In addition to their clinical importance these disorders constitute a remarkable series of 'experiments of nature' that make it possible to study directly the effect of single mutant alleles in terms of their phenotypic effects. And now that it is possible to analyse many of these conditions at the molecular level, they are providing us with a wealth of information about abnormal gene action.

It is becoming clear, however, that the importance of understanding the molecular pathology of single gene disorders may extend far beyond the appreciation of the clinical manifestations

of single gene disorders. Rather, it appears that many common diseases of Western society have a strong genetic basis, although they are probably polygenic in origin, often with an equally strong underlying environmental component. And so, as we come to understand the molecular mechanisms that are involved in the modification of gene action, as evidenced in the genotype/phenotype relationships for the single gene disorders, we can start to apply this information to study variability in the action of genes that make up the polygenic systems that underlie heart disease (see Section 2.7), major psychoses, and autoimmunity. Furthermore, it is becoming apparent that many forms of cancer are associated with mutations, or altered activity produced by other molecular events, that involve critical housekeeping genes, called cellular oncogenes. Thus, as we learn more about these mutations, information obtained from studying the effects of those that are involved in single gene disorders seems likely to help us to understand how acquired mutations may alter the genotype to produce cancer and related disorders of cell proliferation.

Clearly, the study of the molecular basis and phenotype/genotype relationships of the monogenic disorders has important implications throughout pathology and clinical medicine. In this section we shall review briefly the different molecular mechanisms that underlie single gene disorders and examine how different molecular genotypes are reflected in their associated clinical phenotypes.

2.4.2 Historical background

In 1949 Linus Pauling and his colleagues observed that the haemoglobin of patients with sickle-cell anaemia has a different rate of migration in an electric field to that of normal individuals. These workers realized that the different properties of normal and sickle cell haemoglobin reflect a change in their net charges that must, in turn, result from differences in their amino-acid constitutions. The molecular basis for this observation was defined in 1956 by Vernon Ingram, who found that sickle-cell haemoglobin differs from normal haemoglobin by a single amino-acid substitution, valine for glutamic acid. At about the same time it was discovered that this substitution involves one of the pair of globin peptide chains that make up adult haemoglobin, a finding that provided direct evidence in support of the one-gene-one-enzyme (peptide chain) hypothesis proposed earlier by Beadle and Tatum from their work on *Neurospora*.

These studies led to the widespread use of electrophoresis as an analytical tool for examining human proteins, both in health and disease. It was found that nearly all the families of proteins that were studied were remarkably polymorphic and that at least some of this variability was reflected in defective protein function and hence in an abnormal clinical phenotype.

It was soon realized, however, that at least some genetic diseases result from reduced output of a protein and that such protein that is produced is normal in stucture. This led to the notion that some human diseases result from mutations that interfere with the regulation of the rate of protein synthesis. But little further progress was made until it became possible to apply the techniques of recombinant DNA technology to the study of the fine structure of human genes.

In the late 1970s techniques became available for isolating human messenger RNA, for producing gene probes, and for cloning and sequencing human genes. These new tools were soon applied to the study of single gene disorders, notably the thalassaemias and other genetic disorders of haemoglobin production. In a remarkably short time a great deal was learnt about the molecular pathology of monogenic diseases; it seems likely that we already have a relatively complete picture of the repertoire of the types of underlying molecular lesions. It turns out that the majority result from simple mutations that involve structural genes and that interfere with their transcription or with the processing or translation of their products. The 'old' theories, that disorders that result from a reduced output of a protein or enzyme are due to regulatory mutations, have had to be revised; most of these conditions can now be explained satis-

factorily on point mutations or deletions that modify the output from a mutant locus.

2.4.3   Levels of abnormal gene expression

In the previous section we saw how gene action is reflected in a regulated flow of information representing the transcription of structural genes into messenger RNA precursors, a complicated series of steps involving processing of the large precursor molecules into definitive messenger RNAs, and their cytoplasmic translation into a protein product. Although the mutations that underlie single gene disorders must be present in the DNA of the particular structural gene involved, they may manifest themselves by abnormalities at any of these levels (Fig. 2.23). That is, there may be a reduced rate of transcription of a structural gene, a variety of abnormalities involving the processing of messenger RNA precursors, or defects of initiation, translation, or

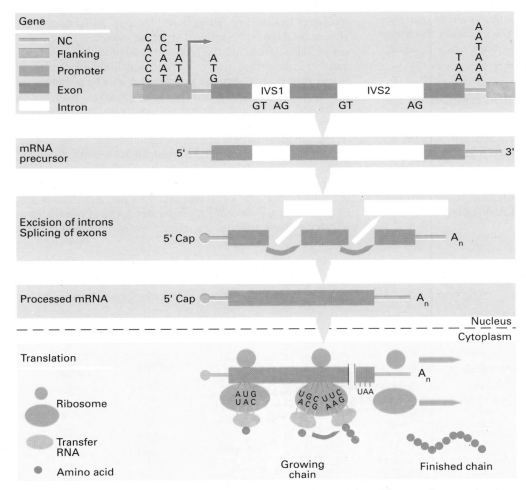

Fig. 2.23 The levels of gene action involved in different point mutations. The mutations can involve transcription of the gene by involving the upstream regulatory boxes, the various steps involved in processing messenger RNA, and, finally, in the various steps involved in translation, including initiation, elongation, and termination. NC = noncoding; A_n = poly A tail.

termination of the synthesis of the protein product on the cytoplasmic messenger RNA template.

By and large, mutations that produce disease are manifest in two different ways. First, a single base substitution or more subtle change in a structural gene may alter the structure of the messenger RNA such that an abnormal protein product is synthesized. If this alters the charge on the protein molecule, it will be reflected by a change in its electrophoretic pattern. However, it should be remembered that many amino-acid substitutions are neutral, that is they do not alter the net charge of the protein and therefore cannot be detected by electrophoresis. The second group of mutations are those that cause a reduction or absence of a particular protein product. It is now apparent that this latter class of disorders may result from mutations that involve transcription or processing of messenger RNA, or which act at the translational level by altering initiation, elongation, or termination.

In the sections that follow we shall consider examples of each of these different types of mutations. Because they were the first to be defined, it will be convenient to start with the structural protein variants that result from point mutations or rearrangements of structural genes. We shall then consider the heterogeneous basis for disorders that result from a reduced output of a protein product.

2.4.4   Monogenic disorders that result from the synthesis of an abnormal protein

The majority of monogenic disorders that result from the synthesis of a structurally abnormal protein reflect single base mutations in structural genes. There are a few examples of structural variants that are caused by much more extensive defects of the structural genes, in particular major rearrangements that lead to the formation of fusion genes that code for novel fusion products.

Point mutations producing abnormal protein products

Much of what is known about the protean manifestations of single base substitutions on human gene function has been derived from the abnormal haemoglobin field. The sections that follow describe the different structural haemoglobin variants that arise from single base substitutions or deletions, and briefly summarize other single gene disorders that have a similar mechanism. The molecular pathology of the haemoglobin variants is discussed in detail by Bunn and Forget (1986) and Weatherall *et al.* (1989).

General considerations

The genetic control of human haemoglobin is summarized in Fig. 2.24. Its structure changes at different stages of development. In adult life the major haemoglobin, haemoglobin A, consists of a pair of α-chains and a pair of β-chains ($\alpha_2\beta_2$). Normal adults also have a minor haemoglobin component consisting of α-chains and δ-chains, haemoglobin A_2 ($\alpha_2\delta_2$). In fetal life the predominant haemoglobin is haemoglobin F, which consists of α-chains and γ-chains ($\alpha_2\gamma_2$). There are two molecular species of fetal haemoglobin that differ only in having either glycine or alanine at position 136 in the γ-chains; these different γ-chains, which are the products of separate loci, are designated $^G\gamma$ and $^A\gamma$ respectively. In embryonic life the α-chains are represented by ζ-chains and the non-α-chains by ε-chains (see Fig. 2.24). The structure of a typical globin gene, including its exons and introns and different regulatory sequences, is summarized in Fig. 2.23.

The genetic disorders of haemoglobin fall into three groups. First, there are the structural haemoglobin variants. Secondly, there are the thalassaemias, which are characterized by a reduced rate of production of either the α- or β-globin chains and which are therefore divided into the α and β thalassaemias. Finally, there is a clinically unimportant group of conditions in which there is a defect in the normal switch from fetal to adult

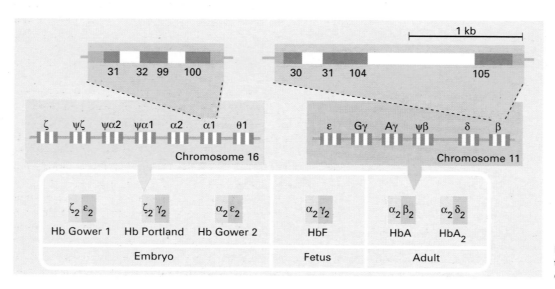

Fig. 2.24 The arrangement of the human haemoglobin genes on chromosomes 16 and 11.

haemoglobin production, hereditary persistence of fetal haemoglobin.

Over 400 human structural haemoglobin variants have been described. Over 95 per cent are due to single amino-acid substitutions in the α- or β-globin chains. All of them described so far are consistent with a single base substitution in the corresponding triplet codon of the globin gene DNA and, of course, in its corresponding messenger RNA sequence. For descriptive purposes it is usual to describe the nucleotide sequence changes created in the transcription product of a gene, that is its messenger RNA. This custom will be adhered to throughout, though it should be remembered that this change will be the result of a corresponding base change in the complementary DNA sequence of the particular structural gene.

In describing the haemoglobin variants it should be remembered that, originally, they were named by letters of the alphabet, but because these were soon used up it has become customary to describe abnormal haemoglobins by their place of discovery. This approach is now extended to most other protein variants. The position of the mutation is described by numbering from the amino-terminal end, i.e. β6 is the sixth residue along the β-chain.

As we have seen, haemoglobin variants usually reflect single base changes in the α- or β-globin-chain gene. For example, haemoglobins Rainier (β145 Tyr→Cys), Bethesda (β145 Tyr→His), and Fort Gordon (β145 Tyr→Asp) can all be explained by a single base substitution in the triplet UAU, which codes for tyrosine at position 145 in the β-globin-chain gene. A few variants have been found that have amino-acid replacements at two different sites on the same globin subunit. Three of these involve the haemoglobin S substitution (β6 Glu→Val). It is believed that these variants arose by one of two mechanisms; a new mutation on a variant (βˢ) gene or a crossover between two variant genes.

It can be calculated that there are 2583 single base substitutions possible for the 141 residues of the α-chain and the 146 residues of the β-chain. Of these, 1690 would result in an amino-acid replacement, but only a third, or 575, would cause a change in charge which would allow the variant haemoglobin to be identified by electrophoresis. Remarkably, about 45 per cent of these variants have already been discovered.

The genetic code shows ambiguity of nucleotide sequences; several different codons can code for any particular amino acid. Interestingly, there are a number of abnormal haemoglobins that suggest that, as judged by the nature of the amino-acid substitution, there is limited ambiguity of the nucleotide sequence of the codons for the human globin genes. For example, haemoglobins Köln and San Diego result from the replacement of valine by methonine at positions 98 and 109 in the β-globin gene, respectively. There is only one codon for methonine, AUG, but there are four possible codons for valine, GUG, GUA, GUC, or GUU. The methonine codon AUG could only derive from a single base substitution in one of the four possible valine codons, GUG, in which the first G is substituted by A. There are many similar examples that suggest there is only limited messenger RNA codon ambiguity. In fact it turns out that most, if not all, individuals share a unique nucleotide sequence for their β-globin genes with little or no variability, or polymorphism, from person to person in the nucleotide sequence at the third position of various codons. Although subsequent sequence analysis of globin genes and their messenger RNAs have shown individual variability, it is, in fact, remarkably small. It is not known whether this rule will apply to most human structural genes.

Consequences of point mutations on protein structure

Most point mutations do not alter the structure of a protein except for a single amino-acid substitution. Although this may profoundly alter the function of the protein, its overall structure only differs from the 'wild-type' protein by the single amino-acid substitution. There are exceptions, however. Occasionally, substitutions may involve the chain termination or initiation codons, or may scramble the genetic code such that either elongated or shortened peptide-chain products are produced. Again, most of the examples that we have so far are from the haemoglobin field.

Elongated peptide chains Studies of the human haemoglobin variants have shown that a few are characterized by elongation of either the α- or β-globin chains. These extended gene products result from one of three different mechanisms; base substitutions in the chain-termination codon, frameshift mutations, or the preservation of the initiator methionine residue.

The first haemoglobin variant with an elongated subunit to be described was haemoglobin Constant Spring (named after the suburb of Kingston, Jamaica, from where the first family to have the variant sequenced came). It is produced in small amounts and its α-chain is elongated at its C-terminus by an additional 31 amino-acid residues. The fact that the elongated portion does not resemble any part of the normal α-chain sequence suggested that this variant did not result from a crossover between two adjacent α-genes. In fact, it results from a single base mutation in the α-chain-termination codon, UAA to CAA which is the codon for glutamine. This substitution would thus lead to the insertion of glutamine instead of the α-globin chain terminating at its usual position at 141. The additional residues attached to the C-terminal end suggest that the α-globin messenger RNA continues to be translated through a region that is not normally utilized until another in-phase stop codon is reached (Fig. 2.25). The result is an α-chain with 31 additional residues at the C-terminal end.

The notion that single base substitutions in a chain-termination codon can give rise to an elongated α-chain has interesting implications. It was predicted, and soon found, that other variants might exist, with different substitutions in the chain-termination codon but with identical residues in their elongated C-terminal ends (Fig. 2.25). For example, haemoglobin Icaria has an identical structure to haemoglobin Constant Spring except that position 142 contains lysine instead of glutamine; this reflects the change UAA→AAA rather than UAA→CAA. In fact, a whole family of elongated α-globin-chain

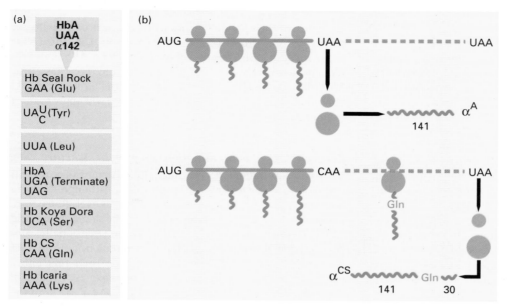

Fig. 2.25 The mechanism for producing elongated α-chain haemoglobin variants by chain termination mutations. (a) Variants, CS = Constant Spring; (b) mechanisms whereby an amino acid replaces the termination codon.

variants has now been discovered, all of which result from single base substitutions in the α-chain-termination codon UAA (Fig. 2.25). The chain-termination mutations are reviewed in detail by Weatherall and Clegg (1975, 1981) and by Bunn and Forget (1986).

Another mechanism for producing an elongated peptide chain followed the discovery of a variant called haemoglobin Wayne. Structural studies showed that this haemoglobin has an elongated α-chain which is identical to normal up to residue 138, after which it differs from normal by having a unique sequence of eight amino acids, thus extending beyond the normal α-chain length by five residues. The mechanism that underlies this variant is illustrated in Fig. 2.26. A deletion of one base, either C at codon 138 or A at codon 139, results in a frameshift, i.e. a single base is lost and the reading frame of the genetic code is completely altered beyond this point. As shown in Fig. 2.26 the α-chain-termination codon, UAA, is now out of phase and thus translation continues until an in-phase termination codon is encountered. There are several other haemoglobin variants in which elongated chains result from frameshifts of this type.

Another haemoglobin variant has been discovered, haemoglobin Grady, in which there is an elongated α-chain but in this case there appears to have been internal reduplication of part of the sequence of the α-globin gene. Between positions 118 and 119 there is the sequence Glu–Phe–Thr which is preceded by an identical sequence, indicating a simple internal reduplication. It seems likely that this has resulted from abnormal and unequal crossing-over between either allelic α-chain genes or between different α-chain loci.

So far, we have considered haemoglobin variants with elongated globin chains that are either extended at their C-terminal ends or in which there has been an internal duplication. How-

ever, it turns out that there are also variants that are elongated at their amino-terminal end (see Bunn and Forget 1986). For example, the abnormal haemoglobin, haemoglobin Long Island, differs for haemoglobin A in two respects; the second position in the β-chain contains proline instead of histidine, and there is a methionine residue at the N-terminal end of the β-chain next to valine which is the usual first residue in this chain; the amino-terminal sequence is thus Met–Val–Pro–Leu instead of the normal Val–His–Leu. Other variants of this type have been discovered. It seems likely that they reflect a defect in processing of newly synthesized globin chains due to a single amino-acid substitution near the amino-terminal end. Methionine is the first residue to be incorporated into a growing globin chain. Normally, during translation of the nascent polypeptide this residue is cleaved, leaving valine as the amino-terminal residue of both the α- and β-chains of haemoglobin. It is thought that, in the case of haemoglobin Long Island, the substitution of proline for histidine in the second position in the chain somehow interferes with this cleavage mechanism so that this variant has both a proline at position 3 in the β-chain and an abnormal methionine preceding the usual amino-terminal valine residue (see later).

Shortened gene products A few haemoglobin variants have shortened globin chains. In all cases one or a few adjacent amino acids are missing from the abnormal chains and the remainder of the subunit is normal. It seems likely that these variants arose from a deletion of one or more intact codons; if an entire codon is lost, the reading frame will remain in phase and the remainder of the amino-acid sequence will not vary from normal. Analysis of the nucleotide sequence of β-globin messenger RNA in the regions where deletions have occurred

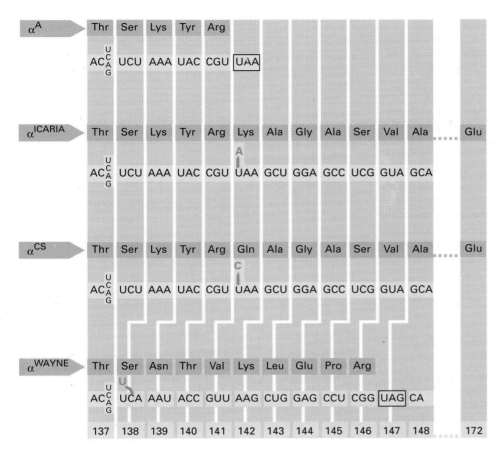

Fig. 2.26 The mechanism for the production of haemoglobin Wayne by a frameshift mutation. U is lost from codon 138 and a new sequence is generated which now puts the termination codon out of phase. The chain-termination mutants, Constant Spring (CS) and Icaria are also shown (see also Fig. 2.25). (Drawn after Weatherall and Clegg 1975, with permission.)

has shown that there is a reiterated nucleotide sequence, from two to eight bases in length. It has been suggested that these deletion mutants may have resulted from misalignment of these sets of sequences during meiosis, with non-homologous crossing-over, such that a segment of the gene of variable length, corresponding to the lost residues, is deleted.

Fusion variants Again, we have to go to the haemoglobin field for the first examples of structural protein variants that appear to have resulted from fusion of different parts of genes, with the production of hybrid globin chains. For example, haemoglobin Lepore has normal α-chains combined with abnormal non-α-chains that have an unusual sequence; the first 50–80 amino acids have the normal amino-terminal sequence of δ-chains, whereas the last 60–90 residues have the normal C-terminal amino-acid sequences of β-chains. The Lepore chain is thus a δβ fusion product. It seems likely that the fusion gene has arisen from non-homologous crossing-over between part of the δ-chain locus on one chromosome and part of the β-chain locus on the complementary chromosome, as shown in Fig. 2.27. It is also clear from Fig. 2.27 that an event of this type should also generate a chromosome containing an 'anti-Lepore' locus which, in addition to carrying normal δ and β loci, would contain a βδ fusion gene, i.e. the mirror image of the Lepore gene. In fact a number of 'anti-Lepore' haemoglobin variants of this type have been found.

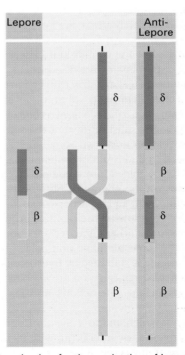

Fig. 2.27 The mechanism for the production of haemoglobin Lepore and other fusion-chain variants.

There is a whole family of human haemoglobin variants due to the production of fusion-chain genes of this type. Presumably this will be a general phenomenon wherever there are gene families with linked loci with rather similar structures that can undergo non-homologous crossovers.

An elegant example of this type of mechanism for the production of individual variability is the molecular pathology of red–green colour blindness. The genes that control colour vision consist of two linked clusters that are involved with the synthesis of red and green pigments, which lie on the X-chromosome, and another set for the blue pigment, which is on an autosome. It has been found that the X-linked form of red–green colour blindness results from an unequal crossing-over event, with the production of varying numbers of genes for the red and green pigments; Lepore-like fusion genes are generated in the process (Nathans *et al.* 1986). We shall return to a discussion of how variation in the number of structural genes brought about by unequal crossing-over can modify the function of a family of genes later in the section.

Structure–function relationships for variant proteins resulting from mutations of structural genes

The results of single amino-acid substitutions in proteins or their subunits vary, depending on the type of amino acid that is substituted and the site of the substitution in the particular protein. It should be emphasized that many amino-acid substitutions have no effect on function; for example, only a handful of the 400 or more human haemoglobin variants cause any clinical disability.

The primary amino-acid sequence of a protein determines whether it will be ordered into some form of secondary structure, such as an α-helix or a β-pleated sheet. Some amino-acid substitutions can shift the equilibrium between α-helix and a random coil in a particular part of a protein. The effect is to cause abnormalities of tertiary structure and to reduce the overall stability of the protein or its subunit. For example, proline cannot participate in an α-helix except as one of the initial three residues. Thus proline substitutions, or the substitution of proline by another amino acid, can sometimes seriously disrupt helical conformation and result in protein instability.

Many proteins are folded into a complex tertiary configuration, so that most of the charged amino acids such as lysine, arginine, glutamic acid, and aspartic acid are found on the surface of the molecule, allowing their ionized groups to be in contact with water. On the other hand, residues orientated towards the interior of the molecule have non-polar groups; thus the inside of the molecule is stabilized by hydrophobic interactions. The substitution of a charged for an uncharged residue can disrupt these important interactions and lead to molecular instability.

Another way in which amino-acid substitution can alter the structure of a protein is by interfering with its function. As we shall see as we examine some of the examples that follow, this can occur in a wide variety of ways.

Structural haemoglobin variants

Studies of the abnormal human haemoglobin variants that cause diseases (see Bunn and Forget 1986) have provided a wealth of examples of abnormal structure–function relationships for protein variants.

The commonest abnormal haemoglobin, sickle-cell haemoglobin results from the substitution of valine for glutamic acid at the 6th position in the β-globin chain. This change somehow stabilizes haemoglobin molecules in the deoxy configuration, such that long linear stacks are formed which cause sickling of the red blood cells and, hence, their premature destruction in the circulation.

There is a family of unstable haemoglobin variants that result from several different molecular mechanisms (Milner and Wrightstone 1981). Some involve amino-acid substitutions in the vicinity of the haem pocket, a hydrophobic crevice in the surface of the α- or β-subunits of haemoglobin in which the haem molecule lies. Amino-acid substitutions in this pocket decrease the stability of the haem-globin linkage, alter the shape of the subunit, and hence lead to molecular instability (Fig. 2.28). Other variants result from disruption of the secondary structure of subunits due to proline substitutions, as outlined above. A third group of unstable haemoglobins is associated with substitutions in the interior of the subunit. Finally, there are several unstable haemoglobins that result from deletions of groups of amino acids leading to instability of subunits, or elongation of globin chains which may also cause instability, in this case by adding a hydrophobic segment to the C-terminal end of the affected chains.

Another group of haemoglobin variants results in hereditary polycythaemia (Charache 1974). In this case amino-acid substitutions interfere with the normal steric changes that occur

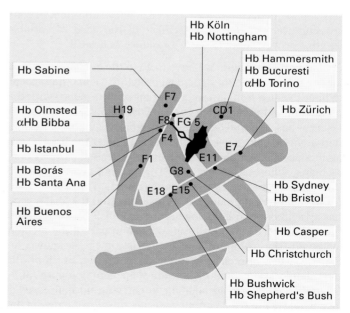

Fig. 2.28 The sites of substitutions of some unstable haemoglobins. (By kind permission of Dr Paul Milner.)

during oxygen delivery and leave the haemoglobin molecules 'fixed' in the oxy configuration. This leads to tissue hypoxia, erythropoietin production, and polycythaemia. The oxygen affinity of haemoglobin also varies according to the intracellular level of 2,3-diphosphoglycerate, a molecule that binds specifically to certain residues in the space between the β-globin chains in the deoxy configuration. Amino-acid substitutions that weaken these interactions also produce high-affinity haemoglobin variants.

There is a family of abnormal haemoglobins that is associated with congenital cyanosis due to methaemoglobinaemia (Bunn and Forget 1986). The iron atom of the haem group of haemoglobin is normally linked to a histidine residue in the haem pocket. Another histidine residue is situated on the opposite side of the pocket, near the sixth co-ordination position of the haem iron, where oxygen normally binds. It turns out that most of the haemoglobin variants associated with permanent methaemoglobinaemia involve substitution of a tyrosine residue for either one or other of the haem-related histidine residues. It seems likely that the phenolic groups of the substituted tyrosine residues are able to form a covalent link with the haem iron, thus stabilizing the atom in the oxidized (Fe^{3+}) state.

These examples of the molecular pathology of the structural haemoglobin variants provide an elegant picture of how single amino-acid substitutions may profoundly alter the stability of function of a protein.

α_1-Antitrypsin

The main inhibitor of trypsin in serum is an enzyme called α_1-antitrypsin (Carrell et al. 1982); it also inhibits chymotrypsin, collagenase, elastase, and some leucocyte proteases. Although this enzyme is not as well studied as haemoglobin, it is becoming apparent that it is the product of a highly polymorphic gene locus and that a number of disease alleles exist, many of which are probably due to single amino-acid substitutions. Currently, at least 25 alleles have been recognized at this locus, which is called PI (for protease inhibitor). The common, or wild-type, form of α_1-antitrypsin is called PI-M. The rare variants have been given letter designations, that run alphabetically from anode to cathode on electrophoresis.

There are two important alleles associated with liver or lung disease, called PI-Z and PI-S. These variants differ from PI-M by single amino-acid substitutions; in the case of PI-Z a glutamate is replaced by a lysine and in PI-S a different glutamate is replaced by valine. It is not yet certain why these substitutions cause a reduced output of the gene products. And it is not absolutely clear why a decrease in α_1-antitrypsin production leads to disease, although it is possible that incompletely inhibited leucocyte proteases and gut proteases may digest lung parenchymal elastin and damage the liver.

A rare variant of PI, PI Pittsburg, has an arginine residue instead of a methionine at position 358; this molecule no longer inhibits elastase but, remarkably, it inhibits thrombin and hence leads to a severe haemorrhagic tendency in heterozygotes.

Defective receptor function

There is increasing evidence that point mutations may have profound effects on receptor function. One of the most elegant stories in this field is the elucidation of the mutations that involve different regions of the low-density-lipoprotein receptor gene, and which lead to the breakdown in the control of cholesterol metabolism and to the clinical picture of monogenic hypercholesterolaemia (Brown and Goldstein 1986; see also Section 2.7).

The low-density-lipoprotein receptor is a cell-surface glycoprotein that is synthesized in the rough endoplasmic reticulum as a precursor. The receptor has a complicated lifestyle which involves travelling to the Golgi complex and thence to the cell surface where it binds two proteins, apo B and apo E. The receptors undergo a remarkable recycling process. They appear on the cell surface in coated pits. Within a few minutes of their formation the pits invaginate to form endocytic vesicles. Multiple vesicles fuse to create larger sacs called endosomes. When the pH of the endosome falls below 6.4 the low-density lipoprotein dissociates from the receptor which then returns to the surface; each receptor makes one round trip about every 10 minutes in a continuous fashion, whether or not it is occupied by low-density lipoprotein.

Monogenic hypercholesterolaemia can result from a variety of mutations of the low-density-lipoprotein gene. At least some of the molecular defects are characterized by a marked reduction in the rate of receptor synthesis and are due to mechanisms that will be described later (see Section 2.7); in some cases no receptors are synthesized at all. A second class of mutations result in a reduced rate of transportation from the endoplasmic reticulum to the Golgi apparatus. A third class is characterized by normal synthesis but failure to bind low-density lipoprotein; several of these mutations involve amino-acid substitutions in the cysteine-rich low-density-lipoprotein binding domain. Finally, there is a class of mutations in which the receptors reach the cell surface and bind low-density lipoprotein but fail to cluster in coated pits. All the mutations that produce the latter abnormality involve the cytoplasmic tail of the receptor that protrudes into the cell cytoplasm; in one case, a single amino-acid substitution, tyrosine for cysteine in the middle of the cytoplasmic tail domain, is involved.

These remarkable studies underline the many ways in which receptor function may be interfered with by point mutations.

Mutations involving post-translational modification of proteins

Some proteins undergo post-translational modification in their structure. A number of point mutations have been described which interfere with this process (Weatherall 1991).

Insulin consists of two dissimilar peptide chains, A and B, linked by two disulphide bonds. However, unlike many other proteins that consist of structurally distinct subunits, insulin is under the control of a single gene locus and chains A and B are derived from a one-chain precursor, proinsulin. Proinsulin is converted to insulin by the enzymatic removal of a segment that connects the amino-terminal end of the A-chain to the carboxyl terminal end of the B-chain, called the C-peptide. A form of familial hyperproinsulinaemia results from mutations of the cleavage sites connecting the A-chains of the C-peptide.

Another example of a defect in post-translational modification is a mutation that is responsible for one form of the bleeding disorder Christmas disease (Bentley *et al.* 1986). Factor IX is synthesized as a precursor that is probably cleaved proteolytically in at least two positions during maturation, during which a prepeptide and propeptide region are removed. One type of Christmas disease results from a single amino-acid substitution at position −4 in the propeptide region; an arginine residue is replaced by a glutamine residue. This change results in the production of a stable, longer protein with 18 additional amino acids attached to the N-terminal propeptide regions. This observation suggests that during the normal maturation of factor IX a signal peptidase cleaves the peptide bond between amino acids −18 and −19, generating an unstable profactor IX intermediate; further proteolytic processing to the mature factor IX molecule must depend on the presence of the normal arginine residue at position −4. Interestingly, this arginine residue is not unique to the factor IX precursor but is also found in factor X and prothrombin, and in many other sequences processed by site-specific trypsin-like enzymes, C3, C4, and C5 of the complement system and tissue plasminogen activator, for example.

As mentioned earlier, haemoglobin variants have been found in which there are elongated globin chains, including some with additional residues at the N-terminal end. These offer some interesting insights into post-translational modification of proteins (Bunn and Forget 1986). The amino-terminal methionine residue, the translation product of the AUG initiation codon, is present only transiently in the nascent peptide chains of most proteins. One haemoglobin variant that has been studied in detail, haemoglobin Long Island, has a methionine residue at the end of the β-globin chain; the third residue is proline instead of histidine. It seems likely that this amino-acid substitution causes either a structural or a charge difference in the nascent β-globin chain, which interferes with the methionine-aminopeptidase mechanism or causes a change in the secondary structure of the messenger RNA of sufficient magnitude to impair the removal of the amino-terminal methionine residue.

In proteins that are secreted or membrane-bound, methionine constitutes the amino-terminal residue of a peptide of about 20 residues in length that may be essential for both protein secretion and its incorporation into membranes. This signal sequence, which is hydrophobic, varies in length and structure but always has methionine at its N-terminal end; it is cleaved by a membrane-bound enzyme in secreted proteins. Indeed, it has been found that the signal sequence is only one of the constituents of an 11S protein termed the signal recognition protein. Clearly, mutations involving such signal sequences may have a profound influence on secreted proteins, although it remains to be established whether the preserved amino-terminal methionine present in these mutant haemoglobins has any effect on their processing or cellular compartmentalization (see Prchal *et al.* 1986).

Developmental mutations

One of the most interesting questions in human biology is how genes are switched on and off at specific times during human development. The globin genes offer a particularly good example because human haemoglobin changes its structure between embryonic, fetal, and adult life (Fig. 2.24). The switch from fetal to adult haemoglobin reflects a change from γ- to β-globin chain production. There is a group of conditions with the general title 'hereditary persistence of fetal haemoglobin' (HPFH), in which there is a genetically determined defect in the normal switch from fetal to adult haemoglobin production. A family of point mutations has been found recently in the region −140 to −202, i.e. in a localized region of about 60 base pairs starting 140 bases upstream from the start of one or other of the γ-globin genes (Weatherall *et al.* 1989). It turns out that these genes function normally during fetal life, but during early development, instead of switching off completely they remain partially open so that adults with these mutations produce variable amounts of γ-globin chains and hence fetal haemoglobin.

These observations raise the interesting possibility that there are critical regulatory regions of DNA upstream from the structural genes which may have a role in interactions with specific proteins that play a part in the suppression of fetal globin genes during adult life. The site of these mutations is summarized in Fig. 2.29.

The mutations that we have just described relate to changes in the developmental pattern of a single gene cluster. However, it seems likely that over the next few years developmental mutations will provide us with information about much more widespread changes in development, such as occur in some serious congenital malformations. For example, it is has been found recently that the homeotic genes of the fruit fly *Drosophila*, which regulate the development of whole body segments, have DNA sequences in common with many other species, including worms, frogs, birds, mice, and man. Homeotic mutations in *Drosophila* result in major developmental abnormalities, including substitutions of one or more segments normally found elsewhere along the body axis. Interestingly, it has been observed recently that transgenic mice who had had the *myc* oncogene (see below) inserted into their genomes, produced offspring with deformities of their limbs. These deformities, and those of other strains of inbred mice, have changes reminiscent of certain homeotic mutations in *Drosophila*. It turns out that the limb deformity gene in mice is on chromosome 2 and that the *myc* gene insert in the transgenic mice with limb deformities is very close to this locus. The isolation of loci of this type, and studies of their mutations, should provide us with some major insights into the developmental genetics of congenital malformation.

Oncogene mutations

Retroviruses that cause cancers carry one or more specific genes that appear to be solely responsible for the neoplastic transforming properties of the virus. Hence they are called viral oncogenes. One of the most remarkable findings of recent years is

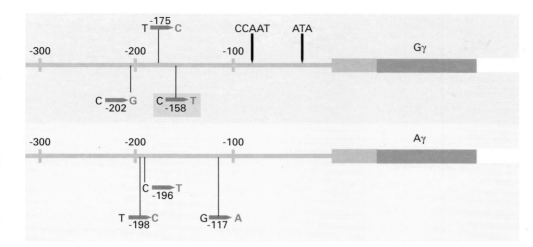

Fig. 2.29 Point mutations upstream from the fetal γ-globin genes associated with persistent fetal haemoglobin production. The boxed mutation is only expressed under conditions of erythropoietic stress.

that, in organisms ranging from yeast to man, genes have been found that are homologous to viral oncogenes; these cellular homologues are called cellular oncogenes (see also Chapter 9). It appears that they are all vital for a cell's normal behaviour and are responsible for the control of proliferation, differentiation, and maturation. The cellular oncogenes are named after their viral counterparts; for example c-*abl* is the cellular homologue of the viral oncogene of the Ableson murine leukaemia virus.

Transfection of DNA isolated from human or other mammalian cells into particular cell lines has turned out to be a valuable analytical tool for studying the action of oncogenes. The cell line used most extensively is a murine fibroblast line (NIH3T3). DNA sequences derived from human and other tumour cells are capable of inducing transformation in these cells, i.e. in causing their disordered growth. By digesting the DNA of these cells with particular restriction enzymes it has been possible to show that the transforming activity is related to specific cellular oncogenes. Although there are a number of ways in which oncogenes can be abnormally activated, it appears that, remarkably, a single amino-acid substitution can confer this property (Bishop 1987). For example, a Ha-*ras* gene cloned from a bladder carcinoma cell line is capable of NIH3T3 cell transformation; it differs from the wild type (non-transforming Ha-*ras* gene) by the substitution of valine for glycine. Point mutations have been found in a variety of oncogenes isolated from tumours, ranging from bladder and colon carcinoma to acute myeloid leukaemia and myelodysplasia; in each case these mutated oncogenes have been shown to have transforming properties.

Although it is still not clear how these point mutations confer transforming properties on oncogenes, some progress has been made. One example must suffice (Bargmann *et al.* 1986). The *neu* oncogene, which is frequently activated in tumours of the nervous system in rats, directs the synthesis of a protein called p185. This is glycosylated and accessible to antisera in intact cells, suggesting that at least part of it is localized on the cell surface. Its gene has sequence similarities to that for the epidermal growth factor receptor. Recent structural studies suggest that it is a transmembrane protein consisting of an extracellular region of about 650 amino acids, a transmembrane domain, and an intracellular portion of about 580 amino acids, part of which consists of a tyrosine kinase domain. It turns out that a single point mutation, valine to glutamic acid, is enough to endow the transforming properties on this oncogene. A possible interpretation of this observation is that this substitution causes the receptor to be active in the absence of ligand and hence to deliver a continuous proliferative signal to an affected cell. This effect might in turn result from clustering of the receptor, stabilization of an interaction between it and its substrate or other effectors in the membrane, or simply by exerting a physical constraint that shifts the receptor slightly inward or outward in the membrane.

It seems likely that as other point mutations are identified at this level it should be possible to determine how they might alter the behaviour of a cell so that it undergoes neoplastic transformation.

2.4.5 Molecular lesions that result in a reduced amount of normal gene product

Many genetic disorders are characterized by a reduced amount of an enzyme or other type of protein; such gene product as is produced is structurally normal. Although it used to be thought that many of these conditions might result from mutations of regulatory loci, recent work has proved that this is not the case. In fact, the majority of them seem to result from simple *cis*-acting mutations that involve the structural genes or sequences in their flanking regions or adjacent areas of DNA (Davies and Robson 1987).

The most spectacular progress in our understanding of the molecular pathology of this class of disorders has followed work on the thalassaemias, the commonest genetic diseases of mankind (Bunn and Forget 1986; Weatherall *et al.* 1989). This heterogeneous group of conditions is characterized by a reduced rate of synthesis of one or more pairs of the globin chains of adult haemoglobin. The commonest types of thalassaemia are α- and β-thalassaemia, which are characterized by defective α- or β-globin-chain synthesis, respectively. This leads to imbalanced globin-chain production; most of the clinical and haematological manifestations can be ascribed to the deleterious effects of the globin subunits that are produced in excess.

The genetic control of haemoglobin and the arrangement of the different globin genes is summarized in Fig. 2.24 (see above). As shown, there are two α-globin genes per haploid genome, but only one β-globin gene. The α-thalassaemias are classified into α^+-thalassaemia, in which there is reduced α-chain production, usually representing the output of only one of the pair of linked α-globin genes, and α^0-thalassaemia in which the output of both genes is defective. The β-thalassaemias are similarly classified; in β^+-thalassaemia there is a reduced output of β-globin chains while in β^0-thalassaemia no globin chains are synthesized.

Sequence analyses of the α- and β-globin genes of patients with α- or β-thalassaemia have provided us with a remarkable picture of the repertoire of human molecular pathology; indeed they have probably shown us most of the mutations that can involve structual genes. In the sections that follow we shall examine the different mechanisms that underlie these conditions and other genetic disorders that are characterized by a reduced output of a particular gene product.

Gene deletions and variation in gene number

There are many examples of partial or complete deletions of genes as the basis for inherited diseases (Table 2.2). Furthermore, we are starting to learn about how such deletional events may have occurred. One field that has been particularly productive in this respect is the analysis of the α-thalassaemias.

As shown in Figs 2.24 and 2.30, there are two closely linked α-globin genes on chromosome 16. In the α^+-thalassaemias there is a deletion involving this chromosome which leaves a single functional α gene. In many forms of α^0-thalassaemia both α-globin genes are lost. The most likely mechanism for the production of a chromosome with a single α-globin gene is non-homologous crossing-over between the two α-globin gene loci after mispairing of homologous chromosomes during meiosis. Duplicated loci, like the α-genes, have arisen by a reduplication event that is mirrored by regions of homology in the flanking regions of the particular genes involved. In the case of the α-globin genes these regions are designated X, Y, and Z. In fact a number of different crossovers have occurred within these homology boxes, resulting in different types of α^+-thalassaemia. If these ideas are correct, the reciprocal product of the crossover event, a chromosome carrying three α-globin gene loci, should be observed. In fact such cases have been found in every human population that has been studied so far. Similar mechanisms are almost certainly involved in the generation of variable numbers

Table 2.2 Examples of the molecular pathology of single gene diseases

Point mutations leading to structural variants:
  Abnormal haemoglobins
  G6PD deficiency
  α_1-antitrypsin deficiency
  Hereditary amyloidosis
  Familial hypercholesterolaemia

Nonsense mutations:
  β-thalassaemia
  Familial hypercholesterolaemia (low-density-lipoprotein receptor)
  Factor VIII or IX deficiency
  Cystic fibrosis

Frame-shift mutations:
  β-thalassaemia
  Familial hypercholesterolaemia (low-density-lipoprotein receptor)
  Factor VIII or IX deficiency
  Cystic fibrosis

Promoter mutations:
  β-thalassaemia

Deletions:
  α-thalassaemia
  β-thalassaemia, HPFH*, $\delta\beta$-thalassaemia
  Growth hormone deficiency
  Anti-thrombin III deficiency
  Factor VIII or IX deficiency
  Elliptocytosis (band 4,1)
  Lesch–Nyhan syndrome (HGPRT)
  Duchenne muscular dystrophy
  Osteogenesis imperfecta
  Familial hypercholesterolaemia (low-density-lipoprotein receptor)
  Chorionic somatomammotropin deficiency
  Retinoblastoma
  Wilms tumour

Inversions:
  $\delta\beta$-thalassaemia

Fusion genes:
  Haemoglobin variants, thalassaemia
  Red/green colour blindness

Initiation codon mutations:
  α-thalassaemia

Termination codon mutations:
  α-thalassaemia

RNA processing mutations:
  Obligatory sequence
    β-thalassaemia
    Phenylketonuria
  Consensus sequence
    β-thalassaemia
  Pseudosplice substitution
    β-thalassaemia
  Cryptic splice site activation
    β-thalassaemia, haemoglobin E
  PolyA addition site
    α-thalassaemia
    β-thalassaemia

Signal peptide mutation
  Christmas disease
  Haemoglobin variants

* Hereditary persistence of fetal haemoglobin.

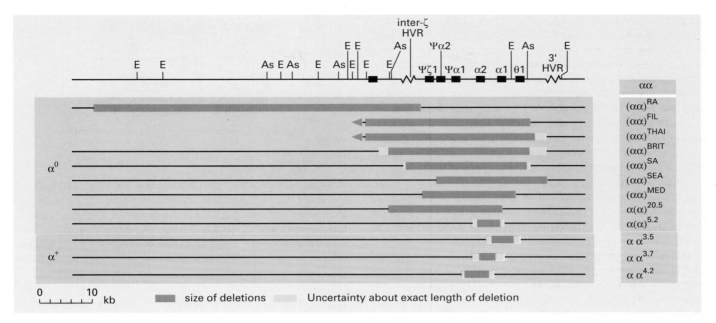

Fig. 2.30 A map of the α-gene cluster and the deletions that underlie the α-thalassaemias. The α and ζ genes are shown as boxes. The letters signify restriction enzyme sites. The red regions indicate size of deletions. Yellow ends indicate uncertainty about exact length of deletions. Superscripts indicate country of origin or size of deletion.

of γ-globin genes on chromosome 11; individuals with one, three, or even four γ-genes have been found.

There are other mechanisms for the production of gene deletions. Recent work on both the α⁰-thalassaemia gene deletions and on long deletions that involve the β-globin gene cluster and give rise to the phenotype of hereditary persistence of fetal haemoglobin (HPFH) have shown some of the breakpoints of the deletions involve sequences with characteristics of *Alu*I repeats. The *Alu*I family, so-called because of the presence of a recognition site for this restriction endonuclease in the centre of the repeat sequence, constitutes a series of repeats of about 300 nucleotides that occur some 300 000 times throughout the human genome. These units, although they have a high level of homology, have no known function despite the fact that at least some of them are transcribed. In addition to the deletions involving the α- or β-globin gene cluster there is an example of a deletion involving the gene for the low-density-lipoprotein receptor in which Alu–Alu recombination has occurred. It is possible that because of their high degree of homology the Alu repetitive sequences serve as 'hotspots' for recombination. On the other hand, at least some of the long deletions which produce HPFH and α⁰-thalassaemia appear to be through non-related sequences; that is they are examples of illegitimate recombination.

Another interesting feature of deletions of the α- and β-globin gene clusters is that in many cases they are of similar length although at different points along the genome (Vanin *et al.* 1983; Nicholls *et al.* 1987). A rather novel mechanism has been suggested to explain these observations. It proposes that the deletions are generated by the loss of chromatin loops at different stages of DNA replication as chromatin moves through specific attachment sites on the nuclear matrix. Following breakage, the two ends of the DNA become reunited with the loss of a loop; recent evidence in favour of this observation has been obtained from the study of an α⁰-thalassaemia deletion in which the gap across the deletion appears to have been filled in by a DNA sequence that is found normally at least 34 kilobases upstream from the site of the deletion. This could only have happened if the deletion had involved a large loop of DNA which brought the 'filler' sequence into the observed site and orientation (Nicholls *et al.* 1987).

It is becoming apparent that many other genetic disorders result from gene deletions. Many X-linked diseases are due to new mutations; a number of different sized deletions have been found to underlie conditions such as haemophilia, Christmas disease, and Duchenne muscular dystrophy. The deletions vary in size from small intragenic lesions to enormous lesions that remove the whole of these very large structural genes. For example, one deletion found in a haemophiliac child removes the whole of the factor VIII gene; this was found to be a *de novo* deletion since it was not present in the boy's mother. Deletions have also been found in some, though by no means all, cases of genetic growth hormone deficiency and antithrombin III deficiency. Some of the other conditions in which gene deletions have been observed are summarized in Table 2.2.

Fusion genes

Another interesting and important result of abnormal chromosomal crossing-over is the production of fusion genes which code for hybrid proteins. The first and best-studied example is haemoglobin Lepore, mentioned earlier, which has normal α-chains combined with non-α-chains which have the N-terminal amino-acid sequence of δ-chains and the C-terminal sequence of β-chains. This variant appears to have arisen through non-homologous crossing-over between part of the δ locus on one chromosome and part of the β locus on the complementary chromosome (see Fig. 2.27). As mentioned earlier, such an event could give rise to two abnormal chromosomes, one with a Lepore gene and the other with its opposite counterpart, an anti-Lepore gene. In fact both these arrangements have been found in a number of patients. A similar mechanism seems to have been involved in the production of one of the sialoglycoproteins of the red cell surface.

Another elegant example of the generation of variation in gene number and the production of fusion genes is provided by recent studies on the molecular genetics of colour vision and colour blindness (Nathans *et al.* 1986). Human colour vision is based on three light-sensitive pigments. The genes for the red and green pigments show 96 per cent identity and lie in a tandem array on the X-chromosome on which there is a single red-pigment gene and variable numbers of green-pigment genes; the blue-pigment gene shows less homology and is on an autosome. Many of the different forms of red/green colour blindness appear to have resulted from unequal crossing-over between the red- and green-pigment genes, with the production of a variety of different fusion genes (see above).

Inversions

There is one example of a gene inversion in man. This has been found in several patients with the phenotype of δβ-thalassaemia, a condition in which there is no δ- or β-chain production from the affected chromosome. The inversion involves a region of DNA between the δ- and γ-globin genes; there is also a small deletion at each end of the inversion. A model has been proposed whereby an inversion of this type is generated by interactions between two chromosomal loops.

Nonsense mutations

A number of point mutations have been described which cause scrambling of the genetic code and hence make it impossible for the translation of a normal gene product. Again, most of these examples come from the thalassaemia field, although similar lesions have been observed as the basis for disorders such as haemophilia, Christmas disease, and several other single gene conditions. The first of these to be identified was a substitution of codon 17 of the β-globin messenger RNA, AAG→UAG, which changes a lysine codon to a premature termination codon. Another premature termination codon of this type is found commonly in patients with β-thalassaemia, in this case an alteration in codon 39, CAG→UAG; CAG codes for glutamine in the normal β-globin chain. Clearly, if there is a chain-termination codon in the middle of messenger RNA, translation will cease prematurely with the production of a shortened and physiologically useless peptide chain (Fig. 2.31).

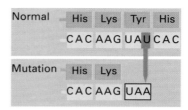

Fig. 2.31 The mechanism of a nonsense mutation.

Frameshift mutations

Another way in which the genetic code can be scrambled is by the generation of a so-called frameshift mutation, the basis of at least seven different forms of β-thalassaemia and some cases of haemophilia and Christmas disease. Since proteins are encoded by a triplet code, the loss or insertion of one, two, or four nucleotides in the coding region of a gene will throw the reading frame out of sequence. As a result a completely anomalous amino-acid sequence will be added to a normally initiated globin chain. Sometimes the altered base sequence generates a new termination codon, leading to premature termination of translation of the abnnormal messenger RNA (Fig. 2.32). Occasionally the messenger RNA may be translatable, and in this case there is a complete change of sequence from normal after the site of the frameshift mutation. As mentioned earlier, at least one form of human haemoglobin variant with an elongated β-chain results from a frameshift mutation; in this case the normal stop codon is rendered out of sequence and therefore the scrambled messenger RNA is translated until another stop codon is produced, so leading to an elongated translation product.

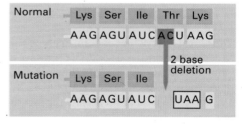

Fig. 2.32 The mechanism of a framesift mutation with the production of a premature stop codon.

Defective processing of messenger RNA

As described earlier (Section 2.3), the primary transcript has to be processed by the removal of introns, joining together of exons, and by polyadenylation. Work in the thalassaemia field has provided a wealth of examples of molecular pathology involving these complex processes (Orkin and Kazazian 1984; Weatherall *et al.* 1989).

We have already discussed how normal splicing of messenger RNA is dependent on having GT and AG dinucleotides at the 5′ and 3′ intron–exon junctions. There are several examples of forms of β⁰-thalassaemia in which a single base substitution in one of these critical sites completely abolishes β-globin chain

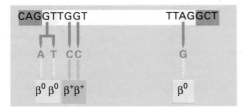

Fig. 2.33 Intron–exon junction mutations. In the β^0-thalassaemia mutations the genes are completely inactivated, while in the β^+-thalassaemia mutations the β-genes are partly inactivated.

production; no normal messenger RNA is produced (Fig. 2.33). These findings underline the critical importance of these sequences for normal splicing. A similar type of lesion is responsible for the form of phenylketonuria that is common in some North European populations.

However, there are much more subtle abnormalities of messenger RNA processing due to point mutations. Several examples are listed in Table 2.2. Single base substitutions within introns may result in preferential alternative splicing of the precursor β messenger RNA molecules at the site of the mutation. For example, a common form of β-thalassaemia that occurs in the Mediterranean population results from a single nucleotide substitution, G→A, at position 110 of the first intervening sequence (IVS1) of the β-globin gene. This change produces an AG sequence that happens to be preceded by a stretch of pyrimidines and thus forms a good 3' acceptor concensus sequence. Thus about 90 per cent of the processed messenger RNA is the result of splicing into this site rather than the normal 3' IVS1 AG (Fig. 2.34). The messenger RNA produced from the

abnormal splicing contains intron sequences and is therefore useless as a template for globin chain synthesis. Because this site is used preferentially more abnormal than normal messenger RNA is produced and therefore there is a severe deficiency of normal β-chain production.

Several other forms of thalassaemia have been described that result from the production of alternative splicing sites within introns. For example, there are two varieties that are caused by single base changes at positions 5 or 6 at the 5' end of the first intervening sequence (Fig. 2.35). Splicing occurs both at the normal site and at the new sites generated by these base changes. The effect of these point mutations are remarkably subtle. Some mutations at position 5 cause a severe defect in β-chain production, while that at position 6 is associated with an extremely mild phenotype. Several other types of thalassaemia have been described in which point mutations in the second intervening sequence cause similar alternate splicing and hence abnormal β-globin messenger RNA molecules.

Perhaps even more remarkable is the fact that mutations have been found in exons of the globin genes that seem to activate 'cryptic' splice sites. One of these is particularly interesting because it is also associated with the production of a structural haemoglobin variant, haemoglobin E. This variant has a lysine for glutamic acid substitution at position 26. This results from a codon change GAG→AAG (Fig. 2.36). The latter seems to activate a 'cryptic' splice site which competes with the normal 5' splice site and hence leads to a reduced output of β-globin

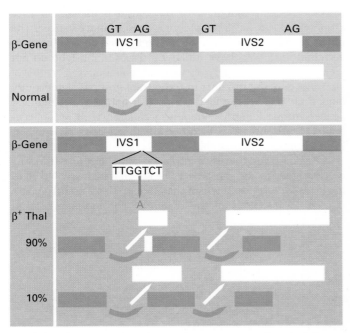

Fig. 2.34 The production of a new donor acceptor splice site in intron 1 as the mechanism underlying a form of β^+-thalassaemia (IVS = intervening sequence).

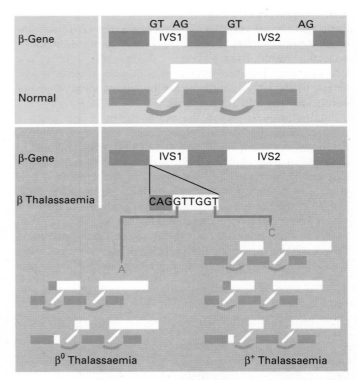

Fig. 2.35 The different phenotypes produced by point mutations in the consensus sequence in IVS1 of the human β-globin gene (see text for details).

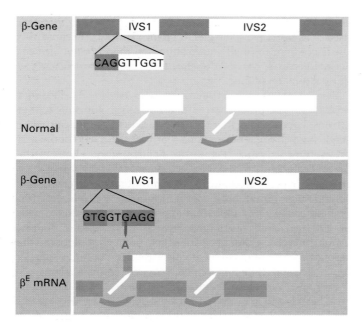

Fig. 2.36 The activation of a cryptic splice sequence in exon 1 as the mechanism for the production of abnormal messenger RNA associated with haemoglobin E (for details see text).

chains. This may be why the haemoglobin E is associated with a β-thalassaemia phenotype.

Several other single gene disorders are now known to result from splicing defects. These include one form of phenylketonuria and several varieties of haemophilia and Christmas disease. Recent studies suggest that one form of factor IX deficiency results from a deletion of an entire exon of the factor IX gene. Despite this an abnormal gene product is produced, presumably by linking the remaining exons together during messenger RNA processing.

Finally, polyadenylation site mutations may also interfere with the normal processing of messenger RNA. For example, the single base change AATAAA→AATAAC, which is found in the α-globin genes of patients with α-thalassaemia in the Middle East and Mediterranean region, seems to almost entirely prevent the production of α-globin chains from the α2-globin gene. Instead of the normal cutting and polyadenylation of the messenger RNA precursor, a long molecule that does not appear in the cell cytoplasm is produced. There may be a small amount of polyadenylated messenger RNA produced, but the overall effect is to almost entirely inactivate the α2-globin gene. It is also possible that this mutation may in some way interfere with the termination of α2-globin gene transcription. A similar polyadenylation site mutation has been observed in the β-globin gene as the basis for one type of β-thalassaemia.

Initiation codon mutations

Several mutations have been observed in patients with α-thalassaemia that involve either the initiation codon itself or the sequences that immediately precede it. As would be expected, these cause a complete absence of normal α-gene product.

Promotor box mutations

Several forms of β-thalassaemia have been described in which point mutations have been found 'upstream' from the β-globin gene (Fig. 2.37), either within or adjacent to the promotor boxes described in Section 2.3. These mutations are associated with a variable reduction in output from the adjacent locus. Their existence underlines the importance of these highly conserved regions of DNA and confirms their likely promotor function.

Recessive genes and cancer

There is increasing evidence that specific gene loci may be involved in retinoblastomas and certain other rare childhood tumours (Cavanee *et al.* 1983; Nyhan 1987; see Chapter 9). It appears that these tumours may be the result of as few as two events, one of which can be inherited as an autosomal recessive trait.

Solid tumours in childhood occur in two types of patients. Some carry a germinal mutation, have multiple tumours (in the case of retinoblastoma the tumours occur in both eyes), and are at increased risk for developing a second primary cancer. The other group is comprised of children who do not carry a germinal mutation, have unilateral disease, and who do not seem to be at risk for carrying a second malignancy. The time of appearance of the tumours in the second group is significantly later than that in the first. These two patterns of childhood cancer are particularly common in children with retinoblastoma but are also seen in other childhood cancers, such as Wilms tumour and neuroblastoma.

The gene locus that is involved in retinoblastoma (Rb) has been assigned to chromosome 13 (13q14). It is closely linked to the locus for esterase D which therefore acts as a useful genetic marker for deletions of the region of chromosome 13 that carries the Rb locus.

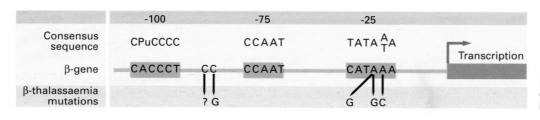

Fig. 2.37 The site of mutations in or near the promotor boxes as the basis for β-thalassaemia.

There is now substantial evidence that the generation of a retinoblastoma requires the loss or inactivation of *both* alleles at the Rb locus on chromosome 13. The first clue that this might be the case came from the study of a family in which a patient was found to have a very small deletion of 13q14 which, although it could not be identified cytogenetically, was suspected because of the reduced amount of esterase D activity in the patient's red cells. When the tumour was examined, although both chromosomes 13 appeared to be cytogenetically normal there was no detectable esterase D activity. This suggested that the chromosome(s) 13 in the tumour cells contained a small deletion of both the RB and esterase D genes. This notion has now been confirmed by restriction endonuclease analysis.

These observations, together with further studies of chromosome 13 in retinoblastomas using restriction enzyme polymorphisms to identify individual members of pairs of homologous chromosomes, have confirmed the idea that the development of retinoblastoma requires two events. The first is inactivation of one Rb locus (Rb$^+$→Rb$^-$). This 'first event' could occur in several ways. In the familial forms of retinoblastoma it would be inherited, whereas in the sporadic unilateral cases it would be acquired as a mutation of the Rb locus in germ or somatic cells. It might also be acquired as part of a deletion of chromosome 13. Whatever the mechanism, a 'second event' is required in a retinoblast such that the other Rb locus is inactivated. Extensive cytogenetic and restriction enzyme analysis of DNA from retinoblastomas has shown that this may occur in several ways. For example, by comparing various restriction fragment length polymorphisms on chromosomes 13 in other tissues with those in the tumour it is apparent that in many cases there is a non-disjunctional loss of one chromosome 13 with duplication of the remaining chromosome 13 in the tumour cells. In other cases there seems to have been mitotic recombination of one chromosome 13, the breakpoint being near to 13q14 and leading to homozygosity at this region (mitotic recombination means that there has been crossing-over between homologous chromosomes during mitosis). A variety of other mechanisms could result in loss of the Rb$^+$ locus, leading to the absence of its gene product and hence to tumour formation. Recent work suggests that the product of the Rb locus is a DNA-binding protein.

An extremely important concept arises from these studies (Murphree and Benedict 1984; Nyhan 1987). It appears that certain tumours arise from the action of recessive cancer 'genes'. We can either be born heterozygous for one of these genes, or acquire one as a germinal or somatic mutation. If things remain like this we can go through life never knowing we have this gene, and we will not develop cancer. On the other hand, if there is a gene rearrangement in a particular tissue that involves the loss of the normal allele, then a cancer will develop. There is increasing evidence that other childhood cancers, such as Wilms tumour, familial renal carcinoma, and neuroblastoma, may have a similar origin (Solomon 1984). For example, the aniridia–Wilms tumour syndrome is associated with a small deletion of chromosome 11 (11p13). As in the retinoblastoma

studies, comparison of the restriction fragment length polymorphism, in this case on chromosome 11, between normal tissues and the tumour shows that the tumour cells are homozygous for the Wilms tumour (WT) locus. These studies illustrate the extraordinary power of restriction enzyme technology in analysing the molecular genetics of certain human cancers.

Mutations that are 'distant' from structural genes

As we have seen, most of the mutations that interfere with the production of peptide chains or enzymes involve either the structural genes themselves or important regulatory sequences in their flanking regions or in 'upstream regulatory boxes'. However, some exceptions are appearing. For example, several deletions have been found in the α- or β-globin gene complex which lie upstream from the α- or β-globin genes and yet appear to switch them off. In one of those, involving the α-globin genes, the deletion ends about 16 kilobases upstream from the α-globin genes yet the latter appear to be completely inactivated. Recent work suggests that these deletions inactivate major control regions called locus control regions (LCRs) which regulate the whole of the α and β globin gene clusters and are responsible for their expression in haemopoietic tissues.

Apart from these positional effects produced by long deletions, there is some evidence, again from the globin field, that unlinked genes may have effects on structural genes. For example, there is one type of hereditary persistence of fetal haemoglobin, in which the genetic determinant appears to segregate quite independently from the globin gene clusters. Whether this represents a true regulatory gene mutation remains to be determined, however; but the bulk of monogenic disorders seem to result from simple *cis*-acting mutations that involve the structural genes or their immediate environment.

2.4.6 Phenotype–genotype relationships for mutations that alter the output of structural genes

Although it is still early days, a start has been made in trying to relate the molecular lesions outlined in the previous sections to associated clinical phenotypes. As might be expected, deletions completely inactivate structural genes. Thus the α^0- and β^0-thalassaemias are associated with a complete absence of adult haemoglobin production and, usually, with a severe clinical phenotype. Similarly, the large deletions that involve the factor VIII or IX genes cause a complete deficiency of the clotting factor products and severe forms of haemophilia or Christmas disease. And deletions of the Duchenne locus on the X-chromosome also produce typical Duchenne muscular dystrophy. It has been established recently that the product of this locus, dystrophin, is a large protein that may be involved in calcium transport.

However, even when a gene is completely inactivated in this way there may be some variation in the clinical phenotype. For example, β^0-thalassaemia is not always severe, and there is increasing evidence that such variability may result from inherited differences in ability to produce the γ-chains of fetal haemoglobin and hence to compensate for defective β-chain production. Similarly, there is variability in the phenotype of the muscular dystrophies; some of the milder forms seem to have deletions that are of similar length to those which are associated with the more severe phenotypes. And, remarkably, it has been observed that there is even clinical heterogeneity in the effect of deletions of the low-density-lipoprotein receptor gene; some cases present with serious vascular disease due to hypercholesterolaemia in the first year or two of life while others seem to survive into adulthood. It seems likely that such heterogeneity will be explained, as in the case of thalassaemia, by the interaction of other genes, the identity of which remains to be determined.

The mutations that involve splicing or the upstream regulatory boxes are associated with a wide variety of clinical phenotypes. Some of them cause a very small reduction in the output of the affected locus and therefore are associated with a very mild clinical phenotype. For example, most of the β-thalassaemias that are due to mutations in or near the upstream regulatory boxes have a mild phenotype. As we learn more about the molecular pathology of single gene disorders we shall be able to describe phenotypes ranging from almost normal to lethal, based on the precise site and action of these point mutations.

The determination of the molecular pathology of single gene disorders also offers insight into the way in which some of these diseases are produced. For example, using restriction fragment length polymorphism analysis it is now possible to define loci for which the gene products are not known. Good examples include Duchenne muscular dystrophy and chronic granulomatous disease. Once the particular genes have been found it is possible to gain some insights into the likely protein products and hence to determine the cause of the disease. This procedure, known as reverse genetics, offers considerable scope for determining the cause of genetic diseases of unknown aetiology. This new field has already led to the identification of the genes involved in Duchenne muscular dystrophy and cystic fibrosis, and has allowed a partial characterization of their products and the identification of many of the mutations which underlie these conditions. It should not be long before the functions of the protein products of these loci are defined and hence the precise aetiology of these diseases determined (Koenig *et al.* 1987; Monaco 1989; Kerem *et al.* 1989).

2.4.7   Implications for the future: polygenic disease

It is clear that we now have a very good idea of the repertoire of molecular defects that can involve structural genes, and that we are already starting to understand how these lesions are manifested in their associated clinical phenotypes. Hence we can start to define a spectrum of effects of these mutations, ranging from a complete absence of a gene product to a very mild reduction in its rate of production. As we define the

different genes involved in polygenic disorders, and we characterize the mutations involved in cellular oncogenes, we shall be able to extrapolate information obtained from studies of the single gene disorders to help us to understand the diverse modifications of gene function that underlie many common polygenic disorders, and the somatic mutations that underlie at least some forms of cancer.

2.4.8   Bibliography

Bargmann, C. I., Hung, M. C., and Weinberg, R. A. (1986). Multiple independent activations of the *neu* oncogene by a point mutation altering the transmembrane domain of p185. *Cell* **45**, 649–57.

Bentley, A. K., Rees, D. J. G., Rizza, C., and Brownlee, G. G. (1986). Defective propeptide processing of blood clotting factor IX caused by a mutation of arginine to glutamine at position − 4. *Cell* **45**, 343–8.

Bishop, M. J. (1987). The molecular genetics of cancer. *Science* **235**, 305–11.

Brown, M. S. and Goldstein, J. L. (1986). A receptor-mediated pathway for cholesterol homeostasis. *Science* **232**, 34–47.

Bunn, H. F. and Forget, B. G. (1986). *Haemoglobin: molecular genetic and clinical aspects.* W. B. Saunders, Philadelphia.

Carrell, R. W., *et al.* (1982). Structure and variation of human alpha$_1$-antitrypsin. *Nature* **298**, 329–34.

Cavanee, W. K., *et al.* (1983). Expression of recessive alleles by chromosomal mechanisms in retinoblastoma. *Nature* **305**, 779–84.

Charache, S. (1974). Haemoglobins with altered oxygen affinity. *Clinics in Haematology* **3**, 357–81.

Davies, K. E. and Robson, K. J. H. (1987). Molecular analysis of human monogenic diseases. *BioEssays* **6**, 247–53.

Kerem, B.-T., Rommens, J. M., Buchanan, J. A., Markiewicz, D., Cox, T. K., Chakravarti, A., *et al.* (1989). Identification of the cystic fibrosis gene: genetic analysis. *Science* **245**, 1073–80.

Koenig, M., Hoffman, E. P., Bertelson, C. J., Monaco, A. P., Feener, C., and Kunkel, L. M. (1987). Complete cloning of the Duchenne muscular dystrophy (DMD) cDNA and preliminary genomic organization of the DMD gene in normal and affected individuals. *Cell* **50**, 509–17.

McKusick, V. A. (1990). *Mendelian inheritance in man* (9th edn). Johns Hopkins University Press, Baltimore.

Milner, P. F. and Wrightstone, R. N. (1981). The unstable haemoglobins: a review. In *The function of red blood cells: erythrocyte pathobiology*, pp. 197–222. Alan R. Liss, New York.

Monaco, A. P. (1989). Dystrophin, the protein product of the Duchenne/Becker muscular dystrophy gene. *Trends in Biochemistry* **14**, 412–15.

Murphree, A. L. and Benedict, W. F. (1984). Retinoblastoma: clues to human oncogenesis. *Science* **223**, 1028–33.

Nathans, J., Thomas, D., and Hogness, D. S. (1986). Molecular genetics of human color vision: the genes encoding the blue, green, and red pigments. *Science* **232**, 193–202.

Nicholls, R. D., Fischel-Ghodsian, N., and Higgs, D. R. (1987). Recombination at the human α-globin gene cluster: sequence features and topological constraints. *Cell* **49**, 369–78.

Nyhan, W. L. (1987). Retinoblastoma—genetic insights into neoplasia. *BioEssays* **6**, 5–8.

Orkin, S. H. and Kazazian, H. H., Jr (1984). Mutations and polymorphisms of the human β-globin gene and its surrounding DNA. *Annual Review of Genetics* **18**, 131–71.

Prchal, J. T., Cashman, D. P., and Kan, Y. W. (1986). Haemoglobin Long Island is caused by a single mutation (adenine to cytosine) resulting in a failure to cleave amino-terminal methionine. *Proceedings of the National Academy of Sciences, USA* **83**, 24–7.

Solomon, E. (1984). Recessive mutation in aetiology of Wilms' tumour. *Nature* **309**, 111–12.

Vanin, E. F., Henthorn, P. S., Kioussis, D., Grosveld, F., and Smithies, O. (1983). Unexpected relationships between four large deletions in the human β-globin gene cluster. *Cell* **35**, 701–9.

Weatherall, D. J. (1991). *The new genetics and clinical practice* (3rd edn). Oxford University Press.

Weatherall, D. J. and Clegg, J. B. (1975). The α chain termination mutants and their relationship to α thalassaemia. *Philosophical Transactions of the Royal Society of London* **271**, 411.

Weatherall, D. J. and Clegg, J. B. (1981). *The thalassaemia syndromes* (3rd edn). Blackwell Scientific Publications, Oxford.

Weatherall, D. J., Clegg, J. B., Higgs, D. R., and Wood, W. G. (1989). The haemoglobinopathies. In *The metabolic basis of inherited disease* (6th edn) (ed. C. R. Scriver, A. L. Beaudet, W. S. Sly, and D. Valle). McGraw-Hill, New York.

Woo, S. L. C., Lidsky, A. S., Guttler, F., Chandra, T. and Robson, K. J. H. (1983). Cloned human phenylalanine hydroxylase gene allows prenatal diagnosis and carrier detection of classical phenylketonuria. *Nature* **306**, 151–55.

Worton, R. G. (1987). Molecular analysis of Duchenne and Becker muscular dystrophy. *BioEssays* **7**, 57–62.

2.5　Storage disorders

E. Beutler

2.5.1　Introduction

In the normal steady state, complex molecules are continuously synthesized and degraded. These processes are enzymatic in nature and multiple enzymes are involved; both synthesis and degradation are stepwise processes. The storage diseases are the result of a genetic lesion affecting one of the degrading enzymes. The modest decrease of enzymatic activity occurring in heterozygotes is not usually sufficient to cause the accumulation of storage material. Thus, storage diseases are either autosomal recessive in nature or, as in Fabry disease or Hunter' syndrome, sex linked.

Table 2.3 summarizes some of the storage diseases, indicating the primary enzymatic defect and the nature of the storage material.

2.5.2　Lysosomal hydrolases

Most of the storage diseases are due to deficiencies in lysosomal hydrolases, and these enzymes have several properties in common. One feature of lysosomal enzymes that plays an important role in their synthesis and targeting to lysosomes is the so-called signal sequence. This hydrophobic stretch of amino acids appears to be essential for the translocation of the enzyme across the endoplasmic reticulum, and is 'clipped' from the enzyme as it is being formed on the ribosome. Lysosomal enzymes are glycoproteins, often containing a high proportion of carbohydrate. The attachment of carbohydrate to the protein is a function of certain sequences in the polypeptide itself and depends upon a number of different glycosyltransferases and glycosylases that fashion the carbohydrate structure of the enzyme. After translocation across the endoplasmic reticulum, lysosomal enzymes undergo glycosylation of selected asparagine residues. A preformed oligosaccharide is transferred to the nascent polypeptide. Some of the sugars are then excised, and the glycoproteins moved to the Golgi apparatus where phosphomannosyl residues are generated by the sequential action of two enzymes. First, a phosphotransferase attaches *N*-acetylglucosamine-1-phosphate to selected mannose residues to form a phosphodiester intermediate. An *N*-acetylglucosamine-1-phosphodiester-α-acetylglucosaminidase removes the

Table 2.3 Some of the storage diseases

Disease eponym	Storage material	Enzyme deficiency
von Gierke	Glycogen	Glucose-6-phosphatase
Pompe	Glycogen	α-1,4-glucosidase (acid maltase)
Cori	Limit dextrin	Amylo-1,6-glucosidase (debrancher enzyme)
Andersen	Abnormal glycogen	α-1,4-glucan: α-1,4-glucan 6-glucosyl transferase (brancher enzyme)
McArdle	Muscle glycogen	Muscle phosphorylase
Refsum	Phytanic acid	Phytanic acid α-hydroxylase
Hurler	Mucopolysaccharide	α-L-iduronidase
Hunter	Mucopolysaccharide	Iduronate sulphatase
Wolman	Various lipids	Acid lipase
Niemann–Pick	Sphingomyelin	Sphingomyelinase
Fabry	Ceramide trihexoside	α-galactosidase A
Gaucher	Glucocerebroside	Acid β-glucosidase
Tay–Sachs	GM$_2$ ganglioside	Hexosaminidase A

N-acetylglucosamine residue to expose a mannose-6-phosphate recognition signal. This signal is required for binding to specific receptors that target the enzyme to the proper location in the lysosomal membrane. This sequence of events is summarized in Fig. 2.38.

The enzymes that catalyse the addition and modification of carbohydrate act on a variety of glycoproteins, and mutations in such enzymes cause multiple protein abnormalities. Thus, in I-cell disease, a deficiency of phosphotransferase results in deficiencies of multiple glycohydrolases. Since hereditary storage diseases are usually caused by the deficiency of a single enzyme, it follows that the defects are in the basic polypeptide backbone of the enzyme itself, not in the pattern of glycosylation. The carbohydrate portion of the enzyme does not appear to play a major role in its catalytic function. Rather, it appears to be involved in proper movement of the enzyme to the lysosome. It has been likened to the 'Zip code' that routes mail to the correct post office. In I-cell disease the affected enzymes are actually synthesized but are excreted from the cell rather than being packaged into lysosomes.

In addition to the removal of signal sequences and attachment and remodelling of carbohydrate of lysosomal enzymes, proteolytic processing may take place. This may include removal of sequences from one end of the polypeptide and the cutting of a large amino-acid chain into two smaller ones, both of which are parts of the completed, mature protein, as in the β-hexosaminidases.

2.5.3　Clinical manifestations

The clinical manifestations of storage disease differ greatly between and within disease states. Different organs are characteristically involved in different disorders. Reticuloendothelial cells serve as the main repository of glucocerebroside and sphingomyelin, so that enlargement of liver and spleen, as well as bone-marrow involvement are characteristic findings in Gaucher disease and Niemann–Pick disease. The distribution of ceramide trihexoside, a glycolipid differing from glucocerebroside in that galactosyl galactose is attached to the glucose of glucocerebroside, is very different. High levels are found in the plasma of patients with Fabry disease, and it tends to accumulate in endothelium and in the cornea of the eye. Patients with this disease often succumb to renal failure or to myocardial infarction.

The morbid consequences of storage diseases are presumably a result of the accumulation of the storage material, but details of pathogenesis are, in general, not known. In Gaucher disease, for example, the liver may undergo a tenfold enlargement, with the liver weight increasing from 1.5 to 10 kg or more. Yet, only 2 or 3 per cent of the liver weight will be the storage glycolipid, glucocerebroside, so that the stored material will only account for less than 0.5 kg of the weight increase. The increase in the liver weight is presumably a reaction to the glycolipid, which includes accumulation of fibrous tissue, water, and many other substances. Similarly, although the accumulation of GM_2 ganglioside in the neuronal cells of patients with Tay–Sachs

disease has been meticulously documented, the biochemical mechanism by which the increased amounts of ganglioside produce functional impairment remains a mystery.

Deficiencies of different enzymes along a series of catabolic reactions may result in accumulation of the same storage material: glycogen accumulation occurs with a variety of enzymatic defects, although the exact nature of the glycogen that accumulates may differ with different enzyme deficiencies. An even greater level of complexity is introduced by the fact that different genetic lesions affecting the same enzyme produce disparate clinical consequences. A striking example is Gaucher disease, in which deficiencies of glucocerebrosidase that appear similar in severity may produce the devastating type II neuronopathic disorder, usually fatal within the first year of life; or the relatively benign type I disease, in which the diagnosis may not even be suspected until the patient is elderly. Both family studies, and studies carried out by cell fusion, indicate that the same gene is responsible for these very different clinical disorders.

2.5.4　Diagnosis

Diagnosis of a storage disease is possible at several different levels:

1. clinical and ancillary laboratory findings;
2. chemical analysis of the stored material;
3. histopathologic patterns;
4. demonstration of the enzyme defect; and
5. demonstration of a specific lesion in DNA.

Clinical patterns

The clinical pattern, together with certain ancillary findings, may be so clear as to make a diagnosis virtually certain. If a Jewish child, normal at birth, shows regression of neuromuscular development with flaccidity, and is found to have a cherry-red spot at the macula on fundosopic examination, it almost surely suffers from Tay–Sachs disease, although another gangliosidosis would remain a remote possibility. A neurologically normal Jewish adult with an enlarged spleen, known to have been present for many years, who is otherwise asymptomatic and whose serum acid phosphatase and angiotensin-converting enzyme activities are markedly increased must have type I Gaucher disease.

Analysis of storage material

Historically, the determination of the structure of the stored material played a central role in the elucidation of the basic biochemical lesions of the storage diseases. In some diseases the concentration of storage material is greatly increased in plasma or in urine, but in many cases material for analysis is not available in the living patient. Moreover, the analysis of the storage material is technically demanding and therefore less readily available than is the estimation of catabolic enzymes. Even today this cumbersome approach may occasionally be useful in problem cases. When diagnosis is in doubt, it is wise to retain for

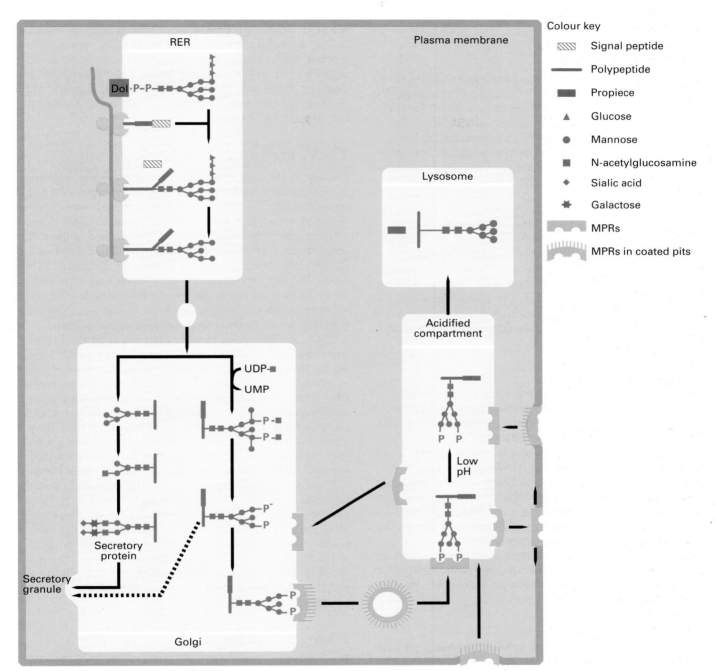

Fig. 2.38 Schematic pathway of lysosomal enzyme targeting to lysosomes. Lysosomal enzymes are synthesized in the rough endoplasmic reticulum (RER) and glycosylated by the transfer of a preformed oligosaccharide from dolichol-P-P-oligosaccharide (Dol). In the RER, the signal peptides are excised. The proteins are translocated to the Golgi where the oligosaccharides of secretory proteins are processed to complex-type units and the oligosaccharides of lysosomal enzymes are phosphorylated. Most of the lysosomal enzymes bind to mannose-6-phosphate receptors (MPRs) and are translocated to an acidified prelysosomal compartment where the ligand dissociates. The receptors recycle back to the Golgi or to the cell surface, and the enzymes are packaged into lysosomes where cleavage of their propieces is completed. The P_i may also be cleaved from the mannose residues. A small number of the lysosomal enzymes fail to bind to the receptors and are secreted along with secretory proteins. These enzymes may bind to surface MPRs in coated pits and be internalized into the prelysosomal compartment. (Drawn after Kornfeld 1986, with permission.)

later analysis frozen samples of affected organs when they become available.

Histopathological diagnosis

The histopathological presentation of many of the storage diseases is sufficiently characteristic that the diagnosis can be established with confidence by tissue examination. The use of histochemical stains for the detection of general classes of compounds, such as lipid, glycogen, etc., is often helpful in linking a clinical and histopathological pattern to a specific storage disease. In living patients, accessibility of the appropriate tissue may pose a problem. Gaucher cells are quite characteristic of Gaucher disease, but their detection requires examination of marrow, spleen, or liver. Some of the glycogen storage diseases present characteristic findings in the liver. Sections of the brain show the characteristic ballooned neurones of Tay–Sachs disease, and in many patients the diagnosis of previously unsuspected Fabry disease is made when a skilled pathologist examines the kidney biopsy obtained from a patient with unexplained renal failure. Although still useful when tissue is available, histopathological diagnosis has become much less important with the discovery of the enzyme defects that cause the storage diseases.

Enzyme assays

With the elucidation of the underlying enzyme deficiency, biochemical detection of specific defects has gradually replaced earlier methods for the diagnosis of the storage disease. In some cases, such as Tay–Sachs disease, Sandhoff disease, or Fabry disease, enzyme levels in the plasma may be diagnostic. Often circulating leucocytes or cultured skin fibroblasts are needed to establish enzymatic diagnosis. The latter have the advantage that they can be stored for repeated study or reference to specialized centres for further investigation even after the patient is no longer available. Red-cell enzyme assays may establish the diagnosis of some of the glycogen storage diseases.

Since pathological changes are usually not present in carriers (Fabry disease being an exception) the enzymatic approach is usually the only means for heterozygote detection to make possible genetic counselling.

DNA analysis

The underlying changes in DNA sequence leading to storage disorders are beginning to be elucidated. Application of this technology makes possible the most specific detection of defects. The high specificity of the technique has some advantages but also some drawbacks. There are literally hundreds of changes in a gene that could cause a deficiency of its product and result in a storage disease. If the most common of these that are known to exist in a population are not found, it does not prove that the disease is not present. On the other hand, finding a defect that has been shown previously to cause a disease is strong evidence that the disease is present.

The ease of application of the techniques of molecular biology to diagnosis of storage disease will change with the available technology. Major gene deletions, as appear to be the cause of the French-Canadian type of Tay–Sachs disease are relatively easy to detect on crude, uncloned DNA, using appropriate restriction endonucleases and probes. Point mutations, as occur in at least one type of Ashkenazi Jewish Tay–Sachs disease and Gaucher disease, can also usually be identified regularly using technology based on the polymerase chain reaction (PCR) (see Sections 2.2 and 30.3.8).

2.5.5   Prevention

Because of the lack of satisfactory treatment for the storage diseases, prevention of the disorders by genetic counselling, and sometimes selective abortion, may be very important. Carrier detection is usually possible through enzyme analysis. In those cases in which the DNA lesion has been defined in the family under study, DNA analysis is becoming a highly reliable means for accurate carrier detection and prenatal diagnosis. In the autosomal recessive disorders, the enzyme activity is usually about one-half normal in carriers. In sex-linked disorders such as Fabry disease and Hunter syndrome, special diagnostic problems exist because of the effect of random X-inactivation.

In the case of diseases that are common in an ethnic group, population-based carrier screening may be very useful. Screening for Tay–Sachs disease in the Jewish community has served as a highly successful prototype for this type of disease prevention. In the case of disorders with a low prevalence, screening is usually limited to family members after the disease has occurred once. Couples at risk are counselled and they then have a number of rational choices. These range from having a child with the disease, in the case of some of the milder disorders, to adoption, to prenatal diagnosis and abortion of affected fetuses.

Prenatal diagnosis has, until recently, depended upon the sampling of amniotic fluid. Enzyme assays are then performed on uncultured or cultured amniotic fluid cells. Since about 1986 the introduction of chorionic villus sampling has made it possible to obtain diagnostic material as early in the pregnancy as the 8th week, and to do so by the vaginal route. The tissue obtained is suitable for study directly or after cell culture, and provides adequate material for either enzyme assay or DNA analysis.

2.5.6   Treatment

Treatment of most of the storage diseases is almost entirely symptomatic in nature. In some of the milder disorders the patients' quality of life can be greatly enhanced by such intervention. For example, splenectomy greatly improves the thrombocytopenia of patients with Gaucher disease and surgical replacement of damaged joints by appropriate protheses can rehabilitate a crippled patient with the disease. Patients with Fabry disease may survive renal failure by virtue of being placed on haemodialysis. Although life may be prolonged in patients with severe neurologic defects by tube feeding and treatment of infections with antibiotics, the results of such intervention are not gratifying.

Because it is possible in some instances (such as Hunter disease) to correct the enzyme defect *in vitro*, there has been much interest in treating this group of diseases by enzyme replacement. Until recently the results of this aproach have been disappointing, but efforts to devise a successful enzyme replacement strategy for some of these diseases has continued. Effective enzyme replacement therapy is now available for patients with Gaucher disease. Organ replacement has also been tried as a treatment for many of the storage disorders. Because the haematopoietic stem cell is the precursor of the storage cell in Gaucher disease, and because the central nervous system is spared in type I disease, bone-marrow transplantation is a particularly rational approach for this disorder. Limited success has been achieved with this procedure, but its hazards have greatly limited its application to a disease that is often as benign as Gaucher disease.

Experiments in which the normal counterparts of genes that are defective in storage diseases are transferred into enzymatically deficient cells have also been conducted. Such studies may ultimately lead to treatment of storage diseases, but the technology required to successfully implement such a strategy has not yet been fully developed.

2.5.7 Further reading

Beutler, E. (1988). Gaucher disease: New developments. *Current Hematology/Oncology* 6, 1–26.

Cline, M. J. (1986). Gene therapy: current status and future directions. *Schweizerische Medizinische Wochenschrift* 116, 1459–64.

Kornfeld, S. (1986). Traficking of lysosomal enzymes in normal and disease states. *Journal of Clinical Investigation* 7, 1–6.

Scriver, C. R., Beaudet, A. L., Sly, W. S., and Valle, D. (eds) (1990). *The metabolic basis of inherited disease*. McGraw-Hill, New York.

von Figura, K. and Hasilik, A. (1986). Lysosomal enzymes and their receptors. *Annual Review of Biochemistry* 55, 167–93.

Walter, P., Gilmore, R., and Blobel, G. (1984). Protein translocation across the endoplasmic reticulum. *Cell* 38, 5–8.

2.6   Genetics of inherited disorders

Bryan Sykes

2.6.1   Introduction

The genome is not completely stable. Evolution by any route depends on this instability as the source of variation and ultimately of new and better genes. When the same instability fails to match an individual to the environment the result is genetic disease.

The fundamental principle of genetic disease is simple. It is that, in any inherited disease, the causal mutation must be contained somewhere within the one-dimensional DNA message. This simplicity is the reason why only a handful of technological innovations over the past decade have been able to bring about what can truly be called a revolution in human genetics. A revolution that realistically promises a complete description of all genetic disease in the foreseeable future. The soundness of the principal has injected the vital ingredient—confidence—to the process. There is a clear sequence of events in understanding the molecular pathology of an inherited disease. First, identify the mutant genetic locus, then the gene product, and, through a detailed description of the mutations, discover how these changes affect the performance of the product and so result in disease. In practice, however, the phenotype (performance of the product) is usually known and the site of mutation is discovered subsequently (see Section 2.7 for further discussion).

2.6.2   Inheritance pattern

Before going on to consider how this sequence is initiated and carried through, it is worth reflecting on what information about the likely outcome can be gleaned from the basic genetics of a disorder. The first is whether the disease behaves as a dominant or recessive trait. Very often a mutation results in a functionless gene product so the effect is to cut the effective output of the locus in a diploid cell by about half. This is the reason why, by and large, enzyme deficiencies are recessive traits because rates of substrate catalysis are maintained at a tolerable level even with a 50 per cent reduction in active enzyme production. Only when both alleles are abnormal is there any sign of disease. Much the same argument applies to inherited hormone and cell-receptor deficiencies which also tend to be inherited as recessive traits. Dominant disorders are more likely to be caused by mutations in genes where the level of output has to be maintained at a high level, so that a 50 per cent reduction cannot be tolerated, or where the polymeric structure of the product serves to amplify the damaging effect of the mutant allele at the expense of the normal counterpart. This is more likely to occur in, for instance, structural proteins whose physical presence in the right amounts is important, or enzymes whose normal level is marginal.

Another consideration is the population genetics of the disorder. Since to cause disease a mutant gene must, by definition, confer a disadvantage at some part of the life-cycle, there have to be good reasons for it to become widespread in a population. In human populations there are three ways for such a gene to achieve a high-enough incidence for it to achieve the distinction of causing an important inherited disease.

Founder effect

Where there has been a rapid population explosion from a few individuals then any traits carried by these founders stand a good chance of becoming relatively common in the descended population, despite being disadvantageous. In recent centuries, colonization of hitherto relatively uninhabited lands by small bands of fecund immigrants has created just these conditions and has led to some remarkably high incidences of inherited traits. For instance, there are now 30 000 Afrikaaners carrying the gene for porphyria variegata, a far higher incidence than in

The Netherlands, all descended from one of a Dutch couple who emigrated to South Africa in the 1680s. From the point of view of the molecular pathology we can be sure that since the sufferers are descended from one individual all the mutant alleles, in this case at the locus encoding the enzyme protoporphyrinogen oxidase, will be identical. This is known as *allelic homogeneity* and is to be expected when the founder effect is operating.

Natural selection

Eventually the effect is diluted by gradual elimination of the mutant allele by selection; so the mutation might only last for a few centuries. Natural selection can also act to increase the incidence of an inherited disease if the disadvantage conferred by the mutant gene is offset by advantage elsewhere. For instance, where the heterozygote carriers of a recessive disorder have a selective advantage over both the normal and the homozygote then selection will increase the frequency of the mutant allele and, hence, of the disorder. This is certainly the explanation for the spread of the β-globin allele carrying the sickle-cell mutation and in this case the selective agent is malaria. Hence the sickle-cell allele is restricted to regions where malaria is, or has been, endemic. Sharp differences in the geographical distribution of an inherited disease point to the action of selection, even though the corresponding selective agent can usually only be guessed at. The significance to the molecular pathology is similar to that of the founder effect. There is a good chance that all the mutant alleles in the population are derived from one, or at any rate a very few, individuals in the distant past, especially if the disorder is racially as well as geographically restricted. Other well-known examples where it is probably natural selection that maintains the high incidence of an inherited disorder are cystic fibrosis in North European Caucasians and Tay–Sachs disease in Ashkenazi (East European) Jews. Partial or complete allelic homogeneity would be expected in both of these.

Mutation

Other disorders, like achondroplasia, haemophilia, osteogenesis imperfecta, and Duchenne muscular dystrophy occur with approximately equivalent frequency in all geographical and racial groupings. The frequency of these disorders is maintained not by founder effect or natural selection but by the third mechanism—mutation. It is very unlikely that the same mutation will have occurred separately in each unrelated family and the disorder will not show allelic homogeneity. However, there is a good chance that all the mutations will have occurred in the same gene so that the disease will show *locus homogeneity*, but this cannot be taken for granted. A high mutation rate in a disorder suggests that the locus is especially vulnerable and there must be reasons for this. Vulnerability to mutation may be an intrinsic property of the gene structure or chromosomal location, as appears to be the case in Duchenne muscular dystrophy where a very large gene is situated in a very unstable region of the X-chromosome. Alternatively, it can be the

consequence of the encoded protein itself, if there are multiple targets for a mutation which will badly damage the structure. Collagen I is an example where substitution of any of the 338 glycine residues will be sufficiently disruptive to result in a lethal form of the bone disease osteogenesis imperfecta.

2.6.3   Finding the mutant locus

The next stage to consider in unravelling the molecular pathology of an inherited disease is the extent of available information or hypothesis about the mechanism. This varies enormously from the well established (factor VIII deficiency causes haemophilia A) through the plausible (collagen defects might cause Marfan syndrome) to the obscure (polycystic kidney disease). Table 2.4 shows how some mutant loci were initially identified.

Candidate genes

Where there is a hypothesis to test, the process is fairly clear. First, the 'candidate' gene is cloned by one of several routes. Usually this is contructed from a normal counterpart of the affected tissue (e.g. liver for factor VIII) via a cDNA library intermediate. These days the clones are often selected by hybridization to a mixture of oligonucleotides of between 15 and 20 bases whose sequences are deduced from the amino-acid sequence of the 'candidate'. Stretches of unusual amino-acid sequence with minimum codon redundancy are preferred, since this reduces the possibility of selecting a clone from the wrong gene and cuts down on the number of oligonucleotides that need to be synthesized to cover all possible alternatives in the cDNA. The cDNA is then used as a probe for genomic DNA libraries, whence the gene can be isolated.

Direct testing for mutations

Whether or not a candidate can be tested directly depends on the nature of the mutation. If it is a large deletion or rearrangement, then hybridization to Southern blots of patient DNA will easily show it. This worked very well in haemophilia B when the factor IX gene was tested against a cleverly selected group of patients who produced high levels of antibodies to injected factor IX during their treatment. It was reasoned, correctly, that this group were more likely to have large deletions leading to complete non-expression of the protein, so that the injected factor IX was immediately recognized as foreign. Techniques for detecting more subtle mutations than these are improving rapidly (see Section 2.4). The acid test for any candidate gene, though, has to be segregation analysis, which also depends on instability within the genome.

Indirect testing—segregation analysis

The human genome is about 6×10^9 bp in length, of which perhaps 5 per cent are coding sequences. Mutations, of course, can occur anywhere, and as well as unfavourable changes leading to inherited disease, normally within or close to coding sequences, mutations in non-coding regions will often have no effect on the phenotype. Random drift will spread some of these

Table 2.4   Identification of mutant loci

Mutant locus identified

From biochemical candidates

sickle-cell anaemia	β-globin
α-thalassaemia	α-globin
β-thalassaemia	β-globin
haemophilia A	factor VIII
haemophilia B	factor IX
α₁-antitrypsin deficiency	α₁-antitrypsin
phenylketonuria	phenylalanine hydroxylase
Lesch–Nyhan syndrome	hypoxanthine-guanine phosphoribosyl transferase
Tay–Sachs disease	hexosaminidase A
combined immune deficiency	adenosine deaminase
adrenal hyperplasia	steroid-21 hydroxylase
hypercholesterolaemia	low-density-lipoprotein (LDL) receptor
hyperlipidaemia	apolipoprotein CII
*osteogenesis imperfecta	collagen I
*Ehlers–Danlos syndrome	collagen I and collagen III
ornithine transcarbamylase (OTC) deficiency	OTC
growth hormone deficiency	growth hormone
*porphyria	uroporphyrinogen decarboxylase
anti-thrombin III (AT3) deficiency	AT3

From chromosomal mapping

chronic granulomatous disease	β-chain of cytochrome b$_{-245}$(Xp)
retinoblastoma (Rb)	Rb protein (13q)
Duchenne muscular dystrophy	dystrophin (Xp)
cystic fibrosis	CF transmembrane conductance regulator (7q)
familial adenomatous polyposis	APC protein (5q)
von Recklinghausen neurofibromatosis	NFI protein (17cen)
Wilms tumour	WT protein (11p)
Marfan syndrome†	fibrillin (15q)
retinitis pigmentosa (autosomal)	rhodopsin (3q)

Mutant locus located

X-chromosome

retinitis pigmentosa	Xp
hypophosphataemia (dominant)	Xp
choroideraemia	Xq
Emery–Driefuss muscular dystrophy	Xq
Hunter syndrome	Xq

Autosomes

von Hippel–Lindau disease	3p
Huntington chorea	4p
*familial Alzheimer disease	21q

* Not all cases due to mutations at this locus.
† Biochemical candidates located by chromosomal mapping.

neutral changes through the population so that there will, for a time at least, be more than one allele at that locus. The ability to distinguish alleles is absolutely fundamental because it serves as a marker system for the locus. In human genetics, the first marker systems were derived from antigenic (e.g. blood groups, HLA antigens) or electrophoretic variants, and were often far from neutral. After decades of valiant service, these have been largely superseded by DNA variants of two kinds. The first depends on variation in nucleotide sequence. On average there is a change in one base per 250–500 between any two chromosomes picked at random. While these could, of course, be detected by nucleotide sequencing, a much cheaper way of finding them, which is good enough for most purposes, is to use restriction enzymes. Allelic sequence differences at restriction sites will give a simple 'cut'/'won't cut' dimorphic variation—

easily displayed on a Southern blot. Most of these have been found simply by comparing the fragmentation patterns of a small number of unrelated individuals. Another source of detectable variation is provided by segments of short direct tandem repeats. A high frequency of unequal crossovers leads to the creation of a set of alleles containing different number of repeats, which can be differentiated as fragments of different sizes. Though less common than restriction site dimorphisms, these length polymorphisms are especially valuable because they allow several alleles to be distinguished rather than just two. Both sources of variation are embraced by the acronym RFLP (restriction fragment length polymorphism).

Genetic distance

A genetic marker acts rather like a flag by which the destination of nearby regions of a chromosome can be traced in a family or in a population. The marker will always be inherited with genes close by on the same chromosome, unless there is a crossover event between them during meiosis. The probability of separation of marker and gene (genetic distance or recombination fraction) correlates roughly with the physical distance between them. The unit of recombination is the Morgan (named after the pioneer of *Drosophila* genetics), with the more useful derivative, the centimorgan (cM). Two loci 1 cM apart on a chromosome have a 1 per cent probability of a crossover occurring between them at each meiosis. The frequency of crossing-over is higher in some regions, such as parts of the X-chromosome and towards autosomal telomeres, and lower in others. The average figure comes out at about 1 per cent per megabase per meiosis, i.e. 1 cM per million bases.

Markers within or close to genes are ideal for testing whether or not a disease is caused by mutations at that locus because the probability of crossover between the marker and the candidate gene is extremely small. Almost by definition, the segregation of a disease in a family must follow precisely the segregation of one (for dominant) or two (for recessive) alleles at the mutant locus. It follows that they must also follow precisely the segregation of very close markers, so that a single example of crossing-over between marker and disease within a pedigree is often enough to dismiss a candidate gene. This approach has been very useful, for example, in sorting out which of the inherited connective tissue disorders are caused by collagen gene mutations. Prior to segregation analysis there was evidence, sometimes good, sometimes bad, that collagen gene mutations were the cause of the Marfan and Ehlers–Danlos syndromes, osteogenesis imperfecta, and some inherited chondrodysplasias, particularly achondroplasia. Only dominantly inherited osteogenesis imperfecta and one variant of the Ehlers–Danlos syndrome survived the rigours of segregation analysis and this has deflected effort on the cause of the Marfan syndrome and achondroplasia away from collagen to other genes.

Linkage

Markers are not, of course, restricted to known genes. Any clone picked from a DNA library, if it can reveal an RFLP, becomes a marker of its immediate chromosomal surroundings. It will therefore segregate with nearby genes in a pedigree, the consistency of segregation depending on the genetic distance. This simple logic means that any disease gene could, given sufficient well-distributed markers, ultimately be located. For the first time, there was a realistic chance of making progress in several major inherited diseases in which biochemical research had failed to suggest a candidate gene. The effect on the scientific community was electrifying and ushered in a frenetic burst of genetic prospecting, still in progress, with spectacular results.

The sex-linked disorders were the first to fall to the onslaught, largely because the mutant loci are, obviously, on the X-chromosome. This had the twin advantages of, first, being able to restrict linkage analysis to markers derived from X-chromosomes, available from libraries made from flow-sorted chromosomes; and, secondly, of simplified tracking of markers through pedigrees because males are, of course, hemizygous for all loci on the X-chromosome (except at the very tip of the short arm).

The pursuit of autosomal disorders, without the inherent advantages of X-linkage, started with the almost miraculous discovery of a marker practically on top of the Huntington chorea gene, one of the first dozen randomly picked from a genomic library. Other voyages of discovery have been more or less favoured by the gods. The polycystic kidney disease (PKD) expedition struck gold soon after launch when a highly variable length polymorphism near the α-globin locus was discovered in the laboratory next door. It was soon found to be only 5 cM from the PKD gene. Others have been saved from the doldrums by observations that focused attention to particular chromosomal regions. Rumours of linkage of the cystic fibrosis (CF) gene to the blood group electrophoretic variants of paraoxonase concentrated an unprecedented burst of activity on 7q, and within weeks the CF gene was shown to be closely linked to DNA markers in the region, and the mutant gene has now been identified. But with neither good clues nor good fortune, searching through the genome for a disease locus can turn into a gruelling slog. Success will always come in the end, as it has for von Recklinghausen neurofibromatosis, but it can be a long job.

2.6.4   'New' genetic diseases

The excitement in human genetics in recent years has had an interesting side-effect. The success, either actual or potential, in understanding the molecular pathology of any Mendelian trait has encouraged a closer look at diseases which have never really achieved Mendelian status. The requirement for large families imposed on any linkage analysis has meant that the first task is always to unearth pedigrees. This has brought to light some truly amazing pedigrees in which disorders, like Alzheimer disease, cleft palate, and bilateral affective disorders (manic depression), which had been thought to be at best only partly genetic, appear as well-behaved Mendelian traits. These diseases are now firmly slotted into the sequence and, as genes are isolated and mutations understood, their impact on unravelling the more usual sporadic cases is eagerly awaited.

2.6.5   Inherited cancer genes

It has been known for some time there are families in which cancers, for example retinoblastoma, Wilms tumour, and multiple endocrine neoplasia (MEN), appear to be inherited. On closer scrutiny it is not the cancer *per se* that is inherited, but the susceptibility to developing it. An example is familial polyposis coli (FPC) which is an autosomal dominant trait where affected invididuals have large numbers of benign polyps in the colon. These polyps can 'spontaneously' transform into malignant tumours. The FPC locus controlling the trait has been located to 5q with linkage markers, in the usual way. That particular chromosomal region was picked for special attention because of visible cytogenetic deletions in occasional individuals with the disease. The same sorts of clues have helped to accelerate the location of the Wilms tumour and retinoblastoma loci.

Although all somatic cells will inherit the trait, only occasionally will cells undergo malignant transformation. One emerging explanation is that a second mutation, this time in a somatic cell, is needed to neutralize the effect of the normal allele which otherwise suppresses tumour growth. The relevant somatic mutation of the normal locus might be complete or partial chromosomal loss by non-disjunction at mitosis or by any of the mutational mechanisms mentioned earlier. When these involve deletion of the normal locus the effect is to make the cells hemizygous for the mutant locus plus any markers in the deleted segment. This establishes a difference between the somatic cells and the tumour cells which can be easily demonstrated on a Southern blot in an individual who is heterozygous for markers in the deleted segment. The somatic cells will have both bands, the tumour cells only one. This kind of observation has shown that about a quarter of sporadic cases of colon cancer are hemizygous at the FPC locus. In these sporadic cases the mechanism must involve at least two somatic mutations, eliminating first one then the other normal allele; whereas in FPC only the second is needed to produce a tumour, the first mutation having already occurred in the germ line of a distant ancestor. Unfortunately, the molecular pathology of cancer cells is more complex than this simple concept would indicate (see Chapter 9).

2.6.6 Prenatal diagnosis

In any inherited disease, once linkage to a marker is established in a pedigree it becomes possible not only to trace the mutant allele retrospectively through other branches but also to predict the outcome of a pregnancy. The precision of such a prediction will depend on the risk of recombination between marker and disease during the critical parental meiosis. Where this is significant, the risk of a false prediction as a result of such a crossover can be reduced by simultaneously following another marker on the opposite side of the mutant locus. If there is no detectable recombination between the two flanking markers then the only risk, a very much smaller one, is that there has been a double crossover between them, in such a way that the two markers remain on the same chromosome while the mutant allele is translocated to the homologue. The usual pattern of events is for the discovery of closer and closer markers which segregate with the mutant allele in meioses which had earlier shown crossovers.

Strictly, linkage and consequent prediction is limited to the disease in that family alone. Expansion to the same disease in another family depends crucially on the degree of locus homogeneity. This can only be firmly established by studying a large number of separate families. Population indicators, mentioned earlier in this section, can imply that a disease is likely to be allelically homogeneous, from which locus homogeneity obviously follows. But in the majority of disorders, especially dominants, the locus homogeneity has to be accurately estimated before a marker can be used for prenatal diagnosis in a new, unrelated pedigree in which linkage has not, for whatever reason, been independently established. The process of estimating locus homogeneity, involving, as it does, studying large numbers of independent families, can delay the routine application of markers for prenatal diagnosis, and has certainly done so in Huntington chorea. In special cases, a limited amount of locus heterogeneity can be accommodated. In osteogenesis imperfecta, for instance, the disease can be linked to either of the two loci (COL1A1 and COL1A2) encoding the subunits of collagen I (see Section 1.4). This was not unexpected since the subunit structure of the candidate protein was well known before linkage studies began. Had it not been, it would certainly have complicated linkage studies with random markers.

Disease-specific haplotypes

Allelic homogeneity is only to be expected when a disease has spread through the population from a single mutation on one chromosome in a common ancestor. As new markers approach closely the mutant locus, the phenomenon of linkage disequilibrium can begin to distinguish the mutant allele from others in the population by preferred combinations of marker alleles which together define a haplotype. These are the relics of the original chromosome in which the mutation occurred or, at least, the chromosome which spread it throuh the population. This phenomenon is already well established in sickle-cell anaemia and regionally homogeneous thalassaemia, and is beginning now to emerge in cystic fibrosis. If the associated haplotype is rare in the normal population, it could be used directly to detect the mutant allele in a fetus or a carrier, thereby avoiding the need for a family study to distinguish the mutant allele(s). Ultimately, of course, detection of the mutation itself will define the mutant allele precisely.

From linked marker to mutant locus

Definition of the mutant gene, and ultimately the causal mutations within it, is the goal of all genetic prospecting. The painful transition from linked marker to mutant gene to causal mutation has exercised some of the brightest minds in molecular genetics. This is not the place for a description of detailed tactics. The strategy is, generally, to redefine a new set of candidate genes physically close to the nearest linkage marker or, even better, between two flanking markers. The candidate genes can be defined as expressed sequences in target tissue (muscle for muscular dystrophy, sweat gland for cystic fibrosis, etc.) or sequences with the characteristics of genes (an open reading frame, sensitivity to DNase in target tissues and not in others, proximity to HPa II tiny fragment (HTF) islands, etc.). Segregation must, of course, be absolutely concordant and must be confirmed in meioses where earlier family studies have detected crossovers between the gene and the closest markers. Eventually, the mutation itself, in allelically homogeneous disorders, or a range of them in disorders showing limited allelic heterogeneity, will be directly detectable using genomic amplification procedures detailed earlier (Section 2.2).

Gene therapy

Whether or not knowing the mutant gene will suggest practical routes to therapy is harder to predict, depending on, as it will, the nature and function of the mutant locus. After all, the precise defect in sickle-cell anaemia has been known for 30 years but this knowledge has not led to a cure. General methodologies of gene replacement, whereby the mutant allele is replaced by the normal counterpart, will need very careful testing before they could be applied safely to embryos or to adults. For the foreseeable future the only realistic scope is essentially preventative—carrier detection and prenatal or preimplantation diagnosis.

2.6.7   Further reading

Caskey, C. T. (1987). Disease diagnosis by recombinant DNA methods. *Science* **236**, 1223–8.

Cooper, D. N. and Schmidtke, J. (1986). Diagnosis of genetic disease using recombinant DNA. *Human Genetics* **73**, 1–11.

Davies, K. E. and Robson, K. J. H. (1987). Molecular analysis of human monogenic diseases *BioEssays* **6**, 247–53.

Gusella, J. F. (1986). DNA polymorphism and human disease. *Annual Review of Biochemistry* **55**, 831–54.

Pearson, P. L. (1987). Recombinant DNA, chromosomes and prenatal diagnosis. *Current Problems in Dermatology* **16**, 30–44.

2.7   Molecular genetic analysis of coronary artery disease: an example of a multifactorial disease

Philippa J. Talmud and Steve Humphries

2.7.1   Introduction

Many of the common disorders that constitute a major part of the health care budget in the Western world are not caused by defects in single genes, although there is a significant genetic component in their aetiology. Early heart attacks (under the age of 55 years), non-insulin-dependent diabetes, hypertension, schizophrenia, and some types of cancers often 'run in families'; but all of these disorders also have a strong environmental component. It appears that there is a genetic predisposition to the development of these disorders but (apart from some rare cases) this is not due to a defect in any single gene. The hypothesis has evolved that variations at a number of different gene loci causing subtle or minor changes in the level of expression or function of these genes, when inherited together, may predispose an individual to development of the disease. These genetic variations may then interact with environmental factors to determine an individual's overall risk of developing clinical symptoms. Molecular genetics should prove useful in dissecting the underlying cause of these disorders. The information gained may in the future be of use in the early detection of individuals who are at risk of developing these multifactorial disorders. Subsequent risk of disease can be modified by environmental changes, such as alterations in diet, life-style, or by appropriate prophylactic drug therapy.

In this section, the study of coronary artery disease (CAD) and, in particular, the genetics of atherosclerosis and hyperlipidaemia will be explored as an example of the approaches that can be used to investigate a multifactorial disorder. We will not attempt to cover all the data published in this field, which has been reviewed elsewhere (Hegele and Breslow 1987; Cooper and Clayton 1988; Humphries 1988; Lusis 1988), rather we will attempt to point out strategies that have been fruitful in the study of this disease and which may prove relevant in the analysis of other multifactorial diseases.

2.7.2   Aetiology of ischaemic heart disease

Atherosclerosis and hyperlipidaemia

A heart attack is usually caused by a thrombotic event in a coronary artery that is already partially occluded by an atherosclerotic plaque (see Section 12.4). All individuals, at least in Western countries, develop atherosclerosis, but it is now clear from animal and epidemiological studies that the rate of progression of these lesions is affected in part by the levels of certain lipids and lipoproteins in the serum. Lesions in the artery wall can be identified, even in very young individuals, as a 'fatty streak'. These lesions contain macrophage-derived cells that have become loaded with cholesterol ester, which causes them to take on a foamy appearance. As the plaque grows, other cells, such as smooth muscle cells, are stimulated to proliferate and also become fat-loaded. Fibrous extracellular matrix components are laid down, and in advanced plaques there are necrotic areas containing dead cells and deposits of cholesterol. These processes have been well documented at the cellular and molecular level (Ross 1986; Section 12.2). From this brief description of factors involved in the aetiology of the disease, a list of 'candidate genes' can be constructed. These include genes involved in blood clotting, genes expressed in macrophages, foam cells, smooth muscle cells and other cells in the wall of the artery, and genes involved in the control of serum lipid levels. Study of all these candidates would be useful, but to illustrate the approach we will focus on the genes involved in determining serum lipid levels.

Cholesterol metabolism

Cholesterol and triglycerides are transported in the blood in protein–lipid particles called lipoproteins (Fig. 2.39). These particles can be distinguished by their buoyant density and by their protein constituents. Following the digestion of dietary fat, the intestine secretes large triglyceride-rich particles called chylomicrons which enter the circulation via the lymphatic system. Triglyceride-rich very-low-density lipoprotein (VLDL) are also secreted by the liver and both chylomicrons and VLDL contain a number of apoproteins, such as apo B, apo E, and apo C pep-

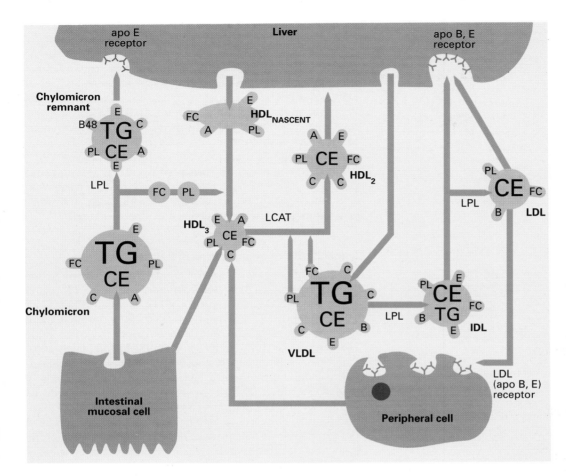

Fig. 2.39 The major steps in cholesterol metabolism. VLDL, very-low-density lipoprotein; IDL intermediate-density lipoprotein; HDL, high-density lipoprotein; A, B, C, and E, apolipoprotein A, B, C, and E; CE, cholesterol ester; FC, free cholesterol; PL, phospholipids; TG, triglycerides; LCAT, lecithin:cholesterol acyl transferase; LPL, lipoprotein lipase. See text for details.

tides. Apo CII is the essential cofactor for the enzyme lipoprotein lipase that hydrolyses the triglyceride core of the lipoproteins. The triglycerides from these particles are metabolized in the muscles as an energy source, or deposited in the adipose tissue. A proportion of the particles (IDL) that are left are removed by the liver via interaction between apo E and specific receptors. A proportion of the VLDL remnants are further metabolized, with loss of all the apoproteins except for apo B, and finally become the cholesterol-rich low-density lipoprotein (LDL) particles. LDL is removed by a specific receptor, the LDL-receptor, on the surface of extrahepatic cells, or more importantly in the liver where the cholesterol can be broken down to bile acids and bile salts and is secreted.

Circulating high-density lipoprotein (HDL) particles are of intestinal and hepatic origin. The apoproteins of HDL are apo AI and apo AII, with some particles also containing apo E and the apo C peptides. HDL functions in 'reverse cholesterol transport', accepting cholesterol from extrahepatic cells or from other lipoproteins. This cholesterol is esterified by the plasma enzyme lecithin:cholesterol acyl transferase (LCAT), with apo AI acting as a cofactor for the enzyme. The HDL, now with a core of cholesterol ester, may be removed by the liver, or the core lipids may be transferred to other lipoproteins by specific transfer proteins (Brown and Goldstein 1986).

Thus the genes encoding the enzymes involved in the synthesis and catabolism of cholesterol and triglycerides, the apoproteins involved in the transport of lipids, and the receptors that remove lipoproteins from the blood are all candidates for study. Many of these genes have been cloned, sequenced, and their chromosomal location determined (Table 2.5). In addition, many common restriction fragment length polymorphisms (RFLPs) of these genes have been reported, and the basic tools for a detailed genetic analysis of predisposition to hyperlipidaemia are therefore available. The initial problem, however, is to determine which of the candidate genes to study first, and how to tell whether genetic variation in any particular gene does indeed contribute to the development of hyperlipidaemia and atherosclerosis.

Table 2.5 Chromosomal localization of the genes involved in lipid metabolism (for references see Lusis 1988)

Gene	Chromosome
apo AII	1p21–qter
apo AI–CIII–AIV	11q13–qter
apo B	2p23–24
apo E–CI–CII	19q
LDL-receptor	19p
Lipoprotein lipase (LPL)	8p22
Lecithin:cholesterol acyl transferase (LCAT)	16q22
Cholesterol ester transferase protein (CETP)	16q
Acetyl:cholesterol acyl transferase (ACAT)	?
HMG–CoA reductase	5q13.1–p14

2.7.3 Identification of candidate genes—inborn errors of metabolism

As with the study of disorders caused by single gene defects, the study of rare inborn errors of metabolism has helped to identify which of the candidate genes involved in lipid metabolism may be most important in the development of hyperlipidaemia and atherosclerosis. Furthermore, in some of these rare disorders other genes, as yet unidentified, are implicated. These genes may also prove important in lipid metabolism and thus in the development of atherosclerosis.

Familial hypercholesterolaemia

About 1 in 20 people who suffer premature heart attacks have familial hypercholesterolaemia (FH), which is an inherited, autosomal dominant trait. Individuals with this disorder have about twice the normal level of serum cholesterol, mainly in the cholesterol-rich LDL fraction. This elevated cholesterol causes the development of premature atherosclerosis, and roughly 50 per cent of men with this disorder will have suffered a heart attack by the age of 55 years if not identified and treated. Women who have inherited the defect also develop high levels of serum cholesterol but are protected from the development of atherosclerosis until after the menopause.

Over the past few years it has been shown by Brown, Goldstein, and co-workers that FH is caused by mutations in the low-density-lipoprotein receptor (LDL-receptor) gene (Goldstein and Brown 1983, Brown and Goldstein 1984). Located on the cell surface, this receptor binds and internalizes cholesterol-rich LDL particles. A reduction in the number of functional receptors leads to an increase in serum and LDL-cholesterol levels and this increases the risk of patients developing premature atherosclerosis and coronary artery disease. The availability of cDNA and genomic clones of the LDL-receptor gene have now made it possible to characterize mutations at the DNA level (Yamamoto et al. 1984; Lehrman et al. 1985). Over a dozen RFLPs of the LDL-receptor gene have been reported, and these can be used to follow the inheritance of the defective gene in familes (Humphries et al. 1985). In some cases serum cholesterol levels in individuals who have inherited a defective LDL-receptor gene may overlap the upper range of normal, or may only become significantly elevated after puberty. In these situations unequivocal identification of affected individuals by RFLP analysis in a family study may be useful.

The LDL-receptor gene is clearly worthy of detailed study. It is possible that as well as causing FH, there may be subclinical defects in the gene that, in combination with variation in other genes, may cause hyperlipidaemia and atherosclerosis.

Familial defective apolipoprotein B-100

Plasma levels of LDL-cholesterol are determined largely by the activity of LDL-receptors, which interact with a specific region of the apo B-100 protein moiety of LDL-particles (Knott et al. 1986; Yang et al. 1986) and remove LDL from the circulation. Reduced removal of LDL could either be caused by defects in the LDL-receptor, as in FH, or by defects in the ligand (apo B-100). Familial defective apolipoprotein B-100 (FDB) is a recently identified, dominantly inherited genetic disorder, which leads to increased serum concentration of LDL-cholesterol with reduced affinity for the LDL-receptor (reviewed by Innerarity, 1990). This disorder is associated with a G to A mutation in exon 26 of the apo B gene (in the putative receptor binding region of the protein) which results in the substitution of the amino acid glutamine for arginine in codon 3500. This mutation has been detected in the USA (Soria et al. 1989), in the UK and Denmark (Tybjaerg-Hansen et al. 1990), and in the FRG (Schuster et al. 1990). So far all individuals identified have been heterozygous for the apo $B(arg_{3500}$-gln) mutation. A crude estimate of the frequency in the general population in the UK is 1/600, or similar to the frequency of FH although this estimate needs to be confirmed in larger studies. The most striking feature of this disorder is that plasma lipid levels and clinical characteristics are similar to those reported for heterozygous FH (Tybjaerg-Hansen et al. 1990; Schuster et al. 1990). In these two studies, about 3 per cent of patients with a clinical diagnosis of FH were heterozygous for the apo $B(arg_{3500}$-gln) mutation, and had normal LDL-receptor activity. Thus, FDB is associated with moderate to severe hypercholesterolaemia with frequencies of coronary artery disease (CAD), of tendon xanthomas and of arcus corneae resembling those reported for FH heterozygotes.

As opposed to FH where more than 40 different mutations in the LDL-receptor give rise to the same phenotype, FDB is caused by one mutation in the apo B gene and can therefore be screened for in the general population as well as in families at risk. However, this is most certainly not the only mutation in the apo B gene causing primary hypercholesterolaemia through reduced binding of LDL to receptors, but is at present the only disorder where the underlying mutation in the apo B gene is known.

Abetalipoproteinaemia

Abetalipoproteinaemia (ABL) is a rare familial disorder where affected individuals have no detectable serum apo B. The obvious candidate gene for this disorder is the apo B gene itself. However, in the few families with abetalipoproteinaemia studied so far, the apo B gene itself appears normal at the gross DNA level, and for some of these patients elevated levels of apo B mRNA have been detected in the liver (Lackner *et al.* 1986). This implies that abetalipoproteinaemia may not be caused by mutations in the apo B gene.

This disorder shows a recessive mode of inheritance. Parents of an affected individual have normal levels of apo B and are obligate heterozygotes. If ABL is caused by a defect in the apo B gene, every affected child in the family should inherit one defective allele from each parent. Thus, using RFLPs the affected children should all have the same apo B RFLP genotype, i.e. they must all have inherited the same apo B allele from both father and mother. Linkage analyses in two families, each with two affected siblings, have recently been reported where, in both families, the children have inherited different apo B alleles from at least one parent (Talmud *et al.* 1988). This is incompatible with the simple model of a mutation in the apo B gene causing the disorder in these families. At the present time the identity of the genetic defect causing ABL is unknown, but the study suggests that there is at least one other important gene, expressed in the liver and intestine, that is vital for the synthesis or secretion of apo B-containing lipoproteins. This gene might be involved in the post-translational modification of apo B, or in the assembly of the lipoprotein particles. If this gene could be identified, it would be a candidate for further study.

Lipoprotein lipase deficiency—familial combined hyperlipidaemia

One of the key enzymes involved in the metabolism of the triglyceride-rich lipoproteins is the enzyme lipoprotein lipase (LPL). Occasionally individuals present, usually in childhood, with severe hypertriglyceridaemia as a result of either deficiency of apo CII or LPL. Several groups have reported investigations into the molecular defects causing apo CII deficiency (Hayden *et al.* 1986; Connelly *et al.* 1987) and for some of these the molecular defect is known (Olivecrona and Bengtsson-Olivecrona 1990). Both of these genes are thus candidates in the study of disturbances in triglyceride metabolism.

Recent studies have, however, indicated that mutations in the LPL gene may also be making a significant contribution to the development of hyperlipidaemia and atherosclerosis in the general population. Homozygous deficiency for LPL occurs at the rate of about one in a million individuals. This means that about 1 in 500 individuals in the population are heterozygous for LPL deficiency—a similar number to those heterozygous for FH. These individuals do not develop very high levels of triglycerides, but recent evidence suggests that they may develop a lipoprotein pattern of mildly elevated cholesterol, and/or elevated triglycerides (Babirak *et al.* 1989). This type of lipoprotein pattern was defined as familial combined hyperlipidaemia (FCH)

in 1973, as a result of family studies (Goldstein *et al.* 1973). This lipoprotein disorder occurs frequently in the general population (1–2 per cent) and in patients with CAD. It is thus possible that a subset of patients with FCH (about one-fifth) may have a defect in LPL, while in the others the defect is in another gene. A very recent study has linked FCH to the apo AI-CIII-AIV gene cluster (Wojciechowski *et al.* 1991).

Tangier disease

An interesting disorder of HDL metabolism suggests an additional candidate gene. Patients with Tangier disease have very low levels of apo AI and HDL, although there is little evidence to suggest that these patients suffer from accelerated atherosclerosis. The defect was originally thought to be in the synthesis of apo AI or in the structure of the apo AI gene itself, but the base sequence of the gene reveals no significant differences compared with the normal apo AI gene (Zannis *et al.* 1984). However, studies have suggested that Tangier-HDL is metabolized at a normal rate when injected into a normal individual, while normal-HDL is rapidly removed from the circulation of a Tangier patient (Brewer *et al.* 1985). Cellular studies have implicated a defect in the way macrophages metabolize HDL from these patients (Schmitz *et al.* 1987). Normally, HDL becomes associated with macrophages (possibly via a specific HDL-receptor), accepts cholesterol from the cell, and subsequently dissociates from the cell. In patients with Tangier disease the macrophages bind and internalize HDL as normal, but then degrade the particle, resulting in low levels of circulating HDL. There may thus be another important candidate gene involved in cellular HDL metabolism that has yet to be identified.

2.7.4   Identification of candidate genes—the 'top-down' approach

Population associations between RFLPs and mutations

One method that has proved useful in the search for candidate genes is to look for 'population associations' between the neutral genetic variation detected by an RFLP, and functionally significant genetic variation in a nearby gene. The approach is to determine the frequency of a particular RFLP in a sample of individuals from the normal population and in a group of patients with a particular phenotype. A difference in frequency suggests that variation at or near this locus is involved in the development of the phenotype studied. The phenotype could be presence or absence of myocardial infarction or coronary artery disease, dyslipoproteinaemia defined as lipid levels above or below the 95th centile for the population, or levels of a lipoprotein or apoprotein above or below a certain cut-off point. We call this the 'top-down' approach (Sing and Boerwinkle 1987).

Ethnic variation and RFLP allele frequencies

It has been known for many years that the allele frequencies of polymorphic markers, such as the ABO blood group or the HLA locus, vary significantly in different populations. Such differences have also been observed using DNA markers, for example at the globin locus (Antonarakis *et al.* 1985), and for many of the apoprotein RFLPs, so far examined, the allele frequencies have also been shown to vary in different populations. For example, the estimates of the rare allele frequency of the apo AI *Sst*I RFLP vary between 0.03 and 0.06 in the UK, 0.15 for an African sample, and 0.35 for a Japanese sample population (Humphries 1988). This variation in frequency may be the result of chance differences in the frequency of the polymorphism in the founders, or it could be due to the fact that the DNA changes causing the variation may have arisen independently in the different populations. It is also possible that these frequency differences may be the result of selection pressure, although it is hard to postulate selection through heart attack risk. Even individuals with severe hyperlipidaemia (e.g. heterozygous FH) have passed reproductive age before the onset of clinical symptoms and, in the sense of reproductive fitness, genetic variation predisposing to any of the hyperlipidaemias is unlikely to have a selective disadvantage. For the 'top-down' approach these observations mean that caution must be exercised to ensure that patient and control groups have the same ethnic origins and in extrapolating results of RFLP frequencies obtained from one population to another.

Haplotype analysis

One approach that has proved fruitful in the analysis of the haemoglobinopathies is to refine the analytical power of the RFLPs by using several of them in conjunction. This 'haplotype' approach is usually only successful in its application within limited geographical areas (Antonarakis *et al.* 1985) or within a particular ethnic group, where a common mutation causing hyperlipidaemia or atherosclerosis may have occurred on a chromosome whose haplotype can be uniquely defined by several RFLPs. There will, however, also be 'normal' individuals in the population with this haplotype but lacking the mutation, and it is unlikely that this approach will be useful for screening the population for individuals at risk of CAD. However, if patients could be subdivided, using haplotypes, into different mutation groups, this may be useful therapeutically if, for example, individuals with different mutations respond best to certain diets or drug treatment.

Apo AI–CIII–AIV RFLPs and atherosclerosis

The genes for apo AI, apo CIII, and apo AIV are tightly clustered on chromosome 11, with only 12 kb of DNA separating the 5′ end of the apo AI gene and the 3′ end of the apo AIV gene. Over 10 common RFLPs have been detected within this gene cluster (Humphries 1988; Lusis 1988) and, since most of these polymorphisms are caused by sequence changes outside the coding regions of the genes, they do not in themselves alter the amino-acid sequence of any of the proteins.

Several investigators have reported that the allele frequency of some of the RFLPs in the AI–CIII–AIV gene region is altered in patients with CAD compared with groups of healthy individuals. The results from some of these studies using the *Sst*I and *Pst*I RFLPs are shown in Table 2.6. These data suggest that

variation in the gene region (genetically close to the RFLPs) is in some way involved in predisposing individuals to develop atherosclerosis. This is not surprising since these genes code for proteins that play an important role in HDL and triglyceride metabolism, and high levels of triglycerides and low levels of HLD are clearly associated with the development of atherosclerosis. Mutations in this gene region predisposing to CAD would presumably act through altering the synthesis or function of one or more of these apoproteins. However, the results from such studies carried out in different laboratories and in different countries are not always consistent. It is possible that the differences in allele frequencies between patients and controls are chance observations due to the small sample sizes involved, and in several instances larger studies have failed to confirm them. Alternatively, differences in the criteria used by different workers to define patients might influence the results and confound comparison. However, the most likely reason for the differences observed between different laboratories is the different ethnic origin of the populations studied.

Apo B gene RFLPs and atherosclerosis

Recently, several groups have isolated DNA probes for apo B and determined the structure of the gene. The structural features and synthesis of the protein and its assembly into lipoproteins have been reviewed (Olofsson *et al.* 1987).

The frequencies of several apo B RFLPs in different groups of patients and controls have been reported by several workers. In a Boston study, the frequency of the rare alleles of the polymorphisms detected with *Xba*I, *Eco*RI, and *Msp*I were all significantly higher in a group of patients who had suffered a myocardial infarction, compared with healthy controls (Hegele *et al.* 1986). Other studies have not confirmed the altered frequency of the *Xba*I RFLP or have reported significant differences in the frequency of only the *Msp*I alleles in CAD patients (Deeb *et al.* 1986). However, a consistent finding appears to be the increase of the frequency of the rare *R2* allele of the *Eco*RI polymorphism in patients with both coronary and peripheral arterial disease (Table 2.7). The *Eco*RI DNA polymorphism is one of the few so far reported where the DNA change also alters an amino acid: codon 4154 is altered from a glutamic acid (common form) to a lysine residue. This will alter the charge of apo B but the protein is so large that this has not been detected as an isoelectric variant. At the present time it is unknown whether this amino acid change has any direct effect on the function of apo B. It is possible that the charge may alter the 'atherogenecity' of the particle by increasing the binding to proteoglycans in the artery wall or to the cellular scavenger receptor. Patients carrying the *R2* allele do not have significantly higher levels of serum cholesterol, LDL, or apo B, thus it is also possible that the polymorphism may be in linkage disequilibrium with a functionally significant mutation elsewhere in the apo B gene.

Linkage analysis explained by evolutionary history

A model to explain these findings, based on evolutionary history, can be proposed (Fig. 2.40). In the original population,

Table 2.6 Reported associations between CAD risk and apoprotein AI RFLPs

RFLP	Sample origin	Number (P/C)	Association	Rare allele frequency (P v. C)	Reference
*Sst*I	London	47/48	Y	0.11 v. 0.02	Ferns *et al.* (1985)
CIII	Seattle	140/101	Y	0.12 v. 0.06	Deeb *et al.* (1986)
	Austria	106/116	N	0.10 v. 0.11	Paulweber *et al.* (1988)
*Pst*I	Boston	88/123	Y	0.17 v. 0.03	Ordovas *et al.* (1986)
Apo AI	London	140/110	Y	0.17 v. 0.06	Wile *et al.* (1989)
	Seattle	140/114	N	0.07 v. 0.10	Deeb *et al.* (1986)
	Austria	106/116	N	0.05 v. 0.06	Paulweber *et al.* (1988)

P, Patients; C, controls.

Table 2.7 Reported associations between CAD risk and Apo B *Xba*I and *Eco*RI RFLPs

RFLP	Origin	Number (P/C)	Association	Relative frequency *X1* allele (P v. C)	Reference
*Xba*I	Boston	84/84	Y	0.64 v. 0.50	Hegele *et al.* (1986)
Codon 2488	Seattle	117/102	N	0.50 v. 0.54	Deeb *et al.* (1986)
	London	124/186	N	0.54 v. 0.47	Gallagher and Myant (pers. com.)
				Relative frequency R2 allele (Pv.C)	
*Eco*RI	Boston	84/84	Y	0.21 v. 0.11	Hegele *et al.* (1986)
Codon 4154	Seattle	108/123	N	0.19 v. 0.14	Deeb *et al.* (1986)
	London	124/186	Y	0.21 v. 0.15	Gallagher and Myant (pers. com.)
	London	200/115	Y	0.20 v. 0.14	Monsalve *et al.* (1988)

P, Patients; C, controls; *X1*, absence of cutting site; *R2*, absence of cutting site.

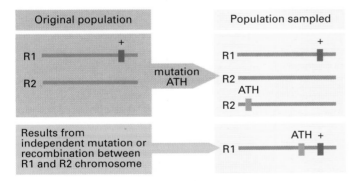

Fig. 2.40 Model to explain the observed population association between the apo B *Eco*RI RFLP and mutation causing atherosclerosis. R1 and R2, chromosomes with and without the *Eco*RI cutting site, respectively (shown as +). ATH, the mutation in the gene causing the development of atherosclerosis.

there were individuals who had chromosomes both with and without the *Eco*RI cutting site. In one individual, a mutation occurred in the apo B gene, and predisposed the individual to develop atherosclerosis (ATH). By chance, the mutation occurred on a chromosome without the cutting site—the *R2*

allele. In the population there were now three types of chromosome, *R1*–normal, *R2*–normal, and *R2*–ATH. This would mean that when the population was analysed many generations later, as a result of its historical association, many people with premature atherosclerosis would have the genotype *R1R2* or *R2R2*, but the *R2* allele would also be found in healthy individuals. We may also find patients with the genotype *R1R1*. This may be the result of an independent mutation occurring on the *R1* allele causing the same or a different mutation, or because of recombination occurring in the region of DNA between them. In general, the rate of recombination between two gene loci is dependent on the distance between them. For the apo B gene, the small genetic distance from one end of the gene to the other (50 kb) means that it will take many hundreds of generations for recombination to lead to the loss of associations between the allele of an RFLP and a mutation within the gene causing atherosclerosis.

As previously discussed for the apo AI gene, the interpretation of case-control studies of this type is complicated by ethnic heterogeneity, differences in selection of patients, and the fact that the development of CAD is influenced by so many genetic and environmental factors. Taking the available data overall, the observations suggest that variation at the apo B locus is involved in the development of some forms of hyperlipidaemia and atherosclerosis, and that the apo B gene warrants further study.

Apoprotein RFLPs and intermediate phenotypes

One of the problems in looking for associations between RFLPs and a clinical endpoint such as CAD, is that there is so much heterogeneity in the determination of the disease. It may therefore be more profitable to study phenotypes that can be better defined, or that are closer to the genes or the gene product. This may also allow us to gain insight into the mechanism by which variation associated with these polymorphisms may be affecting the clinical endpoint. The 'top-down' approach can thus be taken further by comparing the frequency of different apo AI–CIII–AIV RFLPs in groups of individuals with different 'intermediate phenotypes', such as hypertriglyceridaemia or hypoalphalipoproteinaemia (low HDL-cholesterol levels). Both of these phenotypes have been associated, in epidemiological studies, with CAD risk. One of the consistent findings in the field has been that the frequency of the S2 allele of the SstI-apo CIII polymorphism is higher in groups of patients with hypertriglyceridaemia compared with normal individuals (Rees *et al.* 1983). None of the other polymorphisms of this gene cluster shows strong association with hypertriglyceridaemia. Of the three genes known to be in this region, the apo CIII gene is most clearly implicated in triglyceride metabolism. Possibly, variation in the function or level of expression of this gene is part of the explanation for this association, but there are, as yet, no reports to substantiate this hypothesis. A similar approach has been used to study patients with HDL-cholesterol levels below the 5th centile. In these individuals the frequency of the P2 allele of the PstI RFLP was higher than in controls (Ordovas *et al.* 1986). Similarly for apo B, there have been some reports that the frequency of certain RFLPs is altered in groups of patients with particular forms of hyperlipidaemia (Talmud *et al.* 1987).

Although problems of small sample size and ethnic heterogeneity may confound some of the published data, the body of evidence does indicate that variation in the apo AI–CIII–AIV gene cluster and the apo B gene is involved in predisposing some individuals to develop dyslipoproteinaemia and CAD. No such strong association exists with the apo CII gene or the LDL-receptor gene (Humphries, 1988), although as discussed above mutations in both these genes are clearly involved in rare familial cases of inborn errors of lipid metabolism. In view of the heterogeneity and multifactorial nature of atherosclerosis, it is surprising that associations with any RFLPs have been detected. It is possible that within a group of patients there may be a subgroup in which variation at a particular locus may be having a very large effect, whereas in other patients variation in other genes may be the major factor determining CAD risk. The problem is that the 'top-down' approach only gives a limited amount of information about how to locate and identify the mutations associated with the RFLPs, that are contributing to the phenotype. Thus, patients with the same clinical phenotype

of premature atherosclerosis or high serum cholesterol may have different mutations, or even a mutation in a different gene. These problems can best be tackled by other approaches.

2.7.5 Identification of candidate genes—the 'bottom-up' approach

It is most likely that variation associated with an apoprotein RFLP is having an effect on the development of CAD through an effect on the function, or most likely the level, of that apoprotein. It is clear from our knowledge of the metabolism of the lipoproteins that the determination of the serum level of a lipoprotein such as HDL will be affected by genetic variation at a number of different loci, including lipoprotein receptors, enzymes such as lipoprotein lipase, and several apoproteins. Indeed, studies on the heritability of HDL and apo AI levels have indicated a stronger genetic influence on apo AI levels than on HDL levels. It should therefore be easier to use RFLPs to detect genetic variation involved in determining serum apo AI levels rather than HDL levels, although HDL and AI levels are highly correlated. Thus the approach is to take a group of individuals, define their genotype using a number of different RFLPs, of the candidate apoprotein gene, and look at the mean serum levels of the apoprotein in groups of individuals with different RFLP genotypes. This is the 'bottom-up' approach.

Many of the theoretical aspects and appropriate statistical analyses for this approach have been developed by the pioneering work on the apo E protein polymorphisms. It has been known for some time that individuals in the normal population have different apo E isoforms caused by single amino-acid substitutions that alter the charge of the protein. The three isoforms are designated E2, E3, and E4, with E3 being the commonest form (roughly 80 per cent of chromosomes). Individuals with different apo E phenotypes have different levels of serum lipids and apolipoproteins; those with the phenotype E2E2 have the lowest levels, and those with the phenotype E4E4 the highest levels of serum cholesterol (Utermann *et al.* 1984). The contribution of this polymorphism to the total variance in population serum cholesterol levels is about 8 per cent, implying that apo E is one of the polygenes that is having a small effect in determining the variation in normal cholesterol levels (Davignon *et al.* 1988).

The apo AI–CIII–AIV *Pst* I RFLP and levels of apo AI and HDL

This approach has been used to examine a sample of 109 healthy middle-aged men. The individuals with the apo AI PstI genotype P1P2 had a significantly higher mean apo AI level than men with the genotype P1P1 (Kessling *et al.* 1988). The authors estimated that genetic variation associated with the PstI RFLP site accounted for 6.5 per cent of the total variance in serum apo AI levels, but only 0.6 per cent of the total variance in HDL-cholesterol levels. As with the studies in patients, it should be possible to obtain a better definition of the underlying genetic variability by combining information from several

RFLPs. Using the *XmnI*, *PstI*, and *SstI* RFLPs there are 27 possible different genotype classes, although in the sample of men examined only 12 were observed, and many of these classes were represented by only one or two individuals. This immediately raises the problem of how to combine data from different genotype classes, and how to estimate the significance of any observed differences. However, within these limitations, genetic variation in the apo AI–CIII–AIV gene cluster, as defined by these three RFLP haplotypes, accounted for 16 per cent of the phenotypic variance in apo AI concentration, and about 8 per cent of the variance in HDL levels (Kessling *et al.* 1988). A larger study would be needed before extrapolation could be made to the general population, but the data suggest that variation in this gene region is involved in determining the levels of apo AI, and to a lesser extent the levels of HDL-cholesterol in normolipidaemic individuals. These studies also demonstrate that RFLPs can be used to analyse a quantitative trait, and that information from several RFLPs for the same gene, or gene cluster, can be used in conjunction to study genetic variation.

The gene as a polygene

These data also illustrate another concept which is important in the genetic analysis of a quantitative trait. In disorders caused by single gene defects, such as β-thalassaemia, the mutations in the β-globin gene that cause clinical consequences have a drastic effect on the function or level of expression of the β-globin protein. However, there are many potential sites in a gene where a single base change may have only a small effect on gene expression. For example, some sequence changes in the promoter or enhancer region may alter the rate of transcription by only 10–20 per cent. Sequence changes may affect the efficiency of correct splicing of the RNA in the nucleus, or stability of the mRNA, and result in reduced mRNA levels in the cytoplasm. In addition, changes in the amino-acid sequence of the protein may alter its function or the rate of removal. The expression of the candidate gene will therefore be the result of the summation of the effects of sequence variation in and around the gene, with each variation having an additive and interchangeable effect. Different 'mutations' will have occurred at different times in evolutionary history, and thus will occur in several different combinations in the population. The number of combinations will also depend on the rate of recombination at the gene locus, that is 'scrambling' the evolutionary association between the different mutations. The gene thus represents a 'polygenetic system', with expression of the gene being the result of the integrated effect of variation at a number of sites.

This can be illustrated by the data in Fig. 2.41. The effect associated with different haplotypes deduced from three RFLPs on lowering or raising apo AI levels from the mean of the sample, has been estimated by statistical techniques. The *X1P2S1* haplotype is associated with a large increase in apo AI levels, the *X1P1S1* haplotype with a small increase, while the other three haplotypes are associated with a reduction in apo AI levels. This suggests that there may be at least three functionally different haplotypes ('mutations', or combination of variations) that are affecting levels of apo AI in this sample.

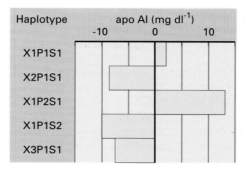

Fig. 2.41 Bar chart to show the effect of five common haplotypes of the apo AI–CIII–AIV genotypes on apo AI levels.

Apo B gene and cholesterol levels

For any one of the apo B DNA polymorphisms, individuals can be divided by genotypes into three classes, and the mean serum total cholesterol, triglyceride, LDL-cholesterol, or apo B level estimated for each group. Several recent reports (reviewed by Humphries 1988) have shown that in the normolipidaemic population, individuals with a particular apo B *XbaI* genotype, designated *X1X1* (Fig. 2.42), have a lower mean serum cholesterol level than individuals with the genotype *X2X2*. In some, but not all, of these studies individuals heterozygous for the polymorphism have intermediate mean serum cholesterol levels. In the same studies two other apo B polymorphisms detected with the enzymes *EcoRI* and *MspI* were not associated with any significant differences in serum cholesterol levels.

The size of the contribution to the sample variance in cholesterol levels can be estimated as for apo AI. In one study (Talmud *et al.* 1987) the estimate is as large as 10 per cent of the total

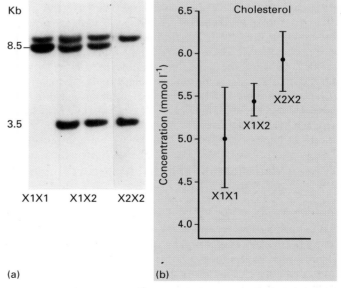

Fig. 2.42 (a) Southern blot hybridization of individuals with different apo B *XbaI* genotypes (*X2* has the cutting site). (b) Analysis of variance of serum cholesterol levels (mean ± SD) in individuals with different apo B *XbaI* genotypes. (With permission, Springer-Verlag, Berlin.)

variance, but this is probably an overestimate, due to several factors, including the small sample size. However, as with apo AI, more information can be obtained by using the RFLPs in conjunction. The *Eco*RI and *Xba*I polymorphisms are in linkage disequilibrium, but when taken together the contribution to the sample variance in cholesterol levels is about double that of the *Xba*I RFLP alone.

These polymorphisms are therefore detecting genetic variation that is involved in determining serum cholesterol levels in or around the apo B gene. The DNA change that creates or destroys the *Xba*I site occurs within the coding region of the gene, but the base change is in the third (wobble) position of a codon and does not alter the amino-acid sequence. Presumably, by a model similar to that proposed earlier (see Fig. 2.40), there is a population association due to evolutionary history, between the *Xba*I polymorphic sites and a mutation due to a DNA sequence change elsewhere in or around the apo B gene. There are two obvious possibilities for the location of this important common sequence variation. First, this change may alter the amino-acid sequence, which may change the functional properties of the protein and perhaps alter its affinity for the LDL receptor. This would result in a high serum LDL concentration because of a catabolic defect. Secondly, the DNA change may affect the level of transcription of the gene and therefore alter the amount of apo B protein produced by the liver. This would result in a higher synthetic rate of apo B and apo B-containing lipoproteins.

Recently, two studies have presented data indicating that variation in the apo B gene itself is affecting the rate of clearance of LDL from serum. In a group of patients with moderate hyperlipidaemia (Demant *et al.* 1988) and a group of healthy men (Houlston *et al.* 1988), there are significant differences in LDL fractional catabolic rate in individuals with different *Xba*I genotypes. Individuals with the genotype *X2X2* have the lowest clearance rate of LDL, and this is compatible with the previous observations that these individuals have the highest mean serum cholesterol. These studies imply that variation in the coding region of the gene, presumably in the region that interacts with the receptor, must be affecting the affinity of the LDL particle for the LDL receptor. The mutations causing these amino-acid sequence changes are in population association with the *Xba*I RFLP.

2.7.6 Identification of individuals carrying a gene 'mutation'

Multiple-unilocus model versus additive polygene model

Having established by one of the approaches described above that a particular candidate gene warrants detailed study, individuals must be identified who, with high probability, carry a 'mutation' in the gene of interest. For disorders carried by a single gene defect such as thalassaemia the question is trivial, but for a polygenic disorder the problem is more complex. The studies in normal or patient populations may have shown that variation at a candidate gene locus is involved in determining a

particular phenotype, such as the elevated lipid levels associated with the apo B *Xba*I genotype *X2X2*. However, not all individuals with the genotype have elevated lipid levels, and some individuals with the genotype and elevated lipid levels may have the phenotype because of variation at other gene loci. This is illustrated in Fig. 2.43, which compares two different models to explain the distribution of lipid levels seen in the population. In the multiple-unilocus model, mutation at one of a number of different loci will elevate lipid levels from the normal into the pathological range; defects in the LDL-receptor causing FH are an example of such mutations. However, in the polygene model, variations in a number of genes have an additive and interchangeable effect on determining lipid levels. The single base change that finally results in the elevation of an individual's lipid levels to above the 95th centile may be in gene *C*, but this 'mutation' is only of pathological consequence when the individual has co-inherited 'mutations' in genes *A* and *B*.

Linkage analysis

The classical way to confirm that variation at a particular gene locus is involved in determining a phenotype is by linkage analysis in a family. All affected relatives in the family should have inherited the same 'defective' allele of the candidate gene, defined by a particular RFLP haplotype, while this haplotype should be absent from all unaffected individuals. When the family size is large enough and the probability of observing the pattern of inheritance by chance alone is very small, linkage is considered to be demonstrated. Classically, an odds ratio of greater than 1 in 1000 (lod score 3.0) is taken to constitute proof of linkage. For the candidate gene approach a recombination event, i.e. an affected relative without the haplotype or an unaffected relative with the haplotype, means the hypothesis of

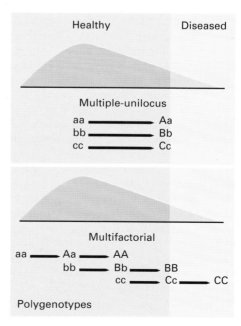

Fig. 2.43 Multiple-unilocus model versus additive polygene model.

linkage is rejected, and the phenotype is not caused by a mutation in the candidate gene. However, for a common multifactorial disorder there are several complicating problems. First, the phenotype may not develop until middle age (e.g. hyperlipidaemia, clinically detectable atherosclerosis, angina, or heart attack). Secondly, where the phenotype is affected by environmental factors, such as diet or obesity, an unaffected individual whose exposure to these environmental factors is reduced may not develop the phenotype at all. With a common disease like hyperlipidaemia, the probability of a spouse bringing in a defective allele causing the phenotype is high, and could result in affected offspring who do not carry the particular haplotype. Conversely, spouses may pass on genes that protect a particular individual from developing the phenotype, even if they have inherited the defective gene.

To date there are few studies that have addressed this problem. As a rule, for a disorder where there is clear bimodality in the distribution of the phenotype, the linkage approach should be feasible. For example, serum cholesterol or LDL-cholesterol levels in the relatives of individuals with FH are bimodal (Kwiterovich et al. 1974), and several studies have demonstrated linkage with the phenotype and RFLPs of the LDL receptor (e.g. Humphries et al. 1985). Patients with the disorder hypobetalipoproteinaemia have serum levels of apo B below the 5th centile, and serum apo B levels in their relatives are either within the normal range, or are very low. One RFLP linkage study in a large kindred has demonstrated co-segregation (lod score > 7.4) of the phenotype and the apo B gene, although even in this family there are individuals, who have inherited the 'defective' apo B allele, whose apo B levels are within the normal range (Leppert et al. 1988). It has been suggested that these individuals have also co-inherited a defective LDL-receptor gene, which causes a reduced clearance rate of LDL, and results in the higher than expected levels of apo B in a patient with hypobetalipoproteinaemia.

An additional complication is that a disorder such as FCH may be caused by mutations in different genes in different families. Therefore, using the apo B probe, co-segregation will be demonstrated in some families and rejected in others. In this situation, analysis will be confused by pooling data from several families, and this can only be overcome by obtaining samples from large multigeneration families. In a family where co-segregation can be demonstrated convincingly (i.e. is unlikely to have occurred by chance alone) it would then be worth isolating the gene of interest for detailed sequence analysis.

Sib-pair analysis

The sib-pair method (Penrose 1935) is based on the relative frequencies of pairs of sibs to be alike or unalike for two traits whose linkage is to be investigated. For example, if hyperlipidaemic sibs share a common apo B haplotype more often than expected by chance alone, this could implicate defects in the apo B gene in the development of the disorder. The method has the advantage that it can detect linkage in the presence of heterogeneity. This approach has been very useful in analysing multifactorial traits, such as diabetes, using HLA markers

(Thomson and Bodmer 1977). Once a concordant sib-pair has been identified, detailed studies on the family can be carried out or the gene involved isolated for sequence analysis.

2.7.7 Identification of 'candidate mutations'

Utilizing the techniques of molecular biology

Once a candidate gene has been identified in a particular individual classical methods can be used for the construction of genomic libraries, and the determination of the sequence of the exons and introns of the gene and its flanking regions. However, the polymerase chain reaction (PCR) technique has revolutionized the study of defined regions of sequenced genes (Saiki et al. 1986). Thus the region of the gene known to contain promoter or enhancer activity can be studied for many individuals in a short space of time. Similarly, regions of the exons known to code for important functions of the protein, such as the region of the apo B gene coding for the amino acids that interact with the LDL receptor, can be analysed. The Taq polymerase that is routinely used for this amplification (see Sections 2.2 and 30.3.8) does introduce occasional errors (estimated to be about 1/5000 base pairs) but any sequence changes detected can be confirmed by re-amplification. The more serious problem is to distinguish which of the detected sequence changes are 'neutral' polymorphisms and which are functionally significant. For promoter or enhancer sequences, alteration of function can be tested by inserting the sequence in the appropriate vector, and studying the ability of the sequence to promote transcription of the chloramphenicol-acetyl-transferase (CAT) gene in a transient transfection assay, for example in the hepatoma cell line HepG2 or in the intestine-derived cell line CaCo2. It is likely that any functionally important sequence change in the promoter region would have its effect through altering the affinity of binding of positive or negative transcription factors, such as the protein SP1. Thus an alternative approach would be to compare the binding of extracts of nuclear proteins to the wild-type and variant sequences using the 'footprint' technique. Such experiments on in vitro induced, single base-pair sequence changes in the promoter region of the LDL receptor have demonstrated the potential of this approach (Dawson et al. 1988).

Sequence changes in exons that may alter the function of the protein can be tested in vitro using synthetic polypeptides, though for a protein as large as apo B, this 'reconstitution' approach may not be feasible. Such sequence changes may, however, be testable using transgenic mice, or by expression in HepG2 cells transfected with the appropriate vector and subsequent isolation of the LDL for further studies.

Other in vitro assays to examine potential variation in splice regions or mRNA stability could be developed in cells transfected with the appropriate gene constructs. The final step in this analysis is to examine the frequency of any detected variations. It may be that a particular mutation may be unique to an individual, or present in a significant proportion of individuals with a particular phenotype. The same mutation may make only a small contribution to the determination of CAD risk, or may be common in patients of a particular ethnic origin and rare in other groups. By analogy with mutations causing thalassaemia, specific mutations are likely to be confined to certain races or ethnic groups in this way.

2.7.8 Implications for understanding pathophysiology and identification of 'at-risk' individuals

The goal of these approaches is to understand how variation in different genes determines the levels of serum apolipoproteins, lipoproteins, and lipids, and so influences the development of atherosclerosis. Taken overall, the published data suggest that variations within the apolipoprotein AI–CIII–AIV and apo B genes do contribute to CAD risk, but the association is weak and may not be the same in different populations. There is greater agreement from the reported studies that many of these RFLPs show allelic population associations with variations in genes that are involved in determining apoprotein, lipoprotein, and lipid levels in both normal individuals and patients. The data, therefore, strongly imply that detailed studies of these genes will lead to the identification of the DNA changes that are causing the different phenotypes such as high serum cholesterol or low HDL levels.

The next stage will be to identify the common mutations in the apoprotein genes by sequence analysis of samples from different individuals. Several questions can then be asked. First, how frequent is any particular mutation in the population or in patients with a particular phenotype? It is important for our understanding of the aetiology of hyperlipidaemia and CAD that we then start to quantify and assign to particular genes the genetic variation responsible for the determination of levels of serum apolipoprotein, lipoproteins, and lipids. Secondly, the effect of interaction between mutations at different loci must be examined. It is possible, because of the metabolic or physiological relationship between the functions of the different apoprotein receptors and enzymes, that combinations of different mutations may have a compensatory, additive, or synergistic effect on lipd levels and CAD risk. For example, a mutation in the apo B gene, such as the apo B3500, that reduces affinity of the LDL for the LDL-receptor may have much more serious consequences if co-inherited with a second mutation in the LDL-receptor gene that affects normal receptor function. It is likely that these sorts of genetic interactions are making a major contribution to the determination of the common forms of hyperlipidaemia and, therefore, CAD risk. The third question that can then be asked is: how do specific mutations affect the response to drugs or diet? Initial approaches to this question can be carried out using RFLPs and a 'bottom-up' approach. The experiment would be to see whether there are differences in the change in serum lipid or lipoprotein levels in response to environment in groups of individuals with different apoprotein RFLP genotypes. The study of variation that distinguishes individuals who respond poorly from those who respond well, is highly relevant to the identification of individuals who are

predisposed to develop hyperlipidaemia and CAD. For those individuals who respond well to a change in diet or drug treatment their environment could be easily modified by the appropriate treatment, to reduce their subsequent risk of CAD.

As more is understood about the genetic factors that are involved in determining serum lipid levels, it may be possible to develop a battery of tests that can be used to identify individuals at risk of developing hyperlipidaemia and atherosclerosis. At the present time the RFLPs of the candidate genes available are not useful for the identification of individuals at risk of CAD since, in the general population, there are healthy individuals who have the particular allele of the RFLP and many patients who do not. However, in the next few years analyses in families, patients, and the 'normal' population should lead to the identification of common mutations in some of the genes involved in lipid metabolism. This information can then be used to develop tests that will be 'mutation specific'; for example, using allele-specific oligonucleotides (Funke et al. 1986) in conjunction with gene amplification. A battery of such tests may be useful for the early identification of individuals with a predisposition to hyperlipidaemia.

DNA tests for diagnosis will only be useful if there is more information at the level of the gene rather than the protein. This may be the case if, for example, the serum level of an apolipoprotein in an individual is genetically predisposed to alter in response to changes in the environment or biological signals. Indeed, the serum levels of many apolipoproteins are altered at puberty, the menopause, and with increasing age, and many forms of hyperlipidaemia only develop in mid-life. Since in any individual the genes involved are fixed at conception, DNA tests may be useful for early detection of this type of genetic predisposition. Secondly, DNA tests may be useful if the 'quality' of a particular apolipoprotein is more important than the 'quantity'. This would be the case if single amino-acid changes cause a subtle alteration in the function or the 'atherogenic potential' of an apoprotein. In theory, it should be possible to detect changes of this kind using specific monoclonal antibodies, but DNA tests may be easier to apply.

The challenge for the next few years will be to move from the imprecise use of RFLPs to the detection and characterization of the underlying DNA changes in the different genes, which collectively predispose to hyperlipidaemia. This should allow the development of precise tests that will have a high degree of accuracy and diagnostic potential.

2.7.9 Bibliography

Antonarakis, S. E., Kazazian, H. H., Jr, and Orkin, S. H. (1985). DNA polymorphism and molecular pathology of the human globin gene clusters. *Human Genetics* 69, 1–14.

Babirak, S. P., Iverius, P.-H., Fujimoto, W. Y., and Brunzell, J. D. (1989). Detection and characterization of the heterozygote state of lipoprotein lipase deficiency. *Arteriosclerosis* 9, 326–34.

Brewer, H. B., Jr, Bojanovski, D., Gregg, R. E., and Law, S. E. (1985). Recent studies on the metabolic defect in Tangier Disease. In *Human apolipoprotein mutants impact on atherosclerosis and longevity* (ed. C. R. Sirtori, A. V. Nichols and G. Franceschini), pp. 129–32. Plenum Press, New York.

Brown, M. S. and Goldstein, J. L. (1984). How LDL receptors influence cholesterol and atherosclerosis. *Scientific American* **251**, 52–60.

Brown, M. S. and Goldstein, J. L. (1986). A receptor-mediated pathway for cholesterol homeostasis. *Science* **232**, 34–47.

Connelly, P., Maguire, G. F., Hoffmann, T., and Little, J. A. (1987). Structure of apo C-II Toronto, a non-functional human apoprotein. *Proceedings of the National Academy of Sciences, USA* **84**, 270–3.

Cooper, D. N. and Clayton, J. F. (1988). DNA polymorphism and the study of disease association. *Human Genetics* **78**, 299–312.

Davignon, J., Gregg, R. E., and Sing, C. F. (1988). Apolipoprotein E polymorphism and atherosclerosis. *Arteriosclerosis* **8**, 1–21.

Dawson, P. A., van der Hofmann, S. L., Westhuyzen, D. R., Sudhoff, T. C. Brown, M. S., and Goldstein, J. L. (1988). Sterol dependent repression of low density lipoprotein receptor promoter mediated by 16-base pair sequence adjacent to binding site for transcription factor SPI. *Journal of Biological Chemistry* **263**, 3372–9.

Deeb, S., Failor, A., Brown, B. G., Brunzell, J. D., Albers, J. J., and Motulsky, A. (1986). Molecular genetics of apolipoproteins and coronary heart disease. *Cold Spring Harbor Symposium on Quantitative Biology* **LI**, 403–9.

Demant, T., *et al.* (1988). The catabolic rate of low density lipoprotein is influenced by variation in the apolipoprotein B gene. *Journal of Clinical Investigation* **82**, 797–802.

Ferns, G. A. A., Stocks, J., Ritchie, C., and Galton, D. J. (1985). Genetic polymorphisms of apolipoprotein C-III and insulin in survivors of myocardial infarction. *Lancet* **ii**, 300–3.

Funke, H. S., Rust, S., Assmann, G. (1986). Detection of apolipoprotein E variants by an oligonucleotide 'melting' procedure. *Clinical Chemistry*. **32**, 1285–9.

Goldstein, J. L. and Brown, M. S. (1983). Familial hypercholesterolaemia. In *The metabolic basis of inherited disease* (5th ed), (ed. J. B. Stanburg. J. B. Wyngaarden, D. S. Fredrickson, J. L. Goldstein, and M. S. Brown), p. 672–712. McGraw-Hill, New York.

Goldstein, J. L., Schrott, H. G., Hazzard, W. R., Bierman, E. L., and Motulsky, A. G. (1973). Hyperlipidaemia in coronary heart disease. I Lipid levels in 500 survivors of myocardial infarction. *Journal of Clinical Investigation* **52**, 1544–68.

Hayden, M. R., Vergani, C., Humphries, S. E., Kirby, L., Shukin, R., and MacLeod, R. (1986). Genetics and molecular biology of apolipoprotein CII. In *Lipoprotein deficiency syndromes* (ed. A. Angel and J. Frohlich), pp. 241–51. Plenum Press, New York.

Hegele, R. A. and Breslow, J. L. (1987). Apolipoprotein genetic variation in the assessment of atherosclerosis suceptibility. *Genetic Epidemiology* **4**, 163–84.

Hegele, R. A., Huang, L.-S., Herbert, P. N., Blum, C. B., Buring, J. E., Hennekeus, C. H., and Breslow, J. L. (1986). Apolipoprotein B-gene DNA polymorphisms associated with myocardial infarction. *New England Journal of Medicine* **515**, 1509–15.

Houlston, R. S., Turner, P. R., Revill, J., Lewis, B., and Humphries, S. E. (1988). The fractional catabolic rate of low density lipoprotein in normal individuals is influenced by variation in the apolipoprotein B gene: a preliminary study. *Atherosclerosis* **71**, 81–5.

Humphries, S. E. (1988). DNA polymorphisms of the apolipoprotein genes—their use in the investigation of the genetic components of hyperlipidaemia and atherosclerosis. *Atherosclerosis* **72**, 89–108.

Humphries, S. E., *et al.* (1985). A common DNA polymorphism of the low density lipoprotein (LDL) receptor gene and its use in diagnosis. *Lancet* **i**, 1003–5.

Innerarity, T. L. (1990). Familial hypobetalipoproteinemia and familial defective apolipoprotein B-100: genetic disorders associated with apolipoprotein B. *Current Opinions in Lipidology* **1**, 104–9.

Kessling, A. M., *et al.* (1988). DNA polymorphisms of the apolipoprotein AII and AI–CIII–AIV genes: a study in men selected for differences in high density lipoprotein cholesterol concentration. *American Journal of Human Genetics* **42**, 458–67.

Knott, T. J., Pease, R. H., Powell, L. M., Wallis, S. C., Rall, S. C. Jr., Innerarity, T. L., *et al.* (1986). Complete protein sequence and identification of structural domains of the human apolipoprotein B. *Nature* **323**, 734–8.

Kwiterovich, P. O., Fredrickson, D. S., and Levy, R. I. (1974). Familial hypercholesterolaemia (one form of familial type II hyperlipoproteinaemia)—A study of its biochemical, genetic and clinical presentation in childhood. *Journal of Clinical Investigation* **53**, 1237–49.

Lackner, K. J., *et al.* (1986). Analysis of the apolipoprotein B gene and messenger ribonucleic acid in abetalipoproteinaemia. *Journal of Clinical Investigation* **78**, 1707–12.

Lehrman, M. A., Goldstein, J. L., Brown, M. S., Russell, D. W., and Schneider, W. J. (1985). Internalization-defective LDL receptors produced by genes with nonsense and frameshift mutations that truncate the cytoplasmic domain. *Cell* **41**, 735–43.

Leppert, M., *et al.* (1988). Inference of a molecular defect of apolipoprotein B in hypobetalipoproteinaemia by linkage analysis in a large kindred. *Journal of Clinical Investigation* **82**, 847–51.

Lusis, A. (1988). Genetic factors affecting blood lipoproteins: the candidate gene approach. *Journal of Lipid Research* **29**, 397–429.

Monsalve, M. V., *et al.* (1988). DNA polymorphisms of the gene for apolipoprotein B in patients with peripheral arterial disease. *Atherosclerosis* **70**, 123–9.

Olivecrona, T. and Bengtsson-Olivecrona, G. (1990). Lipases involved in lipoprotein metabolism. *Current Opinions in Lipidology* **1**, 116–21.

Olofsson, S., *et al.* (1987). Apolipoprotein B: structure biosynthesis and role in the lipoprotein assembly process. *Atherosclerosis* **68**, 1–17.

Ordovas, J. M., *et al.* (1986). Apolipoprotein A-I gene polymorphism associated with premature coronary artery disease and familial hypoalphalipoproteinaemia. *New England Journal of Medicine* **314**, 671–7.

Paulweber, B., Friedl, W., Krempler, F., Humphries, S., and Sandhofer, F. (1988). Genetic variation in the apolipoprotein AI–CIII–AIV gene cluster and coronary heart disease. *Arteriosclerosis* **10**, 17–24.

Penrose, L. S. (1935). The detection of autosomal linkage in data which consist of pairs of brothers and sisters of specified parentage. *Annals of Eugenics* **6**, 133–8.

Rees, A., Stocks, J., Shoulders, C. C., Galton, D. J., and Baralle, F. E. (1983). DNA polymorphism in the apo AI–CIII gene cluster association with hypertriglyceridaemia. *Journal of Clinical Investigation* **76**, 1090–5.

Ross, R. (1986). The pathogenesis of atherosclerosis. *New England Journal of Medicine* **314**, 488–500.

Saiki, R. K., Bugawan, T. L., Horn, G. T., Mullis, K. B., and Erlich, H. A. (1986). Analysis of enzymatically amplified-globin and HLA-DQα DNA with allele-specific oligonucleotide probes. *Nature* **324**, 163–6.

Schmitz, G., Assman, G., Brennhausen, B., and Schaefer, H.-J. (1987). Interaction of Tangier lipoproteins with cholesteryl ester-laden mouse peritonial macrophages. *Journal of Lipid Research* **28**, 87–99.

Schuster, H., Rauh, G., Kormann, B., *et al.* (1990). Familial defective apolipoprotein B-100: comparison with familial hypercholesterolaemia in 18 cases detected in Munich. *Arteriosclerosis* **10**, 577–81.

Sing, C. and Boerwinkle, E. A. (1987). Genetic architecture of interindividual variability in apolipoprotein, lipoprotein and lipid phenotypes. In *Molecular approaches to human polygenic disease*, (ed.

G. Bock and G. M. Collins), pp. 99–127. John Wiley and Sons, Chichester.

Soria, L. F., Ludwig, E. H., Clarke, H. R. G., Vega, G. L., Grundy, S. M., McCarthy, B. J. (1989). Association between a specific apolipoprotein B mutation and familial defective apolipoprotein B-100. *Proceedings of the National Academy of Sciences, USA* **86**, 587–91.

Talmud, P. J., *et al.* (1987). Apolipoprotein B gene variants are involved in the determination of serum cholesterol levels; a study in normo- and hyperlipidaemic individuals. *Atherosclerosis* **67**, 81–9.

Talmud, P. J., Lloyd, J. K., Muller, D. P. R., Collins, D., Scott, J., and Humphries, S. E. (1988). Genetic evidence that the apo B gene is not involved in abetalipoproteinaemia. *Journal of Clinical Investigation* **82**, 1803–6.

Thomson, G. and Bodmer, W. F. (1977). The genetic analysis of HLA and disease associations. In *HLA and disease* (ed. J. Dansset and A. Svejgaard), pp. 84–93. Munskgaard, Copenhagen.

Tybjaerg-Hansen, A., Gallagher, J., Vincent, J., *et al.* (1990). Familial defective apolipoprotein B-100: detection in the United Kingdom and Scandinavia, and clinical characteristics of ten cases. *Atherosclerosis* **80**, 235–42.

Utermann, G., Kindsermann, I., Kaffarnik, H., and Steinmetz, A. (1984). Apolipoprotein E phenotypes and hyperlipidaemia. *Human Genetics* **65**, 232–6.

Wile, D. B., Barbir, M., Thompson, G. R., Ritchie, C. D., and Humphries, S. E. (1989). Genetic variation in apo AI gene RFLPs and association with apo AI and HDL cholesterol in patients with coronary artery disease and healthy controls. *Atherosclerosis* **78**, 9–18.

Wojciechowski, A. P., Farrell, M., Cullen, P., Wilson, T. M. E., Bayliss, J. D., Farren, B., *et al.* (1991). Familial combined hyperlipidaemia linked to the apolipoprotein AI-CIII-AIV gene cluster on chromosome 11q23–q24. *Nature* **349**, 161–4.

Yamamoto, T., *et al.* (1984). The human LDL receptor: a cystein-rich protein with multiple Alu sequences in its mRNA. *Cell* **39**, 27–38.

Yang, C.-Y., Chen, S.-H., Sparrow, J. T., Gianturco, S. H., Bradley, W. A., *et al.* (1986). Sequence, structure, receptor-binding domains and internal repeats of human apolipoprotein B-100. *Nature* **323**, 738–42.

Zannis, V. L., Breslow, J. L., Ordovas, J., and Karathanasis, S. K. (1984). Isolation and sequence of Tangier Apo AI gene. *Arteriosclerosis* **4**, 562A.

3

Cell injury and death

3

Cell injury and death

3.1 Cell death

Andrew H. Wyllie and Edward Duvall

3.1.1 Introduction

Cell death is central to much tissue pathology, being the critical end-point of injury inflicted by hypoxia, virus infection, and many toxins. It is also intrinsic to normal cell and tissue regulation, as in embryonic development, normal tissue turnover, and the selection of appropriate clones in proliferating lymphoid populations. Physiological death of this sort is phylogenetically ancient, and subserves many vital functions in animal development. Death features again at the borderline between pathology and physiology, in the targets of attack by cells of the immune system. In addition, there has been speculation for years about the role of cell death in human ageing. Although cells die in this broad variety of circumstances, the pathways leading from life to death are few. Before discussing these, it is necessary to distinguish cell death from a number of processes with which it is commonly confused.

Identification and measurement of death

In toxicology the 'loss of capacity for cell replication' is frequently regarded as loss of 'survival', and by implication is equated with death. For example, *in vitro* studies of cell 'kill' by cancer chemotherapeutic agents are frequently scored on the criterion of loss of clonal proliferation after treatment. This definition is inadequate in the general case. In terminally differentiated cells, for example, lethal events may be initiated years after replication has ceased. Another index of cell death, widely applied to tumour populations *in vivo*, is the 'cell loss factor'. This is the ratio between the observed growth rate of the tumour, and the growth rate predicted from its cell production rate measured directly by mitotic arrest or similar methods (see Chapter 1.3). Although approaches of this sort have emphasized the importance of cell death in the growth kinetics both of

tumours and normal tissues, they are clearly incapable of elucidating mechanisms, and in any case require cautious interpretation. Certain questionable assumptions are made in the calculation of the cell loss factor, notably that the proliferating cell population is homogeneous and that dead tissue maintain its volume. There is also the more obvious point that 'cell loss' cannot always be equated with cell death, since cells also leave tumours by migration or exfoliation.

It is predictable that these indirect assessments of death should prove unsatisfactory. More surprisingly, conventional direct measurements are also inaccurate in defining the moment of death and may give misleading information about its mechanism. Dye uptake methods have been used for decades in analysing death of cells in suspensions *in vitro*. The methods depend upon failure of membrane homeostasis: lethally injured cells permit entry of dyes such as nigrosine or trypan blue, or the fluorescent DNA-binding molecules ethidium bromide or propidium iodide. As will be shown later, however, cells may exclude such dyes and yet have already initiated the process of death. The same is true for methods that measure loss of radioactive chromium from cells previously charged with it *in vitro*. This chromium release is widely used in studies on immune killing but it evaluates membrane breakdown rather than cell death.

By what standards can the death of cells of different types and in different circumstances be compared? In this section (see also Section 3.2) morphology is taken as a criterion. This is possible because the structure of dying cells alters in a restricted number of ways and two principal sets of changes have been described: necrosis and apoptosis (Table 3.1). Both terms derive from Greek. Necrosis means simply the process of death, and from the same root we have the word necropsy. For many years necrosis was used as a synonym for death but when the distinctive nature of apoptosis was recognized, it was necessary to introduce a new term. Apoptosis means the falling off or away, as of leaves from trees in autumn, hair from balding scalps, or renegade members of holy orders. All share the idea of selective removal of individuals without complete disruption of the rest of the society from which they came.

Necrosis usually results from severely disturbed extracellular environmental conditions, and is associated with uncontrolled

Table 3.1 Comparison of morphology of apoptosis and necrosis

	Apoptosis	Necrosis
Histology	Single cells affected within living tissues	Sheets of cells die together, disrupting tissue structure
Cytology	Pyknotic nuclei, condensed cytoplasm, rounded cell fragments	Cellular oedema Nuclei intact but stain faintly
Dye exclusion tests	Dyes initially excluded	Dyes enter
Ultrastructure		
Cytoplasm	Compacted, intact organelles	Mitochondria show high amplitude swelling and matrix densities
	Dilated ER	Dilated organelle profiles
	Plasma membrane intact	Ruptured plasma and internal membranes
Nucleus	Chromatin condensed in caps and toroids	Coarse chromatin patterns which retain normal distribution
	Nucleolar disintegration	
Circumstances	Often in 'programmed death'	Never physiological Complement
	Atrophy	Hypoxia
	Cell-mediated immune killing	Toxins (high dose)
	Toxins (low dose)	
Tissue effects	No inflammation	Acute inflammation
	Phagocytosis by adjacent cells	Scarring later
	Rapid involution without collapse of overall tissue structure	

cell swelling and rupture. Apoptosis usually—although not invariably—occurs where death is part of a regulated process, and is associated with cell shrinkage and other distinctive morphological changes. A further and much rarer mode of dying involves formation of 'very dark cells' (Harmon 1987). These persist in tissues for long periods, and show greatly shrunken cytoplasm, but nearly normal nuclear outlines. Beyond the information that such cells are metabolically inert, little is known about them or the stimuli for their formation. The rest of this section therefore focuses on the biology of apoptosis and necrosis.

3.1.2 Apoptosis

Incidence

Apoptosis is a developmental process. It occurs in the pre-implantation embryo, during implantation, and at all stages of organogenesis, notably in Müllerian and Wolffian involution, the deletion of interdigital webs, and the genesis of lumina within hollow organs, such as the heart. Cell deletion by apoptosis is particularly well documented in the nervous system, where cells are usually overproduced during development, with subsequent deletion of the surplus. It is also the major recorded mode of death in the involution of tissues during the metamorphosis of amphibia.

Apoptosis contributes to the atrophy of fully developed mammalian tissues, following endocrine and other stimuli. Examples include prostate and adrenal cortex following reduction in trophic hormone stimulation (by surgical or pharmacological means) and the physiological atrophy of post-lactational breast. Probably related in character is the apoptosis of B- and T-lymphocytes after removal of stimulation by trophic cytokines at the end of immunological reactions. Atrophy of the parotid gland after ligation of the main duct is also mediated in part by apoptosis of epithelial cells. Atrophy, of course, also involves loss of intercellular matrix and reduction in volume of the residual living cells, changes which are co-ordinated with, but distinct from, apoptosis.

Apoptosis balances mitosis in the normal turnover of cells within cyclically stimulated epithelia, including the human breast and endometrium. It is responsible for the death of neutrophils after their extravasation into inflamed tissues and is therefore a significant factor in the termination of the inflammatory response. It occurs in the cells of the thymus cortex, where it is related to stimulation by 'self' antigens and is accelerated by glucocorticoid hormones. It is observed in the targets of cytotoxic cells. Apoptosis is also frequently present in tumours, during both their growth and regression. Finally, apoptosis is observed in tissues treated with a variety of toxic stimuli, particularly when these are applied at low dosage (e.g. cytotoxic drugs, hyperthermia, ionizing radiation, and even minor degrees of hypoxia). Under these circumstances, apoptosis can show striking restriction to certain cell types; e.g. the selective death of spermatogonia and conservation of Sertoli cells following testicular irradiation or exposure to radiomimetic drugs (Allan *et al.* 1987).

Morphology

Apoptosis has five cardinal morphological features (Fig. 3.1).

1. There is loss of specialized surface structures, such as microvilli and contact regions, so that the cell adopts a smooth contour, and becomes isolated from is viable neighbours.

2. There is cell volume reduction, associated with compaction of the cytoplasmic organelles, and distortion of cell shape. Frequently the apoptotic cell splits into several membrane-bound bodies (apoptotic bodies), each with its own cluster of organelles (Fig. 3.2).

3. There is conservation of cytoplasmic organelle integrity. In contradistinction to necrosis, mitochondria do not undergo swelling and rupture of internal membranes. However, some unusual features appear: sometimes ribosomes aggregate in semicrystalline arrays, and frequently fascicles of microfilaments can be seen within the cytoplasm, running parallel to the cell surface. Almost always there is a transient dilatation of the smooth endoplasmic reticulum, the dilated cisternae fusing with the cell surface (Fig. 3.3a). Under the

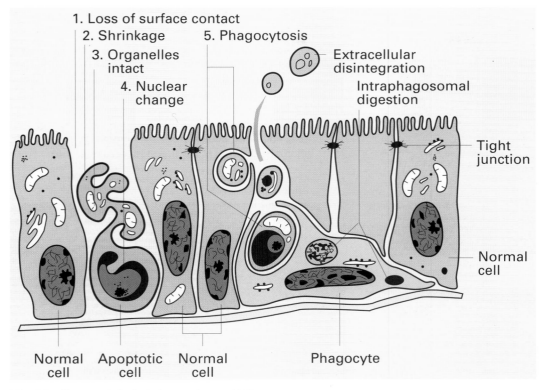

Fig. 3.1 Key morphological changes in apoptosis.

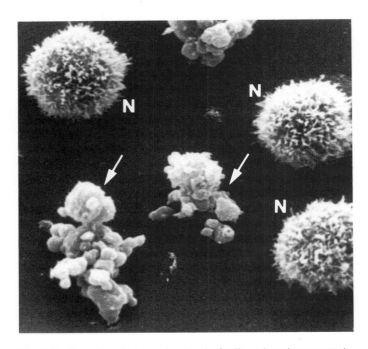

Fig. 3.2 Scanning electron micrograph of cells undergoing apoptosis. In this example the normal cells (marked N) are spherical, with many microvilli. The apoptotic cells (arrowed) are greatly reduced in volume and are undergoing fragmentation to many smooth-surfaced apoptotic bodies. (Reproduced by permission of Academic Press from the *International Review of Cytology*.)

scanning electron microscope, this gives the cell surface a dramatically cratered appearance (Fig. 3.3b).

4. The most striking morphological feature, however, is change in nuclear chromatin configuration. Chromatin condenses under the nuclear membrane, appearing in transmission electron micrographs as densely granular hemilunar caps or complete toroids. Transcriptional complexes are shed from the nucleolus, appearing as a cluster of osmiophilic bodies in the nucleoplasm, whereas the residual nucleolar protein core adopts a characteristic position adjacent to the peripheral marginated chromatin (Figs. 3.3a, 3.4). Nuclear shape undergoes the same distortion as that of the whole cell, and the nucleus frequently breaks up into several fragments, all initially membrane bound. Nuclear pores are concentrated in the few regions where condensed chromatin does not lie adjacent to the membrane.

5. The apoptotic cell is swiftly recognized by its viable neighbours (parenchymal cells or specialized phagocytes) as a target for phagocytosis. The apoptotic cell (and the apoptotic bodies into which it may fragment) undergoes progressive degenerative changes within the phagosome of the ingesting cell. Membranes disappear, organelles become unrecognizable, and ultimately the appearance is that of any large lysosomal residual body (Fig. 3.5). Occasionally apoptotic bodies escape phagocytosis—for example, when apoptotic ductal epithelial cells are lost into the duct lumen. Here they eventually degenerate, losing their high density and

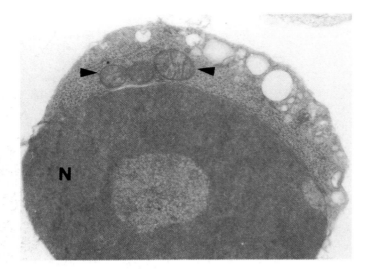

(a)

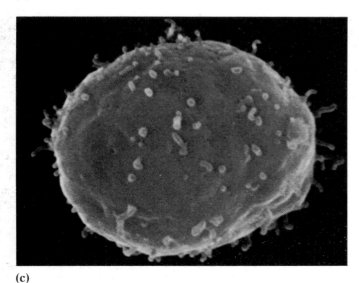

(b)

(c)

showing the membrane breakdown to be described under necrosis.

This description has concentrated on ultrastructural findings, but apoptosis can be recognized under the light microscope. The affected cells appear as clusters of small membrane-bounded, densely eosinophilic cytoplasmic bodies, including either a single highly pyknotic nucleus, or several nuclear fragments. In tissues, because they are quickly recognized and phagocytosed, apoptotic bodies are most commonly seen within large heterophagosomes in the ingesting cells (Fig. 3.6).

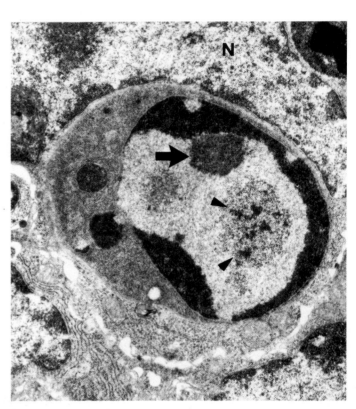

Fig. 3.4 Typical nuclear features in an apoptotic cell lying within the phagosome of an ingesting cell, whose normal nucleus is partially visible (N). Notice the dense peripheral chromatin condensation, the nucleolar fibrillary centre (arrow), and the osmiophilic nucleoplasmic granules (transcription complexes) marked by arrowheads. (Reproduced by permission of Academic Press from the *International Review of Cytology*.)

Fig. 3.3 (a) Transmission electron micrograph of dilated vacuoles of endoplasmic reticulum underlying the plasma membrane of an apoptotic thymus cortical lymphocyte. Notice also the band of condensed chromatin around the periphery of the nucleus (N) and the morphologically normal mitochondria (arrowheads). (Reproduced from the *Journal of Pathology*, with permission.) The bald, cratered surface of a similar cell is seen in the scanning electron micrograph (b), in contrast to the delicate microvillous surface of a normal viable cell (c). (Reproduced from *Immunology Today*, with permission.)

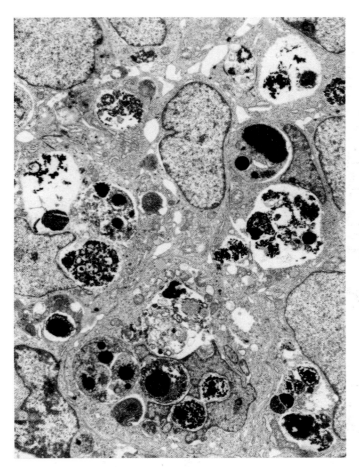

Fig. 3.5 Apoptotic bodies in various stages of degradation lying within the phagosomes of viable cells. The tissue is parotid gland, during atrophy induced by duct ligation. (Provided by Dr N. Walker and Prof. J. F. R. Kerr, Department of Pathology, University of Queensland, Australia.)

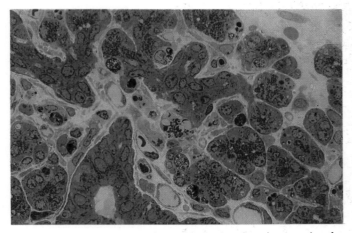

Fig. 3.6 Light micrograph of parotid gland undergoing atrophy after duct ligation. Note the many apoptotic bodies (with dark, homogenous nuclear chromatin) lying within phagosomes. (Reproduced from the *Journal of Pathology*, with permission.)

Kinetics

Time-lapse cinematographic studies show that apoptosis begins abruptly. At a variable time after the onset of the lethal stimulus the affected cell suddenly undergoes shrinkage, blebbing, and bubbling. This phase lasts for only a few minutes, and generates shrunken apoptotic bodies. If the cell is not phagocytosed immediately, it undergoes a gradual loss of cell density, coinciding with loss of membrane integrity, as shown ultrastructurally and by the ingress of dyes. The period for which an apoptotic body, once formed, remains recognizable within a tissue has been variously estimated as between 4 and 9 hours. This coincides broadly with the time-course of complete degradation of other large biological structures within the phagosomes of macrophages. Because this time is relatively short, small increases in the proportion of apoptotic cells seen in tissue sections can conceal large rates of cell loss. For example, in a tissue undergoing atrophy to half its cell complement over 3 days, the increase in apoptosis visible in the light microscope during this time would be less than 5 per cent of the total cell number.

These observations explain much of the obscurity which has, until recently, surrounded this type of cell death, despite the very significant processes for which it is responsible. A further consequence of this obscurity is that the manifestations of apoptosis have been given different names in different tissues. Such names include tingible body macrophages (macrophages containing apoptotic lymphocytes within reactive centres of lymph nodes), Civatte bodies (apoptotic keratinocytes in psoriasis; see Chapter 28), and Councilman bodies (apoptotic hepatocytes; see Chapter 17).

Mechanisms

Alterations in cell shape and size

Early in apoptosis, cells lose about half their volume. There is a concomitant rise in cell density, suggesting selective loss of water and electrolytes with conservation of denser structural elements. This rapid export of water probably takes place into the endoplasmic reticulum, giving rise to transient dilatation, prior to fusion with the cell surface. For many years there was little clue to the biochemical mechanism of this selective fluid loss. Recently, however, a sodium-potassium-chloride co-transporter system has been described, inhibition of which leads to net loss of sodium and water from affected cells (Wilcock *et al.* 1988).

The mechanisms that underlie the striking blebbing and fragmentation of both cytoplasm and nucleus are not known. During this period, however, there is evidence of transglutaminase activity within the affected cells (Fesus *et al.* 1987, 1989). Transglutaminases are enzymes which cross-link proteins, rendering them insoluble even to strong chemical denaturing agents. A rigid shell of transglutaminated protein builds up under the membrane of apoptotic cells. This is likely to cause some of the alteration in cell shape and may be responsible for volume contraction too.

Condensation of chromatin

There are several levels of packaging of normal chromatin. About 180 base pairs of DNA are wound around discoid histone octamers (nucleosomes) with approximately 20 base pairs of linker DNA between them. These discs are often stacked in a solenoid to form a 300 Å diameter filament. Large loops of such filaments are attached at their bases to the protein matrix of the nucleus in association with topoisomerase 2 (Fig. 3.7). The condensation of chromatin seen during apoptosis is due to collapse of this organization through double-stranded cleavage of the internucleosomal linker DNA (Fig. 3.7). A candidate endonuclease activity has been identified. It is active at neutral pH, dependent upon calcium and magnesium, and inhibited by zinc.

Recognition of apoptotic cells

The binding and phagocytosis of apoptotic cells by specialized phagocytes and other viable cells in their neighbourhood requires a specific non-immunological recognition mechanism. Macrophage binding to apoptotic cells is blocked by certain specific sugars (such as N-acetylglucosamine and its dimer N,N'-diacetylchitobiose in rodent cells; glucosamine in human cells). This suggests that a lectin-like receptor molecule on the surface of the macrophage recognizes increased expression of such sugars on the surface of apoptotic cells. Recently, human macrophages have been shown to bind to apoptotic neutrophils and other cells via the macrophage vitronectin receptor—a member of the integrin family previously considered exclusively as a cell adhesion molecule (Savill *et al.* 1990). The nature of the ligand which this receptor recognizes on the surface of the apoptotic cell is not yet clear, nor is it certain that the vitronectin receptor is identical to the receptor binding the sugars mentioned above.

Initiating stimuli

In considering the initiation of apoptosis, two processes must be distinguished. The first is accumulation of the specialist machinery which permits apoptosis to take place. We call this priming for apoptosis. Transglutaminase and the calcium–magnesium endonuclease are examples of enzymes which appear during such priming. The second is the triggering of primed cells into apoptosis itself (Fig. 3.8) Stimuli that trigger primed cells will not initiate apoptosis in unprimed cells, and may induce in them quite different processes. An outstanding example of this is the effect of antigen binding to cells bearing the T-cell receptor. The immature T-cells of the thymus cortex are primed for apoptosis, and receptor occupancy triggers apoptosis in them. In contrast the mature T-cell is not primed, and responds to the same ligand by initiating cell replication. Similarly, the muscle cells of tadpole tails in metamorphosis can be regarded as primed, as they respond to thyroxine by triggering apoptosis, whereas thyroxine is simultaneously a growth stimulus for the muscle cells in the limbs.

Practically nothing is known of the stimuli which prime cells for apoptosis, but there are some clues to the nature of the triggers. Many appear to act by well-known receptor-mediated cellular signalling pathways, involving a sustained, moderate rise in cytosolic calcium of the order of 500–1000 nM (McConkey *et al.* 1990). This is associated with a cascade of induction of new messenger RNA species which include (amongst others of unknown function) c-*fos*, c-*myc*, and certain heat-shock proteins (Buttyan *et al.* 1988). Triggering of apoptosis in primed cells can sometimes be blocked by agents that arrest the rise in cytosolic calcium or inhibit mRNA and protein synthesis. The role of the phosphoinositides and protein kinase C in this pathway is under investigation at present. Phorbol esters (which

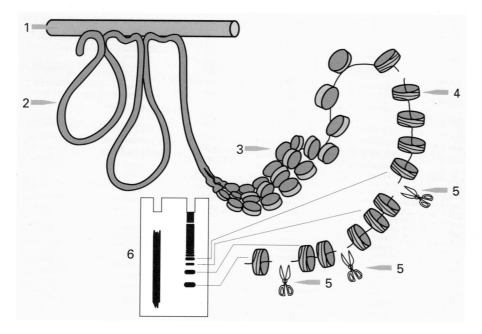

Fig. 3.7 Normal chromatin organization. The interphase nucleus contains a protein matrix (1) to which loops of chromatin fibrils (2) are attached. The chromatin fibril is a contracted solenoid, each turn comprising six nucleosomes (3). Nucleosomes are regularly spaced along the DNA double helix, which is wound twice around each (4). Chromatin DNA is most accessible to cleavage in the linker region between nucleosomes (5). Hence incomplete digestion of chromatin DNA yields a series of fragments differing in length by uniform steps. These separate in gel electrophoresis into a 'ladder' (6). In contrast, naked DNA digests to a complete spectrum of sizes, and appears as a continuous smear on the gel (on the left of the gel).

activate protein kinase C) rescue cortical thymocytes from apoptosis, so that calcium triggering no longer induces apoptosis in them (McConkey *et al.* 1989*a*).

The cytosolic free-calcium concentration in a typical mammalian cell is around 100 nM, whereas that outside is about 10 000-fold greater (1.3 mM). Within the cell there are compartments with relatively high free-calcium concentrations, notably mitochondria and endoplasmic reticulum. The resulting concentration gradients are sustained by several different energy-dependent mechanisms. It is therefore not surprising that mild injury induces increases in free cytosolic calcium and hence triggers apoptosis in appropriately primed cells; see also Section 3.3.

This resolves the paradox that 'programmed' death can be triggered in susceptible cells by unphysiological stimuli (Fig. 3.8). Toxicologists have frequently observed that the regions within tissues where 'spontaneous' apoptosis occurs are also the most sensitive to a variety of xenobiotics. Similarly, some teratogens produce their effects by enhancing the rate of cell loss from regions already showing physiological apoptosis. This concept also explains one of the central features of cell senescence: vulnerability to a progressively broadening spectrum of injurious stimuli.

Priming is reversible. A common strategy in the regulation of cell populations is the production of excess numbers of cells primed for apoptosis, all doomed to die unless rescued by a specific growth factor. The factor involved in this positive selection may be presented on the surface of regulatory cells, or released locally. During immunological reactions, B-cells within germinal follicles are selected in this way through the stimulus of antigen presented on the surface of dendritic cells (Liu *et al.* 1989*a*). Similarly, in the developing central nervous system, motor neurones are generated in numbers substantially greater than the final complement (Williams and Herrup 1988). Those that fail to contact muscle and form an end plate are deleted by apoptosis. It is thought that the rescuing stimulus passes retrogradely across the end plate from the muscle. An analogous situation probably exists in the setting up of interneuronal

networks. The nature of these rescuing signals is poorly understood, but nerve growth factors of great variety, some of them specific for particular neurone type, are known to exist (Walicke 1989). One such factor, neuroleukin, is a 63 kDa protein which supports the survival of dorsal root ganglion cells and other neurones, and also is trophic for B-lymphocytes. It appears to be identical with the glycolytic enzyme phosphoglucose isomerase and the relationship between the glycolytic and trophic functions of the molecule have still to be worked out. Of particular interest in the molecular analysis of neuroleukin is a sequence of 44 amino acids which is homologous to a conserved region of the coat protein gp120 of the AIDS virus, HIV-1. As gp120 causes death of neurones (contributing to, if not accounting for the dementia of AIDS) it is possible that it functions by blocking the neuronal receptor for neuroleukin.

3.1.3 Necrosis

Incidence

Necrosis occurs in circumstances of severely deranged cellular environment, including hypoxia, extremes of temperature, exposure to a variety of toxins, attack by complement, and infection with lytic viruses.

Morphology

The first changes in cells undergoing necrosis are mild cytoplasmic swelling, dilatation of the smooth endoplasmic reticulum, and loss of ribosomes from rough endoplasmic reticulum (Fig. 3.9; see also Section 3.2). A further characteristic change is 'blebbing' from the plasma membrane of cytoplasmic fragments that include cytosol but not the larger organelles such as mitochondria and endoplasmic reticulum.

All these changes, however, can also occur in sublethally injured cells. An important question therefore is the nature of the 'point of no return' at which there is irreversible commitment to necrosis. This commitment coincides closely with two mitochondrial changes seen in the electron microscope: a

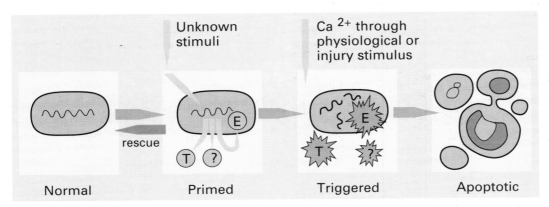

Fig. 3.8 Priming, triggering, and rescue events in apoptosis. During priming, new products such as transglutaminase (T) and the Ca–Mg endonuclease (E) are synthesized, no doubt together with other as yet unknown effectors. Triggering activates these, probably by Ca^{2+}-mediated mechanisms. Apoptosis follows triggering immediately, but the time between priming and triggering may vary.

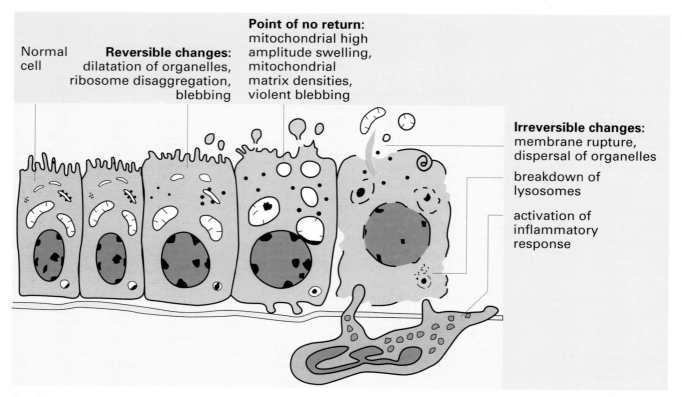

Normal cell

Reversible changes: dilatation of organelles, ribosome disaggregation, blebbing

Point of no return: mitochondrial high amplitude swelling, mitochondrial matrix densities, violent blebbing

Irreversible changes: membrane rupture, dispersal of organelles

breakdown of lysosomes

activation of inflammatory response

Fig. 3.9   Major events in necrosis.

violent dilatation, called high amplitude swelling, and the appearance of matrix densities (Fig. 3.10). The latter are usually flocculent and probably represent denatured proteins, but crystalline densities of calcium phosphates also occur, particularly in hypoxia. The necrotic cell swells rapidly, and both the plasma and internal membranes begin to rupture. Organelles spill out and are found lying in the extracellular space. In contrast to apoptosis, however, nuclear structures remain relatively intact. Although heterochromatin becomes coarser, the normal distinction between euchromatin and heterochromatin is retained, and nuclear pores remain dispersed around the membrane. Eventually, however, the necrotic cell is reduced to an electron-lucent shell containing fragments of membranes and nondescript osmiophilic material.

In the light microscope, the early, reversible changes are difficult to detect. The terms 'hydropic change', 'cloudy swelling', and 'feathery degeneration' probably refer to this phase of cell damage, as perceived in conventionally fixed and stained tissue sections. The rapid changes after the point of no return are more obvious (Fig. 3.11). Cytoplasm loses detail and acquires a homogeneous eosinophilic 'ground glass' appearance. Chromatin patterns in the nucleus are coarser, and eventually nuclear staining is lost ('karyolysis'). Perhaps because necrosis requires major perturbation of the cell environment, and thus frequently results from abnormalities of blood flow, necrotic cells are usually found in contiguous sheets. Unlike apoptosis, necrosis usually induces an acute inflammatory response, with

neutrophil polymorphs prominent around the dead cells. The old terms 'coagulative necrosis' and 'colliquative necrosis' describe the gross appearances of necrosis. The former has a solid and the latter a liquid consistency.

Mechanisms

The endpoint of necrosis is intracellular chaos. It is relatively easy to identify cellular events which are consistently associated with this. It is more difficult to demonstrate causation and so define the biology of the transition from the living to the dead state. We do not know whether the routes to necrosis are many or few. Five major classes of event, however, merit discussion, and some of them appear to fit together in a common pattern (Fig. 3.12).

Ubiquitination of cellular proteins

Ubiquitin is a 76 amino-acid protein found in relatively high abundance in all eukaryotic cells and with highly conserved structure between species. In the presence of ATP, it forms covalent bonds with lysine residues of other proteins. Synthesis of ubiquitin is induced, together with that of another family of proteins called heat-shock proteins (HSP) in cell injury of various types. One role of HSP is to unfold and refold proteins perhaps assisting their movement across organelle membranes or reversing partial denaturation. In contrast, the principal function of ubiquitin seems to be to flag damaged protein for degradation, since ubiquitination sharply reduces protein half-life. In

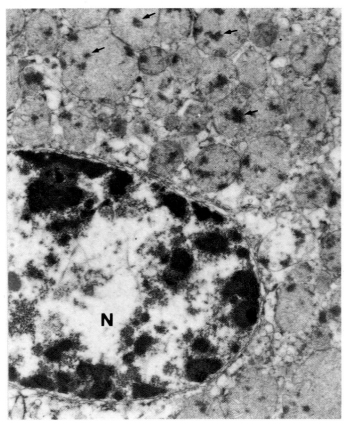

Fig. 3.10 Transmission electron micrograph of a necrotic hepatocyte after the 'point of no return'. Mitochondria are greatly dilated, and contain matrix densities (arrows). In the nucleus (N), although nuclear chromatin patterns are coarse, the general distribution of condensed and decondensed chromatin is similar to normal and very different from apoptosis (see Fig. 3.3).

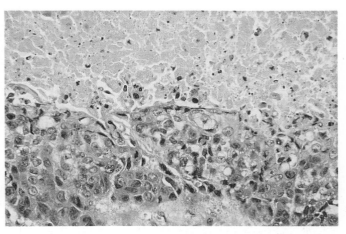

Fig. 3.11 Light micrograph of necrosis, in this case within a poorly differentiated human malignant tumour. Note the ghostly cell outlines and absence of nuclear staining in the necrotic region at the top, in contrast with the band of viable cells below. The vascular stroma lies along the bottom of the figure.

certain degenerating cells of the CNS and elsewhere, however, the ubiquitinated proteins accumulate, forming cytoplasmic inclusion bodies (Table 3.2). These are found in circumstances in which cell death also occurs. There is no evidence, however, that the inclusions cause death. Their accumulation within dying cells probably represents failure of injured cells to cope with the increased concentration of proteins flagged for degradation.

ATP depletion

Dying cells are depleted of high-energy phosphate. This is par-

ticularly true after a hypoxic injury, since the supply of oxygen to the mitochondrial terminal respiratory chain enzymes is necessary for sustained ATP generation. Some ATP derives from anaerobic glycolysis, but this is also inhibited in hypoxia, through accumulation of lactate and NADH. For many years it was considered probable that ischaemic necrosis of myocardial cells was a direct result of this hypoxic depletion of ATP. In support of this was the observation that high amplitude swelling and other indices of loss of cell volume homeostasis appear only as cell ATP levels fall below a critical threshhold (Fig. 3.13). Temporally, however, necrosis and ATP depletion are not so closely linked.

During obstruction to vascular perfusion, tissue ATP falls below the critical concentration yet there are no major structural changes in the myocardial cells. If perfusion with oxygen-rich fluid is restored, necrosis develops with dramatic speed. This is reperfusion injury, a phenomenon discussed in more detail later. Moreover, treatment with agents that inhibit transmembrane calcium flux (such as chlorpromazine) can prevent the development of reperfusion necrosis, although the treated cells show the same low ATP concentrations during their periods of ischaemia. Thus ATP depletion alone is not sufficient to cause necrosis but it may constrain the cell's capacity for recovery by limiting ATP-dependent functions, such as ubiquitination and membrane cation pumps.

Table 3.2 Cytoplasmic inclusion bodies

Disorder	Affected cell type	Ubiquitinated protein species	Pathological nomenclature
Alzheimer's disease	Cortical neurone	Paired helical filament protein	Granulovacuolar degeneration
		Tubulin, neurofilaments	Neurofibrillary tangle
Parkinson's disease	Substantia nigra neurone	Tubulin, neurofilaments	Lewy body
Alcoholic liver disease	Hepatocyte	Cytoskeletal proteins	Mallory body

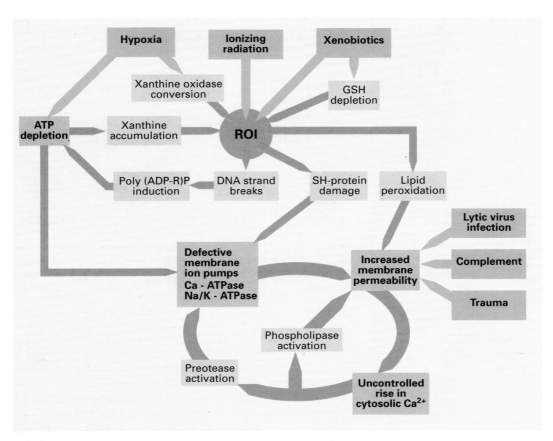

Fig. 3.12 Major processes in necrosis.

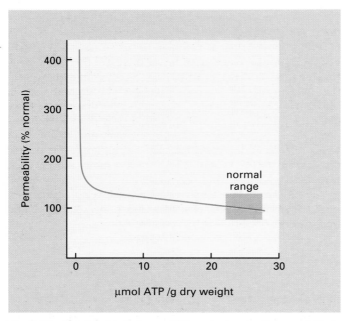

Fig. 3.13 Relationship between ATP content and cell permeability in ischaemic cardiac muscle. Note how the permeability remains essentially the same unless the ATP content falls below about 5 per cent of normal, when it rises uncontrollably.

Reactive oxygen intermediates

Addition of electrons to molecular oxygen leads to the genesis of a series of reactive molecules collectively called reactive oxygen intermediates (ROI). These are capable of injuring tissue and may be responsible for necrosis. Several of the reactive oxygen intermediates are free radicals, that is molecular species containing electrons unpaired in spin. Free radicals are short lived, and this, together with the variety of their potential reactions with cellular components, has made it difficult to be certain of all their biological effects. However, several important principles governing these effects are well established (Halliwell 1989) and are discussed below and in Section 3.3.

Formation of ROI almost certainly occurs continuously Oxygen is present in all living cells, and isolated preparations of mitochondria, endoplasmic reticulum, cytosol and nuclear membranes have all been shown to be sources of ROI. Important molecular sources include agents concerned with oxygen transport and exchange, such as haemoglobin, cytochrome P_{450}, and the mitochondrial electron transport chain. Within cells, however, the damage these would cause is limited by powerful protective mechanisms. Amongst these are anti-oxidants such as α-tocopherol (one component of vitamin E), glutathione, and enzyme systems such as superoxide dismutase, glutathione peroxidase, glutathione synthetase, and perhaps catalase (Fig. 3.14). Inhibition of these protective mechanisms thus constitutes an oxidative stress to the cell, and is likely to result in cell injury.

The most significant ROI These are the superoxide anion (O_2^- ·), the perhydroxyl radical ($HO_2^{\cdot}$), the peroxide ion (O_2^-)—as in H_2O_2 hydrogen peroxide), the hydroxyl radical ($OH^{\cdot}$), and the hydroxyl anion (OH^-). All are generated during the reduction of molecular oxygen (O_2) to water.

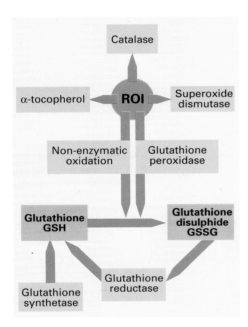

Fig. 3.14 Systems for trapping or destroying reactive oxygen intermediates.

ROI react with themselves and other molecules available within tissues to make further molecular species These are capable of inflicting cell injury in their own right. For example:

$$O_2^- \cdot + H_2O_2 \rightarrow OH^{\cdot} + OH^- + O_2 \qquad (1)$$

This is the Haber–Weiss reaction, and is accelerated by metal ions such as Fe^{2+} in metalloproteins.

$$2O_2^- \cdot + 2H^+ \rightarrow H_2O_2 + O_2 \qquad (2)$$

This is a dismutation reaction, and is accelerated by the enzyme superoxide dismutase.

$$H_2O_2 + Cl^- \rightarrow HOCl + OH^- \qquad (3)$$

This is the myeloperoxidase reaction, used by granulocytes to generate hypochlorous acid which contributes to the killing of ingested micro-organisms. Although this is normally considered a 'beneficial' process it is important to recognize that the toxic ROI are themselves quite non-specific in effect, and capable of inflicting damage on adjacent cells.

ROI and their products differ in their reactivity, half-life, and diffusibility This affects the way in which they interact with cell constituents around the site of their formation. Thus $OH^{\cdot}$ and HOCl (hypochlorous acid) are highly reactive, whereas O_2^- · and H_2O_2, although less reactive, can diffuse further and therefore give rise to additional more reactive species as described above.

ROI interact with lipids Membrane lipids containing unsaturated C=C bonds undergo peroxidation. The lipid hydroperoxides so generated are themselves highly reactive, and hence lipid peroxidation tends to be a self-perpetuating reaction that spreads within the affected membrane. Some of the products of lipid peroxidation (malonaldehyde and 4-hydroxynonenal) increase the permeability and deformability of the membranes in which they are found. Mitochondrial membranes are particularly susceptible to this sort of damage, perhaps because they combine a high risk of ROI-mediated peroxidation (oxygen and metalloproteins are both present in relatively high concentration) with a high content of polyunsaturated C=C bonds.

ROI interact with proteins Thiol-containing proteins are particularly susceptible to peroxidation damage. This may have special relevance in the genesis of disturbed cellular ion homeostasis, since the Ca-ATPase and Na–K ATPases of plasma membranes are both thiol-containing proteins.

ROI interact with DNA This causes strand breaks and has the secondary effect of inducing the enzyme poly(ADP-ribose) polymerase. It has been suggested that the resulting depletion of cellular ADP may be sufficiently severe to reduce total cellular adenine nucleotide (including ATP) to critical levels, as discussed above.

Generation of ROI alters the redox activity of the cell This can have profound secondary effects on enzyme systems sensitive to redox potential. One example of this is depletion of NADPH and generation of $NADP^+$ within mitochondria subjected to oxidative stress. For reasons that are not entirely clear, but perhaps relate to the depletion of intramitochondrial ATP, the change in NADPH–$NADP^+$ ratio results in efflux of calcium from the mitochondria into the cytoplasm. This intracellular ion flux is of great significance in cell injury and is discussed further below and in Section 3.3.

Thus, in summary, ROI may increase membrane permeability, inhibit cation pumps, deplete ATP, and increase cytosolic free calcium. The role of ROI in necrosis is illustrated well by the effects of oxygen therapy in the neonatal lung, paracetamol overdose in the liver, and post-ischaemic reperfusion in the myocardium.

Neonatal respiratory distress syndrome (RDS) In this condition, due to immaturity of the lung at the time of birth, necrosis of pulmonary alveolar lining cells develops. A protein-rich exudate fills the alveoli (Fig. 3.15). One pathogenetic factor is the increased generation of ROI resulting from high concentrations of oxygen, administered therapeutically. Recognition of this has

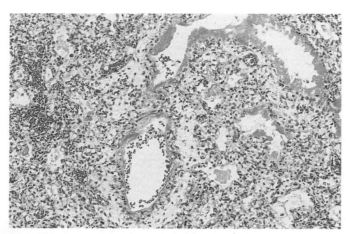

Fig. 3.15 Lung from a neonate who died with respiratory distress syndrome. Notice the pink-staining exudate within the dilated respiratory passages, which represents proteins (including fibrin) that have leaked through necrotic vessel walls. As is characteristic in this condition, the alveoli are largely collapsed. (Provided by Dr J. Keeling, Royal Hospital for Sick Children, Edinburgh.)

led to more circumspect policies in oxygen administration to neonates. Therapeutic oxygen is not the sole factor in the pathogenesis of alveolar cell necrosis, however, another being reperfusion injury.

Paracetamol overdosage This causes hepatocyte necrosis. Free radical scavengers limit the damage, indicating the pathogenetic role of ROI. Metabolism of paracetamol involves the formation of thiolated compounds, the thiol groups being donated by cellular glutathione (GSH). The resulting depletion of GSH leaves the hepatocyte unprotected from oxidative injury (Fig. 3.16). These observations led to the introduction of GSH precursors (e.g. *N*-acetyl-L-cysteine) as antidotes for paracetamol overdosage (Boobis *et al.* 1989). It is probable that many other hepatotoxins cause hepatocyte necrosis by GSH depletion in this way. This is more fully discussed in Section 3.3.

Reperfusion injury The explosive onset of necrosis during reperfusion of ischaemic organs coincides with a burst of ROI generation. An attractive hypothesis attributes this to two simultaneous effects of hypoxia. First, xanthine accumulates from the metabolism of ATP. In the normal aerobic state this is prevented by regeneration of ATP (Fig. 3.17). Secondly, xanthine dehydrogenase, an enzyme found almost exclusively in capillary endothelium, undergoes proteolytic cleavage, altering its activity to that of a xanthine oxidase. When the supply of molecular oxygen is restored by reperfusion the accumulated xanthine is therefore oxidized, a reaction in which ROI are generated. The extent of reperfusion necrosis can be curtailed by treatment with superoxide dismutase (which scavenges ROI), allopurinol (which inhibits xanthine oxidase), or protease inhibitors (which presumably prevent the alteration in xanthine dehydrogenase activity). These interventions therefore have obvious therapeutic potential. This hypothesis, in which endothelial cell damage is an essential intermediate in tissue

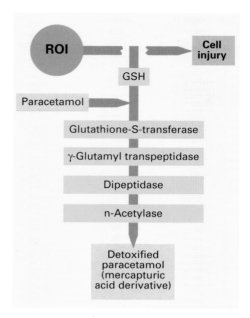

Fig. 3.16 Metabolism of paracetamol (and many other compounds) deflects the glutathione available for scavenging ROI, by using it to form *S*-substituted *N*-acetyl cysteine derivatives (mercapturic acids) via a series of enzymatic reactions. The enzymes involved are abundant in many cells, for example glutathione-*S*-transferase amounts to 10 per cent of cytosolic protein in hepatocytes.

injury, affords a convincing explanation for the profuse extravascular exudate which is characteristic of ischaemic necrosis. The xanthine oxidase hypothesis, however, is only one explanation for ROI generation in reperfusion. One alternative possibility is that during ischaemia iron ions are released from their normal intracellular sites, and so become available for catalysing ROI generation on restoration of the oxygen supply. Another is that the mitochondrial electron transport chain

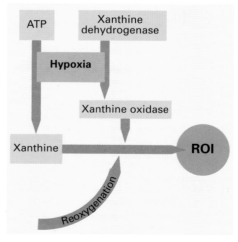

Fig. 3.17 Xanthine oxidase hypothesis for reperfusion damage (see text for details).

becomes 'uncoupled' during ischaemia, and hence on reoxygenation, oxygen intermediates accumulate.

Reperfusion necrosis was first described in the myocardium, but exactly analogous phenomena occur in hypoxic gut, pancreas (for example after severe shock where the pancreatic blood supply is temporarily reduced), and other conditions involving low but fluctuating oxygen supply (as in the pulmonary and intracerebral vasculature of RDS infants). Perhaps more surprising is the fact that xanthine oxidase inhibitors and superoxide dismutase also have a beneficial effect on the pancreatic necrosis which follows non-ischaemic injury, such as ethanol abuse or main duct obstruction. It is possible that ROI are critically involved in the pathogenesis of many conditions where cell damage is not directly related to hypoxia. One explanation of this would be that many types of cell damage reduce the effectiveness of intracellular radical scavenging systems and so subject the cell to oxidative stress.

Loss of calcium homeostasis

Dead cells accumulate calcium. This is to be expected, since during life energy-dependent processes maintain the cytosolic calcium concentration at less than one-thousandth of that of the extracellular fluid, as we have seen earlier. Flux of calcium into dead cells is exploited in nuclear medicine: the size of a myocardial infarct can be visualized by scanning the image generated by a calcium-binding radioactive tracer (technetium-labelled pyrophosphate) (Fig. 3.18). The ultrastructural counterpart of this is the appearance of calcium deposits within mitochondria at the 'point of no return'. The irregular calcium deposits that can often be seen in the light microscope within infarcts are later manifestations of the same phenomenon.

There are reasons to believe, however, that uncontrolled calcium entry can be a cause, as well as a result of, cell death. Thus time-course studies of cytosolic calcium in stressed cells usually show progressive calcium entry before the agonal contortion, blebbing, and swelling (Orrenius et al. 1989). We have already noted that cells can be protected from the toxic effects of many compounds by reducing the extracellular calcium concentration, or by pharmacological inhibition of calcium movement (for example, chlorpromazine). Further, calcium entry appears to activate intracellular mechanisms that initiate a vicious circle of continuing cell damage. Thus calcium-sensitive proteases are activated by lethal stress, and may well be responsible for the destruction of the Ca-ATPases in plasma and endoplasmic reticulum membranes, rendering the cell powerless to return its cytosolic concentration towards more normal levels. The agonal changes in shape in necrotic cells have been attributed to interaction of these proteases with cytoskeletal elements. Calcium-sensitive phospholipases are also activated in lethally stressed cells, and remove phospholipid from plasma membranes, an effect that may render them more permeable to many solutes.

Loss of selective membrane permeability

Loss of selective membrane permeability is an essential feature of necrosis. It is responsible for the dye uptake and chromium

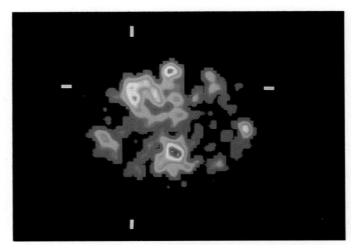

Fig. 3.18 False-colour single photon emission computed tomography image of a myocardial infarction, visualized by localization of technetium (Tc^{99}m)-tagged pyrophosphate, a marker of calcium accumulation. The picture shows a cross-section of the thorax, with accumulation of isotope in the sternum (top), vertebral body (bottom), and a rib (on either side). The yellow and red image on the left ventricle marks the infarct. (Provided by Dr A. Muir, University Medical School, Edinburgh.)

release tests often used to identify cell death. As we have seen, it may be the result of activation of calcium-dependent phospholipases. Direct damage to membranes can result from trauma, freeze–thaw injury, detergents, and biological agents such as complement, perforins (components of cytoxic T-cell granules), and lytic viruses. Complement and the perforins disturb membrane structure by insertion of protein polymers into the lipid bilayer. Lytic viruses also integrate lipophilic molecules into the cell membrane. The molecules concerned—components of the spikes of the viral capsid—are responsible for viral infectivity through insertion into the membrane from the outside. This is associated with a transient change in ion homeostasis of the infected cell. After productive infection, it is presumed that large numbers of newly assembled virus particles insert into the membrane from the inside, causing a more extreme and irreversible change in permeability. In this context, it is of interest that the membranes of hypoxic cells show aggregation of intramembrane particles (IMPs) into patches, in contrast to their usual dispersed array. IMPs consist of transmembrane proteins (either individual molecules or groups) hence the 'patching' in hypoxia creates regions of protein-rich membrane, not unlike the sites of insertion of viral and complement proteins. There thus may be a common mechanism underlying the changes in permeability evoked by agents as diverse as complement, lytic viral infection, and hypoxia.

Reaction to necrosis

Necrosis elicits a local acute inflammatory reaction. It is reasonable to presume that the signals that link necrosis to acute inflammation derive from the dying cells themselves, perhaps from intracellular components released on disintegration of the cell membrane. Recently two specific candidates have been proposed. Leukotrienes, which are known to be important mediators of inflammation, are generated by lipid peroxidation in the membranes of the dying cells. Components of mitochondria have also been shown to be powerful activators of the complement system and hence could initiate acute inflammation (Kagiyama *et al.* 1989). This inflammatory reaction by itself may extend tissue damage, and attempts to limit this underlie some current methods for managing myocardial infarction.

Systemic reactions to necrosis include synthesis and release of acute-phase reactants, a group of proteins that appear in increased concentration in the plasma after injury. The role of these and similar proteins in the systemic reaction to injury is discussed more fully elsewhere (Chapter 4) but two are of particular relevance here. C-Reactive protein (CRP) is a pentameric, 187 amino-acid protein which is synthesized in the liver and appears in plasma at tenfold or greater concentrations above its resting levels following a variety of injuries. It accumulates in necrotic tissue. As it activates the classical pathway of complement, it may exert a role in inducing the inflammatory response to necrosis. A second, structurally similar molecule is serum amyloid-associated protein (AAP). AAP is not an acute-phase reactant, but binds to and opsonizes chromatin (Pepys and Butler 1987), which appears in the plasma after injury, presumably released from necrotic tissue. The fact that AAP is highly conserved amongst animal species suggests that it is important to remove such chromatin from the circulation swiftly.

3.1.4   Cell death in special circumstances

Within tumours and in immunological reactions necrosis and apoptosis frequently occur together. Because of their general importance, these circumstances are considered in more detail.

Cell death in tumours

In most tumours, including the most rapidly growing malignant examples, cells are lost almost as quickly as they are generated. Most of this loss is death, and apoptosis usually co-exists with necrosis (Moore 1987).

Tumour blood supply differs in many respects from the blood supply to normal tissues (Denekamp 1986). The vessels within tumours consist of endothelium lying on basement membrane, with little or no evidence of a muscular wall. The endothelial cells themselves are actively engaged in proliferation: the proportion of cells in S-phase is around tenfold higher than in the endothelium of normal blood vessels. The vascular network is also poorly oriented, so that blood flow within any one channel frequently reverses in direction or undergoes periods of stasis. The result of this irregular flow is that tumours of diameter more than a few millimetres develop zones of profound hypoxia (Tozer *et al.* 1990), compounded by low pH as the acid metabolites of anaerobic glycolysis accumulate. None the less, some regions close to vessels are relatively well perfused and here cell

proliferation continues, the older cells being progressively displaced to the hypoxic zones, where they begin to die. In some animal tumours this process is particularly obvious. The tumour mass comprises a pool of necrosis, surrounded by and contained within a maze of tumour cells, arranged in cords. Each cord consists of a fine axial blood vessel, with a sleeve of viable tumour cells around it. The thickness of these sleeves from the central vessel to the necrotic edge corresponds quite closely with the diffusion distance of oxygen, calculated from theoretical considerations. Human tumours rarely show this complete corded structure, but they commonly contain sheets of viable cells near blood vessels, alternating with zones of necrosis (see Fig. 3.11).

Tumour cells frequently produce angiogenic factors (tumour angiogenic factors, TAFs) which stimulate endothelial growth. The pattern of tumour vasculature described above could well result from failure of the new vessels to match the production rate of tumour cells. This concept is enshrined in the notion that tumours 'outgrow their blood supply'. It is important to realize, however, that hypoxic tumour necrosis of this type is a sign that rapid tumour cell proliferation is continuing. Indeed, in many tumours (notably gliomas and soft tissue sarcomas) the presence of necrosis correlates with poor prognosis.

Factors other than the relative rates of tumour cell proliferation and angiogenesis may also be involved in the pathogenesis of tumour necrosis. Fluctuating levels of angiogenic factors, for example, could induce apoptosis within endothelium, leading to collapse of portions of the vascular network. Tumour necrosis factors (produced by macrophages and lymphocytes within the tumour) may have a similar effect. Both of these may be compounded by formation of microthrombi within the tumour microcirculation, since tumour cells also release procoagulant factors, and the low pH promotes erythrocyte rouleaux formation and hence high viscosity in the perfusing blood.

The distinctive biology of tumour vasculature has only recently been recognized. Since each endothelial cell may be the 'supply line' for up to 2000 tumour cells, there is hope that a therapeutic attack on tumour endothelium may prove a useful method for controlling tumour growth. It appears likely, indeed, that several agents currently used in oncology (for example, hyperthermia) may exert at least some of their effect through an action on tumour blood vessels.

Apoptotic cells within tumours can appear throughout the tumour parenchyma, often intimately admixed with proliferating cells. High local concentrations also occur around the edges of necrotic regions. In the few quantitative studies available in animal or human tumours, the proportion of apoptotic cells varies widely between tumours (from 0.2 to 10 per cent of all cells), and also shows large systematic fluctuations during tumour growth. The relatively high apoptotic proportion of some tumours may aid in their diagnosis. An example of this is the appearance of so-called 'small dark cells' in cervical smears, a feature indicative of endometrial carcinoma. These are apoptotic bodies, produced and released from the carcinoma.

Little is known of the factors responsible for tumour apoptosis, but is seems probable that they include toxic cell injury, activation of internal programmes, and the results of attack by cytotoxic T-cells, natural killer (NK) cells, and macrophages. As discussed above, minor injury may trigger apoptosis in suitably primed cells, and this may account for the apoptosis seen around necrotic regions and as a result of treatment with irradiation, hyperthermia, and various chemotherapeutic agents such as vincristine, 5-fluorouracil, BCNU, and melphalan. The notion that tumour apoptosis may be intrinsically programmed also has interesting implications for therapy and has led to attempts to unravel the regulation of apoptosis in tumour cells. In one such attempt, human *c-myc* or H-*ras* oncogenes were inserted into a rodent fibroblast cell line (Wyllie *et al.* 1987). The resulting cells were tumorigenic but varied in capacity for local invasion and metastasis. All the tumours had high mitotic rates. Those composed of cells that expressed *c-myc* at high levels, however, also had high apoptotic rates and overall tumour expansion was slow. In contrast, *ras*-expressing tumours had low apoptotic rates and were more aggressive. The *ras*-expressing tumours also showed much more necrosis, an observation entirely concordant with the idea that *ras* promotes retention of cells, and tumour necrosis results from the failure of endothelial proliferation to keep pace with tumour cell number expansion.

Immunologically mediated cell killing

Immunological attack induces necrosis and apoptosis. As explained in Chapter 4, complement activation results in polymerization of C9 to form transmembrane channels. These allow the influx of calcium and the initiation of necrosis. All other effectors of immune killing so far studied—cytotoxic T-lymphocytes (CTL), NK cells, antibody-dependent cytotoxic cells (K-cells), and tumour necrosis factors (TNFs)—give rise to apoptosis in their immediate target cells (Flieger *et al.* 1989; Liu *et al.* 1989*b*; Martz and Howell 1989). TNF action upon endothelia might, of course, engender necrosis in the tissues supplied by the vessels under attack.

The patterns of induction of cell death by cytotoxic cells bear remarkable similarities to each other. The process can be divided into three stages: recognition; programming for death; and disintegration. The recognition stage is short ($t\frac{1}{2}$ of 1 min). The characteristic specificity of CTL killing resides largely, if not wholly, in this stage and derives from the immunologically specific recognition mechanisms discussed elsewhere. To permit programming for death, living cytotoxic cells must be present for several minutes ($t\frac{1}{2}$ of 5 min). During this stage the target cell DNA is damaged irreversibly by a process that requires magnesium and calcium ions but is inhibited by zinc. This pattern of ion dependence is the same as that shown by the endonuclease activated in apoptosis of thymocytes. As yet, however, no suitable candidate endonuclease has been identified either in effector cytotoxic lymphocytes or in the target cells. Disintegration takes much longer ($t\frac{1}{2}$ of 100 min). The continuing presence of the cytotoxic cell accelerates the process but is no longer an absolute requirement. During this stage the target cell

membrane becomes permeable to proteins and other large molecules.

The mechanism of cell-mediated immune killing is still a matter of dispute. CTL-indiced apoptosis is unusual in that it does not require RNA or protein synthesis in the dying cell. Rather, it appears that the killing cell transmits a lethal 'package' to its target, and attention has focused on what this package might be.

Cultured CTL and NK cells contain numerous electron dense granules. Initially much excitement was generated by the discovery within them of monomers of a protein, perforin (molecular mass 60–64 kDa), which in the presence of calcium polymerizes to form transmembrane channels with an internal diameter of 16 nm. Perforin has structural, immunological, and functional similarities to C9 (molecular mass 62–66 kDa) which also polymerizes to give a very similar channel of 10 nm in diameter. It thus seemed reasonable to suppose that the cytotoxic cells act by releasing perforin to form a membrane lesion analogous to that produced by C9 (Fig. 3.19).

A paradox arises, however, as cytotoxic cells cause apoptosis, whereas complement induces necrosis. The solution may lie in the fact that perforin is not the only active granule component, and granules themselves may not be the only killing mechanism. Granules isolated from cloned CTL induce both DNA fragmentation and increased cell membrane permeability. Although perforin is essential for granule cytotoxicity, purified perforin induces only the permeability change. This indicates that another factor present in the granules must be responsible for the DNA fragmentation. This factor appears to be a protease, and it has been suggested that its role is to activate a DNAse within the target cell nucleus.

Despite these results from NK cells and cultured CTL lines, the

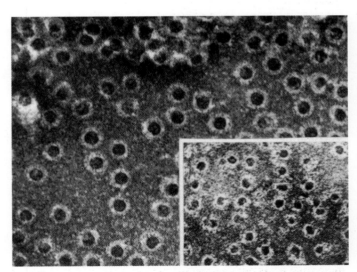

Fig. 3.19 Electron micrographs of transmembrane channels generated by perforin; the lesions induced by complement (at the same magnification) are shown in inset. (Provided by Dr E. R. Podack, New York Medical College, USA.)

role of perforins in cell killing by CTL *in vivo* has been questioned. Anti-perforin antibody blocks NK cell killing but not CTL killing, and several workers have been unable to demonstrate perforin in freshly isolated CTL. It is likely that perforins are important in NK cell killing but their presence in cultured CTL lines may be due to the induction of NK cell-like properties by prolonged exposure to media containing interleukin-2.

A family of at least eight serine proteases ('granzymes') has been identified in CTL granules and NK cells. These may either aid the polymerization of perforin or activate enzymes essential for apoptosis within the target. However, as with perforins, freshly isolated CTL have very low levels of serine protease and these enzymes are also found in cells without demonstrable cytolytic activity.

One argument against the obligate involvement of granule contents in cytotoxicity is the observation that CTL can kill in the absence of extracellular calcium. Under these circumstances exocytosis of granules is blocked and neither perforins nor serine proteases are released. The nature of this killing is, so far, unknown. It is not blocked by inhibitors of protein synthesis. Several of these agents also inhibit the constitutive pathway for secretion of newly synthesized proteins, which bypasses exocytosis of granules. This suggests the existence of a killing mechanism involving neither protein synthesis nor secretion.

Apart from the calcium-dependent exocytosis of granules and the mysterious calcium-independent mechanism, cytotoxic cells secrete a variety of different substances (the leukolexins) that have been shown to induce apoptosis in the absence of calcium. These include lymphotoxin (TNF-β), a protein of 15 kDa molecular mass secreted by stimulated CTL and NK cells. Induction of DNA fragmentation by TNF-β is much slower than in CTL cytotoxicity ($t\frac{1}{2}$ of about 12 h). Killing is faster if TNF-β is introduced directly into the cytoplasm of the target. TNF-β-induced apoptosis does not require protein synthesis in the target cell; indeed, blockade of synthesis of RNA and protein increases the rate of apoptosis. Another leukolexin, TNF-α, is structurally and immunologically related to TNF-β. It is secreted by activated macrophages and induces apoptosis (complete with chromatin cleavage) in certain target cells. A third factor, NK cytotoxic factor, may be a mixture of TNFs and some, as yet, uncharacterized molecules. This cytotoxic factor carries the same restricted target cell specificity as NK cells themselves.

Yet another calcium-independent soluble factor is found in both granules and cytoplasm of mouse CTL. It induces apoptosis at a faster tempo ($t\frac{1}{2}$ of 8 h) than TNF-α or β and is much larger, with a molecular mass of about 50 kDa, although it does bear some antigenic similarities.

Macrophages and polymorphs generate reactive oxygen intermediates capable of damaging microbial cell walls and killing micro-organisms. Although a role for ROI has been suggested in immune effector cell killing, there is little good evidence in support of this. Another mechanism of cell killing, postulated many times but never substantiated, is that the effector cell directly perturbs the target cell membrane.

The observations outlined above indicate that there is no one single killing mechanism employed by all cytotoxic effector cells. It is probable that a cytotoxic cell can call on one or more mechanisms, depending upon circumstances.

3.1.5   Bibliography

Allan, D. J., Harmon, B. V., and Kerr, J. F. R. (1987). Cell death in spermatogenesis. In *Perspectives on mammalian cell death* (ed. C. S. Potten), pp. 229–58. Oxford University Press.

Arfors, K. E. and Del Maestro, R. (1986). Free radicals in microcirculation. *Acta Physiologica Scandinavica* **126** (Suppl. 548).

Boobis, A. R., Fawthrop, D. J., and Davies, D. (1989). Mechanisms of cell death. *Trends in Biochemical Sciences* **10**, 275–80.

Buttyan, R., Zakeri, Z., Locksin, R., and Wolgemuth, D. (1988). Cascade induction of c-*fos*, c-*myc* and heat shock 70k transcripts during regression of the rat ventral prostate gland. *Molecular and Cellular Endocrinology.* **2**, 650–7.

Cowan, W. M., Fawcett, J. W., O'Leary, D. D. M., and Stanfield, B. B. (1984). Regressive events in neurogenesis. *Science* **225**, 1258–65.

Denekamp, J. (1986). Cell kinetics and radiation biology. *International Journal of Radiation Biology* **49**, 357–80.

Duvall, E. and Wyllie, A. H. (1986). Death and the cell. *Immunology Today* **7**, 115–19.

Fesus, L., Thomazy, V., and Falus, A. (1987). Induction and activation of tissue transglutaminase during programmed cell death. *FEBS Letters* **224**, 104–8.

Fesus, L. Thomazy, V., Autuori, F., Ceru, M. P., Tarcsa, E., and Piacentini, M. (1989). Apoptotic hepatocytes become insoluble in detergents and chrotropic agents as a result of transglutaminase action. *FEBS Letters* **245**, 150–4.

Flieger, D., Riethmuller, G., and Zieglar-Heitbrock, H. W. L. (1989). Zn^{2+} inhibits TNF-mediated DNA fragmentation and cytolysis. *International Journal of Cancer* **44**, 315–19.

Halliwell, B. (1989). Free radicals, reactive oxygen species and human disease: a critical evaluation with special reference to atherosclerosis. *British Journal of Experimental Pathology* **70**, 737–57.

Harmon, B. V. (1987). An ultrastructural study of spontaneous cell death in a mouse mastocytoma with particular reference to dark cells. *Journal of Pathology* **153**, 345–55.

Kagiyama, A., Savage, H. E., Michael, L. H., Hanson, G., Entman, M. L., and Rossen, R. D. (1989). Molecular basis of complement activation in ischaemic myocardium: identification of specific molecules of mitochondrial origin that bind human C1q and fix complement. *Circulation Research* **64**, 607–15.

Liu, Y.-J., Joshua, D. E., Williams, G. T., Smith, C. A., Gordon, J., and Maclennan, I. C. M. (1989*a*). Mechanism of antigen-driven selection in germinal centres. *Nature* **342**, 929–31.

Liu, Y., Mullbacher, A., and Waring, P. (1989*b*). Natural killer cells and cytotoxic T cells induce DNA fragmentation in both human and murine target cells *in vitro*. *Scandinavian Journal of Immunology* **30**, 31–7.

McConkey, D. J., Hartzell, P., Duddy, S. K., Hakansson, H., and Orrenius, S. (1988). 2,3,7,8-Tetrachlorodibenzo-*p*-dioxin kills immature thymocytes by Ca^{2+}-mediated endonuclease activation. *Science* **242**, 256–9.

McConkey, D. J., Hartzell, P., Jondal, M., and Orrenius, S. (1989*a*). Inhibition of DNA fragmentation in thymocytes and isolated thymocyte nuclei by agents that stimulate protein kinase C. *Journal of Biological Chemistry* **264**, 13 399–402.

McConkey, D. J., Nicotera, P., Hartzell, P., Bellomo, G., Wyllie, A. H., and Orrenius, S. (1989*b*). Glucocorticoids activate a suicide process in thymocytes through an elevation of cytosolic Ca^{2+} concentration. *Archives of Biochemistry and Biophysics* **269**, 365–70.

McConkey, D. J., Orrenius, S., and Jondal, M. (1990). Cellular signalling in programmed cell death (apoptosis). *Immunology Today* **11**, 120–1.

Martz, E. and Howell, D. M. (1989). CTL: are they virus control cells first, and cytolytic cells second? DNA fragmentation, apoptosis and the prelytic halt hypothesis. *Immunology Today* **10**, 79–86.

Moore, J. V. (1987). Death of cells and necrosis in tumours. In *Perspectives on mammalian cell death* (ed. C. S. Potten), pp. 295–325. Oxford University Press.

Möller, G. (1988). Molecular mechanisms of T cell-mediated lysis. *Immunology Reviews* **103**.

Orrenius, S., McConkey, D. J., Bellomo, G., and Nicotera, P. (1989). Role of Ca^{2+} in toxic cell killing. *Trends in Biochemical Sciences* **10**, 281–5.

Pepys, M. B. and Butler, P. J. G. (1987). Serum amyloid P component is the major calcium-dependent specific DNA binding protein of the serum. *Biochemical and Biophysical Research Communications* **148**, 308–13.

Potten, C. S. (1987). *Perspectives in mammalian cell death*. Oxford University Press.

Savill, J., Dransfield, I., Hogg, N., and Haslett, C. (1990). Vitronectin receptor-mediated phagocytosis of cells undergoing apoptosis. *Nature* **343**, 170–3.

Smith, C. A., Williams, G. T., Kingston, R., Jenkinson, E. J., and Owen, J. J. T. (1989). Antibodies to CD3/T-cell receptor complex induce death by apoptosis in immature T-cells in thymic cultures. *Nature* **337**, 181–4.

Tozer, G. M., Lewis, S., Michalowski, A., and Aber, V. (1990). The relationship between regional variations in blood flow and histology in a transplanted rat fibrosarcoma. *British Journal of Cancer* **61**, 250–7.

Walicke, P. A. (1989). Novel neurotrophic factors, receptors and oncogenes. *Annual Review of Neuroscience* **12**, 103–26.

Wilcock, C., Chahwala, S. B., and Hickman, J. A. (1988). Selective inhibition by bis (2-chloroethyl) methylamine (nitrogen mustard) of the $Na^+/K^+/Cl^-$ cotransporter of murine L1210 leukaemia cells. *Biochemica et Biophysica Acta* **946**, 368–78.

Williams, R. W. and Herrup, K. (1988). The control of neuron number. *Annual Review of Neuroscience* **11**, 423–53.

Wyllie, A. H. (1987). Cell death. In *Cytology and cell physiology* (4th edn) (ed. G. H. Bourne), pp. 755–85. Academic Press, New York.

Wyllie, A. H., Morris, R. G., Smith, A. L., and Dunlop, D. (1984). Chromatin cleavage in apoptosis: association with condensed chromatin morphology and dependence on macromolecular synthesis. *Journal of Pathology* **142**, 67–77.

Wyllie, A. H., Rose, K. A., Morris, R. G., Steel, C. M., Foster, E., and Spandidos, D. A. (1987). Rodent fibroblast tumours expressing human *myc* and *ras* genes; growth, metastasis and endogenous oncogene expression. *British Journal of Cancer* **56**, 251–9.

3.2 Organelle pathology in cell injury

Peter G. Toner, Hassan M. H. Kamel, and

Stuart Cameron

3.2.1 Introduction

In traditional cellular pathology, various abnormalities of cell morphology resulting from sublethal injury were identified by loose terms such as 'cloudy swelling' and 'degeneration'. A more precise definition of such conditions was precluded by the limited resolving power of light microscopy. Electron microscopy has now supplied the missing spatial resolution, but is still far from resolving some of the underlying structural problems relating to cell injury. These include the key issue of the definition of cell death; the distinction between adaptation and cell injury; and the inherent limitations of morphology and the problem of artefact. This section will address these problems, which are partly philosophical, and will then attempt to outline some of the better-documented responses of cellular fine structure to sublethal injury.

Cell death

Death was once a simple concept. Death of the body was deemed to occur when the vital signs of respiration and heartbeat were no longer detectable and life was therefore declared extinct. These simple certainties have now been replaced by complex definitions of 'brain death', with their attendant ethical problems, focused on the concept of the irreversible cessation of brain stem function.

For many years, however, it has been recognized that the physical definition of a 'moment of death' was essentially arbitrary. Beyond any such 'moment', various vital systems of the body can still be sustained by external means for prolonged periods. At the time of disconnection of a life support system from the 'brain-dead' patient, individual organs, tissues, and cells retain the capacity for independent function and cell renewal, a capacity increasingly utilized by the transplant surgeon.

The death of cells has never been simple to define, since the cell has no pulse, no breathing movements, and no brain function to monitor. And yet the cell, like the body itself, has its own vital systems. In health, these systems operate in closely integrated harmony, but in disease, one or more of them may become key targets for pathological change. The best available definition of cell death is the irreversible loss of integrated cellular function. Beyond this point, however, individual subcellular systems may continue for some time to display biological activity, even when integrated function has clearly ceased.

There are arguably three 'vital systems' at the cellular level, concerned respectively with boundary functions, energy metabolism, and protein synthesis. The cell membrane is the homeostatic boundary, controlling all access to the interior of the cell and mediating cellular interactions. The metabolism of the membrane and especially the synthesis and turnover of its component parts are vital for the maintenance of membrane structure. Extensive disruption of the membrane is incompatible with the survival of the cell, as shown by the effectiveness of cell killing through antibody- and complement-mediated lysis of the cell membrane.

Membrane function, however, is itself dependent on energy metabolism. When this is impaired, as in hypoxia or through the action of metabolic poisons on the mitochondria, the consequences are felt throughout the cell. One of the earliest casualties is the sensitive control over fluid and electrolyte balance exercised by cell membrane pumping systems. Cells vary in their sensitivity to hypoxia, but the disruption of energy metabolism through oxygen shortage is one of the commonest mechanisms of cell injury and cell death.

The third vital system is protein synthesis, depending on the ribosomes, often attached to membranes of the endoplasmic reticulum. The half-life of many of the vital proteins of the cell is very short, calling for constant synthetic activity to maintain essential functions. When protein synthesis is halted, whether by specific poisons or by more general metabolic disruption, the irreversible loss of integrated function is not long delayed.

The identification of boundary functions, energy metabolism, and protein synthesis as three key vital functions does not imply that damage to other components of the cell, such as the lysosomes, the nucleus, or the cytoskeleton, can be sustained without the risk of lethal harm. In general, however, these three systems represent the major common pathways through which diverse forms of environmental challenge lead to cell injury and cell death.

The central problem in interpreting such changes at the ultrastructural level lies in the fact that in the cell, as in the body, death is defined in functional, as opposed to morphological terms. A photograph of the recumbent human body will not distinguish between sleep, coma, and death. An electron micrograph is no more able to define the moment of death of an individual cell. In both cases, the fact of death is recognized by its subsequent effects, of which unequivocal morphological change represents the end-result (Fig. 3.20).

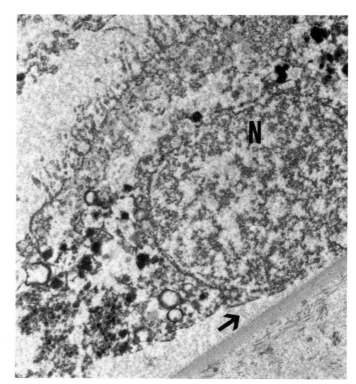

Fig. 3.20 Cell death. Renal tubular cell from a kidney transplant that failed due to blockage of its vascular supply. Note membrane disruption, structural disorganization, dissolution of the nucleus (N), and detachment of the cell (arrow) from its basal lamina. (Micrograph by courtesy of Dr C. M. Hill.)

Adaptation and cell injury

There is a distinction to be drawn between adaptation and cell injury, although this is often difficult to make in practice. Cells are constantly under environmental threat, but are generally capable of maintaining homeostasis by mounting effective adaptive responses to a wide range of challenges. The consequences of challenge are determined partly by the nature of the tissue and partly by the agent concerned. Tissue factors include cell type and relative susceptibility, which in turn reflect specific physiological and metabolic characteristics. Thus cardiac myocytes are more vulnerable to hypoxia than less metabolically active smooth muscle cells. Factors related to the agent include dose, duration of exposure, and mechanism of action.

The range of cell response to a given challenge encompasses several possibilities. There may be no detectable response to a minimal challenge, either in terms of function or of morphology. A more significant disturbance of the environment may lead to an adaptation of cell function, with or without some structural effects. Such adaptations may persist as long as the stimulus remains. It is a matter of judgement and of definition whether changes of this kind are physiological or pathological.

With more severe insults, the adaptive potential of the cell may be exhausted, resulting in unequivocal functional and structural damage. Cell injury may therefore be defined as a failure of the cell, on challenge, to maintain itself within homeostatic tolerance limits. This may be an acute, rapidly developing abnormality, such as the distension of intracytoplasmic membrane-limited spaces, sometimes accompanied by condensation of the intervening cytoplasmic matrix (Fig. 3.21). A more slowly-evolving chronic response may involve the accumulation of secondary lysosomes as evidence of continuing injury. Cell injury such as this may be reparable if the insult is withdrawn. If the cause of injury persists, these acute changes may evolve to a state of adaptation, or may lead to cell death.

Cell death itself is only structurally recognizable after the event, by a degree of disruption of cellular morphology so gross as to be clearly irreversible. This will usually include disintegration of the cell membrane, disorganization of the cytoplasmic organelles, and shrinkage or fragmentation of the nucleus (Figs 3.22, 3.23). The entire cell may become shrunken and condensed, its organelles barely recognizable (Fig. 3.24). Dying cells often become disconnected from their neighbours and detached or extruded from their position, particularly in epithelial sheets (Figs 3.25, 3.26, 3.27), which may in turn lead to disordered function and to the triggering of the defensive mechanisms of inflammation and reparative fibrosis (Fig. 3.28); see also Chapter 5.

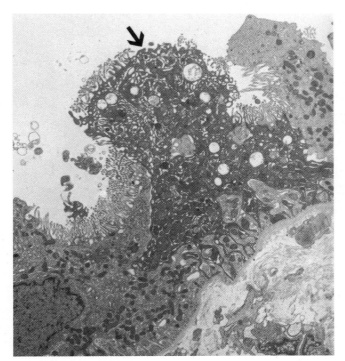

Fig. 3.21 Cell injury in acute renal tubular necrosis, with dilatation of membrane systems and condensation of the cytoplasmic matrix. There is disorganization and partial loss of microvilli (arrow). The cell is becoming detached from its neighbours. (Micrograph by courtesy of Dr C. M. Hill.)

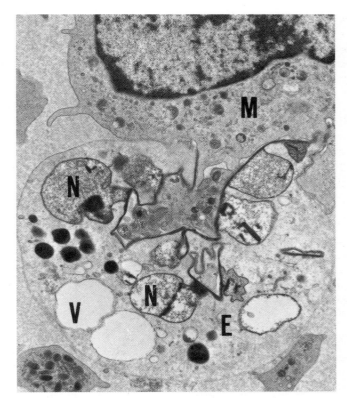

Fig. 3.22 Cell death. A disintegrating eosinophil (E) is about to be phagocytosed by a macrophage (M). The dead cell shows cytoplasmic vacuolation (V), a watery cytoplasmic matrix, and nuclear dissolution (N).

Limitations of morphology

In general terms, cell injury results first in some biochemical or molecular event, followed subsequently by impairment of function. Any associated morphological alterations are likely to occur relatively late in this sequence, once molecular and functional derangement are already well established. Morphology may reflect the extent of cellular damage and the relative sensitivity or resistance of a particular cell type to a particular agent. Characteristic morphological patterns may also reflect a distinct form of insult and may help in understanding its mechanism of action. On the other hand, the knowledge we acquire from morphology is often incomplete, has certain basic limitations and can prove deceptive.

Morphology is limited, because conventional images are static representations of dynamic phenomena and are generally limited to two dimensions, leaving spatial relationships to the imagination, or to cumbersome reconstruction techniques. The technical demands of electron microscopy impose serious limitations on samples, through the need for rigorous protocols for fixation, embedding, sectioning, and staining. Sample size and the effect of plane of section place limits on interpretation. When dealing with human tissues, ethical and practical constraints limit access and dictate the speed, extent, and methodology of sampling and fixation. Most important of all, morphology is limited by the problems of artefact, which can often deceive the incautious observer. As a result, the significance and the underlying mechanisms of various ultrastructurally recognizable forms of cellular alteration often remain poorly understood.

Artefact

Almost any image of tissues or of cells can be considered artefactual, whether in relation to the techniques of specimen preparation, or to the imaging technology itself. Failure to take such factors into account can result in faulty interpretation. The limited resolution of light microscopy may provide a false sense of security, since subcellular detail, never particularly clear, varies only marginally with widely differing techniques. The apparent clarity of an ultrastructural image, however, is a two-edged weapon, since meaningful details and subcellular artefacts are equally clearly rendered in an electron micrograph and may often be difficult to tell apart.

The conventional electron micrograph is a shadow picture of the pattern of heavy metal binding to those features of cellular architecture that are stabilized by fixation and retained in subsequent tissue processing. Delays in fixation, low pH, dissection trauma, variations in the ambient temperature during processing, and changes in the composition of reagents may alter the final image. These morphological artefacts may mimic and are

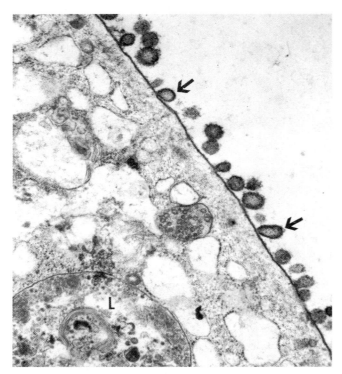

Fig. 3.23 Dying cell. Intestinal epithelial cell prior to shedding from intestinal villus. Note dilated cytoplasmic spaces and a large secondary lysosome (L). The microvillous border has degenerated, leaving a few residual vesicular structure (arrows).

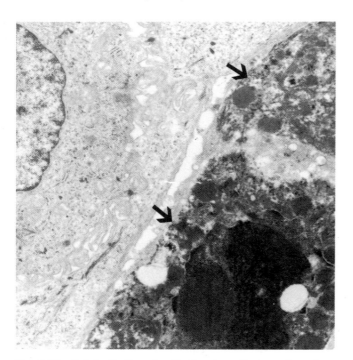

Fig. 3.24 Cell death. Buccal epithelium in graft-versus-host disease. The dead cells (arrows) show nuclear and cytoplasmic condensation with loss of structural detail. (Micrograph by courtesy of Dr A. L. C. McLay.)

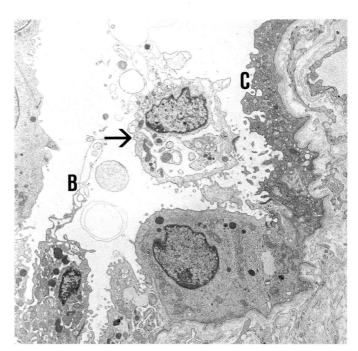

Fig. 3.25 Cell injury. Renal tubular epithelium in acute tubular necrosis. The tubular lining shows an injured cell with a large surface bleb (B), and a surviving attenuated tubular cell (C). A shed cell lies free in the lumen (arrow), with surface blebbing and dilated endoplasmic reticulum. (Micrograph by courtesy of Dr C. M. Hill.)

easily confused with changes produced by a variety of pathological processes. Typical examples include mitochondrial swelling, dilatation of membrane-limited cisternae, nuclear membrane separation, and heterochromatin condensation. Even with optimum handling, the images of certain structures may be either masked or intensified by the use of different fixatives and stains. Failure to take such factors into account can also result in faulty interpretation.

Some confidence can, however, be taken from comparisons between 'well-fixed' tissues and alternative images obtained from less destructive techniques, such as freeze-fracturing, which involves the minimum of chemical intervention. Since cells can survive carefully controlled freezing and thawing, which is more than can be said for any form of fixation, it is reasonable to assume that the frozen cell retains the essential features of the living state. Freeze-fracture images of cell structure reassuringly display surface features, cytoplasmic membrane systems, and patterns of organelles which closely correspond to the images of conventionally fixed and processed tissues. There is, therefore, reason to believe that ultrastructural morphology represents a tolerably close approximation to the structural organization of the living cell.

3.2.2 Cytoplasmic changes in cell injury

The morphological features of cell injury comprise a spectrum ranging from minimal deviation from normality to gross struc-

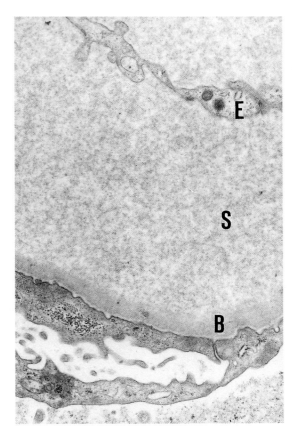

Fig. 3.26 Endothelial detachment. Renal glomerular capillary in polyarteritis showing detachment of endothelium (E) from the renal basement membrane (B). The fluid-filled subendothelial space (S) is analogous to a blister. (Micrograph by courtesy of Dr A. L. C. McLay.)

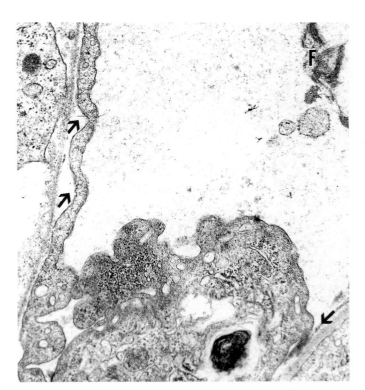

Fig. 3.27 Damaged alveolar lining cells in paraquat poisoning. Parts of damaged type 1 and type 2 pneumocytes are shown, focally detached (arrows) from the underlying basal lamina. Some debris and fibrin strands (F) are seen in the fluid-filled alveolar space.

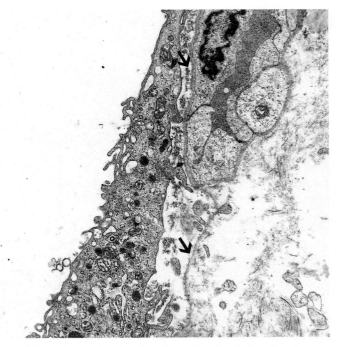

Fig. 3.28 Paraquat poisoning. The alveolar lining has become detached, leaving an exposed basal lamina (arrows) with surface debris. An active macrophage is moving across this surface.

tural disruption. These changes may involve volumetric alterations, qualitative structural alterations, and the appearance of abnormal inclusions. Volumetric alterations resulting from cell injury include any increase or decrease in the relative proportions of the principal elements of normal subcellular structure. Qualitative structural alterations include a wide range of acquired abnormalities in organelle morphology. Abnormal inclusions may be nuclear or cytoplasmic, endogenous or exogenous, and of specified or unspecified composition. In this section, the volumetric and structural responses of the main cytoplasmic organelles to a variety of agents will be described. Sections 3.2 and 3.3 discuss underlying mechanisms.

Changes in cell size

The commonest form of response to environmental stress is cell swelling. This may be induced by a wide variety of chemical, physical, metabolic, or toxic agencies, of which anoxia is perhaps the commonest clinically relevant example. Interference with the balance of cellular energy metabolism leads to acute malfunctions of the energy-dependent pumping systems which maintain the fluid and electrolyte balance of the various compartments of the cell, resulting in abnormal osmotic forces acting across still intact membrane barriers. This causes swelling of the endoplasmic reticulum, the Golgi apparatus, and the mitochondria, due to abnormal accumulation of fluid. Increasing degrees of cell swelling are described on light microscopy as 'cloudy swelling', 'vacuolar degeneration', and 'hydropic degeneration', the cytoplasm progressing from a granular refractile appearance to frank vacuolation. In gross terms, the affected organ is swollen and pale, with a tense capsule, but soft parenchymal consistency.

Other causes of cellular enlargement include an increase in one or more of the major subcellular components. In muscle hypertrophy, this includes the myofilaments, the mitochondria, and the membrane systems of the sarcoplasmic reticulum. Abnormal stored metabolites, such as glycogen or fat, may distend the cell. The abnormal storage of metabolites may reflect either some transient metabolic disturbance or an inborn metabolic error, such as occurs in the various genetically determined storage diseases. These topics are dealt with at greater length below.

A decrease in cell size due to environmental challenge is known as atrophy (see Chapter 8). Prime causes include nutritional deprivation, such as chronic hypoxia, and pathological defunctioning or disuse. The ultrastructure of atrophic cells may show little significant deviation from normality in qualitative terms, although a prominence of secondary lysosomes or residual bodies may reflect the catabolic processes which have contributed to the reduced cytoplasmic mass. The lipid-rich lysosomal residues (lipofuscin pigment) appear as golden-brown granular deposits by light microscopy. Such changes are increasingly common with age. In skeletal muscle, architectural disruption due to trauma may defunction cells which become isolated and trapped in fibrous tissue. These defunctioned cells show marked disorganization of their cytoplasmic ultrastructure, with loss of the normal orderly sarcomere pattern (Fig. 3.29).

Changes in cell surfaces

Since the cell membrane is the first point of contact with any toxic substance, it is not surprising that changes in cell surface morphology often occur at an early stage in the course of cell injury, particularly when the membrane itself, or its metabolism, is specifically targeted. Cell membranes are also secondarily damaged in a variety of pathological states, particularly when there is interference with cellular respiration. Finally, cellular architecture, and thus surface topography, may be distorted as a result of changes in the cytoskeleton. Amongst the most striking examples of abnormal cellular configuration are the various disturbances of red cell morphology, such as the spiky appearance known as acanthocytosis (Fig. 3.30).

Impairment of the energy-dependent sodium pump mechanism of the cell membrane has already been referred to as part of the pathway to cell swelling. Such changes are often reflected in abnormal surface features, such as irregularities of membrane contour and localized blebbing (see Section 3.1). In lethal injury, focal defects, multiple ruptures, and ultimately lysis of

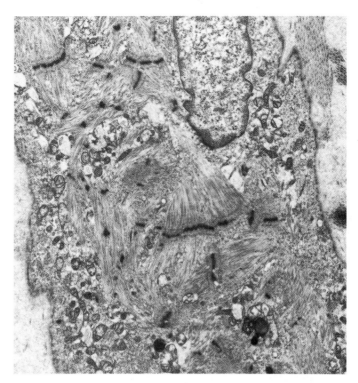

Fig. 3.29 Disarray of skeletal muscle myofibrils. Entrapped defunctioned muscle cell in damaged skeletal muscle shows disorganization of its internal structure, with haphazard sarcomere pattern. (Micrograph by courtesy of Dr I. A. R. More.)

the cell membrane are observed. In contrast, more subtle forms of injury may result in an apparent focal thickening of the cell membrane, such as may be seen at points of attachment of certain micro-organisms to the surface of enterocytes.

Normal surface features of differentiated cells, such as microvilli and cilia, may become swollen, irregular, attenuated, or entirely lost as a result of various forms of cell injury (see Fig. 3.23). Cell surface changes in coeliac disease include degradation of the microvillous border of the enterocyte (Chapter 16). In experimental hyperthermia, rapidly developing changes of contour cause blebbing of the enterocyte surface membrane. Loss of cilia has been described in the epithelium of the respiratory bronchioles after exposure to chemicals such as naphthalene.

The cell coat, or glycocalyx, external to the cell membrane, may also be affected in cell injury. Attenuation and even absence of the glycocalyx occurs in the intestine in cases of salmonella infection, whereas marked thickening of the cell coat of the skeletal muscle cell is seen in *Trichinella spiralis* infection.

Changes in cell inter-relationships

The various specialized intercellular junctions are common targets for toxic agents, which produce their effects by disruption of such contacts. Separation of cardiac myocytes at the inter-

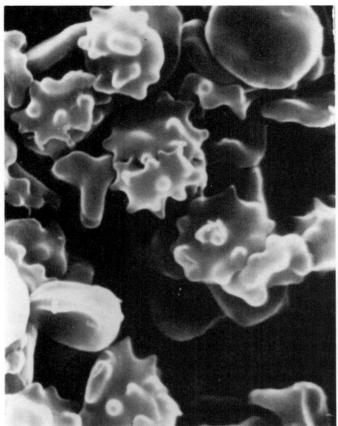

Fig. 3.30 Acanthocytes, or spiky red cells. Surface abnormalities such as these reflect molecular disorders of the cell membrane or of underlying structural proteins. (Micrograph by courtesy of Dr A. L. C. McLay.)

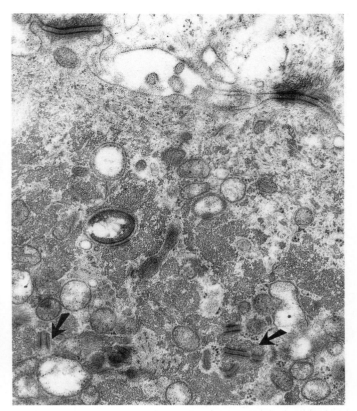

Fig. 3.31 Squamous cell carcinoma. Two normal desmosomes link adjacent cells. Within the cytoplasm a number of other desmosome-like structures are seen (arrows), surrounded by irregular intermediate filament bundles. These internalized desmosomes have no connection with the cell surface.

calated discs occurs in hypoxia, hypothermia, and intoxication by lead and cobalt. Separation and disruption of junctional specializations in the respiratory epithelium has been claimed as a contributory factor in smoking-related disease. In scurvy, the opening of capillary junctions may account for some of the pathological manifestations. Histamine, bradykinin, hyperthermia, and ionizing radiation may have similar effects on endothelium.

An increase in the number of adhesion specializations is an unusual response, but this occurs in arterial endothelium in hypertension, perhaps reflecting some adaptive or compensatory mechanism. In neoplastic cells, both increased and decreased numbers of adhesion specializations are present, along with abnormal and immature forms. The not infrequent finding of intracytoplasmic desmosomes and other internalized junctions in neoplasia may reflect the instability of cell contact relationships in tumours (Figs 3.31, 3.32).

Changes in mitochondria

Mitochondria are particularly sensitive to environmental change, even within physiological limits, so it is not surprising that there is early evidence of mitochondrial damage in response to many types of cell injury. There have been extensive studies of the functional and enzymatic impairments induced in such circumstances, but the complexity of mitochondrial biology makes it difficult, in many instances, fully to explain the observed structural changes.

Impairment of mitochondrial oxidative metabolism and energy generation is the common functional effect of many agents causing cell injury, including hypoxia, various chemicals, and bacterial toxins. This leads to failure of the mitochondrial cation pump (see Section 3.1). These functional events often result in an early stage of mitochondrial condensation and increased electron density, followed by progressive swelling which can ultimately result in mitochondrial rupture. Volumetric changes such as these are frequently accompanied by the accumulation of calcium-related dense bodies in the mitochondrial matrix.

The active role of mitochondria in calcium ion manipulation underlies some of the morphological changes occurring in osteoblasts, osteoclasts, renal, and gut epithelial cells in experimentally induced hormonal hypercalcaemia, although the observed intramitochondrial densities may or may not contain

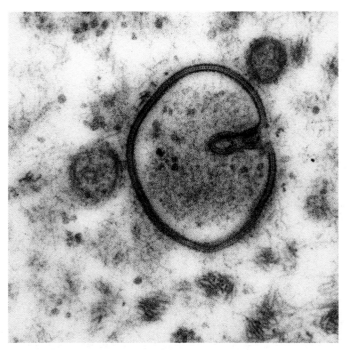

Fig. 3.32 Intracytoplasmic junction. This closed loop has the appearance of a linear contact specialization internalized within the cytoplasm of a tumour cell.

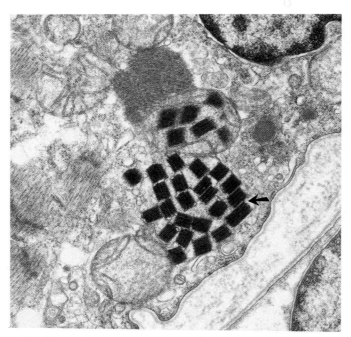

Fig. 3.33 Mitochondrial myopathy. Intramitochondrial crystalline structures (arrow) in skeletal muscle.

high concentrations of calcium. Calcium overloading of mitochondria also occurs in various other pathological conditions. Certain hereditary myopathies are associated with elevated intramitochondrial calcium levels, accompanied by the occurrence of giant mitochondria and disordered configurations of mitochondrial cristae. Distinctive intramitochondrial crystalline inclusions may also be observed (Fig. 3.33).

Mitochondria commonly respond to toxic agents and adverse conditions through variations in size and number. Giant mitochondria occur in hepatocytes after exposure to copper chelating agents and in alcoholic liver injury (Fig. 3.34). Increased mitochondrial size and number occur in the cardiac muscle cells of mice exposed to high altitude conditions and in liver cells in riboflavin deficiency.

An unusual abundance of mitochondria is the explanation of the distinctive eosinophilic granular cytoplasm seen in so-called oncocytic change. This phenomenon occurs, for example, in damaged thyroid follicular cells in auto-immune thyroiditis, or Hashimoto's disease (see Chapter 26). Some tumours display similar features, which has led to the use of the descriptive term 'oncocytoma' (Fig. 3.35). The basis of this is unknown, but presumably reflects some disturbance of control mechanisms which regulate mitochondrial numbers in normal cells.

Reduced numbers of mitochondria have been observed in hepatocytes in starvation and in type 2 pneumocytes in essential fatty acid deficiency. Correction of the underlying defect results in restoration of numbers through mitochondrial multiplication.

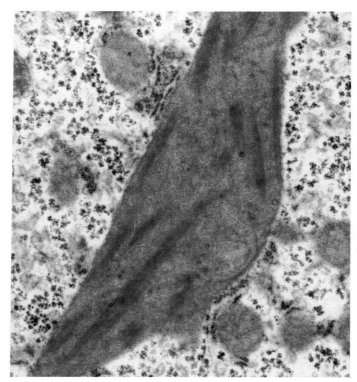

Fig. 3.34 Giant mitochondrion. This bizarre structure contains crystalline inclusions as well as remnants of its normal internal membranes. Several normal-sized mitochondria lie in the surrounding cytoplasm. (Micrograph by courtesy of Dr A. L. C. McLay.)

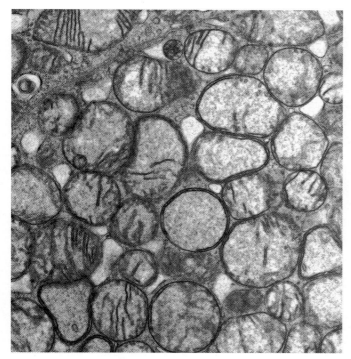

Fig. 3.35 Oncocytoma. The cytoplasm of these thyroid tumour cells contains numerous closely packed mitochondria and little else.

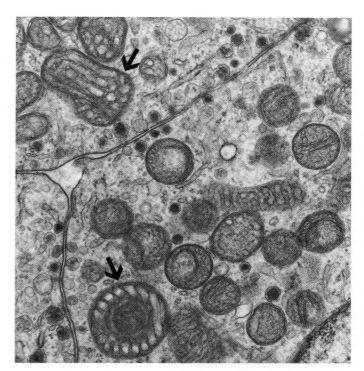

Fig. 3.36 Bizarre mitochondrial configurations (arrows) in a pituitary tumour.

A distinctive configuration and internal pattern of mitochondrial cristae is a consistent characteristic of most differentiated cell types. Disturbances of these patterns may be seen in disease. Loss of mitochondrial cristae is a feature of hepatocytes in diabetics, and abnormally long and narrow, dense mitochondria are common in the hepatocytes of alcoholics. Bizarre mitochondria are commonly seen in tumour cells (Fig. 3.36) and a variety of mitochondrial structural alterations and inclusions have been documented in other less common conditions.

Changes in endoplasmic reticulum and ribosomes

Dilatation of the cisternae of the endoplasmic reticulum is one of the most frequently observed responses to environmental challenge. The endoplasmic reticulum is a system of closed membrane-limited cavities extending throughout the cytoplasm and as such it is susceptible to the action of abnormal osmotic forces. This occurs as part of the complex changes leading to cell swelling. Cisternae may also become dilated through the accumulation of secretory products or abnormal inclusions. In some forms of cell injury (e.g. CCl_4 toxicity) there is structural evidence of disruption of the protein synthetic mechanism, through detachment of ribosomes from the cisternal surfaces of the granular endoplasmic reticulum and disaggregation of polyribosomes into monoribosomes, a change seen also in hyperthermia. The intestinal epithelial cells in starvation, protein deficiency, and kwashiorkor, and the hepatocytes in glutamine deficiency, show a reduction of granular reticulum and associated ribosomes. In contrast, increased numbers of ribosomes are seen in metabolically active and stressed cells and as an initial compensatory response in conditions of impaired protein synthesis. This is seen in pulmonary endothelial cells in hypertension and in capillary endothelium is ascorbic acid deficiency.

Protein synthesis is the main function of the granular endoplasmic reticulum. Smooth-surfaced membrane cisternae have many other roles in cellular metabolism. Proliferation of such membranes, which occurs after exposure to various drugs and chemicals, is an essentially adaptive response, stimulated by the increased functional demand on the associated enzymes required for the metabolism of these agents. The cytochrome P_{450}-linked mixed-function oxidative system, which is involved in these reactions, consists of a series of enzymes manufactured in the endoplasmic reticulum of cells in the liver, kidney, lung, and intestine. In the hepatocyte, proliferation of the smooth endoplasmic reticulum may result in 'ground glass' areas in the cytoplasm after exposure to barbiturates (Fig. 3.37). Similar results are described in type 1 pneumocytes on exposure to 3-methyl indole in cigarette smoke and in skeletal muscle in response to *Trichinella spiralis*.

The formation of concentric membranous bodies represents a particular pattern of proliferation in the endoplasmic reticulum. It is seen in hepatocytes after exposure to various toxic compounds, viral hepatitis, and in some hepatoma cells. The stacks of endoplasmic reticulum membranes form concentric whorls which may occupy much of the cytoplasm, sometimes entangling other structures.

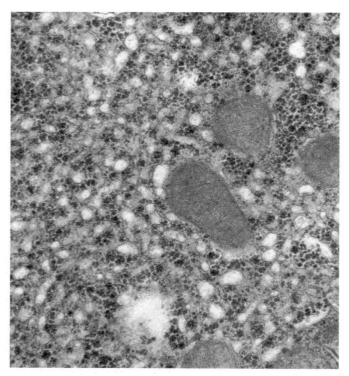

Fig. 3.37 Barbiturate-induced hypertrophy of smooth endoplasmic reticulum in a liver cell. Numerous glycogen particles lie between these membranes.

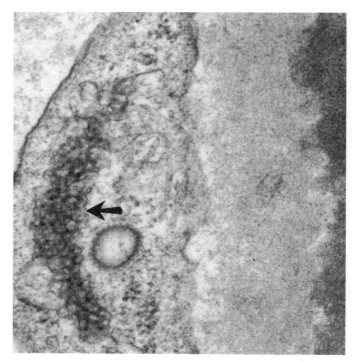

Fig. 3.38 Tubuloreticular inclusion (arrow) in a glomerular endothelial cell in systemic lupus erythematosus (SLE). (Micrograph by courtesy of Dr A. L. C. McLay.)

The accumulation of discrete virus particles and other particulate and paracrystalline inclusions within cisternae of the endoplasmic reticulum have been observed in various circumstances. Examples include the tubuloreticular inclusions observed in cisternae of the smooth endoplasmic reticulum in white blood cells after Epstein–Barr virus infection, in endothelial cells in some cases of systemic lupus erythematosus (SLE) (Figs 3.38, 3.39), and after exposure to certain chemicals. These and other curious structures, sometimes loosely referred to as 'virus-like inclusions', represent abnormal cellular products, but do not themselves provide direct evidence of virus infection. In some infections, however, fully formed virus particles can be demonstrated lying within or budding into the endoplasmic reticulum. Other forms of intracellular parasitization, such as the multiplication of protozoa within the cytoplasm of macrophages in leishmaniasis, appear not to cause immediate lethal cellular injury and are compatible with survival of the cell for some time (Fig. 3.40).

Changes in the Golgi complex

Environmental stress may inhibit or stimulate the functions of the Golgi complex. Inhibition is produced by many chemotherapeutic agents and toxic compounds, particularly those which interfere with protein synthesis and the processing of secretions, with resultant atrophy and collapse of the Golgi cisternae and associated structures. Examples include starvation and protein

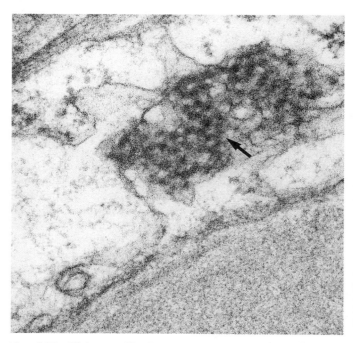

Fig. 3.39 High magnification view of a tubuloreticular inclusion (arrow) in SLE. (Micrograph by courtesy of Dr A. L. C. McLay.)

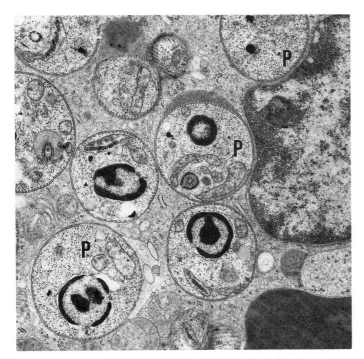

Fig. 3.40 Intracellular protozoal parasites (P) in a splenic macrophage in *Leishmania donovani* infection. The parasites indent the macrophage nucleus but the cell remains apparently viable. The parasites have their own distinctive internal structure. (Micrograph by courtesy of Mr J. D. Anderson, FIMLS.)

deficiency, and the administration of puromycin and cyclo-heximide. In neoplasia, many malignant cells have less well-developed Golgi complexes than their normal counterparts, reflecting functional differences associated with a lesser degree of differentiation. On the other hand, many functionally active tumour cells have correspondingly well-formed Golgi complexes.

Stimulation of synthetic function results in hypertrophy of the Golgi complex, with cisternal dilation. Examples include the response of hepatocytes to steroid hormones, to chlorproma-zine, and to infection with hepatitis B virus. Similar features occur as an initial event after exposure to CCl_4 and actino-mycin D.

Changes in peroxisomes

Peroxisomes and microperoxisomes are vulnerable to a wide range of agencies, including some that interfere with cellular oxidation and fat metabolism. Peroxisomes become increased in number after exposure to hypolipidaemic agents, high fat diet, vitamin D deficiency, and acetylsalicylic acid. Similar effects are seen in the cardiac muscle cells of animals exposed to dietary alcohol. Peroxisomes are reduced in number in fatty liver (Chapter 17) and after exposure to the catalase inhibitor, allyl-isopropylacetamide, and to bacterial toxins from pneumo-coccus.

Changes in microtubules and filaments

There is still uncertainty about the morphology of the cyto-skeleton, not least because of the instability of microtubular structures, which tend to disaggregate at the near-freezing tem-peratures which used to be employed for tissue fixation. Similar effects are produced by certain chemicals such as colchicine and vinblastine which depolymerize tubulin. These changes are often reversible on withdrawal of the toxic agent. The profound disruption caused by these agents in key cellular functions, such as intracellular transport and mitosis, is an indication of the significance of cytoskeletal elements in cellular biology. Beyond this, however, relatively little is known about the sub-cellular pathology of the cytoskeleton. While dealing with microtubules, however, it is worth mentioning the rare occur-rence of an ultrastructural defect involving congenital partial or total absence of dynein arms and radial spokes from cilia throughout the body, a condition known as the immotile cilia syndrome (Fig. 3.41). The resultant functional defects in the respiratory epithelium and in the reproductive system are re-sponsible for a predisposition to chronic respiratory infections, bronchiectasis, and infertility (see Chapter 13). This is an ele-gant example of a gene defect being translated through an ultrastructurally recognizable molecular disorder, resulting ultimately in a complex clinical and pathological syndrome.

Recently, the intermediate filament components of the cyto-skeleton have been intensively studied by pathologists using antibodies to vimetin, desmin, and the various cytokeratins. Such studies, however, have been directed more towards the assessment of tissue differentiation in problem tumours than to the analysis of subcellular morphology. The principal exception is in the field of neurological and myopathic disorders. Distur-bances of desmin metabolism with the formation of intermedi-ate filamentous deposits in myocardial cells have been incriminated in some forms of cardiomyopathy. The formation of neurofibrillary tangles and the proliferation of excessive neurofilaments have been described after various forms of toxic injury. Finally, the release of intermediate filament components from dying cells, as well as by neoplastic epithelium, has been claimed as the origin of some forms of localized amyloidosis (Chapter 5).

In skeletal muscle, myofilament damage is seen in a wide variety of conditions, including denervation, myositis, poly-myalgia rheumatica, malignant hyperthermia, vitamin E defi-ciency, and exposure to clostridial toxins. Disintegration of car-diac myofibrils is observed after adrenaline, or adrenaline and angiotensin injection, while loss of fibrils is reported after lead and cobalt intoxication. In addition to filament disorders, various other abnormal inclusions and deposits are seen in disorders of skeletal and cardiac muscle.

Changes in lysosomes

Phagocytosis, or heterophagocytosis, is the process of engulf-ment of extraneous material by the cell. This may be an entirely physiological process, as in the case of erythrophagocytosis by splenic macrophages (Fig. 3.42), but the same mechanisms

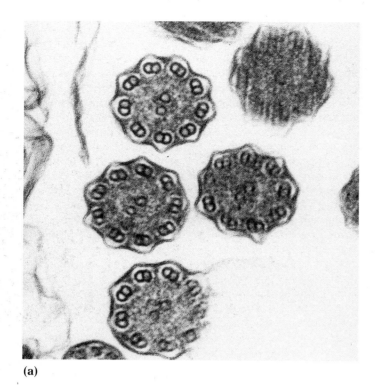

(a)

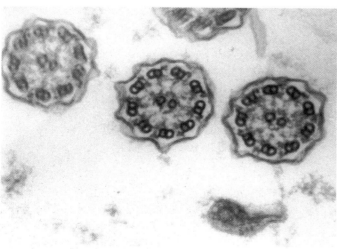

(b)

Fig. 3.41 (a) Immotile cilia. Cross-section of tracheal cilia in the immotile cilia syndrome, showing the preservation of a typical 9+2 tubular structure, but without the dynein arms which are essential for motility. Compare with normal cilia in (b).

operate in pathological circumstances, in response to many types of cell injury. At times, whole cells undergoing shrinkage necrosis or apoptosis (Section 3.1) may be engulfed by their neighbours, forming large round inclusion bodies which then undergo progressive condensation (Figs 3.43, 3.44, 3.45). In this way, potentially harmful debris is enveloped and localized within the lysosomal system, where it is digested, if possible, and any risk eliminated. As well as debris from dead and dying

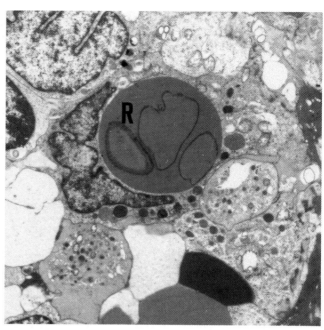

Fig. 3.42 Erythrophagocytosis by a splenic macrophage. The engulfed red cell (R) distorts the macrophage nucleus. (Micrograph by courtesy of Dr A. L. C. McLay.)

cells, infecting organisms or extraneous particulate material will be quickly taken up through heterophagocytosis by surrounding cells and by specialized phagocytes (Fig. 3.46). Phagocytic cells may themselves be damaged during this process and may disintegrate. The spillage of lysosomal enzymes from damaged cells can cause further tissue injury.

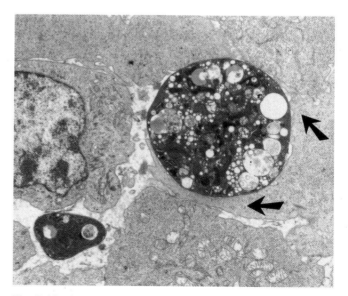

Fig. 3.43 Apoptotic cell in a tumour treated by a cytotoxic drug. The dead cell has rounded off and become condensed, but internal structural detail can still be recognized. An adjacent tumour cell extends processes (arrows) to engulf the apoptotic cell.

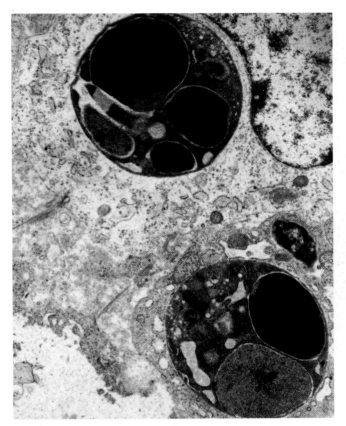

Fig. 3.44 Apoptotic bodies consisting of condensed and shrunken remnants of dead cells, engulfed by neighbours.

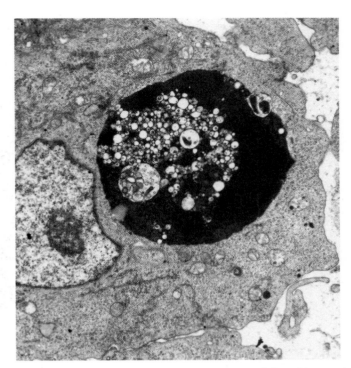

Fig. 3.45 The process of condensation leaves little evidence of structural detail in this apoptotic body.

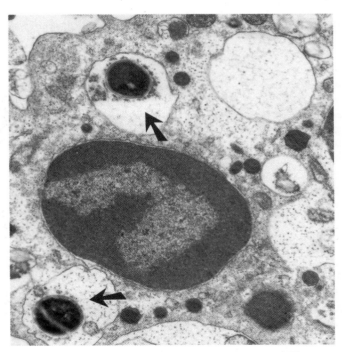

Fig. 3.46 Neutrophil polymorph engulfing staphylococci. The organisms lie with associated debris within phagocytic vacuoles (arrows). Many of the neutrophil granules have been discharged into these vacuoles.

Autophagocytosis is the sequestration of damaged organelles within lysosomes of the same cell. After non-lethal focal cytoplasmic injury (Fig. 3.47), autophagocytosis allows cell damage to be confined and repaired and provides a mechanism for cells to adapt to adverse circumstances by reducing their cytoplasmic mass, and therefore their metabolic burden. This occurs after hypoxia, in nutritional deprivation or metabolic stress, as in septic and haemorrhagic shock, or in severe starvation. Non-lethal irradiation and cytotoxic drug injury have similar effects on susceptible cells.

The ultrastructural appearances of heterophagosomes or autophagosomes will depend on the nature of their content. They are membrane-limited and their contents are usually of variable electron density, with identifiable structures still sometimes recognizable (Figs 3.44, 3.48). These may later be extruded from the cell or may undergo digestion by acid hydrolytic enzymes. Partially digested residues may also be extruded from the cell, or may be retained indefinitely as a dense, ultrastructurally heterogeneous, lipid-rich residual body (lipofuscin).

In a rare defect, the process of fusion of cellular lysosomes with phagosomes does not occur, interfering with one of the major defences against infection. This condition, the Chédiak–Higashi syndrome, is characterized by the presence of large abnormal lysosomes. Various other defects of bacterial killing

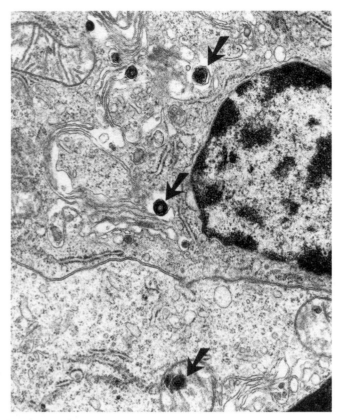

Fig. 3.47 Focal cytotoxic injury in tumour cells. Small dense whorls of laminated material (arrows) are seen around the Golgi apparatus and in a mitochondrion. Areas of focal injury become segrated into lysosomes.

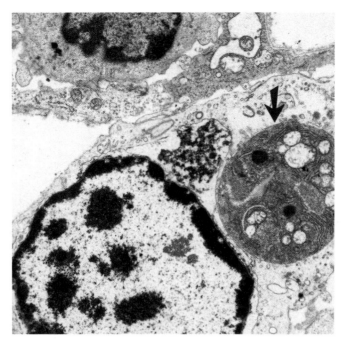

Fig. 3.48 Cytotoxic injury to tumour cell, showing clumping of nuclear chromatin, and a cytoplasmic lysosomal inclusion (arrow) containing recognizable organelles.

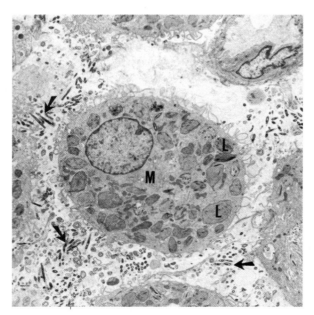

Fig. 3.49 Whipple's disease, showing large macrophages (M) in the lamina propria containing irregularly shaped secondary lysosomes (L), filled with partially digested bacterial residues. Rod-shaped bacteria (arrows) are present in large numbers between the macrophages. (Micrograph by courtesy of Dr I. A. R. More.)

within lysosomes may also lead to chronic granulomatous conditions. The accumulation of partially digested bacterial cell residues in the lysosomes of intestinal mucosal macrophages gives rise to the distinctive histological features of Whipple's disease (Chapter 16), in which electron microscopy provided the first convincing evidence of an infective basis (Figs 3.49, 3.50). There is also evidence that the concentric inclusions of malakoplakia, the Michaelis–Gutmann bodies (Fig. 3.51), may arise by progressive mineral encrustation on incomplete digested bacterial residues (Chapter 19).

There are many other disorders of lysosomal function, reflecting a wide range of genetically determined enzyme defects (see Section 2.5). In each case, the corresponding substrate accumulates within the cells of the body system or tissue exposed to the heaviest metabolic load. The ultrastructural features of such accumulations, such as glycogen, complex lipids, or glycosaminoglycans, may provide a useful aid to diagnosis (Figs 3.52, 3.53). The definitive confirmation of a lysosoal storage disease, however, must ultimately rely on biochemical techniques. Various forms of chronic cellular injury result in an accumulation of secondary lysosomes, but essentially identical appearances are also characteristic of the granular cell tumour (Fig. 3.54), a

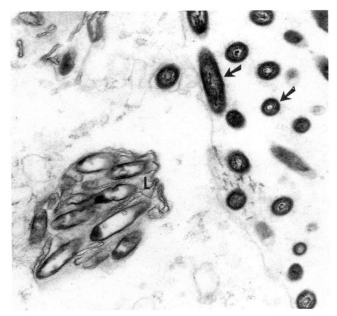

Fig. 3.50 Whipple's disease, showing rod-shaped organisms (arrows) and a secondary lysosome (L) within a macrophage, containing partially digested bacterial residues.

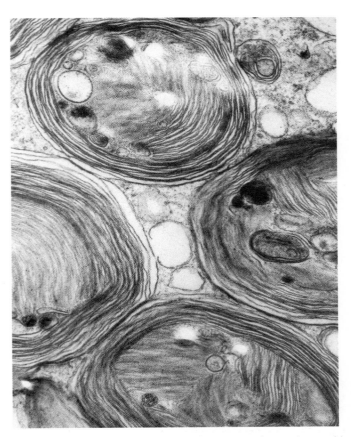

Fig. 3.52 Tay–Sachs disease, showing neuronal cytoplasm with abnormal concentrically laminated accumulations of ganglioside material, which cannot be metabolized owing to a genetically determined enzyme deficiency.

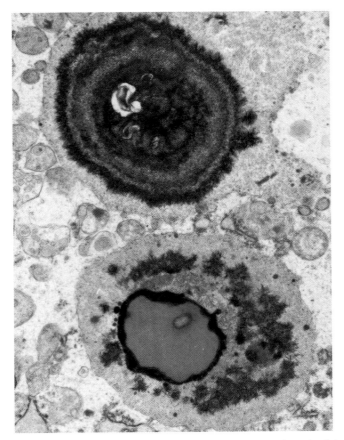

Fig. 3.51 Malakoplakia, showing two concentrically laminated calcified Michaelis–Gutmann bodies.

benign neoplasm generally classified as a nerve sheath tumour. This curious abundance of secondary lysosomes as a feature of tumour cell differentiation raises interesting questions about the underlying mechanism involved.

The morphological end-stage of autophagocytic digestion is the lipid-rich residual body which consists of largely unrecognizable heterogeneous electron dense debris, surrounded by a limiting membrane. On light microscopy, this is yellowish-brown due to oxidation and polymerization of contents originally rich in unsaturated fatty acids. Lipofuscin accumulates most noticeably in stable or permanent parenchymal cells, such as hepatocytes, cardiac muscle cells, and neurones, where its presence is seen as a mark of ageing, although lipofuscin accumulation may be accelerated in certain pathological states. Similarly, the oxidation and polymerization of retained heterolysosomes in macrophages results in residual bodies containing ceroid pigmentation, often characterized on electron microscopy by dense, whorled, laminated inclusions, sometimes referred to as myelinoid bodies.

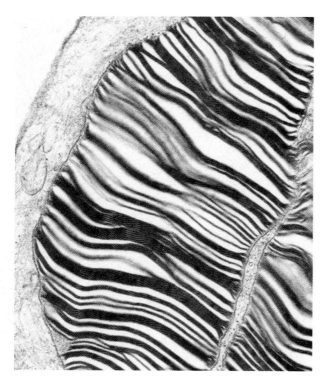

Fig. 3.53 Fabry disease, showing laminated inclusion from renal glomerular epithelium, demonstrating the accumulation of unmetabolized complex lipid. (Micrograph by courtesy of Dr I. A. R. More.)

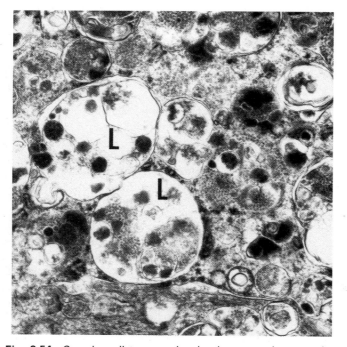

Fig. 3.54 Granular cell tumour, showing large complex secondary lysosomes (L) of uncertain origin.

3.2.3   Abnormal inclusions in cell injury

The previous section dealt largely with volumetric and qualitative changes affecting the cytoplasmic organelles. In this section, attention is focused on various intracytoplasmic inclusions associated with particular forms of cell injury.

Classification of cytoplasmic inclusions

These may be either exogenous or endogenous in origin. Exogenous inclusions represent material engulfed by the cell from the surrounding environment. These include particulate and often mineral-rich foreign bodies, infective agents, or cellular debris. Endogenous accumulations may represent the end-products of cellular catabolism, in the form of lipid-rich lysosomal residues. Alternatively, they may consist of metabolites such as lipid, structural products such as filamentous proteins, or unextruded secretory materials, which have accumulated due to a metabolic block. Lysosomal inclusions have already been dealt with. The following sections are concerned with the other categories of cytoplasmic inclusion.

Mineral inclusions

These include mineral-rich endogenous deposits and particulate material of exogenous origin. Such inclusions are usually visible on light microscopy, or can be demonstrated by special stains or by polarization. On electron microscopy, insoluble mineral-rich inclusions generally appear dense, since they scatter electrons, and may have distinctive morphological features. Their elemental composition can be explored by EM X-ray microanalysis, which reveals an element by a spectral peak of characteristic X-rays emitted by the sample when it is exposed to the electron beam.

Examples of exogenous mineral inclusions range from mineral dust, such as silica or asbestos in pneumoconiosis, to tattoos. The identity of fragmented material from implants and prostheses, the nature of obscure buccal pigmentation of suspected dental origin, and the presence of radiological contrast material in granulomatous reactions (Figs 3.55, 3.56) have all been demonstrated, in clinical situations, by the use of EM elemental analysis. In addition to their scientific value, these techniques have obvious medico-legal applications.

Endogenous electron-dense mineral deposits are usually located in lysosomes. These include iron-rich pigments in haemochromatosis and copper deposits in Wilson's disease (see Chapter 17). Iron storage is usually associated with ultrastructurally identifiable ferritin particles (Fig. 3.57), but the lysosomal accumulation in haemochromatosis may include material of a nondescript dense amorphous appearance. Other endogenous mineral-rich deposits include the needle-shaped crystals seen in calcification, whether physiological, in mineralized bone, or pathological, in other sites (Figs 3.58, 3.59). In all of these instances, X-ray analysis can determine the elemental composition of the tissue deposit.

Lipid inclusions

Small fat droplets are commonly found in many normal cells,

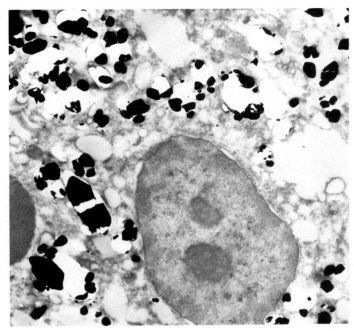

Fig. 3.55 Barium granuloma, showing dense particulate material within a macrophage.

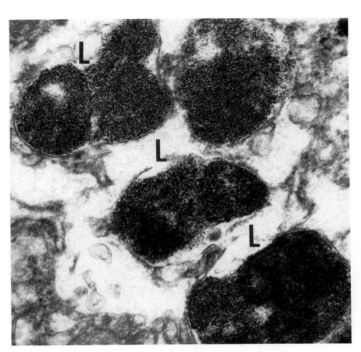

Fig. 3.57 Haemochromatosis, showing liver lysosomes (L) containing finely granular iron-rich material.

but when abnormal triglyceride storage becomes obvious at the light microscopic level, the condition is described as fatty change. This is most commonly seen in the liver (see Chapter 17), in response to hypoxia, alcohol, and a wide variety of toxic and chemical insults (Fig. 3.60). Other sites for fatty change

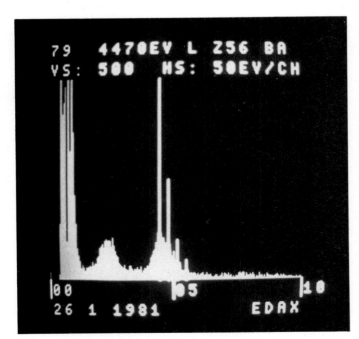

Fig. 3.56 Barium granuloma. X-ray microanalysis displays peaks for barium and sulphur, confirming that the particulate material consists of radiological contrast medium.

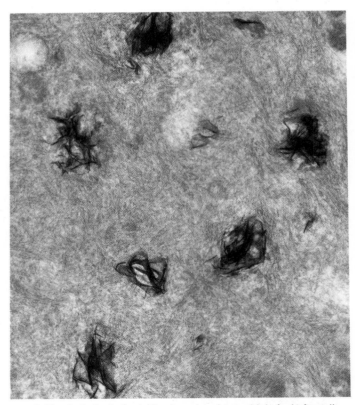

Fig. 3.58 Pathological calcification, showing multiple foci of needle-shaped calcium phosphate crystals deposited amongst keratin filaments in the cells of a pilomatrixoma (calcifying epithelioma of Malherbe) a benign tumour of hair shafts.

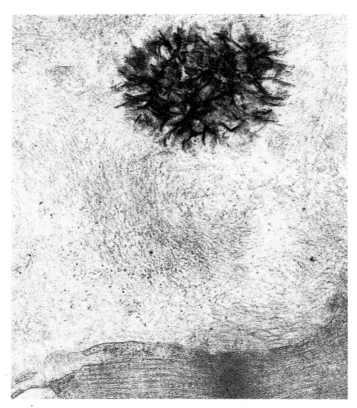

Fig. 3.59 Pathological calcification within a deposit of amyloid in the myocardium.

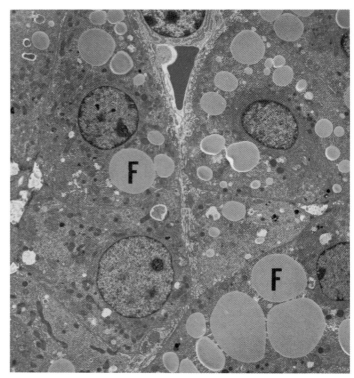

Fig. 3.60 Fatty change, showing numerous fat droplets (F) in liver cells in Reye syndrome.

include the renal tubular epithelium and the myocardium, especially in severe anaemia, with resulting tissue hypoxia.

The ultrastructure of fat droplets varies according to their composition, but in general they are round, of uniform texture, and have quite low electron density. Since triglyceride partitions itself naturally from the aqueous cytosol, fat droplets are not usually surrounded by a membrane, with the exception of lipid taken up by phagocytosis or during intestinal fat absorption. Fat droplets vary from the very small to the very large, in some cases being large enough to fill and distend a hepatocyte, compressing its nucleus to one side.

The extent of lipid deposition is not a reliable guide to cellular malfunction or to the nature or severity of the insult to cellular metabolism. In general, the accumulation of droplet fat reflects a disturbance of the balance of cellular lipid metabolism, whether through input overload, processing malfunction, or output failure. The various causes of fatty change in the liver can be linked with one or other of these basic stages in hepatocyte lipid metabolism. The aetiology and pathogenesis of fatty change are discussed in Chapter 17.

Lipid accumulation occurs also as a result of active phagocytosis of extracellular lipid debris, as in fat necrosis, exogenous lipogranulomas, and some 'histiocytic' tumours (Fig. 3.61). The ultrastructure of lipid-laden macrophages differs from that of the hepatocyte in fatty change. The lipid in a macrophage is

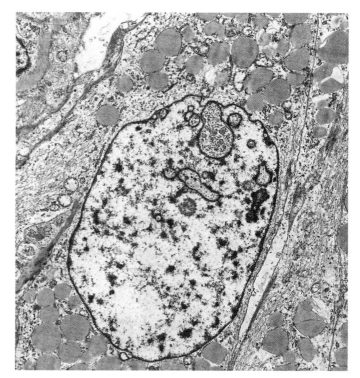

Fig. 3.61 Histiocytic cell in a fibrohistiocytic tumour, containing lipid aggregates which suggest phagocytic activity.

contained within the lysosomal compartment and may show a more heterogeneous morphological appearance. In the case of cholesterol-rich accumulations, the typical clefts appear as empty voids of characteristic shape. As already mentioned, complex lipids in the various forms of lysosomal storage disease have distinctive morphological features (see Figs 3.52, 3.53).

Protein inclusions

The metabolic accumulation of protein deposits is less common than fatty change. When it occurs, it can often be interpreted in terms of the same broad metabolic principles of input overload, processing malfunction, or output failure. A classical example of protein droplet accumulation is seen in the proximal convoluted tubules of the kidney in cases of severe proteinuria (Fig. 3.62). The tubular epithelium normally scavenges any traces of protein which may reach the glomerular filtrate, but this mechanism becomes grossly overloaded when the glomerular filtrate is laden with protein leaking from the plasma across a damaged glomerular basement membrane. Large homogeneous apical droplets, described as hyaline droplets by light microscopy, accumulate within the tubular epithelial cell and are cycled through the lysosomal mechanism (see Chapter 19).

Excess production or reduced output of secretion can also induce the formation of protein inclusions. Immunoglobulin may accumulate in plasma cells (Fig. 3.63), producing refractile eosinophilic hyaline droplets known on light microscopy as Russell bodies. In α_1-antitrypsin deficiency, the enzyme accumulates in large cytoplasmic inclusions in hepatocytes, due to a genetically determined defect which may inhibit its release from the cell (Chapter 17).

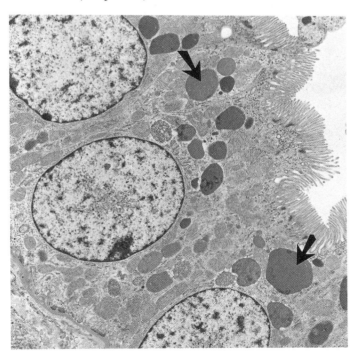

Fig. 3.62 Protein droplets (arrows) in renal tubular epithelium in severe proteinuria. (Micrograph by courtesy of Dr C. M. Hill.)

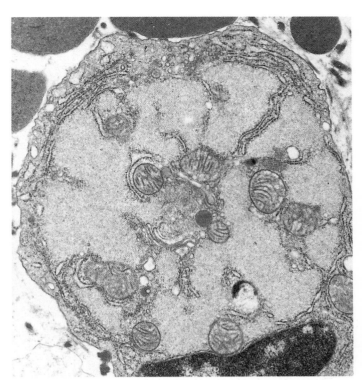

Fig. 3.63 Plasma cell, showing a spherical aggregate of amorphous material within the cytoplasmic matrix. This globular accumulation would be recognizable by light microscopy as a Russell body.

Filamentous inclusions

Abnormal accumulation of cytoplasmic filaments is responsible for Mallory's alcoholic hyaline (Fig. 3.64), a condition traditionally classified as a form of hyaline degeneration. This abnormality may be seen not only in hepatocytes in alcoholic liver disease, but also in some forms of non-alcoholic cirrhosis, Wilson's disease, hepatocellular carcinoma, and various other conditions. Mallory bodies consist of ill-defined, dense aggregates of intermediate filaments, which are largely random in their orientation and which displace the other cytoplasmic components. There is no limiting membrane around these bundles of filaments. Mallory's hyaline is still poorly understood, but may represent a form of disordered partial keratinization in response to injury (see Chapter 17).

Cytokeratin filaments accumulate also in bronchiolar epithelium in chronic smoking, a form of metaplasia associated with an increased risk of malignancy. There is deposition of filaments in hepatocytes in response to colchicine, griseofulvin, and phalloidin, and in tracheal epithelium in vitamin E deficiency. Crooke's hyaline change in the pituitary, a response to prolonged high corticosteroid levels, has a similar morphological basis (Fig. 3.65).

3.2.4 Nuclear changes in cell injury

Subcellular pathology is more difficult to interpret in the nucleus than in the cytoplasm. The various ultrastructural

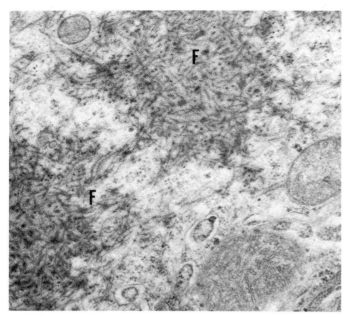

Fig. 3.64 Mallory's alcoholic hyaline, showing filament bundles (F) in liver cell cytoplasm in alcoholic cirrhosis. (Micrograph by courtesy of Dr I. A. R. More.)

disturbances of the specialized cytoplasmic compartments can be represented as the systemic pathology of the cell, but nuclear morphology is less compartmentalized, making it more difficult to correlate structural changes with specific functional effects. The morphological responses of the nucleus to different challenges can often be categorized, therefore, only in the most general of pathobiological terms, as reflecting either increased or decreased nuclear activity. Increased activity encompasses enhanced transcription and synthesis, as in regeneration and neoplasia. Decreased activity implies a decline in nuclear function, as in cellular malfunction generally classified as degenerative and likely to result in cell death. This section attempts to classify and describe some of the commoner ultrastructural changes expressed in the nucleus in cellular injury.

Volumetric changes in the nucleus

These include changes in nuclear number, volume, dimension, and contour. Multinucleation occurs mainly in reactive and neoplastic conditions, ranging from simple binucleation of reactive plasma cells to complex lobulation and multinucleation in high-grade malignant neoplasms. Such changes are usually accompanied by an overall increase in nuclear volume. Nuclei may swell prior to rupture in some forms of lethal injury, but more often the nuclei of degenerating cells become condensed and shrunken (see Fig. 3.44).

Irregularity of contour, increased segmentation, abnormal evagination, or invagination and deep clefting of the nucleus are common findings in cellular pathology, especially in tumours (Fig. 3.66). These changes are often interpreted as a reflection of increased metabolic activity, perhaps associated with increased mechanical and dynamic turbulence within the cell, the irregularity of contour providing an enhanced surface area for nucleo-cytoplasmic exchange. Alternatively, nuclear irregularity may reflect rapid or unbalanced change in nuclear volume following an acute cytotoxic injury. It has also been suggested that such changes might be a consequence of some

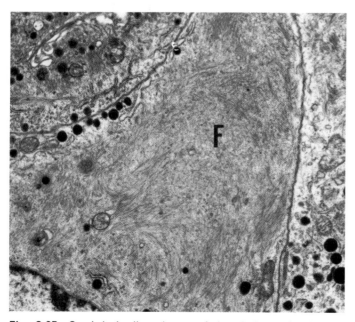

Fig. 3.65 Crooke's hyaline change of the pituitary, showing an irregular whorled mass of intermediate filaments (F).

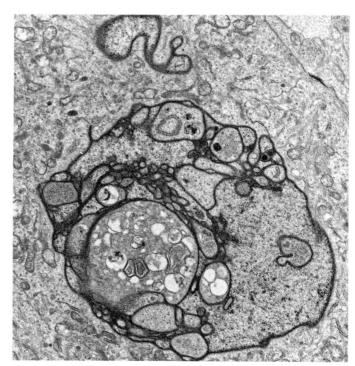

Fig. 3.66 Bizarre nuclear contours in a tumour cell.

primary nuclear defect, perhaps involving a deficiency of nuclear pores. Different explanations may apply in different circumstances.

Prime examples of nuclear irregularity include various types of neoplasm, in some of which the nuclear features are sufficiently consistent as to be almost characteristic. The Sézary cell, a neoplastic T-cell, is the classical example; its nucleus often being cerebriform, owing to its complex contours (Fig. 3.67). Treatment of tumours with cytotoxic agents such as cytosine arabinoside, methotrexate, and fluorouracil may cause nuclear envelope invaginations or protrusions, forming nuclear or cytoplasmic pockets. Irregularity of nuclear contour is also seen in some viral infections and after irradiation.

Changes in the nuclear envelope

In cell swelling, the nuclear envelope, which is functionally continuous with the endoplasmic reticulum, is also susceptible to osmotic damage, resulting in membrane separation and cisternal dilatation. In lethal injury, rupture of the nuclear envelope is a clear indication of irreversible damage, expressed in due course by the light microscopic changes of either karyolysis ('lysis of nuclei') or karyorrhexis ('fragmentation of nuclei'). Thickening, fusion, proliferation, and reduplication of the nuclear envelope are particularly seen in association with viral infections, such as adenovirus and the herpes CMV group. Viral particles may accumulate in pockets and vesicles formed by the proliferating inner nuclear membrane. The nuclear fibrous lamina may become thickened and prominent in various benign tumours, in the myofibroblasts of repaired tissues, and in synovial cells in rheumatoid arthritis. The nuclear pores are said to increase in size and number in neoplasia and to be reduced in states of lowered metabolism, as in the pancreatic acinar cells in cases of kwashiorkor.

Changes in nuclear chromatin

In regeneration and hyperplasia, there is generally a decrease in heterochromatin and a corresponding increase in the proportion of euchromatin. Conversely, an increase in the heterochromatin–euchromatin ratio may be seen in sublethally and lethally injured cells. Heterochromatin condensation characteristically occurs at the periphery of the nucleus and around the nucleolus, producing the peripheral margination and clumping of chromatin often seen in dying and dead cells (Fig. 3.68). There are, of course, exceptions to such general statements. Some rapidly growing tumours may show a high heterochromatin–euchromatin ratio, whereas cell death may be reflected in reduced electron density and a diffuse dissolution of nuclear chromatin (see Figs 3.20, 3.22).

Intranuclear inclusions

True intranuclear inclusions may be distinguished from intranuclear pseudoinclusions, which represents pockets of cytoplasm invaginated into the nucleus, but still retaining a discernible surrounding nuclear envelope (Fig. 3.69). True inclusions, on the other hand, are presumed to have formed inside the nucleus and may or may not have some kind of

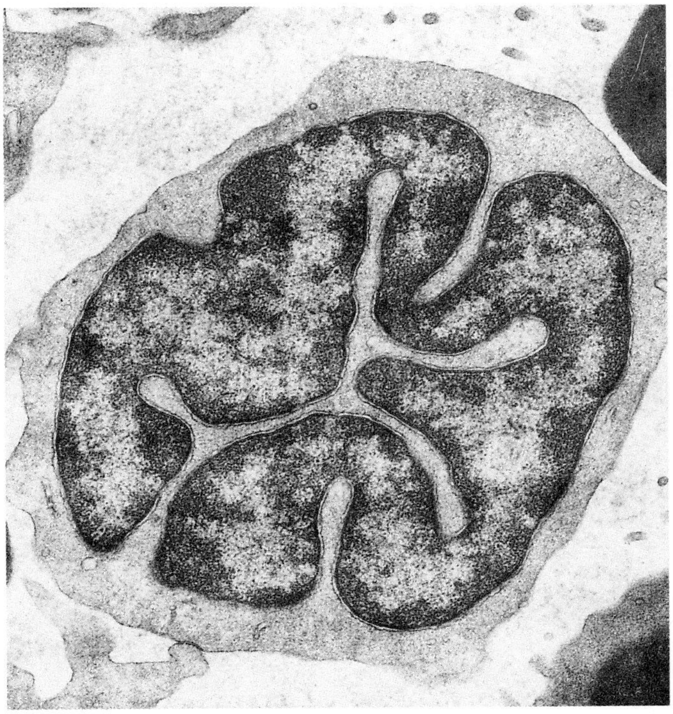

Fig. 3.67 Sézary cell, showing characteristic cerebriform convolution of the nucleus.

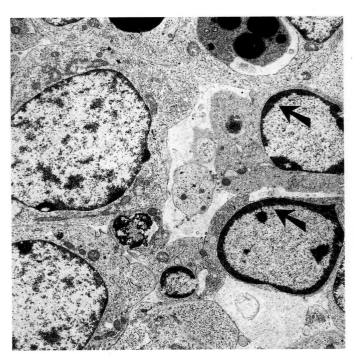

Fig. 3.68 Cytotoxic injury to tumour cells, showing margination of chromatin in dying cells (arrows).

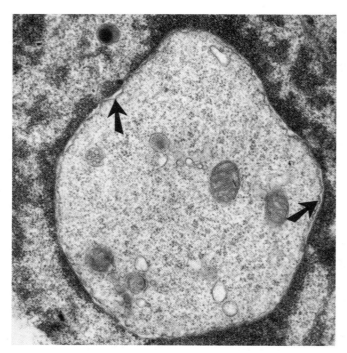

Fig. 3.69 Intranuclear pseudoinclusion, consisting of a pocket of cytoplasm contained within the nucleus and bounded by a normal nuclear envelope (arrows).

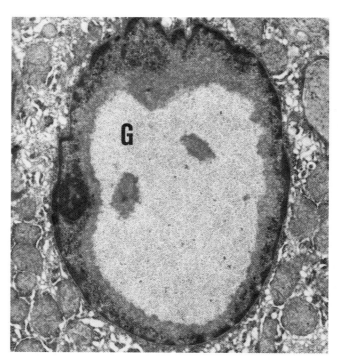

Fig. 3.70 Intranuclear glycogen (G), not demarcated from the nuclear substance.

delimiting boundary. In practice, however, it may be difficult to make this distinction.

A more practical classification of nuclear inclusions is based on the nature of the included material. Specific inclusions are identifiable substances such as glycogen (Fig. 3.70), lipid (Fig. 3.71), haemoglobin in red cell precursors, virus particles (Fig. 3.72)/products, and elemental inclusions (e.g. lead, bismuth). Cytoplasmic organelles and membranes derived from the nuclear envelope may also lie free within the nuclear substance. Unspecified inclusions cannot be categorized in this way, but are given descriptive names, such as nuclear bodies; vermicellar bodies; concentrically laminated inclusions; filamentous, fibrillar, and crystalline inclusions; intranuclear vacuoles, lamellae, tubules, and vesicles; and so forth (Figs 3.73, 3.74).

The diversity of intranuclear inclusions is only matched by our ignorance of their functional significance. Some may represent entrapped cytoplasmic components, whereas others may be by-products of erratic nuclear metabolism. In general, nuclear inclusions are seen most commonly in malignant tumours, in viral infections, after exposure to sublethal cytotoxic insults, and in some metabolic disorders. While some consistent functional associations are clearly recognized, such as the relationship between nuclear bodies and rapidly proliferating cell populations, these and other diverse nuclear inclusions are seen in too many physiological and pathological states to be easily interpretable. Few, if any, of these inclusions can be described as pathognomonic.

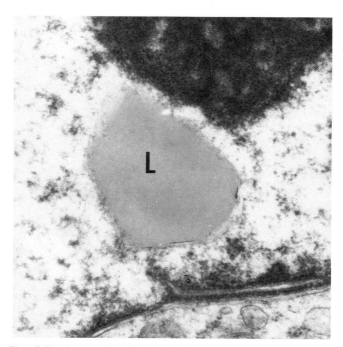

Fig. 3.71 Intranuclear lipid inclusion (L) adjacent to the nuclear envelope and nucleolus.

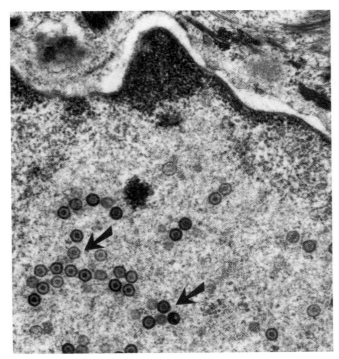

Fig. 3.72 Intranuclear virus particles (arrows) in a herpes virus infection of the skin. (Micrograph by courtesy of Dr A. L. C. McLay.)

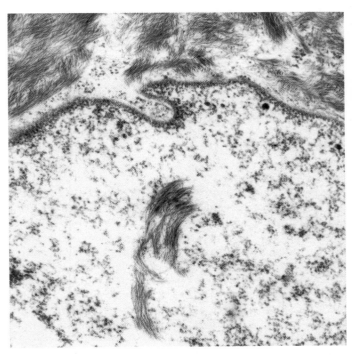

Fig. 3.74 Intranuclear filamentous inclusion in squamous carcinoma.

Changes in the nucleolus

Morphological changes in the nucleolus occur in various pathological states, such as viral infections and neoplasia (Fig. 3.75), and in response to many chemical, metabolic, and cytotoxic agents. Various patterns of volumetric and structural change are described, such as irregularity, enlargement, numerical

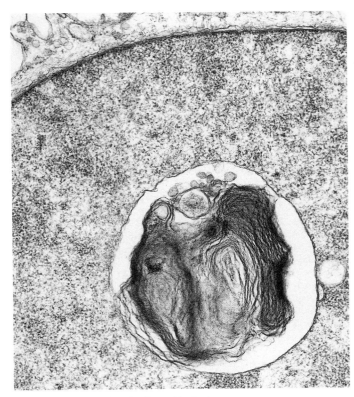

Fig. 3.73 Intranuclear laminated inclusion.

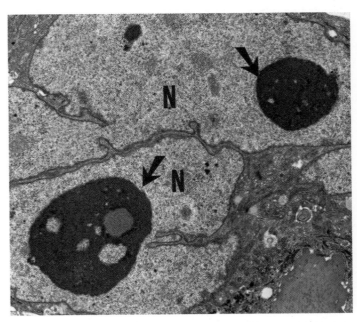

Fig. 3.75 Bizarre nucleus (N) and nucleoli (arrows) in a tumour cell of squamous carcinoma.

increase or decrease, condensation, margination, and segregation.

Certain viral infections induce striking nucleolar alterations. Nucleolar disaggregation occurs in herpes simplex infection, correlating with the gradual inhibition of RNA synthesis. Reticulated, pure fibrillar, and ring-shaped nucleoli occur in adenovirus infections, as do giant nucleoli containing only the granular component. Ring-shaped condensed nucleoli (Fig. 3.76) are seen in aged cells, after irradiation, following treatment with acridine derivatives, and after exposure to hyperthermia.

Nucleolar segregation is characterized by the separation and migration of the fibrillar centres and fibrillar component from the granular component of the nucleolus (Fig. 3.77). This unique morphological pattern is produced by agents that interfere with, or inhibit, DNA-dependent synthesis of ribosomal RNA. Nucleolar segregation is produced by chemotherapeutic and toxic agents such as actinomycin D, amsacrine, mitomycin C, and adriamycin, by carcinogens such as 4-nitroquinoline-N-oxide, and by physical agents such as hyperthermia an irradiation. A reduction or virtual absence of the nucleolar granular component is a hallmark of conditions associated with prolonged inhibition of RNA synthesis.

3.2.5　Conclusions

The morphological manifestations of cell injury are almost endlessly varied, but are often difficult to understand. It must be appreciated that descriptive ultrastructual pathology is still in its infancy and consists largely of a catalogue of random observations of heterogeneous cellular responses, with few common themes. Such observations are hampered by the problems of

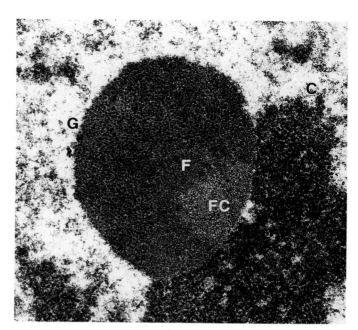

Fig. 3.77 Nucleolar segregation in cytotoxic injury, showing nucleolar-associated chromatin (C) and separation of the structural components of the nucleolus into the fibrillar component (F), the fibrillar centre (FC), and the granular component (G).

artefact and the limitations of ultrastructural interpretation. Nevertheless, many of these phenomena, however poorly understood, are clearly key elements in cellular responses to environmental challenge and demand further study, using the increasingly sophisticated techniques that are now becoming available to the cellular pathologist.

3.2.6　Further reading

Alzelius, B. A. (1981). 'Immotile-cilia' syndrome and ciliary abnormalities induced by infection and injury. *American Review of Respiratory Disease* **124**, 107.

Brandle, E. R. and Gabbiani, G. (1983). The role of cytoskeletal and cytocontractile elements in pathologic processes. *American Journal of Pathology* **110**, 361.

Constantinides, P. (1984). *Ultrastructural pathobiology.* Elsevier, London.

De Robertis, E. D. P. and De Robertis, E. M. F., Jr (1987). *Cell and molecular biology.* Lea & Febiger, Philadelphia.

Dickersin, G. R. (1988). *Diagnostic electron microscopy: A text/atlas.* Igaku-Shoin, New York.

Ganote, C. E. and Van der Heide, R. S. (1987). Cytoskeletal lesions in anoxic myocardial injury: A conventional and high-voltage electron microscopic and immunofluorescence study. *American Journal of Pathology* **129**, 327.

Ghadially, F. N. (1988). *Ultrastructual pathology of the cell and matrix.* Butterworths, London.

Glaumann, H. and Ballard, F. J. (ed.) (1987). *Lysosomes—their role in protein breakdown.* Academic Press, London.

Glew, R. H., Basu, A., Prence, E. M., and Remaley, A. T. (1985). Biology of disease. Lysosomal storage diseases. *Laboratory Investigation* **53**, 250–69.

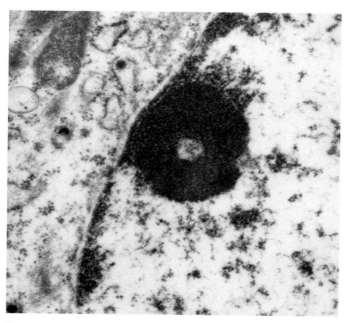

Fig. 3.76 Condensed ring-shaped nucleolus following cytotoxic injury.

Goessens, G. (1984). Nucleolar structure. *International Review of Cytology* **87**, 107–58.

Kamel, H. M. H., Kirk, J., and Toner, P. G. (1990). Ultrastructural pathology of the nucleus. In *Current topics in pathology* (ed. J. C. E. Underwood), Vol. 82, *Pathology of the nucleus*. Springer-Verlag, London.

Katsuma, Y. (1987). Changes in cytokeratin intermediate filament cytoskeleton associated with Mallory body formation in mouse and human liver. *Hepatology* **7**, 1215.

Lazarow, P. B. and Fujik, Y. (1985). Biogenesis of perioxisomes. *Annual Review of Cell Biology* **1**, 489.

Steenbergen, C. (1985). Volume regulation and plasma membrane injury in aerobic, anaerobic and ischaemic myocardium *in vitro*: effects of osmotic cell swelling on plasma membrane integrity. *Circulation Research* **57**, 864.

3.3   Mechanisms of cell injury

Alan R. Boobis, Duncan J. Fawthrop, and

Donald S. Davies

3.3.1   Introduction

Injury to cells leads to a complex sequence of changes to organelles (Section 3.2) and molecular events, frequently culminating in cell death. The commonest consequence of cell damage is necrosis, where cell death is the result of the failure of endogenous protective systems to compensate. However, under certain circumstances, some compounds can initiate programmed cell death (apoptosis—see Section 3.1). However, injury is not always lethal, leading to one of three possible outcomes:

1. temporary impairment of cell function (e.g. secretion, excitation), followed by complete recovery due to the effect of normal homeostatic mechanisms;

2. structural damage to the cell, leading to permanent impairment of function (e.g. in neurones and cardiac myocytes); or

3. damage to DNA, leading to an hereditary alteration in the cell's phenotype (mutation).

An understanding of the mechanisms of cell injury is fundamental to cellular pathology and in the rational design of protective agents or antidotes.

Agents that cause cell injury may be classified into the following categories:

1. mechanical (e.g. silica dust);

2. infectious (e.g. viral, herpes simplex; bacterial, *Listeria monocytogenes*);

3. parasitic (e.g. *Plasmodium falciparum*);

4. immunologic (e.g. auto-antibodies to erythrocyte antigens);

5. metabolic (e.g. thiamine deficiency leading to citric acid cycle inhibition);

6. genetic (e.g. lysosomal storage diseases); and

7. chemical (e.g. paracetamol, paraquat, dimethylnitrosamine).

The interaction of an injurious agent with cells is twofold: there is an effect of the agent on the cell and an effect of the cell upon the agent. In some instances, it is only after the cell has modified the toxin that injury results (metabolic activation). During evolution a variety of systems have evolved to protect the cell from injury and to repair such damage that does occur. These systems include: removal of particulate material (phagocytosis, lysosomes), biotransformation and excretion of exogenous chemicals (biliary and renal excretion, conjugating enzymes, mixed function oxidases), host defence mechanisms (interferons and other cytokines, prostaglandins and other inflammatory mediators), systems for the repair of chemically mediated damage (DNA repair enzymes, antioxidants, thiol-reducing systems), counteraction of biochemical disturbances (calcium-binding systems, anaerobic glycolysis). However, if these protective systems are overwhelmed by the nature or extent of cell injury, permanent damage or necrosis will ensue. Metabolic activation comes about when some mechanisms that are normally protective, such as the mixed function oxidase system, contribute to the injury resulting from certain agents, e.g. paracetamol, by converting them into highly reactive intermediates.

The changes that occur in a cell following injury depend upon the site of injury, the nature and duration of exposure to the injurious agent, the metabolic state of the cell, the supply of oxygen and nutrients to the cell, and the removal of metabolic waste from the cell. In general, metabolically active cells in the centre of organs are the most susceptible to injury. Injurious agents normally cause damage by direct insult to one or more major organelle systems of the cell. However, because of the interdependency of cell structures and functions, direct injury also induces indirect injury. Changes inducing indirect injury include: acidosis resulting from an accumulation of lactate, pressure as a result of cell swelling, and ischaemia due to decreased blood flow. The injury to a cell may be either reversible or irreversible. There is often a reversible, prenecrotic phase, known as hydropic swelling, in which the endoplasmic reticulum becomes dilated and swelling of mitochondria may occur. Irreversible necrotic change is often heralded by an abrupt expansion in the volume of the mitochondria, accompanied by disruption of mitochondrial structure (see Section 3.2).

The plasma membrane, nucleus, mitochondria, endoplasmic reticulum, and lysosomes are all targets for injury (Fig. 3.78). Mechanical damage to cells occurs either due to external trauma, parasite attachment, or as a direct result of the physical movement of cells (such as erythrocytes). When there is severe mechanical damage to the plasma membrane the cells rapidly die. Tears in the cell membrane can repair by indulation and reduplication of the torn margins of the plasma membrane. Damage to cell membranes may also occur as a result of attack on the cell membrane by proteases and phospholipases, either

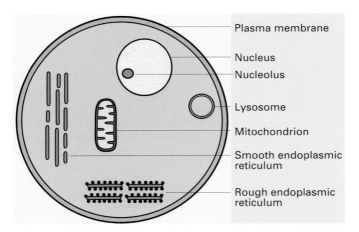

Fig. 3.78   Possible cellular targets for the effects of injurious agents.

externally (e.g. phospholipases in snake venoms, α-toxin of *Clostridium* species) or from within the cell. The organization of the plasma membrane depends upon the integrity of the cytoskeleton. A number of toxic compounds cause cytoskeletal disruption with subsequent damage to the plasma membrane.

The smooth endoplasmic reticulum is often a target of toxic metabolites of agents which are not directly injurious; such compounds are converted to reactive species within the cell by enzymes of drug metabolism. The classical agent in this respect is carbon tetrachloride, which is converted to trichloromethyl free radical by the mixed function oxidase system.

In the nucleus/nucleolus both transcription and translation are potential targets for injurious agents. Cyclophosphamide arylates DNA bases, especially guanine. If cells enter mitosis before being able to repair the damage then cell death occurs. In contrast, the O^6-methylation of guanine by dimethylnitrosamine, if not repaired, leads to mutation and possibly cancer. RNA polymerase in the nucleolus is a target of many toxins, including α-amanitin—the toxic principle of the angel toadstool (*Amanita phalloides*). α-Amanitin inhibits manganese-dependent RNA polymerase which directs the synthesis of mRNA during DNA transcription (Section 2.3).

Cell degeneration can be induced by injury to lysosomes in one of four ways:

1. excessive or incomplete autophagy;
2. hereditary absence of an enzyme in primary lysosomes;
3. failure of phagolysosomal degradation of phagocytosed material; and
4. liberation and activation of lysosomal enzymes.

The role of the lysosome in degrading foreign material renders this organelle particularly vulnerable to certain toxic agents, e.g. gentamicin.

Mitochondria are the sites of the citric acid cycle, electron transport, and oxidative phosphorylation. Any agent that impairs the metabolic pathways of the mitochondria will result in energy deficiency, particularly of ATP, in the cell. Energy is

essential for the maintenance of ionic gradients, particularly those dependent upon the magnesium-dependent, calcium-activated ATPases, and for the transport of essential molecules into (e.g. glucose) and out of (e.g. bilirubin) the cell. Many agents causing cell injury interfere with mitochondrial function, either directly of indirectly.

Identification of the causative events in cell injury has been hampered both by the limitations of the model systems available and the plethora of coincidental changes that occur within a cell upon injury. For example, lipid peroxidation (q.v.) occurs in all dying cells as a consequence of the failure of protective systems. This makes it difficult to identify those situations in which lipid peroxidation might contribute to cell death. Some of the major advances in our understanding of the biochemical mechanisms involved in cell injury have arisen from studies in isolated cells. However, many of these mechanisms have not yet been shown to contribute to toxic injury *in vivo*, often because of the difficulties of devising suitable experiments.

3.3.2   Biochemical changes occurring upon cell injury

The general pattern of biochemical change observed in many cell types injured by a variety of agents is very similar (Fig. 3.79). Early reversible damage to the plasma membrane, either directly or by interfering with metabolic processes on which the plasma membrane depends for its integrity (e.g. ATP synthesis), results in increased membrane permeability. As the concentrations of sodium and potassium are 145 mEq Na^+ and 4 mEq K^+ in the extracellular fluid but 12 mEq Na^+ and 155 mEq K^+ in the intracellular fluid, this increase in the permeability of the plasma membrane leads to the entry of sodium into the cell down its concentration gradient and to a loss of potassium from the cell. These ion movements result in the accumulation of water in the cell, manifest as acute cell swelling. Calcium ions enter the cell down their concentration gradient, aggravating the increase caused initially by release from intracellular stores such as the endoplasmic reticulum and mitochondria. In response to the entry of these ions into the cell, there is enhanced ion pumping via the sodium-activated, potassium-dependent ATPase and the calcium-activated, magnesium-dependent ATPase. The enhanced activity of the ion pumping mechanisms further consumes ATP. The increased consumption of ATP leads to metabolic activation with a resultant increased demand for oxygen and metabolic substrates such as glucose. The depletion of ATP results in activation of phosphofructokinase, which produces fructose-1,6-diphosphate. This activates pyruvate kinase leading to an accumulation of pyruvate. The increase in reducing equivalents in the cytosol following the increased demand for energy in the cell leads to the conversion of pyruvate to lactate. This shift to anaerobic glycolysis results in a decrease of intracellular pH which, together with the increase in the concentration of cytosolic calcium, alters the activity of many intracellular enzymes involved in homeostatic regulation in the cell. There is also a reduction in protein synthesis.

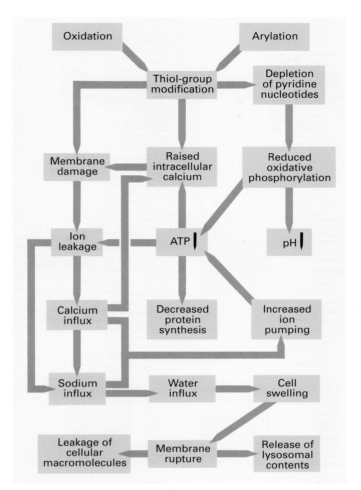

Fig. 3.79 Principal biochemical changes occurring following cell injury.

many cell types is very similar (Table 3.3). One of the earliest events following injury to many cell types is the appearance of protrusions at the surface of the plasma membrane, which have been termed 'blebs' (Section 3.1). Blebbing of the cell surface occurs before any change in membrane permeability is observed and initially it is reversible. At some point, the injury becomes irreversible, although the specific biochemical event that converts reversible injury to irreversible injury is not known. In some circumstances, the rupture of large membrane blebs, with loss of cellular contents, is believed to be the event that finally causes the death of the injured cell.

Table 3.3 Examples of injurious stimuli producing similar biochemical and morphological effects. These include: modification of protein thiols, altered ATP synthesis, disruption of the cytoskeleton, and plasma membrane blebbing

Noxious stimulus	Cell types affected
Adriamycin	Cardiac
Ischaemia/reperfusion	Neuronal/cardiac/endothelial
Mercury	Renal/neuronal
MPTP*	Neuronal
Cyanide	Various
Menadione	Hepatic
Carbon tetrachloride	Hepatic/renal
Paracetamol	Hepatic
Cephaloridine	Renal
Alloxan	Pancreatic
Paraquat	Pulmonary
Rotenone	Pulmonary/gastrointestinal
Primaquine	Red blood cell
Hydrogen peroxide	Epithelial

*1-Methyl-4-phenyl-1,2,5,6-tetrahydropyridine.

Disintegrating organelles release fragments of membrane which aggregate and are phagocytosed by autophagosomes. The breakdown of membrane phospholipids releases arachidonic acid which is a precursor for the formation of eicosanoids. Phospholipids can also participate in reactions leading to the formation of reactive oxygen species, which can cause further damage.

The manifestations of these biochemical changes are dependent upon the nature, status, and location of the cell type affected. Cells that are normally active in ion and water transport show the most prominent swelling following injury to the plasma membrane. Such cells include those of the endothelium, renal tubular epithelium, exocrine cells, epithelium of the intestine and bladder, and cells of the choroid plexus. Metabolically active cells such as neurones are most susceptible to impairment of energy production or of oxygen supply.

Although the injury caused by some agents is due to interference with a specific biochemical pathway of a certain organelle (e.g. saxitoxin inhibition of Na^+ channels), the pattern of biochemical changes caused by many injurious agents and in

3.3.3 The critical biochemical mechanisms involved in cell injury

Interference with endogenous substrates or effectors

Many compounds cause cell injury by competing with, depleting, or inactivating endogenous substrates, receptors, or cofactors (Fig. 3.80). The classic example of such competition is by fluoroacetate. This can participate to a limited extent in the citric acid cycle, serving as a substrate for citrate synthase. However, the product, fluorocitrate, is not a substrate for aconitase and acts as a potent inhibitor of this enzyme, by chelation of the fluorine atom to Fe^{2+} in the active site. This blocks the citric acid cycle and prevents the production of ATP, with the consequences of deprivation described below. This process has been termed lethal synthesis, and is not unique to fluoroacetate but is common to many toxic compounds. Other examples include galactosamine, ethionine, 5-fluorouracil, and carbaryl. The toxic compound may be sufficiently similar to an endogenous substrate to inhibit its enzyme, but not to serve as a substrate itself, for example, eserine inhibition of acetylcholinesterase.

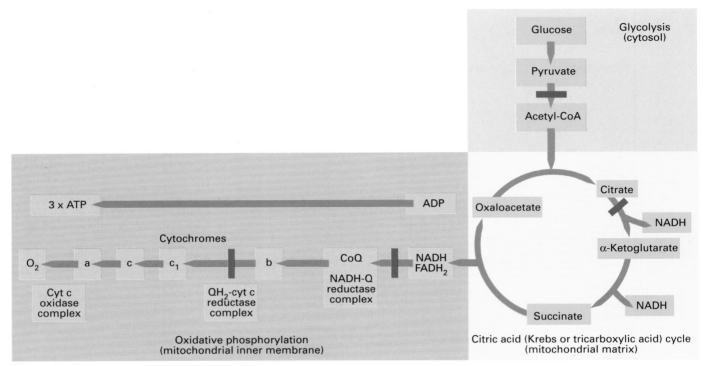

Fig. 3.80 Cell injury by interference with pathways of endogenous substrate metabolism. Compounds may cause injury by acting as pseudosubstrates, impair cofactor supply, or be converted to products that are inhibitors of distal enzymes ('lethal synthesis'). Examples include thiamine deficiency (pyruvate to acetyl-CoA), fluoroacetate (citrate to α-ketoglutarate), rotenone (NADH–Q reductase complex), antimycin A (QH$_2$–cyt c reductase complex), and cyanide (cyt c oxidase complex).

Cell injury can also be a consequence of stimulation or inhibition of receptors, due to structural similarity between the toxin and an endogenous ligand. Much of modern pharmacology is founded on this type of interaction and examples abound. Many natural toxins cause their effect in this way. Examples include curare and nicotine (skeletal muscle nicotinic receptor), muscarine and atropine (stimulation and antagonism of parasympathetic muscarinic receptors, respectively), morphine (enkephalin receptors), and strychnine (GABA receptors). Toxins may also impair signal transduction, for example the ADP-ribosylation of the G_γ subunit by pertussis toxin. In some instances, toxins selectively deplete an essential cofactor, e.g. isoniazid reacts with pyridoxal phosphate to inactivate it, and methotrexate inhibits the synthesis of tetrahydrofolate.

Reactive intermediates

Many of the compounds, or their metabolites, that can cause cell injury are chemically reactive. These can be subject to one or both of two important chemical reactions, dependent upon the chemical nature of the toxin. These reactions are: attack by cellular nucleophiles, determined by the electrophilicity of the compound; and reduction by cellular reducing agents, dependent upon the oxidizing potential of the compound (Fig. 3.81). Some cellular agents can serve both as a nucleophile and as a reductant, for example thiol-containing compounds including a number of proteins and reduced glutathione (GSH).

Electrophilic species will bind covalently to cellular nucleophiles, leading to arylation or alkylation of, for example, proteins. There is an excellent correlation between such covalent binding and tissue necrosis. However, it is important to distinguish between cause and correlation. Thus, the same reactive species may bind to macromolecules and cause necrosis, without any causal association between the two events. Only a small fraction of the cellular protein is involved in those events leading to necrosis. Hence, total covalent binding is not a direct measure of the biochemical lesion. However, it often provides a good measure of the relative amount of the reactive species present in the cell. Oxidizing species will react with susceptible groups in cellular targets and oxidize them, for example reduced thiol groups in proteins will be converted to the disulphide form. This reaction, unlike protein arylation, is readily reversible by both exogenous and endogenous thiol-reducing agents.

Some compounds are subject to enzymic one- or two-electron reduction by cellular reductases (Fig. 3.82). Where such compounds are redox active, i.e. readily participate in an oxidation–reduction cycle, they can themselves act as an electron donor, resulting in the reduction of molecular oxygen and other critical species within the cell. The compound itself is then oxidized back to the parent form, which can be reduced again, thereby cycling between the two redox states and continuously producing active oxygen and other reactive species. This process has been termed 'oxidative stress' and results in the consumption of

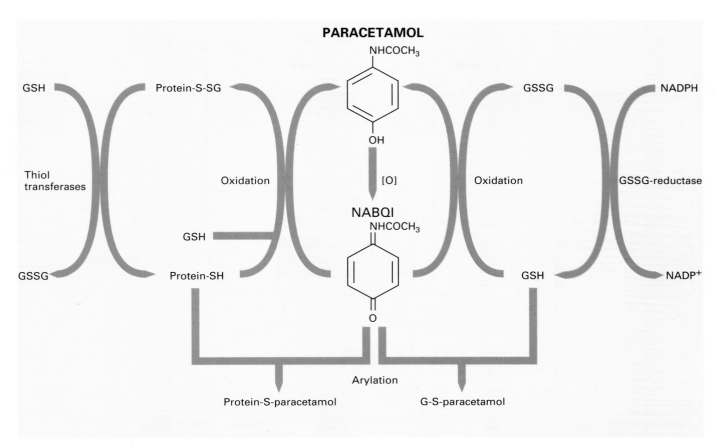

Fig. 3.81 Effects of *N*-acetyl-*p*-benzoquinoneimine (NABQI), the toxic metabolite of paracetamol, on cellular SH-groups. Paracetamol is oxidized ([O]) by the cytochrome P450-dependent monooxygenase system to NABQI. This is both an electrophile, forming adducts with nucleophilic thiol groups (SH) of reduced glutathione (GSH) and proteins, and an oxidizing agent, oxidizing thiol groups of GSH to form the disulphide (GSSG) and of proteins to form mixed disulphides, with both low molecular weight thiols, such as GSH (yielding protein-S-SG) and with the same or other proteins (yielding protein-S-S-protein). Oxidized GSSG is reduced to GSH by the NADPH-dependent enzyme GSSG-reductase, whereas protein mixed disulphides can be reduced by GSH, catalysed by thiol transferases.

the cofactors, usually pyridine nucleotides, for the reductases driving the reaction.

Reduced glutathione is pivotal in protecting the cell against a variety of exogenous toxins. A primary role is the detoxication of many of these compounds, acting either as a nucleophile, forming conjugates with electrophilic compounds, or as a reductant in the metabolism of hydroperoxides, free radicals, and other oxidizing species (Fig. 3.83). The latter reaction results in the oxidation of GSH to its disulphide (GSSG), which can severely compromise host defence. Oxidation of GSH can occur directly, by oxidizing species such as the reactive metabolite of paracetamol, *N*-acetyl-*p*-benzoquinoneimine (NABQI), or secondary to the detoxication of peroxides by glutathione peroxidase and of protein mixed disulphides by thiol transferase (Fig. 3.81). The importance of the peroxidase is evident from the increase in susceptibility to oxidizing agents that occurs in selenium deficiency. Thus, the rate of GSSG formation may serve as an index of free-radical-induced oxidative stress (Fig. 3.82).

The concentration of glutathione in most mammalian cells is

very high (>4 mM), the majority of which is in the reduced form. The synthesis of GSH depends upon the availability of cysteine, the supply of which can be limiting. Following the oxidation of GSH to GSSG it is rapidly reduced back to GSH by NADPH-dependent GSSG-reductase. When the rate of GSSG formation exceeds that of its reduction, or when NADPH becomes rate-limiting, there is accumulation of GSSG. This is then extruded from the cell by a GSSG-stimulated ATPase in the plasma membrane. For example, menadione (see later) causes the oxidation and then depletion of GSH (as GSSG), following which there is a decrease in protein thiols, which is closely related to the occurrence of cell death (Fig. 3.82).

Role of protein-thiol modification

Reactive electrophilic species which interact with proteins (arylating species) do so at nucleophilic centres. Of these, sulphydryl groups (SH) are the most susceptible to such a reaction. For example, the interaction of the reactive metabolite of paracetamol, NABQI, with serum albumin results in the covalent modification of only one site, the sulphydryl group of the single

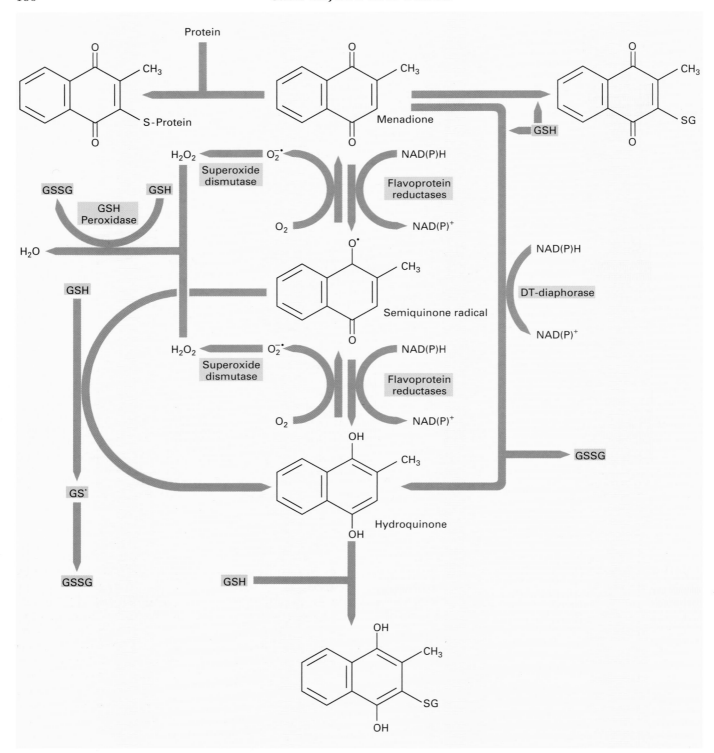

Fig. 3.82 Mechanisms involved in the toxicity of the model quinone menadione. Menadione is subject to sequential one-electron oxidation, leading to the formation of a radical intermediate, the semiquinone. The semiquinone readily reacts with molecular oxygen, producing superoxide anion ($O_2^{-\cdot}$) and menadione. Menadione can thus participate in a redox cycling reaction, in which large amounts of $O_2^{-\cdot}$ are produced. Superoxide dismutes to hydrogen peroxide (H_2O_2), catalysed by superoxide dismutase. However, hydrogen peroxide can react with $O_2^{-\cdot}$ to yield hydroxyl radical $OH^\cdot$, an extremely reactive species (see Fig. 3.83). The metabolism of menadione leads to the consumption of GSH by several mechanisms. These include conjugation of both menadione itself and the hydroquinone, oxidation of GSH to GSSG during the reduction of menadione to its hydroquinone, and in the detoxication of H_2O_2, catalysed by GSH peroxidase, and in both the formation and reduction of protein mixed disulphides (see Fig. 3.81). The redox cycling of compounds such as menadione, with the consequent production of large amounts of active oxygen species, leads to a condition in the cell termed 'oxidative stress'.

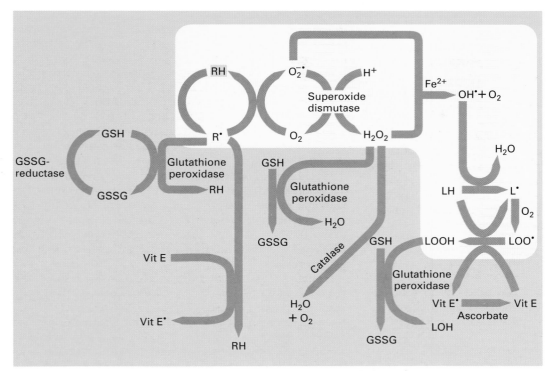

Fig. 3.83 Effects of free radicals in cell injury and cellular defence mechanisms. Many compounds and conditions that lead to cell injury are associated with the formation of free radical species. These can arise from the metabolism of a protoxin (RH) or by the activation of molecular oxygen to OH· radical, in the presence of Fe^{2+}. These radicals have the potential to initiate peroxidation of membrane lipids, producing lipid radicals (L·), which are then converted to lipid peroxy radicals (LOO·) in the presence of oxygen. The reaction of peroxy radicals with further lipid could lead to a cascade with consumption of the membrane lipid. However, a number of cellular defence systems serve to prevent lipid peroxidation. These include the maintenance of free Fe^{2+} at very low concentrations, the detoxication of H_2O_2, lipid peroxides and free radicals (R·) by glutathione peroxidase, detoxication of H_2O_2 by catalase, and termination of radical chain propagation by vitamin E and ascorbate.

cysteine residue in this protein. Sulphydryl groups are irreversibly modified by covalent interaction with arylating species, but they can also be reversibly modified by oxidizing species, such as active oxygen species, NABQI, and quinones. The oxidation of SH-groups results in the formation of either a disulphide cross-linkage or a mixed disulphide, with another protein or with a low molecular weight thiol such as GSH. Thus, following exposure of cells to compounds such as menadione and NABQI, GSH depletion occurs by:

1. direct oxidation of GSH to GSSG;

2. formation of mixed disulphides with protein SH-groups; and

3. conjugation with GSH, which may be enzymic (catalysed by GSH S-transferases) or non-enzymic (Fig 3.81, 3.82).

The modification of free SH-groups in proteins plays an important part in cell injury as free SH-groups are critical determinants in the activity of many enzymes and other proteins. The toxicity of compounds such as paracetamol that are oxidized to potent electrophiles could be due to covalent binding of the reactive intermediate to proteins, particularly to sulphydryl

groups in cysteine residues, and many such cytotoxic compounds do cause a rapid loss of total protein SH-groups. However, in isolated hepatocytes this is due mainly to reversible oxidation.

Direct-acting thiol-reducing agents, such as dithiothreitol, prevent and even reverse the potentially lethal changes, including blebbing, initiated by prior exposure of the cells to compounds such as paracetamol. This demonstrates the importance of the modification of protein thiol groups in cell injury. However, it has been difficult to demonstrate reversible modification of protein thiols *in vivo*. The activity of calcium-stimulated, magnesium-dependent ATPase in plasma membrane fragments from animals treated with paracetamol is reduced irreversibly by about 30 per cent and this correlates with the extent of membrane protein arylation. The difficulty is that the isolation procedure itself causes oxidative impairment of the enzyme. Clearly, cell injury and death can be a consequence of the interaction of reactive electrophilic or oxidizing species with critical cellular sites, but we still do not know precisely which mechanisms are involved, and the relative importance of each process.

Role of lipid peroxidation

Many compounds that can cause cell injury are first metabolized to electrophilic free radicals which can react with molecular oxygen to produce reactive oxygen species, initially
superoxide anion ($O_2^{-\cdot}$), a process that is aggravated if the toxin
can undergo redox cycling (Fig. 3:83). Chemicals that can
generate $O_2^{-\cdot}$ include: alloxan, adriamycin, dialuric acid, paraquat, and streptonigrin. Superoxide anion is highly reactive and
readily participates in a number of metabolic and chemical
reactions. Of particular importance is its dismutation to H_2O_2 by
the enzyme superoxide dismutase. Although this is normally a
detoxication reaction, the H_2O_2 being inactivated by glutathione peroxidase and catalase, at high rates of production, $O_2^{-\cdot}$
and H_2O_2 escape detoxication and generate hydroxyl radicals
($OH^{\cdot}$) by the Haber–Weiss reaction, which is usually catalysed
by chelated iron, e.g. as ADP-Fe^{3+}.

$$O_2^{-\cdot} + H_2O_2 \rightarrow OH^{\cdot} + OH^- + O_2$$

$OH^{\cdot}$ can participate in radical chain reactions to generate
further reactive oxygen species, including singlet oxygen (Fig.
3.83). Protonation of superoxide anion results in the formation
of the hydroperoxy radical ($HOO^{\cdot}$).

Following intoxication by a number of compounds that can
be metabolized to electrophilic free radicals, there is evidence of
lipid peroxidation, the oxidative deterioration of polyunsaturated lipids, either directly or through the formation of reactive
oxygen species (Fig. 3.84). Peroxidation of membrane lipids
results in the formation of lipid peroxy radicals ($ROO^{\cdot}$) which
then produce lipid hydroperoxides ($ROOH$). The peroxy radical
is unstable and readily undergoes decomposition, catalysed by
transition metal ions, particularly Fe^{3+}, to form additional radical products: further lipid peroxy radicals ($ROO^{\cdot}$), lipid radicals
($R^{\cdot}$), lipid alkoxy radicals ($RO^{\cdot}$), and hydroxyl radicals ($OH^{\cdot}$).
Thus, lipid peroxidation is autocatalytic, with propagation of a
peroxidative cascade which may eventually consume much of
the membrane lipid. $O_2^{-\cdot}$-initiated lipid peroxidation may be
mediated by $OH^{\cdot}$, or through the formation of an ADP-perferryl
ion complex (ADP-Fe^{2+}-O_2, ADP-Fe^{3+}-$O_2^{-\cdot}$). Superoxide ($O_2^{-\cdot}$)
may also initiate lipid peroxidation through the intermediate
formation of singlet oxygen. The breakdown of lipid hydroperoxides ($ROOH$) may also liberate singlet oxygen, which will
then react with other unsaturated lipids to form additional lipid
hydroperoxides.

It might be expected that when toxic compounds cause lipid
peroxidation this is a cause of cell death. However, there are a
number of reasons why such lipid peroxidation might be more a
consequence than a cause of cell death. Lipid peroxides and
peroxy radicals are very efficiently detoxified, for example by
glutathione peroxidase and vitamin E (Fig. 3.83). Although
lipid peroxidation leads to the liberation of cytotoxic hydroxyal-
kenals, particularly hydroxynonenal, these are readily detoxi-

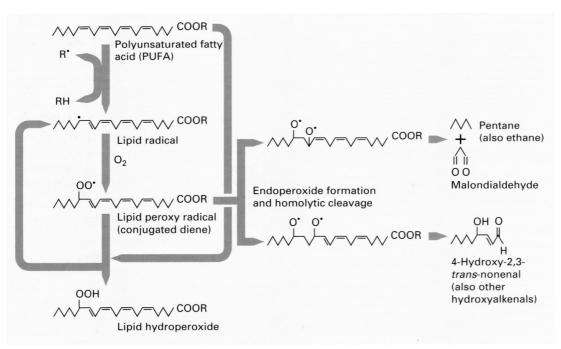

Fig. 3.84 Formation and propagation of lipid radicals, leading to lipid peroxidation. Free radicals which escape
detoxication (see Fig. 3.83) may initiate lipid peroxidation. The peroxy radical formed would react with further
lipid, resulting in radical propagation, with consumption of membrane lipid. The lipid peroxy radical forms a
conjugated diene which is readily detected by UV-spectroscopy, and also undergoes decomposition to produce
volatile alkanes (ethane and pentane), malondialdehyde, and 4-hydroxyalkenals (particularly 4-hydroxynone-
nal), all of which have been used to quantify the extent of lipid peroxidation.

fied by conjugation with glutathione, catalysed by glutathione S-transferases. The redox-active dipyridylium compound, diquat, is readily reduced by reductases, particularly NADPH-cytochrome P450 reductase, to form diquat radical. This radical reacts with O_2 to yield O_2^-· and diquat, which can be reduced again. Diquat thus participates in a redox cycle in which large quantities of active oxygen species are produced. Although this results in extensive lipid peroxidation, it is only when the level of reduced glutathione (GSH) falls substantially that cell death ensues. Similarly, the lipid peroxidation caused by carbon tetrachloride, via the formation of trichloromethyl radical by cytochrome P450, and by compounds such as allyl alcohol, t-butyl hydroperoxide, diethylmaleate, and bromoiso-valeryl urea, does not appear to be responsible for their cytotoxicity. This is probably due to oxidative stress, lipid peroxidation being a consequence of the failure of normal protective mechanisms in dying cells.

Disturbance of calcium homeostasis

The cytosolic free calcium concentration is maintained at very low levels, approximately 0.1 μM in hepatocytes, against an extracellular concentration of 1.3 mM, as calcium plays a key role in the regulation of many cell activities (Fig. 3.85). Maintenance of this gradient is achieved by sequestration of calcium in mitochondria and the endoplasmic reticulum by a Ca^{2+}/Mg^{2+}-ATPase and by the energy-dependent extrusion of calcium by the Ca^{2+}/Mg^{2+}-ATPase of the plasma membrane, an enzyme with a high affinity for Ca^{2+} (K_m approximately 10 nM). In cells such as hepatocytes this translocase is not calmodulin-regulated but is critically dependent on free sulphydryl groups. These Ca^{2+}-transporting ATPases are amongst the SH-dependent enzymes inhibited by thiol-group modification, by cytotoxins such as paracetamol. Their activity can largely be restored by thiol-reducing agents, such as glutathione and dithiothreitol, at least in isolated cells.

Perturbation of cellular Ca^{2+} homeostasis can play an important role in cell injury and death caused by a number of injurious agents in many cell types. On exposure of cells to lethal concentrations of some cytotoxins there is a rapid and sustained rise in cytosolic Ca^{2+} concentration, which correlates well with the subsequent loss of viability. This increase in Ca^{2+} concentration differs from that induced by calcium-mobilizing hormones in that it occurs more slowly, but is sustained for much longer periods and may reach micromolar concentrations. Prevention of this rise in cytosolic Ca^{2+} concentration, or its early restoration to normal levels, prevents cell death.

A number of biochemical processes, including activation of degradative enzymes, are initiated by a sustained elevation of cytosolic Ca^{2+} (Fig. 3.86). However, we do not yet know which of these are directly involved in cell injury and death.

Ca^{2+}-activated proteases

The Ca^{2+}-activated proteases that are active at neutral pH are known as the calpains. These are present in virtually all mammalian cell types and are associated with membranes in con-

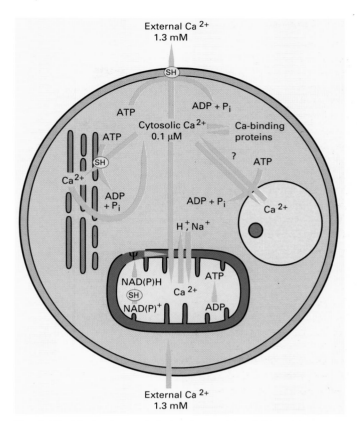

Fig. 3.85 Mechanisms regulating intracellular Ca^{2+} concentration. Ca^{2+} plays a key role in signal transduction and is released from the endoplasmic reticulum following stimulation of some membrane receptors via second messengers. Ca^{2+} can also enter cells via receptor-linked channels. Although the concentration of Ca^{2+} outside the cell is 1.3 mM, the cytosolic concentration is normally maintained at approx. 0.1 μM by sequestration of Ca^{2+} in the endoplasmic reticulum, nucleus, and mitochondrion, and by the active extrusion of Ca^{2+} across the plasma membrane. The Ca^{2+}-transporting systems of the endoplasmic reticulum and plasma membrane are thiol-containing ATP-dependent enzymes. Sequestration of Ca^{2+} in the nucleus also requires ATP. The regulation of mitochondrial Ca^{2+} is complex and is dependent upon the mitochondrial membrane potential (Ψ). This is controlled by the redox state of the cell, particularly the ratio of NAD(P)H to NAD(P)$^+$, itself regulated by thiol-containing enzymes. The mitochondria also influence the regulation of Ca^{2+} indirectly, through the synthesis of ATP, which in turn is dependent on the redox status of the cell. Finally, Ca^{2+} is also involved in exchange processes with Na$^+$ and H$^+$.

junction with their specific inhibitor, calpastatin. There are at least two isoenzymes of calpain, which differ in their requirements for Ca^{2+}. Increased Ca^{2+} autolytically activates the calpains, which break down both cytoskeletal elements and integral membrane proteins, implicated in plasma membrane blebbing. Ca^{2+}-activation of proteases leads to modification of platelet microfilaments and altered physical properties of erythrocyte membranes. The toxicity of some compounds to the liver, myocardium, and platelets can be prevented or delayed by inhibition of these Ca^{2+}-activated proteases.

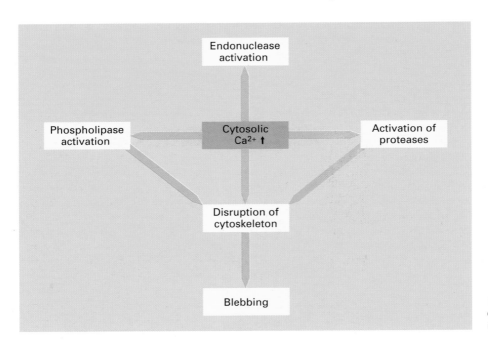

Endonuclease
activation

Phospholipase
activation

Cytosolic
Ca²⁺ ↑

Activation of
proteases

Disruption of
cytoskeleton

Blebbing

Fig. 3.86 Consequences of the increase in cytosolic Ca^{2+} concentrations caused by injurious agents (see text).

Ca^{2+}-mediated alterations in the cytoskeleton

Many cellular processes are dependent upon the normal organization of the cytoskeleton (see Section 1.1). When the cytoskeleton is disrupted directly, by compounds such as cytochalasins and phalloidin, the plasma membrane becomes blebbed. A variety of cytotoxic chemicals and ischaemia also cause plasma membrane blebbing (Fig. 3.86). Calcium may be involved in this process. Treatment of cells with the Ca^{2+}-ionophore A23187 or with other cytotoxins which cause a sustained increase in cytosolic free-Ca^{2+} concentration causes blebbing. Calcium plays an important role in regulating the formation of actin bundles, determining actomyosin interaction, and modulating α-tubulin polymerization. At least two distinct Ca^{2+}-dependent mechanisms are implicated in the toxin-induced cytoskeletal alterations which result in plasma membrane blebbing. Increased cytosolic Ca^{2+} concentration causes a dissociation of actin microfilaments from α-actinin, which serves as an intermediate in the association of microfilaments with actin-binding proteins in the plasma membrane. Calcium can also activate proteases that can cleave actin-binding proteins and lead to dissociation of the cytoskeleton from the plasma membrane. The blebbing, and the loss of viability, caused by certain cytotoxins can be prevented by calpastatin, an inhibitor of Ca^{2+}-dependent neutral proteases. However, for other toxins, the obligatory role of Ca^{2+} in plasma membrane blebbing is less clear. Direct oxidation of thiol-groups of cytoskeletal components may also cause plasma membrane blebbing.

Ca^{2+}-activated phospholipases

Phospholipases are widely distributed in biological membranes and have been divided into several subsets. Some of these, such as phospholipase A_2, are Ca^{2+}-activated. Phospholipase A_2 may be important in the detoxication of phospholipid hydroperox-

ides, by releasing fatty acids from peroxidized membranes. However, it can also degrade the plasma membrane directly by gross hydrolysis of membrane phospholipids and it generates potentially toxic metabolites such as eicosanoids. The sustained increase in cytosolic Ca^{2+} caused by cytotoxic insult can stimulate phospholipase A_2, and cell death in liver and heart caused by ischaemia is prevented by inhibitors of this enzyme. However, the role that this enzyme plays in chemically induced injury is not yet clear.

Ca^{2+}-activated endonucleases and apoptosis

Based on the morphology of dying cells, two distinct patterns of cell death have been identified, which have been termed necrosis and apoptosis. Apoptosis has been described as programmed cell death and is a physiological phenomenon necessary for normal development, maintenance of tissue shape, and cell renewal. Those morphological changes characteristic of apoptotic cells include: blebbing of both plasma and nuclear membranes, compaction of organelles in the cytoplasm, and widespread chromatin condensation (Section 3.1). This condensation of the chromatin is due to the activity of a Ca^{2+}-activated endonuclease which rapidly hydrolyses DNA into characteristic fragments. In addition to its normal physiological role, apoptosis provides a mechanism whereby certain exogenous stimuli can promote cell death. This includes the killing of target cells by cytotoxic T-lymphocytes and the glucocorticoid-induced killing of immature thymocytes. Cytotoxic T-lymphocytes kill their target cells by the insertion of polymeric molecules, which form pores, into the plasma membrane of the target cell, resulting in an increase in membrane permeability leading to Ca^{2+} influx and resultant endonuclease activation. Glucocorticoid hormones cause cell injury and death in thymocytes by the receptor-mediated stimulation of the synthesis of specific proteins that promote the influx of extracellular Ca^{2+}, which activates an endonuclease. Apoptosis can also be stimulated by certain environmental chemicals, in some cell types. For example, the toxicity of the environmental contaminant 2,3,7,8-tetrachlorodibenzo-p-dioxin (TCDD) to thymocytes is due to the stimulation of apoptosis. This is due to the influx of extracellular Ca^{2+}, mediated by a receptor distinct from that stimulated by glucocorticoids. Endonuclease activation may also be responsible for the killing of macrophages induced by oxidative stress. The influx of Ca^{2+}, and consequently endonuclease activation and apoptosis, induced by TCDD and glucocorticoids is due to increased expression of proteins that mediate the influx of Ca^{2+}. The demonstration of chemically induced apoptosis has been confined to a very limited number of cell types, particularly thymocytes. Hepatic nuclei contain an endonuclease that is dependent upon submicromolar concentrations of Ca^{2+} for its activity. However, the rôle that this endonuclease, or apoptosis itself, plays in the chemically mediated killing of hepatic and other cell types is still far from clear. Indeed, the mechanisms by which chemicals kill cells may range from apoptosis at one extreme (e.g. with TCDD) to necrosis at the other (e.g. with rotenone), with many compounds producing features of both, to a varying extent.

Depletion of mitochondrial pyridine nucleotides and ATP

Many cytotoxic compounds alter mitochondrial levels of NAD(P)H. Oxidation or arylation of critical thiol groups in NAD(P)H dehydrogenases results in the oxidation of NAD(P)H. The decrease in the capacity of mitochondria to reduce NAD(P), together with the decline in the NAD(P)H/NAD(P) redox couple, permeabilizes the inner mitochondrial membrane, favouring the release of Ca^{2+} from the organelle and uncoupling oxidative phosphorylation (Fig. 3.85). These effects lead to depletion of ATP. The reduced ATP levels also lead to further impairment of other Ca^{2+} regulating systems, in the plasma membrane and the endoplasmic reticulum. The decrease in NAD(P)H also compromises the activity of GSSG-reductase, and other protective enzymes, further increasing the noxious effects of reactive species (Fig. 3.81).

There is an additional mechanism for the loss of pyridine nucleotides and the depletion of ATP. Exposure of certain cells to reactive species such as hydrogen peroxide and 1,2-dibromo-3-chloropropane, induces single-strand breaks in DNA. This activates a poly(ADP-ribose)polymerase involved in DNA excision repair, which leads to a decrease in NAD^+ levels followed by depletion of ATP, and ultimately to cell death. This might be the basis of a suicide mechanism of cell death to prevent the perpetuation of damaged DNA.

3.3.4 Paracetamol (acetaminophen)

Paracetamol (N-acetyl-p-aminophenol), known in the USA as acetaminophen, was first described as an analgesic and antipyretic by Von Mering in 1893. Studies in the 1940s confirmed its analgesic and antipyretic activities and it was found to be the active metabolite of acetanilide and phenacetin. Unlike the latter two compounds, paracetamol does not cause methaemoglobinaemia. It was introduced world-wide in the mid-1950s as an antipyretic and analgesic drug and since then the number of preparations of which paracetamol is the major component has increased dramatically. The association of severe liver injury in humans with paracetamol ingestion was not recognized until 1966 when two Scottish physicians reported the death of two people following paracetamol overdose.

Adverse effects of paracetamol are extremely rare when it is taken at recommended therapeutic doses. There have been occasional reports linking long-term use of paracetamol with hepatitis. However, it is in overdose that acute lethal injury of hepatocytes can result from paracetamol intoxication, both in humans and in experimental animals. This results in hepatic necrosis which may prove fatal. Following a large overdose of paracetamol, acute renal tubular necrosis also occurs occasionally, but this is usually secondary to fulminant hepatic failure. Mice and hamsters are especially sensitive to the hepatotoxic effects of the drug, which causes centrilobular hepatic necrosis similar to that observed in man. The species differences in susceptibility to paracetamol are due largely to differences in the rate of formation of the toxic metabolite, NABQI. There are also intra-species differences in paracetamol toxicity: in most rat strains paracetamol is primarily hepatotoxic, but in the Fischer 344 strain it is also nephrotoxic.

Within 2–3 h of an overdose of paracetamol the patient feels nauseous and has bouts of vomiting, followed by abdominal pain in the upper right quadrant. Within 24 h, liver dysfunction is present and this reaches a maximum by 4 days after ingestion. At normal doses, paracetamol is readily detoxified, largely by glucuronidation and sulphation in the liver. A small fraction of the dose is oxidized in the liver by the cytochrome P450-dependent monooxygenase system to a highly reactive intermediate, NABQI. This is very effectively detoxified by conjugation with GSH (Fig. 3.81). However, as the dose of paracetamol increases not only the amount but also the proportion of the administered dose that undergoes oxidation to NABQI increases, due to depletion of the sulphate pool. The levels of NABQI increase to an extent such that synthesis of GSH is exceeded, and the intermediate escapes detoxication.

Paracetamol-induced hepatotoxicity can be prevented in experimental animals by inhibitors of cytochrome P450, such as piperonyl butoxide, cobaltous chloride, and acute ethanol. In contrast, induction of cytochrome P450 by compounds such as chronic ethanol, 3-methylcholanthrene, and rifampicin can dramatically potentiate the hepatotoxicity of paracetamol. The reactive metabolite of paracetamol, NABQI, is a strong electrophile which is normally rapidly inactivated by conjugation with glutathione with the formation of the 3-glutathionyl conjugate, which, upon degradation in the intestine and kidney, is excreted in the urine as the mercapturic acid and cysteine conjugates (Fig. 3.81). NABQI is also a potent oxidizing agent so that when it interacts with thiol groups two reactions can occur: the thiol groups can be oxidized to disulphide, one of the mechanisms of detoxication by GSH, at least until the levels of hepatic GSH are low; or they can undergo nucleophilic addition, resulting in arylation (covalent binding) by the reactive metabolite of cellular proteins, particularly at cysteine residues. The relative importance of covalent binding and oxidation of thiol groups in the toxicity of paracetamol has still not been determined. There is a good correlation between the extent of GSH-depletion, covalent binding, and hepatotoxicity of paracetamol in animals treated with agents which modify either the levels of GSH or the activity of cytochrome P450. However, under certain circumstances it is possible to dissociate covalent binding of paracetamol from cell death, both *in vitro* and *in vivo*. Precursors of GSH, such as N-acetyl-L-cysteine and L-cysteine, antioxidants such as promethazine and α-tocopherol, and direct-acting thiol-reducing agents such as dithiothreitol can prevent the toxicity of paracetamol without affecting its covalent binding to protein, even when added after covalent binding has reached a maximum. Some structural analogues of paracetamol, which are unable to arylate thiol groups of GSH or proteins, are not hepatotoxic until GSH is depleted by some means, such as diethylmaleate pretreatment. 3′-Hydroxyacetanilide (3-HAA) is a positional isomer of paracetamol (4′-hydroxyacetanilide) which also possesses analgesic and antipyretic properties. Although 3-HAA binds covalently to hepatic proteins to an extent similar to that of paracetamol, it is not hepatotoxic.

Following intoxication with paracetamol, lipid peroxidation may be observed, which correlates closely with its hepatotoxicity. This, together with the protective effects of antioxidants, might be taken as evidence that lipid peroxidation is involved in the cytotoxicity of paracetamol. However, against this must be weighed the finding that although the administration of iron enhances the lipid peroxidation induced by paracetamol by more than 25-fold, its toxicity is not affected. Lipid peroxidation can be prevented by chelating endogenous iron with desferrioxamine, but this has no effect on the toxicity of paracetamol. Direct-acting thiol-reductants, such as dithiothreitol (DTT), and precursors for the synthesis of GSH, such as N-acetyl-L-cysteine, prevent the cytotoxicity of paracetamol without altering the extent of lipid peroxidation. Lipid peroxidation in paracetamol intoxication, as in the toxicity of many other compounds, is more likely a consequence rather than a cause of necrosis.

In paracetamol toxicity there is a perturbation of cellular thiol-and NADPH-status, and there is indirect evidence, based largely on studies with NABQI, that this leads to a disruption in intracellular Ca^{2+} homeostasis (Figs 3.81, 3.85). The concentration of cytosolic Ca^{2+} in hepatocytes is maintained by active compartmentation in the endoplasmic reticulum and mitochondria, by Ca^{2+}-binding proteins, and by the active extrusion of Ca^{2+} through the plasma membrane (see earlier). Mitochondrial Ca^{2+} homeostasis is regulated by a cyclic mechanism involving the active uptake of Ca^{2+} and Ca^{2+} release by exchange for hydrogen or sodium ions. The release of Ca^{2+} by these exchange mechanisms is modulated by the redox-state of intra-mitochondrial NADPH, as well as by both mitochondrial levels of GSH and the oxidation state of critical membrane-bound thiol groups. NABQI can cause the release of Ca^{2+} from isolated liver mitochondria. Active transport of Ca^{2+} into the endoplasmic reticulum and across the plasma membrane is

mediated by Ca^{2+}-stimulated, Mg^{2+}-dependent ATPases which depend on free sulphydryl groups for their activity. Both microsomal and plasma membrane Ca^{2+}-stimulated, Mg^{2+}-dependent ATPases can be inhibited directly by NABQI. Paracetamol intoxication also leads to inhibition of the ATP-dependent accumulation of Ca^{2+} into isolated microsomal and plasma membrane vesicles, as well as to reduced Ca^{2+}-dependent ATPase activity. The events following paracetamol overdose can be summarized as: depletion of cellular GSH by paracetamol, following which critical protein thiol groups are modified (by arylation and oxidation) and there is perturbation of the NADPH/NADP$^+$ ratio (reflecting mitochondrial redox state). It is believed that these processes lead, in turn, to the disruption of intracellular Ca^{2+} homeostasis, with elevation of the intracellular Ca^{2+} concentration, although this has never been shown by direct measurement. This is followed by membrane blebbing. In isolated cells, over 80 per cent of protein thiol modification following paracetamol exposure is due to reversible oxidation. Thus, the oxidizing ability of NABQI plays a key role in the toxicity of paracetamol to such cells. It has yet to be determined whether this is also the situation *in vivo*.

3.3.5 Menadione

Menadione (2-methyl-1,4-naphthoquinone) is a useful model with which to investigate the mechanisms and consequences of oxidative stress in mammalian cells (Fig. 3.82). Quinones are widely distributed in nature and the quinone nucleus is present in many important antitumour drugs. Quinones are substrates of flavoenzymes and undergo either one- or two-electron reduction to yield the semiquinone or the hydroquinone, respectively. Both microsomes and mitochondria from liver can catalyse the one-electron reduction of menadione, by NADPH-cytochrome P450 reductase and NADH-ubiquinone oxidoreductase, respectively. This produces the semiquinone free radical, which can reduce molecular oxygen to superoxide anion (O_2^-·), with regeneration of the quinone. The quinone continues to redox cycle, there is dismutation of superoxide anion to hydrogen peroxide, with the production of other reactive free radical species, such as OH·, and consumption of pyridine nucleotides with oxidation of GSH to GSSG. These conditions are known as oxidative stress, and are toxic to the cell (Fig. 3.82). The one-electron reduction of quinones to semiquinones is involved in the antitumour and cytotoxic effects of quinonoid drugs. Quinones can also undergo two-electron reduction in the cytosol, catalysed by the flavoprotein NAD(P)H: (quinone-acceptor) oxidoreductase, also known as DT-diaphorase, to form the respective hydroquinone directly, and not via the semiquinone radical. The affinity of DT-diaphorase for menadione is much higher than that of the other flavoenzymes so that the metabolism of menadione, at low concentrations, is solely by the two-electron reduction pathway. This pathway will protect the cell by competing with the one-electron pathway, as hydroquinones are less reactive and more easily excreted than semiquinone free radicals (Fig. 3.82). Inhibition of DT-diaphorase with dicoumarol markedly potentiates the toxicity of menadione.

Only a small proportion of a dose of menadione is excreted as free hydroquinone, the majority being eliminated as conjugates with glucuronic acid, sulphate, and glutathione. The toxicity of menadione can be considerably potentiated by increasing its one-electron reduction, by inducing NADPH-cytochrome P450 reductase with phenobarbitone, or by inhibiting enzymes involved in detoxication reactions, such as catalase and glutathione reductase (Fig. 3.82). Compounds that facilitate the synthesis of GSH reduce the toxicity of menadione. However, oxygen radical scavengers have no effect on its toxicity. GSH depletion, due primarily to the metabolism of hydrogen peroxide by glutathione peroxidase, is the critical event in the initiation of menadione toxicity. Quinones lead not only to the oxidation of GSH to GSSG, but also of protein-thiols to form mixed disulphides. Quinones are also electrophilic, forming conjugates with GSH and arylating protein SH-groups. These processes lead not only to a depletion of GSH but also to a decrease in protein-thiol groups in menadione intoxication. At toxic concentrations, menadione rapidly causes plasma membrane blebbing. As discussed above, such blebbing is often associated with the disruption of intracellular Ca^{2+} homeostasis (Fig. 3.85). Menadione does cause the mobilization and loss of Ca^{2+} from mitochondria, impairing their ability to take up Ca^{2+} by causing the oxidation of pyridine nucleotides, and from the endoplasmic reticulum, by oxidation/arylation of thiol groups critical for Ca^{2+}-stimulated, Mg^{2+}-dependent ATPase activity. There is also inhibition of the Mg^{2+}-dependent Ca^{2+}-ATPase of the plasma membrane. The consequent elevation in intracellular Ca^{2+} concentration could be the critical event in the cell injury caused by menadione. Under certain circumstances, the increased intracellular Ca^{2+} concentration can activate an endonuclease which fragments DNA in a manner characteristic of apoptosis. However, at the present time the role of apoptosis in chemically induced cytotoxicity is not at all clear.

3.3.6 Further reading

Types and general mechanisms of cell injury

Boobis, A. R., Fawthrop, D. J., and Davies, D. S. (1989). Mechanisms of cell death. *Trends in Pharmacological Sciences* 10, 275–80.

Carafoli, E. (1987). Intracellular calcium homeostasis. *Annual Reviews of Biochemistry* 56, 395–433.

Carbonera, D. and Azzone, G. F. (1988). Permeability of inner mitochondrial membrane and oxidative stress. *Biochimica et Biophysica Acta* 943, 245–85.

Dybing, E., *et al.* (1990). Cytotoxicity via interactions with DNA. In *Basic science in toxicology* (ed. G. N. Volans, J. Sims, F. M. Sullivan, and P. Turner), pp. 651–9. Taylor and Francis, London.

Farber, J. L. and Gerson, R. J. (1984). Mechanisms of cell injury with hepatotoxic chemicals. *Pharmacological Reviews* 36, 715–45.

Halliwell, B. and Gutteridge, J. M. C. (1989). *Free radicals in biology and medicine* (2nd edn.). Clarendon Press, Oxford.

Kappus, H. (1987). Oxidative stress in chemical toxicity. *Archives of Toxicology* 60, 144–9.

Lemasters, J. J., Di Guiseppi, J., Nieminen, A.-L., and Herman, B. (1987). Blebbing, free Ca^{2+} and mitochondrial membrane potential preceding cell death in hepatocytes. *Nature (London)*, 325, 78–81.

Mansuy, D. (1990). Reactive intermediates and interaction with biological systems. In *Basic science in toxicology* (ed. G. N. Volans, J. Sims, F. M. Sullivan, and P. Turner), pp. 36–45. Taylor and Francis, London.

Monks, T. J. and Lau, S. S. (1988). Reactive intermediates and their toxicological significance. *Toxicology* 52, 1–53.

Orrenius, S., McConkey, D. J., Bellomo, G., and Nicotera, P. (1989). Role of Ca^{2+} in toxic cell killing. *Trends in Pharmacological Sciences* 10, 281–5.

Poli, G., Albano, E., and Dianzani, M. U. (1987). The role of lipid peroxidation in liver damage. *Chemistry and Physics of Lipids* 45, 117–42.

Raute-Kreinsen, U. and Bleyl, U. (1986). Pathophysiological and morphological aspects of cellular lesions. *Klinische Wochenschrift* 64, (Suppl. 7), 1–6.

Schulte-Hermann, R. and Bursch, W. (1990). Cell death through apoptosis and its relationship to carcinogenesis. In *Basic science in toxicology* (ed. G. N. Volans, J. Sims, F. M. Sullivan, and P. Turner), pp. 669–78. Taylor and Francis, London.

Slater, T. F. (1987). Free radicals and tissue injury: fact and fiction. *British Journal of Cancer* 8 (Supplement), 5–10.

Trump, B. F., Berezesky, I. K., Smith, M. W., Phelps, P. C., and Elliget, K. A. (1989). The relationship between cellular ion deregulation and acute and chronic toxicity. *Toxicology and Applied Pharmacology* 97, 6–22.

Tsokos-Kuhn, J. O., Hughes, H., Smith, C. V., and Mitchell, J. R. (1988). Alkylation of the liver plasma membrane and inhibition of the Ca^{2+} ATPase by acetaminophen. *Biochemical Pharmacology* 37, 2125–31.

Walker, N. I., Harman, B. V., Gove, G. C., and Kerr, J. F. (1988). Patterns of cell death. *Methods and Achievements in Experimental Pathology* 13, 18–54.

Paracetamol

Black, M. (1984). Acetaminophen toxicity. *Annual Review of Medicine* 35, 577–93.

Boobis, A. R., Seddon, C. E., Nasseri-Sina, P., and Davies, D. S. (1990). Evidence for a direct role of intracellular calcium in paracetamol toxicity. *Biochemical Pharmacology* 39, 1277–81.

Moore, M., Thor, H., Moore, G., Nelson, S., Moldeus, P., and Orrenius, S. (1985). The toxicity of acetaminophen and N-acetyl-p-benzoquinone imine in isolated hepatocytes is associated with thiol depletion and increased cytosolic Ca^{2+}. *The Journal of Biological Chemistry* 260, 13035–40.

Prescott, L. F. (1983). Paracetamol overdosage. Pharmacological considerations and clinical management. *Drugs* 25, 290–314.

Tee, L. B. G., Boobis, A. R., Huggett, A. C., and Davies, D. S. (1986). Reversal of acetaminophen toxicity in isolated hamster hepatocytes by dithiothreitol. *Toxicology and Applied Pharmacology* 83, 294–314.

Menadione

Gant, T. W., Rao, D. N., Mason, R. P., and Cohen, G. M. (1988). Redox cycling and sulphydryl arylation: their relative importance in the mechanism of quinone cytotoxicity to isolated hepatocytes. *Chemico-Biological Interactions* 65, 157–73.

McConkey, D. J., Hartzell, P., Nicotera, P., Wyllie, A. H., and Orrenius, S. (1988). Stimulation of endogenous endonuclease activity in hepatocytes exposed to oxidative stress. *Toxicology Letters* 42, 123–30.

Mirabelli, F., *et al.* (1988). Menadione-induced bleb formation in hepatocytes is associated with the oxidation of thiol groups in actin. *Archives of Biochemistry and Biophysics* 264, 261–9.

4

Defence mechanisms

4

Defence mechanisms

4.1 General defence mechanisms

P. G. Isaacson

Like all living things the human body is exposed to all manner of hostile agents in its environment, most of which are micro-organisms keen to gain access to the body's rich pastures; indeed, for some of them entrance to the human body is mandatory for their very survival as a species. Against this myriad of potential invaders, man has developed a variety of defence mechanisms. Some of these are non-specific, others more highly evolved and relatively specific, and still others highly evolved and highly specific. Amongst the first group are included physical and chemical barriers to infection and the second group involves non-specific cellular and humoral responses, including components of the inflammatory reaction. The most sensitive and specific defence mechanism is provided by the immune response.

4.1.1 Non-specific defence mechanisms

Physical and chemical barriers

The importance of the skin as a barrier to infection becomes clear the moment one realizes the ease with which environmental micro-organisms can enter the body through a breach in the skin (a surgical wound for example) unless care is taken to protect the wounded area. Although an effective physical barrier, the skin is by no means impermeable and depends on chemical factors to enhance its function. These include lactic acid and bacteriocidal fatty acids produced by sweat and sebaceous glands.

The respiratory tract relies largely on physical mechanisms to ensure that the air reaching the lungs is sufficiently free of micro-organisms to permit other local defence mechanisms (principally phagocytic macrophages) to render the air sterile. Any particulate matter entering the upper respiratory tract adheres to the mucous coat, which is constantly moving outwards, propelled by the beating action of the cilia. The mechanical effect of the movement of secretions out of organs, whether by ciliary or muscular action, is an extremely important defence mechanism and obstruction of any tubular organ is rapidly followed by infection, whether drainage is external, as in the urinary tract, or internal, as in the biliary system.

Other vulnerable areas for the entry of pathogenic micro-organisms into the body include the eyes, upper gastrointestinal tract, and the external genitalia. The eyes are continuously washed by the tears which, in addition to their mechanical effect, contain lysozyme, an enzyme also known as muramidase. As its names suggest, this substance is powerfully lysogenic for bacteria. Lysozyme is widely distributed in the body, being present in phagocytic cells where it plays an important role in bacterial killing. Lysozyme is also secreted by gastric mucosa where, together with gastric acid, it acts as a chemical barrier to bacterial entry. Chemical factors may also act indirectly by favouring the growth of non-pathogenic saprophytic bacteria and thus preventing pathogenic organisms from establishing themselves. This combination of circumstances is seen in the mouth and female genital tract. The presence of a normal bacterial flora is also one of the most important factors protecting the intestinal tract from infection by 'hostile' micro-organisms.

Cytological and humoral factors

Should the above-described barriers to infection fail, then there is a series of mechanisms that appear to have evolved for the purposes of defence, but which are also components of a wide variety of other important body functions. Phagocytic cells, including polymorphonuclear neutrophils and mononuclear phagocytes (macrophages), aided by complement, indulge in intracellular killing of micro-organisms, while other cells, such as eosinophils and natural killer (NK) cells, can destroy invading organisms by extracellular mechanisms. Complement components can attack the cell membrane of micro-organisms directly, resulting in lysis of the cell, and there are humoral mechanisms, in addition to complement, which either assist complement or act on organisms directly; these include the acute phase proteins and interferon, which inhibits viral replication.

4.1.2   The immune response

While the non-specific defence mechanisms outlined above are highly effective as 'fixed mechanisms' they are no match for living micro-organisms which can call on the resources of evolution to circumvent the body's defence. What is required, therefore, is a defence mechanism that can be adapted to individual organisms and, if necessary, adapt to changes in organisms as they occur. In response to this need there evolved the phenomenon of specific acquired immunity, whereby the powerful destructive mechanisms described above are focused on selected micro-organisms. There is, therefore, a great deal of co-operation and overlap between the immune response and the other defence mechanisms.

B- and T-cells

The immune system has to be able to respond to both extracellular and intracellular organisms and to do this humoral and cell-mediated mechanisms are necessary. These two mechanisms are provided by two variants of the same cell type, namely the B- and the T-lymphocyte. This basic unity of the cellular basis of immunity emphasizes the similarity of the two types of immune response which, superficially, may appear very different.

Humoral immunity

Humoral immunity is effected by antibody, which is the product of B-cells. Through an ingenious molecular biological mechanism, each B-cell that is produced expresses a different antibody on its surface, the repertoire extending to some 100 000 or more antibodies, each capable of recognizing a corresponding antigen. When an antigen-bearing organism comes into contact with a B-cell expressing the corresponding antibody the result is proliferation, with the formation of a clone of B-cells expressing the appropriate antibody. Concomitant with this proliferation, the B-lymphocytes differentiate into plasma cells which are capable of secreting antibody into the tissue fluid and hence the circulation. The role of antibody is essentially to direct the action of complement and phagocytic cells to the antibody-coated organism and also to enhance the effects of their action. Once an antigen has evoked an immune response in this way, the phenomenon of immunological memory comes into play, ensuring an enhanced reaction and, therefore, enhanced protection should that particular antigen be encountered again.

Cell-mediated immunity

Where an invading organism has entered the body and has become sequestered within a cell such as a macrophage, humoral antibody cannot reach it and the process of T-cell-mediated immunity is required to destroy the invader. The surface receptors on T-cells are analogous to the antibody on the surface of B-cells and, while not identical to antibodies in their structure, are similar in many ways. A different receptor molecule is present on each new T-cell produced, so that, once

more, there is a large repertoire of T-cells capable of recognizing antigens present within cells. Contact with the appropriate antigen again results in clonal expansion, but not antibody secretion in this case, since T-cells destroy organisms within cells by cell to cell contact. For this to happen an antigen belonging to the intracellular organism has to be 'presented' on the cell surface. The T-cell can only recognize the antigen in association with certain native molecules belonging to the 'major histocompatibility complex' (MHC) which are already present on the cell wall. The T-cell can then destroy the antigen (and the cell within which it is contained) either by direct cytotoxicity, or indirectly by secreting active substances known as lymphokines and inducing other nearby cells to do the same.

Immunopathology

Clearly, with such a complex system as that responsible for immunity, there is a great deal that can go wrong. Thus there may be deficiencies in one or more parts of the system, leading to a group of diseases known as the immunodeficiencies, of which the acquired immunodeficiency syndrome (AIDS) is the best known. The immune reaction may be so brisk as to damage innocent host cells, a phenomenon known as hypersensitivity, which is responsible for a wide variety of diseases. While the immune reaction is designed to be directed solely against foreign antigens, this specificity may become perverted, resulting in immunity being directed against components of the body itself, leading to the so-called auto-immune diseases.

The sections of this chapter that follow are concerned with a detailed analysis of defence mechanisms beyond the physical and chemical barriers, and the disorders that arise as a result of their dysfunction.

4.2   Antigens and MHC systems

A. J. McMichael

4.2.1   The nature of antigens

Antigens are molecules that interact specifically with antibody or the receptors on T-lymphocytes. Technically there is a subtle difference between antigens which can be used to detect specific immune responses and immunogens which are molecules with the capacity to induce immune reactions. While the two terms are often used interchangeably, the concept of the difference is instructive. While all immunogens are antigens, the opposite is not always true. Thus appropriate antibodies combine to simple chemical molecules such as penicillin, but the chemical itself will not induce an immune response unless coupled to a macromolecule (which may occur spontaneously). Similarly, T-lymphocytes can be shown to recognize simple peptides 10–15 amino acids long, but on their own these often fail to initiate T-cell responses *in vivo* or *in vitro*; again the peptide needs to be part of a macromolecule.

A special feature of the antibody response is its extraordinary capacity to show specificity for a vastly diverse spectrum of antigens: it is possible to raise antibodies to newly synthesized molecules that have never occurred in nature. The range of reactivity appears less for the T-cell receptor because of the special constraint that T-cells only respond to molecules that are bound to the proteins of the major histocompatibility complex (see below). However, the possibility that T-cell receptors might also bind to a wider range of small molecules specifically and directly without activating T-cells has not been excluded.

The size of an antigen binding site in an antibody molecule has been defined using small oligosaccharides or peptides and fits around six sugars or seven or eight amino acids. However, some antigens, such as the dinitrophenyl (DNP) group, are smaller than this and can still bind to specific antibody, so the site does not have to be filled. Small chemicals of this type may be used to measure antibody titre, if radiolabelled or tagged with some other measurable marker. The fact that small antigens may not function as immunogens implies that more is required than simple binding to antibody or T-cell receptor to initiate the immune responses. This requires a macromolecule which will normally have several epitopes, or small antigenic regions. The epitope of interest is called the hapten if it is a chemical grouping, such as DNP, deliberately coupled to the macromolecule, and the latter is called the carrier. The triggering of antigen-specific B- or T-cells requires more than one cell type, including antigen-presenting cells (APCs) and T-helper cells. Thus an antibody response requires B-cells, T-helper cells, and APCs or macrophages. The T-cell response needs APCs and may need other T-cells; some of the cell requirements can be replaced by factors or cytokines such as interleukin-2. The nature of these interactions is described in later sections.

Immunogens may be any kind of macromolecule: proteins, polysaccharides, lipopolysaccharides, and nucleic acids are immunogens. Of these, polysaccharides and proteins predominate. A crucial feature of an immunogen is that it must differ from self. It is a central rule of immunology that lymphocytes do not normally recognize unaltered self macromolecules. Although lipid macromolecules vary little between individuals and rarely if ever trigger antibody responses unless coupled to variable grouping, glycolipids and lipid–protein complexes can be potent immunogens. Carbohydrates and proteins, on the other hand, show sequence variability and genetic polymorphism and so provoke strong antibody responses. Nucleic acids ought to stimulate good immune responses, but rarely do. RNA may be too labile and DNA, which can provoke antibody responses when released, may be protected by its coiling properties and by membranes and nucleoproteins in intact cells. T-cells respond only to antigens bound to MHC molecules and so far these have always been identified as peptides. T-cells do not appear to respond to non-protein antigens.

Polysaccharides present repeating units and as such can trigger B-cells directly. This may be achieved by their ability to cross-link the immunoglobulin receptors on B-cells, which may bypass the need for T-cell help. Alternatively, the carbohydrate, if part of a complex cell surface antigen such as a bacterial cell wall, may obtain help from T-cells specific for other components of the stimulating cell, intermolecular help. In the absence of T-cell help, carbohydrates tend to elicit IgM antibody responses. Natural antibodies to blood group antigens, of great clinical relevance, would fall into this group.

Because of their abundance and great diversity, proteins are the best studied, and probably most important, antigens and immunogens. A key feature that has emerged in the last few years is that antibodies, and therefore B-lymphocytes, frequently react with conformational epitopes that are exposed on the surface of proteins and which can be comprised of non-sequential amino acids. Conversely, T-cells react with epitopes composed of short linear sequences of amino acids. Thus, while T-cell epitopes can easily be mimicked by short synthetic peptides, this is much harder to do for B-cells and antibodies, although the V3-loop of the human immunodeficiency virus-1 envelope appears to be an exception. This has implications for vaccine design where peptides are attractive for safety reasons, but have been disappointing in practice. The reason is simple: B-cells and antibodies react with intact proteins; T-cells interact with processed antigens.

A special type of protein antigen is antibody itself. Each different antibody molecule has unique sequence around the binding site (idiotype) and this can be immunogenic. Anti-idiotype antibodies can therefore neutralize antibody. They can also suppress or sometimes activate B-cells with the same antibody as receptor. This has implications for regulation of the immune response. The network hypothesis of Jerne (1974) suggests that this is a major regulatory feature. The anti-idiotype antibody binding site may mimic the spatial orientation of the original epitope. This is being exploited in attempts to generate vaccines, with some success in animal models.

Similar considerations may apply to T-cell receptors, although this is less clear at present. Antibodies to T-cell receptor idiotypes have been described and can block or activate the relevant T-cell clones according to how they are given. These reagents would have interesting therapeutic potential.

A newly defined class of proteins, mostly bacterial enterotoxins, such as staphylococcal enterotoxins A and B, are known as superantigens. These are able to bind to class II molecules of the major histocompatibility complex and to the variable region of the β chain of subsets of T-cell receptors. In this way they can activate some T-cells. They contribute to toxic shock syndromes where the activated T-cells release lymphokines in large amounts. They are useful experimental tools for exploring T-cell ontogeny and function.

Route of immunization

Various cell types are capable of immunogen presentation. These specialized cells include macrophages, tissue macrophages, dendritic cells in tissues, interdigitating and follicular dendritic cells, and Langerhans cells in skin. In addition, any cell infected by virus may also present virus antigen to cytotoxic T-lymphocytes. The route of immunization as well as the nature of the antigen, ranging from small soluble protein to live virus, can determine which cells are involved. This in turn affects the nature of the response, for instance the relative strength of humoral and cellular immune responses, predominant immunoglobulin isotype, or even epitopes to which the T-cells react.

Another factor that influences immunization is adjuvant, material which can non-specifically enhance immune responses. Potassium alum is used in diphtheria–tetanus toxoid vaccines and probably acts by localizing antigen and producing a non-specific inflammatory response which attracts phagocytic cells and antigen-presenting cells.

Antigen-presenting cells (APC)

Specialized APCs fall into two categories. In lymph nodes the follicular dendritic cells (FDC) are thought to concentrate antigen for B-cells which are then activated in the follicle. They express Fc receptors and complement receptors and thus can collect immune complexes. Pre-existing circulating antibody has been shown to make an antigen more immunogenic. Foreign antigen arrives by afferent lymphatics and percolates through the lymph nodes where some may be trapped in the follicles by FDC to stimulate B-cells.

Dendritic cells are present in the T-cell area of lymph nodes and in many other tissues and express large amounts of MHC class II antigens, making them very efficient at presenting antigen to T-cells. Foreign antigen has to be processed by APCs, which endocytose bound proteins and digest them to fragments which then bind to MHC class II molecules. B-lymphocytes are also effective at this, particularly if they have surface antibody which captures the antigen. Evidence that antigen is processed before presentation to T-cells can be summarized as follows (Schwartz 1985). Helper T-cells respond to (synthetic) peptide fragments of antigen at least as well as to the whole protein. Presentation of whole protein can be blocked by agents which interfere with lysosomal functions, such as chloroquin. Macrophages gently fixed with para-formaldehyde cannot present proteins, but can present the appropriate peptides. The reason why protein has to be processed to peptides is so that it can associate with MHC antigen, the form in which T-cells recognize it.

4.2.2   The major histocompatibility complex (MHC)

MHC proteins play a crucial role in antigen presentation to T-cell receptors (TCR). They also provoke very strong immune responses when they are foreign, i.e. allo-antigens. They were first discovered because of their role in provoking allograft rejection. The basis for their very close relationship with T-cell function lies in the thymus, where immature T-cells are exposed to self MHC antigens: those that respond strongly are deleted while those with weaker or no responses survive. The latter may react strongly with allo-antigens and self MHC which has bound foreign peptide and so appears altered or foreign. There is some evidence that T-cells with receptors that bind weakly to self MHC in the thymus are positively selected and expanded.

Genetic structure

The MHC complex is located on the short arm of chromosome 6. The genes have been grouped into three types, classes I, II, and III, but as more genes are defined in the MHC this classification may need extending. Class I and II products provoke strong allograft rejection and have antigen-presenting functions; class III products are the components of the complement systems C2, C4a, C4b, factor B, and two enzymes, both 21-hydroxylases, that are involved in steroid biosynthesis. Between classes III and I are genes for the cytokines, tumour necrosis factors (TNF) α and β. The MHC is now known to code for many other genes, most of which are non-polymorphic. Some such as the heat shock (hsp70) code for proteins that may be involved in antigen processing. The gene arrangements are shown in Fig. 4.1.

Class I

Four expressed genes have now been defined A, B, C, and G. Of these A and B are highly polymorphic and expressed in virtually all nucleated cells. C is expressed in low amounts and is still somewhat mysterious. G is non-polymorphic and its product is expressed only on trophoblast. Two other genes, E and F, do not appear to code for cell surface molecules. HLA-A and HLA-B each have more than 30 alleles, definable by allo-antisera, antibodies made by individuals exposed to foreign cells, usually pregnant women or blood transfusion recipients. In addition there are further variants of A and B molecules that are definable by T-cell recognition studies, methods such as isoelectric focusing and nucleic acid sequencing. These differ in less than four amino acids only and are quite common, increasing the polymorphism by a factor of two or three and making the MHC extraordinarily polymorphic. The serologically defined A, B, and C antigens are listed in Table 4.1.

The basic structure of an HLA class I molecule is shown in Fig. 4.2. There are three external domains of 90 amino acids, a

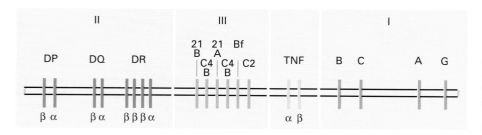

Fig. 4.1 Organization of the known expressed genes in the HLA complex. The class I, II, and III regions are shown, together with the genes. β and α refer to the β- and α-chains. 21B and 21A are 21-hydroxylases B and A. C2, C4, and Bf are the complement components C2, C4, and factor B.

Table 4.1 List of recognized HLA specificities

A	B	C	D	DR	DQ	DP
A1	B7	Cw1	Dw1	DR1	DQw2	DPw1
A2	B8	Cw2	Dw2	DR4	DQw4	DPw2
A3	B13	Cw4	Dw3	DR7	DQw5 (w1)	DPw3
A11	B18	Cw5	Dw4	DRw8	DQw6 (w1)	DPw4
A23 (9)	B27	Cw6	Dw5	DR9	DQw7 (w3)	DPw5
A24 (9)	B35	Cw7	Dw8	DRw10	DQw8 (w3)	DPw6
A25 (10)	B37	Cw8	Dw9	DRw11 (5)	DQw9 (w3)	
A26 (10)	B38 (16)	Cw9 (w3)	Dw10	DRw12 (5)		
A29 (w19)	B39 (16)	Cw10 (w3)	Dw11 (w7)	DRw13 (w6)		
A30 (w19)	Bw41	Cw11	Dw12	DRw14 (w6)		
A31 (w19)	Bw42		Dw13	DRw15 (2)		
A32 (w19)	B44 (12)		Dw14	DRw16 (2)		
Aw33 (w19)	B45 (12)		Dw15	DRw17 (3)		
Aw34 (10)	Be46		Dw16	DRw18 (3)		
Aw36	Bw47		Dw17 (w7)			
Aw43	Bw48		Dw18 (w6)	DRw52		
Aw66 (10)	B49 (21)		Dw19 (w6)			
Aw68 (28)	Bw50 (21)		Dw20	DRw53		
Aw69 (28)	B51 (5)		Dw21			
Aw74 (w19)	Bw52 (5)		Dw22			
	Bw53		Dw23			
	Bw54 (w22)		Dw24			
	Bw55 (w22)		Dw25			
	Bw56 (w22)		Dw26			
	Bw57 (17)					
	Bw58 (17)					
	Bw59					
	Bw60 (40					
	Bw61 (40)					
	Bw62 (15)					
	Bw63 (15)					
	Bw64 (14)					
	Bw65 (14)					
	Bw67					
	Bw71 (w70)					
	Bw72 (w70)					
	Bw73					
	Bw75 (15)					
	Bw76 (15)					
	Bw77 (15)					
	Bw4					
	Bw6					

Specificities in parentheses are earlier specificities that have been split into those shown, e.g. A9 has been split into A23 and A24.

transmembrane region and a short cytoplasmic tail. This heavy chain is associated with β_2 microglobulin which is not polymorphic and is also about 90 amino acids long. The crystalline structure of HLA-A2 has recently been defined by Bjorkman *et al.* (1987a, b) and is shown diagrammatically in Fig. 4.3. The α_3 domains and β_2 microglobulin form a kind of stalk on which the α_1 and α_2 domains form an unusual and interesting structure. The first and second domains fold as an eight-stranded β-pleated sheet over which runs two α-helices with a groove between them. In this groove was found electron density which was probably peptide antigen or a mixture of peptides that had co-crystallized with the HLA-A2. Thus foreign or self peptides demonstrably bind to an HLA class I molecule. This was a very exciting finding because experiments on cytotoxic T-cells had

shown that they recognized complexes of HLA class I antigen plus peptides derived from virus proteins.

Thus, the class I MHC molecules bind foreign peptides and present them as foreign antigen to cytotoxic T-lymphocytes (CTL). It is highly likely that peptides derived from self proteins, as they are degraded, also bind to the cells' HLA class I proteins, and a large part of the alloreactive T-cell response could be directed at these peptide–MHC protein complexes. The peptide binds in the groove which is bounded by the two α-helices where nearly all of the variable amino-acid residues are sited. This suggests that the selective pressure on class I antigens that has generated the extreme polymorphism is the ability of each to bind and present different peptides to T-lymphocytes. It is not yet known how many peptides interact with a single HLA

HLA class I   HLA class II

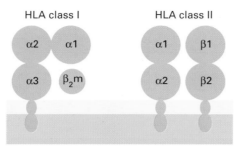

Fig. 4.2 Diagrammatic structure of HLA class I and class II molecules. HLA class I is composed of a heavy chain of three external domains, α_1, α_2, and α_3, each of 90 amino acids, a transmembrane region and cytoplasmic tail. The heavy chain, which is variable in different HLA types, in the α_1 and α_2 domains, is associated with β_2 microglobulin (β_2M). HLA class II is composed of two chains, α and β, each made up of two external domains, a transmembrane region and cytoplasmic tail. The amino terminal domains β_1 (and α_1 in DQ only) vary between different HLA types. Cell membrane is shown in pale yellow.

antigen, but it may be that each peptide will need to have some structural features in common and may thus turn out to be relatively rare. It is known that some HLA molecules are unable to present particular virus proteins, presumably because no peptides are generated which can bind. Extending this, it is possible that rare individuals may fail to generate cytotoxic T-cell responses to certain viruses because of their HLA type. These individuals would be particularly susceptible to those viruses because cytotoxic T-cells play major roles in recovery from virus infections or in keeping persisting viruses, such as the Epstein–Barr virus, under control.

HLA class II

There are three families of class II antigens DP, DQ, and DR. They are coded for by the genes shown in Fig. 4.1. (There are also some pseudogenes in this complex, as there are in class I, but these are not shown in the figure.) All are polymorphic although DP is less so and is still rather poorly understood. Each gene product has the basic structure shown in Fig. 4.2. Like class I, the external parts of each chain can be divided into domains of about 90 amino acids and there is some sequence homology with class I. Both chains cross the membrane and have short cytoplasmic tails.

Although the crystal structure of class II antigens has not yet been determined, they show strong homology with the class I proteins and the N-terminal domains may fold in a similar way. It is known that class II can bind to antigenic peptides and present them to the antigen receptors on T-helper cells and it is expected that they will also have a binding groove with the polymorphic amino-acid residues located around it.

HLA-DR antigens are polymorphic, with the serological types shown in Table 4.1. They share a non-polymorphic α-chain and in most HLA (haplo-) types there are two β-chains expressed, one of which carries the serological specificity that defines DR type and the other confirms further polymorphism

that is less clearly defined serologically, e.g. DRw52 and DRw53.

HLA-DQ antigens were originally divided into three serological types: DQw1, w2, and w3. However, this underestimated the polymorphism. Biochemical techniques have shown that there is considerable polymorphism in the DQ β-chain so that each DQ serological type can be divided into at least three further types. Furthermore, the α-chains are also polymorphic, and as both α- and β-chains are variable it is possible to generate two extra molecules in heterozygous individuals. At the 1987 HLA Workshop this extra polymorphism of DQ was recognized and nine serological types are now definable.

HLA-DP is less polymorphic and seems to be expressed in relatively low quantities. Very little further is known about it at present. While DR and DQ are very closely linked and strong linkage disequilibrium exists between alleles, e.g. between DR2 and DQw1, DP shows little allelic association with DQ or DR. There is probably a recombinational hotspot between DP and DQ.

Class II MHC proteins have restricted tissue distribution and are found on B-cells, dendritic cells, monocytes, Langerhans' cells, thymic epithelial cells, activated T-cells, some endothelium and epithelium, but not other cell types. However, they may be expressed on other cells after exposure to interferon-γ. This may be of some pathological significance; for instance it has been shown that thymocytes and pancreatic islet B-cells undergoing auto-immune attack express HLA class II. It has been argued that this may allow them to present self antigens directly to T-helper cells.

The functions of HLA class II are similar to those of HLA class I, that is to present antigen to T-cells. HLA class II presents to T-helper cells which carry the CD4 glycoprotein. The latter, which is also the receptor for HIV, may bind to HLA class II. HLA class II is normally expressed by antigen-presenting cells such as monocytes, B-cells, dendritic cells, and Langerhans' cells. As described earlier, these cells have been shown to internalize foreign protein antigens and then degrade them to peptides which are then presented, bound to MHC class II. Class II molecules are associated with a third polypeptide, known as invariant chain, after synthesis. This appears to prevent peptide binding until the molecules reach a post-Golgi compartment on their journey to the cell surface. Here invariant chain is removed and degraded and peptides generated in phago-lysosomes bind.

As with class I HLA, different class II MHC molecules present different peptide fragments of foreign antigens. The genes therefore function as 'immune-response genes' controlling the level of helper T-cell response and thus antibody levels to foreign antigens. In fact, class II genes were first identified as immune-response genes in mice, where they determined whether animals would make antibody response to simple synthetic polypeptide antigens.

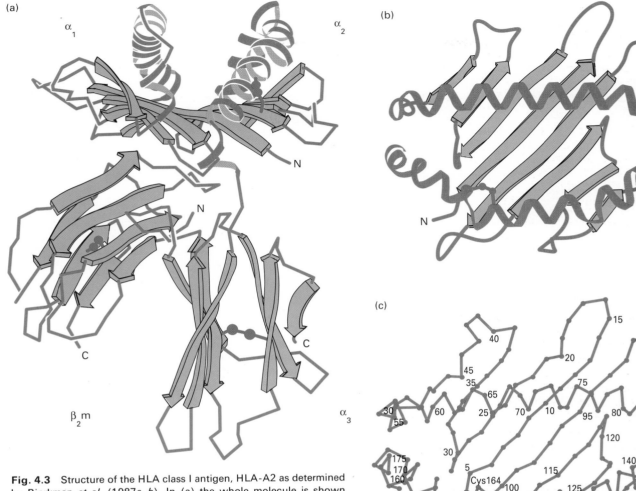

Fig. 4.3 Structure of the HLA class I antigen, HLA-A2 as determined by Bjorkman *et al.* (1987*a, b*). In (a) the whole molecule is shown schematically. Arrows indicate β-pleated sheet and coils indicate α-helices. In (b) the top surface ('T-cell view') is shown with the two α helices lying across an eight-stranded β-sheet. In (c) the amino-acid backbone is traced for the α₁ and α₂ domains; each dot represents an amino acid and every fifth one is numbered. (Redrawn with permission from the Editors of *Nature*.)

HLA and disease

It has been shown that several alleles of the HLA system are associated with susceptibility to diseases, particularly auto-immune diseases. The common associations are listed in Table 4.2.

There are four explanations for the associations, each of which seems possible and may apply to one or more of the diseases. The first is that the disease may be caused by a linked gene. This is true in the case of congenital adrenal hyperplasia, often linked to HLA-B47, in which haplotype there is a deletion of one of the 21-hydroxylase genes. A similar gene deletion or

abnormality may account for the association between idiopathic haemochromatosis and HLA-A3, although the candidate gene has not yet been identified. It might also be true for narcolepsy and ankylosing spondylitis, which have very strong associations with DR2 and B27, respectively, although other mechanisms seem more likely in the latter case in view of the immunological features associated with the disease. Now that it is known that there are many 'housekeeping' genes in the MHC, some of which are involved in antigen processing, the linked gene hypothesis looks increasingly attractive.

The second hypothesis is that there is molecular mimicry between HLA antigens and self antigens or micro-organisms.

Table 4.2 HLA and disease associations[*]

Group	Disease	Markers	Relative risk (percentage association)
Disease not due to chronic auto-immunity	21-Hydroxylase deficiency	Bw47	15
	Idiopathic haemochromatosis	A3	8
Diseases involving auto-immunity	Ankylosing spondylitis	B27	90–350
	Rheumatoid arthritis	DR4 (Dw4)[†]	4–6
	Coeliac disease	B8/DR3/DQw2[‡]	8–11
	Insulin-dependent	B8/DR3/DQw2	3–6
	Diabetes mellitus	B15/DR4/DQw3	2–3
		B7/DR2	0.5–0.25
	Multiple sclerosis	B7/DR2/DQw1	2–5
	Goodpasture's syndrome	DR2	13
Diseases of unknown pathogenesis	Narcolepsy	DR2	100

[*] Only the strongest disease associations are shown in this table.
[†] DW4 is a subtype of DR4.
[‡] Haplotypes are shown as B8/DR3/DQw2.

Some have been described, e.g. between the nitrogenase protein of *Klebsiella pneumoniae* and part of B27. There is also some evidence for serological cross-reactivity between *Klebsiella* and B27 but how this would account for triggering of the disease is not clear. While the homology is undeniable for a sequence of eight amino acids, its significance is very hard to assess at present. It does raise the point, however, that sequence identities, and therefore immunological cross-reactivities, may be much more frequent than previously anticipated because T-lymphocytes react with such small antigenic epitopes.

The third possibility is that particular HLA antigens act as receptors for certain viruses or other micro-organisms. The cell-surface glycoproteins CD4 and CD21 have been shown to be receptors for HIV and EBV, respectively. However, it seems intrinsically unlikely that a virus could be restricted to infecting cells of a single HLA type, given the rapid generation and selection of mutations that occurs in virus replication.

The fourth possibility invokes the natural function of the MHC system in antigen presentation, i.e. the 'susceptible' HLA molecule presents a unique antigen to T-cells. For auto-immune diseases, this might trigger off T-cell clones that cross-react with self antigens. While attractive, this hypothesis has not yet been fully tested for any HLA-associated disease. Another way in which the HLA system's normal role could be involved is highlighted by the association with juvenile-onset diabetes. Here HLA-DR3 and HLA-DR4 occur commonly in patients while HLA-DR2 is almost completely absent. Todd *et al.* (1987) showed that the protective HLA type is the DQw1 molecule and this, and other DQ antigens that appear to protect against diabetes, share a common region of sequence in the β-chain, with an aspartic acid at position 57. The non-obese diabetic mouse, which develops a similar disease, is the only mouse strain so far tested to lack an aspartic acid at position 57 of its IA, DQ equivalent, β-chain. It is possible that self-reactive T-cell clones in individuals with an HLA-DQ β-chain with aspartic acid at

position 57 will be eliminated, and that these T-cells might include those which mediate the auto-immune reaction with β-cells in the pancreatic islets. Alternatively, DQ antigens with asp-57 may present an islet-cell peptide antigen to suppressor T-cells, which then suppress all auto-immune reactions against those cells. These hypotheses can be tested and experiments are currently in progress in several laboratories.

All of the HLA associations so far described are with susceptibility. In view of the key role of the MHC in immune responses and hence infectious disease, particularly virus infections, one might expect to see associations with resistance. Indeed, the HLA polymorphism predicts this, but there have been none demonstrated yet. This may be because of the difficulties of doing such studies, looking for decreased frequencies of already rare alleles in patients. Also, natural selection might already have been so strong as to make fully susceptible haplotypes very rare.

4.2.3 Bibliography

Batchelor, R. and McMichael, A. J. (1987). Progress in understanding HLA and disease associations. *British Medical Bulletin* **43**(1), 156–83.

Bjorkman, P. J., Saper, M. A., Samraoui, B., Bennett, W. S., Strominger, J. L., and Wiley, D. C. (1987a). The foreign antigen binding site and T-cell recognition regions of class I histocompatibility antigens. *Nature* **329**, 512–16.

Bjorkman, P. J., Saper, M. A., Samraoui, B., Bennett, W. S., Strominger, J. L., and Wiley, D. C. (1987b). Structure of the human class I histocompatibility antigen, HLA-A2. *Nature* **329**, 506–11.

Bulletin of the World Health Organization (1988). *Nomenclature for factors of the HLA system.*

Carroll, M. C., *et al.* (1987). Linkage map of the human major histocompatibility complex including the tumour necrosis factor genes. *Proceedings of the National Academy of Sciences USA* **84**, 8535–9.

Jerne, N. K. (1974). Towards a network theory of the immune response. *Annales d'Institute Pasteur Immunologiques* **125c**, 373–89.

Londei, M., Bottazzo, F. G., and Feldmann, M. (1985). Human T-cell clones from autoimmune thyroid glands: specific recognitions of autologous cells. *Science* **228**, 85–9.

Marrack, P. and Kappler, J. (1990). The staphylococcal enterotoxins and their relatives. *Science* **248**, 705–11.

Oldstone, M. A. (1987). Molecular mimicry and autoimmune disease. *Cell* **50**, 819–20.

Schwartz, R. H. (1985). T-lymphocyte recognition of antigen in association with gene products of the major histocompatibility complex. *Annual Review of Immunology* **3**, 237–61.

Todd, J. A., Bell, J. I., and McDevitt, H. O. (1987). HLA-DQβ gene contributes to susceptibility and resistance to insulin-dependent diabetes mellitus. *Nature* **329**, 599–604.

4.3 B-cells and the cellular basis of antibody production

I. C. M. MacLennan

Antibodies are produced by a specialized family of cells known as B-cells. This section will describe the way the B-cell system responds to antigenic challenge with the regulated production of specific antibodies. Details of the structure and function of antibodies themselves will be given in the next section (4.4).

The high level of specificity of antibodies produced in response to infections was already appreciated by the end of the nineteenth century. During the past 25 years much has been learned of the cellular basis for antibody production and the way in which antibody responses are regulated. It has become clear how the genes coding for antibodies give rise to an almost infinite number of different antibody specificities.

4.3.1 B-cells, antibody-secreting cells, and B-cell memory

B-cells carry antigen-specific receptors on their surface. These are antibodies produced by the B-cell and inserted in the cell membrane. Each B-cell only expresses antibodies of a single specificity. If antigen interacts with the antibody on a B-cell's surface, this can initiate its differentiation to an antibody-secreting cell. The specificity of the antibody secreted will be the same as that of the surface antibody on the parent B-cell.

When B-cells are activated by antigen they usually undergo proliferation before becoming antibody-secreting cells. Thus a single B-cell can give rise to many antibody-secreting cells. Proliferating B-cells can also revert to the resting B-cell form when they come out of cell cycle. In this way more B-cells are generated which are capable of binding to the antigen which activated their parent. This is the basis of B-cell memory. This minimal model of B-cell activation and differentiation is summarized in Fig. 4.4. In reality, most antibody responses involve sequential activation of B-cells in a number of different microenvironments. These are associated with a range of activities which will be described later in this section.

4.3.2 The origin of B-cells and the generation of antibody diversity

B-cells are produced throughout life in the bone marrow from pluripotential haemopoietic stem cells, i.e. they share a common precursor with platelets, red cells, granulocytes, macrophages, and T-cells. The stages of primary B-lymphopoiesis are

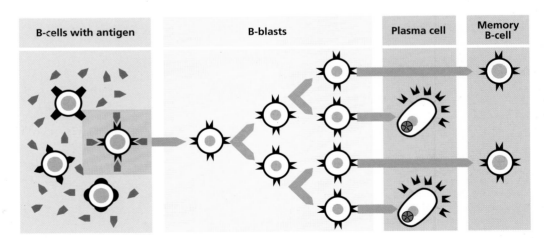

Fig. 4.4 When B-cells bind antigen specifically by their surface immunoglobulin this may result in their becoming antibody-secreting cells. Usually they will require additional signals from other cells for this process to be completed. B-cell activation usually results in the B-cells entering cell cycle. Subsequently some of the cycling B-blasts will enter terminal differentiation and become plasma cells. Others will again become B-lymphocytes, thus increasing the number of B-cells that can respond to the antigen that activated their ancestor.

summarized in Fig. 4.5. As B-cells develop from their stem cells they undergo rearrangement of the genes which encode antibodies. It is by this process of rearrangement that diversity of antibody specificity is generated.

There are six loci encoding antibody or immunoglobulin genes in each haemopoietic stem cell. These are in the configuration found in the fertilized ovum. Each immunoglobulin gene locus is on a different chromosome, one on each of the 2, 14, and 22 chromosome pairs. These, respectively, encode the κ light chains, heavy chains, and λ light chains of immunoglobulin molecules. In any one B-cell only two of its six loci of immunoglobulin genes are transcribed to produce mRNA; one of the four light-chain loci and one of the two heavy-chain loci. The mechanism for exclusion of the other groups of immunoglobulin genes from being transcribed remains uncertain.

Each of the immunoglobulin gene loci can be divided into two sections. One is concerned with programming for the antigen-binding, or V, region of the molecule, the other for the constant region. The heavy-chain V-region genes consist of three sets of exons; V_H segments, D_H segments, and J_H segments. There are a large number of V_H segments, probably between 150 and 300; the precise number still being unclear. In the 3' direction from the last V_H segment there are a series of some dozen D_H segments

and, again 3' to these, five functional J_H segments. The diversity of the heavy-chain V-region genes is created during their rearrangement. In this process one J_H segment becomes joined to one D_H segment, which in turn becomes spliced to one of the V_H segments; the intervening sequences being deleted. The number of possible heavy-chain variable-region structures is therefore the product of the number of V_H, D_H, and J_H segments. In practice the process of splicing these gene segments is not precise. This is referred to as junctional diversity and results in the generation of different codons and hence amino-acid sequences. This greatly increases the number of possible V-region structures that can be produced during immunoglobulin gene rearrangement. Further variability in V-region genes is generated in certain circumstances following B-cell activation by antigen. This results from somatic mutation within rearranged immunoglobulin genes, a process which will be considered later.

The organization of light-chain V-region genes differs only from those of the heavy chains in that they have no D segments; a V_L segment joining directly to a J_L segment. Figure 4.6 depicts the process of rearrangement of immunoglobulin heavy-chain V regions and the production of mRNAs which will be translated to produce immunoglobulin heavy chains.

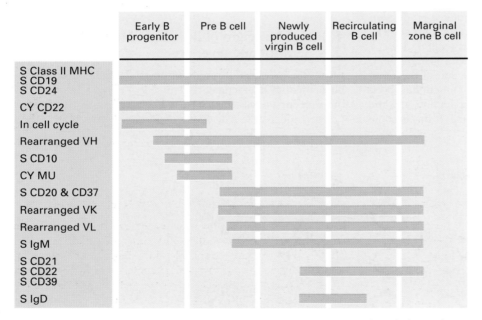

Fig. 4.5 This flow diagram summarizes phenotypic changes occurring during primary B-lymphopoiesis and during antigen-independent recruitment to the peripheral B-cell pools. S, surface-membrane-bound; class II MHC, molecules encoded at the DR and DP loci of the major histocompatibility complex. CD describes a cluster of monoclonal antibodies which bind to the same leucocyte-associated molecule. Different clusters of antibodies identifying different molecules are given a different CD number. For further details of the CD classification see Ling *et al.* (1987). Cy, cytoplasmic; MU, μ immunoglobulin heavy chains; VH, immunoglobulin heavy chain variable region genes; VK, κ immunoglobulin light chain variable region genes; VL, λ immunoglobulin light chain variable region genes. Horizontal lines indicate that the feature listed in the left-hand column is present in the differentiation stages listed at the top of the figure. Note: only a proportion of B-cells have rearranged VL genes.

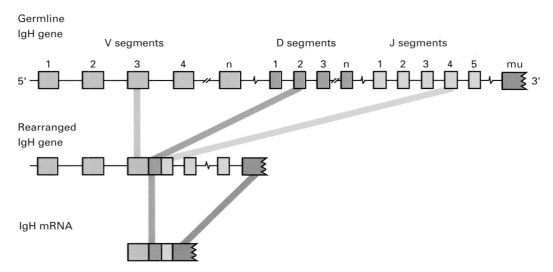

Fig. 4.6 A simplified diagrammatic representation of immunoglobulin heavy-chain variable-region gene rearrangement. Introns are shown as straight lines, exons as boxes. Note, nuclear mRNA includes transcripts of both exons and introns. The intron transcripts are excised before the mRNA becomes associated with ribosomes. The mRNA structure shown in the figure represents ribosomal mRNA encoding IgM heavy chains. The process of immunoglobulin V-region gene rearrangement is outlined in the text.

4.3.3 Conditions for B-cell activation

Interaction between surface immunoglobulin and specific antigen alone is not generally sufficient to push B-cells into cell cycle or to induce them to differentiate to antibody-secreting cells. For this to happen accessory signals must also be received. These can be delivered from a variety of different sources including:

1. T-cells, which have been specifically activated by antigen;

2. macrophages and related cells;

3. specialized cells concerned with antigen presentation, known as follicular dendritic cells (FDC);

4. certain molecules of micro-organisms, particularly the lipo-polysaccharides associated with endotoxin; and

5. the split product of the third component of complement C3d.

The complex triggering systems which control B-cell activation and differentiation are at best only partially understood. But it is clear that they provide a means by which rapid but regulated antibody production can be achieved in response to antigenic challenge. Three basic stages can be identified in the processes which result in a resting B-cell becoming an antibody-secreting cell. The first is associated with resting B-cells becoming receptive to a range of signals that will induce them to start dividing. In the second phase the cells respond to growth factors which drive proliferation. The final stage is where the cells are induced to come out of cell cycle and differentiate into either antibody-secreting cells or memory B-cells. Table 4.3 identifies some of the factors which are known to deliver signals to B-cells during these three stages of antigen-driven B-cell maturation.

4.3.4 The immunoglobulin classes and subclasses

There are five major immunoglobulin classes; IgM, IgD, IgG, IgA, and IgE. In addition, in humans, four subclasses of IgG and two of IgA are recognized. These are described in detail in Section 4.4.2. This section considers the mechanisms which result in different classes and subclasses of immunoglobulin being produced at different stages in response to different classes of antigen.

4.3.5 The three major classes of antigen

It is now apparent that there are three major classes of antigen which induce B-cell-activation in significantly different ways. These differences are of considerable clinical importance for selective deficiencies in responsiveness to these classes of antigen are recognized. These are sometimes present in individuals who have normal immunoglobulin class and subclass levels.

T-cell-dependent antigens

These antigens are only able to evoke antibody responses with T-cell help. They are characteristically proteins or a non-protein antigenic determinant attached to a protein core. An example of the latter is tetanus toxoid, an inactive but immunogenic form of the tetanus neurotoxin. The nerve-binding determinant of this toxin is a carbohydrate side-chain on a carrier protein. The protective antibodies induced by tetanus toxoid, a T-cell-dependent antigen, neutralize tetanus toxin by binding to

Table 4.3 B-cell surface molecules and factors involved in B-cell activation

Primary activators	Proliferation	Differentiation
SIg	IL-4	IL-6
CD20	CD23	α-IFN
IL-4	IL-2	γ-IFN
LPS	LPS	IL-2

Promoters of activation:
CD22, CD40, CD21, CD23

Inhibitors of activation:
CD19, FcIgG

SIg, surface immunoglobulin; for definition of CD see legend to Fig. 4.5; LPS, lipopolysaccharide from *Escherichia coli*; IL, interleukin; IFN, interferon; FcIgG, the two C-terminal domains of IgG. For definition of the three stages of B-cell activation identified in this table see text.

its carbohydrate side-chain, thus preventing the toxin entering nerve cells.

T-cell-independent type 1 antigens (TI-1 antigens)

These antigens typically contain lipopolysaccharides. There are receptors on macrophages and some B-cells for bacterial lipopolysaccharides. Some lipopolysaccharides are able to activate complement by the alternative pathway. This may provide the accessory signals which enable TI-1 antigens to bypass T-cell help. TI-1 antigens characteristically are able to evoke antibody responses before birth and in this respect they differ markedly from TI-2 antigens. Although most TI-1 antigens are based on bacterial lipopolysaccharides, in certain circumstances some pure polysaccharides behave as TI-1 antigens. An example of this is the response to 1,3-dextran in certain strains of mice. The bacterial flagellar protein, flagellin, when highly polymerized also behaves as a TI-1 antigen. It seems likely that these two exceptions have the ability to evoke additional B-cell activation signals to those elicited by most protein or pure polysaccharide antigens.

T-cell-independent type 2 (TI-2) antigens

These antigens are based upon pure polysaccharides. The capsular polysaccharides of *Streptococcus pneumoniae*, *Neisseria meningitidis*, and *Haemophilus influenzae type B* are in this category. These are among the most serious pathogens for hypogammaglobulinaemic (antibody-deficient) patients. IgG antibody against these capsular polysaccharides is highly protective against infection with these bacteria.

TI-2 antigens characteristically fail to evoke IgG antibody responses in infancy, full responsiveness developing only towards the end of the second year of life. Maternally transferred IgG is sufficient to protect during the perinatal period, but children aged between 6 months and 2 years are particularly at risk from these bacteria. It has been estimated that world-wide some five million infants die from infection with this group of encapsulated bacteria each year. Recently it has been shown that young children will produce antibodies against these polysaccharides if they are linked to proteins such as diphtheria toxoid. These modified antigens are capable of evoking T-cell help.

The differences between these three classes of antigen are largely dependent upon the backbone or core structure of the antigen and not on its antigenic determinants. This is demonstrated if small molecules, which can act as antigenic determinants (haptens), are attached to different carrier molecules. For example, the hapten dinitrophenyl conjugated to a protein such as haemocyanin requires T-cell help to evoke an anti-dinitrophenyl antibody response. The same hapten conjugated to lipopolysaccharide from *Escherichia coli* behaves as a TI-1 antigen, while dinitrophenyl conjugated to the polysaccharide Ficoll is a TI-2 antigen. In each case anti-dinitrophenyl antibodies are produced but the conditions required to activate dinitrophenyl-specific B-cells are clearly different for each class of antigen. The cellular and molecular basis for these clinically important differences will be discussed later in this chapter.

4.3.6   The distribution of B-cells and their sites of activation *in vivo*

Most B-cells are located within secondary lymphoid organs, that is to say, the spleen, lymph nodes, the tonsils and other tissue of Waldeyer's ring, Peyer's patches and other gut-associated lymphoid tissue, and the bronchial-associated lymphoid tissue. The primary lymphoid organs are the sites of primary lymphopoiesis, namely the bone marrow and thymus, as well as the liver and splenic red pulp in fetal life. The secondary lymophoid organs provide the principle microenvironments in which B-cells can be activated successfully by antigen. For, in these structures, B-cells, T-cells, and antigen-presenting cells come together. In addition, the secondary lymphoid tissues are strategically placed to receive antigen.

B-cell follicles

A common feature of all secondary lymphoid tissues are collections of B-cells known as follicles (Fig. 4.7). These are centred upon a network of specialized antigen-presenting cells known as follicular dendritic cells (FDC). The origin of these cells is still uncertain; however, they have the ability to take up antigen, which they can hold for long periods. This is the most obvious source of the antigen that is known to be required to drive the long-term antibody production seen during T-cell-dependent antibody responses.

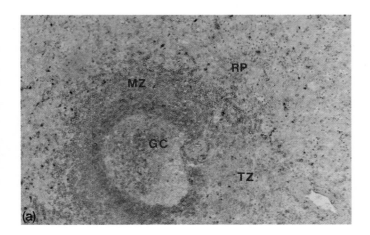

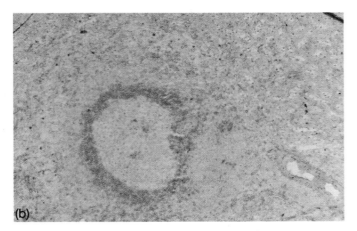

Fig. 4.7 These two figures are photomicrographs (× 100) of the same area of serial sections of spleen stained by indirect immunoperoxidase to reveal IgM (a) and IgD (b). The nuclei of cells in both sections are lightly stained with haematoxylin. Features stained with IgM but not IgD are the marginal zone (MZ) B-cells and IgM-containing immune complex on the follicular dendritic cell-network, which is apparent in the light zone of a well-developed germinal centre (GC). The cells of the dark zone of the GC do not express either immunoglobulin. TZ, T-cell and interdigitating cell-rich zone; RP, red pulp.

In resting or primary follicles, where B-cell activation is not taking place, the spaces between the FDC are filled with small B-cells. Most of these express both IgM and IgD on their surface. During antibody responses to T-cell-dependent antigens in particular, follicles become sites of intense B-cell proliferation. In this situation the proliferating cells hold the central ground in the follicle while the small B-cells are displaced to its outer rim. The central area in an active or secondary follicle is known as a germinal centre, the outer layer of small B-cells the follicular mantle. More detailed consideration of germinal centres is given later.

T-cell-rich areas

Abutting on to follicles are areas which are rich in T-cells. Between the T-cells are cells with relatively short dendritic pro-

cesses, known as interdigitating cells. These cells are derived from haemopoietic cells in the bone marrow. T-cells bind to interdigitating cells *in vitro* and there is a considerable body of experimental evidence to indicate that these cells are important in antigen-specific T-cell activation. The subsequent sections will indicate how B-cells pass into and through these areas where they may also be activated.

B-lymphocyte recirculation

The small B-cells in primary follicles and in the follicular mantles of secondary follicles are in a constant state of non-random migration between the secondary lymphoid organs. By this process, known as recirculation, a B-cell located in a follicle in the spleen one day may be in a popliteal lymph node the following day and a Peyer's patch the day after that. The time between a cell entering one lymphoid organ and the time when it enters the next varies between a few hours and a little over a day.

Recirculating B-cells leave the blood either via specialized small blood vessels known as high endothelial venules or, in the case of the spleen, by the primary blood sinusoidal network of the marginal zone (Fig. 4.7). High endothelial venules are located in the T-cell-rich areas of all secondary lymphoid organs other than the spleen. Consequently, the recirculating B-cells have to pass T-cells and interdigitating cells on their way to the follicles. In the spleen the recirculating B-cells also pass through T-zones on their way to follicles. Experimental immunohisto-logical studies indicate that the T-zones are an early site of B-cell activation in both T-cell-dependent and T-cell-independent antibody responses (Fig. 4.8). There is evidence to indicate that antigen taken up by B-cells via their surface immunoglobulin can be presented to T-cells. This process is likely to occur in these T-cell-rich areas.

Recirculating B-cells, on leaving follicles of all secondary lymphoid organs other than the spleen, pass into the efferent lymphatics. They then travel in the lymphatics to the blood, although they may pass through lymph nodes on the way. Thus B-cells leaving Peyer's patches may migrate through mesenteric nodes. A small number of lymphocytes also pass into non-lymphoid tissues via ordinary capillaries. A schematic representation of lymphocyte recirculation pathways is given in Fig. 4.9. T-lymphocytes recirculate in an equivalent way between the T-cell-rich areas of secondary lymphoid tissues.

The non-recirculating B-cells of the splenic marginal zones and equivalent areas of other secondary lymphoid tissue

The marginal zones of the spleen in man surround the follicles. In tissue sections they are seen as a broad band of intermediate-sized lymphoid cells. Their chromatin is markedly less condensed than that of the follicular mantle B-cells, presumably reflecting more active transcription of their nuclear DNA. Immunohistology reveals that the cells of the marginal zone are B-cells which express IgM on their surface with little or no IgD (Fig. 4.7). The cells of the marginal zone are bathed in a blood sinusoidal system. Arterioles feed the marginal zone sinusoids directly; blood leaves these for the red pulp sinusoidal system

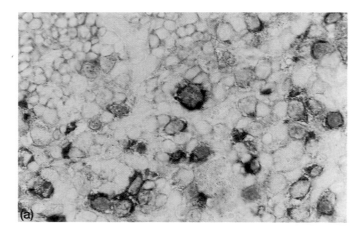

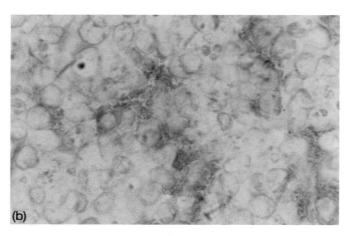

Fig. 4.8 Photomicrographs of the T-zone of spleen. The intense B-blast reaction in a rat spleen 2 days after secondary immunization with the T-cell-dependent antigen dinitrophenyl (DNP)–haemocyanin. DNP-binding B-blasts are stained blue using a DNP–alkaline phosphatase conjugate. T-cells are stained brown using indirect immunoperoxidase with the monoclonal antibody W3/13 which identifies rat T-cells. Cells which have been through the S-phase of the cell cycle in the 2 hours before the spleen was removed are stained red. They are identified immunohistologically by the uptake of the thymidine analogue 5'-bromo-2-deoxyuridine which was given to the rat over this period. This section and those in Fig. 4.12 and 4.13 were prepared by Dr Yong-Jun Liu who kindly gave permission for their inclusion in this chapter. Technical details of the staining procedures used are given in Liu *et al.* (1988). (b) Interdigitating cells in the T-zone of human spleen stained brown by indirect immunoperoxidase which is revealing binding of antibody against DQ class II major histocompatibility molecules. Nuclei are counterstained with haematoxylin.

which perfuses the macrophages on the cords of Billroth. Antigens carried in the blood, therefore, have the opportunity to interact with marginal zone B-cells before encountering the macrophages of the red pulp.

Marginal-zone B-cells do not recirculate but they have been shown to be derived from mature recirculating cells as opposed to newly produced virgin B-cells. Recent experimental evidence

produced in rats indicates that marginal-zone B-cells are a mixture of mature virgin B-cells and memory B-cells. (Virgin B-cells are cells which have never undergone antigen-driven proliferation.) Marginal-zone memory B-cells are generated during responses to T-cell-dependent and TI-1 antigens but not TI-2 antigens. On the other hand, it seems likely that marginal-zone B-cells are capable of being activated to produce antibody by all three classes of antigen, including TI-2 antigens. When activated by antigen they migrate to adjacent T-cell-rich areas and probably follicles before entering the cell cycle. Available evidence indicates that while recirculating B-cells are able to respond to T-cell-dependent and TI-1 antigens they do not respond to TI-2 antigens. These conclusions, drawn from studies in rodents, imply that marginal-zone B-cells and equivalent cells in other secondary lymphoid organs are vital for responsiveness to TI-2 antigens.

Extra-follicular B-cells resembling marginal-zone cells have been identified in other secondary lymphoid organs. Like marginal-zone cells they are located in a good position to encounter antigen. They have been found immediately deep to the dome epithelium which separates Peyer's patches from the lumen of the gut. There are similar cells located at the base of the crypt epithelium in the tonsils and on the inner surface of the subcapsular sinus in lymph nodes.

4.3.7 Newly produced virgin B-cells

It was indicated earlier that B-cells are produced throughout life in the bone marrow. The rate of primary B-lymphopoiesis and the fate of the cells produced in the bone marrow was not considered. In adult mice there is a daily output of B-cells from the bone marrow of some 5×10^7 cells. The number of B-cells in their secondary lymphoid organs is in the order of 2×10^8 cells. It follows that, if all newly produced virgin B-cells were to become mature peripheral B-cells, the average life span of peripheral B-cells would be in the order of 4 days. In reality the life span of follicular mantle B-cells seems to be nearer 4–6 weeks and that of marginal zone cells not much less. It follows that the life span of most newly produced virgin cells must be relatively brief. Kinetic studies of B-lymphopoiesis in man are not available. However, up to 3 per cent of human bone marrow mononuclear cells have the characteristics of committed B-cell progenitors. This makes it likely that the output of newly produced virgin B-cells in man is also substantial.

Analysis of the fate of newly produced virgin B-cells indicates that the high death-rate in these cells cannot be explained by the deletion of autoreactive clones. This has become clear from studies in which the peripheral B-cell pool was depleted while primary B-lymphopoietic capacity was conserved. In this situation the peripheral lymphoid tissues repopulate with B-cells at a rate approaching that of B-cell production in the bone marrow.

Severe depletion of the peripheral B-cell pools in adult rodents can only be reversed fully by the recruitment of newly produced virgin B-cells. After depletion of most peripheral B-cells and all B-lymphopoietic capacity the residual peripheral B-cells are able to respond to antigenic challenge to produce normal antibody

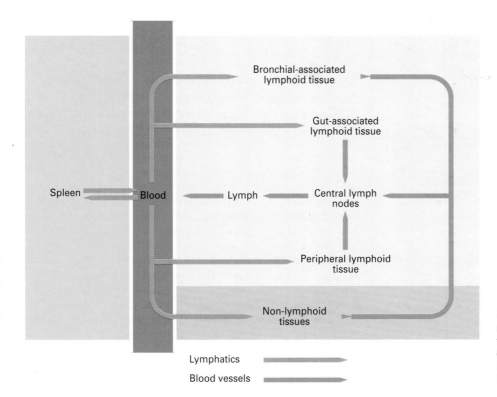

Fig. 4.9 A diagrammatic representation of the main lymphocyte recirculation pathways identified in rats. About a quarter of the recirculating cells leaving the blood pass into the spleen. Probably fewer than 10 per cent enter non-lymphoid tissues.

levels. The memory B-cells produced during these responses, however, are not sufficiently numerous to refill the small B-lymphocyte areas within secondary lymphoid organs. It follows that the mechanisms that control the number of peripheral B-cells are independent of those that regulate the extent of antigen-driven B-cell proliferation. Peripheral B-cells in adult rats show little or no capacity to increase their number by antigen-independent proliferation.

Although in normal circumstances most newly produced virgin B-cells have a short life-span, there is evidence that many of these cells leave the bone marrow and can be activated by antigen. Analysis of this process indicates that both T-cell-dependent and TI-1 antigens are able to activate newly produced virgin B-cells in periods when free antigen is available. During the established phase of antibody responses, however, when free antigen is no longer present, B-cell proliferation appears to be confined to memory B-cells. Studies of B-cell activation by TI-2 antigens suggests that these have little or no capacity to activate either newly produced virgin B-cells or recirculating follicular B-cells. A diagrammatic representation of the relationship of new produced virgin B-cells to peripheral B-cells is given in Fig. 4.10.

4.3.8 B-lymphocytes during ontogeny and CD5⁺ B-cells

B-cells are produced from early in the second trimester of human pregnancy. The first site of B-lymphopoiesis is the fetal liver, and B-cell production also takes place in the fetal spleen as well as bone marrow. Although the phenotype of B-cell pro-

genitors in fetal life is similar to that of progenitors in adult bone marrow, when fetal B-cells arrive in follicles, they express surface molecules that are not found on most adult B-cells. The best characterized of these are the molecules recognized by the CD5, CD1c, and CD10 clusters of monoclonal antibodies. Most peripheral B-cells express these molecules during fetal life and during the first year following birth. During the second year the number of cells with this phenotype declines, so that by the second birthday only around 5 per cent of small B-cells express these molecules.

In some diseases the numbers of CD5⁺ B-cells is markedly raised. These include rheumatoid arthritis and auto-immune thrombocytopenic purpura. The neoplastic B-cells in chronic lymphocytic leukaemia and, to a lesser extent, other low-grade B-cell non-Hodgkin's lymphomas characteristically express CD5 antigen. Analysis of the specificity of antibody on CD5⁺ B-cells has shown that it is often of broad reactivity, including affinity for auto-antigens. The physiological and pathological significance of this subset of B-cells is still relatively unclear.

4.3.9 Responses to T-cell-dependent antigens

Immunogenic and tolerogenic presentation of protein antigens

Although most foreign proteins are immunogenic, if presented in certain ways they may induce a state of specific immunological unresponsiveness (tolerance). This important phenomenon is discussed in Section 4.12. The present section only considers proteins presented in an immunogenic form.

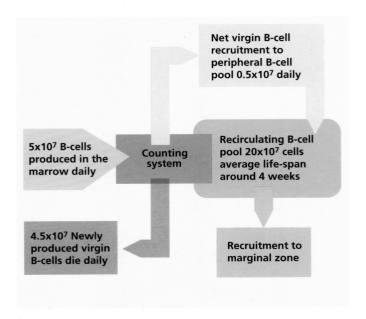

Fig. 4.10 Diagrammatic representation of the relationship between newly produced virgin B-cells and recirculating B-cells and marginal zone B-cells. The numbers given in the figure are based on experimental studies in adult mice. About 10 times as many newly produced virgin B-cells are generated than are required to replenish normal loss from the peripheral B-cell pools. However, if the peripheral pools are severely depleted the rate of their repopulation approaches the rate of primary B-cell production (see text). It is postulated that there must be a 'counting system' which monitors the size of the mature recirculating pool and recruits sufficient newly produced cells to replenish losses. Excess newly produced virgin B-cells must have a short life-span. Marginal zone B-cells are derived from the recirculating pool and not directly from newly produced virgin cells. (Drawn after MacLennan 1987, with permission.)

A single injection of a simple protein antigen into an individual who has not encountered that antigen previously often results in an unimpressive primary antibody response. Serum antibody titres are slow to rise and may not reach high levels or persist for a great length of time. Better responses are obtained when the protein is given in conjunction with a highly immunogenic antigen. Chemically killed *Bordetella pertussis* organisms, the traditional whooping-cough vaccine, is very effective in this respect. Agents acting in this way are known as immunological adjuvants. Even with an adjuvant, primary antibody response against simple protein antigens are relatively slow to develop.

The limiting factor in these primary responses is likely to be the availability of T-cell help. This can be demonstrated in responses to hapten–protein conjugates. If an individual is first primed to the carrier protein to generate carrier-specific T-cell help, then the subsequent anti-hapten response on challenge with the hapten–protein conjugate will be far more rapid than that achieved without carrier-priming (Fig.4.11). In both cir-

cumstances the anti-hapten response is primary, i.e. the availability of hapten-specific B-cells should be the same.

Recruitment of virgin B-cells and persistence of memory B-cell clones during T-cell-dependent antibody responses

It has been possible to investigate both virgin B-cell recruitment and persistence of memory B-cell clones by the transfer of genetically marked B-cells between congenic strains of rats. These experiments indicate that virgin B-cells are recruited into T-cell-dependent antibody responses when free antigen is available. During the established phase of these responses, when antigen is only available bound to FDC, continued B-cell activation is confined to memory B-cell clones. This does not mean that all memory B-cells are being continually activated by antigen on FDC. Memory B-cells which have colonized the marginal zones of the spleen, for example, are not proliferating and are only brought back into cycle if further free antigen becomes available. It seems likely that there is a relatively stable population of memory B-blasts sustained by antigen on FDC. These are likely to be the B-blasts which maintain plasma cell production during the many months of the established phase of T-cell-dependent antibody responses. It is uncertain whether recirculating memory B-cells, which pass though the follicles, are able to displace these blasts.

Sites of B-cell proliferation in T-cell-dependent antibody responses when T-cell help is not limiting

It can be seen in Fig. 4.8 that it is possible to identify the location of hapten-specific B-cells immunohistologically during responses to hapten–carrier conjugates. Using this technique, the sites of specific B-cell activation can be assessed at different stages of immune responses. The conclusions of such a study in rats immunized with hapten–protein conjugates is shown in Table 4.4.

The first site of specific B-cell proliferation in the spleen, following immunization, is the area rich in T-cells and interdigitating cells (Fig. 4.12a). One day after rats, previously primed with protein carrier, are challenged with hapten–protein conjugate, hapten-specific B-cells are seen proliferating in T-zones. This specific B-blast reaction is over within 4 days of immunization.

The follicles are the major site of B-cell proliferation in these responses. Hapten-specific blasts are apparent scattered among the small recirculating follicular B-cells at 36 hours after immunization (Fig. 4.12b). These increase in number dramatically during the next one and a half days. By 3 days after immunization the blasts are confluent in the centre of the follicle and the small recirculating cells are displaced to form a follicular mantle. At this stage the blasts are still expressing surface immunoglobulin. Over the subsequent 24 hours blasts expressing B-lineage antigens but not surface immunoglobulin appear in that part of the follicle nearest the T-zone. These are the centroblasts of the newly formed dark zone of the germinal centre. The centroblasts proliferate rapidly; cell cycle times for these cells in mice being in the order of 6–7 hours (Fig. 4.12c).

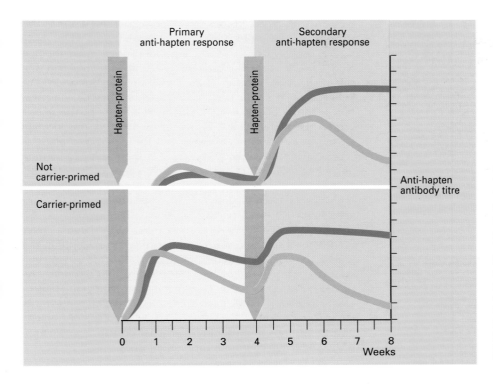

Fig. 4.11 Evidence that the availability of T-cell help is the limiting factor in primary T-cell-dependent antibody responses. Green lines represent IgM anti-hapten antibody titres. Blue lines IgG anti-hapten titres. Purple arrows represent immunization with hapten-protein. The top graph represents anti-hapten responses in a previously unimmunized rat given alum-precipitated hapten–protein antigen with killed pertussis bacteria as adjuvant at time 0 and soluble hapten protein alone 4 weeks later. The lower graph is of responses to soluble hapten–protein given at time 0 and 4 weeks later to rats previously immunized with alum-precipitated protein-carrier to generate carrier-specific T-cell help.

(Their phenotype in human germinal centres and that of other follicular cells is set out in Table 4.5.)

At about the same stage as the appearance of centroblasts in the dark zone, many non-dividing cells start to accumulate in the follicle centre. This area, which until 24 hours earlier was filled with B-blasts, is in that part of the follicle where the FDC network with its supply of antigen is most dense. These non-dividing cells are centrocytes, many of which can be seen to be hapten-binding cells. This area filling with centrocytes is known as the light zone of the germinal centre. At this stage, evidence of massive cell death is apparent within the light zone. This is provided by the characteristic appearance of cells undergoing self-destruction by apoptosis and the presence of nuclear debris resulting from this process within the local macrophages. These are the tingible body, or starry sky, macrophages associated with germinal centres.

The germinal centre reaction peaks within the first week of immunization with hapten–protein antigens in animals

Table 4.4 Sites of hapten-specific B-cell activation in T-cell-dependent antibody response

	Primary response in unprimed rats	Primary response in carrier-primed rats	Secondary response
Response in T-zones	Minimal towards end of first week	Moderate on days 2, 3, and 4	Massive on days 2, 3, and 4
Germinal centre reaction	Small in some follicles only, days 7–21	Large in all follicles, days 4–21	Moderate in most follicles, days 3–10
Marginal zone memory B-cells	Small numbers from day 6	Large numbers from day 3 for months	Lost in first 2 days return in large numbers day 3 and persist for months
Chronic follicular B-blast reaction	Not obvious	Found in centre of some follicles for many weeks	Found in centre of some follicles for many weeks
Red pulp plasma cells	Some, days 4–12	Many, days 1.5–6	Massive numbers days 1.5–6

Results based upon experiments where carrier protein priming was given as an intraperitoneal injection of alum-precipitated haemocyanin with killed pertussis organisms one month before challenge with soluble DNP-haemocyanin given intravenously. Primary responses in unprimed rats were assessed after the injection of alum-precipitated DNP-haemocyanin with killed pertussis organisms given intraperitoneally. Secondary challenge with soluble DNP-haemocyanin was given six weeks after soluble DNP-haemocyanin had been administered to carrier-primed rats. Times in the table refer to the time from the last immunization. Hapten-binding cells were identified as described in Fig. 4.8.

previously primed with the carrier protein (Table 4.4). At this stage most, if not all, follicles in lymphoid organs which have received antigen have active germinal centres. After the first week following immunization the germinal centre reaction subsides and is largely over within 3 weeks of immunization. The final stage of the follicular reaction follows when B-cell activation becomes confined to a cluster of B-blasts in the follicle centres. Hapten-specific B-blasts can be found in this location for many weeks. It seems likely that the established phase of T-cell-dependent antibody responses is the result of persistent antigen on FDC, which maintains proliferation of these blasts.

From the third or fourth day of these responses substantial numbers of hapten-binding B-cells are seen to colonize the marginal zones (Fig. 4.13). Occasional hapten-binding cells are also seen in the follicular mantles. These cells can be shown to have been derived as the result of antigen-driven proliferation but once in the follicular mantles or marginal zones are no longer in cell cycle. They can, however, be recruited into secondary responses following challenge with the same antigen. Hapten-binding memory B-cells have been found in the marginal zones for well over a year following a single injection of hapten–protein into rats primed with the carrier protein. Specific antibody production continues throughout this period.

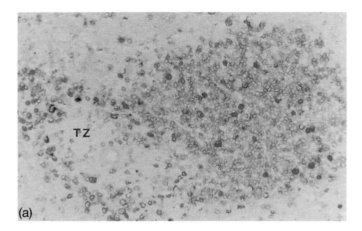

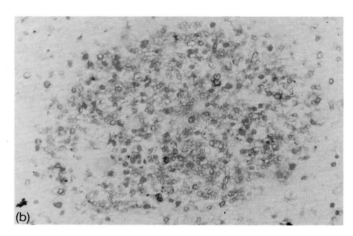

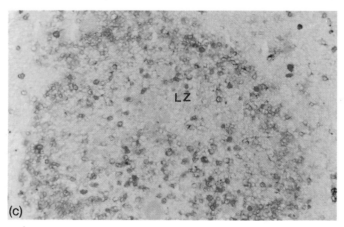

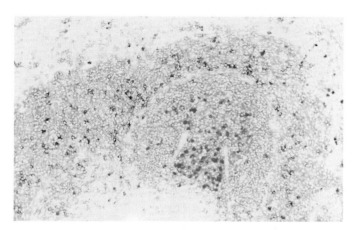

Fig. 4.13 The spleen of a haemocyanin-primed rat 6 weeks after challenge with DNP-haemocyanin (×120). The section was stained as those in Fig. 4.12 except that the brown staining now represents binding of the pan B-cell-reactive monoclonal antibody HIS 14.

Fig. 4.12 Photomicrographs (×160) taken at intervals during the response of protein carrier-primed rats to the hapten–protein conjugate DNP-haemocyanin. Cells stained red have taken up 5'-bromo-2-deoxyuridine in the two hours before the spleen was taken. Cells stained brown are small recirculating B-cells; identified with the monoclonal antibody HIS 22 which does not stain follicular B-blasts, centroblasts, centrocytes, or marginal zone cells. Faint blue staining identifies cells binding DNP–alkaline phosphatase. (a) Taken 24 hours after giving antigen. Some DNP-binding blasts can be identified in the outer layers of the T-zone (TZ). Only occasional blasts are present in the follicle, which is mainly packed with small B-cells. (b) Taken at 48 hours after antigenic challenge. More blasts are now present in the follicle. By 72 hours these blasts will form a confluent follicle centre (not shown). (c) Taken at 96 hours after antigen. HIS 22-positive recirculating B-cells are now confined to the follicular mantle. Centroblasts, which are mostly not hapten binding have formed a dark zone at the base of the follicle. Many of these have been through S phase in the previous 2 hours. The light zone (LZ) contains DNP-binding centrocytes which are generally not in cell cycle. Occasional B-blasts remain in the light zone.

Table 4.5 Phenotypic characteristics of follicular B-cells

Marker	Follicular mantle	Centroblast	Centrocyte
S CD10	−	+	+
S CD19	+ +	+ +	+ +
S CD20	+ + +	+ + +	+ + +
S CD22	+ +	+	+
S CD37	+ + +	+ +	+ +
S CD38	−	+ +	+ +
S CD39	+ +	−	−
S CD76	+ + +	−	−
S CD77	−	+ +	+
S Ig	+ +	−	+ +
In cell cycle	no	yes	no

Definition of the markers referred to in this table are given in the legend to Fig. 4.5.

Sites of B-cell proliferation in true primary responses to T-cell-dependent antigens

The response to hapten–protein in animals not previously primed with the carrier-protein is considerably less dramatic. Small numbers of blasts may be found in the T-cell-rich areas during the first few days following immunization. Proliferation of blasts in some follicles with modest germinal-centre formation is seen from about one week, with the reaction peaking at 10–12 days and subsiding over the next week or so. Some memory B-cells appear in the marginal zones at this time. Persistent B-cell activation in follicles and antibody production in primary responses to soluble antigen may be negligible. Antibody production will be more persistent if the antigen is given in a slow-release form, such as in alum precipitate or in an emulsion. This, in practice, is a primary response leading directly to a secondary response.

Sites of B-cell proliferation in secondary T-cell-dependent antibody responses

Secondary responses to hapten–protein differ quantitatively rather than qualitatively from primary anti-hapten responses in carrier-primed animals. The extrafollicular response is far more marked (Table 4.4). It is associated with memory B-cells passing from the marginal zones via follicles into T-cell and interdigitating cell-rich areas where they enter cell cycle (Fig. 4.8). Proliferation only persists in these sites for 3–4 days after re-exposure to antigen. The follicular response, as before, is much more persistent. But in secondary and subsequent responses to the same T-cell-dependent antigen the formation of mature germinal centres with centroblasts and centrocytes is less pronounced. The significance of this is not certain. It seems likely that both memory and virgin B-cells, activated in follicles, become B-blasts which can give rise to plasma cells and memory B-cells. It is possible that centroblasts are only generated from the blasts formed from virgin B-cells. The germinal-centre reaction is discussed further in relation to affinity maturation of antibody responses.

Sites of antibody production, the life-span of antibody-secreting cells, and the classes of antibodies produced during T-cell-dependent antibody responses

Antibody secretion generally takes place at a site distant from the place where antigen-driven B-cell proliferation takes place. During the first few days of responses to protein antigens in the spleen, antibody production occurs in the red pulp. However, in the established phase of the response antibody production is largely confined to the bone marrow. Similarly for responses in mesenteric lymph nodes, early antibody production is in the medulla of the lymph node whereas in the established response this shifts to the lamina propria of the gut. Table 4.6 lists the sites of antibody production and the classes of antibody produced in association with B-cell activation in different lymphoid organs:

1. in the period immediately following antigen administration; and

2. in the established phase of the response.

The change in site of antibody production during antibody responses is consistent with the hypotheses:

1. that B-cell activation in extrafollicular T-cell-rich areas gives rise to plasma cells which migrate to the medulla of lymph nodes or the red pulp of the spleen; and

2. that activation in follicles results in antibody production in the lamina propria of the gut or the bone marrow.

An additional feature of these two phases of plasma-cell generation is that early antibody production usually includes a substantial proportion of IgM while this is not characteristic of the established response. Also, while most plasma cells in the bone marrow and lamina propria have a life-span of about a month, those of the medulla of lymph nodes and the red pulp of the spleen survive for less than 3 days.

Evidence is now appearing to indicate that different growth and differentiation factors result in a bias of antibody

Table 4.6 Sites of antibody production, plasma-cell life-span, and class of antibody produced following T-cell-dependent B-cell activation in different sites

Site of B-cell activation	Early phase of response	Established response
Mesenteric lymph node	Short-lived plasma cells, mostly producing IgA or IgM, located in medulla of lymph node where B-cells were activated	Mainly long-lived plasma cells producing IgA in lamina propria of the gut
Spleen	Short-lived plasma cells mostly sited in the red pulp of the spleen. All classes of antibody produced but IgM production prominent	Long-lived plasma cells, mainly producing IgG or IgA, located in the bone marrow
Peripheral lymph node	Short-lived plasma cells, producing IgM, IgA, or IgG, in the medulla of the lymph node where the B-cells were activated	Long-lived plasma cells, mainly producing IgG or IgA, located in the bone marrow

This table is not comprehensive. For example, IgE production and antibody production in sites of inflammation are not mentioned. The information in this table is based on the administration of single doses of antigen. The differences between primary and secondary antibody responses set out in the text, Fig. 4.11 and Table 4.4 should be borne in mind when applying the data in this table.

production *in vitro* towards particular antibody classes and sub-classes. It seems likely that this reflects heterogeneity in the types of stimulatory signals which are received by B-cells when they are activated in different microenvironments.

4.3.10 Responses to T-cell-independent type 1 (TI-1) antigens

Although TI-1 antigens, by definition, are able to elicit antibody responses in animals which lack T-cells, in practice many of these antigens are able to elicit T help. In this situation the observed response in normal individuals includes the characteristics of T-cell-dependent responses but has certain additional features. It has already been mentioned that there are receptors for the lipolysccharides associated with most TI-1 antigens on macrophages and neutrophils, as well as on a proportion of B-cells. These lipopolysaccharides are capable of acting *in vitro* as polyclonal activators of B-cells with receptors for lipopolysaccharide. The induction of proliferation in this situation requires signals evoked from macrophages by lipopolysaccharide.

Analysis of the sites of B-cell activation in rodents in response to haptenated lipopolysaccharides indicates that this occurs in conjunction with macrophages and in the T-zones and follicles of secondary lymphoid organs. This macrophage-associated B-cell activation, which is prominent in the red pulp of the spleen, is short lived and produces a substantial proportion of IgM-secreting cells.

4.3.11 Responses to T-cell-independent type 2 (TI-2) antigens

The late onset of responsiveness to TI-2 antigens and the significance of this to infection with encapsulated bacteria have already been discussed. Unlike most TI-1 antigens, many clinically important TI-2 antigens are unable to elicit T-cell help. Responses to these antigens also differ from those to T-cell-dependent antigens in that they are not associated with long-term memory. TI-2 antibody responses can be relatively protracted, probably because of their poor degradation in the body and possibly because of selective localization of these antigens in specialized macrophages of the marginal zones of the spleen. Small numbers of hapten-binding B-blasts can be identified in follicles and in T-zones during TI-2 responses. Germinal-centre formation is not a characteristic of these responses.

In recent years it has become clear that selective deficiency in IgG responses to TI-2 antigens can occur in adults who respond normally to other classes of antigen. For this reason, adults with a history of infection with encapsulated bacteria, but who have normal immunoglobulin levels, should be assessed for their capacity to produce specific IgG antibodies in response to capsular polysaccharides.

4.3.12 Affinity maturation of antibody during immune responses

One of the characteristics of T-cell-dependent antibody responses is an increase in the relative affinity of antibodies produced with time. This cannot be attributed solely to recruitment of rare virgin B-cell clones, since affinity maturation can be seen to continue after the period of virgin B-cell recruitment (Table 4.4). Detailed analysis of the V-region structure of antibodies at different phases during T-cell-dependent antibody responses has shown that antibodies appear which have base-pair substitutions in the genes coding for the V regions. The rate of appearance of antibodies with many mutations in their V-region genes makes it probable that a mechanism is activated which brings about random base-pair substitution in V-region genes. The time of appearance of these mutations during T-dependent antibody responses coincides closely with the germinal-centre reaction. It has been suggested, on the basis of this indirect evidence, that the mutational process is induced in centroblasts and that their progeny, centrocytes, are selected by their ability to be activated by antigen on FDC. In this way the centrocytes with the highest affinity antibody would be most likely to survive. Recent experiments have shown that isolated human germinal centre B-cells kill themselves by apoptosis unless they are activated through their surface immunoglobulin.

4.3.13 Regulation of antibody responses

Antibody responses are regulated by the rate at which B-cells are activated to produce antibody-secreting cells. Several factors will affect this. These are mainly the availability of: antigen, antigen-presenting sites, T-cell help, and antigen-specific B-cells. In primary T-cell-dependent antibody responses the rate-limiting step is likely to be, first, the availability of T-cell help and, later, the availability of antigen. When neither of these two factors is in short supply responses become limited by the number of antigen-presenting sites. In practice this is likely to be the follicular capacity for T-cell-dependent responses.

The requirement for antigen to drive specific antibody responses can be demonstrated with cell transfer experiments between genetically identical animals. If splenic lymphocytes are transferred from an animal during the established phase of a B-cell-dependent antibody response, the recipient will not start to produce antibody against the antigen given to the donor. The recipient will, however, make a full secondary antibody response if given the antigen after cell transfer.

There is evidence that the availability of T-cell help is subject to a series of complex control mechanisms. These will be discussed in detail in the section on T-cell–B-cell interactions. In this section an attempt has been made to present a balanced view of the way in which the B-cell system is organized and how B-cells are activated in a controlled way to produce antibody of different classes at different sites. Many diseases are associated with deficient or disordered antibody production. We are now beginning to understand the cellular basis of antibody production. But this knowledge is still too incomplete to allow us to understand in detail more than a small minority of the defects in this system which result in disease.

4.3.14 Further reading

Organization of immunoglobulin genes

Berek, C. and Milstein, C. (1988). The dynamic nature of the antibody response. *Immunological Reviews*.
Calabi, F. and Neuberger, M. S. (1987). *Molecular genetics of immunoglobulin*. Elsevier, Amsterdam.

B-lymphocyte population kinetics

MacLennan, I. C. M. (1987). In *Mechanisms in B-cell neoplasia* (ed. F. Melchers and M. Potter), p. 63. Editiones Roche, Basle.
MacLennan, I. C. M. and Gray, D. (1986). Antigen-driven selection of virgin and memory B-cells. *Immunological Reviews* **91**, 63.
MacLennan, I. C. M., Liu, Y.-J., Oldfield, J., Zhang, J., and Lane, P. L. J. (1990). The evolution of B-cell clones. *Current topics in microbiology and immunology* **159**, 38–63.
MacLennan, I. C. M., Oldfield, S., Liu, Y.-J., and Lane, P. J. L. (1989). Regulation of B-cell populations. In *Cell kinetics of the inflammatory reaction* (ed. O. H. Iversen), p. 37. Springer-Verlag, Berlin.
Niewenhuis, P. and Opstelten, D. (1984). Functional anatomy of germinal centres. *American Journal of Anatomy* **170**, 421.

Immunohistological methods

Liu, Y.-J., Oldfield, S., and MacLennan, I. C. M. (1988). Memory B-cells in T-cell-dependent antibody responses colonise the splenic marginal zones. *European Journal of Immunology* **18**, 355.

Classes of antigen

Insel, R. A. and Anderson, P. W. (1987). IgG subclass distribution induced by immunization with isolated and protein-conjugated polysaccharide of *Haemophilus influenzae B* and G2m(n) distribution of serum IgG2 in man. In *Clinical aspects of IgG subclasses and therapeutic implications* (ed. F. Skvaril, A. Morell, and B. Perret), p. 128. Karger, Basle.
Mosier, D. E. and Subbarao, B. (1982). Thymus-independent antigens. In *B-lymphocytes today* (ed. J. R. Inglis), p. 70. Elsevier, Amsterdam.

B-cell activation and molecules associated with B-cells

Gordon, J. and Guy, G. R. (1987). The molecules controlling B-lymphocytes. *Immunology Today* **8**, 339.
Ling, N. R., MacLennan, I. C. M., and Mason, D. Y. (1987). B-cell and plasma cell antigens: new and previously defined clusters. In *Leucocyte typing III: White cell differentiation antigens* (ed. A. J. McMichael *et al.*). Oxford University Press, Oxford.
Knapp, W., Dörken, B., Gilks, W. R., Reiber, E. P., Schmidt, R. E., Stein, H., and Borne, A. E. G. Kr von dem (1989). B-cell antigens. In *Leucocyte Typing IV: White cell differentiation antigens, Part 1* (ed. W. Knapp *et al.*). Oxford University Press, Oxford.

Lymphocyte recirculation

Niewenhuis, P. and Ford, W. L. (1976). Comparative migration of T- and B-cells in the rat spleen and lymph nodes. *Cellular Immunology* **23**, 256.

4.4   Antibodies—structure and function

M. W. Turner

Antibody molecules belong to a group of structurally related glycoproteins which are collectively known as immunoglobulins. These proteins are present in the serum and tissue fluids of all mammals and lesser amounts are also found attached to the surface membranes of lymphocytes, macrophages, basophils, and mast cells.

In all higher mammals five major classes (or isotypes) are recognized (see Table 4.7) and in several species, including man, there are recognizable subclasses. The latter appear to have arisen after speciation occurred, since there are clear differences in both the number of subclasses and in their fine structure in different species.

Table 4.7   Nomenclature of human immunoglobulins

Present nomenclature	Shorthand	Previous nomenclature
Immunoglobulin G	IgG	γG-globulin 7Sγ-globulin
Immunoglobulin A	IgA	γA-globulin
Immunoglobulin M	IgM	γM-globulin 19Sγ-globulin
Immunoglobulin D	IgD	—
Immunoglobulin E	IgE	reagin

4.4.1   Basic structure of immunoglobulins

Each immunoglobulin molecule is essentially bifunctional; one region binds to antigen and another is able to express one or more effector functions, such as binding to phagocytic cells, activation of complement, or placental transmission. Some insight into the structural basis of this dual function began to emerge in 1959 when Porter showed that rabbit IgG class antibodies could be split into three large subunits by the plant protease, papain. Using the technique of ion-exchange chromatography, it was possible to show that two of the fragments were identical and retained the capacity to bind antigen (now known as Fab fragments-*fragment antigen binding*) whereas the other portion (Fc-*fragment crystalline*) was distinct and associated with effector function activity (Fig. 4.14).

Subsequently, techniques were developed for separating the peptide chains of immunoglobulins, and in 1962 Porter proposed a basic four-chain structure based on two types of constituent peptide chain. This model is illustrated in Fig. 4.15 and shows two small (*light*) polypeptide chains each with a molecular mass close to 22 000 Da linked to two larger (*heavy*) polypeptide chains having molecular masses greater than 50 000 Da. The structure is stabilized by disulphide bridges between cysteine residues and various non-covalent forces.

The light chain is the common structural feature of all immunoglobulin molecules. Two antigenic forms exist and are known as the κ and λ variants. In any one molecule both light chains are of the same type, although both variants are produced by most individuals.

The heavy polypeptide chain defines the class of a particular immunoglobulin molecule, and there is a distinctive chain characteristic of each class. These chains (γ, α, μ, δ, and ε in IgG, IgA, IgM, IgD, and IgE molecules, respectively) differ considerably in their primary amino-acid sequence and some of these differences underly the antigenic and biological characteristics of the intact molecule.

The advent of rapid amino-acid sequencing and the realization that myeloma proteins are pathological counterparts of normal immunoglobulin, permitted the determination of complete sequences for a number of myeloma proteins in the 1960s, and from such studies it became clear that both light and heavy chains could be divided into two distinct sections known as the *constant* and *variable* regions. In the light chain the constant region (C_L) corresponds approximately to the carboxy-terminal half of the chain, comprising approximately 107 amino-acid residues. In this region there are relatively few amino-acid differences between a set of κ proteins or a set of λ proteins, and such differences as exist are usually allotypic variants. In contrast, the amino-terminal half of the light chain (called V_L) shows a considerable amount of sequence variability from protein to protein. However, this variability is not distributed evenly throughout the region but is particularly clustered into regions which show exceptional variability. These regions are called hypervariable regions, and are present in both κ and λ chains. In the linear sequence numbered from the amino-terminal end of the chain they are located around residues 30, 50, and 95 (see Fig. 4.16).

The hypervariable regions are known to be directly involved in the formation of the antigen binding site and flanking them are numerous highly conserved amino-acid residues, called framework residues, which are believed to create the rigid framework within which the variability can be accommodated.

Heavy chains are also comprised of constant and variable regions. The variable region (called V_H) has approximately 113 amino-acid residues and the regions of hypervariability are found between residues 31–35, 50–65, and 95–102.

Depending on the immunoglobulin class, the constant regions of the heavy chains are either three or four times the length of the light chain constant region. When the amino-acid sequences of heavy chains of the same class are compared there are usually only minimal allotypic and isotypic variants.

In the assembled immunoglobulin molecule the light chain has two intra-chain disulphide bridges formed between cysteine residues—one in the variable and one in the constant region. The heavy (γ) chain of IgG is twice the length of the light chain and has four such bridges. As shown in Fig. 4.17, each bridge encloses a peptide loop of 50–70 amino-acid residues and each constitutes the central part of what is known as a 'homology region' or domain. This reflects the structural homology which has been observed when the heavy-chain sequences are divided

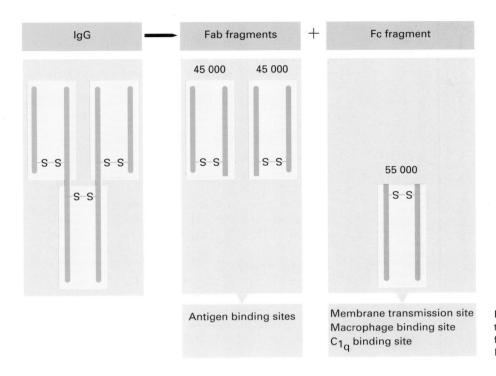

Fig. 4.14 Schematic diagram of IgG showing the effect of papain cleavage to give two Fab fragments (molecular mass 45 000 Da) and one Fc fragment (molecular mass 55 000 Da).

into four regions and the sequences aligned using the disulphide-bridged cysteines. In the light chain the variable and constant regions are called V_L and C_L, respectively. In the heavy chain the variable region is called V_H and the three constant region domains are (from the N-terminal end) C_H1, C_H2, and C_H3. The domain structures of IgG, IgA, and IgD are similar and the homology regions of each protein can be specifically designated on the basis of the heavy-chain letter. Thus, the constant regions of the IgGγ chain are $C_\gamma1$, $C_\gamma2$ and $C_\gamma3$, whereas those of IgA are $C_\alpha1$, $C_\alpha2$, and $C_\alpha3$. Another structural feature common to IgG, IgA, and IgD is the existence of a region of extended peptide chain between the C_H1 and C_H2 domains. This is generally known as the hinge region and is believed to confer some degree of flexibility on the antibody molecules.

IgM and IgE differ from all other immunoglobulin classes in that each has an extra constant region domain (C_H4) and no hinge region.

4.4.2 The three-dimensional structure of antibody molecules

In 1969 Edelman and Gall suggested that each homology region of an immunoglobulin molecule would be folded into a compact globular structure and linked to neighbouring domains by more loosely folded sections of peptide chain. High-resolution X-ray crystallography of several proteins has revealed that the domains do indeed share a basic folding pattern, with several segments of polypeptide chain lying parallel to the long axis of the domain. These parallel sections are arranged in two layers running in opposite directions with many hydrophobic amino-acid side-chains between the layers

(Fig. 4.18). Adjacent domains of the light and heavy chains are paired in the Fab regions, as are the C_H3 domains of the γ-chains. The C_H2 domains of IgG do not interact and are separated by carbohydrate structures (Fig. 4.19).

The variable regions of both light and heavy chains are folded in such a way that the hypervariable regions of both chains come together to create a surface cleft able to bind antigen (see Fig. 4.19). The interaction of antigen with antibody is based on a combination of non-covalent forces, such as hydrogen bonding, electrostatic forces, and van der Waals forces. It is a reversible reaction which can be represented by the equation:

$$Ag + Ab \rightleftharpoons AgAb$$

where Ag represents free antigen, Ab is free antibody, and AgAb is the antigen–antibody complex. The reaction is driven to the right by high-affinity antibodies which form strong bonds with antigenic determinants and result in relatively stable antigen–antibody complexes. Such complexes are more effectively cleared from the body by the concerted actions of the phagocytic and complement systems (see Sections 4.6 and 4.7).

4.4.3 Immunoglobulins as members of a larger family of proteins

The description of the immunoglobulin domain based on two β-sheets of peptide strands forming the characteristic sandwich has been followed by a cascade of reports demonstrating the ubiquity of this structural feature (see Williams 1987). The number of homologous molecules is so great that the collective name 'immunoglobulin supergene family' is now used to denote their presumed common ancestry. A few representatives

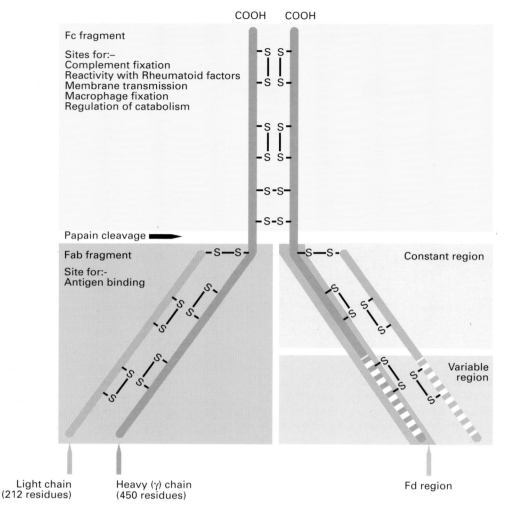

Fig. 4.15 Schematic diagram of human IgG1. The four-chain structure was originally suggested by Porter (1962). The distribution of the inter- and intra-chain disulphide bridges was determined subsequently.

are illustrated in Fig. 4.20, and Table 4.8 indicates that the genes coding for some of these structures are widely distributed on several different chromosomes.

4.4.4 Structure and function of individual immunoglobulin classes

In this section the properties of each class will be discussed separately, but for comparative purposes it is convenient to tabulate much of the data. Physicochemical and metabolic characteristics of human immunoglobulins are summarized in Table 4.9 and some selected effector functions are indicated in Table 4.10.

Immunoglobulin G

In man IgG accounts for 70–75 per cent of the total immuno-globulin pool. It has a heterogeneous electrophoretic mobility

ranging from the γ to the α_2 region. To a limited extent this arises from the subclass profile of the protein. There are four subclasses of human IgG (IgG1–IgG4) and these occur in the proportions of 66, 23, 7, and 4 per cent, respectively. The IgG1 and IgG3 proteins are electrophoretically cathodic, whereas IgG2 and especially IgG4 are relatively anodic and account for much of the material present in the β and α_2 positions.

The four subclasses of human IgG show a high degree of sequence homology and most of the differences are located in the flexible hinge regions of the molecules (Fig. 4.21). There are striking differences in the pattern of inter-heavy-chain S–S bonds and other structural features of this region, which appear to correlate with the expression of certain effector functions (see below).

IgG is, quantitatively, the most important serum immuno-globulin and after prolonged exposure to most antigens, the bulk of the antibody activity is associated with this class. A

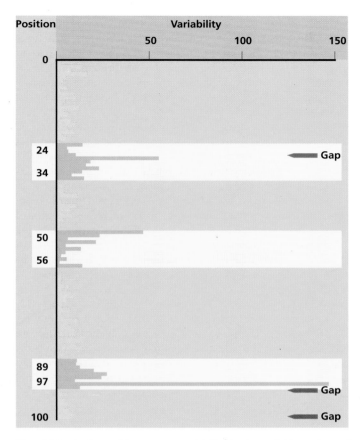

Fig. 4.16 Amino-acid sequence variability in the variable regions of human immunoglobulin light chains. In some sequences extra amino-acid residues occur and in order to maximize the comparison these have been excluded as indicated by the arrows. The three hypervariable regions are shown in brown, with precise ranges indicated by the yellow bands. Amino acid residues are numbered from the N-terminus of the peptide chain. (Derived from Wu and Kabat 1970.)

major function of IgG is the neutralization of bacterial exo-toxins. Most such toxins are relatively small, rapidly diffusing molecules and the ability of IgG to reach the extravascular spaces of the body is clearly advantageous in efficient toxin neutralization.

In most healthy adults, protein antigens generally induce

Table 4.8 Chromosomal location of various loci of the human immunoglobulin supergene family

Locus	Chromosome number
Ig λ light chain	22
Ig κ light chain	2
Ig heavy chain	14
T-cell receptor α-chain	14
T-cell receptor β-chain	7
MHC class I α chain	6
MHC class II $\alpha + \beta$ chains	6
β_2 microglobulin	15

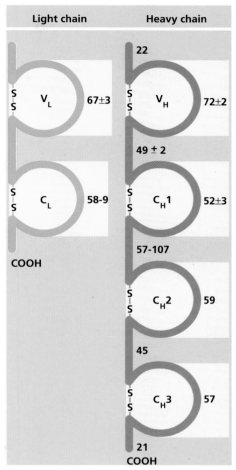

Fig. 4.17 Schematic diagram of human IgG homology regions showing the number of amino-acid residues enclosed by each intra-chain disulphide bridge. The range for the four subclasses is shown.

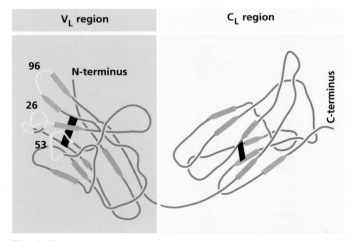

Fig. 4.18 Folding pattern of the polypeptide chain of the variable (V_L) and constant (C_L) region domains of a light chain. Both regions have similar sandwich-like structures with a three-stranded and a four-stranded layer stabilized by a disulphide bridge (black bar) and hydrogen bonds. The hypervariable regions are indicated by the yellow segments with adjacent residue numbers.

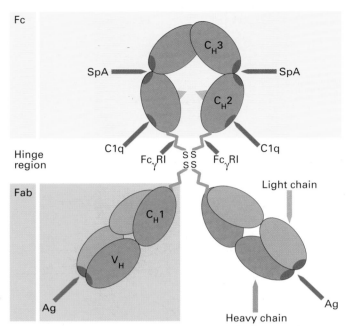

Fig. 4.19 The arrangement of the submolecular domains in human IgG1 and the location of binding sites for antigen (Ag), the complement component C1q the macrophage receptor (FcγRI) and protein A of *S. aureus* (SpA). Note the close pairing of domains except in the C_H2 region. Oligosaccharide groups are shown in dark pink.

IgG1 antibodies with some minor contribution from the IgG3 and IgG4 subclasses. In contrast, polysaccharide structures preferentially induce IgG2 responses, although children appear to produce IgG1 antibodies against both protein and carbohydrate antigens from bacteria. The selective adult pattern of IgG2 responses to carbohydrate structures is established by the early teens.

IgG is synthesized by the fetus as early as 20 weeks of gestation but the levels are insignificant compared to the quantities of maternal IgG which are transferred across the placenta in the last trimester of pregnancy. All four of the human IgG subclasses cross the placenta, although IgG2 may not be transferred as efficiently as the other three subclasses. Thus the newborn infant is provided with a spectrum of IgG molecules of differing antibody specificities and manifesting various effector functions.

The binding of the complement component C1q and the subsequent activation of the classical pathway (see Section 4.7) is one of the major effector functions expressed by IgG. As shown in Table 4.10 the rank order of efficiency is IgG3 > IgG1 > IgG2. IgG4 appears to be inactive, although the isolated Fc fragment of this subclass is able to bind C1q. It is likely that the site involved is located in the $C_\gamma 2$ domain of the molecule (see Duncan and Winter 1988), and the hinge region structure probably modulates the expression of this function. The N-terminal portion of the hinge is responsible for flexibility between the Fab

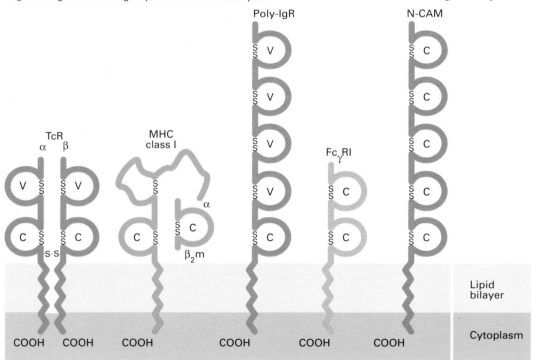

Fig. 4.20 Selected non-immunoglobulin members of the Ig superfamily. TcR is the T-cell receptor which functions as an antigen recognition unit on the surface of T-lymphocytes. MHC (class I) is the class I molecule of the major histocompatibility complex. The poly-Ig receptor is the membrane-bound form of a secretory component which binds specifically to polymeric IgA and IgM molecules. Fc_γ RI is the macrophage Fc receptor which interacts with the Fc regions of IgG molecules. N-CAM mediates adhesion of neural cells. V and C denote homology with either variable or constant region domains of Ig.

Table 4.9 Major physicochemical and metabolic characteristics of human immunoglobulins

Immunoglobulin class	Mean serum concentration (%)	Heavy chain	Molecular mass (Da)	Carbohydrate (%)	Half-life (days)	Distribution (% intravascular)
IgG1	9.0	γ_1	146 000	2–3	21	45
IgG2	3.0	γ_2	146 000	2–3	20	45
IgG3	1.0	γ_3	170 000	2–3	7	45
IgG4	0.5	γ_4	146 000	2–3	21	45
IgM	1.5	μ	970 000	12	10	80
IgA1	3.0	α_1	160 000	7–11	6	42
IgA2	0.5	α_2	160 000	7–11	6	42
Secretory IgA	0.05*	α_1/α_2	385 000	7–11	—	—
IgD	0.03	δ	184 000	9–14	3	75
IgE	0.00005	ε	188 000	12	2†	50

* Higher concentrations in external secretions.
† Molecules bound to mast cells have a longer half-life.

Table 4.10 Selected effector functions of human immunoglobulins

Immunoglobulin class	Complement fixation (C1q binding)	Placental transfer	Binding to mononuclear cells (FcγRI receptor)	Binding to neutrophils	Binding to mast cells and basophils	Binding to staphylococcal protein A
IgG1	+ +	+	+ + +	+ †	−	+
IgG2	+	+	−	−	−	+
IgG3	+ + +	+	+ + +	+ †	−	−
IgG4	−	+	+ +	−	− *	+
IgM	+ + +	−	−	−	−	−
IgA1	−	−	−	+ ‡	−	−
IgA2	−	−	−	+ ‡	−	−
Secretory IgA	−	−	−	?	−	−
IgD	−	−	−	−	−	−
IgE	−	−	−	−	+	−

* Evidence of heterologous interaction with non-human primate cells
† Binding to FcγRII and FcγRIII
‡ Binding to FcαR

regions and the rotational flexibility of each individual Fab region. There is a correlation between the length of this segment and the complement-activating function of the whole IgG molecule. Molecules with restricted flexibility, such as human IgG2 and IgG4, show poor complement activation.

The initiation of classical pathway activation of complement by IgG antibodies leads to the generation of C3b fragments of C3 which through the amplification loop of the complement system generates large quantities of the C3b opsonin. The latter is quantitatively the most important ligand involved in the phagocytosis of micro-organisms by both neutrophils and mononuclear phagocytes. However, IgG antibody molecules are themselves able to function directly as opsonins through interactions with the Fc receptors on phagocytic cells. There is evidence for at least three such Fc receptors: these are the FcγRI, FcγRII, and FcγRIII receptors. The best characterized of these is FcγRI, which is present on the surface of monocytes (density $1–4 \times 10^4$ sites per cell) and binds IgG with high affinity ($K_a = 10^8–10^9$ M^{-1}). The IgG1 and IgG3 subclasses bind more strongly than

IgG4 whereas IgG2 appears not to bind. There is now strong evidence that a leucine amino acid residue at position 235 (in the hinge region) is a major determinant of the IgG binding site interacting with this receptor.

FcγRII and FcγRIII are expressed on a broader range of cells, including neutrophils, eosinophils, and platelets. Their expression and specificity are still the subject of study but IgG1 and IgG3 again appear to interact most strongly with both.

Another interaction of the Fc region of IgG is with protein A of *Staphylococcus aureus*. In Caucasians this binding is expressed by IgG1, IgG2, and IgG4 molecules. IgG3 does not bind because an essential contact residue (histidine at position 435) is replaced by an arginine. In many Mongoloid sera the histidine residue is present and IgG3 is able to bind protein A.

Immunoglobulin A

In man IgA accounts for about 15–20 per cent of the serum immunoglobulin pool, where it exists mainly as a four-chain

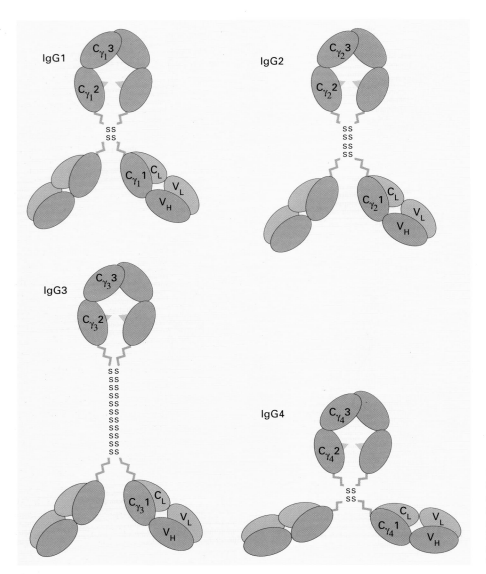

Fig. 4.21 Domain structure of four human IgG subclasses. Oligosaccharide groups are represented by the filled-in symbols. Note the extended hinge region of IgG3 which is believed to correlate closely with its potent effector function activity. The T-shape of IgG4 is suggested by hydrodynamic data and may explain the inability of this subclass to interact with the C1q component of complement.

monomer ($\alpha_2 L_2$) having a molecular mass of 160 000 Da. However, it is now believed that the major role of IgA in the body is to provide antibody activity at or near mucosal surfaces. Seromucous secretions, such as saliva, tracheobronchial secretions, bile, colostrum, milk, and genito-urinary secretions, are particularly rich in IgA. Such IgA exist mainly as a dimer of two monomeric IgA units, covalently linked by J chain and incorporating another peptide chain called secretory component (SC). The J (or joining) chain is a product of the plasma cells secreting polymeric IgA and IgM, and plays a key role in the polymerization of these molecules. The secretory component is a product of epithelial cells and plays an active role in the transportation of IgA into various secretions. The secretory component is now known to be synthesized as a larger precursor receptor molecule (the transepithelial receptor) which is found on the basolateral surface of many glandular epithelial cells. It is a member of the Ig supergene family and probably binds to polymeric IgA through strong *cis* domain–domain interactions.

The complex undergoes endocytosis and is transported across the cell in vesicles before release across the apical cell surface. During transport the receptor molecule is cleaved by a proteolytic enzyme and the portion remaining attached to the immunoglobulin is that which is recognized as secretory component. The structure of secretory IgA is shown in Fig. 4.22.

Most secretory IgA is produced by a population of IgA plasma cells found in large numbers beneath the epithelial surface of the gastrointestinal tract. IgA-secreting cells occur at a density approaching 400 000/mm³ in the lamina propria of the human small intestine. Heremans was the first to suggest that IgA creates an 'antiseptic paint' over the mucosal surfaces of the gastrointestinal, respiratory, and urogenital tracts. It has been demonstrated that the binding sites on the cell walls of pathogenic bacteria are unable to adhere to host oral epithelial cell surfaces after exposure to specific secretory IgA antibody. Secretory IgA has also been shown to inhibit the attachment of *Vibrio cholerae* to the intestinal mucosa, and it is possible that IgA

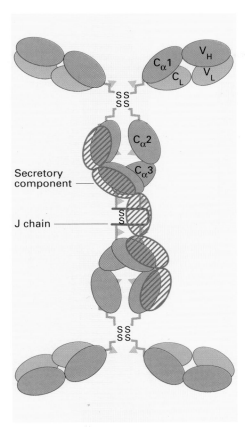

Fig. 4.22 Structure of human secretory IgA showing possible arrangement of IgA monomers, J chain, and secretory component. The details of the pairing between secretory component domains and the α-chains are conjectural. Oligosaccharide groups are shown in dark pink.

antibodies to other enteropathic bacteria and viruses function in a similar manner.

The lymphoid cells of the gut are readily primed by antigen crossing the gastrointestinal tract (see review by Walker 1981) and such lymphocytes have the capacity to migrate to other sites in the mucosal defence system, such as the mammary and salivary glands. Here they subsequently differentiate into plasma cells able to produce specific antibody to enteric antigen. Goldblum *et al.* showed that after pregnant women had been fed living (non-pathogenic) *Escherichia coli* during the last month of their pregnancy their colostrum subsequently contained IgA-secreting plasma cells manufacturing secretory antibody to *E. coli* lipopolysaccharide.

In man two subclasses of IgA have been identified, IgA1 and IgA2. In serum IgA1 seems to predominate (approximately 80 per cent of the total IgA) but in seromucous secretions the two subclasses occur in approximately equal proportions. As in the case of the human IgG subclasses, the major differences between the IgA1 and IgA2 molecules appear to be located in the hinge region.

Immunoglobulin M

In man IgM occurs predominantly in serum as a pentameric structure with a molecular mass of 970 000 Da. Each pentamer is assembled from basic four-chain subunits with two μ heavy chains and two light chains. These come together in association with a single J chain to give a characteristic stellate structure (Figs 4.23, 4.24). Each μ chain has five intra-chain domains (V, $C\mu1$, $C\mu2$, $C\mu3$, and $C\mu4$) and there is no hinge region. The $C\mu2$ domains link the Fab and Fc regions and impose a relative rigidity on the Fab arms which is not seen in IgG and IgA with their hinge regions. Nevertheless, as revealed by electron microscopy, the molecule is able to cross-link bacterial flagellae and often adopts a staple-like configuration when making a multi-point atachment to a single flagellum.

IgM accounts for about 7–10 per cent of the serum immunoglobulin pool and antibodies in this class are frequently the first to be detected following exposure to antigen. The protein has a predominantly intravascular location, and seems to be critically involved in the elimination of micro-organisms from the bloodstream. IgM levels are frequently observed to be high following prolonged periods of exposure to parasites with an intravascular phase, e.g. in malaria and trypanosomiasis.

IgM is synthesized by the fetus and low levels of the protein are demonstrable at birth. A high level of serum IgM in the newborn is usually indicative of intra-uterine infection and occurs particularly in association with rubella, syphilis, toxoplasmosis, and cytomegalovirus infections. After birth the level of serum IgM rises rapidly in response to antigenic exposure as the gut is colonized with micro-organisms. By one year of age most healthy infants have IgM levels close to adult values.

When bound to cell membrane antigens, IgM is a potent activator of complement through the classical pathway and, as such, it is able to promote the lysis of neisserial organisms. More importantly, however, it is able to promote phagocytosis through the generation of C3b fragments from the C3 component. The C3b molecule is the most important opsonic ligand involved in phagocytosis. There are at least three receptors on the cell membranes of phagocytic cells (CR1, CR3, and CR4) which interact with C3b and/or its breakdown product iC3b (see Section 4.7.7). The close interdependence of IgM and C3 is clearly illustrated in individuals with primary C3 deficiency. These patients make normal early IgM antibody responses on primary contact with organisms but in the absence of C3 are unable to opsonize efficiently. Consequently, they suffer from recurrent otitis media, pneumonia, and meningococcal meningitis.

IgM is an extremely efficient agglutinating antibody and, consequently, promotes the formation of large immune complexes which are readily removed by the reticuloendothelial system.

Although IgM antibodies are almost always of low affinity, they have multiple antigen-binding regions (theoretically 10, though the effective valency is almost always less) and are able to maintain their contact with repeating antigenic structures. This so-called *avidity* phenomenon is directly related to the functional multivalency of the molecule.

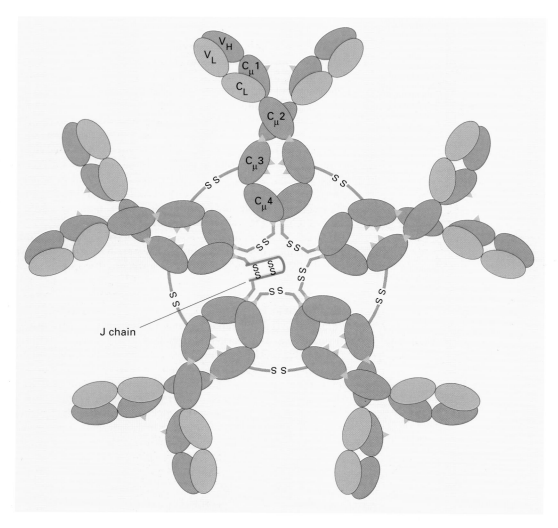

Fig. 4.23 Domain structure of human IgM showing domain interactions, oligosaccharide groups (dark pink), and possible location of J chain.

Immunoglobulin D

IgD is a trace serum protein and accounts for less than 1 per cent of the serum immunoglobulin pool. It is essentially a lymphocyte membrane protein, where it commonly occurs in association with IgM. For this reason it was suggested more than a decade ago by Vitetta and Uhr that the protein plays a role in the differentiation of B-lymphocytes.

IgD is a heavily glycosylated four-chain structure (Fig. 4.25). It has a hinge region which is particularly susceptible to enzymic cleavage, and this property has been linked to the putative role in B-cell triggering. The membrane form of IgD is anchored to the cell surface through an additional C-terminal sequence in the heavy (δ) chains.

There is no selective association of particular antibody responses with IgD and the circulating protein is devoid of all known effector functions.

Immunoglobulin E

Healthy individuals have trace amounts of IgE in their circulation and it is probable that, as with IgD, the bulk of the protein is to be found on cell surfaces, particularly circulating basophils and tissue mast cells.

IgE has a molecular mass of 188 000 Da and exists as a four-chain monomer with two light chains and two ε chains. Structural analysis has revealed four constant-region domains in the ε chain, and the overall molecular structure is somewhat similar to an IgM subunit (Fig. 4.26). This is most apparent in the junction between the Fab and Fc regions, where the hinge region common to IgG, IgA, and IgD is replaced by an intact homology region.

The major effector function of IgE is related to its strong interaction with tissue mast cells and circulating basophils through a site spanning the $C_\varepsilon 2$–$C_\varepsilon 3$ junction in the Fc region. There are

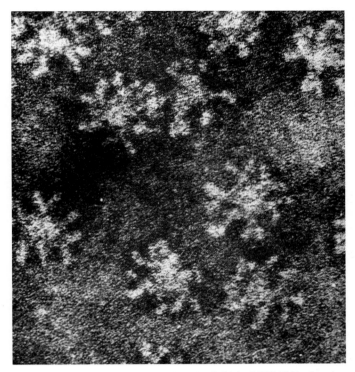

Fig. 4.24 Electron micrograph of murine IgM (× 1 620 000), showing characteristic stellate structure. (Photograph kindly supplied by Dr R. Dourmashkin, Clinical Research Centre, Harrow, UK.)

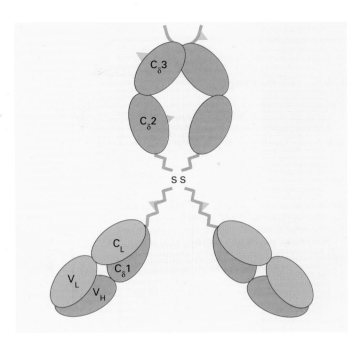

Fig. 4.25 Domain structure of human IgD showing the hinge region and oligosaccharide groups (dark pink).

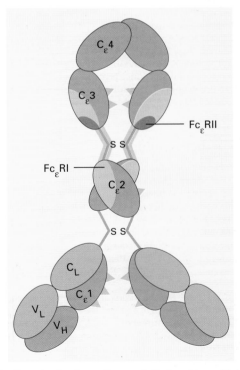

Fig. 4.26 Domain structure of human IgE, showing multiple oligosaccharide groups (dark pink) but the absence of a hinge region. Binding to the $Fc_\varepsilon RI$ receptor of mast cells occurs through a site spanning the $C_\varepsilon 2$ and $C_\varepsilon 3$ domains (green). Binding to the low affinity $Fc_\varepsilon RII$ receptor of eosinophils etc. occurs through a motif in the $C_\varepsilon 3$ domain (red).

many cell surface $Fc_\varepsilon RI$ receptors (10^4 on basophils and 10^6 on mast cells) and when two cell-bound IgE molecules are cross-linked by antigen the cell becomes activated. Such activation results in the release of a large number of potent mediators and factors. For example, the granules of the cell release histamine, various proteolytic enzymes, and a chemotractant for eosinophils. Changes in the lipid bilayer of the cell generate so-called membrane-derived mediators, such as the leukotriene family and various prostaglandins (see Section 4.9.1).

In patients with allergic disease, serum IgE levels are modestly increased (hay fever) or markedly elevated (asthma/atopic eczema). The triggering antigen is frequently a rapidly diffusing protein from a pollen grain (hay fever) or from the faecal particle of the house dust mite (asthma) and the symptoms experienced by the patient will depend on a complex range of ill-understood host factors (see Section 4.9). However, such common hypersensitivity reactions have diverted attention away from the major role of IgE in anti-parasite immunity. It seems to be particularly important in responses to helminths, and patients with such infestations have extremely elevated IgE levels. Work in schistosomiasis by Capron and co-workers has revealed a complex network of interactions involving IgE binding, not only to mast cells but also to platelets and macrophages through a second low-affinity receptor ($Fc_\varepsilon RII$). These interactions, involving a site in the $C_\varepsilon 3$ domain of IgE, lead to the recruitment of eosinophils and parasite killing by release of the major basic protein from the eosinophil granules.

4.4.5 Bibliography

Capron, A., Dessaint, J. P., Capron, M., Joseph, M., Ameison, J. C., and Tonnel, A. B. (1986). From parasites to allergy: a second receptor for IgE. *Immunology Today* **7**, 15–18.

Duncan, A. R., Woof, J. M., Partridge, L. J., Burton, D. R., and Winter, G. (1988). Localization of the binding site for the human high-affinity Fc receptor on IgG. *Nature* **332**, 563–4.

Duncan, A. R. and Winter, G. (1988). The binding site for C1q on IgG. *Nature* **332**, 738–40.

Edelman, G. M. and Gall, W. E. (1969). The antibody problem. *Annual Review of Biochemistry* **38**, 415–66.

Goldblum, R. M., *et al.* (1975). Antibody forming cells in human colostrum after oral immunization. *Nature* **257**, 797–9.

Helm, B., Marsh, P., Vercelli, D., Padlan, E., Gould, H., and Geha, R. (1988). The mast cell binding site on human immunoglobulin E. *Nature* **331**, 180–3.

Porter, R. R. (1959). The hydrolysis of rabbit γ-globulin and antibodies with crystalline papain. *Biochemical Journal* **73**, 119–26.

Porter, R. R. (1962). The structure of γ-globulin and antibodies. In *Symposium on basic problems in neoplastic disease* (ed. A. Gelhorn and E. Hirschberg), p. 177. Columbia University Press.

Vercelli, D., Helm, B., Marsh, P., Padlan, E., Geha, R. S., and Gould, H. (1989). The B-cell binding site on human immunoglobulin E. *Nature* **338**, 649–51.

Vitetta, E. S. and Uhr, J. W. (1975). Immunoglobulin receptors revisited. *Science* **189**, 964–9.

Walker, W. A. (1981). Antigen uptake in the gut. Immunologic implications. *Immunology Today* **2**, 30–4.

Williams, A. F. (1987). A year in the life of the immunoglobulin superfamily. *Immunology Today* **8**, 298–303.

Wu, T. T. and Kabat, E. A. (1970). An analysis of the sequences of variable regions of Bence Jones proteins and myeloma light chains and their implications for antibody complementarity. *Journal of Experimental Medicine* **132**, 211–50.

4.4.6 Further reading

Burton, D. R. (1990). Antibody: the flexible adaptor molecule. *Trends in Biochemical Science* **15**, 64–9.

French, M. A. H. (ed.) (1986). *Immunoglobulins in health and disease*, Immunology and Medicine Series. MTP Press Ltd, Lancaster.

Glynn, L. E. and Steward, M. W. (ed.) (1981). *Structure and function of antibodies*. John Wiley and Sons, Chichester.

Hahn, G. S. (1982). Antibody structure, function and active sites. In *Protein abnormalities*, Vol. 1. *Physiology of immunoglobulins: diagnostic and clinical aspects* (ed. S. E. Ritzmann), pp. 193–304. Alan Liss Inc., New York.

Shakib, F. (ed.) (1986). *Basic and clinical aspects of IgG subclasses*, Monographs in Allergy, Vol. 19. Karger, Basel.

Steward, M. W. (1984). Antibodies: their structure and function. *Outline studies in biology* (ed. W. J. Brammer and M. Edidin). Chapman and Hall, London.

Turner, M. W. (1983). Immunoglobulins. In *Immunology in medicine* (2nd edn) (ed. E. J. Holborrow and W. G. Reeves), pp. 35–58. Grune and Stratton, London.

Williams, A. F. and Barclay, A. N. (1988). The immunoglobulin super-family-domains for cell surface recognition. *Annual Review of Immunology* **6**, 381–405.

4.5   T-cells

P. C. L. Beverley

4.5.1   Introduction

Evidence for subtypes of lymphocytes

Although a great deal was known with regard to the specificity and function of antibody in the early years of the century, the discovery that small lymphocytes were the mediators of immune responses is relatively recent. Only in the 1960s was the first evidence obtained, from experiments relying on anatomical separation, that there were functionally distinct subtypes, of thymus-derived (T) and bone marrow-derived (B), lymphocytes. The subsequent discovery that these subtypes could be separated according to their surface antigen phenotype (the array of glycoproteins carried in the cell membrane) was an important step. Although separation was initially carried out with allo- or heteroantisera, the development of monoclonal antibodies (mAbs) has provided innumerable reagents to investigate the structure and function of the lymphoid system.

T- and B-cells

After the initial separation of T- and B-cells, it soon became clear that while the main function of B-cells was to secrete antibody, T-cells could mediate a bewildering array of functions both *in vivo* and *in vitro* (Table 4.11), posing the question whether there was a single T-cell type or further heterogeneity in the T-cell lineage. Evidence that there were functionally distinct types came once more from experiments using T-cells from anatomically separated sites, but it was impossible to decide whether these represented cells of different lineages, or a single lineage but at different stages of maturation. Figure 4.27 illustrates these possibilities. Clearly, if useful information is to be gained from phenotypic analysis of lymphocytes, it is important to understand the functions of phenotypically distinct cells and their ontogenetic relationships. In this section therefore, I shall

Table 4.11   T-cell function

In vitro	*In vivo*
Help for antibody responses	Protection against infection
Class I and II allo or restricted cytotoxicity	Delayed type hypersensitivity Graft rejection
Unrestricted (LAK) cytotoxicity	Graft versus host response
Proliferation to mitogens, antigens, and alloantigens (MLR)	Tumour immunity
Suppression of antibody and proliferative responses	
Lymphokine production	

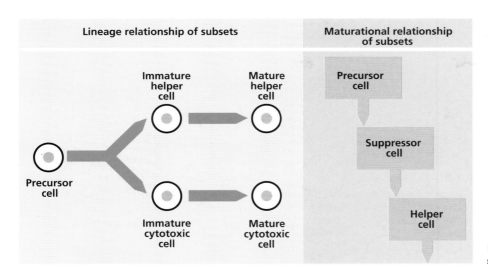

Fig. 4.27 Lineage and maturational relationships of T-cell subsets.

concentrate on discussing how phenotype and function are associated in T-cells and attempt to show which phenotypic markers identify stages of maturation or cell lineage. The discussion will concentrate on human T-cells but, where necessary, data from animal experiments will be included.

Terminology

Monoclonal antibodies have provided reagents for identifying and separating lymphocyte subsets and for characterizing the molecules they express. The large number of mAbs produced necessitated the development of a terminology for the antigens, worked out in three international workshops. In these studies, antibodies are grouped together on the basis of similar reactivity, in blind serological tests carried out in many laboratories, on a large panel of different cell types. Such a Cluster of mAbs defines a leucocyte Differentiation antigen, hence the CD nomenclature. This serological definition is backed up in most cases by biochemical, and frequently molecular genetic, analysis of the antigens.

A limitation of this terminology is that no molecule can be assigned an internationally agreed name until at least two mAbs reacting with it have been produced. There are thus some mAbs in common usage which have still to be referred to by proprietary names. In addition, the terminology is not always logical in dealing with molecular complexes of several polypeptides. Thus, for example, the β-chain of the leucocyte function antigen (LFA) has been assigned to CD18 while the three different α-chains, with which it can associate are termed CD11a, b, and c.

4.5.2   Ontogeny of T-cells

The first cells which express sufficient of the antigens characteristic of T-cells to be recognized as such, are found in the embryonic thymus. Cells able to colonize the thymus (prothymocytes) are found in the yolk sac, fetal liver, and bone marrow, but are virtually absent from the peripheral lymphoid organs. In man, cells expressing cytoplasmic CD3 antigen (cCD3), but not T-cell receptor (TCR) polypeptides, can be found as early as the 7th–9th weeks of gestation. Similar cells are found around the fetal thymic rudiment from the 7th week. Nuclear terminal deoxynucleotidyl transferase (Tdt), an enzyme almost certainly playing a role in the generation of diversity in both immunoglobulins and TCRs, is not seen in thymocytes until much later, at 17–19 weeks. It is not clear what these Tdt-negative cells represent, but they do not appear to be precursors of peripheral TCR $\gamma\delta$ cells since very few thymic $\gamma\delta$ membrane-positive cells are found at any stage in the human thymus.

Following the appearance of Tdt-positive cells, the thymus acquires its characteristic structure and cell populations. Prothymocytes probably enter at the corticomedullary junction and migrate to the subcapsular area which has a specialized epithelium. In this area thymocytes acquire the cortical thymocyte antigen, CD1, and proliferate actively. It is thought that the cells then undergo a sequence of maturation steps while migrating toward the corticomedullary junction. They express both CD4 and CD8, undergo gene rearrangement to generate diverse TCR $\alpha\beta$ heterodimers, and become self-tolerant. Although the details of these selective processes are still not well understood the outcome is that cells able to recognize foreign antigens in the context of self major histocompatibility complex (MHC) antigens are produced (see also Section 4.2). Such functionally mature cells, which are either CD4- or CD8-positive are found in the medulla and presumably represent the survivors of the cortical selection process, since it has been estimated that more than 90 per cent of cells generated in the thymus also perish there. These events are summarized in Fig. 4.28. It is interesting that almost all T-cell tumours, in children, resemble either cortical thymocytes or prothymocytes; both rapidly dividing populations. Thus the most useful markers for the identification of these T-acute lymphocytic leukaemias are cCD3, CD7, and CD2, which appear earliest in T-cell development, and Tdt.

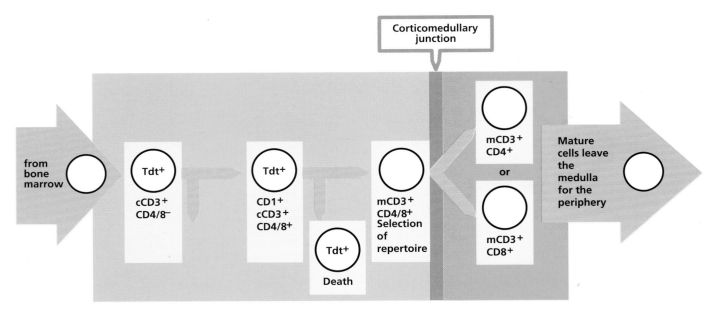

Fig. 4.28 Thymic differentiation.

4.5.3   The T-cell receptor

Structure and genetic organization

For many years the nature of the T-cell receptor for antigen remained obscure until in the early 1980s the use of monoclonal T-cell populations, antibodies, biochemical and molecular genetic analysis, revealed that mature T-cells express a characteristic heterodimer with significant structural similarities to immunoglobulin. The majority of T-cells are now known to express a receptor consisting of α- and β-chains with molecular masses of 45–50 kDa. Human β-chain genes are located at chromosomal position 7q35 and the α-chain genes at 14q11–12. A minority of T-cells express a heterodimer made up of γ- and δ-chains. The γ-chain genes are also coded by genes on chromosome 7 and the δ-chain genes are within the α locus.

As is the case with immunoglobulins, T-cell receptor polypeptides consist of the product of several different genes (Fig. 4.29). Thus human β-chains consist of a V_β segment of 110 amino acids, which has structural similarity to an immunoglobulin V region, a D segment of 3–4 amino acids, a J segment of 15–17 amino acids, and a constant region of ~ 130 amino acids. The constant region includes a hydrophobic transmembrane segment and short (3–5 amino acids) cytoplasmic tail. The general structure of α-, γ-, and δ-chains is similar though not all of these include D segments.

As in the immunoglobulins, each T-cell-receptor gene cluster includes a large number of V genes and smaller numbers of D and J segments, which are assembled to generate large numbers of different VDJ combinations. Additional polymorphism is generated by deletion or addition of nucleotides during VDJ rearrangement. Rearranged VDJ genes are then joined with one of the limited number of constant regions. Table 4.12 shows

Table 4.12   T-cell receptor genes

Receptor chain	Number of genes			
	V	D	J	C
α	>50	0	>100	1
β	>50	2	13	2
δ	>5*	3	2	1
γ	~8	0	5	2

* In theory V_α genes could be assembled with δ chain DJ and C genes but it is not known whether this occurs.

current estimates for the numbers of genes in each of the four gene clusters. The V genes are grouped into several families of related genes. There is evidence from the mouse that expression of V_β gene families is influenced by the MHC allele carried by an individual as well as minor transplantation antigens. Preliminary human data links expression of T-cell-receptor alleles (detected by restriction fragment length polymorphism (RFLP)), analysis with some auto-immune diseases.

Both $\alpha\beta$ and $\gamma\delta$ TCR are invariably expressed only in mCD3-positive cells. Strong evidence suggests that the TCR and CD3 are associated at the cell surface and CD3 may function as a signal transducer for the receptor.

Expression and function of T-cell receptors

The ontogeny of TCR $\alpha\beta$ and $\gamma\delta$ has been described above. In the periphery, most CD4 and CD8 T-cells express $\alpha\beta$ receptors. The TCR functions on these cells as the receptor for antigen, which is recognized in association with Class I or II major histocompatibility complex (MHC) antigens (genetic restriction, see below). Whereas the role of the TCR in determining restric-

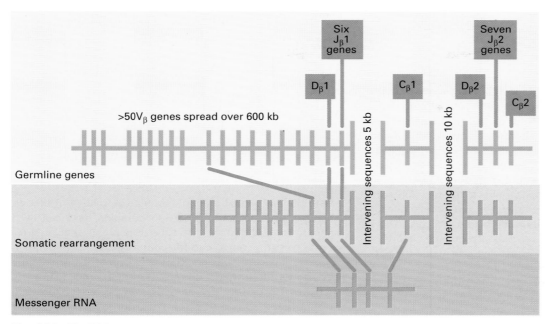

Fig. 4.29 The TCR$_\beta$ gene locus.

tion is not yet clear the CD4 and CD8 molecules themselves certainly contribute to interaction of T-cells with appropriate MHC-bearing target or accessory cells.

More recently it has been observed that the peripheral blood contains a fraction of $\gamma\delta$ T-cells. This is very variable between individuals, generally representing 1–4 per cent of T-cells but in a few individuals up to 20 per cent are seen. These cells are predominantly CD8-positive or CD4/8-negative. While their function remains unclear there is some evidence that they are not restricted by classical class I or II MHC antigens, and that they can act as cytotoxic effector cells. Whether all peripheral $\gamma\delta$ cells are thymus-derived or even thymus-dependent is also a matter of debate.

4.5.4   The human CD4 and CD8 subsets

Function

Early on two major and non-overlapping subsets of T-cells were defined, identified by CD4 and CD8 mAbs. The function of these subsets in man has been extensively investigated *in vitro*. CD4 cells provide help for pokeweed mitogen (PWM) driven immunoglobulin synthesis and for specific antibody responses. While the mechanisms involved in helper function remain imperfectly defined, but probably involve an antigen-specific interaction of T- and B-cells as well as non-specific signals, it is clear that CD4 cells are the major helper subset for antibody production. Less extensive data suggest that CD4 cells are also required for optimal generation of effector cytotoxic T-cell and are the principal subset involved in delayed-type hypersensitivity responses in animals.

In contrast, CD8 cells do not generally provide help for antibody responses and contain both precursors and effectors of cytotoxic cells directed either at alloantigens or virus-infected autologous targets. CD8 cells have also been shown to suppress Ig responses induced by non-specific mitogens or in an autologous mixed lymphocyte response. The properties of the two subsets are summarized in Table 4.13.

Genetic restriction

Although earlier data supported a clear-cut separation into CD4 helper/inducer and CD8 suppressor/cytotoxic subsets, many subsequent experiments have blurred this distinction. CD4 cytotoxic cells are well recognized in both mouse and man, and CD8 helpers have also been described. There are several likely reasons for this. First is the recognition that the most decisive difference between CD4 and CD8 cells is that CD4 cells recognize MHC class II allo-antigen, or specific antigen in association with class II, and CD8 cells MHC class I, or specific antigen in association with class I; the phenomenon of genetic restriction. There is thus no a priori reason that all CD4 cells should be helpers or CD8s killers. However, expression of CD4 or CD8 may bias the function of a cell, as it has been suggested that the CD4 and CD8

Table 4.13   Functions of the CD4 and CD8 subsets

Functions	CD4	CD8
Genetic restriction	MHC II	MHC I
Help for Ig production	+ +	− (+)
Suppression	− (+)	+ +
Cytotoxicity	+	+ +
IL-2 production	+ +	+
IL-4, 5, 6 production	+ +	− (+)
γ-IFN production	+	+

(+) indicates that this is infrequently observed.

antigens guide the two types of T-cells to interact with different cell types.

T-cell-accessory cell interaction

CD4 cells generally interact with class II bearing accessory cells. These are heterogeneous, including macrophages, dendritic cells, and Langerhans cells of the skin, and there is also evidence that many tissue cells, after exposure to γ-interferon (γ-IFN) or other cytokines, can express MHC class II antigens and function as accessory cells. It has been suggested that this is an important mechanism in the pathogenesis of auto-immune disease. In contrast, CD8 cells appear able to interact with any class I expressing target. Direct evidence in support of a role for CD4 and CD8 as guides, which act by binding to class II or I respectively, comes from recent experiments showing binding of CD4-transfected cells to class II expressing cells while the parental CD4-negative cells did not bind.

The outcome of the interaction of the T-cell and accessory cell may vary because 'accessory' cells differ in the way in which they process antigen. Exogenous antigen is most likely taken up by phagocytic cells, degraded, and then displayed in association with class II. Other cell types may more effectively process internal antigen (e.g. derived from polypeptides of a virus infecting the cell) and display it in association with class I. This suggests two distinct intracellular pathways for antigen processing.

A second reason for the overlap between CD4 and CD8 cells is that they share many properties which determine their function. The outcome of the interaction between a T-cell and another cell, e.g. a B-cell, accessory cell, or potential target, probably depends on how the two cells make contact and the range of cytokines produced by both T-cell and non-T-cell. The strength of the cell–cell contact, in turn, depends on the cell surface molecules displayed by both cells. These include the T-cell receptor and several accessory molecules, such as CD4 or CD8, CD18/CD11a (LFA-1), and CD2. These latter interact respectively with MHC antigens, I-CAM 1 and LFA-3 on the non-T-cell. The importance of these accessory interactions may also depend on the affinity of the T-cell receptor for its antigen, as suggested by experiments showing that CD8 cytotoxic clones vary greatly in their susceptibility to inhibition by CD8 antibody.

Lymphokine production

An important consequence of T-cell–accessory cell interaction is the production of lymphokines by the T-cell. It is clear that not all T-cells produce the same spectrum. In man limiting dilution analysis shows that more CD4 than CD8 cells produce interleukin-2 (IL-2) but γ-IFN is produced equally well by both subsets. While there is little data comparing directly the production of putative B-cell stimulatory lymphokines (IL-4, 5, 6) by CD4 and CD8 cells, the fact that CD8 cells only rarely provide help, suggests that the principal producers of these lymphokines are CD4 cells.

4.5.5   The problem of suppressor cells

Suppressor cells remain mysterious and their very existence has been challenged. However, a great number of experiments both in experimental animals and man document suppressive effects. In man much of the data derives from pokeweed mitogen (PWM) driven responses. In such experiments, the addition of CD8 cells to a responding mixture of CD4 helpers and B-cells leads to lowered immunoglobulin production. In similar experiments CD8 cells reduce proliferation in an autologous mixed lymphocyte reaction (AMLR). These human experiments followed earlier mouse work which similarly identified antigen-specific suppressor cells as Lyt-2/3 (CD8).

Both the mouse and human data pose a problem. Although suppressor cells are CD8, suppressor function has often been shown to be restricted by MHC class II, implying that suppressor cells recognize antigen in the context of class II not class I. However, suppression differs from help in that it is frequently restricted by I-E in the mouse or DQ in man while help is restricted by I-A or DR. This paradox may be resolved by data showing that a second CD4 cell type, the suppressor/inducer (see below), is involved in the generation of suppression. In addition, suppressor effectors and suppressor/inducers need not be directed at exogenous antigen but may be directed at TCR idiotypes or other antigens of helper cells. Suppressive T-cell clones which react with autologous helper clones or responding polyclonal T-cell populations have been described. If the specificity and genetic restriction of suppressor and suppressor/inducer cells is unclear, even more so are the mechanisms by which they act. Although a great number of 'suppressor factors' both antigen-specific and non-specific have been described, none of these are well-characterized entities.

4.5.6   Phenotypic heterogeneity of the CD4 and CD8 subsets

In the preceding sections I have alluded to functional heterogeneity within the CD4 and CD8 subsets. This section discusses their phenotypic heterogeneity and how this relates to function. Table 4.14 includes several of the reagents which have been used to further subdivide CD4 and CD8 in man. Most of these antigens are not T-cell specific and the majority further subdivide both CD4 and CD8, so that double-label analysis of cells in suspension or sections may be required in order to identify subsets precisely. There is much more data available relating to the heterogeneity of CD4 than CD8, so this subset will be discussed in more detail.

'Helper/inducers' and 'suppressor/inducers'

Two major subpopulations are identifiable in the CD4 subset. One is termed helper/inducer and characteristically provides help for B-cell antibody responses, whether antigen-specific or mitogen driven. In addition, this subset responds well in proliferative responses to recall antigens. The second subset, termed suppressor/inducer, does not provide help and responds poorly to recall antigens. These cells are required for the development

Table 4.14 Properties of virgin and memory T-cells

	Virgin cells (suppressor/inducers)	Memory cells (helper/inducers)
Phenotype		
CD45RA	+ +	−
CD45RO	−	+ +
CD29	−	+ +
CD44 (Pgp-1)	+	+ +
CD18/CD11a (LFA-1)	+	+ +
CD2	+	+ +
CD58 (LFA-3)	+	+ +
Leu 8	+ or −	+ or −
Other subset antigens further subdivide the memory subset		
Function		
Response to CD2 mAbs	+ / −	+ +
Response to CD3 mAbs	+	+ +
Response to recall antigens	−	+ +
Response to alloantigens	+ +	+ +
Response to mitogens	+ +	+ +
Help for B-cells	−	+ +
IL-2 production	+ +	+ +
γ-IFN production	−	+ +
B-cell factor production	+	+ +

of suppression by CD8 cells, demonstrable in the PWM-driven immunoglobulin synthesis assay or the AMLR. Both cell types are able to proliferate in response to alloantigens or mitogens.

Lineages or stages of maturation?

These data have been interpreted in two ways (Fig. 4.28). On the one hand, the two cell types have been considered to represent stable sublineages of CD4 (akin to CD4 and CD8 themselves) and, on the other, to be sequential stages in T-cell maturation. The former view is suggested by their distinctive functions while the latter is supported by the observations that memory (recall) responses are found in the 'helper/inducer' subset and that 'suppressor/inducer' cells, when stimulated with mitogens or alloantigens, acquire the helper/inducer phenotype. According to the latter view, the 'suppressor/inducer' cells represent naïve or virgin cells, which have not yet encountered antigen in the periphery, while 'helper/inducers' are memory cells.

The phenotype of virgin and memory cells

Many of the mAbs that identify the virgin population have now been grouped into CD45RA. Antibodies to CD45RA identify the two higher molecular mass, 220 and 205 kDa, polypeptides of CD45, the leucocyte common antigen, while several subset mAbs, including the CD29 mAb, 4B4, and UCHL1 against the lowest molecular mass 180 kDa polypeptide of CD45, react with a proportion or all of the reciprocal CD45RA⁻ memory population. The various CD45 isoforms appear to be derived from a single gene by alternative splicing in the extracellular domain of the molecule. The large cytoplasmic domain has recently been shown to have tyrosine phosphatase activity and

is therefore almost certainly involved in transmembrane signalling.

Although the function of the extracellular domains of CD45 is ill-understood, the change in phenotype from CD45RA to UCHL1 (CD45RO) is accompanied by others which are easier to interpret. Thus there is increased expression of CD18 and CD11a (LFA-1), LFA-3, and CD2. These are all molecules important in the interaction of T-cell with other cells, so that it is not surprising that memory cells are more easily triggered by mAbs to CD2 and CD3 (more efficient T-accessory cell interaction) and adhere preferentially to endothelium.

What is suppressor induction?

If the view put forward here is correct, that the CD45RA and CD45RO subsets are steps in peripheral T-cell maturation, at least two major questions remain to be answered. These are, what is suppressor induction and are there further sublineages within CD4? Much of the data on induction of suppression in man is derived from the PWM system. In these experiments both the virgin and memory populations are activated equally by the mitogen. The virgin population is functionally immature, producing mainly IL-2, while the memory population is able to produce at least IL-2, IL-4, and γ-IFN, so that there may be unbalanced cytokine production when both subsets are activated concurrently. Thus, suppressor induction by virgin cells may represent an *in vitro* artefact. Alternately, it may represent an anti-self (perhaps anti-idiotypic) response, a view supported by the observation that CD45RA cells respond well in AMLR while CD29 cells do not.

There is little data available for antigen-specific responses but experiments on the response to *Candida* suggest that suppressor induction in this recall response is mediated by the CD45RA⁻ (memory) subset. In other experiments, in which suppression appears to be HLA-DQ restricted, the cells which induce suppression have not yet been identified phenotypically. Thus, the available evidence suggests that induction of suppression is not always mediated by CD45RA cells and that memory suppressor/inducers may, like other memory cells, express CD45RO.

Heterogeneity of memory cells

Several mAbs indicate further heterogeneity, mainly within the memory compartment of CD4 (Table 4.14). Perhaps the most extensively studied of these is Leu 8. This mAb separates Leu 8⁺ suppressors from Leu 8⁻ helpers but in this case both subsets respond to recall antigens. This, together with double-staining data, indicates that Leu 8 divides memory cells into two subsets. Whether these represent distinct subpopulations or further stages of maturation within the memory compartment is not known. However, in the *Candida* experiments described above, the memory suppressor inducers are Leu 8⁺.

In the mouse, studies of IL-2-dependent T-cell clones indicate that there are at least two major categories of (memory) T-helper cells, which produce different lymphokines. T_h1 cells produce Il-2 and γ-IFN while T_h2 cells make IL-4; both make IL-3 and CSF-GM. As yet these have not been separated by phenotype; however, it may be that Leu 8 or one of the other mAbs listed in Table 4.14 may identify functionally distinct memory or effector CD4 cells.

4.5.7   Heterogeneity of CD8 cells

Much less information is available concerning the heterogeneity of CD8 than CD4. Functionally, two major categories of activity are detected, cytotoxicity and suppression. CD28 mAbs separate MHC class I specific cytotoxic precursor and effector cells from CD11b suppressor cells, most usually assayed in the PWM system. Thus some caution should be exercised in interpreting this data, since the two experimental systems are very different. In addition, not all CD8 lymphocytes express CD3. The nature of these cells is disputed but expression of the CD3/TCR receptor complex is a hallmark of mature T-cells. Since many CD8 cells are also granular lymphocytes and express markers characteristic of natural killer (NK) cells, there is some difficulty

in categorizing these overlapping small subpopulations accurately and in knowing which functions are associated with each phenotype. Table 4.15 gives a simplified summary.

Since CD45RA and CD45RO identify reciprocal populations within CD8 as they do in CD4, this raises the question whether these represent virgin and memory populations here also. As yet only preliminary data are available but these suggest that memory cytolytic cells may indeed express CD45RO.

4.5.8   Distribution of T-cell subsets

The availability of mAbs has provided reagents that can be used to identify cells in tissue sections. This in turn has led to many studies of the distribution of lymphocyte subsets in pathological material. In order to interpret the results it is necessary not only to understand the function of cells identified by different mAbs, but also to know their normal tissue distribution.

The peripheral lymphoid tissues

The major help/inducer and suppressor/cytotoxic subsets occupy distinct microenvironments in the peripheral lymphoid tissues. Thus while both CD4 and CD8 cells are found predominantly in the interfollicular paracortical areas of lymph nodes, there are differences in their localization. In the paracortical areas CD4 cells are frequently found clustered around MHC class II positive interdigitating cells, while CD8 cells do not make such contacts. CD4 cells are also found scattered in the germinal centres of the B-cell follicles (Fig. 4.30). Presumably this distribution reflects the necessity for CD4 cells to interact with class II and their role as helpers for antibody production. Similarly virgin and memory T-cells show differing distributions (Fig. 4.30). In the paracortical areas they are intermingled, but double labelling reveals that there is segregation of each cell type into small clusters, although neither cell type shows a clear association with interdigitating cells. The germinal centre T-cells express CD45RO, indicating that they have encountered antigen and matured into helper cells capable of producing multiple lymphokines.

Gut-associated T-cells

Gut-associated T-cells have unusual phenotypic and functional properties, although in man at least the majority do not appear

Table 4.15   Heterogeneity of CD8

Property	Cytotoxic cells	Suppressor cells	Natural killer cells
CD28	+	−	−
CD3	+	+	−
D44	+	−	+
CD11b	−	+	+
CD57 (Leu 7)	−	+	+
CD16 (FcR IgG)	−	−	+
LGL morphology	−	+	+
CD45RA/CD45RO	Some CD8 cells positive for either		CD45RA

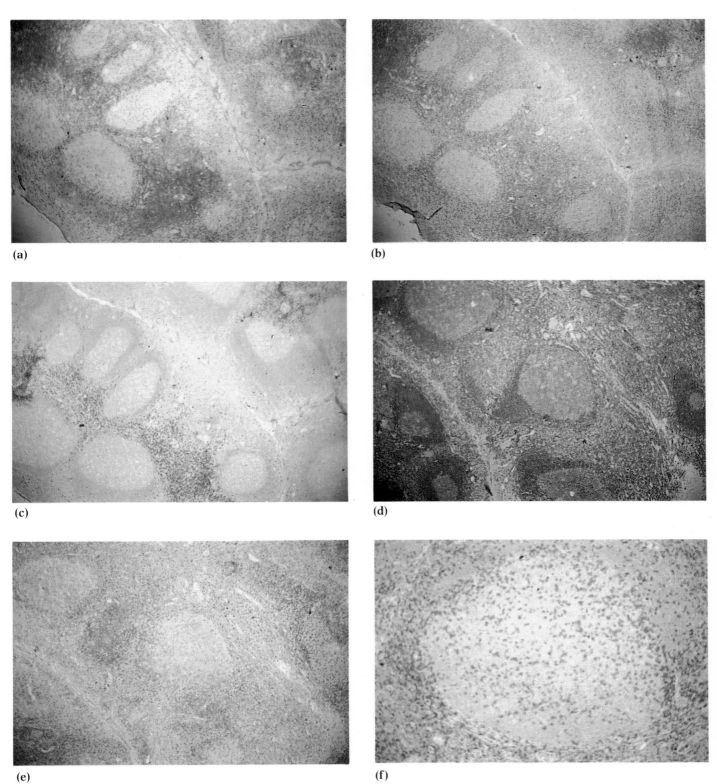

Fig. 4.30 Distribution of T-cell subsets. (a), (b), (c) Low-power views of cryostat tonsil sections stained by the indirect immunoperoxidase technique with CD3, CD4, and CD8 mAbs. (d), (e) Low-power views of cryostat tonsil sections stained with CD45RA and UCHL1 mAbs. (f) Higher-power view of a follicle centre, showing UCHL1⁺ T-cells within the B-cell area.

to express the $\gamma\delta$-TCR as may be the case in mice. In the epithelium the predominant cell population expresses CD8 and CD3. These cells also express CD45 but neither CD45RA nor CD45RO are detectable. In the lamina propria more conventional CD4 and CD8 T-cells are found, of which the overwhelming majority express CD45RO.

4.5.9   Conclusions

In this chapter I have presented a brief survey of the functional and phenotypic heterogeneity of human T-cells. It should be apparent from the discussion that much remains to be elucidated. Because of this, caution should be observed in making assumptions about the function of a cell on the basis of its phenotype, even more so on the basis of staining with a single mAb. Adequate identification of a T-cell requires the use of markers for lineage (CD3/TCR), sublineage (CD4 or CD8), maturation stage (CD45RA or CD45RO), and state of activation (CD25, transferrin receptor, class II). Even then the function of the cell cannot be confidently predicted, since suppressor and cytotoxic cells are not clearly distinguishable and the heterogeneity of CD4 cells is ill-understood. Nevertheless, as the functions of individual molecules are worked out, it will become possible to predict function from phenotype so that the heterogeneity of T-cells will at length become meaningful.

4.5.10   Further reading

Function of molecules of T-cells

Anderson, P., Morimoto, C., Breitmeyer, J. B., and Schlossman, S. F. (1988). Regulatory interactions between members of the immunoglobulin superfamily. *Immunology Today* **9**, 199–203.

Cobbold, S., Hale, G., and Waldmann, H. (1987). Non-lineage, LFA-1 family, and leucocyte common antigens: new and previously defined clusters. In *Leucocyte typing III* (ed. A. J. McMichael *et al.*), pp. 788–803. Oxford University Press, Oxford.

Dustin, M. L., Staunton, D. E., and Springer, T. A. (1988). Supergene families meet in the immune system. *Immunology Today* **9**, 213–15.

Knapp, W., *et al.* (ed.) (1989). *Leucocyte typing IV.* Oxford University Press, Oxford.

Function of peripheral T-cells

Bottazzo, G. F., Todd, I., Mirakian, R., Belfiore, A., and Pujol-Borrell, R. (1986). Organ-specific autoimmunity: a 1986 overview. *Immunological Reviews* **94**, 137–69.

Bottomly, K. (1988). A functional dichotomy in CD4 + T-lymphocytes. *Immunology Today* **9**, 268–74.

Dorf, M. E. and Benacerraf, B. (1984). Suppressor cells and immunoregulation. *Annual Reviews of Immunology* **2**, 127–57.

Sanders, M. E., Makgoba, M. W., and Shaw, S. (1988). Human naïve and memory T-cells: reinterpretation of helper-inducer and suppressor-inducer subsets. *Immunology Today* **9**, 195–9.

Genetic restriction

Bevan, M. J. (1987). Antigen recognition; Class discrimination in the world of immunology. *Nature* **325**, 192–3.

Doyle, C. and Strominger, J. L. (1987). Interaction between CD4 and class II MHC molecules mediates cell adhesion. *Nature* **330**, 256–9.

Mitchison, N. A. and Oliveira, D. B. G. (1986). Epirestriction and a specialised subset of T-helper cells are key factors in the regulation of T suppressor cells (ed. B. Cinader and R. G. Miller). *Progress in Immunology* **VI**, 326–34.

T-cell ontogeny and T-cell receptors

Davis, M. M. and Bjorkman, P. J. (1988). T-cell antigen receptor genes and T-cell recognition. *Nature* **334**, 395–402.

Janeway, C. (1988). Frontiers of the immune system. *Nature* **333**, 804–6.

Janossy, G., Campana, D., and Akbar, A. (1989). Kinetics of T-lymphocyte development. *Current Topics in Pathology* **79**, 59–99.

Posnett, D. N. (1990). Allelic variations of human TCR V gene products. *Immunology Today* **11**, 386–73.

4.6   The mononuclear phagocyte system

S. Gordon

The mononuclear phagocyte system (MPS) consists of a migratory, specialized family of cells derived from haematopoietic precursors, that circulate in blood as monocytes and are widely distributed as macrophages (MΦ) throughout the body normally and in increased numbers in response to tissue injury. By virtue of their specialized plasma membrane receptors and versatile biosynthetic and secretory responses, MΦ play a major role in inflammation, repair, humoral and cellular immunity, and metabolic and neoplastic disease processes. Cells of the MPS help to initiate acute inflammatory responses and predominate in chronic inflammation, locally within granulomatous foci of inflammatory cells, and systemically as a source of mediators that integrate general defence reactions of the host. Their relative longevity, endocytic responsiveness, and ability to generate trophic as well as toxic products make MΦ central actors in many disease processes, contributing to injury, proliferative lesions, and the accumulation of poorly degradable substances in many tissues. Together with polymorphonuclear leucocytes, with which MΦ share many properties, and other leucocytes, they contribute to phagocytosis and resistance to acute infections. Their effector functions in immune responses, combined with those of complement, specific antibodies, and stimulated B- and T-lymphocytes, are vital for resistance to opportunistic and virulent micro-organisms, as shown by the lethal complications of irreversible immunodeficiency. Their role in the induction of immune responses is less clear, since specialized, possibly related, antigen-presenting dendritic cells in lymphoid organs seem to play the major role in primary stimulation of lymphocytes.

The importance of phagocytes in defence against invading

organisms and foreign substances has been appreciated since Metchnikoff, but it has been evident for some time that MΦ are present constitutively in many tissues in the absence of inflammation. The physiological functions of these 'resident' MΦ are not clear. An important MΦ population lines vascular sinuses, e.g. the Kupffer cells of liver, and similar endothelial-like cells, distinct from true endothelial cells, are present in other organs. Phagocytic sinusoidal cells were recognized by Aschoff, among others, to be related to interstitial MΦ and the concept of a reticuloendothelial system (RES) has been in vogue for many years, although the term MPS has been used more recently to emphasize their specialized phagocytic properties. Recent studies with monoclonal antibodies (mAbs), which detect different MΦ-specific differentiation antigens, have confirmed a relationship among many of these cells, but variable expression of marker antigens has indicated that these cells display considerable heterogeneity. Other terms to describe tissue MΦ include histiocytes and microglia, the highly differentiated MΦ in the nervous system.

The boundary between MΦ and closely related lympho-haematopoietic lineages (e.g. Steinman–Cohn dendritic cells, interdigitating, veiled cells, and Langerhans cells) has been difficult to define (Fig. 4.31). This is not surprising, given the adaptibility of these cells and the complex responses to their tissue environment. The concept of lineage-restricted marker antigens has to be treated with caution. Ideally, several independent phenotypic traits should be correlated with life history to indicate a precursor–product relationship between cells, and tissue populations should be isolated and characterized *in vitro*. This poses a problem since tissue MΦ and related cells with extensive plasma membrane processes are deeply embedded, unlike rounded monocyte-like cells or loosely adherent cells in serosal cavities or the alveolar space. Continuous cell migration and turnover make it difficult to deduce the origin and fate of cells

from static observations. However, in spite of marked regional and functional heterogeneity, it is still possible to consider the MPS as a single lineage, capable of extensive modulation, without subsets or clonal diversification, by analogy with T- and B-lymphocytes.

4.6.1 General features of the mononuclear phagocyte system

MΦ and their precursors are found in several compartments within the body, the bone marrow, blood, and peripheral tissues, from which there is little, if any, re-entry into blood (Fig. 4.32). The bulk of MΦ mass is in tissues, where biosynthetically active cells can persist for long periods (weeks to months). Mature MΦ can be conveniently classified according to their functional state (Fig. 4.33): 'resident' cells present in the normal host without an overt inflammatory stimulus; 'elicited' cells, evoked by inflammatory stimuli that do not induce T-lymphocyte-responses; and immunologically 'activated' MΦ, which acquire enhanced cytocidal and microbicidal activities as a result of lymphokine release, particularly γ-interferon. Tissue injury and invasion by inert particulate and other foreign agents induce elicited-type MΦ, persistent infection by intracellular pathogens such as *Mycobacterium tuberculosis* can activate MΦ as part of cell-mediated immunity and delayed type hypersensitivity reactions. Both T-lymphocyte-dependent and independent agents are able to mobilize monocytes to local sites, so that these recruited cells share properties that distinguish them from resident cells in tissues. Monocytes are also recruited to sites such as the arterial wall (e.g. atherosclerosis) or the nervous system (e.g. diabetic neuropathy) in the absence of overt inflammatory or immunological injury, but the phenotype of such cells has not been defined.

Resident tissue MΦ are heterogeneous, depending on their particular local environment (e.g. skin and brain versus lymphoid organs), exposure to plasma or interstitial fluid constituents, and modulation by extracellular matrix and local products of neighbouring cells (Fig. 4.34). Morphologically, cells are rounded (loose or non-adherent) or stellate ('fixed' in tissues, presumably because of adhesion to matrix or other cells). Overall, the MPS therefore includes cells with varied life history and biological properties, that are highly adaptable and responsive to alterations in steady-state conditions. Although MΦ share features with other leucocytes and lymphocytes, their role in tissue homeostasis and host defence is unique.

4.6.2 Production and differentiation of mononuclear phagocytes

Our understanding of MΦ growth and differentiation rests on the development of suitable clonal assays to study haematopoietic regeneration *in vivo* after X-ray irradiation and to cultivate haematopoietic progenitors *in vitro* in the presence of specific colony-stimulating factors (CSF). Mature MΦ derive from haematopoietic stem cells (CFU-S, colony-forming units in

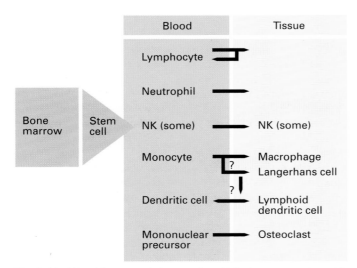

Fig. 4.31 Blood-borne and tissue cells which share properties with cells of the mononuclear phagocyte system. Langerhans cells can give rise to dendritic cells (see text).

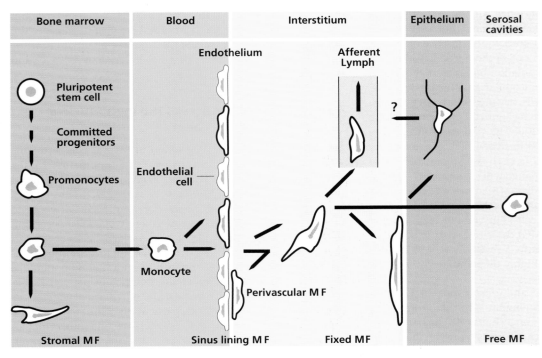

Fig. 4.32   Precursors and distribution of macrophages in different compartments of the body.

the spleen), from committed progenitors (CFU-GM, colony-forming units for granulocytes and MΦ), from promonocytes or more mature MΦ. MΦ production takes place mainly in haematopoietic organs (bone marrow, fetal liver, spleen in some species) and most tissue MΦ derive from blood monocytes. However, local resident MΦ populations, such as spleen and alveolar MΦ, can turn over independently and induced tissue MΦ retain considerable colony-forming potential. Normal cell growth and differentiation depend on specific CSFs (Table 4.16) and recombinant products for several of these are now available for use *in vivo* and *in vitro*. The role of these growth factors in steady-state and induced haematopoiesis within the host is not yet clear. Levels of circulating myelomonocytic cells and their recruitment to tissues can be enhanced by parenteral administration of GM-CSF. However, if production of GM-CSF within the host is massively elevated by overexpressing the gene in transgenic mice or by adoptive transfer of transfected murine bone marrow, novel pathological lesions may accompany MΦ infiltration of tissues such as muscle and eye and result in death.

One natural control which limits over-production of MΦ is the gradually increasing refractoriness to growth factors that accompanies MΦ differentiation. The 'burst size' of the stem cell under optimal culture conditions is thought to be very large, perhaps $> 10^8$ progeny, but this decreases rapidly so that most normal blood monocytes give rise to very few progeny (< 10) and mature resident MΦ divide only infrequently. The mechanism of terminal differentiation is unknown. Specific surface receptors for CSFs are present in differentiated MΦ and mediate other functional responses than growth. Mature resident MΦ are usually refractory to a growth stimulus, whereas alveolar

and induced exudate MΦ give rise to colonies under appropriate conditions *in vitro*. Recent studies on MΦ CSF receptors have clarified mechanisms which bring about loss of growth control. When a normal CSF-1 receptor (c-fms, the receptor for MΦ-specific CSF) is replaced by a viral oncogene product (v-fms), growth is disturbed, resulting in pre- or frank leukaemia syndromes in several animal species. Deletions or other abnormalities of human chromosome 5q, which encodes the CSF-1 receptor and several haematopoietic growth factors, result in myeloid dysplasia.

We know little about other factors which stimulate monocyte production or inhibit their growth and differentiation in the animal. Table 4.16 lists cytokines which influence a range of MΦ activities *in vitro*. Glucocorticoids, retinoids, and microbial products, e.g. lipopolysaccharide (LPS), also influence MΦ production or recruitment by modulating release of cytokines or by direct actions on MΦ. Other genes have been identified that control MΦ responses to various inflammatory stimuli and infections.

MΦ themselves are able to release products that influence production of monocytes (GM-CSF, TGF-β) but it is not known whether mature stromal MΦ in bone marrow play a role in monocytopoiesis (see below). MΦ in bone marrow and elsewhere are a potential source of interleukin-1, an important modulator of early differentiation of many haematopoietic cells, and adhesion receptors on MΦ, other stromal cells, and extracellular matrix control release of haematopoietic cells into the bloodstream.

We have only a rudimentary understanding of the role of

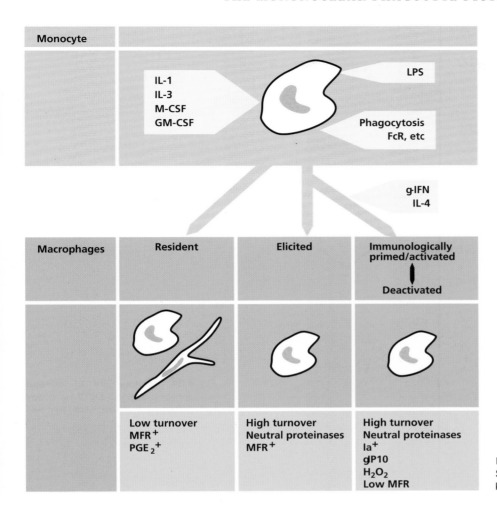

Fig. 4.33 Phenotype of mature macrophages. See Tables 4.16–4.18 for markers and cytokines, and text for further discussion.

cytokines in MΦ differentiation. Growth factors and their specific receptors control differentiation of bipotential progenitors of granulocyte/MΦ, play a role in cell survival, and induce expression of specific traits in mature MΦ. Different CSFs induce a similar, but not identical phenotype in bone marrow culture-derived MΦ. We need to learn more about MΦ gene expression in earlier, less abundant stages of differentiation. Other deficiencies of present cell culture systems include our inability to study commitment of common primary progenitors that give rise to lymphoid and myelomonocytic lineages or to generate Langerhans-type or Steinman–Cohn dendritic cells *in vitro*.

4.6.3   Circulation, recruitment, and turnover

After their production in bone marrow (∼ 7–10 days in man), monocytes are released into the circulation, which they leave after ∼ 1–2 days, even in the absence of an inflammatory stimulus. The reserve pool of monocytes in bone marrow is relatively small, < 5 per cent of nucleated cells, compared with that of polymorphonuclear leucocytes, ∼ 50 per cent, consistent with the acute demands made on the latter. Little is known about sites of constitutive emigration from vessels in the steady state (possibly post-capillary venules), whether monocytes leave the circulation at random, and whether cells for different target tissues are pre-selected, as in the lymphoid system (homing). Induced migration into tissues can be mediated by expression of surface molecules on endothelium at a site of injury or, perhaps, at specialized venular high endothelium (Fig. 4.35). The type 3 complement receptor (CR_3) plays a role in endothelial adhesion and tissue entry of polymorphonuclear leucocytes and monocytes during non-specific and T-cell-induced recruitment of myelomonocytic cells. CR_3 is a member of a leucocyte-adhesion receptor family (Mac-1, LFA-1, p150, 95) that is related to the integrin family of cell-surface glycoproteins involved in adhesion of haematopoietic cells and fibroblasts to various ligands. Inborn deficiency of leucocyte-adhesion receptors results in impaired mobilization of these cells to a site of inflammation. Monoclonal anti-CR_3 antibodies have been isolated that inhibit induced recruitment of myelomonocytic cells within the host, without affecting bone marrow egress or the level of circulating cells. Intravenous administration of such mAb to experimental animals can prevent some of the local deleterious effects of recruited inflammatory cells, e.g. increased vascular permeability in lung, or reperfusion injury in

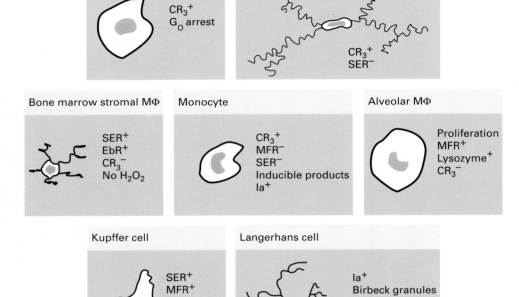

Fig. 4.34 Heterogeneity of resident macrophages. See Table 4.17 for receptors. Where not shown, cell turnover varies.

Table 4.16 Cytokines which influence MΦ growth, differentiation, and activation (for references see Gordon *et al.*, 1988*b*)

Cytokine	Source	Actions on MΦ
M-CSF	Fibroblast, MΦ	Growth and differentiation, urokinase induction
GM-CSF	T-lymphocyte, MΦ, endothelium	Growth, differentiation, and ? activation
IL-1	MΦ, others	Release of IL-1, TNFα, CSF
TNF-α/cachectin	MΦ, T-lymphocyte	Release of PAF, IL-1, PGE$_2$
IL-2	T-lymphocyte	Induction of NK phenotype (with M-CSF)
		Chemotaxis
IL-3	T-lymphocyte	Growth immature stages and differentiation
IL-4	CD$_4^+$ lymphocyte	Fusion, enhanced Ia ag, ag presentation
Interferon α	Leucocyte	Antiviral and modulation of MΦ activation
β	Fibroblast	
γ	T-lymphocyte	Antiviral, MΦ activation, e.g. enhanced Ia ag, respiratory burst, γIP10; down-regulation of MFR
β TGF	Platelet, MΦ	Chemotaxis, growth factor release, MΦ deactivation

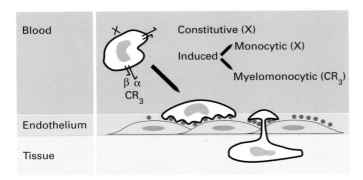

Fig. 4.35 CR$_3$ plays an important role in induced myelomonocytic cell adhesion and emigration. Surface receptors for constitutive and monocyte-specific recruitment are unknown.

heart after induced ischaemia. However, treated animals are unable to contain virulent bacteria, such as *Listeria monocytogenes*, by granuloma formation and become highly susceptible to acute microbial infection. The role of CR$_3$ and other leucocyte-adhesion receptors in constitutive, monocyte-specific emigration has not been defined.

Delivery of monocytes to tissues in the developing and adult animal will be considered below. Monocytes have a unique ability to leave the pool of circulating cells and form a stable, sinus-lining population, e.g. in liver, or to penetrate the blood–brain barrier of the central nervous system. The extent to which these processes continue in the adult under steady-state conditions is unclear and the signals that result in monocyte localization are unknown. Selective adhesion of monocytes occurs in the earliest stages of hypercholesterolaemic injury in walls of major arteries and is thought to contribute to the development of vascular lesions. Endothelial interactions that result in reversible margination of monocytes in different vascular beds have not been defined.

Expression of a local endothelial cell ligand for circulating monocytes must play a role in adhesion and emigration of monocytes/MΦ via endothelial junctions. Migration and turn-over within tissues depend on adhesion to interstitial cells and extracellular matrix, and on the nature of the inducing stimulus, which can vary from inert to highly cytopathic. For example, MΦ in skin tattoos turn over slowly, compared with short-lived monocytes/MΦ in a hypersensitivity granuloma. One difficulty in determining the life-span of MΦ is that ingested particles such as carbon or undegraded inorganic materials are transferred successively from cell to cell. Labelling methods used in experimental animals do not distinguish adequately between resident and newly recruited MΦ.

It is assumed that lymphoid organs are a major graveyard for MΦ entering afferent lymph, since most cells are efficiently filtered out in lymph nodes and do not enter efferent lymphatics or the thoracic duct unless lymph nodes are removed. The spleen, liver, and bone marrow remove senescent or damaged MΦ and other haematopoietic cells from the circulation. The red pulp of spleen is rich in phagocytic MΦ, whereas cells in the marginal zone region may be specialized to capture circulating cells, micro-organisms, or antigens. It is not known how MΦ in tissues recognize dead or effete haematopoietic cells, including dying MΦ.

4.6.4 Cell biology of macrophages

Morphological features of MΦ and related cells are described before considering their modulation in normal and diseased tissues (Figs. 4.36–4.39). Other aspects of MΦ cell biology are considered in Section 4.20. Much of our current knowledge derives from *in vitro* studies with readily available cells from murine peritoneal cavity or human blood. With nucleic acid and antibody probes it is now possible to characterize MΦ functions within the host. Instances of artefactual loss or acquisition of activities in cell culture are well known. It can be misleading to extrapolate from findings made on MΦ-like cell lines and even freshly isolated tissue MΦ tend to acquire a standard cell culture phenotype and do not necessarily retain specialized properties expressed *in situ*.

Mature MΦ do not usually replicate their DNA, but RNA and protein synthesis, lipid metabolism, and other biochemical reactions are prominent throughout their life-span. Metabolic processes are modulated by stimuli such as phagocytosis, LPS, MΦ-activating agents, and various receptor–ligand interactions. The plasma membrane of monocytes and MΦ in cell culture displays continuous ruffling activity, the cells are motile and able to migrate towards a chemotactic gradient. Isolated cells adhere readily to artificial substrata such as glass or tissue-culture plastic. MΦ are able to function in low O$_2$ tension and hypoxia influences their behaviour. The use of O$_2$ as substrate in cytocidal reactions and the respiratory burst will be discussed in Section 4.20. Macrophages consume large amounts of glucose and glutamate in culture, generate abundant lactate, and produce and utilize high levels of ATP to fuel their biosynthetic and other functions, including macromolecular synthesis and continuous membrane flow. They engage avidly in constitutive and receptor-mediated pinocytosis and phagocytosis.

Macrophages express a large repertoire of plasma membrane receptors that mediate specific recognition mechanisms and cellular responses. Receptors for Fc fragments of immunoglobulin subclasses and for cleaved fragments of C$_3$ have been characterized in most detail. Ligands reported to bind to MΦ are listed in Table 4.17 and the role of MΦ receptors in endocytosis and host-cell–pathogen interactions will be considered in Section 4.20.

Membrane flow and recycling are extensive in MΦ and plasma and intracellular membranes undergo continuous, selective remodelling. The cytoplasm contains numerous organelles involved in endocytosis (endosomes, lysosomes, residual bodies), a well-developed cytoskeleton, and abundant cisternal and vesicular elements indicative of active protein synthesis and export. Many secretory products, protein and non-protein in nature, can be generated by MΦ *in vitro* and some of these are listed in Table 4.18. Products include mediators of inflammation and of MΦ defence functions, but also

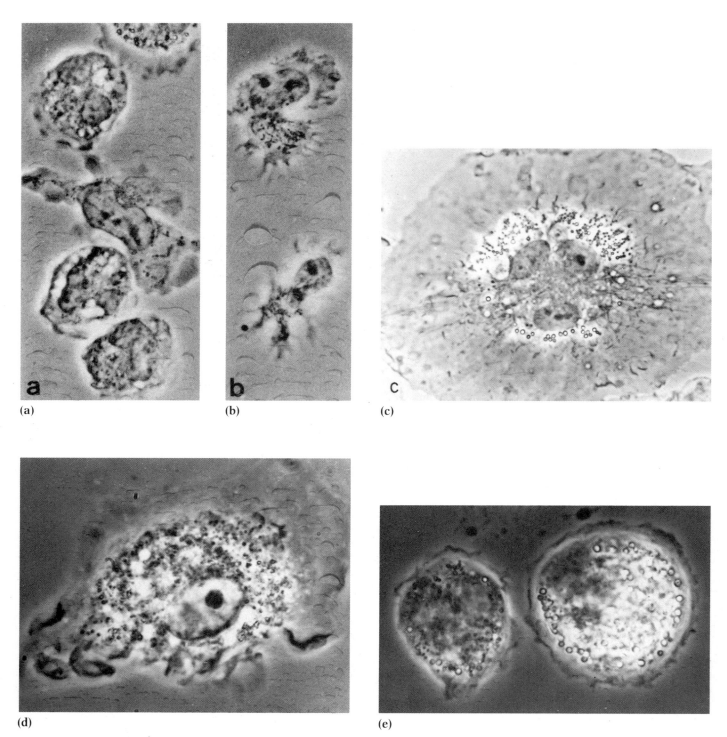

Fig. 4.36 Phase contrast micrographs of mononuclear phagocytes and dendritic cells adherent to glass *in vitro*. (a) A Steinman–Cohn dendritic cell surrounded by four monocytes, which exhibit typical ruffles, lysosomes, and pinocytic vesicles. (b) Enriched dendritic cells after spreading on poly-L-lysine-coated glass. Dendrites extend in several directions and the cytoplasm is rich in mitochondria. (From van Voorhis *et al.* 1982.) (c) Multinucleated mouse peritoneal macrophage. A uniformly well-spread giant cell with refractile lipid droplets. The centrosomal region bordered by nuclei contains lysosomes. Rod-like mitochondria are visible in flattened organelle-free zone. (d) Human macrophage obtained by broncho-alveolar lavage. Note plasma membrane ruffles, numerous phase-dense and phase-lucent vesicles, mainly of endocytic origin and organelle-free zone at leading edge of polarized cell. (e) Rat alveolar macrophages remain rounded. Note ruffles and numerous cytoplasmic vesicles, including refractile lipid droplets.

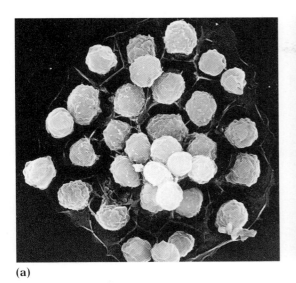

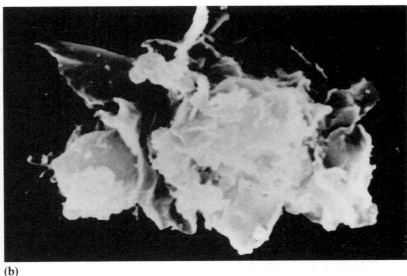

(a) **(b)**

Fig. 4.37 (a) Scanning electron micrograph of a haematopoietic cell cluster isolated from murine fetal liver by collagenase digestion and adherence to glass. Developing erythroblasts are enveloped but not phagocytosed by a single well-spread macrophage with loculated surface folds. (For further details see Morris *et al.* 1987.) (b) Scanning electron micrograph of a mouse lymph node dendritic cell, isolated as in Macatonia *et al.* (1987). Note plasma membrane veils and associated lymphocyte. (Provided by S. Knight and J. Clarke, Clinical Research Centre, Harrow.)

growth and other trophic factors for various cells. Some are typical secreted proteins delivered to the plasma membrane by vesicular transport and exocytosis (the mature MΦ does not contain obvious storage granules of the type found in freshly isolated monocytes) (Fig. 4.39). Unlike granulocytes, MΦ tend to secrete rather than store their products, in keeping with their longer life-span and role in prolonged inflammatory reactions. Other products, such as arachidonate metabolites, are generated from membrane stores by enzymes activated by receptor–ligand interactions and secondary signalling events which have not been well defined. Several MΦ-derived polypeptides (e.g. IL-1) may be released from MΦ membrane-associated forms by proteolysis, or from poorly defined intracellular stores, since they lack a signal sequence for secretion.

4.6.5 Constitutive distribution and functions of tissue macrophages

Studies with mAbs and other markers (phagocytosis, lysosomal enzymes, vital dyes) have demonstrated MΦ in lymphohaematopoietic tissues and most organs of the body (Figs 4.40–4.43). Resident MΦ in normal animals are concentrated at or near portals of entry where they contribute to first-line defence against invading organisms. Immunocytochemical labelling by MΦ-specific mAb such as F4/80, a rat mAb highly restricted to mature mouse MΦ, revealed extensive plasma membrane contacts between MΦ and adjacent cells in bone marrow and other organs. *In situ* studies with various mAbs in mouse and human, and isolation of stromal and other MΦ have revealed novel characteristics and considerable regional heterogeneity among MΦ. There is evidence that resident tissue cells perform trophic,

rather than purely endocytic or cytotoxic functions; stromal MΦ in fetal liver, and adult bone marrow, for example, associate with developing haematopoietic cells and modulate their growth and differentiation. Resident tissue MΦ express properties that make them potential targets for pathogens and for interactions with abnormal host cells.

4.6.6 Ontogeny and distribution of macrophages in the normal adult

Our own observations have been mostly in the mouse, but more limited studies with human material have yielded similar results. In the mouse, MΦ progenitors first appear around day 5 of gestation and mature MΦ are found in the yolk sac at about day 9. Haematopoiesis in the fetus consists mainly of erythroid cells and monocytes, and is initially virtually free of granulocytes. Activity shifts from yolk sac to fetal liver by mid-gestation, then to spleen and bone marrow before birth. Monocytes are delivered to most developing organs from days 10–12. Cells are found relatively early in many mesenchymal tissues and monocytes are recruited to the developing nervous system and lymphoid organs before and after birth. These phagocytic cells remove naturally dying cells, e.g. neurons and axons, and contribute to tissue remodelling. Fetal liver MΦ bind developing erythroblasts via a newly discovered cation-dependent surface haemagglutinin (Fig. 4.37). Before birth, haematopoietic activity ceases in the liver and MΦ assume the appearance of Kupffer cells.

In the normal adult (Figs. 4.40–4.43), large concentrations of MΦ are found in the gut, liver, and spleen, and substantial numbers are present in bone marrow, other lymphoid organs, serosal cavities, and lung. Macrophages are readily detectable

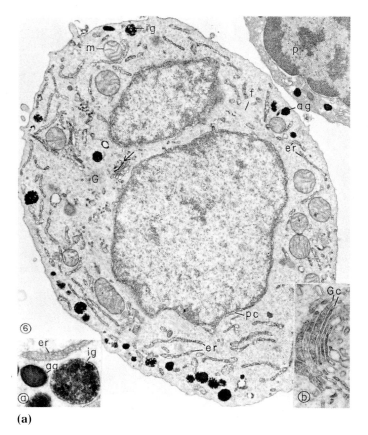

(a)

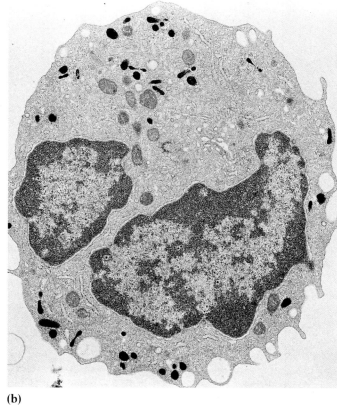

(b)

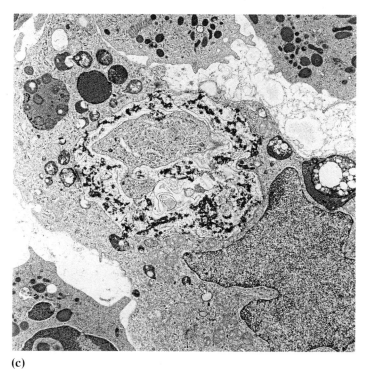

(c)

Fig. 4.38 Electron micrographs of human mononuclear phagocytes at various stages of differentiation *in vivo*. (a) promonocyte from bone marrow, reacted for peroxidase by the Graham and Karnovsky method. Note immature (ig) and mature (ag) granules which contain more reaction product than endoplasmic reticulum (er), Golgi cisternae (Gc), and perinuclear cisterna (pc). The chromatin is dispersed. (From Nichols *et al*. 1971.) (b) Monocyte from blood reacted for peroxidase. Note peroxidase-positive and peroxidase-negative granules and condensed rim of nuclear chromatin. Peroxidase reactivity helps to distinguish monocytes from lymphocytes and dendritic cells. (See Nichols and Bainton 1973.) (c) Mature macrophage from bone marrow shows cluster of developing myeloid cells associated with a stromal macrophage that contains phagocytic inclusions. (See Crocker *et al*. 1990.)

Table 4.17 Ligands reported to bind to macrophage plasma membrane receptors (for references see Gordon *et al.*, 1988*b*)

Opsonins/targeting

Fc IgG (various), IgE, IgA
iC3b, adhesive
C3b
C3d
C1q

Coagulation

Fibrinogen
Thrombospondin
Thrombin
Factor VII, VIIA
Urokinase

Matrix

Fibronectin
Vitronectin Laminin
Sulphated polysaccharide
Hyaluronate

Cell adhesion and recognition

Sheep erythrocytes (sialyl-gangliosides)
Erythroblasts
I-CAM
LFA-1
Endothelium

Other endocytosis and transport

Mannosyl, GlcNAc fucosyl glycoconjugates
Galactosyl particles
β-Glucan (yeast)
Fucosyl glycoconjugates
LDL lipoprotein (various), native, modified (acetyl, malondialdehyde) βVLDL, apoE
Aldehyde-modified proteins
AGE (advanced glycosylation end products)
Transferrin
Lactoferrin
Caeruloplasmin
α_2 macroglobulin
Haemopexin
Mannose-6-phosphate glycoproteins

Growth factors, cytokines, polypeptides

CSF-1
GM-CSF
Interleukin-1
Interleukin-2
Interleukin-3
Interleukin-4
TNFα/cachectin
γ-Interferon
α, β-Interferon
Insulin
Glucagon
Somatomedin
Vasopressin
Parathormone
Transforming growth factor β
C5a

Peptides and inflammatory mediators

fMet-Leu-Phe
Angiotensin
Bradykinin
Substance P
Vasoactive intestinal peptide
Tuftsin
Neurotensin
Leukotriene B4

Pharmacologic

β2 adrenergic
Nicotinic cholinergic
Histamine (H1)
Serotonin
Benzodiazepine
Adenosine
Phorbol myristate acetate/dibutyrate

in kidney, endocrine organs, the urogenital tract, and the nervous system. From a survey of different tissues it is evident that MΦ are either monocyte-like, with few processes, or stellate, with short (e.g. liver) or more exuberant processes (e.g. brain and epithelia). Their anatomic distribution indicates that monocyte entry and migration within tissues are precisely controlled. Monocytes/MΦ line sinusoids or penetrate endothelia, where they often take up a pericapillary location (Fig. 4.32). Others migrate through interstitium towards epithelia, lie beneath, penetrate, or pass through simple or complex epithelia of body surfaces (e.g. skin, bladder) or secretory glands (e.g. prostate, salivary gland). Interactions with adjacent cells, basement membrane, or matrix may involve MΦ receptors for adhesive cellular ligands, fibronectin, or laminin. Specific local interactions result in regional heterogeneity of resident MΦ in different

organs and will be considered in relation to possible functions and role in disease.

Bone marrow

Mature MΦ are a major component of bone marrow stroma and are often associated with erythroblastic islets (Figs. 4.41, 4.42d). *In situ*, these MΦ form an extensive network throughout the stroma, at the centre of erythroid and myelomonocytic cell clusters, that can be isolated from murine bone marrow by collagenase digestion, velocity sedimentation, and adherence to a substratum via their MΦ. Bound haematopoietic cells can be dissociated from stromal MΦ and clusters reconstituted *in vitro*. Two haemagglutinins mediate adhesion of haematopoietic cells to stromal MΦ, the first is a lectin-like receptor for sialylated gangliosides and other glycoconjugates also present on sheep

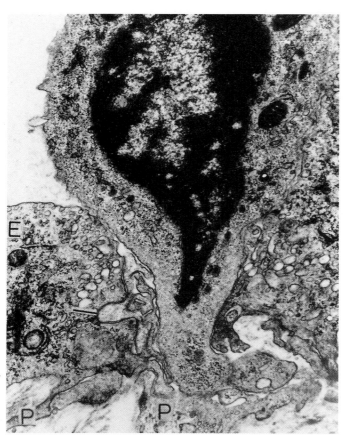

Fig. 4.39 Rabbit monocyte migrating between endothelial cells in response to an inflammatory stimulus (see Marchesi and Gowans 1964).

erythrocytes (the sheep erythrocyte receptor, SER, now termed sialoadhesin), the other a divalent-cation-dependent receptor similar to that on fetal liver MΦ. Both receptors are MΦ-specific, are restricted to 'fixed' tissue MΦ such as those in bone marrow, and are absent or low on circulating monocytes and peritoneal MΦ. Bound haematopoietic cells proliferate on MΦ and are not phagocytosed (Fig. 4.37), although the same MΦ readily take up erythroid nuclei and express other phagocytic receptors, e.g. FcR and mannosyl, fucosyl receptors (MFR) (Fig. 4.38c). The non-phagocytic MΦ haemagglutinins are regulated by distinct mechanisms involving, for sialoadhesin, a species-restricted inducer protein present in homologous plasma. Sialoadhesin has been purified and the isolated receptor shown to bind to ligand-bearing cells. Although its mode of action remains to be established, one possibility is that it modulates haematopoietic cell growth and differentiation directly or through specialized zones of contact. Other interactions between stromal MΦ and haematopoietic cells can also be envisaged involving production of growth factors or inhibitors by MΦ (e.g. GM-CSF, erythropoietin, TGF-β, prostaglandins) and recycling of iron and nutrients from MΦ stores.

Stromal MΦ from marrow display additional characteristics that set them apart from other MΦ and that are relevant to their functions (Fig. 4.33). They lack detectable CR$_3$ antigen and receptor activity, as do Kupffer cells and some MΦ in lympho-haematopoietic organs, and fail to generate a respiratory burst after a phagocytic stimulus, unlike monocytes and activated MΦ. Since they express other clearance and endocytic receptors, this may make them vulnerable to infection. Stromal MΦ could provide a source of infection for other haematopoietic cells and contribute to abnormal haematopoiesis or cell destruction in auto-immune and storage diseases. Through their

Table 4.18 Secretory products of mononuclear phagocytes (for references see Rappolee and Werb 1988)

Polypeptide hormones
  Interleukin-1α and 1β (IL-1)
  Somatotrophin
  Tumour necrosis factor-α (cachectin) (TNF-α)
  Interferon-α (IFN-α)
  Interleukin-6/hepatocyte-stimulating factor/β-cell stimulating factor-2/interferon-β_2
    (IL-6/HSF/BSF-2/IFN-β_2)
  Platelet-derived growth factor(s) (PDGF)
  Substance P
  Fibroblast growth factors (FGF)
  Fibroblast activating factors
  Transforming growth factor-β (TGF-β)
  Insulin-like growth factor-1 (IGF-1)
  Thymosin B4
  Erythropoietin (EPO)
  Colony-stimulating factor for granulocytes and macrophages (GM-CSF)
  Colony-stimulating factor for granulocytes (G-CSF)
  Colony-stimulating factor for macrophages (M-CSF, CSF-1)
  Bombesin
  Erythroid colony-potentiating factor (EPA)/tissue inhibitor of metalloproteinases
    (TIMP)
  Factor-inducing monocytopoiesis (FIM)
  β-Endorphin
  Adrenocorticotrophic hormone

Table 4.18 *Continued*

Plasmacytoma growth factor
Neutrophil-activating and recruiting factors (II-8, MIPIα, β)
Transforming growth factor-α (TGF-α)

Complement (C) components
Classical pathway: C1, C2, C3, C4, C5, C6, C7, C8, C9; active complement fragments
generated by macrophage proteinases; C3a, C3b, C5a, Bb
Alternative pathway: factor B, factor D, properdin
Inhibitors: factor 1 (C3b inactivator), factor H (β-1H)

Coagulation factors
Intrinsic pathway: IX, X, V, prothrombin
Extrinsic pathway: VII
Surface activities: tissue factor, prothrombinase
Antithrombolytic activities: plasminogen activator inhibitor-2, plasmin inhibitors

Proteolytic enzymes
Metalloproteinases: macrophage elastase, collagenase, stromelysin, 92 kDa gelatinase,
68 kDa gelatinase, angiotensin convertase
Serine proteinases: urokinase-type plasminogen activator (UPA), cytolytic proteinease
Aspartyl proteinases: cathepsin D
Cysteine proteinase: cathepsin L, cathepsin B

Other enzymes
Lipases: lipoprotein lipase, phospholipase
Glucosaminidase: lysozyme
Lysosomal acid hydrolases: proteases, lipases, (deoxy) ribonucleases, phosphatases,
glycosidases, sulphatases (approximately 40)
Deaminase: arginase

Inhibitors of enzymes
Proteinase inhibitors: α_2-macroglobulin, α_1-proteinase inhibitor (α_1-P1)/α_1-antitrypsin,
plasminogen activator inhibitor-2 (PA1-2), plasmin inhibitors, tissue inhibitor of
metalloproteinases (TIMP)/collagenase inhibitor/EPA
Phospholipase inhibitor: lipomodulin (macrocortin)

Proteins of extracellular matrix or cell adhesion
Fibronectin
Gelatin-binding protein/92 kDa gelatinase
Thrombospondin
Chondroitin sulphate proteoglycans
Heparin sulphate proteoglycans

Other binding proteins
For metals: transferrin, acidic isoferritins
For vitamins: transcobalamin II
For lipids: apolipoprotein E, lipid transfer protein
For growth factors: α_2-macroglobulin, IL-1
For inhibitors: TGF-β-binding protein
For biotin: avidin

Bioactive lipids
Cyclo-oxygenase products: prostaglandin E_2 (PGE_2), prostaglandin $F_{2\alpha}$, prostacyclin
($PG1_2$), thromboxane
Lipoxygenase products: monohydroxyeicosatetraenoic acids (HETE),
dihydroxyeicosatetraenoic acids, leukotrienes (LT) B4, C, D, E
Platelet-activating factors (PAF): 1-0-alkyl-2-acetyl-sn-glyceryl-3-phosphorylcholine

Other bioactive low molecular weight substances
Oligopeptides: glutathione
Steroid hormones: 1_a, 25-Dihydroxyvitamin D3
Purine and pyrimidine products: thymidine, uracil, uric acid, deoxycytidine, cAMP,
neopterin (2-amino-4-oxo-6-trihydroxyproplpteridine)
Reactive oxygen intermediates: superoxide, hydrogen peroxide, hypohalous acids,
singlet O_2, Hydroxyl radicals
Reactive nitrogen intermediates: nitrites, nitrates, nitric oxide

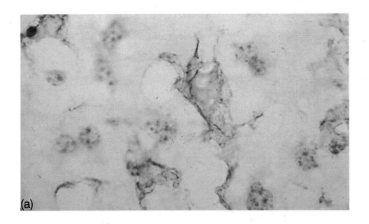

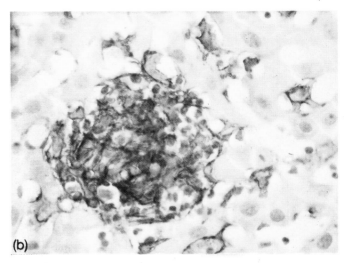

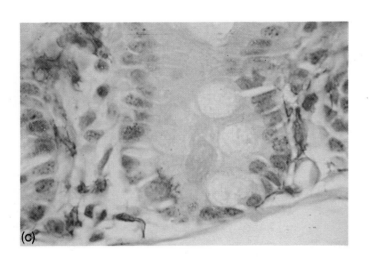

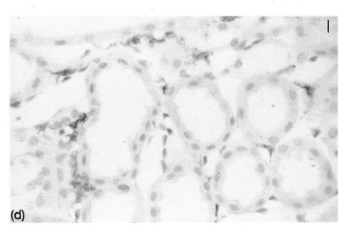

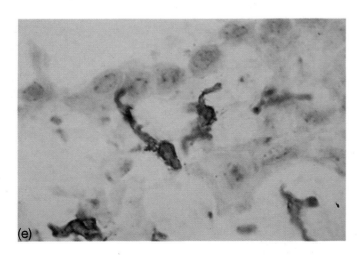

Fig. 4.40 Resident and recruited macrophages in adult mouse tissues detected by F4/80 monoclonal antibody and immunoperoxidase labelling (prepared by D. A. Hume, V. H. Perry, and S. Rabinowitz in our laboratory). (a) Kupffer cells line liver sinusoids. Endothelial cells and hepatocytes are F4/80 negative. (b) F4/80$^+$ recruited macrophages in Bacille–Calmette–Guèrin–induced granuloma in liver. Note increased cell traffic in adjacent sinusoids. A few F4/80$^-$ neutrophils and lymphocytes are also present. (c) Lamina propria of intestinal mucosa, both small and large bowel, contains an abundant population of F4/80$^+$ stellate macrophages, outside the epithelium and closely associated with capillaries. (d) F4/80$^+$ stellate macrophages in choroid plexus are prominent beneath and among F4/80$^-$ epithelial cells bordering on the cerebrospinal space. Contrast the morphology of these cells with that of microglia (Fig. 4.44d). (e) F4/80$^+$ macrophages lie outside the basement membrane of tubular epithelium in the renal medulla.

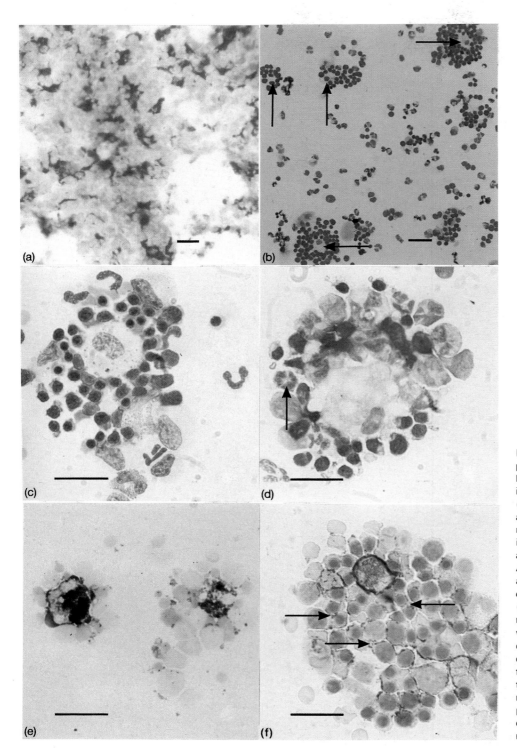

Fig. 4.41 Resident stromal macrophages associate with developing haematopoietic cells *in situ* (a) and after isolation from human bone marrow (b–f). (a) Immunocytochemical staining with anti-macrophage mAb Y–1/82A reveals a network of arborizing macrophages (alkaline phosphatase-anti-alkaline phosphatase stain, haematoxylin counterstain). (b) After isolation and depletion of red cells and other single cells, erythroid clusters contain central stromal macrophage (arrows, Giemsa). (c) Cluster with intermediate and late normoblasts. (d) Cluster with myeloid and erythroid cells, including dividing cell (arrow). (e) Haemosiderin detected by Perl's acid ferrocyanide reaction in bone marrow clusters from multiply transfused patient. (f) Anti-macrophage mAb reveals cell body and extensive plasma membrane processes between central macrophage and attached erythroblasts (see Lee *et al.* 1988).

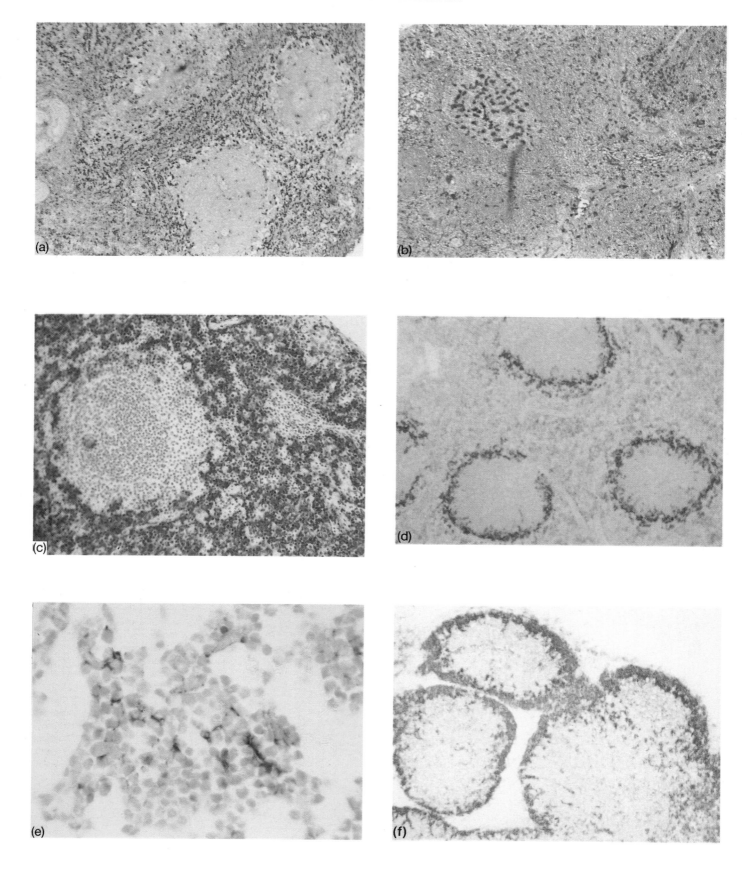

specialized adhesion receptors, stromal MΦ could play a role in trapping of metastatic cells and promote growth of nascent tumour cells.

Liver

Kupffer cells are a major tissue MΦ population involved in clearance and possibly in the release of hormone-like monokines (Fig. 4.40a). They share endocytic receptors (FcR and MFR) with hepatic endothelial cells, reflecting adaptation to a common microenvironment. Because of their location they are exposed to gut-derived microbial products, such as LPS. They lack CR_3 and the ability to generate a respiratory burst after exposure to γ-interferon (Fig. 4.33), although this induces expression of other activation markers such as class II MHC (Ia antigen). It is thought that the respiratory burst is selectively inactivated in Kupffer cells, perhaps sparing adjacent hepatocytes from oxidative injury. These resident MΦ could therefore be vulnerable to infection, so that the host depends on newly recruited monocytes to combat virulent organisms such as *Listeria monocytogenes* that spread to hepatocytes after initial infection of Kupffer cells. Since MΦ-derived mediators potentially play an important role in stimulating hepatocyte plasma protein synthesis it will be important to document *in situ* production of IL-1, TNFα, IL-6 and other monokines by Kupffer cells. Alternatively, these could be generated by recruited monocytes following local encounter with LPS and other microbial and cellular products.

Spleen and other lymphoid organs

The F4/80 antibody reacts strongly with MΦ in mouse spleen red pulp (Fig. 4.42) and with sinus-lining MΦ in lymph nodes, but not with marginal zone MΦ and presumptive MΦ in T-lymphocyte-dependent regions in white pulp, lymph node follicles, and Peyer's patch. Other mAbs react with stromal MΦ in the marginal-metallophil zone or T-cell areas of mouse and man. Phenotypic heterogeneity among resident MΦ populations in lymphoid organs may reflect their unique local microenvironment, resulting from interactions with specialized T- or B-cell populations, cell traffic from blood and lymph, exposure to antigens and organisms, and, in murine spleen, local haematopoiesis.

An important subset of cells in lymphoid organs of bone marrow origin lack F4/80 and other MΦ antigens, but express high levels of class II MHC (Ia) antigens constitutively. This population includes Steinman–Cohn dendritic cells, interdigitating cells, and veiled cells, which are thought to be the major accessory cells involved in primary T-cell responses to foreign antigens (Fig. 4.36, 4.37). Isolated dendritic cells and T-cells form specific clusters when stimulated with antigen in cell culture, resulting in lymphocyte blastogenesis. Dendritic cells constitutively express high levels of Ia antigens and are uniquely potent stimulators of T-cells in primary immune responses *in vitro* (Fig. 4.44). By contrast, requirements for secondary T-cell responses seem to be less stringent and other Ia-bearing cells, including induced MΦ, can then serve as 'antigen presenting cells'. The mechanism of antigen presentation and role of Ia antigen in these cellular interactions are poorly understood. Recent studies have demonstrated binding sites on MHC molecules for small peptides, perhaps derived from native proteins by unfolding or partial proteolysis. MΦ play a better-defined role in the effector limb of cell-mediated immunity, in association with activated T-lymphocytes, as described below. Macrophages and their products, e.g. prostaglandins, also act as powerful inhibitors of lymphocyte blastogenesis *in vitro* and, possibly, in chronic infections associated with acquired immunosuppression.

Apart from their immune functions, MΦ in spleen and other lymphoid organs play a role in turnover of senescent haematopoietic cells (red pulp), phagocytosis of naturally dying cells (thymus) and clearance of particulate agents from the circulation, e.g. infectious organisms and erythrocytes parasitized by *Plasmodium*. Macrophages in the marginal zone selectively endocytose selected polymeric polysaccharides from blood, may be the initial target of infection by certain organisms, and are thought to be involved in triggering of selected B-cell responses. The marginal metallophil macrophages express distinctive surface antigens, including sialoadhesin (Fig. 4.42) but little is known about their origins and functions.

Skin

Numerous MΦ are found in the connective tissue of the dermis and are important in local defences. Langerhans cells in the epidermis are related to MΦ and are important in immune responses to skin-sensitizing antigens. They derive from bone marrow and resemble microglia in their highly dendritic morphology (Figs 4.31, 4.43). Langerhans cells share other properties with MΦ (antigen markers, receptors), but constitutively

Fig. 4.42 Heterogeneity of tissue macrophages in lympho-haematopoietic organs revealed by anti-human (a, b, APAAP method) and anti-murine (c–f, ABC immunoperoxidase method) mAb. All cryostat sections, only (d) perfused through the heart with periodate-lysine-paraformaldehyde. (a) Human spleen. Ab Y2/131 (D. Mason and S. H. Lee, Oxford University) reacts strongly with macrophages in red pulp, as do many other anti-macrophage antibodies, with cells in the marginal zone and with scattered cells (? tingible body macrophages) in the white pulp. (b) Human tonsil. Ab Y1/82A reacts with tingible body macrophages of germinal centre in reactive lymphoid tissue and with scattered macrophages (D. Mason and S. H. Lee). (c) In mouse spleen mAb F4/80 reacts strongly with red pulp but not with marginal zone macrophages or with cells in the white pulp except in association with blood vessels (Crocker). (d) Mouse bone marrow stromal macrophages, but not monocytes, express a haemagglutinin (SER, sheep erythrocyte receptor, mAb SER-4) involved in macrophage-haematopoietic cell interactions. (e) In mouse spleen, SER-4 reacts strongly with a marginal metallophil population of macrophages, weakly with red pulp and not with macrophages in white pulp. (f) Mouse lymph node; subcapsular macrophages express SER-4 antigen-f provided by P. R. Crocker from our laboratory.

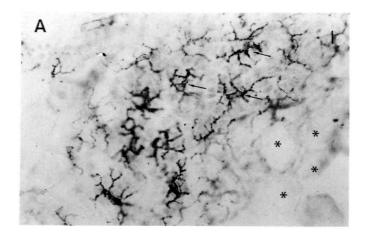

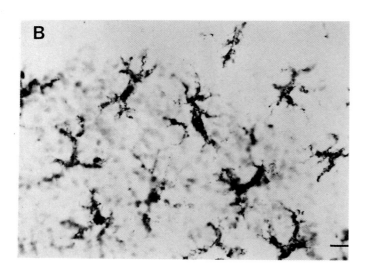

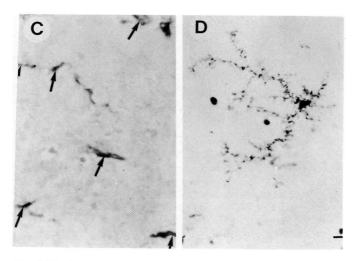

Fig. 4.43 Langerhans cells (A, C) and microglia (B, D) are highly ramified F4/80⁺ macrophages found in murine epidermis (A), stratified epithelia, e.g. oesophagus (C), and in brain (B, D retina). The cells can be distributed in a regular mosaic pattern. (See Hume *et al.* 1983.)

express high levels of Ia antigens unlike most MΦ (Fig. 4.33). They are poorly phagocytic, contain characteristic Birbeck granules not present in MΦ, and share properties with Steinman–Cohn dendritic cells, suggestive of a role in primary antigen responses. After isolation from murine epidermis, Langerhans cells lose some of their MΦ characteristics *in vitro* (e.g. F4/80 antigens) and acquire potent MLR-stimulating activity, indicating that Langerhans cells may be precursors of antigen-presenting cells in lymphoid organs. *In situ*, Langerhans cells form a network of regularly spaced cells at the centre of groups of keratinocytes. Similar highly arborized MΦ are found in other complex epithelia, e.g. oesophagus and cervix. Apart from their possible role in local immune responses, Langerhans cells express receptors for viruses, including herpes simplex and HIV, and these cells, whose phagocytic and respiratory burst activities *in situ* have not been well-defined, may provide an important route of invasion. They are susceptible to ultra-violet irradiation and other forms of local injury, but highly resistant to γ-irradiation.

Gastrointestinal tract

MΦ are normally found in large numbers throughout the gastrointestinal tract within the lamina propria (Fig. 4.40c), outside specialized lymphoid regions, and are well placed for local defence functions. These MΦ are intimately associated with a rich network of capillaries, lymphatics, and nerve terminals. MΦ express plasma membrane receptors for peptides and mediators active in gut (e.g. VIP, bradykinin) (Table 4.17) and release products such as prostaglandins, which in turn could influence cells in their vicinity (Table 4.18). Their possible role in gut physiology and diseases other than infection is unknown.

Lung

Alveolar MΦ are a good example of regionally differentiated resident MΦ that are important in airway defence against invading organisms, particulate substances (e.g. silica, asbestos), and irritants. They are loosely adherent and thus readily obtained for investigation by lavage. Their phenotype is distinct from that of tissue or serosal MΦ (Figs. 4.33, 4.36), but how this arises or is maintained is not known. They respond to local surface-acting stimuli by releasing mediators of inflammation and are thus partly responsible for the influx of other leucocytes, including blood-borne monocytes, after infection or inhalation of irritants such as tobacco smoke. Initial interaction of alveolar MΦ with *Legionella pneumophila*, a MΦ-tropic organism, is critical in determining virulence of this potential pathogen (see Section 4.20). The possible role of alveolar MΦ in other pulmonary functions, e.g. surfactant metabolism, is not clear. Interstitial and other lung MΦ populations are not well characterized, although their proximity to the capillary bed may be important in metabolism of circulating vasoactive peptides such as angiotensin.

Genito-urinary tract

Resident populations of MΦ are found in the interstitium of

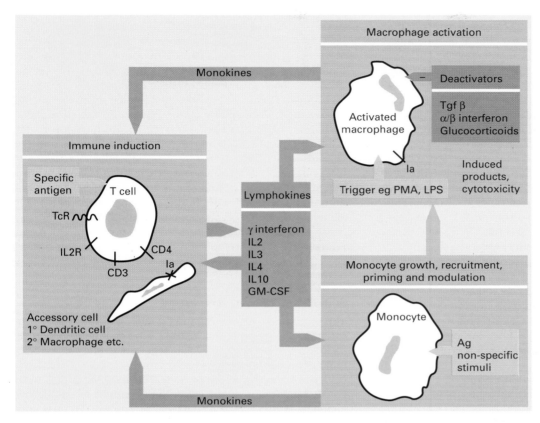

Fig. 4.44 Role of T-helper lymphocytes in immune recognition and monocyte activation in delayed-type hypersensitivity and cell-mediated immunity.

renal medulla (Fig. 4.40e), as part of the juxtaglomerular complex in kidney, and in the lamina propria and epithelium of bladder and prostate. Our own experience is that there are no MΦ in the normal glomerular tuft and that mesangial cells are not related to MΦ. Stellate MΦ in the renal medulla lie close to, but outside, the basement membrane of tubular epithelium, and in the cortex MΦ plasma membrane processes are close to specialized vessels and epithelial cells. Their possible role in control of body fluid balance, pressor activity, and erythropoietin production needs to be investigated. Interstitial MΦ are present in testis and ovary, where fluctuations in cell number and activity occur during the reproductive cycle. MΦ have been noted in the Fallopian tube and are found in the placenta (Hoffbauer cells), but their local properties remain undefined.

Endocrine organs

The adrenal gland contains prominent MΦ in the zona glomerulosa, along vascular sinuses and at the cortico-medullary junction. MΦ are known to respond to glucocorticoids *in vivo* and to metabolize these and other adrenal hormones *in vitro*, but a role in physiologic and pathologic processing of these hormones has not been defined. Both anterior and posterior pituitary contain significant microglial populations. Recent evidence suggests that MΦ/microglia in the posterior pituitary

are part of the pituicyte population, take up neuronal cell fragments and granules with neurosecretory hormones, and possibly modulate hormone release into the circulation. The role of resident MΦ in physiological homeostasis and their contribution to disease processes need further study.

Bone and connective tissue

Numerous interstitial MΦ are found in connective tissue at sites of mechanical stress, and MΦ represent one class of synovial lining cell in joints. Induced MΦ are known to produce various products (growth factors, neutral proteinases, interleukin-1) which influence connective tissue biosynthesis and catabolism, but functions of local resident cells are obscure. Osteoclasts share properties with MΦ (bone marrow origin, blood distribution, giant cell formation, catabolic activities) but lack several MΦ-restricted markers and display unique hormone-responsiveness (Fig. 4.31). They are likely to be a distinct haematopoietic-derived lineage. MΦ in bone retain their markers, as do MΦ giant cells.

Nervous system

After their initial recruitment to the central nervous system during development, monocytes differentiate into microglia and develop elaborate branching processes (Fig. 4.43). Microglia form a regularly spaced network throughout white and grey matter, although certain regions, e.g. the hypothalamus, are particularly densely populated. The morphology and expression of plasma membrane receptors (e.g. CR_3, FcR, CD4) indicate that the phenotype of microglia is influenced by their unique local microenvironment, by the blood–brain barrier, and by their response to local injury ('reactivation'). Microglia in the central and peripheral nervous system differ in appearance and are unlike MΦ in leptomeninges and choroid plexus, which resemble MΦ found outside the nervous system (Fig. 4.40d).

After initial phagocytosis of naturally dying neurons and axons, microglia persist throught adult life and turn over very slowly. The extent of continued recruitment of monocytes to normal adult brain is unknown, although this could play an important role in transporting infectious agents (e.g. human immunodeficiency virus, HIV) to the nervous system by a Trojan horse mechanism. Enhanced recruitment of monocytes to the central and peripheral nervous system following injury may be more significant in this regard and will be discussed below. Resident microglia are down-regulated in expression of many MΦ markers and may retain only a limited phagocytic capacity. Nothing is known about their local functions and responses to ageing, degenerative, ischaemic, or other forms of injury in the nervous system.

Microglia in the nervous system are found on either side of the blood–brain barrier and differential exposure to circulating plasma proteins influences their local functions. For example, their phenotype in circumventricular organs, the subfornical organ and pituitary, differs from that of cells within the blood–brain barrier. The response of microglia in or outside the blood–brain barrier to circulating mediators of inflammation has not been defined, although this could be important in systemic disease processes. Finally, the proximity of MΦ to the cerebrospinal space is compatible with a role in diseases targeted to this site. Apart from their presence in the central and peripheral nervous system, MΦ are also prominent in the autonomic nervous system, although nothing is known about their significance.

4.6.7 Induced recruitment and activation of macrophages: role in host defence, repair, and injury

When local defences are breached and resident MΦ overcome, additional haematopoietic and systemic responses are activated to amplify host resistance, eliminate or contain invading or injurious agents, and initiate repair. Inflammation can comprise antigen-specific humoral and cellular immune processes and a range of immunologically non-specific reactions. Both resident MΦ and recruited monocytes play a role in initiating an acute inflammatory response by releasing mediators after phagocytosis or other stimulation. Monokines and mediators also produced by other cells, e.g. mast cells, endothelium, granulocytes, platelets, and T-lymphocytes, recruit myelomonocytic cells, alter endothelial permeability, activate plasma cascades and platelet reactions, and initiate further systemic

responses. Newly recruited monocytes play a decisive role in host defence through their enhanced cytocidal activities, respiratory burst, and other killing mechanisms, particularly after lymphokine activation (Fig. 4.44). In a murine plasmodial infection model, the number of MΦ in liver and spleen increased 10–20-fold within 1–2 weeks, and similar increases in MΦ mass can be seen during chronic infection by intracellular pathogenic organisms such as *M. tuberculosis* (Fig. 4.40b). Recruitment increases demand on monocyte production and also depends on localized adhesion to endothelium and enhanced extravasation. Macrophages recruited to tissues following infection are heterogeneous and vary in turnover, depending on the nature and persistence of the stimulus. Activated MΦ serve to eliminate invading organisms and stimulate repair, but can cause extensive tissue injury by releasing toxic products and proteolytic enzymes (Table 4.18). We deal here with general aspects of immune and non-specific recruitment and activation of MΦ.

Stimuli for monocyte recruitment

The nature and concentration of a stimulus contribute to the extent and selectivity of leucocyte recruitment. Examples include cell death during development; crush injury to a peripheral nerve; ischaemic injury; sterile irritants, such as thioglycollate broth in the mouse peritoneal cavity; LPS; infections by a wide range of intra- and extracellular pathogenic organisms, including viruses; delayed type hypersensitivity DTH responses; immune-complex deposition; atherosclerotic lesions; metabolic and storage diseases; and certain malignancies. Injury, cell death, microbial infections, and allergic responses tend to elicit recruitment of polymorphonuclear leucocytes and monocytes, with or without involvement of T-lymphocytes, whereas vascular, metabolic, and neoplastic processes evoke more selective mononuclear cell responses. Chemotactic agents for PMN and monocytes include the complement-derived peptides C5a and C3a, leukotrienes and synthetic peptides, e.g. fMet-Leu-Phe. Cytokines such as IL-8, TNFα and β recruit mainly PMN. Chemotactic agents for monocytes alone may derive from fibrin, platelets (TGF-β), T-lymphocytes (MCP-1, Rantes), and other monocytes. Monocytes express plasma membrane receptors for several chemotactic agents (Table 4.17), but their effects on monocyte cytoskeletal, adhesive, and secretory functions are less well characterized than for PMN.

An interesting example of regional differences in recruitment of monocytes is seen in the peripheral versus central nervous system. Section of the sciatic nerve results in brisk inflammatory cell recruitment, uptake of myelin, degeneration of nerve terminals and muscle, and is followed by Schwann-cell proliferation and neuronal regeneration. In contrast, section of the optic nerve results in minimal inflammatory cell invasion which is restricted to the actual site of injury and no distal, Wallerian degeneration or subsequent regeneration. Whether this results from failure to generate or to respond to a chemotactic signal across the blood–brain barrier is not clear. Chemical injury by the excitotoxin ibotenic acid stimulates extensive monocyte recruitment and gliosis in the CNS, but this is highly localized.

Induced MΦ in tissues

Monocyte recruitment is initiated rapidly upon stimulation (hours), but because of the relatively small pools of reserve cells in the circulation and bone marrow, increased numbers of monocyte/MΦ only accumulate in tissues after 1–4 days. These gradually decline in number or persist, depending on the stimulus. Recruited monocytes rapidly acquire new properties upon exposure to endocytic stimuli, lymphokines, microbial products, etc. and are induced to release and synthesize new products (Table 4.18, Fig. 4.33). Exudate MΦ express new plasma membrane antigens, acquire or lose receptor activities, and are able to modulate glycosylation of selected membrane glycoproteins. The pattern of MΦ accumulation depends on the nature of the agent and site of infection, e.g. exudate MΦ are diffusely distributed throughout liver after plasmodial infection, but more focally as granulomata in listeriosis. The well-studied granulomata induced by mycobacterial infection contain T-lymphocytes and several forms of MΦ, including Langhans giant cells and so-called epithelioid cells in human tuberculosis (Fig. 4.45). Epithelioid cells are thought to be poorly phagocytic MΦ, and giant cells result from extensive fusion of MΦ, perhaps induced by the action of lymphokines on cells in which plasma membrane molecules have been modulated by recruitment, microbial products, and other cytokines. Tuberculous and other hypersensitivity granulomata are of the high-turnover type, whereas foreign-body granulomata and MΦ giant cells not associated with activation of T-lymphocytes show little DNA synthesis and cell death. Viruses, e.g. paramyxo- and retroviruses, such as HIV, also directly induce MΦ syncytium formation. Granulomata may contain large numbers of eosinophilic leucocytes (e.g. schistosomiasis), and are usually surrounded by fibroblasts, part of the repair reaction, presumably recruited and stimulated by MΦ-derived growth factors and other products.

Mechanisms of granuloma formation and regression are not fully understood. Particulate, poorly degradable, microbial wall products (e.g. *Corynebacterium parvum*, streptococcal walls) are trapped by Kupffer cells in liver and form a focus of inflammation that initiates T-lymphocyte recruitment and accumulation of monocytes (Fig. 4.44). Nude mice which lack mature T-lymphocytes do not form granulomata in liver in response to these antigens and it is likely that lymphokines, including T-lymphocyte-derived growth factors, play an essential role in monocyte recruitment and focal accumulation. Monokines such as TNFα are also important. Granuloma formation in different organs, e.g. spleen versus liver, is controlled independently by factors such as genetic background of the host and nature of the agent. In experimental listeriosis granuloma formation is needed to localize and contain the infection and the monocyte CR_3 is essential for cell recruitment, granuloma formation, and killing of the organism, as shown by studies with anti-CR_3 mAb which inhibit monocyte/MΦ adhesion to endothelium. In contrast with microbial infections, granuloma formation is uncommon in viral infection, presumably because of spread of organisms between cells and their failure to persist focally.

The spectrum of immune responses seen in human leprosy has provided further insights into DTH and the role of different subclasses of reactive T-lymphocytes in granuloma formation and antimicrobial resistance. CD4$^+$ T-cells are prominent in tuberculoid lesions which contain few surviving organisms, but are inconspicuous in lepromatous lesions in which foamy MΦ are unable to restrict the growth of *Mycobacterium leprae* (Fig. 4.45b, c). Local administration of purified protein derivative (PPD) antigen or recombinant γ-interferon at lepromatous sites induce recruitment and local activation of MΦ. CD8$^+$ cells and a different subset of CD4$^+$ lymphocytes have been shown to control CD4$^+$ helper T-cell responses in models of infection such as experimental leishmaniasis and murine malignancies characterized by immunosuppression, and may play a role in preventing MΦ activation in lepromatous leprosy.

It has been argued on morphological grounds that epithelioid cells in granulomata are highly secretory cells. Indirect evidence indicated that these MΦ secrete high levels of lysozyme, angiotensin-converting enzyme, and probably neutral proteinases which could play a role in antimicrobial resistance and tissue catabolism. Recent *in situ* hybridization studies with nucleic acid probes for human lysozyme cDNA have demonstrated the presence of high levels of lysozyme mRNA in sarcoidosis, tuberculoid reactions in leprosy, and in other granulomatous disease (Fig. 4.46d). It is not known if giant cell formation, *per se*, influences cellular reactivities or whether granuloma MΦ differ from activated MΦ more readily obtained from the peritoneal cavity.

A very different picture is seen in non-infectious conditions such as atherosclerosis or storage diseases (e.g. Fe overload, xanthomata, gangliosidoses) in which local and recruited MΦ accumulate large amounts of endocytosed material, e.g. in vessel walls, connective tissues, lymphohaematopoietic tissues, or the CNS. Lipid-laden 'foam' cells can result from increased uptake, lack of an appropriate mechanism in MΦ to shut down further uptake via low-density lipoprotein (LDL) receptors, or deficiency of lysosomal hydrolases. Lipid accumulation may stimulate secretion of MΦ products, e.g. growth factors for smooth muscle cells, and contribute to the pathogenesis of diseases such as atherosclerosis. Little is known about the mechanisms that selectively recruit monocytes to these lesions.

Properties and modulation of induced MΦ

The phenotype of MΦ varies with the nature of the stimulus, in particular whether different subsets of T-lymphocytes are involved or not, but similar features are induced in MΦ irrespective of the initiating agent or site of stimulation. Unlike lymphocytes, MΦ do not express antigen-specific, clonotypic receptors, but react to class-specific inducers or effector molecules, e.g. LPS, γ-interferon, antibodies, or complement (Fig. 4.45). Induced cells tend to be heterogeneous, express an immature phenotype, high proliferative capacity, and marker changes characteristic of elicited or activated cells. Some of these properties include expression of surface receptors and secretory activities (Fig. 4.33, Tables 4.17, 4.18), important in effector functions. Differences among recruited and resident MΦ

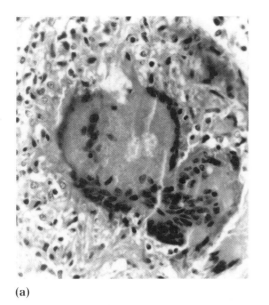

(a)

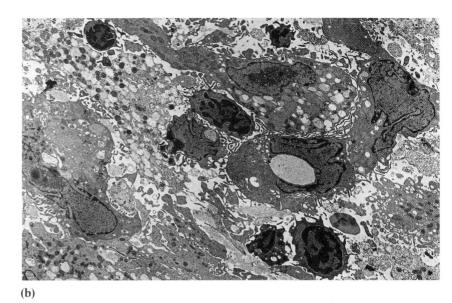

(b)

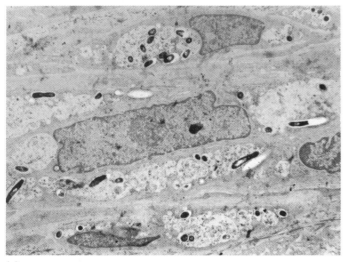

(c)

Fig. 4.45 Heterogeneity in human macrophage morphology and function following granuloma formation in (a) miliary tuberculosis, (b) tuberculoid leprosy, (c) lepromatous leprosy, and (d) toxoplasmosis. (a) Multinucleated Langhans giant cells revealed by haematoxylin and eosin staining and light microscopy. (b) Epithelioid macrophages in contact with activated lymphocytes contain prominent endoplasmic reticulum, vacuoles, and mitochondria, interdigitating plasma membranes, and very few mycobacteria (electron micrograph by G. Kaplan, Rockefeller University, New York). (c) Lepromatous lesions contain few lymphocytes and the macrophages, which lack the abundant organelles seen in (b), are heavily parasitized and foamy in appearance (G. Kaplan). (d) *In situ* hybridization (Chung *et al.* 1988) shows induction of lysozyme message in granuloma macrophages in a reactive lymph node; resident macrophages in most tissues do not contain high levels of lysozyme mRNA or protein (S. Keshav, our laboratory).

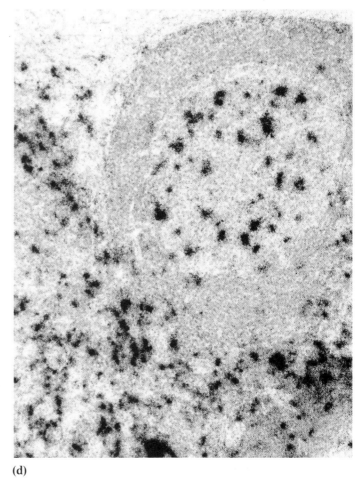

(d)

arise from modulation of MΦ gene expression by the interplay of extrinsic agents and cellular differentiation. Stimuli which modulate MΦ effector functions include micro-organisms, which act on MΦ via phagocytosis or specific wall constituents (e.g. LPS), immune complexes, complement-derived polypeptides, and lymphokines. γ-Interferon is an important MΦ-activating lymphokine and induces many, but not all features associated with MΦ-activation *in vivo*, including enhanced Ia expression and cytotoxicity for intra- and extracellular targets. IC-4, produced by different T-lymphocyte subpopulations, induce Ia, but has distinct modulatory actions on macrophages. γ-Interferon selectively enhances co-ordinate expression of a group of MΦ products, whereas others are down-regulated or unaffected. Some agents synergize with γ-interferon, others, such as glucocorticosteroids which stimulate MΦ to produce lipocortins, oppose its action. α/β-Interferons, derived from non-lymphoid sources including MΦ themselves, induce antiviral resistance and enhanced proteinase release and are able to modify MΦ responses to γ-interferon, but do not induce Ia or prime MΦ respiratory-burst activity. Although acquired immunodeficiency and failure in cell-mediated immunity can usually be ascribed to primary T-cell dysfunction, activated or deactivated MΦ themselves contribute to immunosuppression in a manner which is not yet clear.

Discrete stages of MΦ activation have been defined. It is useful to distinguish a priming stage, e.g. by γ-interferon, from triggering events, e.g. surface stimuli, which localize secretion of a product (Fig. 4.44). The same agent, e.g. LPS, can elicit both stages, although different amounts of an agonist might be required for each step. Macrophages activated within the host by mycobacterial infection display an enhanced response to LPS, compared with resident cells. Massive release of inflammatory mediators and of cytotoxic products such as TNFα can be induced by LPS in such an animal, perhaps reflecting the increased mass of activated MΦ as well as a highly reactive physiological state. Cell activation may be followed by a secondary phase of MΦ deactivation, involving desensitization to specific stimuli and more generalized inhibition of cytotoxic responses, such as the respiratory burst. LPS, TGF-β, and pharmacological agents, such as phorbol myristate acetate (PMA), have been implicated experimentally in these processes. The cellular mechanisms of activation and deactivation, whether at the level of mediator gene transcription and translation, reactivities of surface receptors, or signal transduction, have not been clarified.

Role of induced MΦ in host defence and pathogenesis

The interactions of MΦ with micro-organisms and other targets will be discussed in Section 4.20. Their endocytic activities and secretory products allow induced MΦ to interact with other haematopoietic, vascular, and local cells, and, through effects on hepatocytes, neuronal centres, and endocrine tissues, to co-ordinate systemic responses of the host. These induced MΦ activities are vital for host resistance to injury and infection but, if excessive or persistent, contribute to pathogenesis of disease through cytotoxicity, vascular injury, connective tissue catabolism, hyperplasia, and scarring. Depending on their site of accumulation, they can cause substantial local destruction or dysfunction of cells in their microenvironment. Examples which come to mind include loss of vital tissue functions and fibrosis in lung (tuberculosis, emphysema), joints (chronic destructive arthritis), CNS (HIV encephalopathy), skin (leprosy), and systemic immunosuppression and wasting syndromes associated with persistent infections (trypanosomiasis). Although MΦ are not the only cells involved in these conditions, they are central to the pathogenesis of these diseases.

We know rather less about conditions in which MΦ functions are deficient because of a primary loss of MΦ activity. Direct infection of MΦ by HIV may represent such a situation, although there is also secondary failure of MΦ, associated with T-cell and γ-interferon deficiency. Whatever the mechanism, MΦ failure in advanced acquired immunodeficiency syndrome (AIDS) contributes substantially to the opportunistic infections by intracellular organisms such as *M. avium-intracellulare*. The role of MΦ in chronic diseases such as atherosclerosis, amyloidosis, and neoplasia are less well understood, although they are usually present in these diseases from an early stage. It will be important to develop specific probes to study MΦ functions *in situ* and after isolation of cells in experimental models of disease and in man.

4.6.8 Bibliography

Austyn, J. M. (1987). Lymphoid dendritic cells. *Immunology* **62**, 161–70.

Chung, L. R., Keshav, S., and Gordon, S. (1988). Cloning of the human lysozyme cDNA: Inverted Alu repeat in the mRNA and in situ hybridization for macrophages and Paneth cells. *Proceedings of the National Academy of Sciences, USA* **85**, 6227–31.

Ciba Foundation (1986). *Biochemistry of macrophages. Symposium 118.* Pitman, London.

Cohn, Z. A. (1978). The activation of mononuclear phagocytes: fact, fancy, and future. *Journal of Immunology* **121**, 813–16.

Cohn, Z. A. (ed.) (1988). *Innate immunity.* Current opinion in Immunology. Vol. 1.

Crocker, P. R. and Gordon, S. (1985). Isolation and characterization of resident stromal macrophages and haematopoietic cell clusters from mouse bone marrow. *Journal of Experimental Medicine* **162**, 993–1014.

Crocker, P. R., Morris, L., and Gordon, S. (1988). Novel cell surface adhesion receptors involved in interactions between stromal macrophages and haematopoietic cells. *Journal of Cell Science* Suppl. 9, 185–207.

Crocker, P. R., Werb, Z., Gordon, S., and Bainton, D. F. (1990). Ultrastructural localization of macrophage-restricted sialic acid binding hemaglutinin SER in macrophage-hematopoietic cell clusters. *Blood* **76**, 1131–8.

Furth, R. van (ed.) (1970). *Mononuclear phagocytes.* Blackwell Scientific Publications, Oxford.

Furth, R. van (ed.) (1975). *Mononuclear phagocytes in immunity, infection and pathology.* Blackwell Scientific Publications, Oxford.

Furth, R. van (ed.) (1980). *Mononuclear phagocytes, functional aspects I and II.* Martinus Nijhoff, Dordrecht.

Furth, R. van (ed.) (1985). *Mononuclear phagocytes, characteristics, physiology and function*. Martinus Nijhoff, Dordrecht.

Gordon, S. (1986). Biology of the macrophage. *Journal of Cell Science* Suppl. 4, 267–86.

Gordon, S. (ed.) (1988). Macrophage plasma membrane receptors; structure and function. *Journal of Cell Science* Suppl. 9.

Gordon, S., Keshav, S., and Chung, L. P. (1988a). Mononuclear phagocytes: tissue distribution and functional heterogeneity. *Current Opinion in Immunology* 1, 26–35.

Gordon, S., *et al.* (1988b). *Journal of Cell Science* Suppl. 9, 1–26.

Hogg, N. (1987). Human mononuclear phagocyte molecules and the use of monoclonal antibodies in their detection. *Clinical and Experimental Immunology* 69, 687–94.

Hume, D. A., Perry, V. H., and Gordon, S. (1983). The histochemical localisation of a macrophage-specific antigen in developing mouse retina. Phagocytosis of dying neurons and differentiation of microglial cells to form a regular array in the plexiform layers. *Journal of Cell Biology* 97, 253–7.

Hume, D. A., Perry, V. H., and Gordon, S. (1984). The mononuclear phagocyte system of the mouse defined by immunohistochemical localisation of antigen F4/80. Macrophages associated with epithelia. *Anatomical Record* 210, 503–72.

Kaplan, G. and Cohn, Z. A. (1986). The immunobiology of leprosy. *International Review of Experimental Pathology* 28, 45–58.

Kaplan, G., Luster, A. D., Hancock, G., and Cohn, Z. A. (1987). The expression of a γ-interferon-induced protein (IP-10) in delayed immune responses in human skin. *Journal of Experimental Medicine* 166, 1098–108.

Lang, R. A., Metcalf, D., Cuthbertson, R. A., Lyons, I., Stanley, E., Kelso, A., Konnourakis, G., Williamson, D. J., Klintworth, G. K., Gonda, T. J., and Dunn, A. R. (1987). Transgenic mice expressing a haemopoietic growth factor gene (GM-CSF) develop accumulations of macrophages, blindness and a fatal syndrome of tissue damage. *Cell* 51, 675–86.

Langevoort, H. L., Cohn, Z. A., Hirsch, J. G., Humphrey, J. H., and Spector, W. G. (1970). In *Mononuclear phagocytes* (ed. R. van Furth), pp. 1–6. Blackwell Scientific Publications, Oxford.

Lee, S.-H., Starkey, P., and Gordon, S. (1985). Quantitative analysis of total macrophage content in adult mouse tissues: immunochemical studies with monoclonal antibody F4/80. *Journal of Experimental Medicine* 161, 475–89.

Lee, S.-H., Crocker, P., and Gordon, S. (1986). Macrophage plasma membrane and secretory properties in murine malaria. Effects of *Plasmodium yoelii* infection on macrophages in the liver, spleen and blood. *Journal of Experimental Medicine* 163, 54–74.

Lee, S. H., Crocker, P. R., Westaby, S., Key, N., Mason, D. Y., Gordon, S., Weatherall, D. J. (1988). Isolation and immunocytochemical characterisation of human bone marrow stromal macrophages in haemopoietic clusters. *Journal of Experimental Medicine* 168, 1193–8.

Lepay, D. A., Nathan, C. F., Steinman, R. M., Murray, H. W., and Cohn, Z. A. (1985a). Murine kupffer cells. Mononuclear phagocytes deficient in the generation of reactive oxygen intermediates. *Journal of Experimental Medicine* 161, 1079–96.

Lepay, D. A., Steinman, R. M., Nathan, C. F., Murray, H. W., and Cohn, Z. A. (1985b). Liver macrophages in murine listeriosis. Cell-mediated immunity is correlated with an influx of macrophages capable of generating reactive oxygen intermediates. *Journal of Experimental Medicine* 161, 1503–12.

Macatonia, S., Knight, S. C., Edwards, A. J., Griffiths, S., and Fryer, P. (1987). Localization of antigen on lymph node dendritic cells after exposure to the contact sensitizer fluorescein isothiocyanate. *Journal of Experimental Medicine* 166, 1654–67.

Marchesi, V. T. and Gowans, J. L. (1964). The migration of lymphocytes through the endothelium of venules in lymph nodes: an electron microscope study. *Proceedings of The Royal Society of London B* 159, 283–90.

Metcalf, D. (1984). *The hemopoietic colony stimulating factors*. Elsevier, The Netherlands.

Morris, L., Crocker, P. R., and Gordon, S. (1988). Murine foetal liver macrophages bind developing erythroblasts by a divalent cation-dependent haemagglutinin. *Journal of Cell Biology* 106, 649–56.

Nathan, C. (1987). Secretory products of macrophages. *Journal of Clinical Investigation* 79, 319–26.

Nichols, B. A. and Bainton, D. F. (1973). Differentiation of human monocytes in bone marrow and blood. Sequential formation of granule populations. *Laboratory Investigation* 29, 27–40.

Nichols, B. A., Bainton, D. F., and Farquhar, M. G. (1971). Differentiation of monocytes. Origin, nature and fate of their azurophil granules. *Journal of Cell Biology* 50, 498–515.

North, R. J. (1978). Opinions. The concept of the activated macrophage. *Journal of Immunology* 121, 806–9.

Perry, V. H. and Gordon, S. (1988). Macrophages and microglia in the nervous system. *Trends in Neurosciences* 11, 273–7.

Perry, V. H., Brown, M. C., and Gordon, S. (1987). The macrophage response to central and peripheral nerve injury; a possible role for macrophages in regeneration. *Journal of Experimental Medicine* 15, 1218–23.

Rappolee, D. A. and Werb, Z. (1988). Secretory products of phagocytes. *Current Opinion in Immunology* VI, 47–55.

Rappolee, D. A., Mark, D., Banda, M. J., and Werb. Z. Wound macrophages express TFG-α and other growth factors *in vivo*: analysis by mRNA phenotyping. *Science* 241, 708–12.

Rettenmier, C. W., Roussel, M. F., and Sherr, C. J. (1988). The CSF-1 receptor (c-fms proto-oncogene product) and its ligand. *Journal of Cell Science* Suppl. 9, 27–44.

Rosen, H. and Gordon, S. (1987). Monoclonal antibody to the murine type 3 complement receptor inhibits adhesion of myelomonocytic cells *in vitro* and inflammatory cell recruitment *in vivo*. *Journal of Experimental Medicine* 166, 1685–701.

Schuler, G. and Steinman, R. M. (1985). Murine epidermal Langerhans cells mature into potent immunostimulatory dendritic cells *in vitro*. *Journal of Experimental Medicine* 161, 526–46.

Sherry, B. and Cerami, A. (1988). Cachectin/tumor necrosis factor exerts endocrine, paracrine, and autocrine control of inflammatory responses. *Journal of Cell Biology* 107, 1269–77.

Sieff, C. (1987). Haematopoietic growth factors. *Journal of Clinical Investigation* 79, 1549–57.

Spector, W. G. and Ryan, G. B. (1970). The mononuclear phagocyte in inflammation. In *Mononuclear phagocytes* (ed. R. van Furth), pp. 219–32. Blackwell Scientific publications, Oxford.

Steinman, R. M. and North, R. J. (eds) (1986). *Mechanisms of host resistance to infectious agents, tumors, and allografts*. The Rockefeller University Press, New York.

Steinman, R. M., Inaba, K., Schuler, G., and Witmer, M. (1986). Stimulation of the immune response: contributions of dendritic cells. In *Mechanisms of host resistance to infectious agents, tumors, and allografts*, (ed. R. M. Steinman and R. J. North), pp. 71–97. The Rockefeller University Press, New York.

Voorhis, W. C. van, Hair, L. S., Steinman, R. M., and Kaplan, G. (1982). Human dendritic cells. Enrichment and characterization from peripheral blood. *Journal of Experimental Medicine* 155, 1172–87.

Zucker-Franklin, D., Greaves, M. F., Grosin, C. E., and Marmont, A. M. (eds) (1988). *Atlas of blood cells: function and pathology* (2nd edn). Gustav Fischer, Stuttgart.

4.7   Complement

P. J. Lachmann

Complement was originally defined at the end of the nineteenth century as the heat-labile (at 56 °C) activity of normal human serum that was required in addition to the heat-stable antibody to give rise to the immune lysis of red cells or the killing of bacteria. Over the ensuing decades it has become clear that this activity is the property of a highly complex system of plasma proteins, strongly conserved in vertebrate evolution and with biological functions extending far beyond those originally described, particularly as an enhancer of inflammation.

4.7.1   The components and reaction mechanisms of the complement system

The curious nomenclature of the complement system can be understood only historically. All the original analysis of complement was performed using the lysis of antibody-coated sheep erythrocytes as the test system and those plasma components involved in this reaction are designated by C followed by a number. In general these numbers follow the order in which the components react but the first four components were numbered in the order in which they were described and, for this reason, the reaction sequence begins in the sequence C1, C4, C2, C3. When it was discovered that, using activators other than antibody-coated sheep erythrocytes, these early complement activation stages could be accomplished using an alternative set of proteins, these 'factors' were designated by the letter F followed by other letters. These alternative pathway factors also do not follow a logical sequence of letters since a number of

them, when first named, turned out to be proteins that were already known and named elsewhere in the complement system. There remain Factor B and Factor D as the 'C2-like' and 'C1-like' proteins of the alternative pathway; Factors H and I are two control proteins in this pathway; and Factor P for properdin, the protein originally described by Pillemer in the 1950s.

These many proteins are not a random collection but fall into definite families related to each other by the process of gene duplication and reflect the way that the system has evolved. Figure 4.46 shows the major complement families. Probably the most important is that of the proteins containing the internal thiolester bond (C4, C3, and alpha 2 macrogobulin). C5 is also clearly a member of the same family although it has lost its internal thiolester. The three complement proteins have analogous roles in the classical, alternative, and membrane attack pathways, and C4 and C3 have the capacity to bind to acceptor molecules with either lysine NH_2 groups or sugar hydroxyl groups, forming covalent bonds. These are the essential reactions whereby complement coats micro-organisms or immune complexes and acts as an opsonin.

4.7.2   The reaction pathways of the complement system

There are two quite distinct parts of the complement activation system. The first is a triggered enzyme cascade leading to the cleavage of C3, which is the major complement component, both in quantity and in biological importance. The cleavage of C3 into its two primary cleavage products, C3a and C3bi, is the 'bulk' reaction of the complement system, corresponding to the cleavage of fibrinogen in the coagulation cascade. There are two distinct enzyme cascades giving rise to C3 cleavage: the so-called 'classical' and 'alternative' pathways of C3 activation.

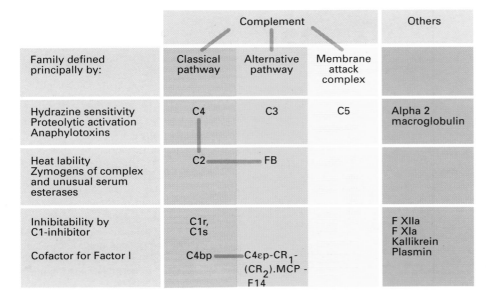

Family defined principally by:	Complement			Others
	Classical pathway	Alternative pathway	Membrane attack complex	
Hydrazine sensitivity Proteolytic activation Anaphylotoxins	C4	C3	C5	Alpha 2 macroglobulin
Heat lability Zymogens of complex and unusual serum esterases	C2	FB		
Inhibitability by C1-inhibitor	C1r, C1s			F XIIa F XIa Kallikrein Plasmin
Cofactor for Factor I	C4bp	C4εp-CR₁-(CR₂).MCP -F14		

Fig. 4.46 Families of complement components. Components joined by lines show genetic linkage in man.

4.7.3   The alternative pathway

It is likely that the alternative pathway is evolutionarily the oldest part of the complement system and it is therefore preferable to describe it first, even though it was worked out much later than the classical pathway. The alternative pathway is essentially a positive-feedback amplification loop in which C3b the principal product of C3 cleavage, itself gives rise to a C3-cleaving enzyme, C3b,Bb (Fig. 4.47). C3b, in the presence of magnesium ions, binds Factor B and this complex is then cleaved to C3b, Bb by Factor D (a serine protease occurring fully active in plasma and which has this as its only known activity). Homeostatic control of this feedback loop is achieved by an analogous cycle in which C3b is further broken down to iC3b which no longer participates in the feedback cycle. Here, C3b binds Factor H and the complex is then cleaved by Factor I (another serine protease occurring fully active in plasma) which cleaves C3b in this complex to C3bi. The extent to which alternative pathway activation proceeds is dependent entirely upon the relative rates of these two opposing reaction cycles and activation of the alternative pathway can be brought about either by mechanisms that accelerate C3b production or those that decrease its destruction. A number of ways in which this can happen are listed in Table 4.19. The most important mechanism is that whereby C3b bound in certain locations is more resistant to inactivation by Factors I and H. These 'protected surfaces' are provided by many particulate polysaccharides, the surfaces of almost all known parasites, and a number of abnormal cells.

This type of dynamic mechanism requires that minimal quantities of C3b are continuously present to keep the system ticking over. It is believed that these are supplied predominantly by the hydrolysis of water of the internal thiolester bond of native C3 to a form designated as C3i which, although it still contains C3a, nevertheless resembles C3b in being able to react in the feedback cycle. It is, however, likely that small quantities of C3b are also generated by other enzymes derived either from the activation of the classical pathway (C42) or from leucocytes (elastase) or from bacteria.

4.7.4   The classical pathway

The classical pathway is more straightforward, being a linear cascade with a definite initiating event, the activation of C1, which is typically brought about by antigen–antibody complexes. The activation of C1 is itself however a far from simple process. C1, as it occurs in plasma, is made up of three separate molecules: C1q, the C1rC1s tetramer, and C1 inhibitor (Fig. 4.48). C1q has six heads capable of reacting with immunoglobulin Fc joined by collagenous stalks to a central region. The molecule has no enzymatic activity and it is believed that conformational changes induced by multiple interaction of the C1q heads with immunoglobulin causes consequent conformational changes in the C1rC1s tetramer, leading to its activation. The C1rC1s tetramer, when isolated from native C1, is a linear molecule having the two C1s molecules peripheral and the two C1r molecules central. Its exact configuration in native C1 remains unknown. It has been suggested both that it is wound around the collagenous arms and that it is held as a ring over the central stalk. The association is fairly loose as is the association with the C1 inhibitor. However, native C1 in the

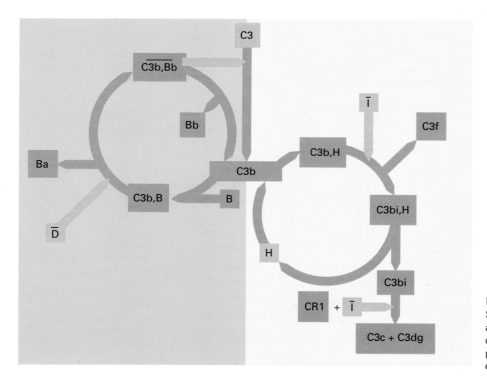

Fig. 4.47 C3b feedback and breakdown. Schematic view of the reaction pathways: Blue arrows indicate conversions; green arrows indicate catalysis. Boxed components are normal plasma proteins; a bar over a component denotes enzymatic activity.

Table 4.19 Initiation of the alternative complement pathway

Tick-over maintained by spontaneous hydrolysis of C3 internal thiolester bond to 'C3b-like' molecule

Tick-over 'fired' by:

1. Mechanisms that increase C3b production
   (a) 'exogenous' C3-splitting enzymes, e.g. $\overline{C4b2b}$
   plasmin
   leucocyte proteases—elastase
   bacterial proteases

   (b) stabilization of $\overline{C3bBb}$
   $\overline{P}$
   Nef
   cp also CVF, Bb

2. Mechanisms that reduce C3b destruction
   (a) fixation on 'protected surface'
   (b) deficiency of Factor H and Factor I
   (c) local sequestration of Factor H

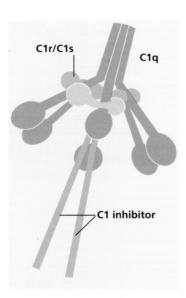

Fig. 4.48 Diagram of the C1–C1 inhibitor complex.

absence of the inhibitor undergoes auto-activation, presumably by an initial 'active-zymosan' activation of C1r (i.e. the pro-enzyme acquiring some activity while still uncleaved) going on to cleave C1s. It requires the presence of C1 inhibitor to prevent this from happening and the real consequence of reacting C1q with an activator is to overcome this effect of the C1 inhibitor. C1s when activated cleaves C4 into C4a and C4b; an analogous split to that of C3 produced by the C3 convertases. The subsequent reactions are entirely analogous to those in the alternative pathway, C3b reacting in the presence of the magnesium with C2 and the complex being split to generate the C3 cleaving enzyme, $\overline{C4b2b}$. However, it is again C1s (or $\overline{C1}$) that cleaves C2 when attached to C4b, so that C1 plays two separate roles in the classical pathway, one initiating the reaction by cleaving C4 (which is not cleaved by either of the C3 cleaving enzymes) the

other taking the role that Factor D has in the alternative pathway. Because calcium is required to hold C1 together, the activation of the classical pathway requires calcium as well as magnesium ions.

4.7.5 The membrane attack pathway

This pathway is the same whether the initial steps are via the classical or the alternative pathway. C3b binds C5; when C5 is so bound it can be cleaved by either of the C3 converting enzymes to give C5a and C5b (again closely resembling C3 and C4 cleavage). Thereafter, the membrane attack complex is non-enzymatic but involves the progressive building up of a multi-molecular complex. C5b combines in its nascent form with one molecule of C6 to give a stable complex C5b6. This complex remains loosely attached to C3b and can elute from it into the supernatant. Normally C5b6 has a very short existence as it immediately reacts with C7, but in certain circumstances (particularly in 'acute phase' plasma) more C5b6 is generated, even in whole plasma, than there is C7 available to react with it and this then gives rise to the formation of free C5b6. C5b6 on its own can be used to initiate the membrane attack complex on cells in the absence of any requirement for other manifestations of complement fixation. This is the procedure known as 'reactive lysis' which has proved very useful in analysing the later stages of complement activation. C5b6 when it reacts with C7 causes the generation of a short-lived binding site, probably on the C7 molecule, which enables the newly formed C567 complex to bind hydrophobically to lipid membranes. This binding is very firm and once the C567 is bound it establishes a long-lived site for the future complement lesion. The sequence is completed by the interaction first of one molecule of C8 and subsequently a variable number of molecules of C9. The C5678 complex itself establishes a small pore through the membrane but a larger and more constantly open pore is established by polymers of C9. The fully formed C9 polymer is circular and contains 12–14 monomers but it is clear that efficient lysis can be produced even in the absence of this circular 'torus' of C9. It is still somewhat controversial whether the membrane lesion produced by complement is wholly a protein-lined channel or whether it is in part also due to the formation of a 'leaky patch' where the inserted membrane attack complex disturbs the lipid bilayer. The full circular polymer of C9 produces the typical electron microscopic lesion of complement (shown in Fig. 4.49).

4.7.6   Membrane proteins limiting complement activation

One of the newer insights into complement function has been that it is not only a plasma system but that a number of cell membrane proteins also participate in the complement sequence. These proteins act at various stages of the complement sequence.

Cofactors of Factor I

Factor I cleaves C3b to C3bi and subsequently to C3dg and C3c (see Fig. 4.50) and cleaves to C4b in an analogous way. In the plasma the cofactor required for C3b cleavage is Factor H but Factor H does not bind C3bi under physiological conditions and so the cleavage to C3dg requires other cofactors. The principal one of these is the membrane complement receptor CR1 which will be discussed in more detail later. CR2 may have a minor reaction of the same kind. There is, however, a further rather shadowy protein—the membrane cofactor protein—which occurs on cells that do not have CR1, which has the same property. All these proteins serve to limit the half-life of C3b bound on cell membranes and therefore serve to limit both the feedback cycle and the initiation of the membrane attack complex.

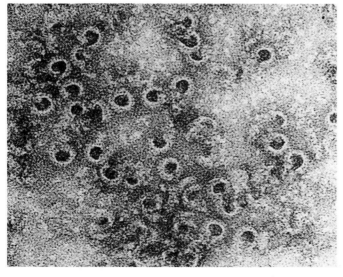

Fig. 4.49 Electron micrograph of complement lesions or bacterial lipopolysaccharide. The lesions are approx 100 Å in diameter. (Micrograph produced by the late Professor J. H. Humphrey.)

Decay accelerating factor (DAF)

There is a further factor on membranes limiting the activation of autologous complement at the C3 convertase stage. This is the decay accelerating factor (DAF), a membrane protein bound through a glycolipid anchor. This acts by preventing the association of C2 with C4b or Factor B with C3b and thereby limits the generation of either C3 convertase. DAF is to some extent species specific in its activity and acts particularly upon autologous complement. Less than a stoichiometric amount of DAF is required for its activity and the molecular mechanisms involved are as yet unknown.

Homologous restriction factors (C8bp and CD59)

There are two other membrane proteins bound through the glycolipid anchor which have a somewhat analogous function to DAF but act at a later stage of the complement sequence. They are the 65 kDa homologous restriction factor C8bp (or HRF) and the 18 kDa CD59 which inhibits the polymerization of autologous C9 and may also limit the activity of autologous C8. They thereby protect cells from lysis by autologous complement.

Paroxysmal nocturnal haemoglobinuria (PNH)

The mechanism generating glycolipid anchors appears to be defective in the clones of cells found in paroxysmal nocturnal haemoglobinuria (PNH). These cells therefore lack both DAF and HRF in addition to acetylcholinesterase, acid phosphatase, and LFA-III. It is the lack of the two complement control proteins that is responsible for the extreme susceptibility of PNH red cells to lysis by their own autologous alternative pathway.

4.7.7   Biological activities of complement

The biological activities of the complement system can be attributed to three kinds of reaction: the interaction of bound complement components, notably C4 and C3, with complement receptors occurring on phagocytic and other cells; production of biologically active fragments, notably the anaphylatoxins C5a and C3a; and the consequences of membrane damage by the membrane attack complex.

The interaction of bound complement components and complement receptors

C3 receptors

The properties and distribution of the four C3 receptors are shown in Table 4.20. It is now clear that they fall into two well-defined pairs. CR1 and CR2 are closely structurally related, both being composed of a series of the typical short consensus repeat found in many proteins that bind C3b (and some others). Nevertheless they show both different ligand binding and a different distribution.

CR1 This is the 'immune adherence' receptor and in primates is present on erythrocytes. It is also found on all phagocytic cells, on kidney podocytes, and on some lymphocytes, notably B-cells. It is known to have two principal functions. The first is

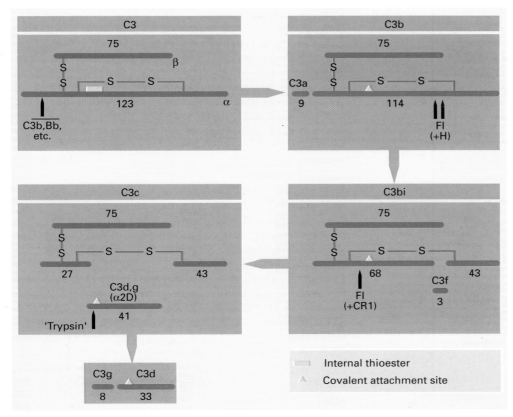

Fig. 4.50 C3 breakdown; figures are molecular masses in kilodaltons.

Table 4.20 Properties and distribution of membrane complement receptors

C receptor type	CD designation	Ligand specificity	Need for divalent cations in ligand binding	Structure (chain mol. wt)	Cell type distribution
CR1	C D 35	C3b, C4b, iC3b	–	Four allotypes: 280K (0.01)* 250K (0.16) 220K (0.81) 140K (0.02) (30+ short consensus repeats)	Erythrocytes, monocyte/macrophages, neutrophils, eosinophils, B-cells, some T-cells, kidney podocytes, dendritic reticulum cells
CR2	C D 21	iC3b, C3dg, C3d EBV	–	140K (16 short consensus repeats)	B-lymphocytes
CR3	C D 11b C D 18	iC3b	+	165K alpha-chain 95K beta-chain	Monocyte/macrophages neutrophils, NK and ADCC effector lymphocytes
CR4	C D 11c C D 18	iC3b, C3dg, C3d	?+	150K alpha-chain 95K beta-chain	Monocyte/macrophages neutrophils, NK and ADCC effector lymphocytes

* Under reducing conditions, allele frequency in brackets; under non-reducing conditions, molecular weights are all approx 30K larger.

The 'short consensus repeats' are sixty-amino-acid domains which are found in most C3-binding proteins (and some others).

as a cofactor for Factor I in the C3b breakdown cycle. In the first step of this reaction, the breakdown of C3b to iC3b, CR1 shares this activity with Factor H. However, in the second and much slower breakdown step of iC3b to C3dg and C3c, CR1 is the only known cofactor. Another major function is that the majority of immune complexes carried in the circulation are bound on red cell CR1 and this plays an important role in the correct handling of immune complexes, discussed below.

CR2 On the other hand, CR2 preferentially binds C3dg and it does not function as a clearance receptor in as much as that red cells coated with C3dg have a normal or supra-normal survival *in vivo*. CR2 is also the Epstein–Barr virus receptor and, as such, is known to be almost wholly restricted in its distribution to B-lymphocyte and B-lymphoblastoid cell lines. Its function seems to be mainly an immunoregulatory one. The interaction of Epstein–Barr virus with CR2 gives rise to the most powerful form of polyclonal activation known in man and requires no collaboration by any other cell type. This polyclonal activation, however, presumably requires steps subsequent to the interaction of the virus with the receptor since it is not found if the virus is inactivated. It has, however, been shown that the interaction of matrixed C3dg, e.g. bound on Sepharose particles, causes B-cell activation while free C3dg has a down-regulatory effect on B-cell activation. Neither CR1 nor CR2 are efficient phagocytic stimulators, although phagocytosis via CR1 can occur on mature macrophages and it is likely that, in synergy with the Fc receptor, CR1 may potentiate phagocytosis.

The other two receptors, CR3 and CR4, belong to the so-called leucocyte-adherance (Leu-CAM) family which also includes LFA-1. These molecules all share a common β-chain and have individual α-chains. CR3 is the principal iC3b receptor on the polymorphonuclear leucocyte. It appears to be wholly specific for iC3b and to have the properties of a lectin since its binding is calcium dependent and can be inhibited by sugars, notably *n*-acetyl-D-glucosamine. CR3 also directly binds yeast cell walls and β-glucan particles. It is a major phagocytic receptor and appears to be the principal receptor responsible for generating a phagocytic superoxide burst in response to complement stimulation. The analogous receptor CR4, which is present in only small amounts on neutrophils, appears to be the major iC3b receptor on the mature macrophage.

Deficiencies of leucocyte-adhesion molecules

Deficiency of the whole family of Leu-CAM molecules has been described in a variety of pedigrees. The abnormality seems generally to be due to a defect in the formation of the β-chain, which leads to an inability to generate the molecules on the cell membrane, and the deficiency is usually subtotal though different pedigrees vary in how severe it is. The clinical consequences of this deficiency are fairly characteristic and of some interest in apportioning importance to the functions of the various receptors.

Typically, the children show delayed separation of the umbilical chord at birth and suffer from an early age from gingivitis with hypertrophy of the gums. They tend to develop skin infections, particularly with staphylococci and these heal poorly, giving rise to 'paper-thin' scars of the type that are associated with polymorph defects. These infections generally respond to antibiotics but a number of children have died of staphylococcal septicaemias which followed upon infections that seemed not greatly different from their previous ones. The deficiency therefore carries a slightly sinister prognosis. Generally, no problems with virus infection, intracellular bacteria, or tumours have been encountered. The syndrome is therefore one that is rather characteristic of neutrophil defect rather than problems with cellular immunity.

On laboratory testing, the characteristic abnormality in these children is their failure to generate a superoxide burst to unopsonized zymosan. It is also possible to demonstrate with monoclonal antibodies that CR3 and CR4 are largely absent on polymorphs and monocytes and that LFA-1 is often more completely absent from lymphocytes. The children show no natural killer (NK) activity, as is to be anticipated from the absence of this group of adhesion molecules, but the same cells that are negative in an NK assay sometimes react, albeit weakly, in ADCC, demonstrating that the problem is mainly in recognition rather than in effector function. This *in vivo* model casts some doubt on the physiological importance of LFA-1 in T-cell functions and emphasizes the great importance of the neutrophil and of CR3 in the host response to bacterial infection.

The anaphylatoxins

The major activation fragments produced in complement activation are C5a and C3a (C4a having similar but very weak reactivity). These fragments are capable of degranulating mast cells, hence their name anaphylatoxins, but they also have striking activation effects on polymorphs and eosinophils and have a direct effect on the microvasculature. C5a is also a potent chemotactic factor. There is no doubt that they can play an important role in anaphylactoid phenomena, though in experimental animals it is necessary to inhibit serum carboxypeptidase B with DL-2-mercaptomethyl-33-guanidioethylthioproanoic acid which destroys the anaphylatoxin *in vivo*, to get the full effect. Animals so treated produced dramatic reactions to complement activation which (in the case of guinea-pigs) may easily lead to death. However, it must be admitted that C5-deficient mice suffer from no very obvious defect that can be attributed to their failure to generate the potent C5a, although they do show some deficiency in response to various infections. Similarly C3-deficient humans, although they show a striking immunity deficiency, show less obvious impairment of inflammatory reactions than one might suppose in subjects who can generate neither anaphylatoxin through the complement system. It is, therefore, still the case that one can attach no particular pathology to an absence of the anaphylatoxins.

The membrane lesions

The most obvious biological effects of the membrane attack system, as demonstrated by the consequences of their deficiency, is in the killing of *Neisseria*. The phagocytosis and intraphagocytic killing of this particular class of micro-organism does not appear to be an effective method for their control, and their destruction in plasma by the complement membrane attack complex seems to be necessary for their adequate control. Deficiencies of the late-acting complement components in man are normally associated only with an increased incidence of neisserial infection, usually meningococcal meningitis, the affected subjects being otherwise quite normal.

4.7.8 Complement, the handling of immune complexes, and the pathogenesis of auto-immune immune complex disease

Deficiencies of the terminal complement components, as stated above, are associated with neisserial infection. Deficiencies of C3, Factor I, or properdin are associated with an immunity deficiency rather similar to that seen in the antibody deficiency states. There is, however, a much less expected association with deficiencies of the early classical complement components, see Table 4.21. These deficiencies are commonly associated with immune complex disease and particularly with systemic lupus erythematosus (SLE). This association is seen, not only with deficiencies of C2 and C4, which are both coded within the MHC, but with deficiencies of C1, which are coded on chromosome 1 for C1q and chromosome 12 for C1r and C1s, and with the secondary deficiencies of C2 and C4 that are seen in hereditary angio-oedema (HAE) due to C1 esterase inhibitor deficiency. This is coded on chromosome 11.

There is, therefore, no possibility of these deficiencies all being linked to a common disease susceptibility gene and there is no reason to question that the increased incidence of these auto-immune immune complex diseases is a consequence of the complement deficiency. Homozygous deficiency of C4 is a (more or less) sufficient cause for the development of SLE and this is almost the only example where a single gene defect is sufficient for the development of an auto-immune disease. It is, however, clearly not necessary since the vast majority of SLE patients are not complement deficient. Further investigation has demonstrated that partial C4 deficiency, and particularly partial deficiency of the C4A isotype (which is the form of C4 that is attached to immune complexes preferentially due to the prefer-

ential formation of amide bonds), also shows an association for SLE, the average relative risk for subjects with a single C4AQ0 allele being in the region of 8. This data is true not only of Caucasians, where the great majority of C4AQ0 is part of a single extended HLA haplotype—the common A1, B8, DR3, C4AQ0 haplotype, but also in oriental populations where the C4AQ0 is not associated with a particular dominant haplotype. This, therefore, suggests that even relatively minor deficiencies of the early components of the classical pathway predispose to these diseases.

While the mechanism for this association is not immediately obvious, the data demonstrate that adequate complement fixation is important for the proper 'handling' of immune complexes. There are probably two ways in which complement fixation influences the fate of immune complexes. The first is that the fixation of C4 and C3 into the antigen–antibody lattice alters the size of immune complex, giving rise to a large number of small complexes as opposed to a small number of large ones. Large complexes formed extravascularly may precipitate locally and cause Arthus reactions but they cannot then give rise to soluble immune complex disease; and it is probable that many pathogenetic immune complexes are formed extravascularly.

The second, and perhaps more important, effect of the presence of C4 and C3 in the immune complex is that such complexes are carried in the circulation predominantly bound on erythrocyte CR1. Under conditions of streamline flow, red cells are in the centre of the vascular stream and the plasma at the periphery. Red cell bound immune complexes should, therefore, not come into contact with endothelial surfaces and should escape transport across endothelia into tissues where they can give rise to inflammation, to the generation of further auto-antigen and to feedback antibody formation.

Red cell bound complexes and antibody-coated erythrocytes are sequestered largely in the liver where there is an efficient macrophage system but no lymphatic tissue and where antigenic material can be removed without feedback antibody formation. To an immunologist this is one of the major functions of the liver. If adequate complement fixation on these complexes fails, they travel in the plasma and can be removed across endothelia into peripheral tissues: the lung, the kidney, the skin, where they can give rise to the problems described above. There is experimental evidence in baboons that in decomplemented animals immune complexes stay in the circulation for a

Table 4.21 Complement deficiencies of early classical pathway components

Component	Chromosomal locus	Number	Healthy	I/C disease (SLE)			Infections (Neisseria)		Other
C1q	1p	17	2	15	(7)	5	(2) skin lesions	(10)	
C1r/C1s	12	9	2	7	(6)	–	–	–	
C4	6p	16	2	14	(12)	6	–	–	
C2	6p	77	15	43	(23)	30	(3)	–	
C1-ina	11	>500	–	2–5%			? not reported (all)		Hereditary angio-oedema

I/C, Immune complex disease; SLE, systemic lupus erythematosus.

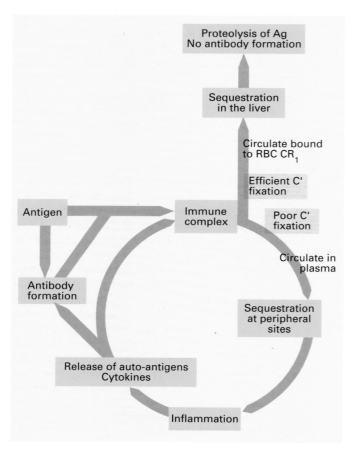

Fig. 4.51 Schema to show the role of complement in immune complex handling and of defective complement function in giving rise to auto-immune immune complex disease.

shorter period of time and are removed at sites other than the liver and spleen. These events are illustrated schematically in Fig. 4.51.

It seems likely that this role of complement in the handling of immune complexes is one of its most important biological activities and one that cannot readily be substituted by other plasma systems. Besides allowing the release of autoantigens at inflammatory sites and promoting antibody formation by the secretion of cytokines, it is possible that the failure to adequately activate complement on immune complexes may also alter immuno-regulation of B-cells through defective C3dg/CR2 interaction.

4.7.9   Further reading

Complement I and II (1983). *Springer Seminars in Immunopathology* **6**, 117–398.

Complement III (1984). *Springer Seminars in Immunopathology* **7**, 93–270.

Lachmann, P. J. (1987). Complement—friend or foe? Heberden Oration 1986. *British Journal of Rheumatology* **26**, 409–15.

Law, S. K. A. and Reid, K. B. M. (1988). *Complement: in focus* (ed. D. Male). IRL Press, Oxford.

Ross, G. D. (ed.) (1986). *Immunobiology of the complement system. An introduction for research and clinical medicine.* Academic Press, London.

Rother, K. and Till, G. O. (eds) (1988). *The complement system.* Springer-Verlag, Berlin.

4.8   Regulation of the immune response

N. A. Mitchison

4.8.1   Control of effector cells by regulatory cells (T–B and T–T co-operation)

Most of the cells in the immune system engage in regulating the activity of other cells, rather than impinging directly on the world outside. This is a feature that the immune system shares in common with the nervous system, and indeed with any system man-made or natural that develops complex homeostatic functions. The principal functions served by the regulatory compartment of the immune system are threefold:

1. tolerance-of-self;
2. epitope linkage; and
3. enabling separate helper and suppressor functions to evolve.

The evolution of a separate regulatory compartment, combined with mechanisms ensuring that effector cells do not normally become activated on their own, has enabled most of the tolerance-of-self functions of the immune system to concentrate within that compartment. This has the enormous advantage of enabling B-cells, as effector cells under regulatory control, to evolve a mechanism of high-rate somatic mutation that would surely not be acceptable in cells that have to take account of self-tolerance. That is not to say that B-cells can never be activated on their own (T-independent responses are discussed below), or that the B-cell compartment never becomes tolerant of self (cell surface allo-antigens such as MHC molecules must induce tolerance of self, as otherwise allo-immunization would generate anti-framework rather than allo-specific antibodies). But several proteins, such as F liver protein and complement component C5, that occur at fairly low concentrations in body fluids have been shown to induce tolerance only within the T-helper cell compartment, and not among B-cells: thus T-cells from C5-deficient mice can co-operate with B-cells from normal mice to make an anti-C5 antibody response.

Epitope linkage is an equally important mechanism. Antigenic structures carry both regulatory and effector epitopes, recognized respectively by lymphocytes of the two compartments. Linkage operates within the immune system in such a way that helper T-cells reacting with a regulatory epitope enable B-cells or the precursor of cytolytic T-cells (Tc-p) to react to effector epitopes, provided that both epitopes form part of the same physical structure. Help of this sort can be intramolecular, with both cells recognizing different parts of the same macromolecule, or intermolecular, involving different macromolecules that form parts of a single antigenic structure, such as a virus or allogeneic cells. The effects of epitope linkage are to facilitate the spread of the response over many epitopes on an antigen, and to minimize the activation of redundant effector cells. Alternatively, epitope linkage can be suppressive, and have the effect of minimizing the spread of the response to new epitopes and thus of canalizing the effector response. The balance between helper and suppressor regulatory cells no doubt determines the balance between the contrary effects of spread and canalization.

Thirdly, there is increasing evidence that the regulatory compartment is split into helper and suppressor subcompartments, and that this has been accompanied by evolution of MHC class II genes so that some specialize in help (*Ir* genes) while others specialize in suppression (*Is* genes). This topic is further discussed below.

4.8.2 The T–B interaction mechanism

Lymphocytes and other cells undergo activation and execute programmed differentiation through fundamentally similar molecular mechanisms. Binding of ligands to receptors transmits a signal to G-proteins that in turn activate membrane-bound nucleotidases, and these in turn generate cyclic nucleo-

tides that act as second messengers to the interior of the cell. Alternatively, or additionally, the phosphatidyl inositol pathway is activated within the membrane, and this generates a Ca^{2+} flux and activation of phosphokinase C, both of which also act as second messages. Lymphocytes can use all three second messages, and these initially drive the cell from G_0 resting condition in to G_1 and then on through the cell cycle. The later stages of activation vary: T-cells start to express IL-2 receptors, secrete lymphokines, and later (in man but not all other mammals) MHC class II molecules. B-cells up-regulate MHC class II expression and subsequently express receptors for the lymphokines that act late in the differentiation programme. Both types of cell, after a series of cell divisions, eventually differentiate, probably at random, into either effector or memory cells.

The first signal received by B-cells is cross-linking of their surface immunoglobulin receptors by antigen. Under physiological conditions this will normally occur at the surface of an antigen-presenting cell, as illustrated in Fig. 4.52. On its own, this signal is not usually sufficient to drive the cell all the way through its differentiation programme to high-rate antibody secretion. Exceptionally, T-cell-independent responses occur, where no further signal is required. There is some evidence for a subpopulation of B-cells that is more likely to perform this type of response, but a more important factor is the nature of the antigen: antigens with repeating epitopes, such as polysaccharides or polymeric proteins such as flagellin, tend to induce

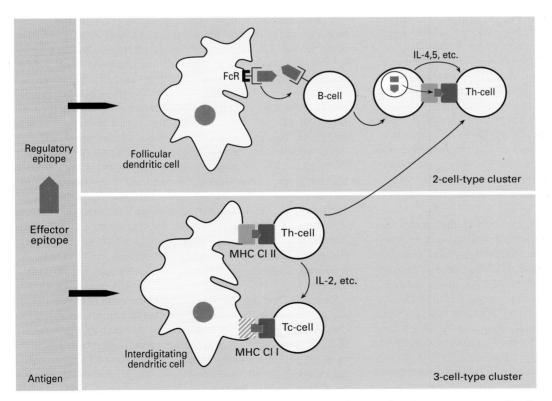

Fig. 4.52 T–B and T–T regulatory interactions. Note (1) at the beginning of the immune response, B cells probably bind antigen directly, not via follicular dendritic cells (2). Accessory and adhesion molecules (not shown) transmit additional signals for T and B cells.

T-cell-independent responses, presumably because they cross-link particularly effectively.

Under *in vitro* conditions cross-linking of Ig-receptors rapidly up-regulates MHC class II expression on B-cells, and this occurs *in vivo* in the mantle zone around lymphoid follicles, where exposure of B-cells to antigen mainly occurs. Meanwhile, as shown in Fig. 4.52, the B-cell is triggered to internalize the receptor–antigen complex in endosomes (receptor-mediated endocytosis) where the antigen is cleaved into peptides able to bind to MHC class II molecules. During the process of degradation the part of the antigen that binds to the Ig-receptor may be protected from attack, and there is evidence that this part is consequently more available to T-cells—the 'protected epitope' hypothesis. Subsequently, some of the peptides bind to MHC class II molecules and then re-emerge on the cell surface, while the immonoglobulin receptors recycle to the surface.

At this point the B-cell is able to make cell-to-cell contact with one or more T-cells, thus forming a 2-cell-type cluster as shown in Fig. 4.52. The contact is mediated by a linked, cognate interaction as illustrated, in which an MHC class II molecule, an antigenic peptide, and a T-cell receptor (TCR) bind to one another to form a trimolecular complex; many such complexes form at the interface between the two cells. In this terminology 'linked' refers to the fact that the epitope recognized by the B-cell that was used to pick up the antigen, and the epitopes finally recognized by the T-cell must be linked together on the same antigenic structure, and 'cognate' refers to the fact that the MHC molecule has to be of the type recognizable by the T-cell. This is an example of the phenomenon of MHC restriction, described in Section 4.2.2. It is worth mentioning that MHC restriction was first discovered in this very context of the T–B interaction, although poorly understood at the time and much clarified by subsequent work on cytolytic T-cells. The interaction that is depicted in the figure has become more vivid now that the three-dimensional structure of an MHC class I molecule is known (see Fig. 4.3). If, as is likely, the same structural principles apply to both classes of MHC molecule, we can expect that the antigenic peptide would bind to a groove on the outer surface of the MHC molecule formed between two α-helices contributed by the two membrane-distal domains (the α_1 and β_1 domains).

The linked, cognate interaction depicted in the figure is not the only force that binds the two cells together. Accessory molecules also take part in the interaction, notably CD4 molecules on the surface of the T-cell that probably bind to the membrane-proximal domains of the MHC molecule (the α_2 and β_2 domains, which are minimally variable in comparison with the distal α_1 and β_1 domains) and thus strengthen the linked, cognate bond. In support of this view, monoclonal antibodies to CD4 inhibit the ability to interact of T-cells believed to have a low-affinity TCR but not those that have a high-affinity one. CD4 molecules also have a signalling function mediated by their cytoplasmic tails. In addition, other glycoproteins on the surface of T-cells, such as LFA-1 and CD2, engage with the B-cell surface prior to and in preparation for the linked, cognate interaction.

An important function of the T–B interaction is to focus the release of lymphokines from the T-cell on to the B-cell, by a process called polarized secretion. Direct microscopic examination of conjugates of T- and B-cells reveals that the Golgi apparatus and the pair of microtubule-organizing centres (MTOCs) of the T-cell become oriented near the nucleus facing the junction, with microtubules running from the MTOCs to the junction. This cytoskeletal structure is reminiscent of the pre-synaptic neurone, where microtubules oriented towards the synapse function as a transport mechanism, bringing vacuoles containing transmitter substances to the presynaptic surface. Quantal release of lymphokines, analogous to that of transmitters by neurones, has yet to be demonstrated.

Recent *in vitro* studies support this view. Cloned T-cells incubate with non-cognate B-cells are able to deliver an activation signal, but they can do so only when the two cell types are crowded closely together, for instance within a tissue-culture well tipped at an angle.

Microscopic examination also indicates that the receptors of the T-cell cluster at the junction. This applies not only to the receptor complex itself, as indicated by CD3 clustering, but also to the CD4 accessory molecules.

4.8.3 Lymphokines that mediate T–B interaction

The lymphokines released by T-cells that interact with B-cells are principally IL-4, IL-5, and IL-6. These are well-defined molecules, with molecular masses respectively of 20 kDa, 18 kDa, and 20 kDa. The DNA sequences of all three structural genes are known. As B-cells go through the processes of activation, proliferation, and differentiation these three lymphokines act more or less in succession, although the details of this sequence are not fully understood. The main factor determining the time of action of each lymphokine is the sequential expression of receptors. Thus, for instance, receptors for the late-acting IL-6 are not present on resting B-cells. In this sequential expression of receptors, B-cells obey the same rules as apply elsewhere in haemopoietic differentiation, for example in the differentiation of macrophages and granulocytes: receptor expression is not exclusive, so that an individual cell can have receptors for and can respond to more than one cytokine. Furthermore, some T-cells have receptors for IL-4, and some B-cells for IL-2, so that the lymphokines are evidently not entirely cell-type specific. Each cell must respond to the balance of the signals that it receives.

In controlling the B-cell response there is no evidence of specialization of T-cells to transmit different signals, in the sense that one T-cell might deliver IL-4 predominantly and another IL-6. Over the question of repetitive linked, cognate interactions by a B-cell, the evidence is equivocal. Certainly, experiments performed *in vitro* demonstrate that a single, brief contact with a T-cell is enough to drive a B-cell to develop into a clone of high-rate antibody-producing cells. Under *in vivo* conditions, responses continue over longer periods and provide opportunity for repetitive interactions, and so the possibility remains open.

Fig. 4.53 illustrates the supposed sequence of action of these lymphokines. IL-4 (previously named B-specific factor I) induces activation of resting B-cells and proliferation, but not differentiation to high-rate antibody production. IL-5 (previously named T-replacing factor, or eosinophil differentiation factor) induces activation (weakly), proliferation, and differentiation. Both the interleukins act also as switch factors, which increase the proportion of IgE-secreting cells; in this process IL-4 induces the switch, while IL-5 selects for B-cells that have switched. IL-5 is also a growth/differentiation factor for mast cells and eosinophils. IL-6 (previously named B-specific factor II or hybridoma growth factor) was first cloned under the name of β2-interferon, but recombinant IL-6 is now known to be devoid of antiviral activity. It promotes the growth and differentiation to high-rate antibody production of B-cells that are already differentiated along this pathway (e.g. hybridoma cells, some EBV-transformed B-cells). It acts also on a variety of other cell types, including astroglia and hepatocytes.

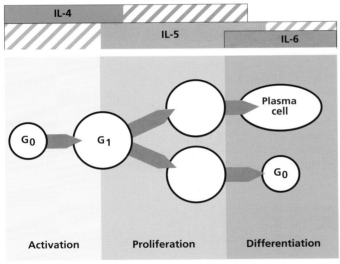

Fig. 4.53 Lymphokine control of the T-cell response.

4.8.4   T–T collaboration

Much can be learned from a comparison of T–B interaction with the interaction between regulatory and effector T-cells. Effector T-cells, cytolytic T-cells (Tc), and also the T-cells that mediate delayed-type hypersensitivity, develop under the control of regulatory T-cells. Thus, cytolytic T-cell responses in the mouse to an antigen such as H-Y are controlled by MHC class II as well as MHC class I immune response genes; IL-2 is a lymphokine that is produced predominantly by CD4 T-cells and is required by many CD8 cytolytic T-cell clones for their growth; *in vitro* cytolytic T-cell responses can be set up in such a way that they depend on extrinsically supplied IL-2; and acquired immunodeficiency syndrome dramatically illustrates an effector T-cell functional deficit brought about by selective loss of CD4 cells.

Under *in vitro* conditions IL-2 often induces an effector T-cell

response without the need for cell-to-cell contact between the lymphokine producer and its target. This is, a priori, unlikely to occur under physiological conditions, as it would lose for the response all the benefits of epitope linkage that were described earlier in this chapter. And, indeed, when the need for epitope linkage in the control of the cytolytic T-cell response has been examined under physiological conditions *in vivo*, in mouse experiments, it is usually evident.

How then is epitope linkage established in this form of cooperative cell interaction? From this point of view vertebrate species divide into two types, those which express MHC class II molecules on T-cells, such as man and chicken, and those which do not, such as mouse. The reason for this difference is not known, although body size has been identified as a possible factor. At any rate, in a species such as the mouse the interaction takes place through the formation of three-cell-type clusters, of the kind illustrated on the right-hand side of Fig. 4.52. In man the situation is slightly different. The presence of MHC class II molecules on T-cells means that two-cell-type clusters, analogous to those formed in the T–B interaction, potentially can mediate T–T interactions; and, indeed, it is hard to imagine what other function MHC class II molecules in that particular location could serve. It is likely that in man T–T interactions involve both types of mechanism, with three-cell-type clusters predominating in at least the initial phase of the immune response.

It is worth summarizing the important information about three-cell-type clusters. First, T-cells can be seen to form clusters around dendritic cells (but not macrophages) *in vitro*. Secondly, when appropriate populations of mouse cytolytic T-cell precursors and regulatory T-cells are combined together *in vivo* by adoptive transfer, their interaction need not be cognate under conditions that do require epitope linkage. This is a negative piece of evidence, so a third point is more telling. In such adoptive transfer experiments, the concentration of antigen can be varied. At low antigen concentration the epitopes recognized by effector–precursor and regulatory cells do indeed need to be linked, presumably because only then will a single host antigen-presenting cell pick up both epitopes, and thus be able to bring the two types of T-cells together. At high antigen concentration the host antigen-presenting cells must have a good chance of taking up both epitopes even when they enter the body on two separate structures, and under these conditions it is, indeed, found that epitope linkage is no longer required for the cell interaction to take place. In terms of ability to work at low antigen concentrations, the three-cell cluster performs almost as efficiently as two-cell ones (i.e. comparing activation of cytolytic T-cells versus B-cells to the same antigen).

4.8.5   The logical structure of the lymph node

The foregoing information about cell clusters provides a framework for discussion of lymph node structure. Various features of lymph node structure and function that previously seemed arbitrary now begin to fit together logically.

Consider first the fact that three-cell-type clusters (T–T)

perform almost as efficiently as two-cell-type clusters (T–B). This is as expected, because some species (e.g. man) can make two-cell T–T clusters while others (e.g. mouse) cannot. When mechanisms vary from one species to another they are unlikely to differ profoundly in efficiency.

Yet T–B interactions never utilize three-cell clusters, or at least no species is known to do so. Probably this is because three-cell clusters work well only when the participating lymphocytes have the same traffic patterns. T-cells and B-cells have different traffic patterns within a node, and therefore require the type of cluster that is easier to form. But this, in turn, raises the question of why these T and B traffic patterns differ.

This difference can reasonably be attributed to differences in antigen presentation. Antigen-presenting cells are of two types: one type that presents to T-cells, and another that presents to B-cells (see Fig. 4.52). The first type degrades antigen and associates it with MHC class II molecules, while the second retains conformationally intact antigen on its surface. The first type comprises interdigitating dendritic cells, and the second follicular dendritic cells. This assignment is based on the presence of conformationally intact antigen in detectable amounts only on the latter type of cell (excepting during the very early phase of the immune response).

In order for the first type of antigen-presenting cell to deliver epitope linkage from three-cell clusters, they must be spaced well apart from one another. This prevents a regulatory T-cell from helping an effector T-cell that is part of another cluster. Histological examination discloses that, as expected, interdigitating cells are indeed spaced well out from one another, whereas follicular dendritic cells form a dense, lacey network.

In order for a follicular dendritic cell to function, a B-cell must be able to steal antigen from the antigen–antibody complex on its surface. To do so it must presumably use a higher affinity antibody than the one that is already part of the complex on the surface of antigen-presenting cell. The maturation mechanism, whereby antibody affinity progressively rises, fulfils that requirement.

As expected, T-cells do not mature in this sense (they lack a hypermutation mechanism). This lack of maturation, and the properties of the interdigitating dendritic cell probably evolved together. There are, of course, other reasons for T-cells to lack hypermutation, notably in order to maintain tolerance of self. Indeed, if proliferation within the micro-environment of a follicle is what causes hypermutation, as the evidence suggests, the difference in traffic pattern would itself ensure that T-cells do not hypermutate. These various properties of the immune system are best thought of as evolving in parallel with one another.

4.8.6   Two populations of regulatory T-cells

There is increasing evidence that CD4 (helper) T-cells can be divided into two main subsets, as indicated in Fig. 4.54. One subset is controlled by *Ir* (immune response) genes that map predominantly to the MHC class II loci HLA-DR in man and H-2A in mouse; mediates resistance to infection; helps in antibody production via release of IL-4, IL-5, and probably also IL-6; is relatively less tightly controlled by the idiotypic network; and is the predominant type of parasite-specific T-cell in animals regressing a leishmaniasis lesion, or vaccinated intravenously with killed parasites. In contrast, the other subset is controlled by *Is* (immune suppression) genes that map predominantly to HLA-DQ and H-2E; mediates protection against

Genetics		Disease resistance		Cell interaction	
Immune response genes (Ir)	Immune suppression genes (Is)	to acute infection	to hyper-sensitivity	Th → B	Th → Ts Th → Tc
Restriction		Id-anti-Id connectivity		Lymphokine secretion (mouse)	
HLA-DR	HLA-DQ	+	++	IL-4 IL-5	IL-2 g-IFN
Markers		In leishmaniasis (mouse)			
CD45R⁻	CD45R⁺ Leu8⁺	T reg. T i.v.	T prog. T s.c.		

Fig. 4.54 Splits in the CD4 immunoregulatory set of T-cells.

hypersensitivity; helps generate suppressor and cytolytic T-cells via release of IL-2 and γ-IFN; in helping generate suppressor T-cells, operates predominantly through the idiotypic network; and predominates in leishmaniasis progressor mice and mice vaccinated subcutaneously.

The potential importance of this split is vast. The balance of activity between the two subsets may determine the outcome of the immune response, in terms of activating T- versus B-effector cells (cellular versus humoral immunity); and also the magnitude of the response, through control of the balance between helper and suppressor activities. These, in turn, can determine resistance versus susceptibility to infection, as well as the level of immunopathological damage in chronic infection and autoimmune disease. Via control of effector T-cells versus mast-cell/Ig-E-mediated mechanisms, the balance between the subsets may determine the nature of hypersensitivity. And, if the MHC class II-specialization hypothesis is correct, the differentiation of these two subsets has played a major role in controlling the evolution of the MHC complex.

The evidence of a split among CD4 T-cells has sharpened recently, particularly in three areas. First, as regards the pattern of lymphokine secretion, the orientation of one lymphokine profile towards T-cell interactions and the other towards B-cells, as outlined above, has found support in an extensive survey of mouse CD4 T-cell clones (IL-6 has not yet been included in this analysis). A terminology of TH1 and TH2 to describe respectively the T- and B-orientated profile is now widely used. Nevertheless, significant problems remain: in particular, studies with human T-cell clones do not support a simple dichotomy.

As regards markers, significant progress has been made through the discovery that many monoclonal antibodies produced in different laboratories do in fact recognize the same molecules of the T200 complex. The T200 gene transcript undergoes alternative splicing so as finally to encode four electrophoretically distinct cell-surface glycoproteins. All four have an identical membrane-proximal domain, and monoclonal antibodies that recognize this domain are grouped together as of type CD45. It is the more distal domain which is subject to alternative splicing, and which is recognized by monoclonal antibodies of type CD45R (R for restricted, to indicate that not all lymphocytes bear this marker). Many antibodies have been made independently that recognize the 2–3 higher molecular weight T200 isoforms. As might be expected, reagents specific for the low molecular weight T200 isoform are harder to make, as they must recognize a new combination at the splice site from an old peptide sequence (or a new conformation), rather than entirely new sequences as is the case for the larger glycoproteins. Only one such reagent is available at present, called UCHL1 (see Section 4.5). All this represents a new insight into the molecular biology of what was previously a confusing group of markers. The CD45R$^-$ condition is a maturation marker, in that most CD4 T-cells have the CD45R phenotype while at rest and convert to CD45R$^-$ upon activation by antigen. This presents a problem, in that the overall split now has to reconcile fixed, lineage-specific characteristics, such as MHC restriction, with this labile marker. At present it is uncertain whether the CD45R glycoproteins engage in some unique molecular interaction while expressed on resting cells, as has been suggested, or alternatively, whether T-cells expressing a particular part of the TCR repertoire occur more frequently in an activation compartment marked by the CD45R$^-$ phenotype, as has also been suggested.

As regards control by the MHC, the evidence has sharpened in regard to *Ir* and *Is* genes, to an extent that merits separate discussion in the ensuing section.

4.8.7   *Ir* and *Is* genes

Procedures for identifying *Is* (immune response) genes are becoming better established, and the list of such genes is growing in man and mouse. Indeed, this may be the best understood part of the whole confusing area of suppression. The standard procedures used now include:

1. at the population level, segregation analysis that can identify an MHC gene (or other gene) mapping as a factor that confers dominant susceptibility to an infection or dominant resistance to a hypersensitivity (or dominant failure to make some other type of immune response);

2. at the family level, concordance in segregation of an MHC gene with similar susceptibility or resistance;

3. *in vitro* analysis of the cellular immune response, usually by proliferation, demonstrating relief of suppression by addition of an MHC-specific monoclonal antibody (referred to as 'reverse titration', as the addition of larger amounts of the antibody has the paradoxical effect of increasing the proliferative response);

4. in the mouse, a distribution of suppression among mouse strains that coincides with deletion or inactivation of the H-2E MHC class II locus;

5. again in the mouse, restoration of suppression by an H-2E transgene.

Note that, in the mouse, familial concordance is made easier to study by the existence of panels of inbred recombinant strains that constitute a sort of frozen family, in contrast to freshly bred animals.

As identified in these ways, *Is* genes map without exception to MHC class II loci. This activity is not distributed at random among class II genes, but tends to focus at one specialized locus for each species, namely HLA-DQ in man and H-2E in the mouse. By now there are many such examples in the mouse, and no clear-cut exceptions except where the E locus is inactive, in which case suppression may or may not switch to H-2A. In man the following responses have been identified as provoking HLA-DQ-linked suppression: to *Cryptomeria* pollen, to a schistosome antigen, to *Mycobacterium leprae*, and auto-immune insulitis; and tuberculin hypersensitivity is suspected of doing so. This specialization of loci is by no means complete, as for instance H-2E can also serve as an *Ir* gene in the immune response to foreign cytochrome C. Nor is it consistent in evolution, for H-2E and HLA-DQ are not homologous genes.

This kind of loose bias in function can be viewed as largely a consequence of evolutionary selection by chronic infection, rather than as fulfilling a supposed need for homeostatic balance within the immune system. According to this view parasites are under selective pressure to generate immunopathology, as this will put pressure on the host to develop *Is* function, which will in turn benefit the parasite. In support of this view, fitness of the host is generally reduced less by parasitization *per se* than by immunological conflict between host and parasite that generates immunopathology. Hypersensitivity to parasites is a major feature of tropical disease. When parasite and host engage in this kind of collusion, neither is under selective pressure to escape through polymorphism, and *Is* function will tend to focus at one locus so as to leave the other free to develop the high level of polymorphism that is associated with *Ir* function. This may explain why it is the less polymorphic loci H-2E and HLA-DQ that exercise *Is* function, even though they are not homologous.

4.8.8 T-helper and T-suppressor factors

Immunologists do not at present know what to make of antigen- or idiotype-specific helper (ThFs) and suppressor (TsFs) factors produced by T-cells. The body of experimental data supporting the existence of such factors cannot be avoided, but progress with molecular characterization has been slow, and this area has largely dropped out of current research. At one time it was hoped that this research would provide a way into the molecular biology of T-cell receptors, but progress made elsewhere has superseded that motivation. More importantly, the new information that has been acquired concerning lymphokines, cells clusters, and cell-to-cell functions tells us that ThFs are not a necessary part of the cell interaction machinery, although it does not exclude the possibility that they are an optional extra. Nor does it exclude the possibility that ThFs and TsFs may find valuable applications in therapeutic manipulation of the immune response. A few immunologists hold high hopes for the use of such factors in the control of allergy and in prevention of transplant rejection, and studies to those ends are still being pursued. Success in those endeavours would undoubtedly rekindle general interest in these factors.

ThFs and TsFs are either extracted from T-cells or collected from their supernatant *in vitro*. They fall into two broad categories: Fc_ε R-like molecules that can be shown to regulate the IgE response, and molecular complexes of MHC class II and TCR molecules (or fragments of these molecules) that bind to antigen-presenting cells and regulate the activity of helper T-cells. In neither case has the possibility that these molecules are simply cleaved off the surface of T-cells under artificial conditions been entirely excluded. Some of these factors are active not only in *in vitro* assays but also upon transfer into experimental animals, but there is no convincing evidence that they are actually released under physiological conditions *in vivo*. Such evidence may be very difficult to obtain, as the long history of debate over candidate neurotransmitters has shown.

4.8.9 The idiotypic network

Thus far this account of the immune system has been couched in the usual terms of a system at rest until it 'responds' to an external 'challenge' in the form of an antigen. There is an alternative view, first formulated by N. Jerne, that focuses on idiotype–anti-idiotype (id–anti-id) interactions that maintain the system in a constantly active equilibrium until that equilibrium is perturbed by antigen.

Every antibody has a structure of its variable region that is more or less unique, and which can be recognized as such by other antibodies able to combine with it. The antigenic determinants that these other antibodies recognize are termed 'idiotopes', and the set of idiotopes defines the 'idiotype' of the original antibody. Note that the relationship between an anti-idiotypic antibody and the idiotope that it recognizes is completely symmetrical; each binds to the other, and each can induce the other. Hence the term 'network', for presumably these interactions ramify indefinitely. Note also that the theory as originally formulated for antibodies applies equally well to T-cell receptors, and indeed there is some irony in the contemporary view that it is among the T-cell receptors that the strongest evidences of network control are to be found.

Network interactions that can ensue as a consequence of antigenic challenge are shown in Fig. 4.55. An antigen enters the immune system, and induces a rise in the concentration of Ab1 antibodies. These antibodies were previously present at too low a concentration to perturb the system, i.e. they induced neither immunity nor tolerance, but now they begin to provoke an anti-idiotypic response. The anti-idiotypic antibodies are termed by convention types Ab2α and Ab2β. Ab2β antibodies recognize the binding site for the original antigen on the Ab1 set and, therefore, jointly constitute an 'internal image' of the antigen, while Ab2α antibodies recognize those parts of the Ab1 idiotype that fall outside the combining site. The Ab2 sets give rise to a further Ab3 set, as shown, and so on indefinitely.

As noted above, the network theory can be formulated in an alternative way. Instead of starting with an antigenic challenge, we consider the immune system as it develops, and suppose that

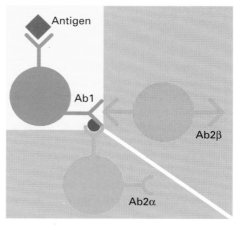

Fig. 4.55 The idiotypic network.

antibodies at their unperturbed concentrations are able to stimulate other lymphocytes via id–anti-id interactions. More realistically, we may assume that only some antibodies can do so, most probably the germ-line-encoded ones that are known to be formed in quite large amounts in the absence of antigen. The whole system will then tend to develop as a network, with a multitude of activating and suppressive connections. According to this view, the effect of conventional, extrinsic antigen will be to perturb the network, making and breaking the established connections, and this is what somehow generates the conventional immune response.

Although this represents a radical reappraisal of the way the immune system works, its mechanisms are not really very different in detail. Effector and regulatory compartments would still interact much as before, and antigen presentation work in much the same way. Indeed there is growing evidence, for instance, that idiotypic antigens work most effectively if presented by dendritic cells.

4.8.10   An assessment of the importance of the network: CD5 B-cells

Several studies have shown that network interactions during the first few weeks of life are particularly important in moulding the B-cell repertoire of the mouse. Thus, for example, treatment of a mouse with antibodies to the major germ-line idiotype of anti-1, 3-dextran antibodies, or to that of anti-phosphorylcholine antibodies, induces a profound perturbation, so that for the rest of its life the mouse becomes unable to make these idiotypes. In an even more convincing demonstration of network control, it has been possible to induce similar perturbations not with the anti-id itself, but with an anti-anti-id (Ab3). Indeed, as more becomes known of the germ-line-encoded repertoire, it is becoming possible to predict exactly what the impact will be made on a given anti-id further along the network.

It transpires that most of these germ-line encoded antibodies in the young mouse are made by a subset of B-cells bearing the CD5 marker, a structurally well-characterized cell surface glycoprotein of unknown function (the gene sequence suggests that it may be a receptor for a growth factor). From the network viewpoint these constitute a central subset, which is tightly connected by network interactions, which gradually expands during the life of a mouse driven only by id–anti-id interactions, and which influences through network connections the repertoire of conventional B-cells and also of T-cells, as illustrated in Fig. 4.56. Thus while conventional B-cells upon adoptive transfer die out unless stimulated extrinsically with their specific extrinsic antigen, CD5 B-cells gradually expand independently of extrinsic stimulation. According to this assessment, then, the network is critically important, but only for a limited part of the immune system.

In the normal adult mouse, and probably also in man, CD5 B-cells contribute less than 10 per cent of the antibody response to most conventional antigens, with the rest coming from conventional B-cells. CD5 B-cells contribute a larger proportion of

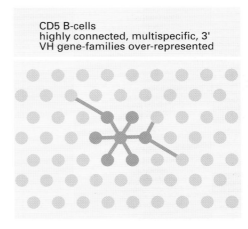

CD5 B-cells
highly connected, multispecific, 3'
VH gene-families over-represented

Fig. 4.56   A central set of B-cells.

some of the antibodies important in immunopathology, particularly certain auto-antibodies in rheumatoid arthritis. Their normal function is less clear: their principle role may be in moulding the repertoire expressed by other lymphocytes; alternatively, or additionally, they may form an early developing, first-line, constitutive defence against microbial infection, as the presence of antibacterial antibodies such as anti-dextran and anti-phosphorylcholine in their repertoire suggests.

4.8.11   A further assessment of the network: epirestriction of T-cells

Another aspect of the immune system where control through the idiotypic network operates is in the influence exercised by immunoglobulin V genes on the T-cell repertoire. The mechanism of this control is outlined on the left-hand side of Fig. 4.57. An immunoglobulin molecule is expressed on the surface of a B-cell, where it can be recognized by the receptor of a T-cell through an id–anti-id interaction. Consequently this T-cell becomes activated, and in turn interacts with a second set of T-cells, whose receptors will jointly form an internal image (as defined above) of the V region of the original immunoglobulin molecule. The intermediate T-cell has been termed a 'conductor' cell, and its effect is to select the second population of T-cells strongly in favour of those that form the internal image. So strongly can this selection operate that, in the extreme case, T-cells become unable to make id–anti-id interactions with T-cells of unrelated individuals that have been exposed via this pathway to the products of other immunoglobulin genes.

This selection is responsible for the following remarkable phenomenon in the field of suppression. Certain types of suppressor-effector T-cells (indeed perhaps all such cells) require an obligatory id–anti-id interaction with a suppressor-inducer cell in order to become activated. It has been observed several times that these suppressor-inducer and suppressor-effector cells become unable to interact with one another if they come from mice which differ only at the *IgVH* genes. For many years this phenomenon was misinterpreted in terms of involvement of

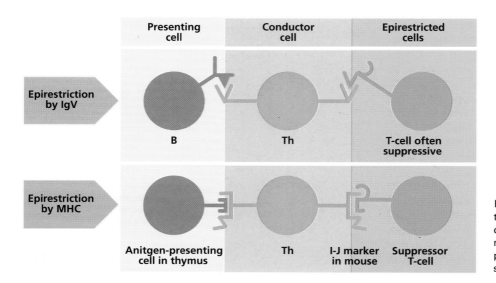

Fig. 4.57 Indirect control of T-cell receptors through the idiotypic network. The TCRs depicted here as directly recognizing Ig or TCR molecules in fact probaby mainly recognize peptides derived from these molecules, presented by MHC molecules.

an *IgVH*-linked gene product on the surface of the suppressor cells, but it now seems highly probable that the mechanism depicted in Fig. 4.57 is responsible. The phenomenon was termed *IgVH* restriction, by analogy with MHC restriction which it closely resembles. Note, however, that the two T-cells recognize one another here through their usual T-cell receptors, without involving an immunoglobulin. So the gene that operates the restriction does not itself encode the product that is recognized by the restricted cells. Hence the term 'epirestriction' that has been coined for this phenomenon.

Several other lines of evidence support the view that the T-cell repertoire is strongly influenced by immunoglobulin V genes. Thus:

1. *IgVH*-encoded idiotypes are expressed in T-cell populations, and in genetic crosses of mice these T-cell idiotypes cosegregate with *IgVH* genes;

2. in other genetical experiments in mice, *IgVH* genes profoundly influence the fine structure of T-cell responses to allo-antigens; and

3. treatment of young mice with anti-IgM antibodies has a profound effect on T-cell responses.

In this last type of experiment, *IgVH*-epirestriction as defined above can be altered or lost; and an *IgVH*-encoded idiotype that is normally expressed by helper T-cells has been made to disappear from the treated animal. In these experiments it is particularly significant that the mice need to be young, and that treatment of older mice has little effect: once again, the CD5 B-cell is implicated, this time as the B-cell depicted at the top of Fig. 4.57.

The right-hand side of Fig. 4.57 illustrates a more controversial pathway, but one for which there is some evidence. Through essentially the same mechanism as is described above for epirestriction by *IgVH* genes, MHC molecules expressed in the thymus likewise appear to generate their internal image within the T-cell repertoire. This internal image is important in

interpreting certain findings concerned with suppression, concerning the puzzling I–J marker of the mouse. The salient facts about I–J are that this antigen is controlled but not encoded by MHC class II genes; that interactions of suppressor-effector cells with both their inducers and their targets behave as though epirestricted by I–J; that the I–J phenotype of a T-cell is determined not by the genotype of that cell but by the thymus with which the cell matured; and that I–J switches to donor phenotype in an H-2E⁻ mouse bearing an H-2E transgene. These observations can best be explained by the epirestriction scheme shown in the figure.

In this admittedly murky area of T-cell network control what stands out is the major impact that epirestriction has on suppressor T-cells. Here, and from other evidence as well, these cells seem to be more highly connected through the idiotypic network than other T-cells. Naturally, the question arises whether suppressor function may be a direct consequence of connectedness; perhaps a cytolytic T-cell that interacts with its target via id–anti-id binding, thereby exerting a suppressive effect? Until more is known about the mechanism of suppression this question is likely to remain unanswered. In the meanwhile, a high degree of connectedness can be numbered with justification among the characteristic features of suppressor T-cells, as shown in Fig. 4.55.

4.8.12   Further reading

Allen, D., *et al.* (1987). Timing, genetic requirements and functional consequences of somatic hypermutation during B-cell development. *Immunological Reviews* **96**, 5–22.

Griffiths, J. A., Mitchison, N. A., Nardi, N., and Oliveira, D. B. G. (1987). F protein. In *Immunogenicity of protein antigens: repertoire and regulation*, Vol. II (ed. E. Sercarz and J. Berzofsky), pp. 35–41. CRC Press, Florida.

Kieber-Emmons, T. and Kohler, H. (1986). Towards a unified theory of immunoglobulin structure–function relations. *Immunological Reviews* **90**, 29–48.

Lanzavecchia, A. (1987). Antigen uptake and accumulation in antigen-specific B-cells. *Immunological Reviews* 99, 39–51.

Miller, A. and Sercarz, E. (1987). The choice of T-cell epitopes utilized on a protein antigen depends on factors distant from, as well as at, the determinant site. *Immunological Reviews* 98, 53–73.

Mitchison, N. A. and O'Malley, C. (1987). Three cell type clusters of T-cells with antigen presenting cells best explain the epitope linkage and non-cognate requirements of the *in vivo* cytolytic response. *European Journal of Immunology* 17, 1579–83.

Mitchison, N. A. and Oliveira, D. B. G. (1986). Epirestriction and a specialised subset of T-helper cells are key factors in the regulation of T-suppressor cells. In *Progress in immunology VI* (ed. B. Cinader and R. G. Miller), pp. 326–34. Academic Press, London.

Slaoui, M., *et al.* (1986). Idiotypic games within the immune network. *Immunological Reviews* 90, 73–91.

Swain, S. L. and Dutton, R. (1987). Consequences of the direct interaction of helper T-cells with B-cells presenting antigen. *Immunological Reviews* 99, 263–80.

Vitetta, E. S., *et al.* (1987). Interaction and activation of antigen-specific T- and B-cells. *Immunological Reviews* 99, 193–239.

Takemori, T. and Rajewsky, K. (1984). Mechanism of neonatally induced idiotype suppression and its relevance for the acquisition of self-tolerance. *Immunological Reviews* 79, 103–17.

4.9 The hypersensitivity reactions

S. T. Holgate and T. J. Hamblin

The classification of hypersensitivity reactions into four types, as originally proposed by Gell and Coombes, represented a milestone in the understanding of how exaggerated immune responses could be tissue damaging and how these destructive events related to known clinical diseases. With a clearer understanding of the complexities and the interrelationships between the various areas of the immune system, the strict application of any one of the four categories of hypersensitivity response has become increasingly difficult. Nevertheless, for clinical purposes the Gell and Coombes classification is helpful in providing a framework upon which to broadly base examples of hypersensitivity responses.

4.9.1 Type I immunological damage

The type I or immediate hypersensitivity response is most frequently associated with the IgE response and the involvement of mediator secreting cells, such as mast cells and basophils. In a previously sensitized subject, exposure to allergen produces a bronchopulmonary or vascular response, taking seconds to minutes to reach maximum, being sustained for approximately 60 minutes, and then gradually recovering. Such immediate responses are observed following the intradermal injection of allergen or challenge of the bronchi in atopic subjects, and is the catastrophic event underlying systemic anaphylaxis. Allergic asthma, rhinitis, conjunctivitis, and urticaria are examples of type I reactions localized to individual organs.

In the airways, contraction of smooth muscle together with some mucosal oedema is responsible for the acute symptoms of cough and wheeze on exposure to allergen, while vascular leakage at the level of the post-capillary venules is the main feature of urticaria, angio-oedema, conjunctivitis, and rhinitis. These events, together with the stimulation of afferent nerve endings, result from the action of an array of pharmacological mediators derived from mast cells and basophils (see p. 334). The major broncho- and vaso-active mediator are histamine, acting through its H_1-receptors; PGD_2 and its metabolite 9α, 11β-PGF_2; and the sulphidopeptide leukotrienes, LTC_4, LTD_4, and LTE_4. Other mast cell mediators, such as tryptase, chymase, and the acid hydrolases, promote disaggregation of tissue ground substance and serve to extend and prolong the immediate response. Another system recruited to exaggerate the type I response is a component of the afferent nervous system comprising non-adrenergic non-cholinergic nerves. When stimulated these non-myelinated 'C' fibres release an array of neuropeptides, such as substances P, neurokinin A, calcitonin gene-related peptide (CGRP), and neuropeptide Y, all of which have potent pharmacological effects on blood vessels, smooth muscle, and inflammatory cells.

As discussed in Section 4.19 mast cells are activated to release their preformed and newly generated mediators by an allergen signal presented to the cell via IgE bound to high-affinity FcRI receptors. This mechanism underlies most of the acute symptomatology experienced in rhinitis, conjunctivitis, and urticaria, and it is therefore not surprising that in these disorders histamine H_1-receptor antagonists and 'anti-allergic' drugs such as sodium cromoglycate are effective treatments.

In diseases such as asthma and chronic rhinitis prolonged immunological stimulation recruits other effector cells into the response. Approximately 70 per cent of atopic asthmatics challenged with inhaled allergen experience a prolonged phase of bronchoconstriction at 3–12 hours, associated with a progressive increase in responsiveness of the airways to a wide variety of 'non-specific' stimuli, e.g. histamine, cold air, exercise, water vapour, sulphur dioxide. This hyperresponsiveness is an important component of clinical asthma and its symptomatology. During the late-phase response eosinophils are selectively recruited into the airways, where they exhibit features of activation and mediator secretion. At one time eosinophils were considered to be protective in the type I response, but recent work would suggest that they have the capacity to secrete a wide array of potent tissue-damaging mediators (Fig. 4.58). Since eosinophils are observed in the tissue of many reactions involving type I hypersensitivity, it is likely that they play an important pro-inflammatory role in prolonging tissue inflammation. The capacity of these cells to interact with fibroblasts and secrete mediators which are basophil and mast cell activators emphasizes their potential role as initiators of more chronic inflammatory events (Fig. 4.59).

Cytokine-secreting T-4 lymphocytes, monocytes, and activated macrophage also contribute to type I allergic responses. Their capacity to be activated via their low-affinity IgE FcRII receptors renders them susceptible to allergen stimulation.

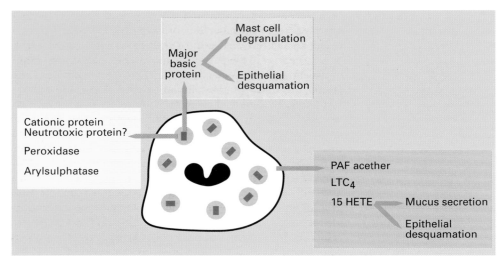

Major basic protein

Mast cell degranulation

Epithelial desquamation

Cationic protein
Neutrotoxic protein?

Peroxidase

Arylsulphatase

PAF acether

LTC$_4$

15 HETE

Mucus secretion

Epithelial desquamation

Fig. 4.58 Schematic representation of the known preformed and newly generated mediators of inflammation released by activated eosinophil.

There is increasing evidence that mononuclear cells with their capacity to secrete potent cytokines, such as the family of interleukins (especially IL-4, IL-5, and IL-10), granulocyte macrophage colony stimulating factor (GM-CSF), tumour necrosis factor, and nerve growth factor, are important cells in extending the tissue damage initiated by a type I response. These cells are found in abundance in the bronchial mucosa of patients with asthma and exhibit the characteristic phenotypic markers of cell activation. Through the elaboration of cytokines, mononuclear cells share with mast cells the ability to secrete molecules that promote endothelial leucocyte interaction and chemotaxis, two events fundamental for the recruitment of secondary polymorphonuclear in such diseases as asthma and rhinitis (Fig. 4.58).

Another form of the type I reaction is acute anaphylaxis, which is most widely recognized with hymenoptera venom and drug reactions. The catastrophic fall in blood pressure, coronary vasoconstriction, and reduced cardiac output occur from the activation of basophils within the vascular compartment and mast cells within the walls of blood vessels and heart. The responsible chemical mediators are those with predominant effects on the endothelium and smooth muscle of capacitance vessels, namely histamine, PGD$_2$, LTC$_4$, and platelet-activating factor.

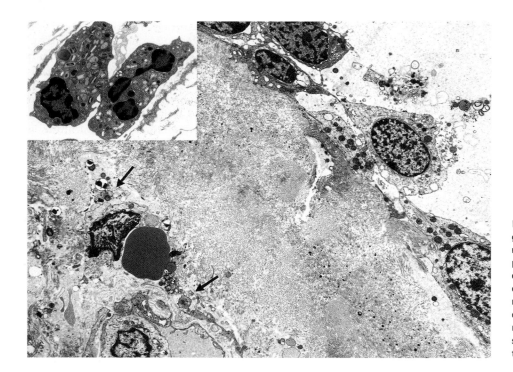

Fig. 4.59 Transmission electron micrograph of the epithelium and sub-epithelial regions of an endobronchial biopsy from a patient with mild atopic asthma. Note the epithelial disruption, subepithelial collagen deposition, and infiltration of the submucosa with eosinophils (arrows). The inset demonstrates an 'activated' eosinophil and neutrophil within the lumen of a bronchial submucosal venule prior to their chemotactic recruitment.

One-third of the population of the Western world exhibit the enhanced capacity to generate IgE directed to common environmental allergens (atopy) and yet, while common, the prevalence of allergic diseases does not follow this distribution. For most conditions, such as asthma, a relationship with atopy has been clearly established, but is far from absolute. Other factors, both genetic and environmental, are required to determine a target organ response in the presence to atopy, although knowledge concerning this aspect is still rudimentary.

4.9.2 Type II immunological damage

Type II immunological damage is caused by the reaction of antibody with surface antigen. The combination of antibody with antigen, in itself innocuous, invokes effector mechanisms that are lethal to the cell under attack. Antibodies of IgM, IgG1, and IgG3 subclasses fix complement via the classical pathway. In some (rather rare) circumstances generation of the C5b6789 membrane attack complex occurs, causing direct cell lysis, but more commonly, deposition of C3b on the cell surface induces immune adherence of neutrophil polymorphs and mononuclear phagocytes.

Activation of complement causes the release of the anaphylotoxins C3a and C5a. Although these are normally promptly inactivated by serum, rapid infusion of either foreign antigen or antibody, e.g. an incompatible blood transfusion or treatment with a monoclonal antibody, may cause such speedy generation of anaphylotoxins as to swamp the inhibiting mechanism and mimic type I hypersensitivity reactions with bronchospasm and increased vascular permeability. Furthermore, even in its inactivated form, C5a is chemotactic for neutrophils and monocytes and able to initiate inflammatory mechanisms. These include the release of interleukin-1, which mediates some of the clinical effects (such as fever) noted in severe type II reactions.

The fixation of complement is not necessary for cell death since a variety of effector cells (neutrophils, monocytes, natural killer (NK) cells, and platelets) carry receptors for immunoglobulin Fc and may adhere opsonically to target cells.

Transfusion reactions may occur against a variety of red cell antigens, but those against ABO groups are the most important. Human serum contains naturally occurring isoagglutinins of IgM type, which fix complement and lead to intravascular haemolysis. Severe reactions cause fever, hypotension, low back pain, a feeling of tightness in the chest, nausea, and vomiting. The released red cell contents may lead to acute tubular necrosis of the kidney. Almost all other transfusion reactions involve IgG antibodies. Red cell destruction takes place in the spleen and to a lesser extent in liver and bone marrow, and the major clinical effects are anaemia and jaundice.

Haeomolytic disease of the newborn is caused by an anti-red-cell allo-antibody present in the maternal bloodstream crossing the placenta and destroying fetal red cells. The presence of these IgG antibodies implies prior sensitization of the mother, which usually occurs during childbirth due to a leak of fetal red cells into her circulation. In mild cases the baby suffers anaemia and jaundice but more severe cases develop cardiac failure, oedema, and ascites (*hydrops fetalis*).

The ability of an antibody to cause immunological damage in the fetus after crossing the placenta is a good indication that a type II reaction is taking place. Other antibody-mediated diseases transmitted transplacentally include immune thrombocytopenia, myasthenia gravis, and thyrotoxicosis.

Auto-immune haemolytic anaemias caused by both IgM and IgG antibodies are well recognized. Antibodies which do not fix complement cause red cell destruction mainly in the spleen and thus may be treated by splenectomy. With antibodies which fix C3b to the red cell, haemolysis also occurs in the liver. Immune thrombocytopenia is also antibody mediated, destruction occurring in the spleen; and antibodies to granulocytes or erythroblasts, respectively, lead to neutropenia and pure red cell aplasia. In some auto-immune cytopenias the antibody reacts with a drug acting as a hapten on the surface of the cell.

In Goodpasture's syndrome antibodies to renal basement membrane cause complete complement activation leading to a local inflammatory reaction which causes destruction of glomeruli. The antibody cross-reacts with pulmonary basement membrane and the clinical syndrome produced consists of acute renal failure together with pulmonary haemorrhage.

In myasthenia gravis an auto-antibody reacts with acetylcholine receptors of the motor end plate and leads to their disappearance and therefore to a failure of neuromuscular transmission. The exact mechanism by which the receptors disappear is unclear, but it may involve antigenic modulation with antibody-induced aggregation of the receptors within the membrane, followed by pinocytosis of the complexed receptor.

In thyrotoxicosis an auto-antibody mimics the action of thyroid stimulating hormone on thyroid cell receptors, activating adenylate cyclase so as to stimulate secretion of thyroxine. This type of antibody-induced reaction (sometimes called type V) may operate in other systems.

Auto-antibodies have been implicated in the destruction of gastric parietal cells in pernicious anaemia and of pancreatic islet cells in diabetes mellitus, although in neither case is the mechanism clear. Other auto-antibodies found in the sera of patients with auto-immune disease, such as anti-smooth-muscle antibodies in chronic active hepatitis, seem not to be implicated in the disease process.

4.9.3 Type III immunological damage

The inflammatory reaction that results from the deposition of immune complexes in the tissue is known as a type III hypersensitivity response. As with type II reactions, complement activation plays an important part in the initiation of inflammation. The characteristic histological picture is of a small-vessel vasculitis.

The formation of immune complexes is an everyday occurrence whenever antibody meets antigen. It normally leads to no harm as the complex is rapidly cleared by the reticuloendothelial system. In antibody excess, complexes are precipitated at the site of introduction of the antigen. In moderate to marked antigenic excess, small soluble complexes are formed to which C3b binds, preventing the formation of large insoluble aggregates. The small soluble complexes bind to the CR_1 receptor on red cells and are transported to Kupffer's cells where they are phagocytosed.

Local exposure to an extrinsic antigen in the presence of high-titre antibody, or prolonged systemic exposure to an antigen of either extrinsic or intrinsic origin may lead to a type III response.

An experiment performed by Maurice Arthus provides a model for the type of reaction. Soluble antigen injected intradermally into hyperimmunized rabbits produced redness and swelling 3–8 hours later. In the Arthus reaction immune complexes are precipitated within the nearest venule, leading to infiltration of granulocytes, platelet aggregation, and the release of inflammatory mediators.

Similar reactions have been held to occur within the lung in response to the inhalation of a wide variety of extrinsic antigens by individuals with high-titre precipitating antibodies. The characteristic picture of extrinsic allergic alveolitis is seen in farmer's lung in which the inhalation of thermophilic actinomycetes present in mouldy hay by sensitized individuals leads to fever, malaise, cough, and dyspnoea within 6–8 hours. However, lung biopsy tends not to show the characteristic features of an Arthus reaction, but more commonly a lymphocytic infiltrate with non-caseating granulomas, suggesting a type IV response. Lung biopsies are seldom available early in the illness so that, as with most immune mechanisms, there may be a mixture of antibody-induced and cell-mediated effects.

Type III responses have also been held responsible for a variety of reactions to the local release of large quantities of antigen from an infectious agent in individuals with high-titre antibodies. Examples include the inflammatory reaction around lymphatic obstruction and elephantiasis, erythema nodosum leprosum in leprosy patients treated with dapsone, and the Jarish–Herxhiemer reaction seen in patients with syphilis treated with penicillin.

Serum sickness is the best recognized model for circulating immune complex disease. Originally seen as a complication of the treatment of infectious diseases with horse serum, it occurs some eight days after the injection of the foreign protein and is characterized by fever, lymphadenopathy, generalized urticaria, and arthraglia associated with a low serum complement and transient albuminuria. The clinical features are the result of inflammatory reactions produced by the deposition of appropriately sized complexes in the walls of small blood vessels.

For circulating immune complexes to become pathogenic there must be a breakdown in their normal clearance. In rare cases a genetic deficiency of C2 or C4 limits complement binding to small complexes, and allows larger insoluble complexes to form. Such individuals frequently develop lupus-like syndromes. More commonly, exhaustion of the clearance system can be demonstrated, with poor expression of CR_1 receptors on erythrocytes, slow clearance of heat-damaged red cells from the circulation, and down-regulated mononuclear phagocytic

function. The cause of this exhaustion appears to be overload. Increased generation of immune complexes occurs in two circumstances:

1. persistent chronic infection with, for example, *Streptococcus viridans* in subacute bacterial endocarditis, *Plasmodium malariae* in the nephrotic syndrome of quartan malaria, or hepatitis B in some cases of polyarteritis nodosa; and

2. auto-immune diseases such as systemic lupus erythematosus.

Secondary deficiency of serum complement is common in immune complex diseases and this tends to perpetuate the syndrome.

Deposition of immune complexes in the tissues is triggered by an increase in the vascular permeability induced by complement activation and release of vaso-active peptides. Deposition is likely at sites of high blood pressure or turbulence, such as glomeruli, the choroid plexus, and arteriolar junctions. Exactly why different organs are targeted in different diseases in unclear but it may be related to the nature of the antigen. In certain types of acute nephritis it is believed that the antigen (e.g. DNA) has a high affinity for collagen in the basement membrane and that immune complexes form locally rather than being filtered from the blood.

4.9.4 Type IV immunological damage

Type IV reactions are characterized by a delayed response to antigenic challenge which is mediated by cells rather than serum. The best known example is the Mantoux reactions obtained by injecting tuberculin into the skin of an individual previously infected by *Mycobacterium tuberculosis*. Erythema and induration appear after several hours and are maximal at 24–48 hours. Histologically, there is an infiltration of lymphocytes and monocytes extending outwards from blood vessels disrupting the organization of the collagen bundles of the dermis.

The cellular basis of the reaction is for sensitized T-cells to recognize antigen together with MHC class II molecules on an antigen-presenting cell. Stimulated T-cells undergo blastic transformation and release lymphokines, which attract and activate macrophages and cytotoxic T-cells. If the reaction becomes chronic, the accumulation of large numbers of macrophages gives rise to arrays of epithelioid cells, some fusing to form giant cells leading to the formation of granulomas.

This sort of reaction forms part of the body's defences against a number of infections and infestations, including tuberculosis, leprosy, leishmaniasis, listeriosis, blastomycosis, and schistosomiasis. In these conditions the intradermal injection of the appropriate antigen leads to a tuberculin type of reaction.

A similar reaction is seen with contact hypersensitivity, which is characterized by an eczematous area of skin at the site of contact of the allergen. Most commonly, haptens such as nickel (in jewellery clasps) or *p*-phenylene diamine (in hair dyes) becomes conjugated to cellular proteins to form new antigens, which are presented by the MHC class II rich Langerhans cell.

Contact hypersensitivity occurs predominantly in the epidermis, whereas tuberculin hypersensitivity occurs in the dermis.

In some forms of auto-immune disease there is a dense mononuclear cell infiltrate of the affected organ, which has led to the suggestion that a type IV response is implicated in the destruction of tissue. In auto-immune thyroiditis there is an inhibition of leucocyte migration by thyroid microsomes, and in patients with ulcerative colitis T-cells will kill normal colon cells in tissue culture. However, there is no firm evidence that cell-mediated immunity is implicated in the pathogenesis of any auto-immune disease, and the cellular infiltrates seen in Hashimoto's disease and pernicious anaemia may simply be effector cells in antibody-dependent cellular cytotoxicity.

4.9.5   Further reading

Type I immunological damage

Barnes, P. J. (1986). Neural control of human airways in health and disease. *American Review of Respiratory Disease* **134**, 1289–314.

Britton, W. J., Woolcock, A. J., Peat, J. K., Sedgwick, C. J., Lloyd, D. M., and Leeder, S. R. (1986). Prevalence of bronchial hyper-responsiveness in children: the relationship between asthma and skin reactivity fo allergens in two communities. *International Journal of Epidemiology* **15**, 202–9.

Gerblich, A. A., Cambell, A. E., and Schuyler, M. R. (1984). Changes in T-lymphocyte subpopulations after antigenic bronchial provocation in asthmatics. *New England Journal of Medicine* **310**, 1349–52.

Goetzl, E. J., Wasserman, S. I., and Austen, K. F. (1975). Eosinophil polymorphonuclear function in immediate hypersensitivity. *Archives of Pathology* **99**, 1–4.

Holgate, S. T. and Finnerty, J. P. (1988). Recent advances in understanding the pathogenesis of asthma and its clinical implications. *Quarterly Journal of Medicine* **149**, 5–19.

Type II immunological damage

Chenoweth, D. E. (1986). Complement mediators of inflammation. In *Immunobiology of the complement system* (ed. G. Ross), pp. 63–86. Academic Press, Orlando.

Patrick, J. and Lindstrom, J. M. (1973). Autoimmune response to acetyl choline receptor. *Science* **180**, 871–2.

Salmon, C. (1982). Autoimmune hemolytic anemia. In *Immunology* (ed. J. R. Bach), pp. 770–93. John Wiley, New York.

Wilson, C. D. (1979). Immunopathology of antibasement membrane antibodies. In *Mechanisms of immunopathology* (ed. S. Cohen, P. A. Ward, and R. T. MacClusky), pp. 181–207. John Wiley, New York.

Type III immunological damage

Arthus, M. (1903). Injections répétées de serum de cheval chez le lapin. *Comptes Rendus des Seances de la Societe de Biologie (Paris)* **55**, 817–20.

Border, W. A. (1984). Glomerular acceptors: new thoughts about the pathogenesis of immune complex glomerulonephritis. *Plasma Therapy* **5**, 395–402.

Davis, A. E. (1985). The efficiency of complement activation in MHC-linked diseases. *Immunology Today* **4**, 250–2.

Dixon, F. J., Vazquez, J. J., Weigle, W. O., and Chochrane, C. G. (1958). Pathogenesis of serum sickness. *Archives of Pathology* **65**, 18–28.

Type IV immunological damage

Calnan, C. D. and Turk, J. L. (1975). Allergic contact dermatitis. In *Clinical aspects of immunology* (3rd edn) (ed. P. G. H. Gell, R. R. A. Coomb, and P. J. Lachmann), pp. 1019–42. Blackwell, Oxford.

Turk, J. L. (1975). The mechanisms and mediators of cellular hypersensitivity. In *Clinical aspects of immunology* (3rd edn.) (ed. P. G. H. Gell, R. R. A. Coomb, and P. J. Lachmann), pp. 847–57. Blackwell, Oxford.

4.10   Inherited and 'primary' immunodeficiency syndromes

A. D. B. Webster

There are about eight well-recognized defects that specifically affect lymphocyte function, and at least 10 other inherited diseases that affect both lymphocytes and other cell types. Most of these disorders affect cellular immunity, with variable effects on antibody production. Although the commonest causes of antibody deficiency are chronic lymphatic leukaemia and myeloma, there are about 600 patients in the UK with 'primary' hypogammaglobulinaemia of unknown aetiology (Table 4.22), with probably a larger number of milder cases where the defect is less clinically significant.

It is customary to subgroup immune deficiency syndromes into those where the defect mainly involves either B-cells leading to a number of antibody deficiency syndromes, T-cells, or both. Accessory cells (macrophages or antigen-presenting/dendritic cells) may also be compromised in some cases, but defects in these cell types are technically difficult to define.

4.10.1   X-linked agammaglobulinaemia (XLA)

Genetics

The defective gene has been mapped to the Xq21-22 region on the proximal segment of the long arm of the X-chromosome (Fig. 4.60). DNA probes recognizing restriction fragment length polymorphisms (RFLPs) close to the *XLA* gene are available to diagnose most heterozygous carriers provided extended families can be studied. Using the same techniques, it is technically possible to make a prenatal diagnosis by probing the DNA from cultured amniotic fluid cells.

Immunopathology

DNA probes recognizing the active X-chromosome in obligate heterozygous carriers have been used to show that all the circulating B-cells use the normal X-chromosome. This implies that the defect is intrinsic to B-cells. Phenotyping with monoclonal antibodies shows that there is a block in B-cell differentiation

Table 4.22

Defects in cellular immunity	Antibody deficiency syndromes

Selective T-cell defect
  Thymic aplasia (Di George's syndrome)
  Purine nucleoside phosphorylase deficiency*
  Cartilage hair hypoplasia*
	Inherited
	  X-linked
	    Agammaglobulinaemia (XLA)
	    Hypogammaglobulinaemia IgG >1 g/l
	    With raised IgM
	  X-linked lymphoproliferative syndrome

Combined immunodeficiency
  Clinically severe (SCID)
    Adenosine deaminase (ADA) deficiency*
    X-linked
    Bare lymphocyte syndrome*
    Omenn's syndrome
    Reticular dysgenesis*
	Acquired
	  'Common variable' hypogammaglobulinaemia (CVH)†
	    Subgroups: (a) With circulating B-cells
	            (b) Without circulating B-cells
	    Thymoma and hypogammaglobulinaemia

Clinically mild/moderate
    Wiskott–Aldrich (X-linked)
    Ataxia telangiectasia*
    Bloom's syndrome*
    Chediak–Higashi disease*
	Selective isotype deficiencies
	  IgA
	  IgA with IgG2
	  Selective IgG (1–4) deficiencies*
	  IgM

General metabolic disorders affecting the immune system
  Orotic aciduria*
  Biotin-dependent carboxylase deficiency*
  Acrodermatitis enteropathica*
  Transcobalamin II deficiency*

* Autosomal recessive inheritance.
† Classified under common variable immunodeficiency (CVI) by WHO.

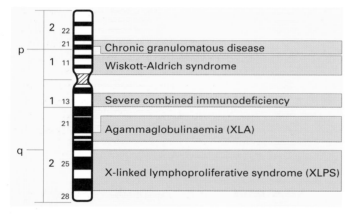

Fig. 4.60 Localization of the genetic defects in the X-chromosome causing immunodeficiency.

soon after the expression of the CD10 (CALLA) surface antigen, causing an accumulation of CALLA-positive cells in the bone marrow. The block is not absolute, and sometimes a few B-cells may differentiate further and appear in the circulation; such cells can be stimulated by Epstein–Barr virus *in vitro* into IgM-secreting lines. Very little, if any, immunoglobulin is produced *in vivo*, and there is atrophy of germinal centres in the tonsils, lymph nodes, and appendix.

Cellular immunity is intact, but there are subtle changes in the circulating T-cells which may reflect an immature phenotype. This is probably secondary to the B-cell defect and is clinically insignificant.

Clinical features

Recurrent infections become a problem when the maternal IgG disappears, usually at about 6 months. Affected children are prone to infection with some bacteria, particularly non-typeable *Haemophilus influenzae*, mycoplasmas, and enteroviruses. However, they recover uneventfully from the common childhood viral infections (e.g. varicella, mumps).

Diagnosis

Agammaglobulinaemia (i.e. IgG < 0.5, IgA < 0.1, and IgM < 0.1 g/l) in a six-month- to two-year-old male child is virtually diagnostic of XLA. However, some children with retarded development of humoral immunity may have very low levels which then recover over the subsequent few years. Unlike XLA children, these have normal numbers of circulating B-lymphocytes as well as visible tonsils.

Treatment

Intramuscular gammaglobulin (25 mg/kg) weekly should be given to infants as soon as possible after diagnosis. Antibiotics should be used liberally at the first sign of infection. Intravenous gammaglobulin (200 mg/kg every two weeks) should be substituted as soon as the child's veins are of adequate size to permit regular infusions. For those diagnosed later in life, intravenous gammaglobulin should be used from the outset.

Diagnosis and management of unusual infections

Enterovirus CNS disease

Headaches, eighth nerve deafness, convulsions, and fibrosis of the limb muscles is characteristic of chronic echovirus disease. The diagnosis is confirmed by growing viruses from the CSF, which has a slightly raised protein and lymphocyte count. The disease is insidious and usually progresses to death within five years. The progression can be halted by giving infusions of specific antibody against the relevant echovirus serotype, but the patients often relapse after treatment is discontinued.

XLA patients are probably prone to poliomyelitis, and have been demonstrated to secrete vaccine strains for long periods in their stools. They should therefore not be immunized with live viral vaccines.

Mycoplasma arthritis

Septic mycoplasma arthritis is probably more common in XLA patients than bacterial (pneumococcal, *H. influenzae*) arthritis and is difficult to diagnose. Any one of at least three mycoplasma species can be involved, some being commensals in the urinary and respiratory tracts. There is an overgrowth of these organisms on mucosal surfaces in the absence of antibody, and it is thought that they are then carried within phagocytes to joints. Serology is inappropriate in these patients, so the organisms must be cultured in special laboratories. In practice, mycoplasma arthritis is very likely if routine culture is sterile; the patient should then be treated with a combination of high-dose tetracycline and erythromycin.

Chronic diarrhoea

Diarrhoea and malabsorption is usually due to *Campylobacter jejuni*, giardiasis, and occasionally *Salmonella*. About 10 per cent of patients have watery diarrhoea which is not apparently related to bacterial or protozoal infection. Ileal and/or colonic inflammation can often be demonstrated and symptoms usually improve with elemental diets.

4.10.2 Other X-linked antibody deficiency syndromes

X-linked hypogammaglobulinaemia

Affected brothers in a few families have been described with a clinically less severe disease than those with XLA. Serum IgG levels are above 1 g/l. The molecular basis of this disorder is probably different to that in XLA.

X-linked hypogammaglobulinaemia with hyper-IgM

Affected children have a very low serum IgG, absent IgA, and elevated IgM, although their ability to make functional IgM antibodies is partially impaired. They are prone to recurrent infections and usually need gammaglobulin replacement therapy.

X-linked lymphoproliferative syndrome

This very rare disease is due to a failure to control Epstein–Barr virus replication, the relevant gene being on the distal segment of the long arm of the X-chromosome. Affected males may present with either B-cell lymphomas, hypogammaglobulinaemia,

or die from fulminant infectious mononucleosis. Neither the failure to control EBV, or the antibody deficiency, is understood.

4.10.3 Primary (common variable) hypogammaglobulinaemia (CVH)

This is an acquired disease with no obvious familial predisposition. There are rare instances of a parent and child being affected, but the majority of cases are sporadic and show no geographical clustering. The peak incidence is in the third decade of life, but it can occur in the first few years of life or in the elderly. The condition is probably caused by a number of separate defects in the immune response, and affects about 600 people in the UK.

Immunopathology

Most patients have some circulating immunoglobulin, usually about 1 g/l of IgG and about 0.1 g/l of IgM, but lack any serum or secretory IgA. About 20 per cent of patients lack circulating B-lymphocytes, while the rest have normal numbers; these cells express surface IgM and in about half the patients can be induced *in vitro* to make some IgM with various stimuli. It is not clear whether this is due to an intrinsic B-cell abnormality or to suppression by other cells.

Unlike XLA, at least one-third of patients show evidence of a defect in cellular immunity, with absent delayed hypersensitivity skin tests and poor *in vitro* T-cell proliferation with mitogens. Such patients are usually lymphopenic ($<1000/\mu l$) but have normal relative numbers of T-cells. However, the majority show normal T-cell help for *in vitro* antibody production, with a minority (about 10 per cent) showing enhanced suppressor T-cell activity for *in vitro* immunoglobulin production in pokeweed-driven systems. It is not clear whether these suppressor T-cells have any *in vivo* significance.

Clinical features

Splenomegaly is common and is usually associated with lymphopenia. Hypersplenism sometimes occurs with neutropenia and thrombocytopenia.

CVH patients are prone to the same spectrum of infections as those with XLA, although echovirus and mycoplasma infections are less common (see Fig. 4.61). About 5 per cent of patients develop chronic central nervous system disease manifested by ataxia and/or dementia; culture of CSF for viruses has so far been negative in these cases.

Some patients develop auto-immune blood dyscrasias, usually auto-immune haemolytic anaemia or neutropenia, and may require immunosuppressive treatment. In contrast to XLA, achlorhydria with atrophy of the antral gastrin secreting cells is common in CVH patients and is probably one factor responsible for the increased incidence of gastric carcinoma. Intestinal submucosal lymphoid nodules (nodular lymphoid hyperplasia) occur in about 20 per cent of patients but do not cause gastrointestinal symptoms.

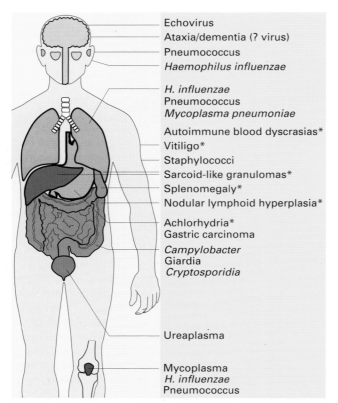

Echovirus
Ataxia/dementia (? virus)
Pneumococcus
Haemophilus influenzae

H. influenzae
Pneumococcus
Mycoplasma pneumoniae

Autoimmune blood dyscrasias*
Vitiligo*
Staphylococci
Sarcoid-like granulomas*
Splenomegaly*
Nodular lymphoid hyperplasia*

Achlorhydria*
Gastric carcinoma

Campylobacter
Giardia
Cryptosporidia

Ureaplasma

Mycoplasma
H. influenzae
Pneumococcus

Fig. 4.61 Infections and other complications in hypogammaglobuli-naemic patients. * Only in CVH patients.

Association of retroviruses with CVH

HIV-1 has been isolated from two heterosexual CVH patients with no risk factors for HIV-associated disease; both remained hypogammaglobulinaemic, one dying early from opportunistic infections and the other from lymphoma seven years later. These patients may have been infected by contaminated gammaglobulin used in their treatment.

In contrast, three homosexual CVH patients have seroconverted to HIV-1, becoming hypergammaglobulinaemic and recovering their ability to make functional antibodies against a range of organisms. These confusing findings have not yet been explained but there is evidence that some HIV strains stimulate antibody production *in vitro* while others depress. There may also be genetic factors which determine the effect on immune regulation.

Treatment and prognosis

About two-thirds of CVH patients require intravenous gammaglobulin therapy, with the remainder progressing satisfactorily on intramuscular injections. Spontaneous recovery of antibody production is extremely rare, but can occur.

Thymoma and hypogammaglobulinaemia

This rare association is considered to be a separate disease, possibly with an auto-immune mechanism. It nearly always occurs in patients over 40 years of age, and is usually associated with a benign, well-encapsulated spindle cell thymic tumour, the removal of which has no effect on the hypogammaglobulin-aemia. There may be associated auto-immune blood dyscrasias or pure red cell aplasia. In contrast to XLA and CVH patients, pre-B-cells are often absent in the bone marrow.

4.10.4   Selective immunoglobulin class and subclass deficiencies

About 1 in 700 healthy individuals in the West lack both serum and secretory IgA. There is no prevalence data for the Third World but the rarity of IgA deficiency suggests that this isotype may be an important survival factor. There is no convincing evidence that IgA deficiency is associated with a susceptibility to recurrent respiratory infection, although the numerous anecdotal reports suggest that it is a risk factor. There are a few reports of familial IgA deficiency, but most IgA-deficient subjects have an acquired defect which is sometimes temporary. It is important to remember that gold, penicillamine, phenytoin, and sulphasalazine can induce selective IgA deficiency, and this probably accounts for the raised incidence of the defect in patients with Still's disease and rheumatoid arthritis.

IgG subclass deficiency

Patients with deficiencies in one or more of the four subclasses of IgG have received much attention over the past few years, but there is still no consensus as to the clinical relevance of these defects. There were early claims that IgG2 deficiency, particularly when associated with IgA deficiency, predisposed to respiratory infections. The fact that most healthy children under two years of age have very low levels of both IgG2 and IgA casts doubt on this suggestion. Furthermore, healthy subjects have been described with deletions of two of the IgG subclass heavy-chain genes, indicating that other subclasses can compensate. Attention is now being focused on whether IgG1 sometimes fails to compensate for IgG2 deficiency in young children with recurrent infections.

Other selective deficiencies

Selective IgM deficiency is rare and is usually associated with lymphoid malignancy. Selective IgE deficiency has been reported but is clinically insignificant.

4.10.5   Thymic aplasia (Di George's syndrome)

This rare intra-uterine malformation of the fetal third and fourth pharyngeal pouches leads to absence of the parathyroid glands and thymus. Associated anatomical abnormalities include a fish-shaped mouth, cleft palate, abnormalities of the larynx, great vessels of the thorax and the heart. Hypocalcaemic convulsions and/or severe heart disease may be the presenting features.

Diagnosis

The thymic shadow is absent on a lateral chest X-ray, and there are very low numbers of circulating T-cells with a relative expansion of B-cells. Many affected infants make antibodies after vaccination. Recurrent respiratory infections may be a problem, particularly in those with complete thymic deficiency. Those with some residual thymic tissue do well and there is usually a gradual recovery in the numbers of circulating T-cells over the first few years of life. The hypocalcaemia can be effectively controlled with alfacalcidol.

4.10.6 Purine nucleoside phosphorylase (PNP) deficiency

This autosomal recessive condition is caused by mutations in the coding gene for PNP on chromosome 14. The substrates for PNP, deoxyguanosine, and guanosine, are toxic for T-cells by an unknown mechanism. Most affected children present soon after birth with severe T-lymphopenia, although some have residual T-cell function at birth which wanes over the first few years. Susceptibility to infection is variable but chronic cytomegalovirus and varicella infection may be a problem. Affected children are prone to auto-immune blood dyscrasias and some have neurological complications manifested by hypotonia, tremor, or spasticity. It is not clear whether the CNS complications are directly related to the enzyme defect or to a secondary viral infection.

Diagnosis

The presence of deoxyguanosine in urine is diagnostic, and PNP deficiency can be confirmed by assaying for the enzyme in red cells.

4.10.7 Cartilage hair hypoplasia

An autosomal recessive condition, prevalent in the Old Order Amish, characterized by short-limbed dwarfism, a variable susceptibility to recurrent upper and lower respiratory tract infections and severe varicella. Humoral immunity is normal but T-cell proliferation is impaired. Affected patients are not prone to malignancy, possibly because natural killer (NK) cytotoxicity remains intact. The mechanism of the disease is not understood.

4.10.8 Severe combined immunodeficiency (SCID)

Adenosine deaminase (ADA) deficiency

An autosomal recessive condition caused by mutations in the coding gene for ADA on chromosome 20. One of the substrates for ADA, deoxyadenosine, kills resting T-lymphocytes and prevents their activation *in vitro*; this is thought to be the cause of the severe T-lymphopenia. There is no antibody production, probably due to the toxic effects of deoxyadenosine on B-cells and accessory cells, particularly macrophages.

Diagnosis

The finding of deoxyadenosine in the urine is diagnostic, and ADA deficiency can be confirmed by measuring the enzyme in red cells.

Treatment

Red cell transfusion may help in the short term by metabolizing the excess deoxyadenosine and regular injections of ADA linked to polyethylene glycol (ADA-PEG) shows promise in recent trials. However, bone marrow transplantation is required for long-term recovery. Gene therapy may soon be available.

X-linked SCID

The abnormal gene has been mapped to the long arm of the X-chromosome and DNA probes recognizing regions (RFLPs) close to the gene can be used to diagnose carriers in extended families. Affected infants present soon after birth with failure to thrive and infection and require bone marrow transplantation for survival.

Bare lymphocyte syndrome

This is a very rare autosomal recessive disease caused by a defect in the expression of class I and/or class II antigens on lymphocytes. Most affected infants are North African, some lacking only class I while others lack class II in combination with a partial deficiency of class I. There is a severe defect in both cellular and humoral immunity but, in contrast to other types of severe combined immunodeficiency, there are usually normal numbers of circulating T-lymphocytes which proliferate with mitogens *in vitro*. However, their lymphocytes will not respond to specific antigens. Survival depends on a successful bone marrow transplant, and it may be necessary to use DNA probes for class I and class II genes to type the blood lymphocytes prior to searching for a compatible donor.

Ommen's syndrome

Infants with this autosomal recessive condition present with erythrodermia, diarrhoea, hepatosplenomegaly, lymphadenopathy, and eosinophilia. There is usually a profound T- and B-cell lymphopenia and the patients require bone marrow transplantation for survival. Similar features may occur in infants with other types of severe combined immunodeficiency who have graft versus host disease (GVHD) due to the transfer of maternal lymphocytes to an immunocompromised fetus. This can be excluded by a lack of hyperkeratosis and proliferation of Langerhans cells in the skin.

Reticular dysgenesis

An autosomal recessive defect in an early stem cell of the white cell series causes severe neutropenia, monocytopenia, and lymphopenia at birth. Survival depends on the success of an early bone marrow transplant.

Other inherited metabolic disorders causing immunodeficiency

There are a number of inherited metabolic defects which affect lymphocyte function as well as other cell types (Table 4.23). These should be considered in infants presenting with failure to thrive and infection.

4.10.9 Syndromes associated with immunodeficiency and lymphomas

DNA repair defects

Ataxia telangiectasia (AT)

This is a relatively rare autosomal recessive condition with about 1 per cent of the population being heterozygote carriers. The disease is characterized by telangiectasia on exposed areas of skin and on the bulbar conjunctivae, progressive cerebellar atrophy, and a variable predisposition to recurrent upper and lower respiratory tract infections. Most patients are confined to wheelchairs by their early teens, and those who survive beyond adolsescence usually develop lymphomas or other malignancies.

AT patients have a defect in DNA repair, particularly the repair of gamma-radiation damage to nucleotide bases. Their lymphocytes have a high frequency of chromosomal breaks and translocations, particularly involving sites on chromosomes 14 and 7, which contain the genes for the T-cell antigen receptor. This may explain the subtle defects in cell-mediated immunity involving cytotoxic T-cell responses. There are also subtle defects in antibody production, with about half the patients having low or absent serum and secretory IgA, and the majority having low serum IgG2 levels, although the severity of these defects does not correlate with predisposition to infection. A few AT patients develop severe hypogammaglobulinaemia and require replacement gammaglobulin therapy.

Bloom's syndrome

This autosomal recessive syndrome is due to defects in the enzyme(s) which ligate DNA in the final stages of DNA repair. There are variants within the syndrome, some patients having severe defects in cellular immunity with low numbers of T-cells which show functional abnormalities *in vitro*. Growth retardation, elf-like features, cutaneous light sensitivity, and increased fragility of their chromosomes *in vitro* are characteristic features. IgA deficiency, and sometimes low IgM, can occur, leading to a susceptibility to recurrent infection. Lymphomas are common in those who survive beyond puberty.

Wiskott–Aldrich syndrome

This is an X-linked disorder, the relevant gene being located on the proximal part of the short arm of the X-chromosome. The main problem is recurrent bleeding due to thrombocytopenia, the platelets being smaller than normal and having a low level of a membrane glycoprotein (the von Willebrand's factor recep-

tor) which is involved in platelet adhesion. There are also subtle functional T-lymphocyte defects, which are probably responsible for the failure to make IgM antibodies to polysaccharides and for the high serum IgE levels and associated atopy. The T-cells lack membrane sialophorin (CD43), but this is not the primary cause of the disease. B-cell lymphomas are common in those surviving beyond puberty.

Chediak–Higashi disease

Affected children are particularly attractive, with silver hair and blue sclera due to the associated albinism. There is also a defect in the formation of white cell cytoplasmic lysosomal granules in this autosomal recessive condition. Large vacuoles form in the cytoplasm which interfere with the mobility of neutrophils and lead to a susceptibility to bacterial infections. T-cell function and antibody production are not significantly impaired, but NK cytotoxicity is very much reduced. This probably accounts for the high frequency of lymphoma and leukaemia, which often appear to follow a chronic lymphotropic viral infection.

4.10.10 Further reading

Akeson, A. L., Wiginton, D. A., States, J. C., Perme, C. M., Dusing, M. R., and Hutton, J. J. (1987). Mutations in the human adenosine deaminase gene that affect protein structure and RNA splicing. *Proceedings of the National Academy of Sciences USA* **84**, 5947–51.

Asherson, G. L. and Webster, A. D. B. (1980). *Diagnosis and treatment of immunodeficiency diseases.* Blackwell Scientific, London.

Businco, L., *et al.* (1987). Clinical and immunological findings in four infants with Omenn's syndrome: a form of severe combined immunodeficiency with phenotypically normal T-cells, elevated IgE and eosinophilia. *Clinical Immunology and Immunopathology* **44**, 123–33.

Grierson, H. and Purtilo, D. T. (1987). Epstein–Barr virus infection in males with the X-linked lymphoproliferative syndrome. *Annals of Internal Medicine* **106**, 538–45.

Malcolm, S., *et al.* (1987). Close linkage of random DNA fragments from Xq 21.3–22 to X-linked agammaglobulinaemia. *Human Genetics* **77**, 172–4.

Morgan, G., Levinsky, R. J., Hugh-Jones, K., Fairbanks, L. D., Morris, G. S., and Simmonds, A. (1987). Heterogeneity of biochemical, clinical and immunological parameters in severe combined immunodeficiency due to adenosine deaminase deficiency. *Clinical and Experimenal Immunology* **70**, 491–9.

Polmar, S. H. and Pierce, G. F. (1986). Cartilage hair hypoplasia: immunological aspects and their clinical implications. *Clinical Immunology and Immunopathology* **40**, 87–93.

Roder, J. C., *et al.* (1980). A new immunodeficiency disorder in humans involving NK cells. Nature **284**, 553–5.

Willis, A. E., Weksberg, R., Tomlinson, S., and Lindahl, T. (1987). Structural alterations of DNA ligase 1 in Bloom's syndrome. *Proceedings of the National Academy of Sciences USA* **84**, 8016–20.

Zegers, B. J. M. and Stoop, J. W. (1988). Metabolic causes of immunodeficiency—mechanisms and treatment. In *Immunodeficiency and disease* (ed. A. D. B. Webster), Immunology and Medicine Series. MTP Press, London.

4.11 Acquired immunodeficiency and the acquired immunodeficiency syndrome (AIDS)

Anthony J. Pinching

4.11.1 Introduction

In building up a picture of the immune system and its function, two essentially complementary, though overlapping, approaches are used. The basic scientific approach is to propose ways in which it could function and to test these hypotheses by designing appropriate experiments. On the other hand, clinical science observes pathological processes as 'experiments of nature' and deduces normal physiology from how things go wrong. The latter rather resembles the building up of a jigsaw puzzle by identifying the shape and probable image of the bits that are missing. The two approaches are interdependent: parts of the overall picture deduced from clinical observations can be subjected to basic scientific test, while the hypotheses derived from basic scientific analysis are frequently challenged by pathological events.

Immunodeficiency and opportunist infection

Immunodeficiency disease provides one of the clearest examples of the contribution of clinical pathology to the understanding of the normal function of the immune system, the absence of immune defence leading to events that reveal implicitly the normal physiological role of the part of the system that is deficient. The principal events seen clinically in immunodeficient patients are known as opportunist infections. These are infections that occur when a micro-organism takes advantage of a defect in host defence to cause disease that it would not produce in a normal person. Opportunist organisms are not, as is commonly supposed, a particular breed of organisms, but rather any organism that has its intrinsic pathogenicity enhanced by the presence of a defect in the host's defence. The type of infection seen in particular immunodeficiencies is determined by the loss of specific host mechanisms normally involved in protection against the causative organism. These range from infections due to organisms that are not normally pathogenic, through those that cause mild, self-limiting disease in the normal host, to others that are serious human pathogens. In the immunodeficient host, these organisms have heightened pathogenicity, causing more severe, more disseminated, more persistent infections and, in some cases, different patterns of disease from those seen in the immunocompetent host. In an analogous manner, patients with immunodeficiency may develop tumours that behave as opportunist tumours, emerging characteristically in hosts with impaired immune defence. The tumours seen are of particular and unusual types, often ones in which viral oncogenesis is known or suspected. Their occurrence implies that host mechanisms are involved in their control.

4.11.2 Acquired immunodeficiencies

Until recently, the best examples of immunodeficiency were the congenital immunodeficiencies discussed in Section 4.10, where the failure to develop a specific constituent part of immune defence leads to characteristic clinical and immunological consequences. Acquired immunodeficiencies resulting from disease or drug therapy generally cause multiple abnormalities in several host defence systems, so that it is not usually possible to discern a precise component defect. For example, the leukaemias lead not only to disorders of the primary tumour lineage in cells of the immune system, but also to secondary changes in other systems resulting from marrow or tissue infiltration by tumour; the picture is also soon modified by therapeutic interventions, including cytotoxic chemotherapy and the breaching of skin or mucosal defences. Similarly, the immunosuppressive properties of high-dose corticosteroid therapy are due to effects mediated on many different parts of immune defence: these include defective tissue localization of neutrophils, decreased receptor expression and function in cells of the monocyte–macrophage lineage, altered lymphocyte traffic, and impaired responses of cells to signals from regulatory cytokines. The complex pattern of susceptibility to infection resulting from these acquired immune defects is an amalgam of several processes that have only been fully understood by reference to more precise experimental systems or to the defects seen in congenital immunodeficiency.

4.11.3 Acquired neutropenia

Severe depletion of neutrophils has long been recognized as a major cause of increased susceptibility to infection. Neutropenia usually results from the suppression of marrow production, whether by disease or, more commonly, by cytotoxic drug therapy used in the treatment of malignant or other disease. Occasionally severe neutropenia is the result of peripheral destruction of neutrophils by, for example, hypersplenism or auto-immune destruction. Many studies have shown that when the circulating neutrophil count falls below $0.5–1.0 \times 10^9$ per litre, susceptibility to infection is greatly increased. Levels between $0.5–1.0 \times 10^9$ per litre are associated with increased susceptibility in some patient groups. It is notable that monocyte counts are also depressed in neutropenic patients, so this cell population is not able to act as a back-up phagocyte population. Recent studies have shown that patients with more profound monocytopenia are more susceptible to infection than those with similar neutrophil counts and near normal or normal monocyte counts. Thus 'neutropenia' as a cause for immunodeficiency could be perhaps more accurately termed phagocytopenia.

The pattern of infection seen in these neutropenic patients closely resembles that seen in congenital neutropenias and congenital defects of neutrophil function. The major infecting organisms include *Staphylococcus aureus* and *S. epidermidis*, *Escherichia coli*, *Klebsiella*, *Pseudomonas*, *Proteus*, *Bacteroides*,

Candida albicans, and *Aspergillus*. Most cannot only cause localized tissue infection but also tend to cause bacteraemia or fungaemia, and hence disseminated infection. They may present as fever with few, if any, localizing signs. The lack of neutrophils and their precursors means that infections are associated with little formation of pus, of which neutrophils are the bulk constituent, but rather a thin serous exudate. In addition, these infections are not associated in such patients with a rise in neutrophil count as they would be in the normal host. Rather the count falls as the few circulating cells are recruited to tissue sites and the marrow is unable to replace these or recruit others. Candidal infection in the neutropenic patient is generally seen as fungaemia, infection of foreign bodies such as intravenous cannulae, or as abscesses, whereas in patients with defective cell-mediated immunity it presents as mucocutaneous candidiasis, indicating that different host mechanisms are responsible for the control of these different aspects of infection with a single organism. *Aspergillus* presents as invasive tissue disease, often eroding into vessels in, for example, lung, in contrast to the aspergilloma seen in patients with lung cavities, etc.

Susceptibility to infection in neutropenic patients is frequently exacerbated by damage to other host defence systems. For example, skin or mucous membranes may be damaged by disease (e.g. graft versus host disease) or by the placement of, for example, intraveous cannulas or urinary catheters, which allow organisms to gain ready access to blood or tissues, where the lack of neutrophil defence means that infection easily results. The use of broad-spectrum antibiotics to treat infective episodes may eradicate the normal protective mucosal microbial flora, allowing pathogens to colonize more readily; in the absence of neutrophil defence, such colonization is more likely to lead to systemic infection.

4.11.4   Malnutrition

Severe protein–calorie malnutrition causes predominantly defective cell-mediated immunity, where collaboration between T-cells and macrophages and the induction of cytotoxic cellular immunity is defective. Children are affected commonly and are especially susceptible to severe and often fatal measles and chicken-pox infection. Other infections normally controlled by cellular immunity are particularly common or severe, such as tuberculosis and *Pneumocystis carinii* pneumonia.

4.11.5   Immunosuppression in other disease states

A number of disease and metabolic states are associated with defective immune mechanisms. For example, patients with lymphoblastic leukaemia show increased susceptibility to infections associated with cell-mediated immunity, such as *Pneumocystis carinii* pneumonia. Patients with Hodgkin's lymphoma may present with shingles, a reactivation of latent varicella zoster virus. Increased susceptibility to viral and fungal infections is notable in patients with systemic lupus erythematosus,

even without therapy, suggesting that these patients have some degree of cellular immunodeficiency as part of their disordered immune regulation. Patients with Hodgkin's disease and alcoholism have increased susceptibility to staphylococcal infection, apparently related to the presence of inhibitors of endogenous chemotactic factor generation. Acquired neutrophil functional defects are seen in patients with hypophosphataemia, a state often seen in acutely ill patients, and this may be due to defective energy supply for neutrophil metabolism; this may increase susceptibility to infection with staphylococci and Gram-negative bacteria. Patients with diabetes have multiple host defence defects, including those due to impaired microcirculation. In addition they show neutrophil functional defects, especially in those with poorly controlled diabetes; this and the vascular damage result in increased infection with *Staphylococcus aureus*, notably affecting the feet. However, defective cell-mediated immunity is also apparent with increased susceptibility to tuberculosis; the pathogenesis of this is unclear. Some infections themselves cause defective immune defence, of which the best recognized are defective neutrophil function induced by influenza, leading to increased susceptibility to *Staphylococcus aureus* pneumonia, and cell-mediated immunosuppression by measles, cytomegalovirus, and (congenital) rubella.

4.11.6   Corticosteroids

Patients receiving high-dose corticosteroids, for example in the treatment of auto-allergic disease or the prevention of graft rejection, are rendered susceptible to a wide range of infections as a result of multiple effects on host defence mechanisms. Such patients commonly develop infection with staphylococci, Gram-negative bacilli, *Aspergillus*, and systemic candidiasis, all of which point to a neutrophil defect. On the other hand, they are also susceptible to the whole range of infections associated with defective cell-mediated immunity, including *Pneumocystis carinii*, tuberculosis, cytomegalovirus, herpes simplex and zoster, *Listeria*, *Legionella*, and mucocutaneous candidiasis.

Corticosteroids have been shown to have numerous effects on various assay systems *in vitro* and the literature has been confused by the use of suprapharmacological doses and inappropriate model species. Neutrophil locomotion, chemotaxis, receptor expression, phagocytosis, and intracellular killing do not show significant defects at the doses used therapeutically. However, the major effect on this cell type is a reduction of neutrophil tissue localization. This results from a defect in neutrophil–endothelial interactions, with the effect that neutrophils are unable to leave the circulation or to migrate through endothelium at sites of tissue injury or inflammation. A good marker for this effect of corticosteroids is a rise in the blood neutrophil count. This is due to release of marginated neutrophils into the circulating pool. Thus the steroid-treated patient is rendered functionally neutropenic (in tissues), while seemingly having plentiful neutrophils in circulation, where they are unable to mediate useful defence. Monocytes, although they are able to localize in tissues, show reduced locomotion, chemotaxis, and notably Fc and C3b receptor expression, with consequently reduced phagocytosis of opsonized organisms. They cannot therefore act as a back-up phagocyte population.

The defective cell-mediated immunity appears to be largely because steroids reduce the expression of a number of important surface molecules on macrophages. In particular they show reduced responsiveness to macrophage-activating lymphokines such as γ-interferon as well as reduced expression of HLA class II antigens. These effects will impair T-cell–macrophage co-operation in the induction of immune responses and, more importantly, in the elimination of facultative intracellular pathogens by macrophage activation. Additional effects are seen on lymphocyte traffic, because steroids affect the migration of lymphocytes through high-endothelium venules of lymph nodes. This results in reduced circulation of T-cells, especially CD4$^+$ 'helper' cells, but the significance of this effect in impairing cell-mediated host defence is unclear.

4.11.7 Hyposplenism

The spleen is a central component of the normal immune response and compromise of its function leads to immunological defects, the extent of which is partly dependent on the age of the patient when hyposplenism occurs. The causes of hyposplenism are listed in full in Section 24.7.4, but the most common and important cause of hyposplenism is splenectomy. The spleen is important in the defence against encapsulated bacteria and also seems to be particularly important in mounting an immune response to antigens not previously encountered, that is the formation of the initial IgM antibodies which precede the formation of those of IgG class. Patients, especially children, who have undergone splenectomy may develop overwhelming septicaemic infections with *Streptococcus pneumoniae* (particularly the more rare subtypes) and, less often, *Haemophilus influenzae* and other organisms such as *Staphylococcus aureus* and *Neisseria meningitidis*. There appears to be failure both of the formation of appropriate opsonizing antibody and of phagocytosis by splenic macrophages. These infections are more common in the first two years after splenectomy and thereafter their frequency gradually decreases.

4.11.8 The acquired immunodeficiency syndrome

In the early 1980s, the acquired immunodeficiency syndrome (AIDS) emerged as a novel and epidemic form of immunodeficiency disease with a highly characteristic clinical profile. This profile suggested that AIDS resulted from a defect in immune responsiveness with a specificity more reminiscent of those seen in congenital immunodeficiencies. The elucidation of its aetiology (HIV, the human immunodeficiency virus) and its pathogenesis over the past few years have shown that AIDS does indeed result from a very precise immunopathological process, albeit one that has widespread secondary immunological consequences. The exploration of the clinical and biological characteristics of AIDS has not only revealed mechanisms that are particular to this remarkable disorder, but has also shed light on the normal interactions in human immune responses, advancing our understanding considerably and posing new questions for basic science.

4.11.9 Clinical profile of AIDS and HIV infection

Clinicians in the early 1980s noticed that young, previously fit young men were developing a constellation of infections and tumours that strongly implied the presence of a profound defect in cell-mediated immune defence. The pattern of infections and tumours was similar in many respects to that seen in congenital and acquired immunodeficiencies that had already been identified; it was this pattern recognition that led to the recognition of AIDS as an immunodeficiency disease. In the ensuing years, the detailed clinical profile has been established, identifying some opportunist events that are especially common in AIDS as compared with other immunodeficiencies and others that are not seen. Some of these reflect the particular immunological defect of AIDS while others are a consequence of the different microbiological context in which AIDS occurred. The major opportunist infections and tumours seen in AIDS and HIV-associated immunodeficiency are given in Table 4.23.

The opportunist infections characteristic of defective cell-mediated immunity seen in AIDS comprise fungal, protozoal, viral, and bacterial pathogens that cause similar infections in

Table 4.23 The major opportunist infections and tumours seen in AIDS and HIV-associated immunodeficiency

Infections reflecting cell-mediated immune defect
  Pneumocystis carinii pneumonia
  Oral and oesophageal candidiasis
  Hairy oral leukoplakia
  Mucocutaneous herpes simplex ulceration
  Multidermatomal herpes zoster (shingles)
  Molluscum contagiosum
  Extensive trychophyton skin infection
  Mycobacterium tuberculosis (pulmonary, gastrointestinal, or disseminated)
  Salmonella enteritis and septicaemia
  Toxoplasma gondii cerebral abscess/encephalitis
  Cryptococcal meningitis or disseminated cryptococcosis
  Chronic intestinal cryptosporidiosis
  Chronic intestinal isosporiasis
  Disseminated histoplasmosis
  Visceral leishmaniasis
  Extraintestinal or invasive strongyloidiasis
  Disseminated or localized cytomegalovirus infection
  Disseminated atypical mycobacterial infection (especially avium-intracellulare)
  Progressive multifocal leucoencephalopathy

Tumours reflecting cell-mediated immune defect
  Kaposi's sarcoma
  B-cell lymphoma (cerebral or disseminated)
  Hodgkin's lymphoma

Infections reflecting associated immune defects
  Pneumococcal pneumonia
  Haemophilus influenzae bronchopulmonary infection
  Bramhanella catarrhalis bronchopulmonary infection
  Staphylococcal pneumonia and skin infection

patients with congenital T-cell immunodeficiency or those on immunosuppressive drugs, such as corticosteroids used for organ transplantation or the suppression of auto-immune disease. Many of them are known as facultative intracellular pathogens (mycobacteria, *Toxoplasma*, *Histoplasma*, *Salmonella*, and probably *Pneumocystis* and *Cryptosporidium*), or are organisms eliminated by similar mechanisms, which involve co-operation between CD4$^+$ (helper/inducer) T-cells and macrophages. The normal containment of the herpes viruses (herpes simplex and zoster and cytomegalovirus) may involve similar mechanisms together with the action of CD8$^+$ (cytotoxic) T-cells, which are induced by CD4$^+$ lymphocytes, and natural killer cells, whose recruitment and function is dependent on the interferons produced by CD4$^+$ lymphocytes and macrophages. The normal control of the opportunist tumours is thought also to be a function of natural killer cells. However, the infections with capsulated bacteria, which have become increasingly recognized as a part of the spectrum of opportunist infections seen in AIDS or HIV infection, especially in children, are more characteristic of absolute or functional immunoglobulin deficiency, and the background to these is discussed later.

Prevalence of opportunist organisms

The unusually high prevalence in AIDS of some of these infections reflects the fact that the causative opportunist pathogens are commonly encountered by people at risk for AIDS, for example sexually transmitted infections such as cytomegalovirus. The epidemiology of Kaposi's sarcoma strongly suggests that it is due to an oncogenic organism, presumably a virus, that is sexually transmissible. Other infections are especially common in certain geographical areas: for example, tuberculosis is a particularly common manifestation of AIDS in tropical countries and histoplasmosis affects people who have resided in endemic areas for this infection, such as the mid-West of the USA or parts of the Caribbean; visceral leishmaniasis is now emerging among AIDS patients in areas endemic for this organism and, rarely, disseminated strongyloidiasis is also seen.

Many of the opportunist pathogens are ones that establish latent or dormant infection earlier in life, with or without symptomatic disease, and re-emerge from latency when immunodeficiency supervenes. Examples of these include *Pneumocystis*, the mycobacteria, *Histoplasma*, *Toxoplasma*, and the herpes viruses. Others are ubiquitous (e.g. *Candida*) or are readily acquired from the environment (e.g. *Salmonella* and *Cryptosporidium*).

Of equal biological interest are those organisms that are widely prevalent in affected hosts or their environment but which do not appear to be major pathogens in AIDS, despite their association with other similar immunodeficiencies. These include *Listeria monocytogenes*, the prototype facultative intracellular pathogen, and *Legionella pneumophila*, which is believed to be resisted by the same defence mechanism. The fact that these infections occur rarely in AIDS suggests that other defence mechanisms which are unaffected by HIV but which are affected by, for example, corticosteroid therapy can contain them. Thus the clinical profile of AIDS is a clear biological statement of the nature of the host defence defect, not only through the opportunist pathogens that do cause infection but by the absence of others that might have been expected to do so from experience of other similar immunodeficiencies or from a knowledge of basic host defence mechanisms.

Biological clues from opportunist events

The infections that do arise in AIDS and the less severe immunodeficiency of AIDS-related complex (ARC, see below) provide an *in vivo* marker of the severity of immune deficiency in the patient. In essence, the higher-grade pathogens cause disease early in the course, when immunodeficiency is least marked, while the later stages of AIDS are typified by the occurrence of infections due to low-grade pathogens that can only cause disease when host cell-mediated immunity is profoundly impaired. The former are exemplified by mucocutaneous candidiasis, herpes simplex and zoster, *Mycobacterium tuberculosis*, and *Pneumocystis carinii*, while the latter include the atypical mycobacteria, cryptosporidium, and disseminated cytomegalovirus infection. Along the same lines it is apparent that Kaposi's sarcoma occurring in isolation represents a much less severe immune defect than that seen in some ARC patients with infection and AIDS patients with major opportunist infection. However, because it is such a readily identified disease marker, it has become part of the surveillance definition of AIDS.

The presenting symptoms, signs and laboratory abnormalities that are characteristic of most infections in normal hosts result as much from the host response to the infecting organism as from the organism itself. As this host response is notably deficient in AIDS, the clinical presentations, radiological, and pathological features of opportunist infections in AIDS are generally blunted; clinical presentations are more subtle and insidious in onset and tissue responses are less evident. This is an important factor in the clinical assessment of such patients but it also provides valuable biological clues as to the relative contribution of host response and microbial pathogenicity to clinical and pathological manifestations in both the normal and the compromised host.

Other HIV-associated clinical syndromes

Soon after the recognition of AIDS, it became apparent that other clinical events could be identified that were occurring in the same affected populations, in some cases preceding the development of AIDS. Over the past few years these clinical entities have become increasingly well characterized and their relationship to the same causative agent (HIV) established. It was clear that AIDS is a late consequence of HIV infection, occurring some 2–7 years or more after HIV infection. Another major disease consequence, typically occurring in people with AIDS and presenting after the onset of overt immunodeficiency, was HIV encephalopathy, presenting as a progressive decline in cerebral function with dementia and motor defects. These disorders clearly reflected the major pathogenetic processes engendered by HIV that are described below.

Initial HIV infection is typically symptomless but in some patients there is an acute, glandular fever-like illness with fever, malaise, transient lymphadenopathy, arthropathy, rash, headache, and sometimes an acute meningoencephalitis. Whether or not such a discernible illness occurs, antibodies against HIV proteins are detectable from this stage and a symptomless phase of HIV infection follows, lasting several years in most instances. In some patients, persistent enlargement of peripheral lymph nodes is seen, described as persistent generalized lymphadenopathy (PGL), but is not associated with systemic symptoms. Symptomless patients may remain so for as long as they have been followed, but a substantial proportion show progression to symptomatic disease, AIDS, or encephalopathy (see section 4.11.14).

Symptomatic disease may consist of weight loss, fever, diarrhoea, oral candidiasis, oral hairy leukoplakia, shingles, and/or other minor opportunist infections, constituting a syndrome known as the AIDS-related complex (ARC); lymphadenopathy may be present but is usually less marked than in PGL. Patients with ARC have a high risk of progression to AIDS itself and already have evidence of some degree of immunodeficiency, as judged by the occurrence of minor opportunist infections.

4.11.10 The cardinal immunological abnormalities in AIDS

From the very earliest clinical reports on AIDS, it was apparent that the most characteristic immunological abnormality in AIDS is a profound depletion of CD4 lymphocytes, both in circulation and in the tissues. This is associated with reduced production of the lymphokines normally elaborated by CD4 lymphocytes, such as interleukin-2 (T-cell growth factor) and the macrophage-activating lymphokines, notably γ-interferon. The function of CD4 lymphocytes is also abnormal, including impairment of mitogen- or antigen-induced proliferation, T-cell help for immunoglobulin production, and induction of antigen-specific responses in T- and B-cells. In vivo tests of cell-mediated immunity are abnormal, as shown by anergy on delayed-type hypersensitivity skin testing. These immunological abnormalities strongly suggested, as did the clinical profile, that the primary defect of AIDS is a loss of CD4 lymphocyte numbers and function, together with associated defects of cellular functions (macrophages, natural killer cells, cytotoxic cells, and B-cells) that are dependent on CD4 lymphocytes.

Another notable change seen in AIDS is polyclonal hypergammaglobulinaemia resulting from non-specific stimulation of B-cells. This predominantly affects the immunoglobulins IgG1, IgG3, IgA, IgD, IgE and, in children, IgM. The production of IgG2, which is of particular importance in the response to defence against capsulated bacteria, is typically reduced. This, combined with the failure of B-cell responses to neoantigens, seems to account for the susceptibility to bacterial infections previously associated with humoral immune defects, such as congenital hypogammaglobulinaemia.

4.11.11 Epidemiology of AIDS

Although AIDS was initially identified in sexually active homosexual and bisexual men in the United States, it soon became apparent that it and the underlying HIV infection also affected intravenous drug users, recipients of blood and blood products (particularly factor VIII used for the treatment of haemophilia), sexually active heterosexuals, including those in sexual contact with other groups at risk, and children of women at risk from AIDS. In developed countries the bulk of the epidemic affected homosexuals, bisexuals, and intravenous drug users, while in developing countries, such as those of Central and East Africa and parts of the Caribbean, the spread was predominantly among sexually active heterosexuals; in South America, the two patterns coexisted. The different patterns of spread seem to reflect different patterns of social and specifically sexual anthropology, with the added influence of drug misuse in developed countries. The transfusion of HIV-contaminated blood or blood products was another vector in all areas.

These observations clearly pointed to the notion that AIDS and related conditions were due to a sexually transmissible and blood-borne infection that could also be transmitted transplacentally or at parturition. This has subsequently been shown unequivocally to be the retrovirus, human immunodeficiency virus (HIV), mainly by epidemiology, serology, and virus isolation. Risk of HIV infection increases with the number of sexual contacts or sharing of needles and especially with sexual or blood exposure to those at higher risk of HIV infection.

4.11.12 Aetiology of AIDS

Human immunodeficiency virus (HIV)

The human immunodeficiency virus (HIV) is a retrovirus, which is an enveloped RNA virus that has the capacity to make a DNA copy of itself through its characteristic enzyme, reverse transcriptase. This enzyme reverses the normal process of gene replication and enables this virus group to establish latency similar to that seen for the DNA viruses, such as herpes viruses, the DNA transcript being spliced into the host genome and acting as the template for further viral RNA replication. Thus HIV establishes a life-long infection.

Many animal retroviruses were already known which could cause a wide variety of diseases including tumours, immunodeficiency, chronic encephalopathy, arthritis, anaemia, and bone disease. One other human retrovirus disease had been recognized, adult T-cell leukaemia, which had been shown to be caused by the human T-cell leukaemia virus Type I (HTLV-I). This virus is a transforming virus causing unrestrained T-cell proliferation, similar in some respects to the oncogenic or tumour viruses of animals.

When HIV was identified and characterized it was found to have important differences from HTLV-I in its genetic makeup. It lacks transforming potential but is a cytopathic or cell-damaging virus. In addition to the usual structural, polymerase, and envelope genes common to retroviruses, HIV has a number of regulatory gene sequences that serve to enhance HIV gene transcription selectively over the normal host gene products. As well as these regulatory genes, other host and viral signals can act to enhance HIV replication. As a result of these factors, new virus particles are being produced much of the time after infection, causing an infected person to be potentially infectious, by the above routes, life-long. In addition, the continuing viral replication leads to cell-to-cell transmission of HIV within the body, increasing the viral load and thereby infecting an increasing proportion of its target cells.

The HIV genome

The principal genes of HIV are called *gag*, *pol*, and *env*, encoding respectively the structural proteins (p24 and p18), polymerase proteins (reverse transcriptase, endonuclease, and protease), and the envelope proteins gp41 (transmembrane) and gp120 (outer envelope); the gp41 transmembrane protein appears to be important in cell fusion. At each end of the gene sequence is a long terminal repeat (LTR) and at the 5′ end is the site at which most of the regulatory genes and other influences act to enhance or decrease viral transcription. The transactivating sequence, *tat*, acts on this LTR to increase replication, and the same site can respond to the transactivating genes of other viruses including HTLV-I and the herpes viruses. In addition T-cell and macrophage activation appear to cause enhanced HIV replication by acting at this site. Several *in vitro* studies have shown that T-cell activation or stimulation of cells of the macrophage lineage by cytokines will enhance the production of new HIV virions and possibly cytopathogenicity. Clinical studies on natural history (see below) indicate that these effects of host or other viral gene activators contribute to disease progression. The *rev* gene enhances the production of HIV structural proteins post-transcriptionally. There are two open reading frames in the HIV genome, one of which, *vif*, appears to confer viral infectivity, while the other, *nef*, seems to downregulate replication. Two other genes, *vpr* and *vpu*, have been identified but their role is unclear.

Target cells of HIV

Like a number of other viruses, HIV has specificity for particular host cells. As could be predicted from the clinical and laboratory characteristics of the immunodeficiency, the major target for cytopathic effects is the CD4 (T4) helper cell. In addition the virus establishes latency in cells of the macrophage lineage, including monocytes, Langerhans cells, dendritic cells, microglia, and follicular dendritic cells of lymph nodes. Elegant studies *in vitro* using different cell lines as targets for HIV infection and using monoclonal antibodies to block infection have shown that the CD4 antigen itself acts as the virus receptor for HIV on target cells. The CD4 antigen is a major surface molecule characterizing T-helper cells but is also found on cells of the macrophage lineage. The CD4 molecule has an important role in cellular communication between cells of the immune system, being the cellular binding site for HLA class II molecules on collaborating or target cells.

It has since been shown that the virus envelope protein gp120 contains a number of highly conserved sites which serve as the CD4 binding site, attaching to a major part of the CD4 molecule. Following binding to this receptor, HIV is internalized releasing viral RNA into the host cell. Thereafter reverse transcriptase production by HIV RNA leads to the formation of a DNA copy, which is then spliced into the cell genome. From this further RNA transcripts are produced. Virus proteins are then assembled at the cell surface and new virions are produced by budding from the host cell surface. The cytopathic effects of this and consequences of immune recognition of virus-infected cells are discussed below. However, it is important to note that, whereas CD4 cells are destroyed after HIV infection, macrophages are generally not, so they serve as the major cellular reservoir of virus in the infected host; they are also the main site of infection in the nervous system. Recent data show that macrophages can be infected via Fc or C3b receptors, as well as by CD4.

During budding the virus acquires its envelope, which is derived from the host cell membrane. It is this envelope that determines the physical properties of HIV, its relative fragility and susceptibility to inactivation outside the body. The transmission characteristics of HIV described above largely result from these physical features and are unaffected by genetic variation, which is characteristic of RNA viruses and which is well exhibited by HIV, especially in its envelope proteins.

4.11.13 Pathogenesis of AIDS

Viral cytotoxicity

The characteristic feature of AIDS is the loss of CD4 cells in blood and tissues. Several potential mechanisms for the loss of these cells have been proposed and it seems likely that several are involved. Direct virus cytotoxicity has been shown, involving lysis or syncytium formation or both. Syncytia are formed by the fusion of several cells into multinucleate giant cells and these may incorporate both infected and uninfected CD4 lymphocytes. Such syncytia will die prematurely or be eliminated by host mechanisms.

Host-mediated cytotoxicity

However, it is probable that some of the destruction of HIV-infected CD4 lymphocytes is due to those host mechanisms that eliminate virus-infected cells, a major defence against viral infection. These may be mediated by antibody-dependent cellular cytotoxicity, whereby killer T-cells lyse cells that are recognized by antibody, or by HLA-restricted cytotoxic CD8 lymphocytes that kill cells bearing host HLA in association with viral antigens. Both of these have been shown to be present in HIV-infected subjects, with or without disease. While such mechanisms are designed to defend the host against virus infection, they can obviously contribute to pathogenesis by destroying HIV-infected target cells, especially if HIV infection of such cells is widespread and their regeneration is impaired. As well as destroying infected cells, these mechanisms could also damage uninfected cells, if they have free HIV gp120 attached to CD4 antigen. The loss of CD4 cells and the reduced production of

CD4 lymphokines, such as γ-interferon and interleukin-2, can account for many of the observed defects in AIDS.

HIV products and immune defects

However, there is also evidence that the few remaining CD4 cells, which are largely uninfected, are functionally defective. This could result from selective loss of subsets of CD4 cells, for which there is some evidence, or from other immunosuppressive effects of HIV. HIV gp120 appears to be immunosuppressive to T-cells in its own right. It also acts as a potent polyclonal activator of B-cells, and B-cell activation is probably responsible, together with the loss of T-cell regulation, for hypergammaglobulinaemia and the unresponsiveness to neoantigens. In addition, abnormal macrophage function, presumably due to latent infection is also seen, over and above the effects of the loss of CD4 lymphokine signals. Natural killer cells also show impaired function, largely due to the lack of interferons and IL2, which are of major importance in the recruitment and cytotoxic activity of these cells. Thus, the typical clinical and laboratory defects seen in AIDS can be readily explained in terms of the known biological consequences of HIV on cells of the immune system.

Neuropathogenesis

The pathogenesis of HIV encephalopathy is less well established. Most of the infected cells and in the nervous system are microglia or perivascular macrophages; endothelial, glial, or even neuronal infection have been suggested but are less evident and their role is less clear. Defects of neuronal function and a cytopathic effect on glia or neurones may result in large part from HIV products or from factors released from HIV-infected macrophages.

4.11.14 The natural history of HIV infection

Rates of progression

Cohorts of HIV-infected subjects have been followed up for up to 10 years and about 35 per cent remain symptomless, with or without PGL, at this stage; the remainder have developed AIDS (50%) or ARC (15%). More studies have been performed on subjects infected for 3–5 years; they suggest that progression to AIDS occurs in about 15–20 per cent at 3 years and 25–30 per cent at 5 years. While the long-term outcome for the whole group remains speculative, there are still individuals with long-standing infection who develop the disease after many years. It is thus uncertain whether some symptomless individuals have developed true protective immunity or are insusceptible or whether the varying natural history simply reflects differing rates of immune destruction.

Cofactors

Cohort studies and anecdotal evidence have, however, suggested that the rate at which disease develops may be influenced by intercurrent events and other host factors. Sexually transmitted infections and possibly co-infection with HTLV-I and other systemic infections seem to enhance progression. This can be explained readily in terms of T-cell or macrophage activation and a consequential increase in HIV replication. Similarly, having more than one HIV positive pregnancy, which would also repeatedly activate T-cells through the maternal response to the paternal antigens on the fetal graft, seem to enhance progression. Infants with HIV infection also show more rapid progression than adults and this may be the result of activation by the many responses to exogenous antigens occurring in early life. Other cell-mediated immunosuppression, such as that with therapeutic immunosuppressive drugs, other viral infections, and malnutrition can also enhance the effects of HIV in an additive manner. Given the very similar natural history of encephalopathy, this may be subject to similar cofactors. Genetic factors in the host may also contribute to relative or absolute susceptibility, as with other infections, but these have yet to be clearly delineated. Recent evidence indicates that the HLA haplotype A1, B8, Cw7, DR3 is associated with increased risk of disease progression.

4.11.15 Immune responses to HIV

In natural infection

Although the foreign antigens of HIV are recognized by T- and B-cells, eliciting T-cell responses against HIV and HIV antibodies, these mechanisms appear to afford little evident protection against disease, being found in patients with disease as well as in those that remain symptomless. It is possible that some of the latter have true protective immunity but its nature and mechanism have not been established. Neutralizing antibodies are formed, though in relatively low titre, but these will serve largely to limit fluid-phase transmission of virus within the host. There is little to suggest that neutralizing antibodies are protective. It now seems likely that much of the cell-to-cell transfer of HIV occurs by direct contact, where antibodies will have limited efficacy. Some patients show an association between the loss of p24, p17 (p18), and anti-reverse transcriptase antibodies and progression. However, this may not be due so much to the loss of protective antibodies as to the loss of these antibodies in immune complexes secondary to increased viral replication. Similarly, antibodies involved in cellular cytotoxicity are present whether or not progression occurs. These and HLA-restricted cytotoxic mechanisms may not be protective but rather could contribute to continuing cellular destruction and pathogenesis as discussed above.

Vaccine strategies

Attempts are being made to prepare vaccines to protect uninfected individuals against primary HIV infection. Although envelope proteins presented on a variety of vectors can elicit a detectable antibody and T-cell response in chimpanzees and humans, subsequent HIV challenge of chimpanzees (which are susceptibile to HIV infection, though not to disease) has shown that they are not protected. Whether other immunogens or immunizing schedules will afford protection remains to be established.

4.11.16   Therapeutic strategies in AIDS

Treatment of opportunist events

Given the extraordinarily rapid development of our understanding of the aetiology, pathogenesis, and consequences of AIDS, it is not surprising that a wide variety of approaches to treatment have been developed. While many of these can produce useful clinical benefits, they fall well short of providing a truely effective treatment and none can be construed as even approaching a 'cure'. The most immediate priority in any patient, and the strategy that has formed the mainstay of therapy for AIDS, is the treatment of opportunist infections and tumours. Despite the underlying immunodeficiency, antimicrobial therapy and the treatment of tumours with radiation or chemotherapy have proved extremely useful and can lead to resolution of these intercurrent problems. Treatment is most likely to be effective if initiated early for infections, but maintenance therapy to prevent recurrence is usually required. On the other hand, over-aggressive therapy of tumours can precipitate more severe immunodeficiency and care must be taken in the choice and timing of such regimes. In addition, an active programme of nutrition and the avoidance of other cofactors can improve the outlook for patients with AIDS.

Immunorestoration

Immunorestorative approaches seemed logical and many have shown limited benefit, although the extent has been generally disappointing. Early approaches included the use of T-cell lymphokines such as interleukin-2 and γ-interferon. While immunological tests on treated patients showed that some of the defects were less evident, clinical benefits were few. The use of bone marrow transplantation seemed an even more logical strategy in replacing the cells that had been lost. Although successful engraftment occurred (usually done in identical twins), benefit was soon lost. This seemed to be the result of HIV infection of the donor cells.

Antiretroviral therapy

It became increasingly evident that the most important priority was to find an effective antiretroviral agent to stem HIV replication. This could reduce or prevent further damage to the cells of the immune and nervous system and could perhaps allow some immune reconstitution to occur. Or it could be combined with immunorestorative approaches in immunodeficient patients. Given the presence of integrated viral DNA in host cells, the ideal agent is readily administered (preferably orally), safe and well-tolerated in life-long use, and able to achieve levels in blood and tissues, especially the nervous system, that can totally suppress HIV replication without interfering with normal host cellular mechanisms.

The only agent so far shown to be effective *in vivo* falls short of some of these expectations. This is zidovudine (AZT), a reverse transcriptase inhibitor, which thereby uses a virus-specific enzyme as its target. It certainly reduces HIV replication *in vivo* although it does not totally inhibit it. The rate of immune decline in patients with AIDS or ARC is slowed and as a consequence the frequency and severity of infections is reduced; this leads to lower immediate mortality, although in due course progressive immunodeficiency is still seen. Encephalopathy may be improved in some patients and may be prevented when zidovudine is given before it develops. However, the drug has major bone marrow toxicity, causing anaemia, and ultimately leucopenia and occasionally, thrombocytopenia in a high proportion of patients, even though it is symptomatically well tolerated. A mitochondrial myopathy develops in some patients treated for long periods.

Whether zidovudine can prevent the development of immunodeficiency or neurological disease by use in early HIV infection and whether toxicity is less in this setting remain to be established; early results in asymptomatic HIV positive individuals with subnormal CD4 lymphocyte counts are encouraging. The considerable benefits seen with zidovudine in late disease indicate the potential of this approach. This drug should be regarded as a prototype. Other drugs are under development that act either at the same point in viral replication or at other sites; it is to be hoped that similar or more effective drugs with lower toxicity and good long-term tolerance can be developed in due course. Combinations of antivirals with different sites of action or of antivirals with immunorestorative approaches in advanced disease seem the most hopeful approach to this devastating disease.

4.11.17   Conclusions

AIDS and HIV infection have presented an unparalleled challenge to basic science and clinical medicine, quite apart from their wide-ranging social and personal impact. In a relatively short time, the aetiology and pathogenesis have been largely established, illustrating clearly the cellular and molecular mechanisms underlying clinical disease. While much remains to be done in developing specific preventive and treatment strategies, early progress in the latter is encouraging and already exceeds the options available for many long-established diseases. Furthermore, AIDS and HIV infection have served to illuminate many aspects of the basic biology of both host and virus and have advanced our understanding in an unprecedented manner. It is to be hoped that the phoenix that arises from the ashes of this extraordinarily destructive process in human pathology will help to equip us for the control of many other current and future diseases. It has certainly illustrated clearly the way in which clinical observations can challenge and advance basic scientific understanding.

4.11.18   Further reading

Chandra, R. K. (ed.) (1983). *Primary and secondary immunodeficiency disorders*. Churchill Livingstone, Edinburgh.

Friedland, G. H. and Klein, R. S. (1987). Transmission of the human immunodeficiency virus. *New England Journal of Medicine* **317**, 1125–35.

Gottlieb, M. S., Jeffries, D. J., Mildvan, D., Pinching, A. J., Quinn, T. C., and Weiss, R. A. (eds) (1987). *Current topics in AIDS*, 1. John Wiley, Chichester.

Gottlieb, M. S., Jeffries, D. J., Mildvan, D., Pinching, A. J., Quinn, T. C., and Weiss, R. A. (eds) (1989). *Current topics in AIDS, 2.* John Wiley, Chichester.

Ho, D., Pomerantz, R. J., and Kaplan, J. C. (1987). Pathogenesis of infection with human immunodeficiency virus. *New England Journal of Medicine* **317**, 278–86.

Levy, J. A. (ed.) (1989). *AIDS—pathogenesis and treatment.* Marcel Dekker, New York.

Pinching, A. J. (1985). Laboratory investigation of secondary immunodeficiency. *Clinics in Immunology and Allergy* **5**, 479–90.

Pinching, A. J. (ed.) (1986). AIDS and HIV infection. *Clinics in Immunology and Allergy* **6**, 441–687.

Pinching, A. J. (1988). Factors affecting the natural history of human immunodeficiency virus infection. *Immunodeficiency Reviews* **1**, 23–38.

Pinching, A. J., Weiss, R. A., and Miller, D. (eds) (1988). AIDS and HIV infection: the wider perspective. *British Medical Bulletin* **44**, 1–234.

Seligmann, M., *et al.* (1984). AIDS—an immunologic reevaluation. *New England Journal of Medicine* **311**, 1286–92.

Seligmann, M., *et al.* (1987). Immunology of HIV infection and AIDS—An update. *Annals of Internal Medicine* **107**, 234–42.

4.12 Immunological tolerance and self non-responsiveness

M. Feldmann

4.12.1 Introduction

Immunological tolerance is the acquired non-responsiveness towards an antigen, consequent upon prior exposure to that antigen. The form of antigen which induces immunological tolerance is often termed a 'tolerogen', in contrast to the immunogenic form of antigen, or the 'immunogen'. Functionally and operationally, tolerance is the converse of immunity.

The fundamental importance of tolerance towards self antigens was recognized by Ehrlich, early in the development of immunological concepts. Auto-immunity may be envisaged as a failure of the mechanisms of self non-responsiveness, leading to an immune response against self antigens. Thus the mechanisms of self non-responsiveness need to be understood as these are the conceptual bases underpinning ideas about the genesis of auto-immunity and, in this section, various postulated mechanisms of self non-responsiveness are considered.

In the 1920s the experimental induction of immunological tolerance was reported, using bacterial antigens, such as pneumococcal polysaccharide or diphtheria toxoid. Large doses were found to suppress the immune response, which would normally be elicited by smaller concentrations of antigen. Subsequently it was found that exposure to antigen in embryonic life led to the development of immunological tolerance. An early example of this was provided by Owen in 1945 who found that dizygotic cattle twins (which are genetically non-identical) were sometimes tolerant of each other's tissue cells. This occurred if they had exchanged embryonic blood during placental fusion and were thus stable chimeras, with haemopoietic cells derived from both animals. The chimeras were tolerant, being unable to reject skin grafts from the twin. This form of immunological tolerance was reproduced experimentally in 1956 by Billingham, Brent, and Medawar, who injected live adult mouse spleen cells into newborn mice of a different strain. Subsequently the newborn mice were shown to be specifically tolerant to the skin of the mouse strain from which the injected spleen cells were derived.

These studies led to a variety of further experiments which demonstrated that both in neonatal and adult mice, rats, and other species, tolerance could be induced with a wide range of antigens, including proteins, carbohydrates, and cellular antigens by the administration of supra-immunogenic concentrations of antigen. There were differences, however, in the ease of induction of immunological tolerance, which was much easier to induce in immature mice, and with antigens of a particular type and structure. A variety of experimental studies have suggested mechanisms to account for different forms of immunological tolerance, but no single mechanism is considered to account for the diverse phenomena encompassed in 'immunological tolerance'.

Analysis of the immune competence of spleen or lymph node cells from tolerant animals, for example by adoptive transfer into irradiated mice or in tissue culture, revealed that the lymphoid cells were unable to respond, and that tolerance was due to a lack of functional precursor cells. Thus tolerance was considered to be a 'central' phenomenon, inherent in the immunocompetent cell pool, and not a 'peripheral' event due to the manner in which antigen is presented or delivered to the precursor cells.

4.12.2 Mechanisms of self non-responsiveness

Immunological tolerance, as conceived in the 1960s is not the only mechanism of self non-responsiveness. Other mechanisms include suppressor cells and anti-idiotypic antibodies; although both of these mechanisms may closely resemble immunological tolerance, and indeed may be involved in pathways towards immunological tolerance, e.g. high concentrations of antigen may induce suppressor T-cells. However, these regulatory pathways of suppression and anti-idiotypic antibodies may be entered by other ways, and contribute to forms of immune regulation not necessarily related to self-tolerance. There is also evidence for self non-responsiveness to certain antigens, which is not due to a lack of precursor T-cells.

Understanding the mechanism of immunological tolerance depends on understanding the mechanisms of immunity, as tolerance could occur due to a block at any step in the immune response. Regrettably, there are many details of the mechanism of immunity which are still unclear, and consequently this imposes limitations on our understanding of immunological tolerance.

Types of tolerance

'Partial' tolerance refers to antigen-induced reduced responsiveness, in contrast to complete tolerance which refers to antigen-induced unresponsiveness. There was discrimination between the two forms of tolerance in the past but these are now considered to be different degrees of the same process.

In some systems, unresponsiveness of the antibody-producing system has been detected together with a concomitant normal or even heightened delayed-type hypersensitivity response. This has been termed 'split' tolerance, and emphasizes the need to consider tolerance in both the T- and B-cell pool, and raises the possibility that these may have different mechanisms.

Comparison of tolerance in T- and B-cells

Studies with protein antigens, such as deaggregated human gammaglobulin (dHGG) have shown that the kinetics of tolerance in T-cells and B-cells differs significantly. Thus it was found that T-cell tolerance is induced more rapidly, with lower concentrations of antigen, and last longer than B-cell tolerance. The differences noted with dHGG were quite substantial, e.g. 10 μg needed to induce T-cell tolerance cf. 1 mg for an equivalent degree of B-cell tolerance. Virtually complete T-cell tolerance occurred within 24 hours, whereas B-cell tolerance took almost a week. There was recovery from B-cell tolerance in ~50 days whereas T-cell tolerance lasted 6 months or more. The duration of tolerance is related to antigen persistence, and thus it has been found that poorly degraded antigens, such as polysaccharides or polymers of D amino acids, are very good tolerogens.

Tolerance in B-cells

Due to the greater ease of experimental analysis, relatively more is known about B-cell tolerance than T-cell tolerance, although in physiological terms it is likely that T-cell tolerance is of much greater significance, due to the requirement of T-cell help for optimal B-cell function. B-cell tolerance is necessary, though, because of the somatic mutations possible in IgG, with consequent change of specificity towards self-reactivity.

B-cell tolerance can be induced very readily in immature B-cells. This will occur in the presence of low concentrations of monomeric antigens and, as clones of B-cells with that antigenic specificity do not develop, was termed 'clonal abortion'.

Stimulation of adult B-cells with immunogenic doses of T-independent antigen may cause all the mature B-cells capable of responding to a given antigen to differentiate into antibody-forming cells. This has been termed 'clonal exhaustion'.

Functional inactivation of B-cells may occur with either T-dependent, or T-independent antigens. With T-dependent antigens, if there is no T-cell help, B-cells recognizing antigen may become inactivated. T-independent antigens at supra-immunogenic concentrations may also induce B-cell inactivation. This process is termed 'clonal anergy'. This can be clearly demonstrated in vitro.

Active antibody-forming cells may also be switched off by high concentrations of antigen, especially multivalent T-independent antigens. This phenomenon, termed 'antibody-forming cell blockade' is rapidly reversible and so is unlikely to be of significance in self-tolerance.

Tolerance in T-cells

Unlike B-cells, T-cells recognize and are activated by cell-bound antigens, usually peptide determinants in association with MHC antigens: usually T-helper cells recognizing antigen associated with MHC class II and T killer cells recognizing antigen associated with class I antigens. This difference between T- and B-cell recognition must also imply differences in mechanisms of tolerance.

Bretscher and Cohn proposed a simple scheme in which recognition of antigen in itself was a tolerogenic signal, while recognition in the presence of a 'second signal' was immunogenic. While initially suggested for B cells, prior to understanding the molecular nature of T-cell receptors and their peptide MHC targets, a variant was proposed, implying that T-cell recognition of antigen in the absence of MHC was tolerogenic, whereas in the presence of MHC, it was immunogenic. However, experimental analysis by Lamb and Feldman showed that T-cell tolerance, like immunity, required MHC co-recognition.

Mechanisms of tolerance in T-cells are not fully understood, but a number of recent experimental models have shed some insight. There is experimental evidence for clonal abortion or deletion as postulated for B-cells, based on analysis of T-cell receptor gene usage during the maturation of thymocytes. Using a monoclonal antibody to a V_β family (V_β17a) it was found by Kappler, Roehm, and Marrack that in mouse strains which did not express this receptor gene family in their peripheral T-cells, but which possessed the structural gene for it (as they were F_1 crosses), immature thymocytes (high Thy 1 cells) bearing V_β17a were present, but not mature thymocytes low in Thy 1. The expression of V_β17a receptors on immature cells but their deletion or failure to develop in mature T-cells is strongly suggestive of the operation of a mechanism of clonal abortion.

Functional abrogation of T-cell reactivity has been observed in experimental systems *in vitro*. Exposure of human activated T-helper cell clones (which express class II antigens) to supra-optimal concentrations of peptide antigens (which do not need processing) leads to a state of antigen-induced unresponsiveness, which is not due to cell death, as the cells can still respond to interleukin-2 (IL-2). This type of unresponsiveness is prolonged, and can also be induced in murine T-cell clones, which do not express HLA class II, provided that fixed antigen-presenting cells are present in co-culture together with high concentrations of antigen. This form of tolerance is now termed 'clonal anergy'.

The involvement of T-suppressor cells in antigen-induced unresponsiveness has been demonstrated in a variety of ways using different antigenic systems. By far the most reproducible demonstrations have been *in vivo*, which does not permit refined analysis about mechanisms. *In vitro* analysis of suppression has led to a variety of conflicting and inordinately complex formulations, the validity of which is not unequivocally established.

4.12.3 Maintenance of self non-reactivity

Self non-reactivity can occur as a consequence of a variety of mechanisms, which may occur either within the immunocompetent cell pool, or before antigen interacts with the immunocompetent cells.

Lack of exposure to antigen

There is a certain threshold of antigenic concentration beneath which immune responses are not elicited. Thus it is possible that lack of antigenic exposure may be responsible for some forms of self non-responsiveness, especially if the antigen is rare, and not exposed to the immune system. This concept of 'immunologically privileged sites' has never been firmly established. However, it is likely that it applies to sites without vessels or lymphatics, such as the cornea. Grafts of foreign corneas do not elicit immune responses without the need for immune suppression, and are by far the commonest and most successful type of graft. However, they are rejected if the cornea has been vascularized, following inflammation, for example.

Inoculation of antigens into the brains of experimental animals has been reported not to elicit immune responses. There is a barrier to the trafficking of molecules from the blood to the brain, the 'blood–brain barrier', which, together with the absence of lymphatics in the central nervous system apart from the meninges, may be responsible for the inaccessibility of brain antigens to the immune system.

Lack of effective antigen presentation

Since T-cells cannot recognize free antigenic molecules, but require them to be 'presented' to T-lymphocytes on the surface of cells expressing MHC molecules, the latter cells are termed 'antigen-presenting cells'. These cells include macrophages, monocytes, dendritic cells, Langerhans cells, Kuppfer's cells, B-cells, and in certain circumstances T-cells also. Thus, a very wide range of cells under appropriate circumstances may act as antigen-presenting cells. Conceivably this function may be mediated by any cell which has the appropriate surface MHC molecules, although with varying degrees of efficiency. The relative efficiency of different antigen-presenting cells is well documented, although the reasons for it are not fully understood: amounts of class II antigens, expressed at the surface, or interleukin-1 (IL-1) production do not appear to explain these differences adequately.

Protein antigens (and possibly cell surface antigens also) need to be 'processed' in order to be presented effectively. Conceivably certain antigens may not be recognized by the immune system due to a failure of antigen presentation. Thus, failure of antigen presentation could occur at any of the three well-recognized processes (class II expression, IL-1 production, antigen processing).

Table 4.24 Possible mechanisms of self non-responsiveness

Afferent
    Lack of antigen exposure
    Lack of antigen-presenting capacity (class II⁻)
Central
    Clonal abortion or deletion
    Clonal anergy
    Suppressor T-cells
    Idiotypic regulation

Idiotype regulation

The variable (V) region of antibody molecules or of T-cell receptors may in themselves act as antigens which are recognized by antibody or T-cell receptors and thus elicit the formation of antibody molecules. These are termed 'anti-idiotypic' antibodies, and can interact with the surface of cells bearing the appropriate V-region molecule. These antibodies interacting with the receptors may mimic antigen and initiate immunological events—immune induction or perhaps immunological tolerance. There is evidence that such antibodies have the potential to influence immune responses (see Section 4.8.9), but whether they do so in the majority of immune responses is not clear.

Experimentally it has been found that anti-idiotypic antibodies raised to the receptor of T-cells recognizing an allo-antigen may prevent response to that allo-antigen. The exact mechanism by which the anti-T-cell receptor antibodies prevent responsiveness to the corresponding allo-antigen is not known. The most obvious is by blocking receptors of T-cells or B-cells. However, this mechanism does not seem to be efficient, as high concentrations of antibody would be needed to maintain a long-lasting and efficient inhibition. Since to most antigens there are a number of responding T-cell (and B-cell) clones with different idiotypes, it would also be inefficient as there would be the need to have a whole panel of such antibodies operating if the anti-idiotype response were to be effective.

There are other mechanisms which may permit anti-idiotype antibodies to work more efficiently. If the specificity is for a family of cells, e.g. a cross-reactive Ig idiotype or a TCR anti-V_α or V_β family, fewer distinct antibodies would be required. Another possibility is that the anti-receptor antibodies may not act directly, but in conjunction with other effector mechanisms. Opsonization by phagocytes may cause antibodies to yield irreversible damage. Cytotoxic cells with Fc receptors, e.g. natural killer (NK) cells, may be armed to deliver a lethal hit to cells reacting with the appropriate anti-receptor antibody. Cytotoxic cells recognized by the anti-receptor antibody may lyse helper cells recognized by the same anti-receptor antibody. This latter mechanism is very efficient and may be an important mechanism to prevent clonal overgrowth. At present the significance of idiotypic regulation is still debated.

Consequences of self-tolerance

Tolerance to self antigens, by whatever mechanism it is caused—clonal abortion, clonal deletion, or suppression—causes a loss of immune potential. The incapacity to respond to the self antigen (in association with HLA) causes a 'hole in the repertoire' of the antigenic universe that an individual can recognize and hence respond to. These 'holes in the repertoire' mean that certain complexes of HLA and extrinsic antigens, which would mimic the complex of HLA (not necessarily the same determinant) and self antigen cannot be recognized. Thus there is a 'penalty' for self tolerance, and this loss of recognition capacity is one of the causes or mechanisms of MHC-associated genetic control of the immune response. In view of the large number of self antigens, each with multiple epitopes, and the large number of HLA antigens with which they could associate, there must be a limit to the extent of self-tolerance if there is to be a functional repertoire capable of effectively recognizing extrinsic antigens such as potential pathogens.

According to this concept it is not possible to have effective self-tolerance to all self antigens without a loss of immune potential, and thus there is a risk of auto-immunization. There is also the likelihood that forms of self non-responsiveness that do not irretrievably influence the host's immunocompetence will be employed for antigens which are less likely to be immunogenic, i.e. present at low concentrations or present on cells not expressing class II antigens. Thus mechanisms such as lack of antigen presentation may be important in the overall scheme of self non-responsiveness (see below).

Characteristics of antigens involved in immunological tolerance

The nature of the antigens involved in the induction of B-cell tolerance *in vivo* and *in vitro* has been investigated in order to obtain insights into the mechanism of tolerance induction. It was noted that the most potent B-cell tolerogens were large polymeric antigens, polysaccharides such as levan or dextran, or proteins such as polymerized flagellin. Reducing the size of these antigens led to a loss of tolerance induction, suggesting that the capacity to cross-link receptors may be important in tolerance induction (reviewed Howard 1985). This conclusion was supported by studies analysing tolerance to haptenic determinants conjugated to a polymeric backbone. It was found that if the haptenic determinants were present at very low density, neither tolerance nor immunity could be induced, at intermediate levels immunity but not tolerance, subsequently both, and at the highest determinant density only tolerance. These results indicated that whereas cross-linking of B-cell receptors was of importance in both processes, a high degree of cross-linking favoured tolerance. Analogous studies have not yet been performed for T-cell tolerance, and would be difficult to interpret in view of the fact that co-recognition of MHC is also involved, and

the density of MHC antigens would clearly be as relevant as that of extrinsic antigen.

T-cell suppression and immunological tolerance

The relationship of T-cell tolerance and suppression is complex, because many of the stimuli which favour one also favour the other. However, there is clear evidence that in certain circumstances tolerance does not involve the obligatory participation of suppressor T-cells, even though these may be present.

Thus, it has been found that T-helper cell depletion may occur more rapidly than the induction of T-suppressor cells. Tolerance is induced more readily in the presence of drugs, such as cyclophosphamide, which abrogate suppressor cell induction. Furthermore, tolerance can be broken *in vivo* by normal lymphocytes, as in parabiosis experiments. Thymectomy delays the recovery from T-cell tolerance, suggesting that recruitment of new precursors is a key step in recovery. The above observations are from *in vivo* experiments, where conclusions are not direct. *In vitro*, much more direct experiments have been performed. A clone of T-helper cells can be tolerized by antigen, in the absence of any other cells. Thus tolerance can be induced in the absence of suppressor cells.

However, T-suppressor cells are of importance in certain types of tolerance, especially that induced in adult life. A particularly interesting type of tolerance is induced by the multiple injection of sub-immunogenic concentrations of antigen, over a period of weeks. This has been termed 'low-zone tolerance'. Prior to the discovery of suppressor cells, this was a difficult phenomenon to understand. It was found that low-zone tolerance was transferred by T-cells, and thus this is a prime candidate example of tolerance mediated by suppressor cells.

Immunosuppressive drugs have been reported to facilitate the induction of tolerance with antigens which are highly immunogenic. Such drugs include cyclophosphamide, which facilitates tolerance in both T- and B-cells. Suppressor cells have been reported, but it is also likely that other mechanisms operate, e.g. cyclophosphamide would be expected to delete clones of dividing cells responding to antigen; and there is evidence that the re-expression of Ig surface receptors in B-cells is inhibited by cyclophosphamide.

Cyclosporin A is a drug that has received widespread attention due to its successful use in clinical transplantation, e.g. of kidney, heart, and liver. The exact mechanism of action of cyclosporin A remains elusive, despite much endeavour. Actions on T-, B-, and accessory cells have all been reported and facilitation of the induction of suppressor cells has been noted. Production of IL-2 and other lymphokines (e.g. γ-IFN) is inhibited by cyclosporin A. Lack of IL-2 may be of particular relevance in promoting tolerance, as it would prevent the growth of specifically activated T-cells. There is recent evidence that excess IL-2 may block the induction of tolerance, or lead to reversal of tolerance *in vivo* and *in vitro*, and hence the lack of IL-2 production during cyclosporin treatment may be critical to its tolerogenic effects.

Anti-lymphocytic serum has also been used to treat graft

rejection episodes. This has a multitude of effects, e.g. opsonization, and suppressor-cell induction has also been reported. Suppressor cells have also been induced in regimes which induce tolerance to delayed-type hypersensitivity.

Despite the importance of suppressor cells in a variety of immune regulatory phenomena, their properties are poorly defined, partly because they do not grow readily under the conditions which permit T-helper and cytotoxic cells to be cloned efficiently. Thus, there are few reports of cloned suppressor T-cells. It is striking that among those few reports, two describe suppressor cells that were specific not for antigen, but for the antigen-specific receptors of helper cells, i.e. they recognized idiotypic determinants. This it is possible that idiotypic regulation may be very important at the T-cell level.

4.12.4 Bibliography

Banerjee, S., Haqqi, T. M., Luthra, H. S., Stuart, J. M., and David, C. S. (1988). Possible role of V_β T-cell receptor genes in susceptibility to collagen-induced arthritis in mice. *Journal of Experimental Medicine* **167**, 832–9.

Billingham, R. E., Brent, L., and Medawar, P. B. (1956). Actively acquired tolerance of foreign cells. *Nature* **172**, 603–6.

Bretscher, P. and Cohn, M. (1970). A theory of self–nonself discrimination: paralysis and induction involve the recognition of one and two determinants on an antigen, respectively. *Science* **169**, 1042–9.

Feldmann, M., Zanders, E. D., and Lamb, J. R. (1985). Tolerance in T-cell clones. *Immunology Today* **6**, 58–62.

Howard, J. G. (1985). Immunological tolerance. In *Immunology* (ed. I. M. Roitt, J. Brostoff, and D. K. Male), pp. 12.1–12.12.

Jerne, N. K. (1974). Towards a network theory of the immune system. *Annals of Immunology* **125**(C), 373–89.

Kappler, J. W., Roehm, N., and Marrack, P. (1987). T-cell tolerance by clonal elimination. *Cell* **49**, 273–80.

Lamb, J. R. and Feldmann, M. (1982). A human suppressor T-cell clone which recognizes an autologous helper T-cell clone. *Nature* **300**, 456–8.

Lamb, J. R. and Feldmann, M. (1984). Essential requirement for major histocompatibility recognition in T-cell tolerance induction. *Nature* **308**, 72–4.

Nossal, G. J. V. (1983). Cellular mechanisms of immunologic tolerance. *Annual Review of Immunology* **1**, 33–62.

Owen, R. D. (1945). Immunogenetic consequences of vascular anastomoses between bovine twins. *Science* **102**, 400–1.

4.13 Auto-immunization

M. Feldmann

4.13.1 Introduction

The presence of auto-antibodies does not indicate that an auto-immune disease is present. In recent years it has become apparent that auto-antibodies can be present in serum as part of the normal repertoire of Ig, without causing any disease, both in men and mice. Such 'normal' auto-antibodies are chiefly IgM, occur early in life, and have been studied effectively by making hybridomas of B-cells from fetal or neonatal mice.

Later in life, auto-antibodies, chiefly IgG can also be detected with routine clinical tests in a percentage of individuals which increases with age, with females more likely to have auto-antibodies than males. These results suggest that the process of auto-immunization is not rare, and is far more frequent than the development of clinical auto-immune diseases which is characterized by high titre IgG antibodies. The concept that clinical auto-immunity does not necessarily follow from auto-immunization makes it essential to understand the predisposition towards auto-immunity, both genetic and environmental, and how this influences the pathogenesis of the disease process.

Autoimmunization can encompass both the humoral and the cell-mediated response, and the same helper T-cells and antigen-presenting cells participate in both responses.

4.13.2 Precursors of autoreactive lymphocytes

There is abundant evidence that B-lymphocytes reactive to a number of auto-antigens are found in normal individuals and animals. They have been detected using radiolabelled antigens, such as myelin basic protein or thyroglobulin. Mitogen stimulation, for example with LPS, of normal mouse spleen cells leads to the formation of auto-antibodies of many specificities, thus indicating that precursors were present. Recently a subpopulation of B-cells which bears the CD5 (Ly1, T1) antigen, and is the majority of B-cells in early fetal development has been described in man and mouse. B-cells of young mice (fetal liver, neonatal spleen) have revealed a high degree of connectivity, with their Ig reacting with a lot of Ig idiotypes. Hybridomas made from adult spleen cells do not show the same frequency of reactivity with Ig idiotypes. CD5 B-cells in both mouse and man have been shown to make a lot of auto-antibodies—anti-DNA, anti-RBC, anti-Ig rheumatoid factors, etc.

The above findings make it clear that the B-cell repertoire, while not necessarily complete, does contain many autoreactive precursors, and thus clonal abortion or deletion at the B-cell level cannot be the sole means of maintaining self non-reactivity at the B-cell level. It is of interest that mitogenic stimulation does not yield antibodies to all antigens, e.g. no anti-albumin, and so it is likely that clonal abortion/deletion does occur for some antigens (see Section 4.12).

At the T-cell level, there is evidence of autoreactivity but of a different type. All T-cells recognize antigens in association with MHC antigens, and this is more appropriately considered elsewhere. *In vitro*, it is possible to demonstrate T-cells recognizing autologous HLA class II positive cells. This reaction is termed the autologous mixed lymphocyte reaction, commonly abbreviated 'AMLR' but its significance is unclear. There is a school of thought that considers that the AMLR is of fundamental immunological significance, and that recognition of self HLA class II keeps the immune system functioning effectively, with the T-cells releasing lymphokines such as γ-interferon needed for maintenance of immune competence, e.g. by inducing HLA class II on macrophages. However, there is another school of thought that considers the AMLR to be an *in vitro* artefact, due to the co-recognition, along with HLA class II of serum protein or plastic-derived antigens. At present there is no proof that the AMLR fulfils a critical role *in vivo*.

T-cells precursors which recognize self antigens in association with HLA have also been detected with certain antigens such as myelin basic protein and so it is likely that they also occur with other antigens. This is an important consideration in the context of auto-immunity as it indicates that abnormalities in the normal mechanism controlling the activation and clonal growth of these precursors would predispose significantly to the development of auto-immunity.

4.13.3   Auto-antibody formation and function

Auto-antibodies can be detected in a wide variety of clinical tests, e.g. immunofluorescence for detecting islet cell antibodies in diabetics, haemagglutination for detecting antibodies to thyroglobulin in thyroid auto-immunity, radioimmunoassay (RIA), or enzyme-linked immunoassays (ELISA) for detecting anti-DNA antibodies, etc. As the relevant auto-antigens become characterized and purified the assays tend to become more quantitative, such as ELISA assays for the Ro and La proteins in Sjögren's syndrome.

Auto-antibodies arise against both intracellular components and cell surface proteins. The former are particularly common, and in the rheumatic and connective tissue diseases many of the auto-antibodies define cytoplasmic and intranuclear ribonucleoprotein complexes. Some of these are described in Table 4.25. It is interesting that auto-antibodies develop to particles with very important functions in cell biology, e.g. U1 and U2 ribonucleoproteins are essential for the correct splicing of heterogeneous nuclear RNA to form functional messenger RNA capable of directing protein synthesis.

Currently it is not known whether antibodies to intracellular (I/C) components can bind to, and influence their targets *in vivo*, with intact cells. It would be expected that antibodies are too large to get into cells in an intact manner. However, there are some studies (a minority) that suggest that this may not always be the case. There is no evidence that auto-antibody to intracellular components can explain the manifestations of the disease, e.g. how would anti-Jo-1 antibody, selective for myositis, which reacts with histidinyl transfer RNA, explain the onset or specificity of myositis?

In certain instances antibodies react with auto-antigens which were considered to be cytoplasmic, but have subsequently been demonstrated to be present at the cell surface also. An example would be antibodies to the thyroid microsomal–microvillar antigen, now known to be the thyroid peroxidase enzyme involved in the iodination of thyroglobulin, necessary for the production of active thyroid hormones.

It is apparent that antibodies to cell surface structures could be of major significance in the development of auto-immunity. This has been clearly demonstrated, for example, in myasthenia

gravis, where the auto-antibodies against the acetylcholine receptor lead to a receptor aggregation and a diminished half-life of the receptor, with consequently a reduced number on the cell surface. Some antibodies also block transmitter function, leading to a more rapid and dramatic effect. Other potential pathogenic effects of antibodies to cell surface components would be complement-mediated lysis, or antibody-dependent cell-mediated cytotoxicity (ADCC), involving either natural killer cells or macrophages as the effector cells.

The significance of auto-antibodies is twofold. In all instances if at high titre, these are markers of disease, and sometimes the levels of antibody may be of prognostic significance, correlating with the severity of the clinical process. In some instances these antibodies may be of diagnostic use, discriminating between diseases with similar clinical manifestations, e.g. chronic hepatitis of the postviral and auto-immune type. In some diseases, as described above for myasthenia gravis and acquired haemolytic anaemia, the antibodies are directly involved in the pathogenesis of the disease process, although even in these, it should not be assumed that antibodies are solely responsible for disease manifestations.

4.13.4   Predisposition to auto-immunity

Clinical studies have documented that there are both genetic and environmental predispositions to auto-immune disease, which differ between diseases, although many diseases have common predisposing features, e.g. female gender.

Sex

In the majority of auto-immune diseases there is an excess of females. In RA the F:M ratio is ∼3:1, in diabetes 2:1, in SLE ∼8:1. This excess of females applies to both humans and other animals, and as it can be abrogated by castration or the administration of sex hormones, appears to be dependent on the latter.

The mechanism of female preponderances is not clearly understood, but it is probably relevant that females (human or other animals) produce higher antibody titres, to a variety of antigens, and thus the greater likelihood of auto-immunization may be a reflection of a wider propensity to respond efficiently to antigen.

Age

Certain auto-immune diseases have typical ages of onset. Insulin-dependent diabetes mellitus has a typically young onset, maximal at 12–13 years. High predisposition to multiple sclerosis depends on the geographical latitude of individuals before the age of 15. The early onset of many auto-immune diseases is reminiscent of the age of onset of infectious disease, rather than late onset of degenerative-type disease, such as those which may occur once immune function diminishes. However, other diseases have a later onset, e.g. RA.

Genetic predisposition

Family studies in the majority of auto-immune diseases have

Table 4.25 Immunoreactive polypeptides in non-organ-specific auto-antigens

Antigen	Molecular mass (kDa)	Disease association (prevalence, %)
Serologically defined antigens		
Sm	28, 16	Systemic lupus erythematosus SLE (25%)
nRNP	68, 33, 20	Mixed connective tissue disease MCTD (100%); SLE (30%)
La (SS-B)	45	SLE (18%); Sjögren's syndrome. SS (63%)
Ro (SS-A)	55, 60	SS (80%)
RANA (EBNA-1)	80	Rheumatoid arthritis, RA.
(Scl-70) (DNA topoisomerase I product)	70	Scleroderma
Scl-86	86	Scleroderma (59%)
Jo-1 (tRNA-his synthetase)	50	Polymyositis/dermatomyositis, PM/DM (30%)
PL-7 (tRNA-threo synthetase)	80	PM/DM (<5%)
PL-12 (tRNA-ala synthetase)	110	PM/DM (<5%)
Ki (Ku, Pl-9)	86, 66	SLE
SL	(32)	SLE (7%)
Functionally defined small antigens		
DNA topoisomerase I	95	Scleroderma
Histone H1, H2B (trypsin-sensitive regions)		SLE
Histone H2A, H2B (trypsin-resistant regions)		Procainamide-induced lupus
Histone H3, H4 (trypsin-resistant regions)		Hydralazine-induced lupus
RNA Pol I	120	SLE
RNA Pol I	65	RA
RNA Pol I	42	MCTD
Lamins A, C	70, 60	Linear scleroderma
Lamin B	68	SLE
Proliferating cell nuclear antigen (PCNA, cyclin)	33	SLE (3%)
Vimentin	57	Acute hepatitis: A, B and non-A, non-B
Functionally defined assemblies		
Mitochondrion	70, 50, 45 72, 45	Primary biliary cirrhosis (90%) Scleroderma (13%)
Human mitochondrion	46	Idiopathic hypoparathyroidism
Nucleolus	93, 92, 69 37, 35	Scleroderma (73%)
Large ribosomal subunit	38, 16, 15	SLE (10%)
Centromere	140, 80, 17	CREST (70%)
Signal recognition particle	54	Polymyositis

made it clear that there is a genetic predisposition. However, these studies have also indicated that non-genetic factors also have an important role, as identical twins have a concordance rate (both twins having the disease) of ~50 per cent or less, usually 30–40%. The exact nature of genes involved in various diseases have been the subject of intense study, without as yet any conclusive answers as to how genetic traits are converted into disease susceptibility.

HLA

The advent of HLA typing has elucidated that essentially all auto-immune diseases are HLA associated. A cluster of the diseases are associated with HLA-B27 but the others are associated with HLA-DR or DQ. Systemic lupus erythematosus appears to be more closely associated with the class III (complement) genes, especially C4 null alleles. There is evidence that in some disease, the 'haplotype' (cluster of linked genes in the HLA region) is more important than a single gene. HLA and disease associations are illustrated in Table 4.26.

Table 4.26 HLA class II associations and auto-immune disease, with the relative risks, DR type of the patients analysed (modified from Todd *et al.* 1988)

Class II antigen	Relative risk
Coeliac disease	
DR3	8–12
DR7	
DQw2	
Insulin-dependent diabetes mellitus	
DR3	4–6
DR4	4–6
DR3, 4	20
DR2	0.25
Rheumatoid arthritis	
DR4	4–6
DR1	
Multiple sclerosis	
DR2	4
Pemphigus vulgaris	
DR4	24
DRw6	1.5
Systemic lupus erythematosus	
DR2	1–3
DR3	2–3

The known function of the HLA component with which a given disease is associated would be expected to provide clues towards the mechanism of the disease susceptibility or the disease process. Thus associations with C4, which is involved in solubilizing immune complexes, would suggest that complexes are of importance in systemic lupus erythematosus.

Associations with HLA-DR and DQ, the HLA class II elements co-recognized with antigenic peptides by CD4 T-cells which have helper-inducer or suppressor-inducer function suggests that CD4 T-cells have a major role in these diseases. However, this role is not understood—CD4 T-cells could be involved in recognizing a viral peptide more efficiently in association with a certain DR or DQ allele, thus implying a role in the early events. However, it is possible that CD4 T-cells may be involved in the recognition of an auto-antigenic peptide, suggesting a role of DR or DQ after the triggering events, and in the maintenance of the disease. In principle these two possibilities may be distinguished by an analysis of the DR/DQ recognition spectrum of autoreactive T-cells. If these are heterogeneous, it is likely that the simple HLA genetic predisposition reflects an early triggering event, and not the recognition of auto-antigens. It may also reflect changes in the TCR repertoire.

With developments in DNA sequencing it became possible to ask whether diseased individuals with a certain HLA type have the same sequences at their polymorphic regions as non-diseased individuals with the same serological HLA type. This has been performed for HLA-B27, and no difference detected between those with ankylosing spondylitis and those without.

A fine analysis of the role of HLA class II molecules in the development of auto-immunity has become possible with the development of the polymerase chain reaction by Henry Ehrlich permitting the rapid sequencing of HLA class II molecules from a variety of individuals with or without disease. It has thus been found that, in general, there are no disease-specific class II molecules. Thus sequences found in patients are not different from those in some healthy individuals, although the frequency of certain sequences can be very high in some patient groups, compared to healthy individuals. Several studies are of interest. In insulin-dependent diabetes, it has been found that patients have a neutral amino acid at position 57 of the DQ β-chain, whereas aspartic acid is very rare in diabetes but common in the population. In certain populations of patients with pemphigus (Israeli Jews with DRw6), there is also a gross overrepresentation of a certain DQ allele, e.g. /DQw1.9, whereas in controls it was only found in 1 of 13 controls (DRw6 DQw1 Israelis). These studies suggest that these sequences are associated with the disease process but in themselves are not sufficient to cause the disease.

In rheumatoid arthritis, it is known that DR4 and DR1 populations have an increased risk of developing the disease, whereas other DR types have a reduced risk. With DR4, only certain 'DW types', are at risk. Sequence analysis of the DR4 DW types has revealed that the types at risk differ in amino acid positions 70/71 of the DR β-chain.

Immunoglobulin

Associations of auto-immune disease such as with immunoglobulin Gm allotypes suggest that the Ig gene cluster is involved in the disease process. The most likely Ig genes to be involved are those determining recognition specificity, i.e. V, D, or J genes. The exact analysis of which Ig genes confer heightened susceptibility to a given disease is a difficult task. However, recent family studies using Ig gene probes has confirmed a role of the Ig gene cluster, by restriction fragment length polymorphism (RFLP) analysis.

T-cell receptor genes (TCR)

Restriction fragment length polymorphism (RFLP) studies using T-cell receptor Cβ and Cα probes have been performed, but the data so far is not conclusive, and there are conflicting claims. In terms of the TCR, what matters is the repertoire which is expressed and finds itself at the site of the disease process. Such studies are in progress, and the results so far in human auto-immunity suggest that autoreactive T-cells are not uniform in their use of TCR genes.

However, a recent analysis of murine clones recognizing the myelin basic protein N-terminal peptide (1–8), which is encephalitogenic in mice, revealed that the majority of clones used the same V_α and V_β genes, and also the same J_α. This study suggests that possession of certain T-cell receptor genes is necessary to develop autoreactive T-cells. A similar conclusion has been reached in murine collagen arthritis, as strains have lost certain V_β genes they did not develop the disease.

Acetylator status

The discussion of genetic predisposition has so far concentrated on genes controlling immune responsiveness, HLA-DR/DQ, Ig, or TCR. However, other types of genes may also be involved, and one that has been discussed is the capacity to acetylate and thus inactivate drugs. Acetylator status is thus relevant to drug-induced auto-immunity, and slow acetylators are at risk of developing lupus with, for example, treatment with hydralazine and phenyl hydantoin.

There is a possibility that other drug clearance systems, which are polymorphic, e.g. cytochrome P450s, could also be involved.

Environmental factors

Drugs have been implicated in the induction of certain type of lupus. This is one of the clearest demonstrations that environmental factors can be extrinsic precipitating causes.

Viruses and bacteria

A number of infectious organisms have been associated with 'auto-immunity'. A clear example is post-streptococcal carditis where the immune response to *Streptococcus* group A generates an immune response which cross-reacts with the endocardium, leading to long-term disease. This 'rheumatic fever' has become rarer in recent years with the advent of antibiotics and better sanitation. Now rheumatic fever is rare in the Western world, but not in other parts.

There are a number of diseases associated with arthritis: Reiter's syndrome, currently believed often to be precipitated by chlamydial infection. A high percentage of affected individuals are HLA-B27$^+$. Exactly how an infection provokes an auto-immune response is not clear. However, sequence homologies between infectious agents and auto-antigens have been found and so molecular mimicry is a popular, but unproven concept.

4.13.5 Cellular mechanisms of auto-immunization

Histological and immunohistological analysis of the sites of auto-immunity have revealed appearances consistent with active immune responses. In rheumatoid arthritis (RA), for example, dense cellular infiltrates of mononuclear cells, nodular around vessels and diffuse elsewhere, are typical with thickening of the lining layer of cells and the formation of finger-like processes. High endothelial cells as in lymph nodes are seen.

Immunostaining reveals that many of the cells are T-lymphocytes, with abundant monocytes/macrophages. In the nodules the CD4 T-cells abound and three are few B-cells,

but many plasma cells. HLA-antigen expression is augmented, both for class I (HLA-A, B, or C) but especially for class II. The majority of the cells in an active RA joint express HLA-DR (Fig. 4.62).

The features described above are typical of local auto-immune reactions, and are probably not very different from inflammatory sites generated in other ways. Of particular interest is the capacity of cell types which do not normally express HLA class II to do so during auto-immune reactions. This is seen clearly in thryoiditis and in diabetes. This process was termed 'aberrant' expression. In both Graves' and Hashimoto's thyroiditis the epithelial cells express HLA-DR, DP, and DQ, the former at higher levels than the latter. In insulin-dependent diabetes mellitus, of the islet cells only the β (insulin-producing) cells express class II. This is of particular interest as only these cells are damaged during the auto-immune process. In contrast, all three types of islet cells become strongly class-I positive during the active phase of diabetes, but after the loss of the β-cells the remaining cells lose their class I expression. These observations are most compatible with the induced expression of HLA class I and class II during the auto-immune process (Fig. 4.63), and indicate the close linkage between class II expression and

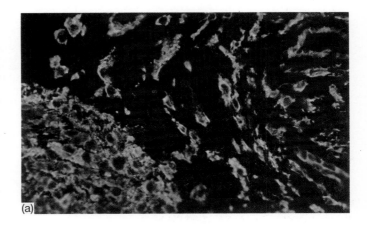

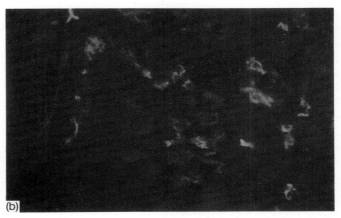

Fig. 4.62 Comparison of HLA-DR expression on (a) rheumatoid arthritis and (b) osteoarthritis joints.

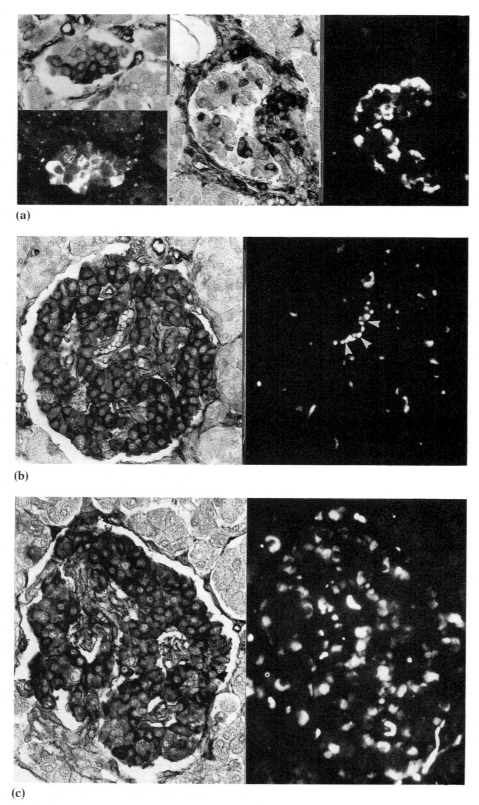

(a)

(b)

(c)

Fig. 4.63 Selective expression of HLA-DR on islet β-cells in insulin-dependent diabetes mellitus.

tissue damage. This would be interpreted as implying a major role for CD4 cells (recognizing class II) in the disease process.

Based on these immunohistological observations and current immunological concepts it was suggested that local activated T-cells produce molecules which induce the target tissues to express class II antigens, and hence could act as antigen-presenting cells and stimulate autoreactive T-cells. These in turn produce molecules capable of maintaining class II expression, and of activating the immune mechanisms involved in mediating the tissue damage of auto-immunity. This concept is schematically illustrated in Fig. 4.64, and was initially proposed for endocrine auto-immunity by Bottazzo *et al.* in 1983, although it became apparent subsequently that similar considerations applied to non-endocrine local auto-immune diseases, such as rheumatoid arthritis. This working hypothesis makes a number of testable predictions which are discussed in the next section.

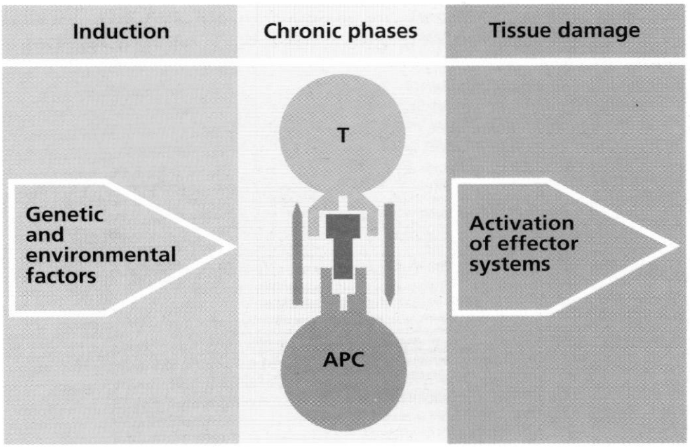

Induction	Chronic phases	Tissue damage
Genetic and environmental factors	T APC	Activation of effector systems

Fig. 4.64 Scheme of the development of autoimmunity. T, T-cells; APC, antigen-presenting cells.

4.13.6 Hypothesis of auto-immunization

Products of activated T-cells induce class II in auto-immune target tissues

For thyroid epithelial cells γ-IFN sufficed to induce class II expression, in the order noted *in vivo* (DR > DP > DQ). However, analogous studies with human islet cells did not reveal class II induction it was eventually found that a mixture of γ-IFN and either lymphotoxin (LT) or tumour necrosis factor (TNF) was capable of inducing class II expression on human islet cells. These molecules can all be produced by T-cells and so this was compatible with a role of T-cells in inducing the class II expression in the target tissues. In rodents different results have been obtained. γ-IFN may induce class II weakly in mouse islets, and in genetically predisposed BB/W rats. The latter results are not necessarily discrepant with those in the human as it is possible that the BB/W rats may have been exposed to TNF or LT *in vivo*.

HLA class II expressing target cells act as presenting cells

Thyrocytes from Graves' disease operative specimens were used to determine whether aberrantly expressing cells were capable of acting as antigen-presenting cells (APC). Thyrocytes are highly adherent and so can only be incompletely purified. However, it was found that T-cell clones that recognize influenza virus haemagglutinin and peptides of that sequence were found to be stimulated by histocompatible thyrocytes using peptides as antigen, but not live or dead virus. This is in contrast to results using irradiated blood mononuclear cells as antigen-presenting cells, which were able to present both peptides and virus. Thus the selective presentation of peptide was indicative that the thyrocytes were capable of presentation.

Thyrocyte antigen-presenting function was also noted using autoreactive T-cell clones from Graves' disease infiltrates. Autologous but not heterologous thyrocytes were capable of restimulating the clones, demonstrating that they were functional APC, also bearing the relevant auto-antigen. The need for class II expression for APC function in this (as in all systems) was shown by the inhibitory capacity of anti class II monoclonals.

Autoreactive T-cells infiltrate auto-immune lesions and can be restimulated by target cells

If autoreactive T-cells are being restimulated by target cells, then clearly there must be autoreactive T-cells in the lesions. These can be examined most thoroughly by cloning them. This has now been performed in a number of diseases, initially in Graves' disease, and as described above, autoreactive clones were found in all instances. The frequency varied from individual to individual, perhaps reflecting the severity or stage of the disease. Commonly 10 per cent or so of the cells cloned as described were thyroid specific (Fig. 4.65). A small percentage (~ 5 per cent) were AMLR cells.

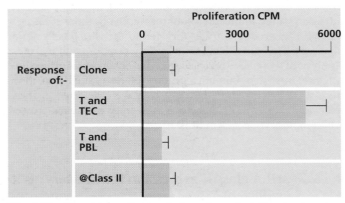

Fig. 4.65 Thyroid-specific T-cell clones from the infiltrating lymphocytes of Graves' disease. Specific stimulation by autologous thyrocytes but not blood cells, inhibited by anti class II antibodies. (Drawn after Londei *et al.* 1985*a*, with permission.)

Autoreactive T-cells produce mediators required for perpetuating the disease

It would be predicted, according to the hypothesis discussed (Fig. 4.65), that for the maintenance of the presenting capacity autoreactive T-cells must be capable of producing the mediators necessary for class II induction. This has been established with clones derived from Graves' disease, Hashimoto's thyroiditis, and rheumatoid arthritis. The majority of clones produce γ-IFN and TNF. The later finding was unexpected, as it was previously considered that TNF was a product of macrophages/monocytes. As discussed γ-IFN suffices for inducing class II in some cell types, but TNF is also necessary for others. In many cell types there is a synergy between γ-IFN and TNF in class II induction.

Induction of auto-immune manifestations by IFN or IL-2 therapy

If the induction of class II target cells is necessary for auto-immunity, then it would be predicted that infusion of molecules capable of inducing class II may be sufficient to induce auto-immunity, provided the homeostatic processes are not sufficient to overcome the stimulus. The therapeutic infusion of IFN for cancer therapy provided an opportunity to determine the effects of these potent molecules on the auto-immune process. A number of studies have shown a markedly augmented frequency of auto-immunity after α-interferon treatment at high concentrations. Auto-immune reactions against thyroid, parotid glands, and epididymis have been noted.

This result may appear paradoxical, but it can be readily explained: NK type cells, which infiltrate auto-immune sites, may be triggered by α-IFN, and release γ-IFN locally. This 'ripple effect' induction of one mediator by another is a marked feature of the cytokine network and makes it difficult to predict effects of mediators *in vivo*.

Recently it has been found that IL-2 therapy (lymphokine-activated killers) precipitates thyroid auto-immunity of the Hashimoto's type. This is consistent with the scheme in Fig. 4.64.

Transgenic mouse technology has permitted the direct testing of the idea that local production of T-cell cytokines such as inteferon γ may induce auto-immunity. Using the insulin promoter, IFNγ production was targeted to the islet β cells of the pancreas. This caused an inflammatory response and diabetes. Analysis of these mice revealed that the diabetes was of immune origin. Thus islets but not pituitary gland grafted into these mice were destroyed, cytotoxic T-cells were detected in these mice, and there was no diabetes if these mice were back-crossed with lymphocyte-deficient SCID mice.

4.13.7   HLA class II expression is necessary: is it sufficient?

Discussion so far has centred on the essential role of HLA class II in the maintenance of the auto-immune disease process. The obvious question becomes whether it is sufficient. In principle it could be sufficient, if there was no tolerance towards the relevant self-antigens, and a lack of effective suppression.

Whether class II expression was sufficient was investigated by comparing thyrocytes and infiltrating lymphocytes from an auto-immune disease, Graves' hyperthyroidism, and another non-auto-immune disease, non-toxic goitre. In the latter disease, there is infiltration by lymphocytes, as well as class II on an appreciable percentage of thyrocytes.

Thus experiments were performed to determine whether thyrocytes from non-auto-immune patients could, if induced to express class II, act as APC, for example in a mixed lymphocyte reaction. They were able to do so, but unlike Graves' thyrocytes not without γ-IFN pretreatment. The capacity of infiltrating lymphocytes to respond to autologous class II expressing thyrocytes was tested. Only the auto-immune yielded any response. These results suggest that the presence of autoreactive lymphocytes is critical to the generation of the auto-immune process (Fig. 4.66). The expression of class II, and the infiltration by T-cells is not sufficient in the absence of autoreactive T-cells. Thus a major question to be answered is how self non-reactivity

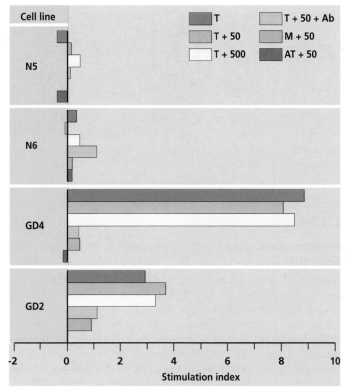

Fig. 4.66 Specificity of intrathyroidal T-lymphocytes after four weeks expansion with OKT3 and IL-2, from non-toxic goitre (T-cell lines N5 and N6) and from Graves' disease (T-cell lines GD4 and GD2). Proliferative responses after a 4-day co-culture of presenter and responder cells. Boxed insert: T, thyrocytes; 50, 50 μ/ml γ-IFN; Ab, anticlass II monoclonals; M, macrophages; AT, allogeneic thyrocytes. (Drawn after Grubeck-Loebenstein *et al.* 1988, with permission.)

is lost. The possibilities for this were discussed in Section 4.12. However, which possibilities are involved in a given disease is not yet known.

4.13.8 What are the molecular mediators of the auto-immune process?

This problem can be divided into two questions: which mediators are involved in the perpetuation of the disease process, and which mediators are involved in the tissue damage and inflammation? While there is a fundamental difference in immuno-pathological terms between the two, in practice the same molecules (e.g. γ-IFN) may be involved in both; for example, inducing class II is important for perpetuation, and activating mononuclear cells to release reactive oxygen metabolites and radicals is important in tissue damage. The significance of knowing which of the potential mediator molecules are present is due to the fact that therapeutic intervention directed against these may be more effective than current therapies based on totally empirical grounds, or the blockage of symptoms by reducing inflammation.

Since the appropriate assays for determining which molecules are present in auto-immune tissues have only been available for a short period of time, a complete description of any disease is not possible and so a composite picture has been drawn from rheumatoid arthritis, where the most data is available, and thyroiditis, where there is less data, but controls are available, by investigating operative samples from non-toxic goitre (NTG). Normal joint tissue is virtually acellular and so cannot be used as controls.

Interleukin-1 (IL-1)

IL-1 is involved in the induction of T- and B-cell responses and so its presence in auto-immune sites is expected. In RA, IL-1α protein and mRNA were found at higher levels than anticipated from prior studies in activation of blood mononuclear cells, which produce ∼ 16-fold more IL-1β than α. In RA the ratio was ∼ 1 : 1. IL-1 induces inflammation, e.g. PGE_2 release, fever, acute phase proteins, loss of cartilage and bone, and so it is considered that excess IL-1 may be of considerable relevance to the pathogenesis of RA. IL-1α and β were also found in Graves' disease, although it is not clear whether they are only produced by the infiltrating cells or also by thyroid follicular cells.

Interleukin-2 (IL-2)

This is the strongest activator of T-cells, especially of T-cell growth, and in auto-immune disease, with evidence of T-cell proliferation, IL-2 would be expected to be produced. There is recent evidence for abundant IL-2 mRNA production in active RA joints. However, free IL-2 protein has not been detected, possibly due to the presence of free IL-2 receptors or to the presence of IL-2 inhibitors. The lack of free IL-2 in synovial fluid does not indicate that it is lacking in the synovial tissues where the cells are concentrated.

Interleukins-3, 4, and 5

Little information is available on the presence of these entities in auto-immune sites, or their relative expression.

Interleukin-6 (IL-6)

This entity has been disovered and described under many other names: B-cell stimulating factor-2 (BSF-2), interferon-$β_2$, hybridoma growth factor, 22K, IL-1 inducer, hepatocyte stimulating factor (HSF). Many of these properties would be relevant to the manifestations found in auto-immunity, and it was noted that patients with certain tumours (e.g. cardiac myxoma) develop many of the manifestations of auto-immunity, e.g. auto-antibodies such as antinuclear factors, rheumatoid factors, and elevation of acute phase proteins. These tumours were found to produce IL-6 and the auto-immune manifestations were abrogated after extirpation of the tumour. In RA, high levels of IL-6 production were detected, which could account for the elevated acute phase proteins, the rapid differentiation of B-cells into plasma cells, and partly the production of auto-antibodies.

Tumour necrosis factor (TNF) and lymphotoxin (LT), also sometimes termed TNFβ

These molecules have closely related functions, interacting with the same receptor. These functions overlap closely with those of IL-1, partly because these entities induce IL-1 production in a number of target tissues. The capacity of TNF/LT to induce cartilage and bone degradation make these molecules of potential importance for the tissue catabolism of RA, and also in certain tissue tumours.

In acute rheumatoid joint tissues, both RNF and LT mRNA can be detected in the majority of instances. The relative amounts vary but, on average, the amount of LT is greater than that of TNF, a rather surprising result, since activated blood mononuclear cells make much more TNF than LT, and so do T-cells cloned from RA joints. Since the only known source of LT is lymphoid cells, these results suggest that plasma cells maybe also be producing LT mRNA in vivo. However, at the protein level there is far more IFNα than LT produced.

LT and TNF have the potential to act as inducers of inflammation, and as cytotoxins. They could thus be important especially as these effects are markedly enhanced by γ-IFN. This synergy is also important in HLA class II induction, and the synergy may compensate for the relatively low levels of γ-IFN detected in RA joints. In Graves' disease, the production of TNF and LT is much greater than in NTG. In rheumatoid arthritis the use of antibodies to TNFα revealed that it is a 'dominant' cytokine in the network, as anti-TNFα IL-1 production, GM-CSF production, adhesion, etc.

γ-Interferon (γ-IFN)

γ-IFN is the most potent inducer of macrophage activation and of HLA class II induction. Thus its presence in auto-immune tissues such as rheumatoid arthritis is anticipated. γ-IFN mRNA is found in RA, but at relatively low levels, compared to those anticipated from activated blood cells or relative to IL-2. When RA joint cells were placed in culture in the absence of any extrinsic stimulus, they were found to produce augmented levels of γ-IFN mRNA, suggesting that *in vivo*, there was a regulatory mechanism inibiting γ-IFN production. This sort of observation suggests that what is detected in a lesion is not necessarily the result of the 'pro-inflammatory' response, but could be part of the homeostatic mechanism tending to inhibit the tissue damage or to repair it.

In Graves' disease, there is considerably more γ-IFN mRNA than in NTG, consistent with the involvement of γ-IFN in the pathogenesis of the auto-immune process. A summary of the cytokines detected in RA joints is presented in Table 4.27.

Table 4.27 Cytokine gene expression in RA

Cytokine	Expression		Duration mRNA expression
	mRNA	protein	
IL-1α	+ +	+	prolonged
IL-1β	+ +	+	prolonged
IL-2	+ +	controversial	prolonged
Il-3	?		
IL-4	?		
IL-5	?		
IL-6	+ + +	high	prolonged
α-IFN		+	
β-IFN			
γ-IFN	+	low	increases in culture
TNF	+	+	
LT	+	low	
GM-CSF	+ +	+	prolonged
M-CSF	+	+	
G-CSF	+	+	
TGFβ_1	+	+	
TGFβ_2	?		
PDGF-A	+ +		prolonged
PDGF-B	+		prolonged
aFGF	?		
bFGF	?		

4.13.9   Conclusions

Current analyses and ideas provide a good account of the mechanisms occurring during the active phase of the auto-immune response. There is increasing evidence that T-cells participate actively in the generation of many if not all auto-immune diseases. These T-cells recognize auto-antigens, and so the essential mechanisms of auto-immunity are not very different from those of the immune response to auto-antigens.

However, there are many gaps in our knowledge of what happens in the very early stages of the generation of an auto-immune disease, the counterplay between genetic and extrinsic influences which result in the breakdown of 'self tolerance'. This is a fertile field for future research.

4.13.10   Acknowledgements

The author thanks Dr D. Williams for preparing Table 4.25, Dr A. Foulis for the photographs in Fig. 4.62 and P. Wells for preparing the manuscript.

4.13.11   Bibliography

Banerjee, S., Haqqi, T. M., Luthra, H. S., Stuart, J. M., and David, C. S. (1988). Possible role of V_β T cell receptor genes in susceptibility to collagen-induced arthritis in mice. *Journal of Experimental Medicine* **167**, 832–9.

Bottazzo, G. F., Pujol-Borrell, R., Hanafusa, T., and Feldmann, M. (1983). Hypothesis: Role of aberrant HLA-DR expression and antigen presentation in the induction of endocrine autoimmunity. *Lancet* **ii**, 1115–19.

Buchan, G. S., Barrett, K., Fujita, T., Taniguchi, T., Maini, R. N., and Feldmann, M. (1988). Detection of activated T cell products in the rheumatoid joint using cDNA probes to interleukin 2, IL-2 receptor and Interferon γ. *Clinical Experimental Immunology* **71**, 295–301.

Feldmann, M. and Brennan, F. M. (1991). Cytokine assays: role in evaluation of the pathogenesis of autoimmunity. *Immunological Reviews* (in press).

Grubeck-Loebenstein, B., Londei, M., Greenall, C., Pirich, C., Kessal, H., Waldhause, W., and Feldmann, M. (1988). Pathogenic relevance of HLA class II expressing thyroid follicular cells in nontoxic goiter and in Graves' disease. *Journal of Clinical Investigation* **81**, 1608–14.

Janossy, G., Panayi, G., Duke, O., Bofill, M., Poulter, L, W., and Goldstein, G. (1981). Rheumatoid arthritis: a disease of T lymphocyte/ macrophage immunoregulation. *Lancet* **ii**, 839–41.

Londei, M., Bottazzo, G. F., and Feldmann, M. (1985a). Human T cell clones from autoimmune thyroid glands: specific recognition of autologous thyroid cells. *Science* **228**, 85–9.

Londei, M., Lamb, J. R., Botazzo, G. F., and Feldmann, M. (1985b). Epithelial cells expressing aberrant MHC class II determinants can present antigen to cloned human T cells. *Nature* **312**, 639–41.

Maini, R. N., Plater-Zyberk, C., and Andrew, E. (1987). Autoimmunity in rheumatoid arthritis: an approach via a study of B lymphocytes. *Rheumatic Disease Clinics of North America* **13**(2), 319–38.

Oldstone, M. B. A. (1987). Molecular mimicry and autoimmune disease. *Cell* **50**, 819–20.

Pujol-Borrell, R., *et al.* (1987). HLA class II induction in human islet cells by interferon-γ plus tumour necrosis factor of lymphotoxin. *Nature* **326**, 304–6.

Saiki, R. K., *et al.* (1988). Enzymatic amplification of β-globin genomic sequences and restriction site analysis for diagnosis of sickle cell anemia. *Science* **230**, 1350–4.

Todd, J. A., *et al.* (1988). A molecular basis for MHC class II-associated autoimmunity. *Science* **240**, 1003–9.

Tournier-Lasserve, E., Hashim, G. A., and Bach, M. A. (1988). Human T cell response to myelin basic protein in multiple sclerosis patients and healthy subjects. *Journal of Neuroscience Research* **19**, 149–56.

Turner, M., Londei, M., and Feldmann, M. (1987). Human T cells from autoimmune and normal individuals can produce tumour necrosis factor. *European Journal of Immunology* **17**, 1807–14.

Urban, J. L., *et al.* (1988). Restricted use of T cell receptor V genes in murine autoimmune encephalomyelitis raises possibilities for antibody therapy. *Cell* **54**, 577–92.

4.14 Mechanisms of graft rejection

P. J. Morris

4.14.1 Introduction

The rejection of a tissue allograft (see Table 4.28 for terminology) is complex and is surprisingly still poorly understood despite the current success of clinical organ transplantation. However, the development of more specific immunosuppressive therapies will depend on a much more precise knowledge of the complex cellular and humoral responses that inevitably result in rejection of an allograft in an unmodified host, and indeed not infrequently in clinical practice despite immunosuppression. The cellular interactions that are involved in the recognition of antigen and the induction of the immune response to that antigen have been fully described in this section already, and are obviously relevant also in the immune response to an allograft. But as well as the accepted wisdom that host antigen-presenting cells present foreign histocompatibility antigens of the donor organ in association with host class II MHC antigen to host T-helper cells (MHC restriction), there is almost certainly an additional form of recognition of allografts by the recipient that is not MHC restricted. For allogeneic class II MHC antigen expressed on passenger leucocytes (dendritic cells) and on endothelium within the graft can be recognized directly by host T-helper cells randomly passing through the vascularized graft. This is possibly the more important form of antigen recognition in the case of a vascularized organ allograft such as the kidney, whereas in a free graft, such as skin, induction of the immune response probably takes place in the usual way.

A number of factors are important in the induction of an immune response to an allograft (the afferent limb) as well as in the effector arm of the response (the effector limb) which gener-

---

Table 4.28 Terminology

Autograft (autologous):
   Transplantation of an individual's own tissue to another site, e.g. the covering of third-degree burns with skin from unburnt areas or a saphenous vein femoropopliteal graft

Isograft (isogeneic or syngeneic):
   Transplantation of tissues between genetically identical members of the same species, e.g. kidney transplant between monozygotic identical twins or skin grafts between mice of the same inbred strain

Allograft (allogeneic):
   Transplantation of tissues between genetically non-identical members of the same species, e.g. a cadaveric renal transplant or a skin graft between mice of different inbred strains

Xenograft (xenogeneic):
   Transplantation of tissues between members of different species, e.g. a baboon kidney transplanted into a human

---

ally will result in rejection of an allograft if not modified (Table 4.29). For simplicity it is easier to discuss the mechanism of rejection separately under these two main headings, namely the afferent and effector limbs.

Table 4.29 Factors influencing rejection of a tissue allograft

Afferent limb
   Major histocompatibility complex (MHC)
   Minor histocompatibility antigens
   Recognition of foreignness
   Site of sensitization
   Privileged sites and tissues
   Genetic control
Effector limb
   Specificity
   Specific T-cells
   (a) T cytotoxic cell
   (b) T-helper cell
   (c) T-suppressor cell
   Non-specific cells
   Antibody
   Target cells

4.14.2 Afferent limb

Major histocompatibility complex (MHC)

Incompatibility for antigens of the MHC is in general essential for rejection of a graft to occur. The importance of the MHC in man (HLA) in clinical organ transplantation is illustrated by the superior survival of renal transplants in siblings that are identical for HLA in comparison to that of parent-to-child transplants (one haplotype identical), and both in turn have an overall better graft survival than cadaver grafts. The biochemistry and genetic control of MHC systems have already been described in detail and are remarkably similar in all mammalian species. Rejection of a graft in experimental models will occur in the presence of class I or class II MHC incompatibilities, but class II incompatibilities provide a greater immunogenic stimulus than class I incompatibilities for the reasons given in the introduction. This also provides an explanation for the apparently much greater influence of compatibility for one of the class II antigen series, namely HLA-DR, in clinical renal transplantation than compatibility for other components of the HLA complex (Table 4.30).

It also appears that MHC antigens of themselves are not immunogenic unless recognized by the recipient on the surface of a viable cell, and perhaps only a lymphoid cell, but as already suggested endothelium may also fill this role, at least in the human. Presentation of MHC antigen in the form of a soluble membrane extract will not lead to an immune response, and indeed presentation of MHC class I antigens on cells which do not express MHC class II antigen in general fails to give rise to a response, suggesting that class II MHC antigens must be present on cells of the immunizing tissue allograft for induction of the alloreactive immune response to take place. However, it is

Table 4.30 HLA-DR mismatches and the outcome of patient and cadaveric graft survival in Oxford in patients treated either with azathioprine or cyclosporin

Number of HLA-DR mismatches	Number of patients	Percentage success		
		1 year	3 years	5 years
Graft survival				
0	132	80	74	66
1	199	66	57	50
2	104	59	55	52
Patient survival				
0	132	95	95	89
1	199	95	89	86
2	104	90	87	83

known that congenic strains of mice differing only for class I MHC antigens can reject a skin allograft, so that incompatibility for class II antigens is not essential for the induction of the immune response to a graft, which can still occur by the conventional pathway.

Minor histocompatibility antigens

Minor histocompatibility antigens may play a prominent role in graft rejection where donor and recipient are compatible for the MHC but the recipient has been presensitized against donor minor antigens. This presumably explains the not uncommon acute rejection episodes that occur in HLA-identical sibling renal transplants. Furthermore, it has been clearly demonstrated in a mouse cardiac allograft model that multiple minor histocompatibility differences can cause rejection of the graft in a non-sensitized recipient in the presence of MHC identity. Although over 30 minor histocompatibility antigen systems have been identified in the mouse (and there may be as many as 300), little is known about such systems in man, as they cannot be detected serologically (in the mouse they are determined by their ability to cause allograft rejection). However, several systems in man have now been identified by cellular assays and these appear to play a role in the occurrence of graft-versus-host reactions after bone marrow transplantation between HLA-identical siblings.

Recognition of foreignness

Although it is clear that incompatibility for MHC antigens stimulates the immune response to the foreign graft, it seems, as mentioned in the introduction, that there is a special mechanism by which the graft is recognized as foreign apart from the conventional presentation of incompatible MHC antigen by the host antigen-presenting cells. And that is by recognition of incompatible class II MHC antigen present on a specialized cell widely distibuted through all tissues and known as a dendritic cell (Fig. 4.67). Phenotypically this cell is not of the macrophage nor the T-cell lineage and is a potent stimulator of allogeneic cells in a mixed lymphocyte reaction. That such a cell could be important in inducing the immune response to an organ allograft has been recognized for a long time, the cell

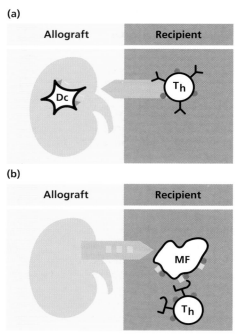

Fig. 4.67 Two possible methods of sensitization to a vascularized renal allograft. (a) T_h cells of the recipient randomly enter the kidney where incompatible class II antigen in the donor organ is presented by the dendritic cell to the host T_h. (b) Antigen leaves the kidney and is processed in the usual way by host antigen-presenting cells such as the macrophage ($M\Phi$) and presented to the T_h in the conventional way (MHC restriction). ▲, Donor class II antigens; ■, donor class I antigen; ●, recipient class II antigen; Ⴗ, Υ, receptors for class I and class II antigens. (Drawn after Dallman and Morris 1988, with permission).

being known previously for want of any identification as a passenger leucocyte. Experiments in the rodent in selected strain combinations were able to show that removal of the passenger leucocytes led to prolonged survival of organ allografts. This has important implications in clinical transplantation if the passenger leucocyte, now identified as a dendritic cell, has an equally important role in man as demonstrated in many, but not all, rodent strain combinations. However, one major difference exists between the rodent and man in that endothelium does not express class II MHC antigen in the rodent, whereas it does in man. Furthermore, if class II antigen on endothelium can be similarly recognized as on the dendritic cell, then attempts to remove the dendritic cell population from the graft before transplantation in order to reduce the immunogenicity of the graft are likely to be fruitless.

Site of sensitization

This may differ depending on whether the allograft is primarily vascularized, as is the case with an organ allograft such as the kidney, or secondarily vascularized, as in the case of a free graft such as skin. In the case of the vascularized organ allograft recognition of foreignness and the induction of the immune response probably takes place primarily in the graft as T-helper lymphocytes randomly enter the graft and recognize allogeneic antigens on the donor dendritic cells or, perhaps, donor endothelium. While in the case of the free skin allograft, donor histocompatibility antigen, or possibly donor dendritic cells (in the skin these are the Langerhans cells), pass via host lymphatics to central lymph nodes and sensitization occurs centrally. The important role of the lymphatic drainage of the bed of a skin allograft has been demonstrated clearly, for if the bed of the graft is maintained on a vascular pedicle alone with no lymphatic drainage, a skin allograft will show markedly prolonged survival (Fig. 4.68). In contrast, the lymphatic drainage of an organ allograft plays little role in the induction of the immune response to that graft.

Privileged sites and tissues

Tissue allografts placed in certain sites, such as the anterior chamber of the eye, the brain, or the cheek pouch of the hamster, may not evoke an immune response, and survive for a prolonged time. What such sites have in common is the absence of a lymphatic drainage. If the recipient animal is sensitized beforehand to the allograft, then it will not survive in the privileged site.

Certain tissues are also less susceptible to rejection. Cartilage is one such tissue, and fetal skin allografts show prolonged survival in certain mouse strain combinations, as do certain endocrine tissues such as ovary and parathyroid tissue.

Genetic control

There is good evidence in the rat and the mouse that the immune response to an allograft is genetically controlled by immune response (*Ir*) genes linked not only to the MHC but also to non-MHC antigen systems. There is also some evidence in clinical renal transplantation suggestive of an MHC-linked *Ir* gene influence on graft rejection, although it has proved difficult to substantiate.

4.14.3   Effector limb

Specificity

The immune response to an allograft tends to be highly specific and involves memory in that following rejection of an allograft, a subsequent allograft from the same donor will be rejected in an accelerated manner, whereas a third-party allograft will be rejected in a normal fashion. However, there are a variety of effector mechanisms both specific and non-specific, all of which may result in tissue destruction. These include the cytotoxic T-cell and complement-dependent antibody on the specific side, while on the non-specific side, there are activated macrophages, natural killer cells, and antibody-dependent cell-mediated cytotoxicity, all of which in theory can destroy an allograft.

In addition there is a cellular response which, given the right circumstances, can down-regulate the effector limb, and in experimental models of organ allografts in the rodent lead to permanent acceptance of a graft. This aspect of the response to a graft is mediated also by T-lymphocytes (T-suppressor cells), and the final outcome of an allograft, at least in the experimental model, depends on the dominance of one or other of these two interdependent responses.

Specific T-cell

The T cytotoxic (T_c) cell

For many years the T_c cell has been considered the main cell responsible for rejection. However, in the last few years experimental rodent models depleted of all lymphoid cells by irradiation and then reconstituted with different lymphocyte populations, have been used to show that in many instances T_c cells in the absence of T-cells of the helper phenotype (T_h cell) will not reject a graft, thus suggesting that the T_h cell is the key cell involved in rejection rather than the T_c. However, the recognition that some cells of the T_h phenotype may also be cytotoxic has confused the issue still further, as has the demonstration that T_c cells which show donor-specific cytotoxicity *in*

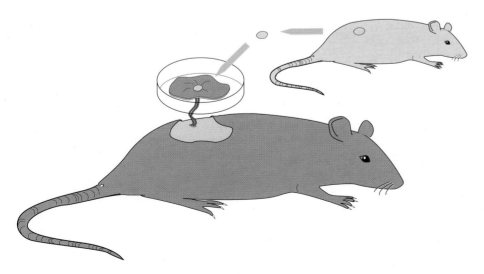

Fig. 4.68 In this model, a skin allograft has been placed on a flap of skin raised from the host and nurtured by a single artery and vein, but separated from the host by a plastic dish such that lymphatic ingrowth is prevented. (Drawn after Dallman and Morris 1988, with permission.)

vitro may be extracted from a renal allograft in the rat which is not undergoing rejection. Nevertheless at present the T_c cell must still be considered as having a major role in the rejection reaction.

The T-helper (T_h) cell

The experiments referred to above provide strong support for the role of the T_h cell in rejection and support a long-held view that rejection of an allograft is a delayed type hypersensitivity reaction in which the initial effector part of the response is mediated by the T_h cell and then, after the release of various lymphokines, the rest of the rejection reaction is mediated by non-specific cells such as macrophages and natural killer (NK) cells. However, although there is no doubt that the T_h cell is an important and perhaps the most important cell in the effector limb of the response to an allograft, it has proved extremely difficult to demonstrate any significant role for macrophages and NK cells in this arm of the response, at least at an early stage of the rejection reaction, although they are present in substantial numbers in the late stages of a rejecting graft.

The T-suppressor (T_s) cell

The T_s cell probably composes a hierarchy of T-cells, which have the ability to both suppress the induction of the immune response (this cell being of the T_h phenotype), as well as maintain the graft in place (these cells being of the T_c phenotype). The latter cell is able to transfer suppression specifically from a rodent with a long-surviving allograft to a syngeneic recipient, usually lightly irradiated, such that an allograft of the same specificity as that in the long-surviving animal is not rejected by the recipient of the suppressor cells. The role of such cells in clinical transplantation and their mechanism of action is unknown, although the evidence that such cells must exist is now quite compelling in a variety of experimental allograft models. Indeed, these cells appear to be responsible for most examples of adult tolerance produced in such models.

Non-specific cells

The macrophage certainly must play a role in rejection as it is present in such substantial numbers in a rejecting graft, but it is probably at a late stage of the reaction that it serves its role. NK cells certainly exist in allografts undergoing rejection but it has not proved possible to demonstrate that they play a role in the reaction, for these cells can be extracted from kidneys undergoing rejection, as well as from kidneys with quite stable function. Similarly, in the case of the K cell, which is the cell responsible for the *in vitro* killing of target cells via the Fc receptors of specific antibody attached to the target, so-called antibody-dependent cell-mediated cytotoxicity (ADCC), it has not proved possible to show convincingly that this *in vitro* phenomenon has any *in vivo* relevance.

Antibody

Preformed antibodies directed at donor MHC antigens and resulting from prior exposure to MHC antigens (e.g. a previous transplant or pregnancy) may undoubtedly cause immediate (hyperacute) rejection of a renal allograft in man. This fierce reaction is accompanied by the deposition of antibody and complement within the graft and a widespread infiltration by polymorphonuclear leucocytes, followed by generalized arteriolar and glomerular thrombosis. Such an event is prevented now in clinical practice by the lymphocytotoxic crossmatch between the serum of a sensitized recipient and donor lymphocytes. The role of antibody in acute or chronic rejection is unclear. Many of the changes seen in acute rejection, such as glomerular capillary thrombosis, interstitial haemorrhage, and fibrinoid necrosis of arteriolar walls, have been considered to be due predominantly to antibody, and indeed deposition of IgG and IgM can be demonstrated more frequently in kidneys undergoing acute rejection. Similarly, the obliterative intimal fibrosis of arterioles and arteries seen in organs undergoing chronic rejection is considered probably to be due to antibody. On the other hand, the appearance of donor-specific cytotoxic antibodies in a human recipient of a renal allograft does not always precede rejection nor indeed is it necessarily associated with rejection at all. To confuse the picture further, it is possible in the rat to passively transfer donor-specific cytotoxic antibodies to a recipient of a renal allograft at the time of transplantation and produce complete suppression of rejection and prolonged survival (passive enhancement). The rat is thought to have a relatively defective complement system and hence complement fixation and antibody-mediated destruction of the graft does not occur. Nevertheless, despite the difficulty in defining a clear role for antibody in rejection of an allograft (apart from that in hyperacute rejection) it would be surprising if donor-specific antibody did not have an important role in the rejection reaction.

Target cells

It seems probable that in a vascularized organ allograft it is the endothelium that bears the primary brunt of the immune response, the parenchymal cells being secondarily affected. In general, the target antigen will be MHC antigens, either class I or class II or both. In this respect it is particularly relevant to note that in the past few years it has been shown that virtually all cells in an allograft undergoing rejection express more class I MHC antigen, and there is also a marked increase in class II expression not only by cells that normally do express it but also in cells that normally do not (Fig. 4.69). The augmented expression of MHC antigen is under the control of γ-interferon, one of the lymphokines released by activated T_h cells. This increased expression of MHC antigen would, of course, markedly increase the density of the target antigen for the ongoing immune response, thus amplifying the potential for destruction.

4.14.4 Conclusions

It can be seen from what has been said that the immune response to a tissue allograft, which will generally result in rejection of an allograft in an unmodified host, is a complex interaction between both the specific and non-specific cellular components of the response together with antibody. It is likely

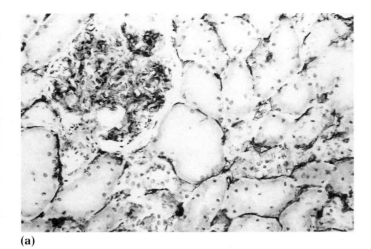

(a)

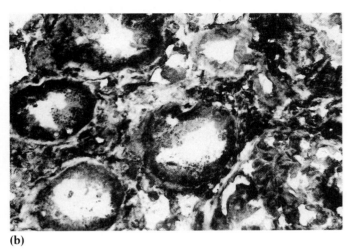

(b)

Fig. 4.69 (a) Biopsy of a kidney at the time of transplantation labelled with a monoclonal antibody to HLA class II antigen (immunoperoxidase), showing staining of intertubular capillaries, dendritic-like cells, and mesangial cells only. (b) The same kidney during an acute rejection episode three weeks after transplantation, showing widespread induction of class II antigen on proximal tubules.

that there is no single mechanism of rejection and that furthermore, given the right stimulus, the response may be downregulated by a suppressor-cell response. However, the mechanism of rejection of tissue allografts is slowly being unravelled in experimental models, while in man the use of monoclonal antibodies is allowing a more precise description of the cells involved in human graft rejection, although this does not of course necessarily relate to function. As patterns of rejection are defined, more precise methods of prevention, diagnosis, and treatment will follow in clinical organ transplantation.

4.14.5 Further reading

Austyn, J. M. and Steinman, R. M. (1988). The passenger leucocyte: a fresh look. In *Transplantation Reviews* (ed. P. J. Morris and N. L. Tilney) 2, 139–76. Grune and Stratton, New York.

Baldwin, W. M., Paul, L. C., Claas, F. H. J., and Daha, M. R. (1986). Antibody mediated events in transplantation: challenges to past dogmas and hopes for the future. In *Progress in transplantation*, Vol. 3 (ed. P. J. Morris and N. L. Tilney), pp. 85–114. Churchill-Livingstone, Edinburgh.

Dallman, M. and Morris, P. J. (1988). The immunology of rejection. In *Kidney transplantation: principles and practical* (3rd edn) (ed. P. J. Morris), pp. 15–36. Saunders, New York.

Fuggle, S. V., Carter, N. P., Ting, A., and Morris, P. J. (1986). Sequential analysis of HLA-class II antigen expression in human renal allografts: induction of class II antigens and correlation with clinical parameters. *Transplantation* 42, 144–9.

Hutchinson, I. V. (1986). Suppressor cells in allograft rejection. *Transplantation* 46, 547–55.

Kissmeyer-Nielsen, F., Olsen, S., Petersen, V. P., and Fjeldborg, O. (1966). Hyperacute rejection of kidney allografts associated with pre-existing humoural antibodies against donor cells. *Lancet* 1, 662–5.

Lafferty, K. J., Gill, R. G., Babcock, S. K., and Simeonovic, C. J. (1986). Activation and expression of allograft immunity. In *Progress in transplantation* vol. 3, (ed. P. J. Morris and N. K. Tilney), pp. 55–84. Churchill-Livingstone, Edinburgh.

Mason, D. R. and Morris, P. J. (1986). Effector mechanisms in graft rejection. *Annual Review of Immunology* 4, 119–45.

Morris, P. J. (1988). *Kidney transplantation: principles and practice* (3rd edn.). Saunders, New York.

Peugh, W. N., Superina, R. A., Wood, K. J., and Morris, P. J. (1986). The role of H-2 and non-H-2 antigens and genes in the rejection of marine cardiac allografts. *Immunogenetics* 23, 30–7.

Ting, A. and Morris, P. J. (1978). Matching for B-cell antigens of the HLA-DR (D-related) genes in cadaveric renal transplantation. *Lancet* i, 575–7.

Ting, A. and Morris, P. J. (1985). Current status of crossmatching in clinical transplantation. In *Progress in transplantation*, Vol. 2 (ed. P. J. Morris and N. L. Tilney), pp. 44–68. Churchill-Livingstone, Edinburgh.

Williams, G. M., Hume, D. M., Hudson, R. P., Morris, P. J., Kano, K., and Milgrom, F. (1968). Hyperacute renal homograft rejection in man. *New England Journal of Medicine* 279, 611–18.

4.15 Morphology of graft rejection

D. G. D. Wight

4.15.1 Introduction

Modern immunosuppressive drugs are so effective that it is now possible successfully to transplant not only kidneys but also most of the other major parenchymal organs such as the liver, heart, heart–lung, and pancreas. One-year survival for each of these organs can now, in the best centres, be expected to be in the range 70–90 per cent. Although technical factors such as difficulties with organ preservation and with reconstruction of vascular and other anastomoses were responsible initially for a significant number of graft failures, as experience has increased they have become less and less significant. The two major complications that therefore remain are rejection and infection, the main aim of clinical management being to keep rejection suppressed while maintaining adequate defences against opportunistic pathogens. Rejection is an important cause of morbidity and loss of organ grafts; it can only be monitored by morphological means.

4.15.2   Monitoring graft outcome

In clinical practice, both tissue biopsy and fine-needle aspiration biopsy (FNAB) can be used to monitor the progress of the graft. FNAB, which produces a cytological preparation, has the advantage that it has a very low complication rate and thus can be frequently repeated. The technique is particularly useful for monitoring the cellular infiltrate in rejection. Tissue biopsy in essential when an assessment of architectural changes in needed, for example when irreversible lesions are suspected. The kidney and the liver can both be readily sampled by blind needle core biopsy, while forceps biopsies are obtained from the lung and the right ventricle, by the transbronchial and transjugular routes, respectively. In contrast, because of the risks of enzyme leakage, the pancreas can only be sampled at open operation.

With the widespread availability of monoclonal antibodies, it is now also possible to study the cellular expression of framework antigens of the major histocompatibility complex (MHC) since these are thought to be the principal targets of rejection. Most cells express class I antigens (HLA-A, B, and C) but there is some variation in different tissues and between species. Class II antigens (HLA-DQ, DP, and DR) are expressed mainly on CD4-positive T-helper (T_h cells) and the cells with which they interact, namely macrophages and other antigen-presenting cells (such as dendritic cells) and B-lymphocytes. Class II antigens are also found on some vascular endothelia in normal tissues where they may also play a part in antigen presentation.

4.15.3   Classification of rejection

Organ grafts differ from the classic skin grafts of Medawar in that they are vascularized from the time of insertion, allowing both the process of sensitization and subsequently that of rejection to occur promptly. The pattern of rejection of organ grafts by unsensitized recipients and without any immunosuppressive treatment has been well documented in a variety of experimental animals. Immunosuppression, which produces mainly quantitative rather than qualitative changes in the pattern of response, is, of course, mandatory in the clinical setting and thus the descriptions that follow refer to patients receiving standard treatment.

The main targets of rejection are antigens expressed upon the surface of accessible cells; those which have been defined are antigens of the HLA system and blood group antigens of the ABO system. Matching of the blood groups of donor and recipient is simple and standard, but until relatively recently HLA matching of donor with recipient has not been practicable since it takes many hours. The improvement of organ preservation techniques and the development of national schemes for organ

sharing, however, now mean that a kidney harvested in one centre can be transplanted into the recipient with the best HLA match wherever he lives. Close matching of this type appears to have caused about a 10 per cent improvement in graft survival. With the development in the past few months of new perfusion fluids it will soon become possible to match other organs but, interestingly, retrospective studies have not shown any improved survival of grafts when the match happened to be close.

The effector mechanisms may be antibody alone, lymphocytes alone, or the two in combination. Traditionally, rejection is classified according to the speed of onset into three types.

4.15.4   Hyperacute rejection

Hyperacute rejection is due to the presence of preformed circulating antibodies directed against donor-specific antigens within the graft. Those of the ABO blood groups are of course innate, while pre-sensitization to HLA antigens can occur not only from a previous graft, but also as a result of blood transfusion or pregnancy. Its incidence has been greatly reduced by careful matching of the blood group and, in the case of the kidney, use of an *in vitro* crossmatch assay which uses donor lymphocytes to detect antibodies in the recipient's serum. The few remaining cases are due either to antibodies directed against antigens not expressed on lymphocytes, and therefore undetected by the crossmatch, or to technical errors.

The preformed antibody binds to target antigen, which in a vascularized organ graft is mainly the donor endothelium, where it binds complement leading to endothelial cell destruction, chemotaxis of neutrophil polymorphs, lysosomal enzyme release, and subsequent deposition of platelets and fibrin. The changes are initially centred on capillaries which become engorged with fibrin–platelet aggregates and neutrophil polymorphs. The changes rapidly spread to involve arterioles and arteries which then show frank fibrinoid necrosis of their walls and thrombotic occlusion of their lumina. Damage to the integrity of the small vessels results in widespread interstitial haemorrhage. Ultimately many or most of the major vessels become occluded by thrombi, and so the pathology of hyperacute rejection eventually becomes that of ischaemia.

The onset of damage may be almost instantaneous, and certainly soon enough for it to be recognized by the surgeon before completion of the operation. Rarely, onset may be delayed for hours or even days (so-called 'accelerated' rejection), possibly a reflection of antibody of lower titre or lower affinity. The course of hyperacute and acelerated rejection is quite uninfluenced by therapy and thus nephrectomy (or graft replacement) is always required.

In the case of the liver, hyperacute rejection is rare, and indeed is extremely difficult to induce even in pre-immunized experimental animals. The liver has therefore been successfully transplanted in the presence of ABO incompatibility.

Predictably, immunohistochemical staining of all allografts with hyperacute or accelerated rejection reveals widespread linear/granular deposition of IgG and of C3, especially in the walls of capillaries and other small vessels.

4.15.5 Acute rejection

Acute and chronic rejection are distinguished mainly by the speed of the rejection process both morphologically and in terms of deterioration of graft function. However, acute rejection is dominated by cellular processes (which are potentially reversible) whilst chronic rejection appears to be mainly humoral (and essentially irreversible).

Most acute rejection episodes occur within 2 months of transplantation, and changes frequently commence within 4–5 days of surgery. The patient may become febrile with an enlarged and, in the case of the kidney, tender graft (easily palpable in the iliac fossa). There may also be clinical evidence of disordered function, for example elevated serum creatinine or, in the case of the pancreas, hyperglycaemia. Sometimes, rejection may be clinically silent until changes are irreversible; this is the main reason for taking elective biopsies.

Histological findings

Interstitial cellular infiltration is a constant finding and generally commences in and around capillaries, arterioles, and venules (Fig. 4.70). Mononuclear cells appear first in the lumen, where they adhere to the endothelium. Subsequently they may also be seen infiltrating beneath the endothelium and migrating into the adjacent interstitium, which also becomes oedematous. Initially the cells are predominantly small lymphocytes, but soon macrophages, and larger lymphocytes, frequently in mitosis, are seen. Eosinophils, important markers of rejection in FNAB specimens, basophils, and plasma cells are also quite numerous (Fig. 4.71). The intensity, cell composition, and distribution of the cellular infiltrates vary according to the phase and severity of rejection, and to the organ involved.

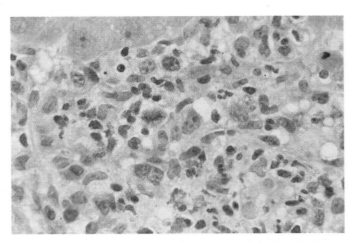

Fig. 4.71 Liver graft, 7 days. Portal area showing acute cellular rejection. The infiltrate includes a large proportion of transformed cells with occasional mitotic figures. Note also the eosinophils.

In the kidney, changes start in the peritubular capillaries and small arteries of the cortex (Fig. 4.70). These cells subsequently extend into the interstitium and often invade adjacent tubular structures, producing the so-called tubulitis. Similarly, in other organs such as the heart, lung, and pancreas there is invasion of the parenchyma to a variable degree. Severe rejection may be associated with tissue necrosis, due partly to damage to vessels and subsequent thrombosis, and partly to direct cell-mediated attack, for example in the heart. In the liver, the cellular infiltration is nearly always confined to the vicinity of the hepatic venules and the interstitium of the portal tracts. Direct involvement of the parenchyma, either at the limiting plate or adjacent to the hepatic venules, is unusual, an observation which may be explained by the pattern of expression of the HLA antigens (see below). Of particular interest is the fact that bile duct epithelium is a target of the infiltrating mononuclear cells in human (but not rat) liver allografts. In comparable fashion, the epithelium of small bronchioles is a target of attack in the lung. The involvement of biliary and bronchiolar epithelium to some extent determines the nature of the complications of chronic rejection (see below).

Cellular rejection responds well to increased immunosuppression, usually in the form of a standard three-day course of soluble methylprednisolone and resolution of the infiltrate can be monitored by repeat biopsy. There is often residual post-inflammatory fibrosis, which is proportional to the intensity of the initial rejection reaction.

With monoclonal antibodies it is possible to characterize the infiltrating cells. At the onset of rejection there is an influx of CD3-positive T-cells and macrophages with smaller numbers of natural killer (NK) cells (large granular lymphocytes) and B-cells. NK cells may actually precede T-cells. Initially the T-cells appear to be inactive precursors, predominantly of the T_h (CD4) lineage, with smaller number of $T_{c/s}$ (CD8) cells. Subsequently the T-cells display activation markers, such as the

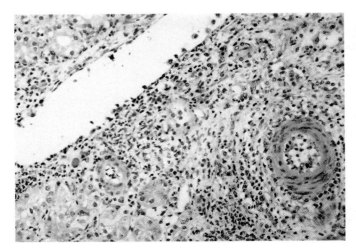

Fig. 4.70 Renal biopsy, 8 days after transplantation, showing acute cellular rejection. Mononuclear cells can be seen adhering to and infiltrating beneath the endothelium of a large venule (left) and a small artery (right). There is also extensive interstitial infiltration.

IL-2 and transferrin receptors. Macrophages, too, may display activation markers.

There thus seems no doubt that T-cells are the principal effector cells in cellular graft rejection, but the relative importance of the two subtypes remains unresolved. Most of the evidence points to direct cytotoxic action by $T_{c/s}$ cells, with T_h cells being concerned with the activation and proliferation of specific $T_{c/s}$ cells. However, the involvement of T_h cells in a type of delayed hypersensitivity reaction, where the graft killing is mediated by lymphokines, cannot be totally ruled out. Indeed, it is possible that both mechanisms may operate at different times and in different patients. This would help to explain the widely differing proportions of T_h and $T_{c/s}$ cells found by different authors in their own material.

Concomitantly, there may also be humoral damage caused by antibody induced by antigens within the graft (although this may occur in any organ, it is most common in the kidney and pancreas and least common in the liver). The damage takes the form of fibrinoid necrosis of the walls of arterioles or small arteries, frequently associated with neutrophil infiltration. It may be segmental or circumferential and may coexist with cellular rejection in a single vessel. The more severely affected arteries may become thrombosed. Immunoglobulin, complement, and fibrin can all be detected in affected vessels. Humoral damage does not respond to increased immunosuppression.

Prognosis

Clearly it would be advantageous to be able to predict the likely outcome of a graft in an individual patient, especially to assess the usefulness of further aggressive therapy when graft function fails to respond to a first course of high-dose steroids. Various complicated scoring schemes, based on quantitative and qualitative assessment of conventional histological features, have been devised but generally they have not been found to be successful. Thus, very severe acute rejection may be fully reversible with increased immunosuppression. The only true predictors of graft failure, therefore, are those which already indicate the presence of irreversible changes, such as vascular necrosis, infarction, or thrombosis of small vessels.

Many authors have attempted to correlate outcome with staining patterns with monoclonal antibodies. The numbers of T (CD3) lymphocytes correlate with the presence but not the prognosis of acute rejection. However, in the kidney, increased numbers of $T_{c/s}$ cells, especially when infiltrated diffusely through the graft or confined to the glomeruli, are associated with a poor response to immunosuppression and an increased risk of graft loss. No consistent pattern has been found with other organs.

During rejection of all organs there is increased expression of both class I (up to 25-fold) and of class II (up to eightfold) HLA antigens on the tissues which normally express them, with, in addition, new expression of class I antigen on hepatocytes and cardiac myocytes, and of HLA-DR on vascular endothelium. The increased expression of HLA-DR on tubular epithelium has been correlated by some authors with irreversible rejection, but others have found no correlation between HLA expression and graft outcome. There have been similar conflicting observations with other organs. The liver is interesting and unusual because class I antigens are not normally expressed on the surface of hepatocytes, but during rejection there is usually intense staining. In general, the intensity of staining correlates with the intensity of rejection, suggesting that it may merely be the consequence rather than the cause of rejection. This view is supported by the relative sparing of parenchymal cells during rejection, and the observation that similar induction of class I antigens occurs in many other conditions. The heart is very similar.

4.15.6 Chronic rejection

This is a heterogeneous group characterized by progressive organ failure occurring some months after engraftment and which affects from 10 to 30 per cent of long-surviving grafts. The distinction from acute rejection is imprecise, but the balance shifts from cellular infiltrates and fibrinoid necrosis towards proliferative stenosing lesions of arteries (Fig. 4.72) which result in varying degrees of graft ischaemia. Since chronic rejection is wholly unresponsive to medical measures, the only rational treatment is graft replacement.

Kidney

In the kidney there is progressive impairment of renal function often accompanied by persistent proteinuria. Serial studies have shown that the arterial changes follow repeated deposition of platelets and fibrin which are subsequently covered by endothelium and incorporated into the intima. Lipids released from platelets are taken up by macrophages which become foam cells. This is followed by a loose myxoid concentric proliferation of collagen fibrils and myointimal cells. With the passage of time

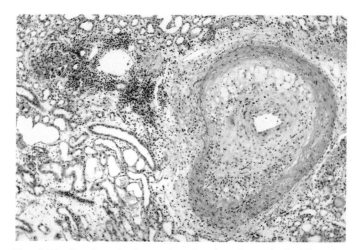

Fig. 4.72 Renal graft, 4 months, showing the typical obliterative lesion of chronic rejection in an arcuate artery. The lumen is greatly narrowed by myointimal fibrous thickening. Note also the foam cells (above) and the medial extension (left).

organization occurs and the thickened intima gradually becomes replaced by relatively acellular collagen and smooth muscle, leading to severe compromise of the lumen (Fig. 4.72). Focal disruption and fragmentation of the media is quite common and may represent extension of the process into the media or previous fibrinoid necrosis during the acute phase.

The vessels most affected are the interlobular and arcuate arteries, which may be obviously thickened when excised kidneys are examined with the naked eye. The resulting renal ischaemia is initially patchy and so atrophic nephrons alternate with those which have undergone hypertrophy, but ultimately the graft becomes uniformly small and shrunken.

The second component of chronic rejection, interstitial fibrosis, is probably the consequence of organization of the interstitial oedema occurring in the acute phase, although there is recent evidence that cyclosporine toxicity may contribute, at least to late fibrosis. Initially there may also be scattered foci of small lymphocytes and plasma cells, but ultimately the fibrosis becomes compact and relatively acellular.

Apart from ischaemic glomerular damage, a true transplant glomerulopathy occurs in some patients (up to 40 per cent in some series). The pathogenesis of this lesion is far from clear, although it has been linked with cytomegalovirus (CMV) infection, but its main significance is that it is wholly irreversible. It must also be distinguished from recurrence of primary disease.

Heart

Vascular lesions are particularly common in heart grafts (as many as 30 per cent of one-year survivors may have significant changes on arteriogram) where they are referred to as accelerated or transplant atherosclerosis. They do, however, differ from spontaneous atherosclerosis in a number of ways. They tend to be concentric rather than eccentric and are much more diffuse so that the penetrating intramyocardial arteries are involved as well as the large epicardial vessels. Indeed, early occlusion of the former may lead to sudden death in the presence of an apparently normal arteriogram. Since the biopsy is taken from the endocardial aspect of the ventricle and thus does not include significant sized vessels, the changes may also be unapparent on biopsy. It has not been possible to find any correlations with conventional atherosclerosis risk factors such as age, sex, or serum lipid profile, nor is there evidence that the incidence is reduced by prophylactic treatment with platelet inhibitors such as dipyramidole. As with renal grafts, there is no clear correlation with severity or distribution of preceding acute rejection.

Liver

Some 10–20 per cent of patients develop a progressive cholestatic syndrome which leads to graft failure within 3–9 months. Examination of these grafts reveals three major features in addition to canalicular cholestasis. Many medium-sized and larger arteries are narrowed or even totally occluded by the same type of obliterative lesion. Only rarely are small arteries and arterioles affected and so, as with the heart, the changes are rarely

seen in biopsies. Some, but not all, patients with arterial lesions develop the second major feature, progressive bile duct loss (the 'vanishing bile duct syndrome') (Fig. 4.73a). This is diffuse and affects primarily the interlobular and smaller ducts. The third feature, a variable degree of liver cell loss and sinusoidal dilatation around hepatic venules, is also fairly constant and is

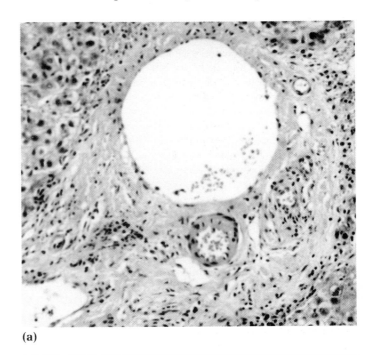

(a)

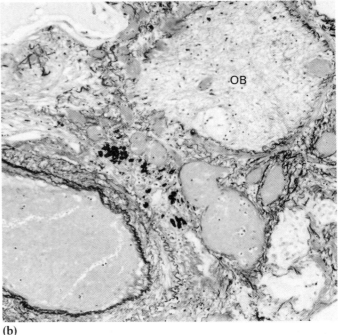

(b)

Fig. 4.73 The late result of chronic rejection in the liver (a), which shows loss of the bile duct in this medium-sized portal tract; and lung (b), which shows obliterative bronchiolitis (OB).

probably due to ischaemia caused by the narrowed arteries. If the graft is left in place there is progressive centrilobular collapse and fibrosis which, in 1–2 years, leads to a true cirrhosis.

There are no satisfactory animal models of chronic rejection of the liver and thus experience is almost entirely based upon human grafts. The pathogenesis of the arterial lesions is thought to be the same as in the kidney, but sequential changes have been difficult to study because of the inaccessibility of the affected vessels. Bile duct loss is much easier to study. In an individual patient it may be possible to follow, in serial biopsies, a progression from cellular infiltration during acute rejection to epithelial vacuolation and distortion and then gradual disappearance of individual cells. Ultimately the whole duct disappears (Fig. 4.73a). There is usually accompanying post-inflammatory fibrosis so that the portal tracts eventually contain only vascular structures embedded in an acellular fibrous stroma. The bile duct loss may be one of the factors responsible for cholestasis.

This sequence suggests that the bile duct loss is due to cell-mediated attack, and, as the target antigen disappears, so do the aggressor T-cells. There has therefore been much interest in the pattern of expression of the HLA antigens. Class I antigens are strongly expressed on normal bile duct epithelium whereas class II antigens are generally absent, although they are easily induced by a variety of stimuli such as infection and bile duct ligation as well as transplantation. Although the rat liver is very similar with regard to class II antigen expression, there is normally only very weak expression of class I antigens on biliary epithelium, which might explain why rat grafts do not develop vanishing bile duct syndrome.

In common with the kidney, biopsy changes are poor predictors of chronic rejection; the likelihood is related neither to the intensity nor the distribution of acute rejection. It may be, therefore, that mismatch of specific HLA antigens will ultimately prove to be more important in predicting outcome in an individual than the intensity of expression on the various cell types. So far, however, this has been difficult to prove.

Lung

The small airways of the lung are in many ways comparable to the bile ducts, since they, too, are a target for invasion by inflammatory cells during acute rejection. The inflammatory infiltration leads to an ulcerative bronchiolitis, which often becomes infected. The subsequent repair in these tiny airways often leads to their total obliteration (Fig. 4.73b) and thus a serious functional deficit. Other late changes in lung grafts include interstitial and pulmonary fibrosis as well as the characteristic obliterative arterial lesions.

Pancreas

Pancreas grafts have a higher technical complication rate than other grafts and thus rejection is relatively less important. Chronic vascular lesions are seen in long-surviving grafts, but graft failure, and in particular islet-cell failure, may, in some cases, be due to a different mechanisms. For example, there is often lymphocytic infiltration of islets even in grafts from HLA-identical twins, suggesting that the immunological attack may be directed against a β-cell, non-HLA antigen.

4.15.7   Further reading

Billingham, M. E. (1987). Cardiac transplant atherosclerosis. *Transplantation Proceedings* **XIX**, 19–25.

Colvin, R. B. (1988). Clinical application of monoclonal antibodies in renal allograft biopsies. *American Journal of Kidney Diseases* **XI**, 126–30.

Herskowitz, A., *et al.* (1987). Histological predictors of acute cardiac rejection in human endomyocardial biopsies: A multivariate analysis. *Journal of the American College of Cardiologists* **9**, 802–10.

Imbasciati, E., Banfi, G., Egidi, F., Tarantino, A., and Ponticelli, C. (1987). Morphologic patterns of renal allograft rejection. *Contributions to Nephrology* **55**, 105–22.

Sale, G. E. (ed.) (1990). *The pathology of organ transplantation*. Butterworths, Boston.

Sibley, R. K. and Sutherland, D. E. R. (1987). Pancreas transplantation. An immuno-histologic and histopathologic examination of 100 grafts. *American Journal of Pathology* **128**, 151–70.

Steinhoff, G., Wonigeit, K., and Pichlmayr, R. (1988). Analysis of sequential changes in major histocompatibility complex expression in human liver grafts after transplantation. *Transplantation* **45**, 394–401.

Wight, D. G. D. and Portmann, B. (1987). Pathology of rejection. In *Liver transplantation* (2nd edn) (ed. R. Y. Calne). Grune & Stratton, Orlando.

Yousem, S. A., Burke, C. M., and Billingham, M. E. (1985). Pathologic pulmonary alterations in long term human heart–lung transplantation. *Human Pathology* **6**, 911–23.

4.16   Graft versus host disease

I. A. Lampert

4.16.1   Introduction

A syndrome originally termed 'secondary disease' a wasting disease associated with infections was originally described by Barnes and Loutit as a cause of mortality in irradiated mice after transplantation with allogeneic haemopoeitic cells. Long-term survival could only be achieved in recipients of syngeneic grafts. The aetiology of this syndrome was at first unclear and a viral cause was initially sought. Further studies showed that secondary disease occurred in F_1 hybrid recipients given parental marrow but not in parental recipients given F_1 hybrid marrow. These observations led to the conclusion that secondary disease was the consequence of a donor-mediated host reaction and not the result of a host-mediated donor reaction, and thereafter it was known as graft versus host disease (GVHD).

The requirements for classical graft versus host disease were formulated by Billingham as follows:

1. Genetically determined histocompatibility differences between donor and recipient.
2. The presence of immunocompetent cells in the graft which can recognize foreign histocompatibility antigens of the host and mount an immunological reaction.
3. The inability of the host to react to or reject the graft.

4.16.2 Conditions associated with GVHD

In experimental animals GVHD can be induced both on the basis of differences at any of the major histocompatibility antigens and also on the basis of minor histocompatibility loci. In clinical marrow transplants it is the preferred option to employ marrow from close relatives which is compatible at all MHC loci, this still leaves minor histocompatibility antigenic differences. If these donor sources are not available, a variety of other sources have been employed, i.e. relatives with MHC differences and unrelated donors compatible at the MHC loci. These other sources have an increased liability to cause GVHD.

Table 4.31 Conditions associated with graft versus host disease

Allogeneic bone marrow transplantation
   Indications: aplastic anaemia
              malignancies and leukaemia
              inborn errors of metabolism etc.
Transfusion of viable blood products to immunosuppressed or immuno-incompetent recipients
Liver and gut transplants
Autologous and syngeneic marrow transplants

Agents employed in the treatment of malignancy, particularly cytotoxic drugs, are highly immunosuppressive. Patients in this state confirm to the Billingham criteria for GVHD and infusion of fresh blood can and does frequently cause severe and at times fatal GVHD. In such patients it is necessary to irradiate the blood to eliminate immunocompetent lymphocytes. A similar syndrome is seen in neonates.

The gut contains a vast reservoir of lymphocytes and is probably the largest lymphoid organ of the body. GVHD has been observed in experimental gut transplants.

4.16.3 Syngeneic and autologous GVHD

Clinical syndromes resembling GVHD were seen in bone marrow grafts between identical twins. Histological examination of the tissue revealed features identical to those seen in classical skin and gut GVHD (see below). Subsequently, similar lesions were seen following autologous marrow transplants and minor forms of the disease have been reported in 10 per cent of such transplants. A similar disease has been produced in syngeneic rats treated with the immunosuppressive drug cyclosporin A during bone marrow transplantation. The mechanism of this disease process is at this time a subject of conjecture. It is thought to arise from two possible mechanisms. Either as a consequence of the failure of the orderly elimination of auto-reactive T-cells in the thymus or due to an imbalance between autoreactive T-cells and their corresponding suppressor cells.

4.16.4 Acute and chronic GVHD

Two distinct forms of GVHD, acute and chronic, have been recognized in humans and in animal models of the disease (Table 4.32). Acute and chronic GVHD have different onset as well as different clinical and pathological manifestations. Inflammatory destruction of the epithelial cells in the skin, liver, and gastrointestinal tract represents the characteristic feature of acute GVHD, whereas chronic GVHD is characterized primarily as increased collagen deposition resulting in fibrosis. Evidence from murine models that closely resemble the human disease have suggested that acute and chronic GVHD represent two separate pathophysiological entities rather than different phases of a single pathological process. T-cell clones recovered from spleens of mice with chronic GVHD due to non-MHC disparities were non-cytotoxic L3T4$^+$ cells which showed proliferative responses specific for autologous class II MHC antigens and produced factors that produced collagen synthesis. T-cell clones recovered from spleens with acute GVHD on the basis of non-MHC differences were heterogeneous. A large proportion were cytotoxic Lyt-2$^+$ cells which showed MHC-restricted responses specific for recipient minor histocompatibility antigens.

Animals studies have shown that depletion of marrow of mature T-cells prevents the development of GVHD and allows the development of chimerism. Unfortunately, depletion of the marrow of T-cells across histocompatibility barriers allows graft rejection. This phenomenon, first discovered in F$_1$ hybrid

---

Table 4.32 A comparison of acute and chronic graft versus host disease

	Acute	Chronic
Onset	Up to day 100	After day 100
Organs involved	Limited—skin, liver, GIT	Widespread
Primary pathology	Destruction of epithelium	Mixed epithelial and mesenchymal lesions
Inflammatory responses	Mild	Often marked

strains, has often been termed hybrid resistance and is thought to be due to the action of radio-resistant natural killer (NK) cells. This has been overcome by a series of therapeutic manœuvres. Subsequently, it has been found in clinical bone marrow transplantation (BMT) that depletion of the marrow of T-cells is associated with a higher incidence of recurrence of underlying malignancy such as leukaemia; this and other experimental evidence demonstrates that GVHD may have a therapeutic effect, the so-called graft versus leukaemia effect.

In the effort to overcome the ill-effects of T-cell depletion and to further identify the nature of the pathogenesis of GVHD, considerable efforts have been made to identify the nature of the T-cells responsible for GVHD, hoping thereby to selectively deplete the marrow of these specific T-cell subsets.

On the basis of a variety of functional studies, T-cells were formerly characterized into a variety of groups, e.g. helper, inducer, suppressor, cytotoxic, etc. Attempts were made to correlate function with antigenic markers on the surfaces of the T-cells. In mice the marker L3T4 (corresponding to the CD4 markers in man) was found generally, but not exclusively, to correlate with helper function, and Lyt-2 (CD8 in man) to correlate, again not exclusively, with suppressor and cytotoxic functions. Subsequently it has been found that these cell markers correlate with other functional properties. T-cells cannot recognize antigen without the assistance of antigen-presenting cells (APCs), and the T-cells are restricted in that they must be compatible with the MHC on the surface of these APCs. L3T4 T-cells must have APCs compatible at the class II MHC loci and Lyt-2 cells at the class I MHC loci. Murine studies have shown that GVHD caused by class I MHC differences are mediated exclusively by Lyt-2 cells, and those caused by class II MHC differences are mediated exclusively by L3T4 cells.

Currently most allogeneic BMTs in man are conducted when host and donor are compatible at all MHC loci (so far as can be determined) and thus the majority of cases of GVHD must be due to non-MHC histocompatibility differences. These correspond to GVHD in mice due to minor histocompatibility antigen differences. In these studies it has been found that for these minor histocompatibility antigens the infused T-cell are class I MHC restricted and that in the majority of cases the critical cells are the Lyt-2 cells; however, in a small number of strain combinations L3T4 cells can cause GVHD. Thus there is no evidence that depleting marrow selectively on the basis of CD4 or CD8 antigens will prevent GVHD.

4.16.5   Acute GVHD

Clinical manifestations

Acute GVHD in humans typically develops in the first 60 days after marrow transplantation and usually manifests as a characteristic dermatitis, accompanied in its more severe forms by a hepatitis and enteritis. Skin involvement often appears initially as pruritic macular exanthem of the palms and soles with moniliform lesions on the extremities, trunk, and face. In progressive disease the lesions become confluent, leading to

generalized erythroderma, bulla formation, bacterial super-infection, and exfoliation. Liver involvement is indicated by an increase in serum bilirubin and alkaline phosphatase. Hepatic failure can occur in very severe cases. Liver biopsy can be helpful but GVHD has to be distinguished from veno-occlusive disease which often results from therapy of the underlying disease.

Gastrointestinal involvement is indicated by watery diarrhoea and malabsorption and in more severe cases by crampy abdominal pain, anorexia, nausea and vomiting, and haemorrhagic ileus. In certain cases it is difficult to distinguish GVHD from viral enteritis.

Pathological manifestations

See Table 4.33.

Table 4.33   Features of acute GVHD

1.   Limited organ involvement
2.   Epithelial destruction
3.   Epithelial proliferation
4.   Accessory factors, e.g. Langerhans cells and effects of interleukins 1 and 2
5.   Lymphokine effects

Cutaneous GVHD

Acute GVHD is typically a lichenoid skin eruption (Fig. 4.74). Major features are basal cell vacuolation and destruction associated with apoptotic bodies (acidophil bodies) found throughout the epidermis. The degree of lymphoid infiltration is always suprisingly light in view of the extensive keratinocyte destruction. With increasing severity there is bullus formation and in the most severe cases total necrosis of the epidermis. This is the basis for the grading of GVHD.

Morphometric studies have shown that the rete ridges are the

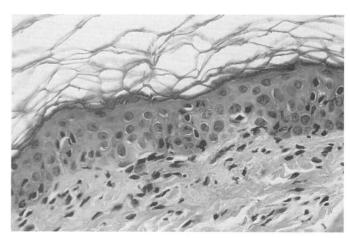

Fig. 4.74   Skin in acute graft versus host disease. There is hyperkeratosis and death of individual keratinocytes with surrounding lymphocytes (Satellitosis).

primary site for damage in the epidermis. This is believed to be associated with the fact that these are proliferating cells. These cells are also the main focus for damage associated with chemotherapy and ionizing radiation, necessary prerequisites for the treatment of the underlying disease and for preparation for engraftment. Thus the pathological diagnosis of cutaneous GVHD is difficult in the first 2–3 weeks after transplantation because these forms of therapy also produce basal vacuolation and death.

It has been found that in various immune disorders involving epithelia, the epithelial cells express class II MHC antigen or HLA-DR. This is due to the secretion of the lymphokine γ-interferon by T-lymphocytes. The earliest manifestation, therefore, of GVHD in the skin can often be the expression of HLA-DR; however, it is to be noted that GVHD skin lesions can occur in the absence of class II expression.

Lymphoid analysis of the skin in graft versus host disease reveals a mixture of CD4$^+$ and CD8$^+$ lymphocytes, and in the early phase of the disease the dominant cell in the epidermis is the CD8$^+$ lymphocyte.

The skin lesions of GVHD are graded into four grades according to the severity of the disease:

Grade I Non-specific epidermal vacuolation accompanied by mononuclear cell infiltration around the superficial venules in the dermis and into the epidermis.

Grade II As above, together with acidophil bodies, distinctive individual cell death—apoptosis—in the basal or supra-basal layer. These degenerative cells sometimes are associated with lymphocytes, giving the appearance of satellitosis.

Grade III Characterized by bullus formation.

Grade IV Total destruction of the epidermis resembling toxic epidermal necrolysis and resulting in sloughing.

Hepatic GVHD

Hepatic GVHD is characterized by cholestatic hepatitis with the degeneration and paucity of small bile ducts. Although hepatic GVHD may resemble viral hepatitis and drug-related injury, in drug GVHD there is cytoplasmic eosinophilia of bile duct cells and segmental necrosis of bile ducts. Portal tracks often show infiltration of lymphocytes.

Gastrointestinal GVHD

In the gastrointestinal tract individual crypt cell necrosis with lymphocytic cell infiltration unaccompanied by widespread necrosis is the hallmark of GVHD. These are evident in rectal biopsies (Fig. 4.75). The maximal damage to the mucosa in both the small bowel and in the large bowel is in the base of the crypts, i.e. in the region of maximal cell proliferation; similarly in the stomach the area of maximal damage is in the neck of the glands, i.e. in the region of maximal cell proliferation. In more severe disease lesions extend to the surface of the epithelium, eventually leading to epithelial denudation.

A curious feature of GVHD is not only its selectivity of cell in-

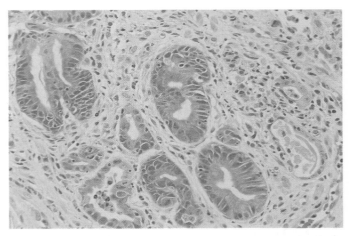

Fig. 4.75 Rectal GVHD. The characteristic features of gut GVHD are single-cell death or apoptosis of the crypt epithelial cells, disintegration of glands, with accumulation of cell debris in the lumen and fibrosis of the lamina propria.

volvement but also of organ involvement. Thus the brain is never involved and neither are the endocrine organs such as the thyroid, adrenals, and parathyroid. Skeletal muscle involvement is not usually a feature of acute GVHD.

Pathogenesis of GVHD

Ultrastructural studies of GVHD have indicated that lymphocytes are the effector cells, extending broad pseudopods that indent but do not appear to breach the membranes of cells that appear to be necrotic. Immunohistochemical studies have identified CD4$^+$, CD8$^+$, and NK cells infiltrating the gut in GVHD.

The issue of which particular T-cell function, cytolysis, or lymphokine release, accounts for GVHD is continually debated. Ultrastructural studies referred to above suggest that direct T-cell cytolysis is responsible, this is confirmed by studies that indicate that compatible skin implanted on to a vulnerable host is spared. On the other hand, it has been shown that if gut compatible with the infused lymphocytes is placed under the renal capsule it will be damaged in the ensuing GVHD—demonstrating the so-called 'bystander' effect. This suggests that lymphokines released by the activated T-cells stimulate accessory cells and NK cells to destroy the tissue. The fact that antibodies against anti-sialo-GM1, a marker for NK cells in mice, can prevent GVHD on the basis of minor MHC differences provides support for the latter point of view.

Prognostic factors in acute GVHD

Certain prognostic factors have been related to the development of clinical GVHD after allogeneic bone marrow transplantation. These are:

1. HLA disparity is the clearest factor for acute GVHD.

2. A striking effect of age on the risk of acute GVHD has been observed in many studies; the reason for the increased risk is

not explained; a possible role for reduced thymic function of patients is suspected.

3. A germ-free environment has been observed to reduce GVHD-induced mortality in certain murine and human cases of acute GVHD. The mechanism for this is not known; however, the same effect can be observed in certain animal models of GVHD with bowel sterilization and the effect nullified by the introduction of Gram-negative organisms, suggesting the effect of endotoxin.

4. Cytotoxic treatment of the recipient increases the severity of acute GVHD.

5. Chimerism. Complete chimeras have a higher incidence of GVHD than mixed chimeras, suggesting that the persistence of host cells will suppress the alloreactive cells.

6. Sex mismatching.

4.16.6   Chronic GVHD

This has been described as a syndrome with a spectrum of clinical manifestations resembling naturally occurring collagen diseases such as Sjögren's syndrome, polymyositis, lichen planus, scleroderma, and primary biliary cirrhosis with involvement of skin, liver, gut, and eyes. Initial manifestations of the disease generally occur by day 100 but can appear at day 70. In most patients the disease follows acute GVHD either in direct progression or with an intervening quiescent period. In 20–30 per cent of patients this arises *de novo* without prior acute disease.

The disease in the skin clinically following the manifestations of acute GVHD differs from that of acute GVHD and often occurs in sun-exposed areas with a pseudo-follicular rash, sometimes violaceous in colour, affecting the face and extensor surfaces (resembling lichen planus) or becomes generalized with dermal thickening and epidermal atrophy (resembling scleroderma). Mouth lesions identical to those seen in lichen planus are present frequently, together with loss of papillae of tongue and oral ulceration. The condition is associated with a sicca syndrome leading to xerostomia and xerophthalmia. Nail dysplasia, chronic exfoliative dermatitis, and alopecia also occur. The condition may progress to a generalized scleroderma particularly affecting the skin, exocrine glands, and gastrointestinal tract. Malabsorption and weight loss can become major complications. The liver may also become affected, with progressive portal fibrosis associated with a vanishing bile duct syndrome leading to fatal liver failure. Lung involvement can result in obstructive airways disease.

Chronic GVHD is associated with a variety of abnormalities of the immune system such as auto-immune haemolytic anaemia and auto-immune thrombocytopenia. There is a profound depression of cell-mediated and humoral immunity, this facilitates the development of opportunistic bacterial and fungal infections and the reactivation of viral infections, principally with herpes zoster and cytomegalovirus.

Pathological features of chronic GVHD

Skin

In generalized GVHD the early phase shows epidermal hypertrophy and hyperkeratosis with a lichenoid infiltrate in the dermis associated with basement membrane thickening. There is inflammation of the pilar units and the sweat glands and subcutaneous fat. These lead to atrophy of the pilar units and squamous metaplasia in the sweat ducts. In advanced cases there is epidermal atrophy and fibroplasia of the dermis, producing lesions similar to those of scleroderma (Figs 4.76, 4.77).

Digestive system

In a similar fashion, in the oesophagus there is inflammation leading to submucosal fibrosis leading to stricture formation. In

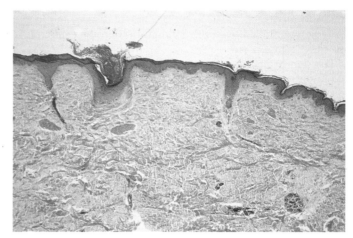

Fig. 4.76 Skin from chronic GVHD (day 400 post-transplantation). The skin appendages have been destroyed. The epidermis is thinned, remaining hair follicles plugged with keratin. The normal dermal collagen is replaced with thick coarse fibres entrapping the sweat glands.

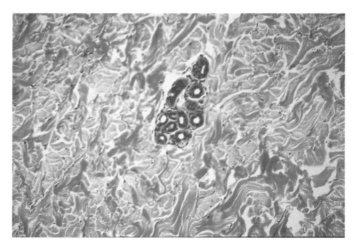

Fig. 4.77 Sweat gland coils in chronic GVHD. Normally sweat gland coils are placed at the dermo-epidermal junction and are surrounded by fat. As a consequence of the dermal fibrosis this fat is lost. The features are identical to those of sclerodermatous skin disease.

liver the changes of acute GVHD progress, leading to fibrosis and loss of small bile ducts, producing a histological picture resembling primary biliary cirrhosis. The salivary glands and lacrimal ducts show similar features, and there is lymphoid infiltration of the ducts, resulting in cell destruction and squamous metaplasia.

Respiratory tract

In the lung the effect of chronic GVHD is concentrated on the bronchiolar epithelium and consists predominantly of a lymphocytic infiltrate, although polymorphs may be seen in some cases. The consequence is oedema and connective tissue proliferation, squamous metaplasia in some cases. Functionally this results in narrowing of the lumen and the development of obstructive airways disease.

Cellular mechanisms in chronic GVHD

Although the aetiology of chronic GVHD is identical to that of acute GVHD, there is evidence that the disease process follows a separate pathogenetic pathway. In experimental studies it has been shown that if animals are allowed to progress to chronic GVHD after developing acute GVHD their lymphocytes, injected in irradiated recipients, result in the direct development of chronic GVHD without passage through an acute phase. As mentioned in chronic GVHD caused by minor histocompatibility antigenic differences, in contrast to acute GVHD T-clones isolated from these animals, all antigens were I-A reactive L3T4$^+$ cells.

The circulating cells of patients with chronic GVHD, even in the absence of overt immunodeficiency, are able to inhibit the mixed lymphocyte response to irradiated third-party cells. This is non-specific suppression and is mediated by CD8$^+$ lymphocytes. Similar non-specific suppression is seen in animal models of chronic GVHD. The mechanism leading to this non-specific suppression induced by chronic GVHD is unknown. Both acute and chronic GVHD have an overall mortality of 10 per cent. GVHD continues to bedevil clinical marrow transplantation, particularly with the tendency to employ marrow from non-related and mismatched donors. This complication has stimulated much immunological research which may unravel pathological processes in other diseases, such as the collagen diseases which GVHD so resembles in the chronic phase.

4.16.7   Further reading

Korngold, R. and Sprent, J. (1987). T cell subsets and graft versus host disease. *Transplantation* **44**, 335–9.

Martin, P., Hansen, J. A., Storb, R., and Thomas, E. D. (1987). Human marrow transplantation: an immunological perspective. *Advances in Immunology* **40**, 379–438.

Sale, G. E., Shulman, H. M., Galluci, B. B., and Thomas, E. D. (1985). Young rete ridge keratinocytes are preferred targets in cutaneous graft-versus-host disease. *American Journal of Pathology* **118**, 278–87.

Santos, G. W., Hess, A. D., and Vogelsang, G. B. (1985). Graft-versus-host reactions and disease. *Immunological Reviews* **88**, 169–92.

Shulman, H. M., *et al*. (1988). Chronic graft-versus-host syndrome in man: a long term clinicopathologic study of 20 Seattle patients. *American Journal of Medicine* **69**, 204–17.

Simonsen, M. (1985). Graft-versus-host-reactions: the history that never was, and the way things happened to happen. *Immunological Reviews* **88**, 5–24.

Thomas, E. D., Storb, R., and Clift, R. A. (1975). Bone marrow transplantation. *New England Journal of Medicine* **282**, 832.

4.17   Neutrophil leucocytes

A. W. Segal and M. J. Walport

4.17.1   Introduction

Polymorphonuclear leucocytes provide a major component of the body's resistance to microbial infections and an important mechanism for the removal of autologous and exogenous debris from sites of inflammation. Their vital role in host defence is illustrated by the consequences of deficiencies of neutrophil activity. The resulting immunodeficiency state is characterized by recurrent infections with bacteria that are usually associated with the formation of pus, i.e. pyogenic bacteria, and these include Gram-positive cocci such as staphylococci and streptococci, and Gram-negative rods such as *Escherichia coli*, *Klebsiella*, and *Serratia*. Patients with neutropenia are also at risk of opportunistic fungal infections with *Candida* and *Aspergillus* species. A very similar spectrum of bacterial infection is seen in association with deficiency of antibodies or of certain complement proteins; this illustrates that the normal pathway of defence against these microbes is opsonization with antibody and complement, followed by phagocytosis and intracellular killing by neutrophils. Abnormal function of any of the links in this chain therefore causes a similar impairment of host defence. In addition to their antimicrobial activities, neutrophils play an important role in the removal of exogenous and endogenous debris. Absence of this function results in the accumulation of this material in the tissues.

4.17.2   Ontogeny and normal life cycle

Mature granulocytes are derived from pluripotential stem cells located in the bone marrow. The development of mature neutrophils with segmented nuclei takes about 7 days within the bone marrow and these mature cells normally spend about 4 days within the marrow before entering the circulation. Differentiating stem cells and their products are subject to the influence of several growth factors, named colony-stimulating factors (CSFs), of which four have been identified in humans and their genes cloned: multi-CSF (IL-3), granulocyte and macrophage CSF (GM-CSF), granulocyte CSF (G-CSF), and macrophage CSF (M-CSF). As their names imply, these growth factors exert their differentiation and growth effects on progressively more committed stages in the maturation of leucocytes. It is believed that the physiological activities of these growth factors include both the normal regulation of production of leucocytes and also the dramatic changes in granulocyte kinetics and activities that follow inflammatory stimuli *in vivo*.

Cell-labelling experiments have shown that the life-span of neutrophils in the circulation is short, with a half-life of approximately 7 hours. The number of neutrophils in the circulation in a resting subject is approximately 5×10^9 per litre. The implication of these figures is that the turnover of neutrophils in the circulation is massive and, indeed, the rate has been measured to be 1.63×10^9 cells/kilogram/day. The fate of aged neutrophils is not established but it seems probable that there are specific recognition mechanisms for the uptake of aged cells, possibly by macrophages. Similarly, the view that neutrophils disintegrate at sites of inflammation, releasing all their toxic contents, is probably incorrect, and here also it is likely that macrophages remove senescent or exhausted neutrophils.

There are two pools of neutrophils within the circulation, a circulating pool and a 'marginated' pool of cells. The marginated pool is believed to consist of neutrophils sequestered within the microvasculature of many organs, of which the most important may be the lungs and spleen. These two pools of cells are in dynamic equilibrium. Following infection, the number of neutrophils within the circulating pool may increase within 24–48 hours by up to tenfold. This increase is mediated by transfer of cells from the marginated pool, by accelerated release of neutrophils from the bone marrow, and by stimulated maturation of immature neutrophils by CSFs.

4.17.3 Structure

Neutrophils are members of the granulocyte family of leucocytes. The members of this family, which comprises neutrophils, eosinophils, and basophils, all contain cytoplasmic granules which are storage pools for intracellular enzymes, cationic proteins, receptors, and other proteins. The second characteristic morphological feature of neutrophils is a multilobed nucleus.

Receptors

The interaction of neutrophils with the external milieu is mediated through the binding of extracellular ligands to specific cell surface receptors. Many such receptors have been partially characterized, although this work is in its early stages. Four major classes of neutrophil receptors have been recognized and are classified below according to their ligands.

Receptors for inflammatory mediators and bacterial products

There are two types of receptors on neutrophils which bind to products of inflammation. The first type have as ligands peptides produced by triggered enzyme cascades, such as the complement system, and lipid mediators, produced by metabolism of cell membrane phospholipids. Examples of these are the receptors for the anaphylatoxin, C5a, produced by the cleavage of C5 by the complement C5 convertase enzymes, and for leukotriene B4, derived from the metabolism of cell membrane arachidonic acid by lipoxygenase enzymes. Another important lipid mediator that activates neutrophils is platelet-activating factor (PAF), but the receptor for this molecule has not been characterized. The second type of neutrophil receptor binds directly to peptides derived from bacteria, the formyl-methionyl-leucyl-phenylalanine (f-Met-Leu-Phe) receptor. The supernatants of many bacterial cultures contain molecules with potent chemotactic activity for neutrophils. This finding, coupled with the observation that the initial sequence of many bacterial proteins is formyl-methionyl-, led to the synthesis of a series of small peptides with chemotactic activity for neutrophils, of which the most potent was f-Met-Leu-Phe.

Receptors for lymphokines and monokines

The lymphokines and monokines: interleukin-1, tumour necrosis factor -α and -β, and γ-interferon, have each been shown to activate neutrophils in a very similar manner, discussed below. Specific receptors for these molecules have yet to be characterized but it is probable that several neutrophil surface receptors will be responsible for ligation of these products of activated cells of the immune system.

Opsonic receptors

A general mechanism for the removal of foreign antigens from the circulation and from tissues is the binding of antibodies and/or complement proteins to the foreign substance. Clearance of these coated (opsonized) substances is then mediated by specific receptors on phagocytic cells. Neutrophils play an important part in these clearance mechanisms and bear receptors with specificity for the Fc portion of antibody (Fc receptors) and for the major cleavage fragments of C3 (C3b and C3bi) and C4 (C4b). Two such complement receptors have been characterized on neutrophils: complement receptor type 1 (CR_1), whose ligands are C3b, C3bi, and C4b, and complement receptor type 3 (CR_3), whose ligand is C3bi. CR_3 also binds to non-complement ligands, possibly through a second binding site, and the other activities of this receptor are discussed below.

Receptors for endothelium and proteins of the tissue matrix

The fourth major group of receptors on neutrophils is the molecules that mediate the attachment of neutrophils to tissues. Egress of neutrophils from vessels is initiated by their adherence to endothelial cells and to proteins of the tissue matrix at sites where the endothelium is damaged. The receptor CR_3 and the closely related protein p150,95 are thought to be important in these adherence reactions, together with other as yet uncharacterized molecules. A receptor for laminin, a basement membrane glycoprotein, has recently been identified on neutrophils. This may allow the binding of neutrophils to basement membrane underneath damaged endothelium.

Granules

The cytoplasmic granules (Fig. 4.78) consist of an outer membrane surrounding the contents of densely packed proteins assembled in a mucopolysaccharide matrix. The granules are heterogeneous with at least two, and probably several more, different types (Table 4.34).

Azurophil (primary) granules

These are the densest of the granules and are characterized by their content of myeloperoxidase. They also contain a diverse group of degradative enzymes.

Myeloperoxidase This is an abundant protein making up about 5 per cent of the total cellular protein. It is responsible for the characteristic green colour of these cells, which in turn impart it to pus. Its function has not been fully defined. It might utilize hydrogen peroxide produced by the respiratory burst to generate toxic oxidized halide derivatives, or it might play an important protective role against oxygen free radicals. Deficiency of this enzyme is not uncommon and is not generally associated with an obvious predisposition to infection.

Bactericidal/permeability-increasing protein (BPI) This 60 kDa protein is potently bactericidal towards a broad range of enteric Gram-negative bacteria but is ineffective against Gram-positive organisms. It binds to the surface of Gram-negative organisms and permeabilizes their outer membranes.

Defensins and cationic proteins A variety of highly cationic proteins were described in neutrophils which were very plentiful and found to have a direct antimicrobial role at neutral and alkaline conditions. Subsequently a group of small proteins

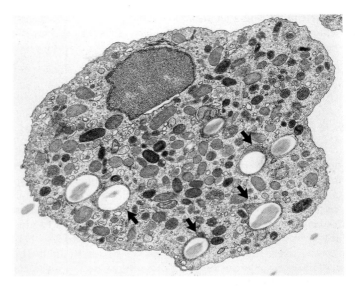

Fig. 4.78 Transmission electron micrograph of a human neutrophil, showing the considerable heterogeneity of the cytoplasmic granules. The cells were fixed 10 seconds after the addition of IgG-coated latex particles which had been partially dissolved from within phagocytic vacuoles during fixation. Fusion of the cytoplasmic granules with these vacuoles can be seen clearly (arrowed).

(< 4 kDa) have been identified, which appear to be the pure components of these fractions. They consist of between 32 and 34 amino acids, of which six are cystines, and 4–10 arginines accounting for their positive charge. They are cidal to a wide range of microbes at neutral pH, but their mechanism of action is unknown.

Table 4.34 Constituents of granules of neutrophils. There are subtypes of each granule enriched in particular components (see text; adapted from Gallin *et al.* 1988, with permission)

	Primary (azurophil) granules	Secondary (specific) granules
Microbicidal enzymes	Myeloperoxidase Lysozyme	Lysozyme
Neutral serine proteases	Elastase Cathepsin G Proteinase 3	
Metalloproteinases	Collagenase	Collagenase Gelatinase
Acid hydrolases	N-Acetyl-β-glucosaminidase Cathepsins B and D β-Glucocuronidase β-Glycerophosphatase α-Mannosidase	
Cationic microbicidal peptides	Defensins	
Other		Alkaline phosphatase Lactoferrin Vitamin B_{12}-binding protein Cytochrome b-245
Membrane receptors		f-Met-Leu-Phe receptor CR_3 p150,95 Laminin receptor

Cathepsin G This is a chymotrypsin-like 25–29 kDa neutral proteinase that kills both Gram-positive and Gram-negative organisms at neutral pH.

Elastase This is a neutral non-specific proteinase which is capable of cleaving a wide range of human proteins, including elastin and collagen, at physiological pH. Of importance within the neutrophil as a general digestive enzyme, it is also of considerable relevance in connection with the destruction of normal tissues once it has escaped from the cell (see below).

Lysozyme This enzyme is distributed equally between the azurophil and specific granules. It is also found in many secretions, including tears and saliva. The cell wall of most bacteria consists of long carbohydrate chains composed of alternating *N*-acetyl muramic acid and *N*-acetyl galactosamine residues linked by short peptide chains. Lysozyme cleaves the bond between these sugars, disrupting the chains and lysing the cell wall. It is very effective in destroying the cell wall of organisms such as *Micrococcus lysodecticus*, possibly accounting for their lack of pathogenicity, but other organisms, such as *Staphylococcus aureus* in which the sugar chains are more tightly packed and the susceptible bonds unexposed, are resistant to its action.

Specific granules

These granules are less dense than the azurophil granules, and the following proteins have been localized to them:

Membrane proteins The membranes of these granules contain components of the electron transport chain described below, CR_3 and other adhesion glycoproteins, and a variety of other receptors (see Table 4.34). When these cells are stimulated to phagocytose, not only do these granules fuse with the phagocytic vacuole, releasing their contents into its lumen, but they also fuse with the external plasma membrane. This results in the secretion of their contained proteins to the exterior, in addition to replenishing the membrane and membrane proteins that have been utilized in the formation of the wall of the phagocytic vacuole.

Lysozyme About half the cells' complement of this enzyme is located in these granules (see above).

Lactoferrin This protein has a very high ability to chelate iron and, to a lesser extent, copper. Its function has not been fully established. It might have a bacteriostatic effect by depriving microbes of important metal growth factors. It probably also has an important function in relation to free radicals (see below). Neutrophils generate superoxide and hydrogen peroxide that can react, in the Haber–Weiss reaction, to produce the very toxic hydroxyl radical, which could cause damage to the neutrophil and adjacent cells. This reaction is greatly accelerated in the presence of free metal ions and an important function of lactoferrin might be to chelate these and protect against uncontrolled oxidant damage.

Vitamin B12-binding protein As its name predicts, this protein binds cobalamin with a very high affinity. Its function is

unknown, it could deprive bacteria of this essential growth factor and inhibit cobalt-dependent free radical reactions.

Other granules There are a heterogeneous variety of granules in addition to those described above. The lysosomes, containing acid hydrolases, probably constitute a distinct group, and a gelatinase-containing tertiary granule has also been identified.

4.17.4 Neutrophil activation

Following ligation of one or more types of surface receptors on neutrophils, a number of activation steps occur. These stimulate the adherence of neutrophils to vascular endothelium and emigration of neutrophils through vessel walls towards sites of inflammation in tissues. During this process secondary granules are mobilized to the cell surface with the release of proteases. The cells undergo a shape change, in part due to translocation to the surface of the membranes of the granules which bear an additional pool of presynthesized receptors, including CR_3. Several receptors are activated, probably mediated by phosphorylation of the receptor, and this enables the cell to phagocytose particles bearing appropriate ligands. The respiratory burst of the neutrophils is triggered, with release of free radicals and myeloperoxidase. These activation steps are described individually in the following paragraphs.

Receptor activation and signal transduction

The activity of neutrophil surface receptors is highly regulated. For example, a resting neutrophil bears approximately 5000 CR_1 molecules. Ligation of these by particles bearing C3b is followed by binding and, if the particle is small, by absorptive endocytosis of the particle through clathrin-coated pits, described below. In contrast, an activated neutrophil bears 50 000 CR_1 and ligation of these receptors by large C3b-coated particles (e.g. C3b-coated erythrocytes) now results in respiratory burst generation and phagocytosis of the particles. The mechanisms of receptor activation are only just beginning to be understood and only the general principles will be enunciated here.

Surface receptor numbers appear to be regulated in two general ways. Increased numbers of many receptors can be rapidly expressed by their translocation from the membrane pools of specific granules, as described above. Occupation of receptors by ligands may result in a decrease in surface receptor expression caused by absorptive endocytosis of receptors. The f-Met-Leu-Phe receptor and CR_1 both show these mechanisms for numerical up- and down-regulation.

A second level of receptor regulation is modulation of the affinity of the receptor for its ligand. The f-Met-Leu-Phe and the LTB_4 receptors both exist in high- and low-affinity forms, with about a fiftyfold variation in binding constant between the two affinity states. Ligation of the receptors in their low-affinity state leads to release of lysosomal enzymes and to stimulation of the respiratory burst, and in their high-affinity state to chemotaxis and to increased adherence. The mechanism of conversion of the receptors between these two states is only partially understood, but is believed to involve the interaction of the receptors with guanine nucleotide-binding regulatory proteins (G proteins).

The third level of complexity in the regulation of the consequences of neutrophil receptor ligation is mediated via the intracellular 'second messengers', diacylglycerol (DAG) and inositol 1,4,5-triphosphate ($1,4,5$-IP_3). The production of these messengers is stimulated by activation of the enzyme, phosphoinositide-phospholipase C, by activated G-proteins. This enzyme catalyses the cleavage of a phosphorylated product of phosphatidylinositol, inositol 4,5-biphosphate, into the two intracellular 'second messengers', inositol 1,4,5-triphosphate ($1,4,5$-IP_3) and diacylglycerol (DAG). $1,4,5$-IP_3 stimulates a rise in intracellular Ca^{2+} by releasing it from an intracellular pool located in endoplasmic reticulum and by stimulating a secondary Ca^{2+} influx from outside the neutrophil. DAG stimulates the activation of protein kinase C. This activated enzyme phosphorylates a variety of intracellular proteins, possibly including certain cell surface receptors. There is preliminary evidence that activation and deactivation of neutrophil CR_1 and CR_3 is accompanied by reversible phosphorylation of the receptors. The mechanism of receptor activation by these second messengers is not understood but may involve differential coupling of the receptors to cytoskeletal proteins.

The effects of ligation of these receptors can be mimicked using chemical stimuli and analogues of various molecules of the signal transduction pathways. For example, the calcium ionophore, A23187, causes shape changes and specific granule release similar to that induced by chemoattractants. Certain synthetic analogues of diacyl glycerol and phorbol esters, such as phorbol myristal acetate, activate protein kinase C directly and sequentially activate and deactivate CR_1 and CR_3 for phagocytosis of opsonized particles. Incubation of neutrophils with phorbol myristyl acetate and thiophosphate, a false substrate for protein kinases, leads to irreversible thiophosphorylation of proteins and CR_1 and CR_3, and prolonged activation of both receptors.

Adherence

Resting neutrophils are located predominantly in the intravascular pool. From here they may be mobilized quickly to sites of inflammation. The initial step in this process is margination and adherence of neutrophils to vascular endothelium. This process is dependent on cations and involves activation steps in both neutrophils and endothelial cells. A large number of stimuli have been recognized which increase neutrophil adhesiveness and these include f-Met-Leu-Phe, the anaphylatoxins of complement (C3a and C5a), leukotriene B4, tumour necrosis factor-α, phorbol myristal acetate, and the calcium ionophore A23187. The activity of these two molecules in the process suggests that at least one of the mechanisms for transducing the signal mediating neutrophil adherence involves the opening of membrane calcium channels, and activation of the enzyme, protein kinase C. Neutrophils from patients with inherited deficiencies of the glycoprotein family, CR_3, p150,95, and LFA-1, fail to adhere to endothelium and to artifical substrates. This defect

can be mimicked by treating normal neutrophils with monoclonal antibodies to CR_3 and to p150,95, both of which are expressed on the surface of neutrophils. These experiments suggest that these molecules probably play a direct role in the binding of neutrophils to endothelium. The surface expression of CR_3 and p150,95 on resting neutrophils is low and increases up to twentyfold following activation of neutrophils by each of the molecules, described above, which promote adherence. The intercellular pool for CR_3 and p150,95 is located within the membrane of specific granules and this is translocated to the cell surface rapidly after neutrophil activation. The ligand for these molecules on endothelial cells has not yet been identified.

Neutrophils adhere especially to endothelium that is adjacent to sites of inflammation within tissues and, although this may partly be determined by chemotactic factors diffusing from the inflammatory site, there is also evidence that there are inducible endothelial factors promoting adherence of neutrophils. Several molecules have been characterized which interact directly with endothelial cells to enhance neutrophil adhesion. These include interleukin-1, LTC4, tumour necrosis factor-α (which also act directly on neutrophils), and thrombin. Monoclonal antibodies to CR_3 and to p150,95 do not inhibit the enhanced adherence of neutrophils to stimulated endothelium and this suggests the involvement of a further, uncharacterized, ligand–receptor interaction between neutrophils and endothelial cells. Thrombin has been shown to stimulate release of the lipid mediator, platelet activating factor (PAF), from endothelium. PAF, in addition to platelet activation, has also been shown to activate neutrophils in vivo. This illustrates the complexity of the mechanisms of the interactions between neutrophils and endothelium.

Chemotaxis

Neutrophils change their shape following activation and their cell membrane takes on a ruffled appearance. This change coincides with release of the contents of the specific granules and is believed to be mediated by incorporation of the granule membranes into the cell membrane causing it to increase its surface area.

In response to chemotactic agents, neutrophils orientate in the direction of the concentration gradient by advancing a lamellipodium and crawl along supporting surfaces towards the source of the chemotactic agent (Fig. 4.79). The mechanism for directed movement involves detection of concentration gradients of chemotactic agents, which is mediated by differential occupancy of receptors along the length of the cells. The mechanism of movement involves the cytoskeletal proteins, of which actin and myosin are prominent components. At the leading edge of the neutrophil degranulation of specific granules occurs and the membrane of the specific granules is incorporated into the advancing cell membrane. Conversely at the trailing edge (uropod) of the cell, membrane is internalized by the process of pinocytosis.

Endocytosis and phagocytosis

The external membrane of neutrophils is not a fixed structure

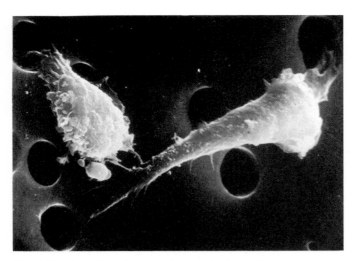

Fig. 4.79 Scanning electron micrograph of two human monocytes migrating through 5 μm pores of a polycarbonate filter in response to a chemotactic lymphokine (from Snyderman and Goetzl 1981, with kind permission; copyright 1981 by the AAAS).

but instead equilibrates continuously with internal membrane pools. This is an extremely active process: an amount of membrane equal to that of the external cell membrane may be turned over every 30 minutes. Membrane is endocytosed in the form of vesicles containing a small quantity of plasma and this uptake of plasma is known as pinocytosis. A remarkable structural protein, clathrin, is involved in vesicle formation; these start life on the cell surface as 'coated pits' and become 'coated vesicles'. The process of recycling the cell membrane selectively includes certain cell membrane proteins, such as CR_1 and Fc receptors, which are believed to bind to structural proteins associated with clathrin. Cross-linking of these receptors by ligands stimulates their uptake within coated vesicles, a process known as endocytosis. Within the cytoplasm, the receptor–ligand complex becomes dissociated, the ligand is proteolysed, and some of the receptor may be actively recycled to the cell membrane.

The process of phagocytosis involves the selective uptake of particles of sizes up to several microns. Sequential steps in phagocytosis include:

1. specific recognition of the particle by neutrophil receptors;
2. adherence of the neutrophil membrane to the particle;
3. invagination of the neutrophil membrane about the particle;
4. pinching off the cell membrane at the neck of the phagocytic vesicle (phagosome); and
5. fusion of the phagosome with both primary and secondary neutrophil granules to form a phagolysosome.

Killing and digestion of the particle is accomplished within phagolysosomes. Neutrophils are messy eaters and, during the process of phagocytosis, some release of both primary and secondary granule contents occurs, mediated by fusion of granules with phagosomes which are formed incompletely.

Respiratory burst

The professional phagocytic cells, neutrophils, monocytes, macrophages, and eosinophils, demonstrate a very unusual process when they engulf microbes. They rapidly consume a relatively vast amount of oxygen. This 'extra respiration of phagocytosis' is not used for the normal purpose of generating energy by mitochondrial oxidative phosphorylation, for which the bulk of our inhaled oxygen is used. The energy required for the ingestion of organism is produced by glycolysis, phagocytosis occurring quite normally in the absence of oxygen, and the respiratory burst is not inhibited by mitochondrial poisons such as cyanide or azide. The oxygen consumption of the respiratory burst is required to produce the optimal conditions for the killing of most common bacterial and fungal pathogens as well as a variety of commensals. Cells deprived of oxygen engulf but fail to kill some microbes efficiently. The same deficiency of killing is seen in the syndrome of chronic granulomatous disease (CGD), the hallmark of which is complete absence of this respiratory burst in cells that appear to be functionally normal in all other respects.

The oxidase system

The overall reaction transfers electrons from the high energy state of glucose to oxygen. The electrons from glucose are first incorporated into the low potential, high energy, reduced pyridine nucleotide, NADPH. The microbicidal oxidase of phagocytes is made up of an electron transport chain with a very unusual cytochrome b, called cytochrome b_{-245} because of its mid-point potential of -245 mV, as its terminal component. This cytochrome is located in the membrane of the specific granules of neutrophils and in the plasma membrane of these cells and of the other phagocytes, and is incorporated into the wall of the phagocytic vacuole as this forms. The other components in the chain remain to be defined but almost certainly include a flavoprotein interspersed between NADPH and the cytochrome, because cytochromes are unable to receive electrons directly from NADPH.

Microbicidal mechanism of respiratory burst

There are three main mechanisms by which this respiration might promote killing, any one of a combination of which may be physiologically important.

Free radical generation The addition of a single electron to oxygen results in the formation of superoxide which dismutates to form hydrogen peroxide. The discovery of this phenomenon led to speculation that these reduced oxygen species, and other radicals like the hydroxyl radical produced by their interaction, may themselves be toxic to the organisms because they can be strong oxidizing and reducing agents. However, it is now clear that in addition to these reduced oxygen molecules there is a requirement for the granule contents for the killing process to occur.

Myeloperoxidase-mediated halogenation Myeloperoxidase (MPO) has the potential to use hydrogen peroxide as substrate to oxidize halides such as chloride and iodide to chlorine and iodine, their hypohalous acids, with the generation of long-lived chloramines. However, it is not established that the generation of these molecules is a physiological function of MPO, which has a number of other possible reactions within the vacuole. It can react with superoxide, and might be present to mop up free radicals and prevent them producing local cellular and tissue damage. Large numbers of symptomless subjects have been identified whose cells are completely devoid of this enzyme.

Alkalinization of the phagocytic vacuole The neutrophil granules contain proteins, particularly a group which are strongly cationic, that are potently microbicidal *in vitro*. The anomaly is that the same proteins are much less effective when released on to the organism within the environment of the phagocytic vacuole in anaerobic cells or in the condition of CGD. This must indicate a difference within this environment. The oxidase causes a rise in pH to about 7.8–8.0 within the phagocytic vacuole by pumping electrons, unaccompanied by protons, into this compartment. Granule proteins that are active at this pH are then able to kill and digest the microbe.

4.17.5 Inherited deficiencies

Disorders of neutrophil adherence and mobility

Failure of neutrophils to reach sites of infection, because of very low circulating numbers or because of defects such as the absence of adhesion glycoproteins, allows spreading bacterial infections with little in the way of pus formation. The only well-defined disease entity in this category of defects is the leucocyte adhesion protein deficiency. The others are ill-defined clinical groupings with poorly documented functional abnormalities in which the molecular nature of the lesion is unknown. The lazy-leucocyte syndrome exemplifies this descriptive classification in which a predisposition to infection is associated with reduced mobility without any characteristic diagnostic features.

Leucocyte adhesion protein deficiency

During recent years a rare, inherited, immunodeficiency syndrome has been described that has given considerable insight into the physiological activities of the family of molecules containing CR_3, LFA-1, and p150,95. The disease usually becomes manifest in the neonatal period with delayed separation of the umbilical cord. This is followed by recurrent, severe, cutaneous, and deep infections with pyogenic bacteria. The skin infections ulcerate and show no infiltrate of neutrophils on microscopic examination. The ulcers heal with the formation of dystrophic scars. Patients suffer from recurrent severe gingivitis usually leading to early loss of teeth. Examination of the peripheral blood shows persistent neutrophil leycocytosis because these cells are unable to bind to the endothelium and migrate out of the vasculature, and these cells behave abnormally in both *in vivo* and *in vitro* assays of adherence and chemotaxis.

The first structural abnormality to be clearly defined on the

neutrophils of affected patients was a deficiency of a protein of approximately 165 000 Da molecular mass on analysis of surface proteins using polyacrylamide gel electrophoresis. This molecule was later characterized as the complement receptor, CR_3. This molecule shares a common β-chain with LFA-1 and p150,95 and it was found that the underlying molecular defect responsible for expression of the disease was abnormal synthesis of this β-chain preventing normal surface expression of the whole family of heterodimeric molecules. Although this family of molecules is represented on most lineages of cells derived from the bone marrow, including lymphocytes, monocytes, macrophages, and neutrophils, the main clinical features of the immunodeficiency state derive from inadequate neutrophil function. Antibody production in most patients is not severely impaired, nor is host defence against viral infections.

Specific granule deficiency

A small number of patients have been identified with a congenital deficiency of neutrophil specific granules. These subjects suffer from recurrent bacterial infections. Their granules are morphologically abnormal and the cells are deficient in all of the constituents of specific granules. Their neutrophils show reduced chemotaxis and this may be correlated with their inability to up-regulate the level of surface expression of the receptors normally contained within the membranes of specific granules.

Disordered intracellular killing

Chronic granulomatous disease (CGD)

Clinical manifestations Classical infections that should alert the clinician to the possibility of this condition include cervical and inguinal lymphadenitis, liver abscesses, osteomyelitis, and fungal pneumonia. Infections of the skin and respiratory tract are also common. Children can also get unusual gastrointestinal manifestations such as pyloric stenosis, and intestinal lesions that mimic Crohn's disease and ulcerative colitis.

Although the molecular defect is congenital and constant, the frequency and severity of infection is surprisingly variable from patient to patient, and although infections manifest themselves in most individuals in infancy or childhood, it is not uncommon for major infection to first present in the second decade or later. Staphylococci are the commonest organisms, but some very unusual microbes, such as *Serratia marcescens* and fungi, can quite often be responsible.

The molecular basis of CGD The unifying defect in this very heterogeneous condition is an abnormality of the function of the oxidase electron transport chain. CGD is a syndrome with heterogeneous causes and the patients may be classified into different subgroups, depending upon which of the components of the electron transport chain is at fault. There are a variety of atypical and partial defects: the two main subgroups of the syndrome will be dealt with here.

1. Inherited on the X chromosome. The largest subgroup of the disease is inherited in an X-linked manner, with affected

males and heterozygote carrier females. The molecular basis of the lesion in the vast majority of these patients is the absence of cytochrome b-245 from their phagocytes, with a mosaic of normal and completely defective cells in heterozygote carriers. The genetic lesion in these patients has been identified on the X chromosome in the gene coding for the 76–92 kDa β-subunit of the cytochrome.

2.   Autosomal recessive inheritance. The molecular defect is very different in these subjects. Although their cells contain normal amounts of the cytochrome, and its properties and subcellular distribution appear normal, electrons cannot be transferred on to it. This suggests an abnormality of the activation processes or of a proximal link in the electron transport chain. The majority of these patients fail to phosphorylate a 47 kDA protein that is missing from their cells. The identity and function of this molecule await characterization.

Mechanism of defect   The common unifying abnormality in CGD is failure of electron transport to oxygen in the phagocytic vacuole. Reduced oxygen molecules are not generated and the pH in this compartment falls precipitously. Whatever the primary mechanism of the defect, this results in a diminished ability to kill certain microbes. In addition, the abnormal conditions pertaining in the vacuole impair digestion of engulfed organisms as well as autologous debris. It is this defect of digestion that accounts for the diffuse granulomata responsible for the name accorded to this condition and the hepatosplenomegaly that sometimes develops in these patients.

Myeloperoxidase deficiency

This is a relatively common autosomal recessive disorder resulting in partial (prevalence 1 in 2000) or complete (1 in 4000) deficiency of this enzyme. Although this results in mildly impaired killing of bacteria and fungi *in vitro*, these subjects do not have an increased incidence of infection. The abnormal gene is located on chromosome 17 and appears to result in a genetic defect that affects post-translational processing of an abnormal precursor protein.

Chediak–Higashi

This is a rare autosomal recessive condition. Analogous abnormalities have been described in Aleutian mink, partial albino Hereford cattle, albino whales, and beige mice. The most obvious abnormality in these subjects relates to the function of cytoplasmic granules in a wide variety of cell types.

In the leucocytes giant cytoplasmic granules are apparent. The phagocytic cells appear to be in a state of constant activation and these giant granules are in fact secondary lysosomes produced by the inappropriate fusion of specific and azurophil granules to form large inclusions containing sequestered, functionless, granule proteins. It seems probable that this constant state of activation and sequestration of granule protein is responsible for the loss of functional reserve of these cells that is manifest by an increased frequency of infection, gingivitis, and

periodontal disease. Defective function of pigment cells accounts for the oculocutaneous albinism. The hair often has an unusual silvery appearance which may be patchy. Absence of pigment from the iris and retina causes photophobia and nystagmus. These patients may also develop a peripheral neuropathy. This chronic disease is often interrupted in adolescence by an accelerated lymphomatous phase characterized by anaemia, pancytopenia, and splenomegaly. The current treatment of choice is bone marrow transplantation, providing a suitable donor is available.

4.17.6   Acquired deficiencies

Acquired, secondary, deficiency of neutrophil numbers and/or function is much commoner than the primary deficiencies described above, but is not usually associated with catastrophic immunodeficiency unless the marrow is severely damaged. myeloid stem cells may themselves be diseased, caused by toxins (commonly drugs), auto-antibodies, or malignancy. Infiltration of bone marrow by tumours and in certain inherited diseases (e.g. glycogen storage disorders) may reduce the space for stem cell proliferation. Severe neutropenia is a common sequel to therapy with cytotoxic drugs, and bacterial infection of immunosuppressed patients is a common cause of death.

Neutrophil function may be impaired following burns and major trauma. Cells from such individuals show reduced chemotaxis and phagocytosis, loss of lysosomal enzymes, and reduced respiratory burst. The explanation for these multiple defects may be that systemic activation of neutrophils has occurred, mediated by release of chemotactic peptides, such as C5a, from sites of tissue injury. These activated neutrophils are rendered incapable of responding to further stimulation, for example arising from foci of infection. Neutrophils which have been activated systemically by mediators released from sites of major trauma may be important contributors to the condition of 'shock lung'. In this lethal condition, which is a complication of major trauma, burns or sepsis, activated neutrophils adhere to pulmonary endothelium and cause inflammation through release of enzymes, cationic proteins, and possibly also oxygen radicals.

4.17.7   Deleterious effects of neutrophils in disease

Although the general role of neutrophils is protective, there are certain situations when neutrophils themselves may play a major pathogenetic role in human disease. Recruitment of neutrophils to sites of persisting inflammation results in extensive local tissue damage, by the mechanisms cited above. If the stimulus to this inflammation is inappropriate, then the net result for the host may be deleterious. A clear example of this is in auto-immunity, where inappropriate antibody- or cell-mediated responses to autologous tissues result in chronic inflammation which is partially mediated by neutrophils.

α_1-Antitrypsin deficiency

The consequences of uncontrolled activity of neutrophil elastase is seen most dramatically in individuals with inherited deficiencies of α_1-antitrypsin. This protease inhibitor, secreted mainly by the liver, is the major physiological inhibitor of neutrophil elastase. It is a member of the Serpin (*serine proteinase inhibitor*) supergene family of molecules and has been renamed α_1-proteinase inhibitor, a less misleading name which reflects its capacity to inhibit serine proteinase enzymes other than trypsin. Subjects with inherited deficiencies of α_1-proteinase inhibitor develop severe pulmonary emphysema with alveolar destruction. This becomes a symptomatic problem in non-smokers in their fifth and sixth decades, but in smokers the process is accelerated and patients may die in their thirties of emphysema and secondary pulmonary hypertension. This 'experiment of nature' formally shows that the constituents of cigarette smoke cause pulmonary damage in part by mechanisms mediated by neutrophils.

Glomerulonephritis

Neutrophils are a prominent feature of the inflammation seen in glomeruli in tissue derived from patients with post-infectious nephritis, diffuse proliferative nephritis, and Goodpasture's disease (mediated by auto-antibodies to basement membrane). The role of neutrophils in causing inflammatory damage to glomeruli was established by a number of classical studies in rabbits. Rabbits infused with sheep anti-rabbit glomerular basement membrane antibodies developed a nephritis with proteinuria which was histologically similar to Goodpasture's disease in humans. Animals in which complement was depleted by prior injection of cobra venom factor were largely protected from the development of nephritis, and their glomeruli showed no influx of neutrophils. Similarly, experimental depletion of neutrophils, by injections of nitrogen mustard, abrogated most of the nephritis. When neutrophils were infused into such animals, full-blown glomerulonephritis with proteinuria was restored. These and other experiments showed that the sequence of events in this form of nephritis was:

1. binding of antibody and fixation of complement to glomerular basement membrane;

2. attraction of circulating neutrophils by complement-derived peptides (probably mainly the anaphylatoxin, C5a); and

3. exocytosis of neutrophil granule contents and stimulation of the respiratory burst, leading to damage to the glomeruli.

4.17.8 Conclusions

Neutrophils contain powerful mechanisms for killing bacteria and for degradation of the debris of inflammatory reactions. These activities are normally beneficial but can cause extensive, harmful, tissue necrosis at sites of inappropriate stimulation of neutrophils. Much has been learnt about the normal, physiological, activities of neutrophils by the study of the fate of subjects with inherited and acquired deficiency of neutrophil numbers or function.

4.17.9 Acknowledgements

We would like to thank the Welcome Trust, the Medical Research Council, and the Arthritis and Rheumatism Council for support.

4.17.10 Further reading

Badwey, J. A., Curnutte, J. T., and Karnovsky, M. L. (1979). The enzyme of granulocytes that produces superoxide and peroxide. An elusive pimpernel. *New England Journal of Medicine* **300**, 1157–60.

Clark, S. C. and Kamen, R. (1987). The human hematopoietic colony-stimulating factors. *Science* **236**, 1229–37.

Gallin, J. I., Goldstein, I. M., and Snyderman, R. (1988). *Inflammation: Basic principles and clinical correlates*. Raven Press, New York.

Graziano, M. P. and Gilman, A. G. (1987). Guanine nucleotide-binding proteins: mediators of transmembrane signaling. *Trends in Pharmacological Sciences* **8**, 478–81.

Klebanoff, S. J. (1971). Intraleucocytic microbial defects. *Annual Review of Medicine* **22**, 39–62.

Klebanoff, S. J. (1975). Antimicrobial mechanisms in neutrophilic polymorphonuclear leucocytes. *Seminars in Hematology* **12**, 117–42.

Klebanoff, S. J. and Clark, R. A. (eds) (1978). *The neutrophil: Function and clinical disorders*. North Holland, Amsterdam.

Malech, H. L. and Gallin, J. I. (1987). Neutrophils in human diseases. *New England Journal of Medicine* **317**, 687–94.

Pearse, B. M. F. (1987). Clathrin and coated vesicles. *EMBO Journal* **6**, 2507–12.

Pike, M. C. and Snyderman, R. (1984). Leucocyte chemoattractant receptors. In *The receptors* (ed. P. M. Conn), Vol. 1, pp. 223–59. Academic Press, New York.

Putney, J. W., Jr. (1987). Calcium-mobilizing receptors. *Trends in Pharmacological Sciences* **8**, 481–6.

Rossi, F. (1986). The O_2^--forming NADPH oxidase of the phagocytes: Nature, mechanism of action and function. *Biochimica et Biophysica Acta* **853**, 65–89.

Segal, A. W. (1989). The electron transport chain of the microbiridal oxidase of phagocytic cells and its involvement in the molecular pathology of chronic granulomatous disease. *Journal of Clinical Investigation* **83**, 1785–93.

Snyderman, R. and Goetzl, E. J. (1981). Molecular and cellular mechanisms of leucocyte chemotaxis. *Science* **213**, 830–7.

Wright, S. D. and Griffin, F. M., Jr. (1985). Activation of phagocytic cells' C3 receptors for phagocytosis. *Journal of Leucocyte Biology* **38**, 327–39.

4.18 Eosinophil leucocytes

C. J. F. Spry

Eosinophils are inflammatory cells that are produced in the bone marrow, and migrate through the blood to the tissues, where they carry out a wide range of functions. Some of these are protective, but others contribute to tissue injury and pathological processes. They are present in all vertebrates and their production is greatly increased in response to several factors released in response to infection and allergic stimulation. These factors are G-CSF, GM-CSF, interleukin-3, and interleukin-5. Eosinophils are derived from a stem cell in common with basophils and possibly some lymphocytes. Although they show some structural similarities with neutrophils and are able to respond to similar stimuli in tissues, their constituents and properties show that they have evolved to carry out separate functions.

4.18.1   Structure and cell biology

Eosinophils contain one type of granule which alters in appearance as the cells develop and degranulate (Fig. 4.80, Table 4.35). Primary granules are formed in the bone marrow and mature into crystalloid granules. Small granules are remnants of crystalloid granules which have undergone partial secretion and are present especially in tissue eosinophils. Crystalloid granules contain large amounts of storage proteins, which are released into endocytic vacuoles or secreted to the outside of the cell. Newly formed components, which are produced in mature eosinophils in response to stimulation, include products of unsaturated fatty acid metabolism and reactive oxygen species. The eosinophil has a marked capacity to take up oxygen and glucose, and is one of the most metabolically active cells in inflammatory lesions.

4.18.2   Receptors and activation

As eosinophils mature and move into tissues, they are stimulated to develop receptors for complexed immunoglobulin and complement (Table 4.36). They are also responsive to a wide

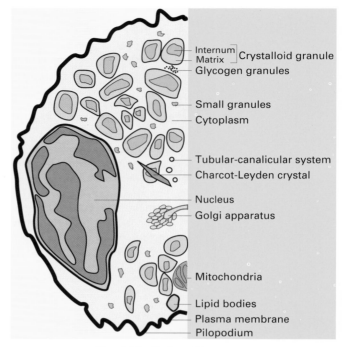

Fig. 4.80   Eosinophil structure.

range of activating signals (Table 4.37), which increase their metabolic and functional capacities to take part in inflammatory reactions. Some of these signals are derived from adjacent tissues and cells, such as endothelial cells and macrophages and others from parasites. Products from damaged tissues also increase the functional capacities of eosinophils.

4.18.3   Degranulation and secretion

After stimulation by activating factors or complexed immuno-

Table 4.35   Eosinophil constituents

Crystalloid granules
    Internum: major basic protein, 12 kDa, basic
    Matrix: eosinophil ribonucleases:
                eosinophil cationic protein, 18.5–22 kDa, basic
                eosinophil neurotoxin, 17–20 kDa, basic
           peroxidase, 75 kDa, basic
           histaminase
           phospholipase D
           lysosomal enzymes
           acid phosphatase, masked
           collagenase
           zinc

Small granules
    arylsulphatase B
    acid phosphatase, unmasked
    peroxidase
    eosinophil cationic protein

Other constituents
    lysophospholipase (Charcot–Leyden crystal protein), 13 kDa, acidic
    phospholipid exchange protein

Table 4.36 The eosinophil plasma membrane

Receptors for
  IgG: Fc_γ, high affinity
  IgE: Fc_ε IIG, low affinity
  sIgA Complement components: CR_1, CR_3
  Steroids
Membrane antigens
  HLA antigens
  Membrane proteins involved in secretion
  Antigens shared with neutrophils
  Antigens shared with preB-cells and platelets (CD9)

Table 4.37 Eosinophil-activating factors

Endogenous factors
  T-lymphocyte-derived factors
    IL-2, T-ECEF
  monocyte/macrophage-derived factors
    M-ECEF, EAF
  eosinopoietic factors
    GM-CSF, G-CSF, IL-3, IL-5
  endothelial cell-derived factors
  platelet-activating factor
  tumour necrosis factor
  interferons

Parasite-derived factors

Effects on eosinophils
  reduce cell surface charge
  increase glucose metabolism
  decrease cell density
  affect oxygen metabolism
  increase cytotoxicity to target cells/parasites
  increase granule protein secretion
  increase LTC_4 production
  increase receptors for immunoglobulins, complement

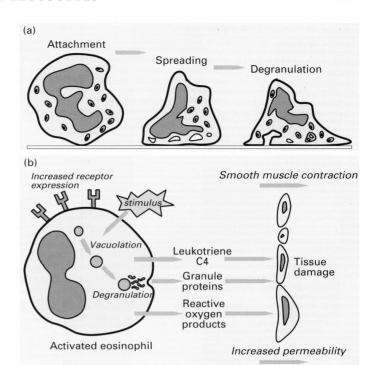

Fig. 4.81 (a) Stages in eosinophil-dependent killing of schistosomulae *in vitro* (from Vadas *et al*. 1980). (b) Mechanisms of eosinophil-induced injury to tissues.

globulin with complement, eosinophils secrete their storage proteins, and generate membrane-derived mediators of inflammation, including leukotriene C_4, and platelet-activating factor. Secretion starts within a few minutes and can continue for several hours. As eosinophils may survive in culture (and in tissues) for several days, or weeks, these effects may be prolonged. Eosinophils have a small biosynthetic capacity, but following degranulation, or in the absence of eosinopoietic factors, they undergo apoptosis and die and are replaced by newly arrived eosinophils which have localized along altered endothelium in the sites of inflammation.

4.18.4 Protection and injury

Eosinophils probably evolved 25–40 million years ago to protect against metazoan parasitic infections. They are particularly effective at killing nematode and trematode life cycles at their point of entry into the body, but are less effective against parasites that have reached their definitive sites in the body. The principal effector mechanisms are the secreted basic proteins and products of oxygen metabolism (Fig. 4.81a).

These effector mechanisms can also damage normal tissues (Fig. 4.81b). In patients with a persistently raised blood eosinophil count, chronic release of eosinophil granule proteins and other components produce thromboembolic lesions, tissue necrosis especially affecting the endocardium, and the deposition of fibrous tissue. IgE stimulation of eosinophils can produce vascular permeability changes that are reversible. The type and degree of tissue injury depends on the nature of the stimuli applied to eosinophils and the products which they secrete. Eosinophil secretion products damage the bronchial epithelium and also activate the complement and the intrinsic coagulation systems, and cause mast cells and basophils to degranulate. This forms the basis of an eosinophil-dependent cascade of tissue injury, which amplifies their initial effects on adjacent structures.

4.18.5 Functions in disease

Eosinophils take part in such a wide variety of diseases (allergic, vasculitic, granulomatous, parasitic, neoplastic, drug hypersensitivity, etc.) that it has not proved possible to provide a single unifying concept of the role of eosinophils in disease, despite earlier attempts to do so. As their main functions appear to be in immunity to certain parasite stages and to produce acute and chronic tissue injury, it is likely that they have multiple effects in disease. Some of these roles are protective but others give rise to further tissue damage.

4.18.6   Further reading*

Beeson, P. B. and Bass, D. A. (1977). The eosinophil. *Major Problems in Internal Medicine* 14, 1–269.

Butterworth, A. E. (1984). Cell-mediated damage to helminths. *Advances in Parasitology* 23, 143–235.

Capron, M., Capron, A., Joseph, M., and Verwaerde, C. (1983). IgE receptors on phagocytic cells and immune response to schistosome infection. *Monographs in Allergy* 18, 33–44.

David, J. R., *et al.* (1980). Enhanced helminthotoxic capacity of eosinophils from patients with eosinophilia. *New England Journal of Medicine* 303, 1147–52.

Gleich, G. J. and Adolphson, C. R. (1986). The eosinophilic leukocyte: structure and function. *Advances in Immunology* 39, 177–253.

Hamann, K. J., *et al.* (1990). Structure and chromosome localization of the lumen eosinophil-derived neurotoxin and eosinophil cationic protein genes: evidence for intronless coding sequences in the ribonuclease gene superfamily. *Genomics* 7, 535–46.

Spry, C. J. F. (1982). The hypereosinophilic syndrome: clinical features, laboratory findings and treatment. *Allergy* 37, 539–51.

Spry, C. J. F. (1988). *Eosinophils. A comprehensive review and guide to the scientific and medical literature.* Oxford University Press.

Vadas, M. A., *et al.* (1980). Interactions between human eosinophils and schistosomula of *Schistosoma mansoni.* I. Stable and irreversible antibody-dependent adherence. *Journal of Immunology* 124, 1441–8.

* An indexed and fully searchable DOS-based reference and abstract database is available. It is updated regularly and contains over 8,500 references to this topic. Spry, C. J. F. (1991). *EOS-REFS database of scientific references on eosinophils and eosinophilic diseases.* Business Simulations, London SW1A 1HB, UK.

4.19   Basophil polymorph and mast cells

S. T. Holgate

4.19.1   Introduction

Mast cells, basophils, and eosinophils develop from the same precursor stem cell in the bone marrow. Under the influence of specific colony-stimulating factors, each of the cell types takes on its individual characteristics which are completed once the cell reaches its destination and comes under the influence of the microenvironment. In rodents, and probably in humans also, the predominent growth factor for mast cells is interleukin-3 (IL-3), although the newly recognized IL-10 may also be important. Similar cytokines are probably involved in basophil differentiation and maturation, although this cell has more characteristics in common with the eosinophil.

There is convincing evidence that mammalian mast cells are heterogeneous with respect to ontogony, structure, and function. At mucosal surfaces such as the gastrointestinal and respiratory tracts, mast cells take on the characteristics of relatively immature IL-3 stimulated cells. These 'mucosal type' mast cells differ markedly from mast cells localized to connective tis-

sue sites, in which final maturation occurs by an interaction between mast cells and fibroblasts. Table 4.38 highlights some of the differences between human mast cells isolated from mucosal and connective tissue sites. Mast cell hyperplasia at mucosal surfaces occurs in response to a particular type of antigenic stimulus characteristic of allergic and parasitic reactions and involving proliferation of a subset of sensitized T4-cells capable of releasing mast cell growth factors. Mast cells at connective tissue sites also proliferate in the early stages of fibrotic reactions, e.g. fibrosing alveolitis, scleroderma, and wound healing.

4.19.2   Mast cell and basophil mediators

Involvement of the mast cell in Type I (immediate) hypersensitivity reactions and parasite elimination stems from its capacity to secrete a wide variety of biologically active mediators of inflammation. In addition to histamine and heparin (the proteoglycan that imparts metachromatic staining properties to the secretory granules), mast cells synthesize and store a large number of other preformed mediators in their lysosomes (Table 4.39). One important product of human mast cells is tryptase, a four-chained neutral protease of molecular mass 135 kDa that comprises approximately one-third of the protein content of the lung mast cell. In addition to substantial amounts of tryptase, connective tissue mast cells contain a single-chain protease, human chymase (30 kDa), which clearly separates these cells from those found at mucosal surfaces. The difference in neutral protease content of the granules accounts for the characteristic ultrastructural features of scrolls for mucosal mast cells (MC_T) and gratings and lattices for connective tissue mast cells (MC_{TC}). Basophils contain reduced amounts of heparin mixed with chondroitin sulphate and only trace amounts of tryptase.

When appropriately stimulated, mast cells mobilize arachidonic acid which is oxidized by the cyclo-oxygenase pathway to prostaglandin (PG) D_2, smaller amounts of thromboxane (TX) A_2, and by the 5-lipoxygenase pathway, to the sulphidopeptide leukotriene, LTC_4, a major component of slow-reacting substance of anaphylaxis (SRS-A). Subsequent cleavage of the 6-sulphidopeptide glutathione adduct by extracellular enzymes leads to the other components of SRS-A, LTD_4, and LTE_4. Basophils do not express PGD_2 synthetase activity and oxidize arachidonic acid predominantly to LTC_4. All of these newly formed mediators have potent vaso- and broncho-active properties and, along with the preformed products of the secretory granules, interact to produce the tissue responses characteristic of the initial phase of the Type I response.

4.19.3   Activation signals for mast cells and basophils

The identification of IgE as the reaginic molecule responsible for the passive transfer of acute allergic response led to the identification of high-affinity Fc receptors (FcRI) on mast cells and basophils. These receptors are quite different from the low-

Table 4.38 Comparison of human mast cell subtypes

	Mast cell source	
	Lung (mucosal)	Skin (connective tissue)
Size	5–18 μm	5–18 μm
Formaldehyde fixation	mainly sensitive	mainly resistant
Staining	mainly alcian blue	mainly safranin O
MC$_{TC}$ (%)	<5%	<95%
Proteoglycans		
heparin	65%	100%
chondroitin sulphate E	9%	?
Histamine	3–5 pg/cell	4–8 pg/cell
Prostaglandin D$_2$	++	++
Leukotriene C$_4$	+++	+
Activated by		
IgE-dependent	yes	yes
compound 48/80	no	yes
substance P	no	yes
poly-L-lysine	no	yes
Effect of sodium cromoglycate		
inhibited	yes	no

affinity (FcRII) IgE-receptors on platelets, eosinophils, macrophages, monocytes, and lymphocytes. In the presence of low antigen concentrations, interaction with cell-bound IgE through the Fab portion enables two or more IgE molecules to be bridged, thereby linking adjacent FcRI receptors to provide the transduction signal for mediator release.

In a calcium- and energy-dependent process, IgE-triggered activation secretion coupling involves a complex series of biochemical events (Fig. 4.82). One of the earliest of these is the exposure of serine esterase activity in relation to the receptor protein. This is followed by stimulation of the phosphatidylinosital cycle within the cell membrane. These processes are intimately associated with the exposure of channels allowing a transmembrane influx of calcium ions, mobilization of intracellular calcium (probably through the action of the polyphosphoinositides) and the phosphorylation of a number of perigranular proteins (Fig. 4.82). Some of these proteins are probably involved in the transport of water and anions into the granule matrix to initiate solubilization of the preformed mediators prior to their secretion. Others are involved in the myosin–actin coupling that promotes intracellular granule fusion and exocytosis of their membrane-bound mediators. Mobilization of calcium from intra- and extra-cellular sources activates phospholipase A$_2$ and diglyceride lipase, which mobilize arachidonic acid from membrane and cytoplasmic phospholipids. The by-products of monoacylglycerol and lysophospholipids serve to promote granule fusion with each other and with channels that extend to the surface of the cell. Release of preformed mediators into the extracellular milieu is finally completed by chemiosmosis and ion exchange of individual mediators associated with the glycosaminoglycan chains of heparin with extracellular sodium ions

at rates dependent upon the isolectric point of the individual mediators. Thus, molecules such as histamine are released rapidly while highly cationic molecules such as tryptase and carboxypeptidase are leached away from the heparin complex slowly.

Cross-linkage of IgE-FcRI receptors also produces a short-lived stimulation of adenylate cyclase. The resultant increase in cellular cyclic AMP concentrations serves to switch off the coupling of activation to secretion by activating protein kinase A. One function of this enzyme is to phosphorylate myosin light-chain kinase, an enzyme crucially involved in intracellular transport of granules.

In addition to an IgE stimulus, mast cells and basophils may be activated by a wide variety of other secretory signals. Mast cells from different sites vary in their responses to the non-immunological stimuli and this represents another level of mast cell heterogeneity. Similarly, basophils differ from mast cells in their sensitivity to some of these agents. Basic substances such as substance P, morphine, compound 48/80, and poly-L-lysine activate connective tissue mast cells through a common activation site that exhibits low specificity and might well be a y-protein. Moreover, compared to an IgE signal, the time course and profile of mediator released by these cationic stimuli differ in that the latter produces explosive histamine secretion which is essentially complete within 10 seconds and is accompanied by only minimal generation of PGD$_2$ and LTC$_4$. The importance of these non-IgE stimuli for activating mast cells is only just being appreciated in relation to the y-protein transduction mechanisms, as is their potential role as mediator-secreting cells in such disorders as delayed hypersensitivity reactions, tumour-associated angiogenesis, physical urticarias, and fibrogenesis.

Table 4.39 Preformed mediators of human mast cells

Mediator class	Mediator	Physiochemical characteristics	Functions
(1) Biogenic amines	Histamine	2–5 pg/cell	H_1 and H_2 receptor mediated effects on smooth muscle, endothelial cells, and nerves
(2) Neutral proteases	Chymase	300 000 Da	Cleavage Type IV collagen, glucagon, neurotensin, fibronectin
	Tryptase	Tetramer $\alpha_2 \beta_2$ 134 000 Da	Cleavage of C3, fibrinogen, precollagenase, fibronectin
	Carboxypeptidase B	30 000–35 000 Da	Converts angiotensinogen to angiotensin
	Dipeptidase	?	Converts LTD_4 to LTE_4
	Kininogenase	?	Converts kininogen to bradykinin
	Hageman Factor inactivator	13 000 Da	Inactivation of Hageman Factor
(3) Acid hydrolases	β-d-Hexosaminidase	Tetramer 108 000 Da	Removes β-linked hexosamines from complex carbohydrates
	β-d-Glucuronidase	Lysosomal form, Tetramer 75 000 Da	Hydrolyses β-linked glucuronic acid
	β-d-Galactosidase	Type A 72 000 Da	Hydrolyses β-linked galactose
	Arylsulphatase	Isoenzyme B	Hydrolyses aromatic sulphate esters
(4) Oxidative enzymes	Superoxide dismutase	?	Converts O_2^- to H_2O_2
	Peroxidase	?	Converts H_2O_2 to H_2O, inactivates leukotrienes, generates lipid peroxides
(5) Chemotactic factors	Eosinophil chemotactic factors (ECF-A)	Heterogeneous oligopeptide (?cytokines)	Eosinophil chemotaxis and priming
	Neutrophil chemotactic activity (NCA)	Glycoprotein (?IL-8) >700 000 Da	Neutrophil chemotaxis and priming
(6) Protease	Heparin	60 000 Da	Anticoagulant anticomplimentary modifies activities of other preformed mediators

4.19.4 Biological activities of mast cell and basophil mediators

Henry Dale was the first to draw attention to histamine as a potent vaso- and broncho-active mediator which, when injected into animals, reproduces many of the features of anaphylaxis. Three receptor subtypes have now been described and are designated H_1, H_2, and H_3 in accordance with their order of discovery. Most of the pharmacological activity of histamine that manifests in IgE-dependent reactions are mediated through the H_1 receptor. These include bronchoconstriction, vasodilatation, vascular leakage, and stimulation of afferent nerves.

Tryptase, the major neutral protease of human mast cells exhibits wide ranging biological activities. These include cleavage of fibrinogen, conversion of C3 to the anaphylatoxin C3a, activation of collagenase, degradation of fibronectin, and conversion of kininogen to bradykinin. In concert with an accompanying highly basic enzyme, carboxypeptidase B, tryptase contributes towards the breaking down of intracellular tissue ground substance. Other proteases localized to mast cells, which include chymase, elastase, a plasminogen activator, and a dipeptidase, probably participate in this process, but have not been studied in detail.

A variety of peptides and proteins with chemokinetic and chemotactic properties when exposed to neutrophils and eosinophils have been attributed to mast cell granules. Eosinophil chemotactic factor of anaphylaxis (ECF-A) was at one time considered to comprise a series of tetrapeptides, but these are now known to be protease cleavage products from larger molecular weight oligopeptides, probably cytokines GM-CSF and IL-5. A high molecular mass (>650 kDa) chemotactic factor for neutrophils that has long been associated with mast cell responses *in vivo* may well be an aggregation product of a lower molecular mass species derived from IgE-triggered T-lymphocytes rather than from mast cells (possibly IL-8). Human mast cells do not have the capacity to secrete the potent lipid chemotaxins, LTB_4, and platelet-activating factor (PAF).

A variety of other enzymes are released from activated mast cells. The acid hydrolases β-glucuronidase, β-galactosidase, β-hexosaminidase, and arylsulphatase are lysosomal enzymes that, along with the neutral proteases, serve to degrade complex glycoproteins and proteoglycans. Superoxide dismutase converts superoxide generated by the mast cell to hydrogen peroxide. Human heparin is a proteoglycan of relatively low molecular mass (60 kDa), whose highly charged glycosaminoglycan side-chains serve to inactivate and package the other

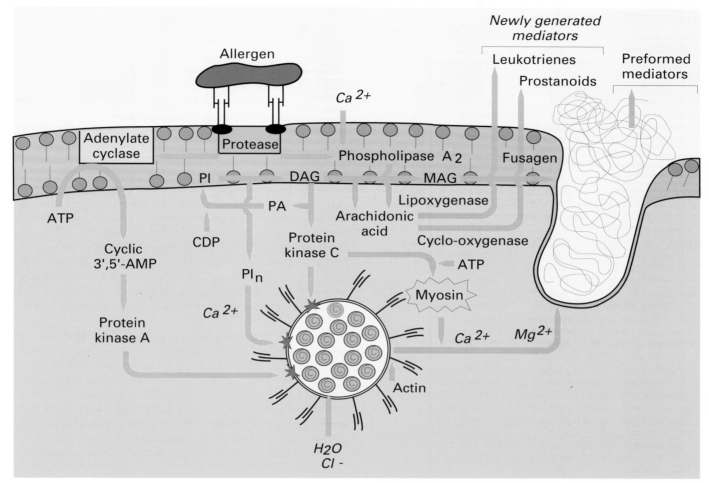

Fig. 4.82 Schematic diagram to illustrate some of the known biochemical events of mast cell activation secretion coupling. (Abbreviations: PI, phosphatidylinositol; DAG, diacylglycerol; MAG, monoacylglycerol; CDP, cytidine 5'-diphosphate.)

preformed mediators within the mast cell granules economically. It is released from activated mast cells as a complex with the proteases tryptase, chymase, and carboxypeptidase. As an extracellular mediator it modifies the substrate specificity of tryptase, increases the activity of histaminase, binds other basic proteins such as eosinophil major basic protein, is anticoagulant through its selective binding of antithrombin III, and also inhibits the alternative pathway of complement activation. Human basophils also contain heparin but in lower concentrations and mixed with proteoglycans containing chondroitin sulphates.

Of the mediators newly generated by mast cells, PGD_2 and LTC_4 are produced most abundantly and are the most biologically active. Both eicosanoids are potent contractile agonists for human airways smooth muscle, being approximately 30 and 100–1000 times more potent than histamine, respectively. Prostaglandin D_2 and its immediate metabolite 9α, 11β-PGF_2 are also vasodilators and in high concentrations increase vascular permeability. Lekotrienes C_4, LTD_4, and LTE_4 are vasoconstrictor and also increase vascular permeability. Once released, these mediators, along with those of the granules, interact in creating events that characterize the immediate phase of the Type I response.

4.19.5 Pharmacologic modulation of mediator release

Sodium cromoglycate, β_2-adrenoceptor agonists, and xanthines inhibit the preformed and newly generated mediator release from IgE-triggered mast cells. Sodium cromoglycate and the more potent drug nedocromil sodium are commonly referred to as anti-allergic drugs, although their range of pharmacological activities extends far beyond the mast cell to include platelets, macrophages, and eosinophils, but not basophils. β_2-agonists and xanthines inhibit mediator release through their capacity to elevate cellular levels of cyclic AMP. Corticosteroids have an indirect suppressive effect on mast cells which is mediated through the suppression of mast cell growth factors from T-lymphocytes. By contrast, corticosteroids are able to directly suppress mediator release from activated basophils.

4.19.6 Further reading

Befus, D., Goodacre, R., Dyck, N., and Bienenstock, J. (1985). Mast cell heterogeneity in man: I. Histologic studies of the intestine. *International Archives of Applied Immunology* **76**, 232–6.

Church, M. K. (1986). Is inhibition of mast cell mediator release relevant to the clinical activity of anti-allergic drugs. *Agents and Actions* **18**, 288–93.

Craig, S. S., Schechter, N. M., and Schwartz, L. B. (1988). Ultrastructural analysis of human T and TC mast cells identified by immunoelectron microscopy. *Laboratory Investigation* **58**, 682–91.

Dvorak, A. M., *et al.* (1985). Immunoglobulin E-mediated degranulation of isolated human lung mast cells. *Laboratory Investigation* **53**, 45–56.

Haig, D. M., McKee, T. A., Jarrett, E. E., Woodbury, R., and Miller, H. R. P. (1982). Generation of mucosal mast cells is stimulated *in vitro* by factors derived from T-cells of helminth infected rats. *Nature* **300**, 188–90.

Holgate, S. T., Robinson, C., and Church, M. K. (1988). Mediators of immediate hypersensitivity. In *Allergy: principles and practice* (ed. E. Middleton Jr., C. E. Reed, E. K. Ellis, N. F. Adkinson Jr., and J. W. Yunginger), pp. 135–63. C. V. Mosby, St. Louis.

Levi-Schaffer, F., Austen, K. F., Gravallese, P. M., and Stevens, R. L. (1986). Coculture of interleukin 3-dependent mouse mast cells with fibroblasts results in a phenotypic change of mast cells. *Proceedings of the National Academy of Sciences* **83**, 6485–8.

Lowman, M. A., Rees, P. H., Benyon, R. C., and Church, M. K. (1988). Human mast cell heterogeneity: histamine release from mast cells dispersed from skin, lung, adenoids, tonsils and intestinal mucosa in response to IgE-dependent and non-immunologic stimuli. *Journal of Allergy and Clinical Immunology* **81**, 590–7.

Peters, S. P., *et al.* (1984). Arachidonic acid metabolism in purified human lung mast cells. *Journal of Immunology* **132**, 1972–9.

Schick, B. A. and Austen, K. F. (1987). The biochemistry of mast cells and basophils. In *Allergy: an international textbook* (ed. M. H. Lessof, T. H. Lee, and D. M. Kemeny), pp. 105–35. John Wiley & Sons, London.

4.20   Monocytes/phagocytes

S. Gordon

4.20.1   Introduction

Monocytes (MΦ) are adaptable, relatively long-lived phagocytic cells and express a variety of plasma membrane receptors (Table 4.17) and secretory products (Table 4.18) that contribute to their central role in host defence and disease. Here we deal with the cellular processes involved in phagocytic recognition and endocytosis and consider killing mechanisms and interactions with intracellular organisms that help to determine the outcome of host infection. Recognition mechanisms and responses resemble those displayed by polymorphonuclear and other leucocytes as discussed elsewhere in Sections 4.17–19.

4.20.2   Phagocytic recognition and endocytosis

Interactions between MΦ and a wide range of ligands (molecules, cells, micro-organisms, particulate substances) are specific and highly selective. For example, MΦ are able to discriminate among glycoproteins according to their terminal cabohydrate residues, distinguish minimally denatured proteins and damaged cells versus their normal counterparts, and recognize different foreign invaders by a range of specific plasma membrane receptors (Fig. 4.83). These act alone or in concert with other receptors to bind, ingest, and destroy some targets, whereas other cells with which MΦ interact trophically are bound at the surface without ingestion. Expression of potential entry receptors by MΦ provide obligate or facultative intracellular organisms with an uptake pathway which, combined with various strategies for evasion of MΦ-cytocidal activities, can result in successful parasitism. The balance tilts towards the host if MΦ are immunologically activated by T-lymphocyte products (see Section 4.6), especially γ-interferon, or interact with specific antibodies and complement, activated by the classical or alternative pathway, to restrict growth of pathogens.

Phagocytic and pinocytic receptor-mediated endocytosis are related processes by which substances are transported into the cell via the plasma membrane (heterophagy). Differences in uptake mechanism can be accounted for by the size of ligand (peptide to large particulates), the bulk of membrane involved, and the need for cytoskeletal activation and energy. Binding to specific plasma membrane receptors enhances uptake of ligands considerably, compared with uptake of unbound solutes via fluid phase pinocytosis, a constitutive activity of isolated MΦ. The vacuolar apparatus of MΦ is shown schematically in Fig. 4.84 and consists of interconnected acidic intracellular compartments, the early and late endosomes and secondary lysosomes. Organelles involved in secretion and exocytosis (endoplasmic reticulum, Golgi complex, storage granules, and primary lysosomes) are less well defined in mature MΦ than in other cells. Storage granules with myeloperoxidase, lysozyme, and other constituents are present in blood monocytes, but are not a feature of MΦ once endocytic activity has commenced.

It has been difficult to isolate and characterize intracellular organelles of MΦ, except for secondary lysosomes laden with exogenous particles such as latex. The composition of the MΦ plasma membrane and its derivatives and precursors differ in spite of the continuous and extensive flow, sorting, and recycling that accompanies fusion and fission of membranes. Little is known about the molecules, some of which may span the membrane, which control these processes. MΦ lysosomes are rich in acid hydrolases and the cells are able to modulate the levels of enzymes according to physiological circumstances, e.g. after a phagocytic meal. The fate and turnover of the contents of MΦ phago- and pinolysosomes play an important role in regulating cellular biosynthesis and secretion. Low molecular weight digestion products (amino acids, some dipeptides, bases, monosaccharides) readily diffuse across the lysosomal membrane, whereas non-degradable substances accumulate in swollen

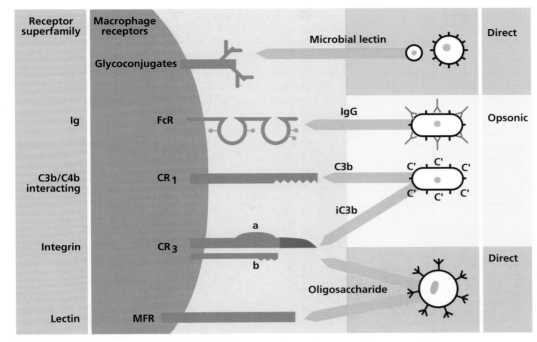

Fig. 4.83 Phagocytic recognition mediated by macrophage plasma membrane receptors.

vacuoles or in residual bodies. There is no evidence that MΦ regurgitate phagocytic debris, although retro-endocytosis of fluid accompanies *in vitro* uptake of solutes such as sucrose. Low molecular weight products reaching the cytosol diffuse freely from the cell (e.g. thymidine, because of low levels of salvage pathways) or, in the case of certain organic anions (? bilirubin) and dyes (e.g. lucifer yellow), are pumped from the cell by plasma membrane and lysosomal transporters. The proton

pumps that play a role in acidification of endosomes and lysosomes have not been well characterized in MΦ.

4.20.3 Mechanism of phagocytosis

Plasma membrane receptors for the Fc fragment of certain IgG subclasses (FcR) and for cleaved C3 (C3b, CR_1, iC3b, CR_3, together referred to as C3R) are the major cell surface molecules

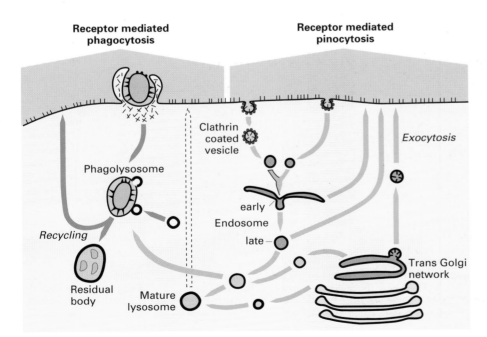

Fig. 4.84 Vesicular transport within the macrophage vacuolar apparatus (prepared by S. Rabinowitz in our laboratory).

involved in opsonin-mediated phagocytosis (Figs 4.83–4.85). Their mechanism of function has been studied by Silverstein and his colleagues in a series of experiments with isolated murine peritoneal MΦ. Binding and ingestion of an opsonized particle are discrete events. Phagocytosis proceeds by a zipper-like mechanism in which MΦ receptors in a local segment of membrane interact with ligands on the surface of the particle. Sequential receptor–ligand interactions guide the MΦ plasma membrane over the surface of the particle (Fig. 4.85a). Plasma membrane fusion occurs if this continues around the complete circumference of a target and ingestion is brought about by contraction of actin filaments, anchored to receptors in the membrane (Fig. 4.85d). Ingestion does not take place if the flow of MΦ plasma membrane is interrupted. This mechanism applies to a wide range of targets taken up by opsonic and non-opsonic phagocytosis.

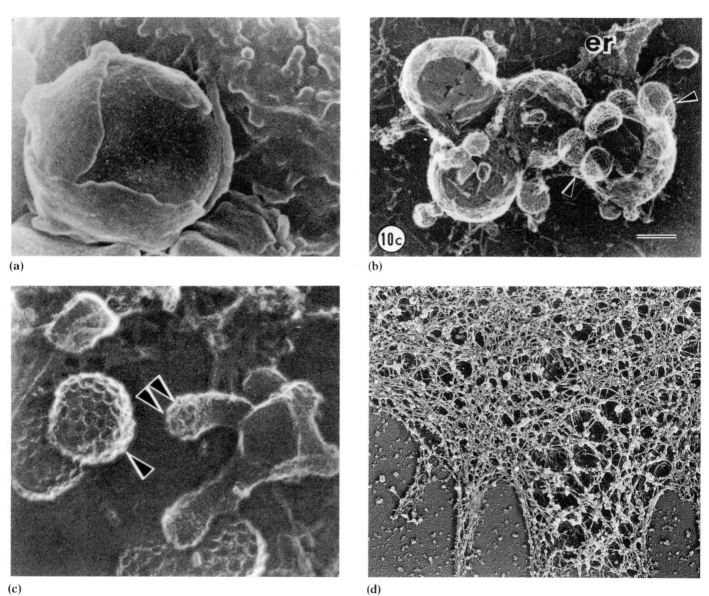

(a)

(b)

(c)

(d)

Fig. 4.85 Morphology of phagocytosis in macrophages. (a) Scanning electron micrograph showing progressive circumferential envelopment of an opsonized erythrocyte by macrophage plasma membrane, compatible with the zipper hypothesis of phagocytosis. (See Sheldon and Orenstein 1977 for further details.) (b) High-resolution electron micrograph of a platinum replica of the cytoplasmic surfaces of latex bead phagosomes viewed from inside broken-open macrophages. Clathrin-coated vesicles are shown (arrowheads) budding off from phagosomes. (From Aggeler and Werb 1982). (c) Replica of the cytoplasmic surface of the adherent bottom of a phagocytosing macrophage showing coated pit formation and vesicles (arrowheads). Note basketwork of clathrin coat. (From Aggeler and Werb 1982.) (d) Electron micrograph showing the organization of filaments at the periphery of a Triton X-100 insoluble cytoskeleton of an adherent rabbit alveolar macrophage. The proteins were fixed with glutaraldehyde, rapidly frozen, and freeze dried. (For details of actin skeleton structure see Yin and Hartwig 1988.)

Other determinants that play a role in controlling ingestion include the physiological state of the cell and the nature of the receptors involved. For example, resident peritoneal murine MΦ bind and ingest antibody-coated targets readily via FcR, but complement-opsonized particles are bound without ingestion by these unstimulated MΦ. The CR_1 and CR_3 receptors for complement exist in functionally different states in different MΦ, and stimulation of the MΦ (e.g. by thioglycollate broth intraperitoneally) or activation of receptors (e.g. by phorbol myristate acetate) is required to induce phagocytosis. The molecular basis for modulation of receptor function is unclear, although density and distribution (free or clustered) of receptors and ligands, receptor phosphorylation and interactions with cytoskeleton are likely to contribute.

The analysis of MΦ complement receptor function illustrates the importance of receptor interactions in phagocytosis. Different receptors co-operate to stabilize weak receptor–ligand interactions directly involved in opsonization, or interact with one another by an indirect mechanism, whereby receptors not involved in binding of a target influence the function of other opsonic receptors at a distance. FcR and C3R synergize in particle uptake at low concentrations of ligand. An example of indirect receptor collaboration is demonstrated by substratum-bound fibronectin, which activates complement receptor function at the free surface of adherent MΦ. Adhesion to an artificial substratum, such as polystyrene, does not activate CR function or actin assembly in a manner analogous to phagocytosis, whereas adhesion through integrin-receptors to fibronectin or other matrix components activates CR and the cytoskeleton and resembles attempted ingestion.

MΦ bind and ingest many targets in the absence of an exogenous opsonin such as antibody or complement (Fig. 4.84). The CR_3 is a member of a leucocyte family of integrin-related adhesion receptors (CR_3/LFA-1/p150,95) that share a common β-chain and express distinct α-chains (see Section 4.17). The CR_3 plays a role in myelomonocytic adhesion to inflamed endothelium, interacts directly with ligands expressed on yeast walls (zymosan), *Leishmania* promastigotes, and certain microorganisms, e.g. *Salmonella* and *Legionella*, and contributes to divalent cation-dependent binding to artificial substrata such as polystyrene plastic. These adhesive interactions involve a receptor epitope that is distinct from the iC3b binding site. A tripeptide sequence (Arg-Gly-Asp, RGD) is often present in ligands that interact with integrin-related receptors, but adhesion by particular receptor molecules is made selective by other structural determinants that are not well defined. Many of the ligands for CR_3 are able to activate the alternative pathway of complement, and MΦ in culture can secrete the complement proteins needed to assemble cleaved C3 on such targets, but it is not clear whether MΦ-derived complement proteins (see Section 4.6) are necessarily involved in these interactions. Carbohydrate residues contribute to phagocytic recognition in several ways. Micro-organisms and parasites recognized by MΦ contain sugar moieties which activate the alternative pathway, interact with CR_3 directly, or can be recognized by MΦ lectin-like receptors.

MΦ express carbohydrate-binding plasma membrane receptors with specificity for several different terminal saccharides, but the best-defined endocytic receptor is that for mannosyl, fucosyl glycoproteins or particulates (the MFR). The MFR is found on MΦ and some endothelial cells, is modulated on MΦ by maturity and lymphokines, and mediates phagocytosis and pinocytosis of appropriate ligands such as mannan-rich yeast walls or artificial glycoconjugates, e.g. mannosylated albumin. The MFR has been purified and cloned and is related to an acute-phase, circulating, mannose-binding protein produced by hepatocytes and possibly involved in opsonic clearance. Even the well-known FcR system, which has served as the prototype for phagocytic defence functions, may include circulating Fc-binding components that contribute to host defence.

The molecular aspects of MΦ receptor structure and function are currently under investigation. MΦ phagocytic receptors are transmembrane glycoproteins that belong to several gene superfamilies (Fig. 4.83) and display structural and functional heterogeneity. The cytoplasmic domains of different receptors vary, an indication of possible interactions with clathrin (Fig. 4.85b, c) and cytoskeleton, and thus are important in the link between ligand-binding and endocytosis or other cellular responses. Coupling of plasma membrane receptors to the cytoskeleton initiates polymerization of actin (Fig. 4.85d) and interactions with other components that generate the contractile forces needed for membrane flow and particle ingestion. Phagocytic cells are rich in proteins such as gelsolin and others that regulate actin assembly and disassembly and confer sensitivity to changes in intracellular Ca^{2+} levels. The fungal metabolite, cytochalasin B, selectively inhibits particle ingestion, but not pinocytosis, by depolymerizing actin.

The contents of the endosome are rapidly and progressively acidified once internalization of plasma-membrane-derived vesicles has occurred, probably by activation of a H^+ pump in the membrane. Partial hydrolysis occurs in endosomes, although most hydrolases are delivered and activated after fusion with primary or secondary lysosomes, which are able to undergo repeated rounds of fusion with incoming membrane. Endocytic vesicles move centripetally towards the centrosomal region and display saltatory movements as a result of their interaction with microtubules. Intracellular fusion is controlled by organelle motility and is highly selective among different organelles. Contents of digestion are disposed of as discussed above, whereas membrane molecules turn over at different rates, dependent on their selective internalization and retrieval, and on the presence or absence of specific ligands which accelerate destruction of receptors. For example, valency of the ligand and pH-stability of receptor–ligand complexes influence the rate of dissociation of FcR and bound antibody in endosomes. Monovalent antibody fragments and bound FcR can be recycled to the surface, whereas multivalent interactions direct the delivery of immune complexes to lysosomes and result in their destruction. The FcR are then similarly degraded.

This complex and dynamic intracellular pathway is regulated by appropriate balance of inflow, outflow, and compartment size. It has been estimated that MΦ in cell culture internalize the equivalent of their total surface area every 30 min, yet fluid and membrane balance are maintained by reflux and recycling, as well as net synthesis and outflow from the Golgi complex (Fig. 4.84). These processes are highly sensitive to cell injury, toxicity, and invasion by pathogenic organisms, all of which are able to induce the formation of abnormal vacuoles. Well-defined examples include agents that increase internalization of molecules from the plasma membrane (lectins, e.g. wheatgerm agglutinin), inhibitors of endosome–lysosome fusion (concanavalin A, microbial wall constituents), and inhibitors of acidification (weak bases, e.g. chloroquine). Other examples of pathological changes induced by infectious agents within the MΦ vacuolar system will be considered below.

4.20.4   Killing mechanisms and receptor-mediated secretion

In Section 4.6 we described how cellular defence mechanisms and secretory responses are enhanced by priming of monocytes and MΦ by T-cell products, especially γ-interferon. Surface-active agents, such as immune complexes or LPS, trigger activated MΦ to release cytotoxic and inflammatory mediators of local and systemic host defence and repair. Cytokines and extrinsic stimuli induce selective and co-ordinate changes in the expression of a programme of genes involved in MΦ activation, details of which are still under investigation. Here we place some of these cellular events in perspective.

Only selected plasma membrane receptors trigger product release by primed MΦ. These include several distinct FcRs, which are differentially expressed by activated and non-activated MΦ, and the MFR, which contributes to the efficient stimulation of MΦ responses even by unopsonized zymosan. CR$_3$ involved in adhesion and phagocytosis of opsonized and unopsonized targets does not trigger a respiratory burst or release of TNFα or of arachidonate metabolites by MΦ. Pharmacological agents such as PMA are efficient agonists of secretion by MΦ, as in many other cells.

Activated MΦ do not necessarily display enhanced phagocytic activity. FcRs, and probably other receptors, trigger cytotoxic responses in primed/activated MΦ (e.g. BCG-induced peritoneal MΦ) upon contact with their ligand and these MΦ kill extracellularly, rather than by ingestion. This process resembles antibody-dependent cellular cytoxicity (ADCC) by related leucocytes. Intracellular killing does occur, however, as shown by lymphokine (γ-interferon) treatment of MΦ containing *Trypanosoma cruzi* or other internalized organisms, which sterilizes parasitized cells. Acid hydrolases are involved in degradation of dead organisms, not in the primary killing process.

A substantial body of evidence suggests that activated MΦ express potent O$_2$-dependent killing mechanisms that are responsible for much, but not all, cellular cytotoxicity. BCG and other activated MΦ can be triggered by PMA or other stimuli to release relatively large amounts of H$_2$O$_2$ and other reactive oxygen intermediates (superoxide anion, hydroxyl radicals, singlet oxygen). These are generated by activation of an electron transport chain present in the plasma membrane of the MΦ (see Section 4.17 for further discussion). It is not clear whether intracellular storage granules deliver components of this system to the cell surface, as in granulocytes. The respiratory burst complex in myelomonocytic cells includes an NADPH-dependent oxidase, a novel b-type cytochrome, and possibly a flavoprotein. Membrane preparations of leucocytes retain the ability to take up O$_2$ and generate O$_2^-$, but the oxidase system has not been fully characterized. The cytochrome has been purified and cloned, and mutations and other inborn errors are known to give rise to autosomal and X-linked forms of chronic granulomatous disease (CGD). Although rare, CGD patients are susceptible to microbial infections because of the inadequate respiratory burst by PMN and monocytes, and studies of their leucocytes have been instructive in establishing the importance of this system in host defence.

The cytotoxic and antimicrobial effects of H$_2$O$_2$ can be considerably enhanced by the Klebanoff reaction in which myeloperoxidase (MPO) (see Section 4.17.4) uses H$_2$O$_2$ as substrate to generate highly reactive halide radicals, that halogenate and kill a wide range of targets. Genetic deficiency of MPO does not result in major susceptibility to infections, perhaps because of alternate killing mechanisms. Microbial targets and MΦ vary in their resistance to reactive oxygen intermediates and free radical injury, depending on complex scavenger and enzymatic mechanisms, such as catalase, glutathione, and the ability to regenerate reducing equivalents within the cytosol.

Lysozyme is a bulk product of induced MΦ and contributes to lysis of various microbial targets, especially if saccharide substrates are exposed to enzyme access by antibody and complement. It is not clear whether activated MΦ generate other specific cytotoxic proteins able to inflict direct injury on cellular and microbial targets. Cytolytic esterases and cationic polypeptides/proteins are candidate cytotoxins but have not been defined in MΦ, compared with other leucocytes and cytolytic lymphocytes. Endotoxin-challenged and activated MΦ release high levels of tumour necrosis factor-alpha (TNF-α) which has direct effects on a range of cellular targets and also contributes to enhanced cytotoxicity by several indirect mechanisms. TNF-α is essential for host resistance to virulent pathogens such as *Listeria monocytogenes* and is a potent stimulus of the respiratory burst of PMN and possibly monocytes under appropriate *in vitro* conditions. A large part of the cytopathic action of TNF *in vivo* is mediated by its effects on vascular endothelium that give rise to ischaemic injury and local necrosis, e.g. in organs such as the bowel, and possibly in tumours.

Interferons represent an important family of antiviral proteins produced by MΦ (α/β), T-lymphocytes (γ), or other cells (α/β). Interferons act on MΦ to induce an antiviral state and enhance surface properties (e.g. MHC class I, II expression) that promote immune cellular interactions. Different interferons bind to distinct surface receptors and induce complex metabolic effects on MΦ. They interact among themselves to modulate activation of MΦ, together with glucocorticoids, lipocortins, and other cytokines, e.g. TGFβ (see Table 4.16). The colony-stimulating factors M-CSF, GM-CSF, interleukin-3 influence MΦ cytotoxicity indirectly by their actions on growth and differen-tiation, but do not prime MΦ in the same way as γ-interferon. Interleukin-4, originally defined as a B-cell stimulating factor, also activates certain MΦ effector properties.

Apart from reactive O_2 intermediates, MΦ are able to gener-ate other low molecular weight metabolites and to release various proteins following stimulation (see Table 4.18). The arachidonate metabolites (prostaglandins, leukotrienes, throm-boxanes) generated by the cyclo-oxygenase and lipoxygenase pathways are mainly products of resident-type MΦ and play a role as acute mediators of inflammation. Nitrogen metabolites are also produced by stimulated MΦ and act on endothelium and possibly other targets. Elicited and activated MΦ generate a range of neutral proteinase activities (plasminogen activator, elastase, collagenase) that activate plasma proteinase cascades (fibrinolysis, kinin generation, and complement activation) and contribute to connective tissue catabolism. The MΦ plasmino-gen activator is of the urokinase-type and may be involved in cell migration and tissue repair. The active enzyme is generated by complex intra- and extracellular mechanisms (transcrip-tional and translational controls, interactions with specific in-hibitors) and much of its proteolytic activity is generated close to the surface of the cell, by local activation of plasminogen. Extracellular inhibitors (e.g. anti-plasmin, α-macroglobulin) and clearance of urokinase, alone or as inhibitor complexes, regulate proteolysis in the vicinity of the MΦ.

Monokines such as interleukin-1, interleukin-6, and TNF-α exert multiple hormone-like effects on cells throughout the body. These products of stimulated MΦ modulate and integrate a range of local and systemic metabolic and host defence mech-anisms, such as fever, hepatocyte acute phase protein syn-thesis, and catabolism of muscle, fat, and connective tissue. These and other monokines have also been implicated in growth of haemopoietic cells, blood vessels, and connective tissue. However, regulation of their sources, release mech-anisms, and actions within the host are poorly defined and require further study.

4.20.5 Interactions of macrophages and pathogenic organisms

A wide range of organisms is able to enter and establish them-selves within MΦ by utilizing physiological entry mechanisms (Figs 4.86, 4.87). Virulence for the host depends on the survival strategy of the organism and the response of the MΦ. Study of the cellular biology of MΦ–pathogen interactions has helped to elucidate the normal pathway of endocytosis and has revealed mechanisms of pathogenesis of a major group of infectious dis-eases. Observations have been made with microbial agents (mycobacteria, *Legionella*, *Listeria*), viruses (HIV, flaviviruses), parasites (*Trypanosoma cruzi*, *Toxoplasma*, *Leishmania*), fungi (*Histoplasma*, yeasts), and *Chlamydia*, examples of agents which invade MΦ. Although there is considerable variation in their mode of entry and survival within MΦ, it is useful to treat their interaction with MΦ in general terms to illustrate common themes of intracellular parasitism.

4.20.6 Binding and recognition, the cellular basis for macrophage tropism

Pathogen and phagocyte both express specific surface mo-lecules that determine the range of cells that can be infected and of organisms that can be recognized. Expression of several plasma membrane receptors that mediate recognition and uptake of opsonized (e.g. FcR, CR) and unopsonized targets (e.g. CR, MFR) is restricted to MΦ and related cells and thus contrib-utes to tropism of some organisms for MΦ. The fate of antibody and complement-coated organisms within MΦ is very different from that of unopsonized organisms and leads to destruction of the organism and degradation in lysosomes. Lymphokine ac-tivation of MΦ also renders the MΦ more resistant to invasion and enhances cytocidal mechanisms. Organisms can be des-troyed by immunologically activated MΦ during entry or after uptake, when dead or dying pathogens are sequestered within secondary lysosomes by a process which resembles autophagy. However, the initial encounter with a pathogen may involve resident-type tissue MΦ in lymphoid organs and liver, rather than elicited or activated monocytes and recruited MΦ, so that host cell–pathogen interactions are heterogeneous. The resid-ent Kupffer cells in liver, for example, express a different profile of endocytic receptors (low CR_3, high levels of MFR) and altered defence capabilities (deficient respiratory burst and refractori-ness to priming by γ-interferon for a respiratory burst) and may therefore be vulnerable to infections, e.g. in listeriosis and vis-ceral leishmaniasis (Section 4.6). MΦ heterogeneity has not been adequately taken into account in studies that have clari-fied recognition mechanisms and responses by MΦ in culture.

Studies with *Leishmania* illustrate some of the requirements for entry into MΦ of promastigotes, the flagellated form, but do not account for uptake of amastigotes, which enter efficiently by an unknown mechanism. The promastigote form of *L. donovani*, for example, expresses specific surface glycolipids and glycopro-teins which interact with CR_3 directly, after opsonization with alternative pathway proteins, and/or with MFR-like receptors (Fig. 4.84). It is possible that these receptors function concur-rently in pathogen entry. The extent to which either receptor is utilized depends on the physiological state of the organism (growth versus stationary phase) as well as receptor expression by monocytes (MFR, CR_3) or tissue-type MΦ. It is possible that other parasites and organisms that show restricted entry into MΦ (e.g. *Histoplasma*, mycobacteria) utilize the same receptors for entry. The relative contribution of each receptor during entry will also influence an organism's ability to evade killing, since the CR_3, unlike MFR, is not thought to trigger a respirat-ory burst. For example, *Toxoplasma gondii* enters MΦ without triggering a burst, but the receptors involved have not been defined.

Another entry receptor documented on MΦ is the CD4 mo-lecule, which binds and promotes entry and syncytium forma-tion by human immunodeficiency virus (HIV). CD4 expression by MΦ is independently regulated from that by T-lymphocytes and the mechanism of viral entry is not clear. Gp120, a cleavage product of HIV env glycoprotein, plays a key role in infection of both cell types, although alternate entry receptors (e.g. FcR) have not yet been excluded for MΦ (see discussion of antibody-mediated enhancement of virus infection below).

4.20.7 Internalization, penetration, and persistence of intracellular organisms

Mycoplasma replicates on the surface of MΦ and other infected cells, but many organisms need to be internalized and to transport their nucleic acid across the endosome or lysosomal membrane to initiate replication. Others avoid killing mechanisms upon entry into the cell and replicate within the vacuolar apparatus (Fig. 4.86). Parasites are known that inhibit endosome acidification (e.g. *Legionella*), interfere with endosome–lysosome fusion (e.g. *Mycobacteria*, *Toxoplasma*), replicate within parasitophorous vacuoles (e.g. *Leishmania*), or escape

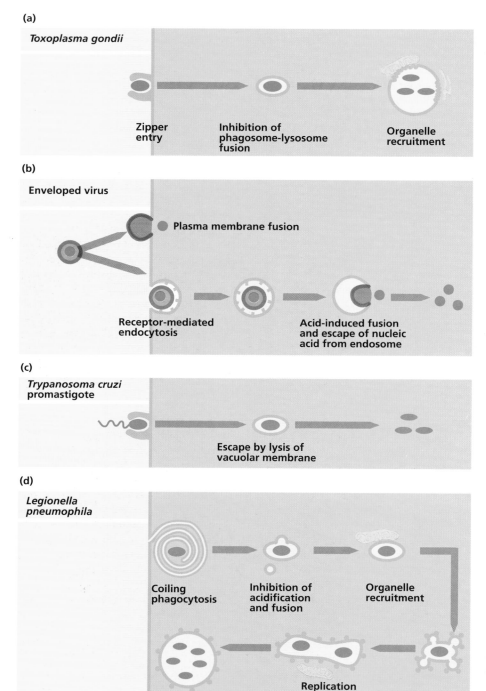

Fig. 4.86 Strategies by which pathogenic organisms penetrate macrophages. [(a) After Jones and Hirsch 1972; (b) after Helenius *et al.* 1983; (c) after Nogueira and Cohn 1976; (d) after Horwitz 1983.]

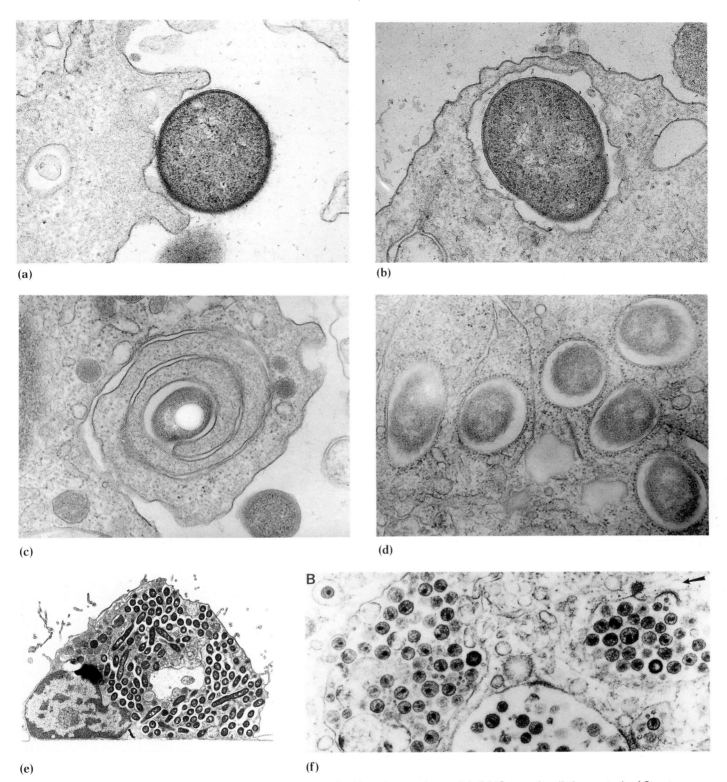

Fig. 4.87 Entry and growth of pathogens in human monocytes and cultivated macrophages. (a), (b) 'Conventional' phagocytosis of *Streptococcus pneumoniae* (Horwitz 1984). (c)–(e) *Legionella pneumophila* enters by coiling phagocytosis, resides in a phagosome surrounded by ribosomes and proliferates extensively in vacuoles. (For further details see Horwitz *et al.* 1980, Horwitz 1983.) (f) HIV-1 replicates in cytoplasmic vacuoles in human blood monocytes cultivated *in vitro* in the presence of CSF-1 (see Orenstein *et al.* 1988). Mature virions are shown, and budding, immature forms. Coated vesicles are associated with the vacuole membrane (arrow). Intravacuolar virions far exceed those associated with the plasma membrane.

into the cytosol by disrupting vacuolar membranes (*Trypanosoma cruzi*, *Listeria monocytogenes*). The mechanisms of these interactions are unknown, although lytic molecules may be involved, as recently identified for *Listeria*. *Legionella* enters MΦ by an unusual coiling structure rather than by a zipper-mechanism (Fig. 4.87c–e). This is thought to be mediated by a porin in the wall of the living organism. Once within the cell, *Legionella* exhibits other unusual features apart from its effects on acidification and fusion. Its presence in MΦ elicits clustering of rough endoplasmic reticulum and mitochondria around the vacuole (Fig. 4.87d). The benefits derived from organelle recruitment by the organism are not known. These changes are a striking feature of invasion by *Legionella*, but MΦ display similar, although less marked changes after invasion by other intracellular pathogens (Fig. 4.86). As with other invaders, the MΦ can be activated by γ-interferon to kill *Legionella*, and the unusual cytological features are then lost.

Reoviruses contain a double-stranded RNA genome that survives uncoating in MΦ lysosomes, but many viruses transfer their nucleic acid across the endosomal membrane by an acid-catalysed envelope-fusion reaction similar to that defined in other cells. In the case of HIV and other viruses, fusion can occur at neutral pH at the plasma membrane. The interactions of flaviviruses with MΦ illustrate the importance of the relative rate of endosomal escape versus transfer to lysosomes in determining the outcome of an infection, and the paradoxical effects of certain antiviral antibodies in enhancing, rather than neutralizing virus infection. Poorly neutralizing cross-reactive antisera or monoclonal antibodies are able to enhance binding of virus to MΦ-FcR and greatly increase subsequent virus replication, effectively making such a virus tropic for MΦ. It is not clear whether the FcR provides an alternate receptor for enhanced entry of virus [the receptor(s) for flaviviruses are not known] or enhances binding to its natural receptor. More efficient escape from endosomes is thought to contribute to the mechanism of enhancement. The CR₃ has also been implicated as a receptor that can mediate enhanced infection or neutralization.

Once established within a macrophage, an organism can replicate free in the cytosol or within a membrane-bound organelle, including elements of the vacuolar apparatus (Fig. 4.87e). Budding of enveloped viruses such as HIV-1 may be predominantly intracellular (Fig. 4.87f), rather than exclusively from the plasma membrane.

In addition to antiviral antibody and complement, activated by classical or alternate pathway mechanisms, virus–MΦ interactions are modified by MΦ activation, cell maturity, and host genetic differences. In experimental animals strain differences that influence host cell–pathogen interactions include MHC and several non-MHC loci, several of which act at the level of MΦ. Different genes determine host susceptibility to a variety of infectious agents, including flaviviruses, influenza, herpes simplex virus, and non-viral micro-organisms. One common locus is involved in resistance to several organisms (BCG, *S. typhi*, and *Leishmania*), but its mode of action in host resistance is unknown. Finally, the effects of parasitism on MΦ biosynthesis remain poorly understood, but include initial events that accompany entry and infection, and subsequent secretory and other responses associated with persistence of an organism within the cells. Together with altered expression of MΦ plasma membrane molecules (MHC class I, class II, and CD4) these may influence MΦ interactions with other immune cells (T-helper and cytotoxic cells) and facilitate the elimination or survival of the organism, with profound and prolonged effects on the host.

4.20.8   Further reading

Aggeler, J. and Werb, Z. (1982). Initial events during phagocytosis by macrophages viewed from outside and inside the cell: membrane-particle interactions and clathrin. *Journal of Cell Biology* **94**, 613–23.

Anderson, D. C. and Springer, T. A. (1987). Leukocyte adhesion deficiency: an inherited defect in Mac-1, LFA-1, and p150,95 glycoproteins. *Annual Review of Medicine* **38**, 175–94.

Blackwell, J. M., Ezekowitz, R. A. B., Roberts, M. B., Channon, J. Y., Sim, R. B., and Gordon, S. (1985). Macrophage complement and lectin-like receptors bind *Leishmania* in the absence of serum. *Journal of Experimental Medicine* **162**, 324–31.

CIBA Foundation (1982). *Membrane recycling, Symposium 92*. Pitman, London.

D'Arcy Hart, P., Young, M. R., Jordon, M. M., Perkins, W. J., and Geisow, M. J. (1983). Chemical inhibitors of phagosome-lysosome fusion in cultured macrophages also inhibit saltatory lysosomal movements. *Journal of Experimental Medicine* **158**, 477–92.

Ezekowitz, R. A. B. and Stahl, P. D. (1988). The structure-function of vertebrate mannose lectin-like proteins. *Journal of Cell Science* Suppl. 9, 121–34.

Ezekowitz, R. A. B., Dinauer, M. C., Jaffe, H. S., Orkin, S. H., and Newburger, P. E. (1988). Partial correction of the phagocyte defect in patients with X-linked chronic granulomatous disease by subcutaneous interferon gamma. *New England Journal of Medicine* **319**, 146–51.

Griffin, F. M., Jr., Griffin, J. A., Leider, J. E., and Silverstein, S. C. (1975). Studies on the mechanisms of phagocytosis. I. Requirements for circumferential attachment of particle bound ligands to specific receptors on the macrophage plasma membrane. *Journal of Experimental Medicine* **142**, 1263–82.

Havell, E. A. (1987). Production of tumor necrosis factor during murine Listeriosis. *Journal of Immunology* **139**, 4225–31.

Helenius, A, Mellman, I., Wall, D., and Hubbard, A. (1983). Endosomes. *Trends in Biochemical Science* **8**, 245–50.

Ho, D. D., Pomerantz, R. J., and Kaplan, J. C. (1987). Pathogenesis of infection with human immunodeficiency virus. *New England Journal of Medicine* **317**, 278–86.

Horwitz, M. A. and Silverstein, S. C. (1980). Legionnaires' disease bacterium (*Legionella pneumophila*) multiplies intracellularly in human monocytes. *Journal of Clinical Investigation* **66**, 441–50.

Horwitz, M. A. (1983). Formation of a novel phagosome by the Legionnaires' disease bacterium (*Legionella pneumophila*) in human monocytes. *Journal of Experimental Medicine* **158**, 1319–31.

Horwitz, M. A. (1984). Phagocytosis of the Legionnaires' disease bacterium (*Legionella pneumophila*) occurs by a novel mechanism: engulfment within a pseudopod coil. *Cell* **36**, 27–33.

Hynes, R. O. (1987). Integrins: a family of cell surface receptors. *Cell* **48**, 549–54.

Jones, T. C. and Hirsch, J. G. (1972). The interaction between *Toxoplasma gondii* and mammalian cells. II. The absence of lysosomal fusion with phagocytic vacuoles containing living parasites. *Journal of Experimental Medicine* **136**, 1173–94.

Klebanoff, S. J. and Clark, R. A. (1978). *The neutrophil: function and clinical disorders*. North Holland Publishing, Amsterdam.

Law, A. (1988). C3 receptors on macrophages. *Journal of Cell Science* Suppl. 9, 67–98.

Mellman, I., Mellman, I., Koch, T., Healey, G., Hunziker, W., Lewis, V., Plutner, H., Miettinen, H., Vaux, D., Moore, K., and Stuart, S. (1988). Structure and function of Fc receptors on macrophages and lymphocytes. *Journal of Cell Science* Suppl. 9, 45–66.

Nogueira, N. and Cohn, Z. A. (1976). Trypanosoma Cruzi: Mechanism of entry and intracellular fate in mammalian cells. *Journal of Experimental Medicine* **143**, 1402–20.

Ohkuma, S. and Poole, B. (1981). Cytoplasmic vacuolation of mouse peritoneal macrophages and the uptake into lysosomes of weakly basic substances. *Journal of Cell Biology* **90**, 656–64.

Orenstein, J. M., Meltzer, M. S., Phipps, T., and Gendelman, H. E. (1988). Cytoplasmic assembly and accumulation of human immunodeficiency virus types 1 and 2 in recombinant human colony-stimulating factor-1-treated human monocytes: an ultrastructural study. *Journal of Virology* **62**, 2578–86.

Sheldon, E. and Orenstein, J. M. (1977). Membrane phenomena accompanying erythrophagocytosis. A scanning electron microscope study. *Laboratory Investigation* **36**, 363–74.

Silverstein, S. C., Steinman, R. M., and Cohn, Z. A. (1977). Endocytosis. *Annual Review of Biochemistry* **46**, 669–722.

Steinman, R. M., Mellman, I. S., Muller, W. A., and Cohn, Z. A. (1983). Endocytosis and the recycling of plasma membrane. *Journal of Cell Biology* **96**, 1–27.

Unkeless, J. C., Scigliano, E., and Freedman, V. H. (1988). Structure and function of human and murine receptors of IgG. *Annual Review of Immunology* **6**, 251–81.

Wright, S. D. and Detmers, P. A. (1988). Adhesion-promoting receptors on phagocytes. *Journal of Cell Science* Suppl. 9, 99–120.

Yin, H. L. and Hartwig, J. H. (1988). The structure of the macrophage actin skeleton. *Journal of Cell Science* Suppl. 9, 169–84.

4.21   Natural killer cells

P. C. L. Beverley

4.21.1   Introduction

Natural killer (NK) cells were discovered more than 15 years ago. Early experiments identified cytotoxic activity against certain target cells that was not dependent on prior immunization, was not T-cell mediated, and was later shown not to be major histocompatibility complex (MHC) restricted. The activity was shown to be associated mainly with a subset of large granular lymphocytes (LGL), lacking most T-cell markers and surface immunoglobulin but expressing Fc receptors for IgG.

These early studies raised numerous questions. Among the more important are: what is the function of NK cells, what is their origin and lineage relationship to other cell types, and how do they recognize other cells? More recently, the recognition that activated lymphocytes frequently acquire non-specific cytotoxic activity and may have therapeutic potential, has

raised questions of the relationship of activated killer cells to NK cells and of the *in vivo* traffic of NK and NK-related cells.

4.21.2   Terminology

The use of the term NK cell for the population of non-T/non-B lymphocytes that carry out MHC unrestricted lysis is traditional. However, it is well recognized that cells capable of mediating this activity are heterogeneous and that 'NK' cells are also capable of a variety of other non-cytotoxic functions, so that the term is not an entirely logical one. Nevertheless, since other terms have not gained wide acceptance, I shall continue to use NK in this review. For the related cells generated in culture I shall use the terms activated killers (AK) or LAK when lymphokines are the stimulus.

4.21.3   Phenotypic definition of NK cells

Since the first recognition of natural (i.e. not requiring prior immunization) killer activity, a great deal of effort has been devoted to the identification of the effector cells. They have been defined as effector cells with spontaneous cytotoxicity against various targets, lacking the properties of classical macrophages, granulocytes, T- or B-lymphocytes. The cytotoxicity is MHC unrestricted. These properties are associated with a small (about 5 per cent) population of mononuclear cells found in peripheral blood. These cells have a low buoyant density, are of medium to large size and characteristically exhibit cytoplasmic azurophilic granules. However, closer examination indicates that this is an oversimplification. Even before the development of monoclonal antibodies (mAbs), it was shown that NK cells expressed receptors for sheep red blood cells, a property of T-cells, and Fc receptors for IgG, a property of myeloid cells. Analysis with mAbs has confirmed both these observations but has provided in addition several reagents that are helpful in identifying NK cells (Table 4.40).

At present the most useful reagents are HNK-1 (Leu 7), CD16 (Leu 11, the low-affinity receptor for IgG), and NKH-1 (CD56). Even with these mAbs caution is necessary since HNK1 is not present on all cells with NK activity and is expressed on some T-cells, CD16 is present on granulocytes and on a very small number of T-cells, while NKH-1 is also not expressed on all NK active cells. Thus at present the most satisfactory phenotypic definition of an NK cell is a CD3$^-$, CD16$^+$ mononuclear cell, which may be heterogeneous for a variety of other markers, including CD2, CD8, CD11b (OKM1), HNK-1, NKH-1, granules, and cytolytic activity.

4.21.4   Origin of NK cells

The phenotypic data discussed above does not provide a definitive answer to the problem of the lineage of NK cells, indeed it has been taken to imply a relationship to T-cells, to the myelomonocytic lineage, or that NK cells are a third lineage of non-T non-B lymphocytes. More clearcut are cell transfer experiments showing the bone marrow origin of NK cells and that NK

Table 4.40 The phenotype of NK cells

Property	Cytotoxic/suppressor T-cells	NK cells	Monocytes	PMN
CD3	+	−	−	−
CD8	+	+/−	−	−
CD11b	−/+	+	+	+
CD16 (Fc$_\gamma$R)	−/(+)	+	−	+
CD57 (Leu 7)	−/(+)	+/−	−	−
CD56 (NCAM)	−	+/−	−	−
LGL morphology	−/+	+	−	−
Adherence	−	−	+	+
ADCC	−	++	+	−
Memory	+	−	−	−

(+) Indicates that a small minority of the population expresses the property. −/+ Indicates that a substantial proportion of the population expresses the property.

activity is undiminished in nude mice, which lack a functional thymus. This data implies that although NK cells may be pre-T cells, they do not require thymus processing and are not thymus dependent. Furthermore, the CD3⁻, CD16⁺ population does not show rearrangement of T-cell rceptor (TCR) αβ genes. Evidence that NK cells are monocyte related rests on data showing cytolytic activity of promonocytes obtained from bone marrow and on the sharing of certain phenotypic markers. However, most mononuclear cells can mediate cytotoxicity under appropriate conditions and monocytes are distinguishable from NK cells by several antigens. Thus, at present it is not possible to decide on the lineage relationship of NK cells, although it is reasonable to suggest that they may represent a third lymphocyte population.

4.21.5 Function of NK cells

Although NK cells were originally defined on the basis of their cytolytic properties, it has since become apparent that they have broader functional capabilities. In particular, a wide variety of immunoregulatory effects have been described. Thus, in human *in vitro* experiments, the addition of NK cells can suppress or amplify both humoral and cell-mediated responses and regulate haemopoietic stem-cell proliferation and differentiation. *In vivo* experiments in animals suggest the involvement of NK cells in tumour immunity, resistance to infection, and in hybrid resistance to bone marrow grafts as well as graft versus host disease (summarized in Table 4.41). What remains unclear, as in the case of T-cells, is how many different types of cell mediate these varied functions. However, three main subtypes have been distinguished, NK cells, natural cytotoxic (NC) cells, and natural suppressor (NS) cells. The former two are principally distinguished by differences in their specificity for cytotoxic targets while NS cells are non-cytotoxic in conventional assays. The three cell types cannot be clearly distinguished on phenotypic criteria and it is not clear whether they represent distinct cell types or different stages in the maturation or activation of a single type.

Table 4.41 The functions of NK cells

Tumour immunity
  inhibition of primary tumour development
  inhibition of metastases
  in vitro cytotoxicity
Transplantation immunity
  hybrid resistance
  graft versus host disease
  organ transplant rejection
Cell regulation
  up- or down-regulation of antibody reaponses
  up- or down-regulation of cell-mediated responses
  natural suppression
  control of haemopoiesis
Infection
  protection against viral, fungal, parasitic, and bacterial infection

4.21.6 Lymphokines and NK cells

The diverse activities of NK cells and their relatives can perhaps be best accounted for on the basis of two properties; their ability to produce and respond to diverse lymphokines, and the way in which they recognize other cells (see Section 4.21.8). Both fresh LGL and cloned NK cells have been shown to produce at least interleukin-1, 2, and 4, NK cytotoxic factors (including lymphotoxin), interferons (IFN) α, β, and γ, and colony-stimulating factors. There is some evidence that these may be produced by different LGL subsets and preferentially induced by different stimuli.

NK cells not only produce lymphokines but also respond to them. γ-IFN has long been known to be a potent inducer of NK activity, increasing both the number of LGL able to form conjugates with their targets and the number of lytically active cells. However, some NK cells and NC cells appear to be resistant to the effects of IFN. NK cells also respond to interleukin-2 (IL-2), both by proliferation and by increased cytolytic activity. Thus NK cells are involved in many immune responses because they respond to lymphokines produced by T-cells and modulate responses of other haemopoietic cells by virtue of their own cytokine production.

4.21.7 Activated killer cells

It has been known for several years that *in vitro* activation of lymphocytes by a variety of agents is capable of inducing non-specific cytolytic activity. The advent of monoclonal antibodies and recombinant lymphokines made it possible to analyse this phenomenon. The use of IL-2, in particular, was shown to induce high levels of cytotoxicity *in vitro* and the effector cells have been termed lymphokine-activated killer (LAK) cells. These cells have been shown in a variety of model systems to have therapeutic effects against established tumours and to protect against metastases. The nature of the effector cells has, however, been disputed, perhaps because it now appears that many cells can mediate non-specific cytotoxicity when appropriately activated. The dominant population in a culture will depend on the starting population, the nature and dose of the stimulus, and the time of culture. Thus in cultures of peripheral blood mononuclear cells (PBM) stimulated with IL-2 the predominant effector type is a $CD3^-$, $CD16^+$ cell, which appears early in the culture. In contrast, after longer culture periods or in the presence of phytohaemagglutinin (PHA), $CD3^+$ effectors are generated. Irrespective of the stimulus, AK cells have a broader range of cytolytic activity than resting NK cells, being able to kill a range of tumour cell lines and fresh tumour cells that are resistant to the latter. It is this broad range of tumour cytotoxic activity that has aroused interest in LAK cells as a therapeutic modality.

4.21.8 Antigen recognition by NK and AK cells

Cold target inhibition studies on fresh NK cells and analysis of the range of target cells killed by NK clones, suggest that most NK and LAK cells can kill more than one target cell in an MHC unrestricted fashion. Different clones show varying specificities, some being restricted to one or a few targets while others may kill many different cell types. Since many NK clones are $CD3/TCR^-$, their specific reactivity cannot generally be attributed to recognition via this receptor. Inhibition studies with a variety of mAbs show that several molecules appear to be involved in NK/target cell interaction (Table 4.42). Since ex-

Table 4.42 Target recognition structures of NK cells

Antigen on NK cell	Ligand on target
CD2	CD58 (LFA-3)
TCR$\alpha\beta$/$\gamma\delta$	antigen
CD8	MHC I
CD16	IgG or Ig-like structures
CD11a/CD18 (LFA-1)	CD54 (ICAM-1)
CD45	not known
laminin	laminin receptors

Other less well-characterized molecules have been described as receptors and targets.

pression of many of these is heterogeneous on NK and LAK cells and the ligands for these structures will also be expressed heterogeneously on potential target cells, the specificity of NK/LAK recognition of targets may depend on the mosaic of surface recognition structures present on both cells.

4.21.9 Conclusions

In spite of a great deal of work, NK cells remain enigmatic. It is in fact much easier to say what they are not, rather than to assign them a definitive lineage relationship and function. What is clear is that they do not express TCRs or surface Ig, nor do they possess another characteristic of T- and B-cells, that of memory. It seems most likely, therefore, that their role may be in modulating the responses of other cell types, rather than in initiating responses.

4.21.10 Further reading

Hersey, P. and Bolhuis, R. (1987). 'Nonspecific' MHC-unrestricted killer cells and their receptors. *Immunology Today* **8**, 233–7.

Maier, T. Holda, J. H., and Claman, H. N. (1986). Natural suppressor (NS) cells, members of the LGL regulatory family. *Immunology Today* **7**, 312–17.

Ortaldo, J. R. and Herberman, R. B. (1984). Heterogeneity of natural killer cells. *Annual Review of Immunology* **2**, 359–94.

Reynolds, C. W. and Ortaldo, J. R. (1987). Natural killer activity: the definition of a function rather than a cell type. *Immunology Today* **6**, 172–6.

Rosenberg, S. A. and Lotze, M. T. (1986). Cancer immunotherapy using interleukin-2 and interleukin-2-activated lymphocytes. *Annual Reviews of Immunology* **4**, 681–709.

5

The response to injury

5

The response to injury

5.1 Introduction

Nicholas A. Wright

There are many occasions when organisms encounter injury: such events can be caused by physical or chemical agents and, of course, there are numerous instances in which organisms are themselves assailed by other organisms, viral, bacterial, fungal, or indeed protozoal.

In the response to all such primary injuries, a common thread of events can often be discerned. This section describes and analyses the acute response to injury, how the damage produced is repaired, and the events which ensue if such damage cannot be adequately repaired, or, indeed, if the repair process itself goes wrong in some way.

5.2 Acute inflammation

N. C. Turner

Inflammation is the most common biological reaction to a variety of noxious stimuli and to local injury; it is the process by which serum proteins and phagocytic cells gain access to areas of damaged tissue, infection, or foreign material. The first description of inflammation was made almost 2000 years ago, by Celsus, who identified redness, heat, swelling, and pain as characteristics of the reaction. In the nineteenth century Virchow added loss of function to this list, and together these characteristics comprise the five cardinal signs of the inflammatory reaction.

Inflammatory reactions can be triggered by physical or chemical trauma (burns, radiation, caustic substances), invading organisms, antigen–antibody reactions, and is often exacerbated by the resultant cell damage. During this complex response plasma enzyme systems (complement, kinin, clotting) may be activated, cells resident in the tissue (mast cells, macrophages) may be stimulated, and circulating cells recruited.

In general, the overall inflammatory process is dependent on the generation of vasoactive and chemotactic agents which diffuse from the site of initiation to the blood vessels. Local vasodilatation increases regional blood flow to the affected area and, together with an increase in microvascular permeability, results in loss of fluid and plasma proteins (exudation) into the tissues. Concomitantly, chemotactic mediators stimulate the adherence of circulating cells to the vascular endothelium and their migration into the inflamed site. At the site of the inflammatory focus these recruited cells accumulate and become activated. Phagocytic cells ingest foreign material and cell debris, release hydrolytic and proteolytic enzymes, and generate reactive oxygen species designed to eliminate and digest invading organisms and cell debris, thus limiting tissue damage (Figs 5.1, 5.2). Paradoxically, the release of lysosomal enzymes and reactive oxidants into the extracellular medium may also contribute to cell injury.

Thus, returning to the cardinal signs: the *redness* of inflammation is due to dilatation of the vascular beds within the injured area. *Heat* results from the increased blood flow, delivering blood at core temperature to areas, such as the skin, which are normally at a lower temperature. The exception to this, of course, being when the inflammatory reaction is also associated with fever. *Swelling* is a consequence of oedema formation caused by accumulation of fluid and plasma proteins in the extravascular spaces. *Pain* in inflammation is poorly understood, but may involve increased firing of sensory afferents in the effected area and as a result of increased pressure in the tissues, secondary to oedema formation. Additionally, some inflammatory mediators can directly cause pain or sensitize peripheral pain receptors to other stimuli. *Loss of function* probably arises from pain and swelling in the affected area.

These fundamental features may arise directly through damage to elements of the vascular system, through release of potent chemical mediators from cells resident in or recruited into the tissue, or activation of the complement cascade (Table 5.1). Indeed, as will be seen, the inflammatory response often involves the interaction between these cellular and enzyme systems (Fig. 5.1).

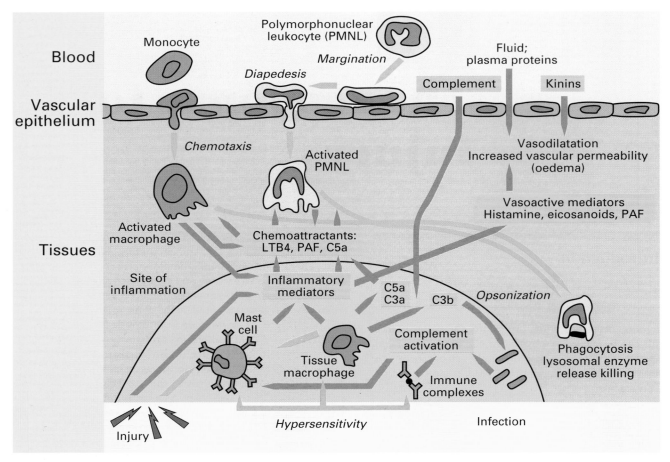

Fig. 5.1 Salient features of the inflammatory reaction. Following the primary stimulus (injury, hypersensitivity reactions, or infection) mast cells may be stimulated to release mediators, either directly in the case of sensitized mast cells or indirectly via the release of macrophage products or complement fragments and/or complement activated via the alternate pathway. These mediators induce local inflammation and stimulate the migration of circulating or marginated phagocytes into the tissues. These recruited cells move up the concentration gradient of chemotactic agents and accumulate at the site of inflammation. The secondary release of oxygen metabolites, granular enzymes, and inflammatory mediators, including chemotactic agents, serves to amplify the overall reaction. At the same time the increase in vascular permeability introduces plasma enzyme systems into the tissues which in association with cellular mediators facilitates the inflammatory reaction. Clearly if this process were uncontrolled, it could be self-generating, and may be so in chronic conditions. While the processes that control the resolution of inflammatory reactions remain poorly understood, however, neutrophil death and removal by macrophages are likely to be important.

5.2.1   Cells of the inflammatory reaction

As indicated above, the principal function of inflammatory reactions is the delivery of phagocytic cells to sites of trauma or immunological stimulation. The function of these cells is to eliminate particulate matter (bacteria, viruses, cell debris) through the process of phagocytosis. These effector cells originate from a common pluripotent stem cell in the bone marrow, where they proliferate and progress to terminal differentiation prior to release into the circulation. During inflammatory reactions the circulating phagocytes (polymorphonuclear neutrophils, monocytes, and macrophages) respond to chemotactic stimuli and selectively migrate into the inflamed tissue. The predominant cell in the early stages of acute inflammatory reactions is the neutrophil (Fig. 5.3) while in the later stages the

macrophage predominates (Fig. 5.4). In some special circumstances, particularly in allergic reactions or helminth infections, eosinophils may be present in large numbers, while in others (delayed hypersensitivity reactions) lymphocytes may predominate. To these cells we can add those normally resident in the tissues such as the mast cell, and also fibroblasts and fixed tissue macrophages, which are believed to be associated with progression to a more chronic state.

Neutrophils

Neutrophils (PMNLs) are normal constituents of the blood, representing about 60 per cent of the leucocyte pool. The bone marrow itself, however, is the major store of mature neutrophils and it has been calculated that approximately 10^{11} neutrophils

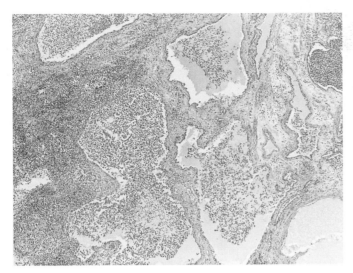

Fig. 5.2 An acute inflammatory lesion in bovine prostate gland. The exudate in the tissue and filling the gland is rich in plasma proteins and neutrophils. Macrophages can also be seen in some areas of the lesion.

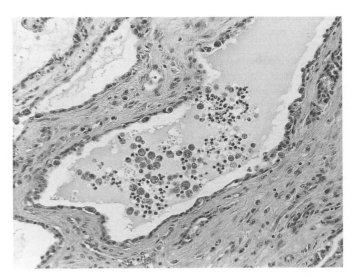

Fig. 5.4 A protein rich inflammatory exudate can be seen in the gland, with both neutrophils and macrophages present.

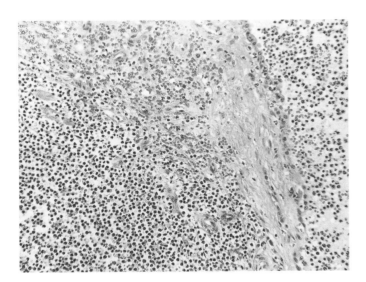

Fig. 5.3 At higher magnification neutrophils can be clearly identified in the tissues and there is evidence of haemorrhage.

Table 5.1 Principal mediators of the inflammatory reaction

Effect	Mediator
Vasodilatation	histamine PGI_2, PGD_2, PGE_2, PAF, C3a, C5a bradykinin
Increased microvascular permeability	histamine, PAF, LTC_4, LTD_4, bradykinin, C3a, C5a
Chemotaxins	PAF, LTB_4, C5a mast cell peptides
Cellular activation	PAF, IL-1, TNF

are released into the circulation each day. The mature circulating neutrophil is an end-stage cell with a short circulating half-life (about 8 h). Of those neutrophils in the circulation, over 50 per cent are adherent to the vascular endothelium. These adherent cells make up the marginated pool and are available for rapid release into the circulation or migration into the tissues. It is the appearance of these cells in the tissues which is a characteristic of acute inflammatory lesions.

During neutrophil maturation, in the bone marrow, the cell synthesizes myeloperoxidase, forms and packages azurophilic granules, and develops the capacity for movement and phagocytosis. Morphologically the mature neutrophil is characterized by its multilobed nucleus and granule-rich cytoplasm. Two main types of granule have been identified histochemically and by enzyme profiling. Large, dense primary azurophilic granules have characteristics of lysosomes and contain many enzymes, including acid hydrolases, myeloperoxidase, and lysozyme. The secondary, or specific, granules are smaller and, although they contain lysozyme and lactoferrin, their relative importance in killing and digesting micro-organisms is uncertain.

The primary granule constituents have the capacity to both kill and digest micro-organisms. Acid hydrolases are the predominant granular enzymes. They are involved in the hydrolysis of polysaccharides, mucopolysaccharides, and glycoprotein oligosaccharides into their constituent monomers, the breakdown of DNA and RNA into mononucleotides, and degradation of complex proteins, peptides, and lipids into smaller units. It has been suggested that these enzymes, as well as neutral proteases, may not be important in cell killing but are important for full digestion of the endocytosed particle. These enzymes are active only at acid pH and lysosomal pH is maintained at near 5 by an hydrogen-ion pump in the lysosomal membrane.

The cell-killing potential of the neutrophil is achieved through the action of other enzyme systems and generation of toxic oxygen metabolites. Myeloperoxidase is an abundant neutrophil constituent and is considered one of the principal cytotoxic elements of the neutrophil. In the presence of hydrogen peroxide and halides it catalyses the production of hypohalite ions which are toxic to bacteria, viruses, and mammalian cells. Other enzymes with bacterocidal activity include lysozyme and lactoferrin. The superoxide generating system is also associated with the lysosomal membrane.

In addition to the release of granular enzymes, neutrophils metabolize arachidonic acid through both the cyclo-oxygenase and lipoxygenase pathways. The principal product of neutrophil arachidonate metabolism is leukotriene B_4 (LTB_4) which, together with neutrophil-derived platelet-activating factor (PAF), may be involved in further amplification of neutrophil function and continued recruitment.

Neutrophils express membrane receptors for IgG subclasses, complement fragments, and chemotactic peptides and lipids, enabling them to respond, by migration or phagocytosis, to agents in their environment. Furthermore it is now quite clear that the state of neutrophil activation is up-regulated by agents in their environment and that this is crucial to the inflammatory response.

Since they are end-stage cells, neutrophils die in the tissues, and whole neutrophils as well as neutrophil debris are removed by macrophages. Indeed, it has been suggested that neutrophil death may act as a stimulus for the resolution of the inflammatory response.

Monocyte–macrophages

Cells of the monocyte–macrophage lineage play an essential role in host defence, not only because of their ability to phagocytose foreign or host material but also as a support to lymphocyte proliferation and antigen presentation.

Like the neutrophil, macrophages are derived from precursor cells in the bone marrow; indeed it is thought that both cell types are ultimately derived from a common progenitor myeloid cell. Mature monocytes are released into the circulation with a circulating half-life of about 1 day. Unlike neutrophils, however, there is no bone marrow store of monocytes and there is little evidence for the existence of a marginated pool. Circulating monocytes are slightly bigger than lymphocytes and appear to be a heterogeneous cell population, although this heterogeneity may simply reflect developmental differences in the circulating cells. Ultimately the destination of these cells is the tissues, where they transform into macrophages. It has been estimated that the pool of monocytes which have recently moved into the tissues is approximately 25 times greater than those circulating and there now is little doubt that these cells are destined to maintain the macrophage population. Migration into the tissues appears random, unless directed by local inflammation, and once resident their half-life is in the order of months. Both monocytes and macrophages share common morphological and membrane characteristics: a highly developed Golgi complex, many cytoplasmic granules, surface receptors for IgG–antibody complexes or monomers, low-affinity receptors for IgE, CR_1 and CR_3 receptors for complement components, receptors for cytokines and growth factors, and

receptors for chemotactic stimuli. Both cell types are actively phagocytic, produce reactive oxygen species, and have a spectrum of lysosomal enzymes, which are similar to those of the neutrophil, but which differ in the type of peroxidase present. They also metabolize arachidonic acid through both cyclo-oxygenase and lipoxygenase pathways, predominantly to thromboxane A_2 (TXA_2) and LTB_4, respectively.

The resident macrophage is a somewhat bigger cell than the circulating monocyte, has a greater rate of metabolic activity, and expresses greater numbers of membrane receptors. An important functional characteristic of the macrophage is its conversion from the resting state to that of the activated inflammatory macrophage. This activation is brought about by agents in its external environment. The activated cell is larger than the normal resident cell, has increased numbers of lysosomal granules, and more mitochondria. It has a greater capacity to phagocytose opsonized particles, shows increased rates of spreading and attachment to surfaces, forms more pseudopodia (suggesting increased mobility), and has an increased number of pinocytotic vesicles. In addition, the activated cell has increased levels of hydrolytic enzymes and a greater capacity to generate superoxide anions. These changes convey the activated cell with a greater antimicrobial capacity and ability to kill cells. Although the activated cell may be derived from the resident cell it now seems likely that they develop from more newly recruited monocytes.

The ability of the activated cell to phagocytose both large and smaller soluble molecules (pinocytosis) is, of course, well known, but in addition it also secretes a wide spectrum of inflammatory stimuli such as interleukin-1 (IL-1), tumour necrosis factor (TNF), PAF, and other factors which are chemotactic for and activate neutrophils, and which stimulate the degranulation of mast cells. They are also an important source of complement components. Interestingly, the spectrum of activities of macrophage products raises the possibility that at inflammatory sites they are self-activating.

Eosinophils

Eosinophil recruitment is not a usual characteristic of acute inflammatory lesions but is associated with allergic conditions, such as asthma, and during parasitic infestation. They are highly granulated cells with a greater capacity to produce superoxide anions than their close relative, the neutrophil. The eosinophil has a relatively poor phagocytic capability and degranulation usually proceeds via lysosomal fusion with the plasma membrane. Granular contents and superoxide are thus released outside the cell. In this respect eosinophil products, including cytotoxic cationic proteins, are involved in the killing of organisms too large for phagocytosis. The extracellular release of toxic species also suggests that eosinophil products may contribute to host cell destruction and dysfunction. It has been suggested that eosinophils also release substances that inhibit neutrophil recruitment and activation, but this needs to be clarified. Eosinophils are, in addition, major sources of leukotriene C_4 (LTC_4) and PAF.

Mast cells

Mast cells are present in great numbers in connective tissue and in mucosal membranes. They are a heterogeneous cell population, as defined by their enzyme and glycosaminoglycan content, and together with their circulating correlate, the basophil, are the main cellular source of histamine. They degranulate in response to a variety of stimuli, including basic polyamines, complement components, and physical, thermal, and chemical trauma. Mast cell membranes have high-affinity receptors for IgE, and dimerization of these receptors by interaction between cell-bound IgE and antigen is also a potent stimulus to degranulation. Mast cell products include histamine, prostaglandin D_2 (PGD_2), the leukotrienes, acid hydrolases, and chemotactic factors. Its reactivity to trauma and immunological stimuli implicate this cell in the initiation of inflammatory events.

5.2.2 Vascular changes in inflammation

Alterations in flow

Ultimately the means of delivery of inflammatory effectors to an inflammatory site is the vasculature, and observations of the microvasculature have identified alterations in blood flow through the area of insult as one of the earliest events of an inflammatory reaction. Blood flow through the microvasculature is largely determined by the inflow resistance of the pre-capillary arterioles and the outflow resistance through the post-capillary venules. In resting tissues only a few capillaries are involved in tissue perfusion.

Immediately following an inflammatory insult there is usually a transient vasoconstriction of the arterioles feeding the damaged tissue. This is thought to be a consequence of direct stimulation of vascular smooth muscle by the injury. This rapidly resolves and is invariably followed by a local vasodilatation and hyperaemia (erythrema). These changes can be observed, quite clearly, following mechanical abrasion of the skin; the so called Lewis triple response, where local flushing is followed by oedema formation and a more disseminated flare. The local flush is most likely due to release of vasodilator mediators, while the flare involves a neuronal reflex.

The changes in microcirculatory flow are brought about by alterations in the tone of arteriolar smooth muscle and opening of pre-capillary sphincters. Thus, following arteriolar dilatation there is a considerable increase in the size of the capillary bed being perfused. Capillaries have little or no smooth muscle and do not dilate, and there is probably little change in venular tone, although larger veins may contract. Blood flow rapidly increases and pressure in all vessels rises. First fluid and later plasma proteins are lost into the extravascular space; consequently there is an increase in the viscosity of the blood flowing through the capillary bed and vascular congestion (Fig. 5.5). This, coupled with the increased margination of PMNLs and platelets on to the vessel wall, may result in obstruction of microvessels by neutrophils and a slowing of capillary flow. In some instances, this ultimately leads to stasis, and nutritional

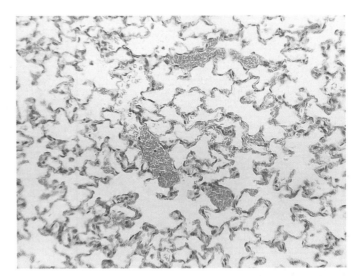

Fig. 5.5 A dilated alveolar vessel in guinea-pig lung showing gross vascular congestion after a mild inflammatory stimulus; note the integrity of the alveolar walls.

supply to the tissues may become so compromised that tissues become ischaemic or even necrotic.

Increased vascular permeability

All blood-vessels are lined by a continuous layer of endothelial cells which, in addition to having a metabolic function, provide a passive diffusion barrier, permitting water and solute flow while restricting the movement of larger molecules such as plasma proteins. Endothelial cells are joined by tight junctions but have pinocytotic vesicles distributed throughout their cytoplasm, giving them the ability to absorb macromolecules. It is thought that normal microvascular permeability to water is determined by the existence of small aqueous pores penetrating the membrane. Permeability to larger molecules might be accounted for by larger intercellular slits and the pinocytotic vesicles. In addition, in capillaries and post-capillary venules there is substantial endothelial thinning (fenestrations) and this may account for the increased passage of water and solutes that occurs at the venous end of the vascular bed. Furthermore, while tight junction structure is thought to be under the control of cytoskeletal elements, they may be less complex and therefore more permeable in small venules.

In normal conditions fluid loss through a vascular bed is governed by the balance between hydrostatic and oncotic pressures in the plasma and tissues, with fluid tending to be lost at the arterial end and reabsorbed at the venular end. The increase in capillary hydrostatic pressure resulting from the local vasodilatation after an inflammatory injury drives fluid out of the vascular compartment and into the extravascular spaces at a rate that is too rapid for reabsorption by the lymphatics to prevent the resulting oedema formation and tissue swelling (Fig. 5.6). This mechanism of fluid loss, however, does not explain the protein-rich exudate seen in inflammation. Thus simultaneous

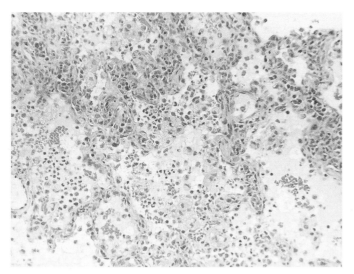

Fig. 5.6 Guinea-pig lung following a more severe inflammatory reaction. Neutrophils have migrated into the tissue and the inflammatory exudate has caused alveolar congestion.

with the changes in blood flow, an increased permeability of the microvasculature to larger molecules must occur. Such changes can be readily observed during *passive cutaneous anaphylaxis* (PCA). This is an experimental condition in which the dermis is passively sensitized and antigen and Evans blue dye is injected intravenously. This dye binds to plasma proteins and extravasation of the dye at the site of passive sensitization allows a measurement of leakage of plasma proteins to be made. The experimental use of colloidal carbon has localized the site of leakage to the junctions between endothelial cells.

It is now agreed that protein loss occurs following the opening of intercellular tight junctions, particularly those of the post-capillary venules. Why these junctions open remains poorly understood. Endothelial cells contain contractile elements (actin, myosin, troponin) and there is evidence that endothelial cells contract in response to inflammatory mediators. Loss of plasma proteins into the interstitium delivers plasma enzyme systems into the injured tissue and also increases extravascular oncotic pressure, pulling more fluid out of the vascular compartment. Generally, the intercellular tight junctions close again after 15–30 min. Frequently, however, there is a delayed opening of the junctions which may last for periods of hours, depending on the stimulus.

The changes in permeability may be brought about by the direct action of inflammatory mediators or through the secondary recruitment of effector cells. Interestingly, no humoral stimulus has yet been discovered that affects the permeability of capillaries: all stimuli analysed to date exert their effects on venular endothelium. In some types of inflammation, however, particularly that associated with burns, gross changes in capillary permeability are seen. The mechanisms underlying these changes remain unknown but most likely reflect direct damage to the vascular bed. The importance of increased blood flow to oedema formation, however, should not be underestimated.

Thus studies in which agents such as the vasoconstrictor peptidoleukotriene have been injected into the skin have clearly shown that oedema formation is substantially increased if they are co-injected with vasodilators.

5.2.3 Cellular accumulation

Inflammatory reactions which last more than a few hours are characterized by cellular accumulation within the area of insult.

Chemotaxis

Chemotaxis is the mechanism through which circulating cells gain access to the tissues, and can be defined as the directional movement of cells along a chemical gradient. This unidirectional movement of cells may also be accompanied by a chemokinetic response, namely an increase in speed of motion of the cell and in its frequency of directional changes. These responses are brought about by agents in the environment called *chemotaxins*. Thus the response of the cell to the local release of chemotactic agents is an integrated increase in motility of the cell coupled to its directed migration into the tissues up the concentration gradient of the released substance or substances.

During this chemotactic response there is a characteristic change in morphological orientation of the cell, be it neutrophil or macrophage. It loses its classic rounded appearance and becomes wedge shaped. At the leading edge pseudopodia extend, the nucleus is located towards the rear of the cell, the cytoplasm and lysosomal granules lying between the nucleus and advancing pseudopod. The morphological reorientation also involves the increased polymerization of microtubules which are involved in orientation and in determining the direction of movement. In addition, microfilament arrays become localized in the pseudopod. Movement of the cell is amoeboid, the phagocyte using the contractile elements actin and myosin within the advancing pseudopod to pull the rest of the cell behind it.

Essentially the chemotactic stimulus serves to attract cells, particularly marginated neutrophils into the tissue where they can phagocytose foreign particles or damaged host cells. Phagocytes, particularly neutrophils, are exquisitely sensitive to chemotactic agents, responding to changes in concentration of as little as 1 per cent over their length. In addition, following stimulation there is a movement of receptors for the chemotaxin to the leading edge of the cell and an increased expression of, and conformational change in, the receptors involved in adhesion to the vascular endothelium.

Interaction between circulating cells and the endothelium

The migration of cells out of the circulation with their accumulation at sites of inflammation is clearly a prominent feature of the inflammatory process. The interaction of mononuclear cells and PMNLs with the vascular endothelium, therefore, plays a central role in the movement of cells into the tissues.

Adherence of cells to the endothelium is the initial step in

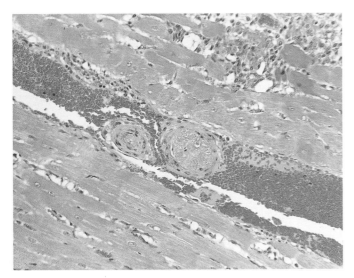

Fig. 5.7 Section of rat heart showing polymorphonuclear leucocytes marginated on to coronary vessels. The inflammatory lesion is in the right-hand corner of the plate with the PMNLs adherent to the side of the vessel adjacent to the lesion. Many neutrophils have migrated to the site of tissue damage.

their movement out of the vascular compartment (Figs 5.7, 5.8). This is achieved through altered expression and conformational changes in specific cell-surface glycoproteins (adhesion molecules) in response to the chemotactic agent. Using monoclonal antibodies, directed against specific leucocyte/lymphocyte surface antigens, a related family of three adhesion glycoproteins (*the CD11/CD18 receptor complex*) has been identified as being important for cell adhesion. This complex is a heterodimer composed of a common β subunit (CD18) but which differs in its α subunits. These 3 adhesion molecules termed LFA-1 (CD11a/CD18), Mac-1 (CD11b/CD18), and p150,95 (CD11c/CD18) are present on phagocytes and the expression and conformational state of these glycoproteins is necessary for adhesion of circulating cells to the vascular endothelium and subsequent migration into inflamed tissues. Indeed patients who are genetically deficient in this family of adhesion molecules frequently develop severe infections in which accumulation of PMNLs at the inflamed site is severely impaired. In addition CD11b is also the CR3 receptor for C3bi. Furthermore, while normal neutrophils express few adhesion molecules on their surface, they appear to be rapidly increased following exposure to chemotaxins such as C5a, FMLP, or LTB$_4$, probably through cycling from an intracellular pool.

The endothelial cell also expresses adhesion molecules, although these differ from those of circulating cells. Two main subclasses of receptor have been identified and are classified as *intercellular adhesion molecules* (ICAM 1 and 2) and *endothelial cell–leucocyte adhesion molecule* (ELAM-1). These adhesion molecules are increased in number by cytokines, through a process that probably involves synthesis of new proteins, and are thought to interact with the CD11/CD18 complex.

Endothelial cells also have the capacity to synthesize and release factors that may have pro- or anti-inflammatory functions. One such factor, discussed in more detail in a later section, is PAF which has potent inflammatory activity. In addition, a number of stimuli (shear-stress, activated neutrophils, peptidoleukotrienes, histamine) release a product from endothelial cells, probably prostacyclin (PGI$_2$), that reduces granulocyte adherence. The balance between these two factors may therefore play a pivotal role in regulating feedback cycles which determine the severity of some inflammatory reactions.

Following adhesion to the endothelium, the responding cell

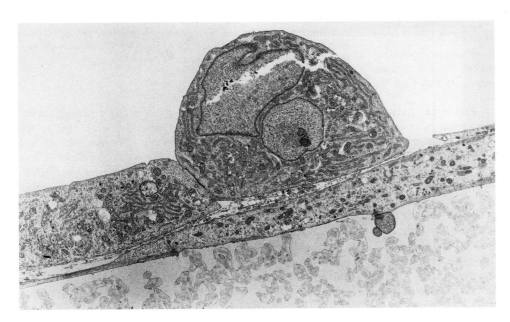

Fig. 5.8 Electronmicrograph of a blood monocyte adherent to a vascular endothelial cell *in vitro* prior to migration through an endothelial cell monolayer.

extends pseudopodia into the tight junction between adjacent endothelial cells and pushes between them by amoeboid motion (a process termed emigration). The mechanism by which the cell penetrates the basement membrane is obscure, but may involve release of lysosomal elastase and collagenase. Disruption to the basement membrane is transient and rapid repair mechanisms maintain its integrity. The neutrophil is the first cell type to be recruited to the site of damage or immune reaction, perhaps reflecting the large number of these cells marginated on arteriolar or capillary endothelium. As the cell approaches the inflammatory focus there is an increase in concentration of chemotactic factors in the cells microenvironment. This stimulates the recruited cells to aggregate, localizing them to the damaged area, and there is stimulation of the exocytotic release of inflammatory mediators and degranulation. The ultimate function of the recruited cells is to engulf and destroy foreign material and to remove damaged cells and debris. The process by which this occurs is termed *phagocytosis* (Fig. 5.9).

Phagocytosis

Neutrophils and macrophages have an inherent capacity to recognize and engulf foreign particles through recognition of surface carbohydrates via cell-surface receptors for mannose and fucose. The exposure of foreign material to serum proteins, however, greatly enhances this phagocytic capacity. The process by which particles are coated with serum proteins, to render them more readily phagocytosed is called *opsonization*. The opsonins which prepare the foreign material for phagocytosis are well known and comprise antibodies against the particle (principally IgG) and activated complement fragments (C3bi). As mentioned previously, neutrophils and macrophages have receptors on their surface that recognize the different subtypes of IgG, attaching to the Fc portion of the immunoglobulin and also receptors recognizing complement components. The first stage of phagocytosis is therefore attachment of these receptors to their respective ligands. It has now become clear that the expression of these receptors is subject to immunological regulation and can be increased by exposure to chemotactic agents. Furthermore, if both IgG and C3bi opsonize the particle, phagocytosis is greatly enhanced.

When the PMNL or macrophage has bound to the particle there is a localized contraction under the point of contact, resulting in the formation of a cup-shaped invagination. Pseudopods adhere to the opsonized area and enclose it within a vacuole. Contraction of microfilaments at the plasma membrane results in closure of the vacuole and formation of the phagosome (Fig. 5.10). The cell only interacts with areas of the foreign object that have bound ligand: thus if only part of the particle is opsonized then the cell only interacts with this area and there is no phagosome formation.

Movement of the phagosome towards the granule-rich areas of the cytoplasm results in fusion of the phagosome with nearby lysosomes. Lysosomal contents are discharged into the phagosome and its membrane is incorporated into the vacuole

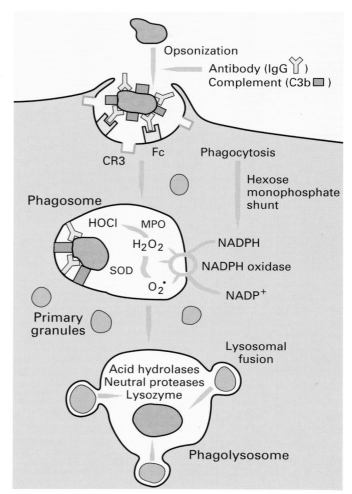

Fig. 5.9 The primary events of phagocytosis. The opsonized particle is enclosed within a vacuole and internalized. This process activates the hexose monophosphate shunt which ultimately transfers electrons into the phagosome. The sequential action of superoxide dismutase (SOD) and myeloperoxidase (MPO) results in formation of hypochlorite anions. Lysosomal fusion with the phagosome releases granular enzymes into the phagolysosome and digestion of the internalized particle occurs.

membrane; the resulting organelle is called *a phagolysosome*. Generally, release of lysosomal enzymes is restricted to the phagolysosome. When phagolysosome formation occurs in a granule-rich area of the cytoplasm, however, discharge of lysosomal enzymes may occur prior to closure of the phagosome. Under these conditions lytic enzymes and reactive oxygen species can escape into the extracellular space causing damage to host cells in the vicinity. Similarly, if the phagocyte attempts to engulf a particle that is too large, frustrated phagocytosis occurs and there is gross extracellular release of lysosomal contents.

Ultimately, the objective of phagocytosis is killing and digestion of bacteria and cell debris. This is achieved by release into the phagolysosome of lytic enzymes that break down the extracellular matrix, cell proteins, and lipids. Indeed, the battery of

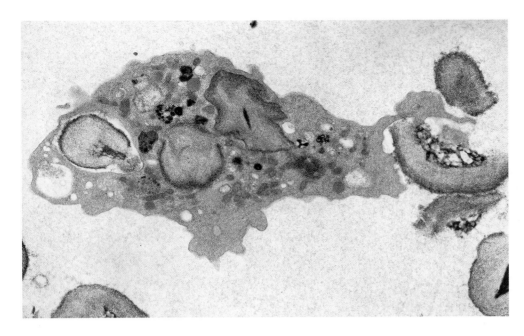

Fig. 5.10 Electromicrograph of a neutrophil showing many cytoplasmic granules and phaocytosed particles.

enzymes and cationic proteins released is capable of breaking down most cellular constituents (see Table 5.2). In addition, phagocytosis is associated with a burst of metabolic activity. Activation of the hexose monophosphate shunt generates NADPH, there is an increased activity of the membrane-associated enzyme NADPH oxidase and reduction of molecular oxygen to its superoxide anion. The release of this cytotoxic species is vectored to the outside of the membrane which during phagocytosis is, of course, into the phagolysosome. A series of sequential reactions are also activated. In neutrophils, superoxide is converted to hydrogen peroxide (by superoxide dismutase) and in the presence of the granular enzyme myeloperoxidase and halide this is converted to highly reactive and toxic hypohalite ions; indeed the HOCl anion is thought to be the final oxidant produced.

Products of the degranulation process are transported into the cytoplasm and incorporated into macromolecules or metabolized further. Indigestible material is maintained in the phagosome, and lysosomal membranes are recycled through the plasma membrane.

Inactivation of lysosomal fusion and generation of oxidants is poorly understood. The oxygen burst is short-lived (15–30 min) and myeloperoxidase may be involved in inactivation of superoxide-generating systems. Lysosomal enzymes may be inactivated by autolysis.

5.2.4 Mediators of the inflammatory reaction

Historically, observations of local inflammatory reactions have led to suggestions that they are humorally mediated. In 1910 Sir Henry Dale demonstrated that histamine could mimic many

Table 5.2 The principal secretory products of phagocytic cells

Oxidants
Superoxide anion (MNE)
Hydrogen peroxide (MNE)
Hypochlorous acid (MNE)
Hydroxyl radicals (MNE)

Enzymes
Lysozyme (MNE)
β-Glucuronidase (MNE)
N-Acetyl glucosaminidase (MN)
Collagenase (MNE)
Elastase (MN)
Cathepsins (MN)
Peroxidase (M)
Eosinophil peroxidase (E)
Myeloperoxidase (N)
Aryl sulphatase (E)

Cytotoxic proteins
Eosinophil cationic protein E
Major basic protein (E)
Eosinophil neurotoxin (E)
Tumor necrosis factor (M)

Inflammatory mediators
Platelet activating factor (MNE)
Leukotriene B_4 (MN)
Leukotriene C_4 (E)
Thromboxane A_2 (MN)
Prostaglandins (MN)
Complement fragments (M)
Interleukin-1 (M)

M = macrophage product, N = neutrophil product, E = eosinophil product.

of the features of acute anaphylaxis, and in 1927 Sir Thomas Lewis suggested that histamine or a histamine-like substance might account for wheal and flare reactions in the skin. The effects of histamine, however, were more transient that those seen in most inflammatory reactions, implicating other agents in their generation and maintenance. In the intervening years the involvement of multiple mediators in immune and inflammatory reactions has become well established and the list of endogenous chemicals that can minic some or all of the characteristic signs of inflammation is now extensive, as is the list of chemicals identified in inflammatory exudates (Table 5.1). It should be emphasized, however, that although discussed here in isolation, the overall response is determined by interaction between multiple inflammatory mediators and systems. Thus, as will be seen in the following sections, few mediators have a spectrum of activity that can encompass all inflammatory events. Furthermore, inhibition of the synthesis or action of single mediators, while attenuating some inflammatory signs, is poorly effective in preventing all aspects of the inflammatory response.

Histamine

Derived from the essential amino acid histidine via the action of the enzyme histidine decarboxylase (Fig. 5.11), histamine is widely distributed throughout the body and is a normal constituent of most tissues. While the tissue content is high, the level of free histamine in body fluids is low and this is achieved by its storage as an inactive macromolecular complex. Its major site of storage in tissues is the mast cell, whereas its correlate in the circulation is the basophil. It is stored as a complex with either heparin or chondroitin sulphate in granules that also contain proteolytic enzymes and acid hydrolases. Histamine has potent effects on smooth muscle, eliciting contraction of some structures, notably the airways, gut, and large blood-vessels, and relaxation of others, such as arterioles. Its effects are mediated by interaction with at least two specific receptor types, designated H_1 and H_2, as characterized by specific antagonism by compounds such as mepyramine and cimetidine, respectively. The actions of histamine in local vascular beds parallels those seen in early inflammatory reactions and include transient (10–15 min) vasodilatation and increased vascular permeability. The vasodilator properties of histamine are mediated by both H_1 and H_2 receptors, while changes in vascular permeability are a consequence of interaction with H_1 receptors alone.

Histamine is also chemokinetic for PMNLs and exerts an

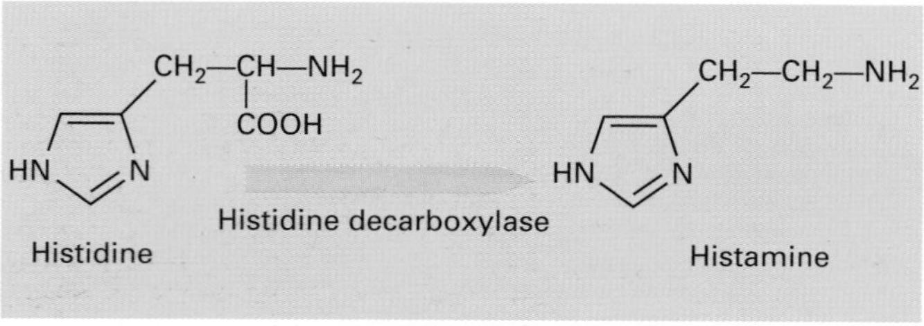

Fig. 5.11 Histidine metabolism to histamine.

immunomodulatory role, suppressing a variety of lymphocyte responses and its own release from mast cells.

Histamine release has been demonstrated in man during a variety of inflammatory conditions, including anaphylaxis, urticaria, and following thermal injury. However, although erythema and oedema formation can be reduced by histamine antagonists, this is largely restricted to early inflammatory changes and even then a non-histamine component persists.

Lipid mediators

Eicosanoids

Eicosanoids do not exist preformed in cells but are synthesized *de novo* following inflammatory stimuli or through the secondary action of other mediators (Fig. 5.12). Both the prostaglandins and leukotriene families of eicosanoid mediators are derived from the 20-carbon, polyunsaturated, essential fatty acid arachidonic acid. The concentration of free arachidonate in the cell is low but it is liberated, largely from phosphatidylcholine and phosphatidylinositol following hydrolysis by phospholipase A_2 or phospholipase C, respectively. The arachidonic acid so released can then be enzymatically oxygenated via two independent pathways or re-esterified into membrane phospholipids.

The cyclo-oxygenase pathway Fatty acid cyclo-oxygenase is a microsomal enzyme which adds molecular oxygen as a peroxide linking C9 and C11 and as a hydroperoxide at C15, yielding the cyclic endoperoxide PGG_2. It also catalyses the conversion of this intermediate to the C15-hydroxy product PGH_2, which is the pivotal precursor for the pathway leading to synthesis of the classical prostaglandins through a series of synthetase and isomerase enzymes (PGI_2, TXA_2, PGD_2, PGE_2) or by reduction ($PGF_{2\alpha}$). While most cells have the capacity to generate most, if not all, of these products, there is some selectivity, with platelets and macrophages producing predominantly TXA_2 and endothelial cells PGI_2. PGD_2 is the principal prostanoid produced by mast cells and PGE_2 by the microvasculature. In the circulation the prostanoids have short half-lives and there is almost quantitative metabolism in a single pass through the pulmonary circulation.

Prostaglandins have been shown to be released in response to a variety of inflammatory stimuli and show a spectrum of biological activities. In the vasculature, prostaglandins of the E series, PGI_2, and PGD_2 are predominantly potent vasodilators (PGI_2 also being anti-aggregatory for platelets), whereas TXA_2 is a vasoconstrictor and stimulates platelet aggregation.

Although there is some evidence for a direct effect of PGEs in increasing microvascular permeability, they are relatively ineffective. It is well established, however, that PGE_1 and PGE_2 are able to potentiate microvascular leakage to other agents. Despite their well-documented effects on platelet function, prostanoids are only weak chemotactic agents.

The pro-inflammatory activity of the prostanoids, however, is complicated by immunoregulatory effects on some inflammatory cells. Thus some prostaglandins increase cAMP levels and, as a consequence, inhibit platelet-release reactions, lysosomal

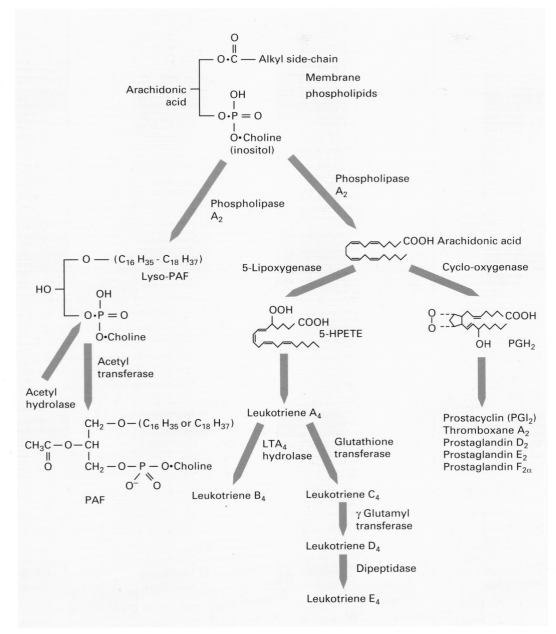

Fig. 5.12 The pivotal role of membrane phospholipids in the formation of three potent classes of inflammatory mediator.

enzyme release from PMNLs, and inhibit mast cell and basophil histamine release. In addition some prostanoids, particularly PGE_2 and stable analogues of PGI_2, are potent cytoprotective agents protecting hepatocytes and the gastrointestinal tract against the effects of a number of noxious stimuli.

The potency of aspirin and other non-steroidal anti-inflammatory agents in suppressing or reducing the severity of a variety of inflammatory conditions correlates well with their efficacy as inhibitors of fatty acid cyclo-oxygenase, suggesting

that the prostanoids play an important role in some acute inflammatory conditions.

The lipoxygenase pathway The second pathway for oxygenation of arachidonic acid leads to the formation of leukotrienes (LTs) and mono-eicosatetraenoic acids. The family of lipoxygenase enzymes (primarily 5-, 12-, and 15-lipoxygenases) oxygenate arachidonic acid to yield hydroperoxy intermediates. The product of the 5-lipoxygenase pathway (5-HPETE) can undergo enzymatic dehydration to yield LTA$_4$. Further metabolism proceeds in two directions: enzymatic hydrolysis to give LTB$_4$; or addition of glutathione at C6 yielding the peptidoleukotriene LTC$_4$, sequential loss of glutamine and glycine residues resulting in formation of LTD$_4$ and LTE$_4$, respectively. It is now well established that these three moieties express the biological activities once attributed to the so-called slow-reacting substance of anaphylaxis. The peptidoleukotrienes are a potent family of inflammatory mediators, being approximately 100–1000 times more potent than histamine as smooth-muscle spasmogens. In animals, leukotrienes C$_4$ and D$_4$ have profound effects on the cardiovascular system, producing rapid contraction of arteries and microvascular vessels: injection into the skin resulting in immediate blanching. These agents are also potent inducers of microvascular leakage, although this effect (particularly to LTC$_4$) is often masked by the reduction in blood flow following the local vasoconstriction. In man they have been reported to elicit both wheal and flare; the mechanism of the flare, however, is uncertain. Plasma leakage, however, is markedly potentiated by vasodilator prostaglandins.

Whereas the peptidoleukotrienes are potent spasmogens, leukotriene B$_4$ shows different biological activity. It is a powerful chemoattractant for neutrophils and stimulates PMNL aggregation and lysosomal enzyme release. It has also been reported to increase plasma leakage, although this is secondary to PMNL activation. Administration of LTB$_4$ *in vivo* into the lungs, skin, or peritoneal cavity results in accumulation of PMNLs, confirming that its principal action at inflammatory sites is recruitment of circulating cells.

Leukotriene release into inflammatory exudates and body fluids during a number of inflammatory conditions (asthma, antigen challenge, blister fluids, urticaria, psoriatic lesions) has been established and, clearly, the spectrum of biological activities of lipoxygenase products is consistent with them having a major role in inflammatory diseases. Furthermore recent studies in animal models using selective leukotriene antagonists have indicated that peptidoleukotriene, along with histamine, play a significant part in mediating the increase in microvascular leakage associated with airway and cutaneous hypersensitivity reactions. The current development of specific receptor antagonists and 5-lipoxygenase inhibitors will help to elucidate a functional role for these agents in human inflammatory disease.

Platelet-activating factor (PAF)

In the early 1970s a factor released from leucocytes that caused platelet aggregation was described by a number of research groups. This factor, identified as a phospholipid, was consequently termed platelet-activating factor (PAF). PAF, like the eicosanoids, is not stored within cells and is synthesized on cell activation (Fig. 5.12): hydrolysis of membrane phospholipids, by the enzyme phospholipase A$_2$ yields both arachidonic acid and a substance, lyso-PAF, that is both the precursor and metabolite of PAF. In general, most cells and organs release much greater amounts of lyso-PAF than PAF itself. This may be due to rapid conversion of PAF, by the highly active cytosolic enzyme

acetyl hydrolase, back to lyso-PAF, or alternatively rapid release of lyso-PAF into the extracellular medium, making it unavailable to the transferase enzyme. It does seem likely, however, that much of the PAF generated by inflammatory cells remains cell-associated. While PAF itself is one of the most potent biological moieties known, lyso-PAF is largely devoid of activity. Lyso-PAF (along with PAF itself), however, is cytotoxic and is rapidly inactivated by acylation, with incorporation of arachidonate back into the molecule and reintegration into the plasma membrane.

PAF is synthesized by a variety of cell types, including platelets, leucocytes, macrophages, endothelial cells, and has been detected in a number of biological fluids following inflammatory stimuli. Its spectrum of biological activities also strongly indicates its involvement in a variety of inflammatory conditions, such as bronchial asthma, endotoxic shock, immediate and delayed hypersensitivity reactions, and ischaemic disease.

In animals, when injected intravenously, PAF elicits bronchospasm, hypotension, reductions in circulating platelet and neutrophil numbers, and increases microvascular permeability. Direct administration into the airways triggers an inflammatory response involving oedema formation and recruitment of macrophages, PMNLs, and platelets. Injection into the skin similarly results in plasma leakage and cell accumulation. In man, intradermal PAF injection produces an immediate wheal and flare reaction which can be potentiated by vasodilators. In addition, some authors have reported that PAF elicits dual responses that are reminiscent of those seen after antigen challenge in allergic subjects, and an associated recruitment of monocytes and eosinophils.

Interestingly, cells that release PAF are also activated by it and PAF therefore has the capacity to stimulate its own release. As mentioned previously, PAF is one of the most potent promoters of microvascular leakage, causing endothelial cell retraction and blebbing. PAF also induces PMNL and monocyte recruitment and activation and is a potent chemoattractant for eosinophils.

Perhaps one of the more interesting activities of PAF is its ability to augment the effects of other agents. Aerosols of PAF produce long-lasting increases in airway reactivity to other spasmogens. *In vitro*, PAF amplifies superoxide and leukotriene release from PMNLs, amplifies interleukin-1 and tumour necrosis factor production by macrophages and monocytes, leukotriene release from eosinophils and granulocyte–macrophage colony-stimulating factor (GM-CSF) release from endothelial cells. One of the functions of PAF may, therefore, be to 'prime' cells, resulting in enhanced responses to other inflammatory stimuli.

Recently, potent and specific PAF antagonists have become available and will help to clarify the potential central role of PAF in inflammatory reactions. In animals, bronchoconstriction due to aerosolized antigen and endotoxin or immune shock are attenuated by PAF antagonists. In addition, hypotension, oedema, and neutropenia following immune complex or antigen administration, also to animals, is reduced by PAF antagonists, as is ischaemic damage to the heart and gastrointestinal tract. Although their involvement in clinical inflammatory conditions remains to be clarified, PAF antagonists have been reported to reduce allergic wheal and flare reactions in man.

Plasma enzyme systems

Complement

Complement is the term given to a complex enzyme system which is crucial to host defence. Simplistically, activation of the complement cascade, with its localization to membranes and particulate surfaces, followed by sequential activation of the next proteinase precursor in the sequence, gives rise to a stable unit (*the membrane attack complex*) that causes membrane disruption and cell lysis. The cytolytic effects of the system, however, are localized by virtue of their association with cell membranes or immune complexes. In addition to the cytolytic activity, components of the complement cascade have a more disseminated effect and cause a number of inflammatory responses.

The complement system can be activated by antigen/antibody complexes (the classical pathway) or by a non-specific process (the alternative pathway) that bypasses the initial events in the classical pathway (Fig. 5.13). The two activation paths, however, both result in the production of enzymes that convert C3 to an active product C3b and yields another enzyme, the C5 convertase which catalyses the conversion of the fifth complement component to yield C5a.

Opsonization, the coating of particles, whether they be bacteria or inert, with C3bi, is a major function of the complement system. Receptors for this complement fragment are found on the surface of a variety of phagocytic cells, including macrophages, neutrophils, and eosinophils. The binding of C3bi, therefore, is a pivotal event in the ingestion of foreign particles by phagocytes, enhancing their adherence and promoting phagocytosis.

The complement fragments C3a and C5a, the so-called anaphylatoxins, also exert powerful pro-inflammatory effects, although C5a is approximately 20 times more potent than C3a. Both agents cause smooth-muscle contraction and increase venular permeability, the latter being thought to require the presence of PMNLs. Additionally, C5a is a chemoattractant for neutrophils and stimulates mast cell degranulation and neutrophil superoxide generation.

Kinins

Kinin formation can occur in plasma and in extracellular fluids through the activation of proteolytic enzymes called *kallikreins* and the subsequent cleavage of high molecular weight precursor proteins (*kininogens*) to biologically active nona- and decapeptides (*bradykinin* and *kallidin*, respectively). Contact of blood with negatively charged surfaces (such as collagen, basement membranes, and bacterial cell walls) or activation of the clotting cascade results in conversion of plasma pre-kallikrein to the active form of the enzyme. Alternatively, kallikrein can be directly released from activated mast cells. Once cleaved from the precursor kininogen, the active peptides have short tissue and circulating half-lives and are rapidly inactivated by the enzyme carboxypeptidase N.

Injected or infused intravenously, bradykinin produces a short-lived fall in blood pressure as a result of a reduction in total peripheral resistance. In the peripheral circulation, local administration of bradykinin intravenously produces arteriolar dilatation, increased capillary flow, contraction of veins, and increased plasma leakage into the tissues. Not surprisingly, therefore, when injected into the skin, bradykinin produces a classical wheal and flare reaction. In addition, bradykinin also produces pain when administered locally through stimulation of peripheral pain receptors.

While kinin formation and kallikrein release have been demonstrated in a variety of inflammatory conditions, including local antigen challenge and reactive hyperaemia, their importance to the inflammatory reaction remains uncertain until specific receptor antagonists become available.

Cytokines

Of particular importance in the control of cell proliferation, differentiation/activation and crucial to host defence, are a diverse group of glycosolated proteins, collectively called *cytokines*.

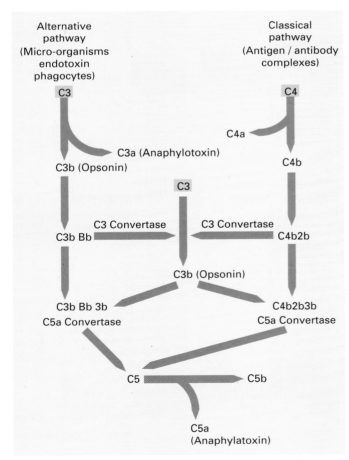

Fig. 5.13 The complement pathway.

These agents regulate the interaction between cells involved in immune or inflammatory reactions and act on progenitor cells in the bone marrow to increase release of some cell types into the circulation or to induce maturation of others.

Interleukins are a family of related glycopeptides, of approximately 130–270 amino acids. Interleukin-1 (IL-1α and β) is released predominantly from activated monocytes and macrophages, although a number of other cell types, including endothelial cells, epithelial cells, and neutrophils, have been shown to generate IL-1-like activities. IL-1 exerts a number of important effects on T-cell, macrophage, and neutrophil functions. T-helper cells are stimulated to release IL-2 and to increase expression of IL-2 receptors; furthermore it has been suggested that IL-1 is a required factor supporting T-cell activation and clonal expansion. IL-1 is also a co-stimulant, supporting B-cell proliferation and antibody production. In addition to its effects on the immune system, IL-1 also increases neutrophil release from the bone marrow, is chemotactic for neutrophils and monocyte/macrophages, stimulates degranulation and superoxide release from these cells, and increases expression of adhesion molecules by endothelial cells. In addition IL-1 is the major endogenous pyrogen.

Interleukin-2, released from T-cells is primarily a T-cell growth factor and augments B-cell proliferation and antibody production. Interleukins 3–6 are a group of T-cell factors which affect differentiation and proliferation of cells having inflammatory and immune functions. IL-3 is a multi-lineage colony-stimulating factor stimulating increased neutrophil and macrophage formation. It is, in addition, thought to be essential for mast cell proliferation. IL-4 and IL-6 are differentiation factors for B-lymphocytes, while IL-5 induces myeloid progenitors to differentiate into eosinophils.

Interferons (IFN) were identified by virtue of their ability to inhibit viral replication; IFNγ, however, also induces receptor expression on antigen-presenting cells and augments lymphokine activities. It has been shown to increase T-cell expression of IL-2 receptors, enhance T-cell cytotoxic activity, induce TNF production and to prime macrophages, so enhancing their phagocytic potential. INFγ also enhances B-cell proliferation, induces or enhances immunoglobulin production, and synergizes with IL-2.

Tumour necrosis factor (TNF), is produced by activated lymphocytes and macrophages and exerts a number of activities important to inflammatory and immune responses. It was first identified because of its cytotoxic and antitumour activity but has since been shown to interact synergistically with IL-1 and IFN to induce expression of leucocyte and endothelial adhesion molecules and in PMNL activation.

Thus the cytokines are highly potent factors released principally from lymphocytes and monocytes/macrophages following immunological stimulation, or non-specifically following phagocytosis or cell injury. IL-1 and TNF are considered of particular importance in inflammation and their biological activities are wide ranging; however, their effects on cell proliferation and activation indicates that they may serve to amplify and prolong inflammatory reactions.

Neurogenic influences

In 1927 Lewis attributed the disseminated flare seen after skin abrasion to neuronal influences, and it is thought that this is a result of substance P (SP) release from non-adrenergic non-cholinergic nerve fibres (NANC). Nearly all blood-vessels and other smooth muscles are innervated by SP-containing nerves, and when injected into the skin SP produces a wheal and flare reaction. In addition *capsaicin*, the extract of hot peppers, when injected intradermally also causes local vasodilatation through a mechanism that involves sensory fibre firing and SP release.

Recently, SP has been shown to be co-stored with the potent vasodilator *calcitonin gene-related peptide* (CGRP). This substance, when injected into the skin of animals, also causes a very long-lasting and widespread flare and potentiates SP-induced oedema formation (wheal reaction), suggesting possible synergism between these two neuropeptides, although this needs to be confirmed in man.

SP responses in the skin are attenuated by H_1-receptor antagonists and SP is a well-documented stimulus to mast cell degranulation, suggesting that some of the inflammatory effects of neuronal activation may be indirect and a result of local histamine release. In addition, inflammatory events still occur in denervated tissues and in the presence of local anaesthetics. Therefore, it is likely that although neuronal stimulation can mimic the early features of inflammatory reactions, its contribution to the overall response is small compared to those of the humoral mediators.

5.2.5   Consequences and resolution of the inflammatory reaction

By definition, acute inflammatory reactions resolve within a matter of a few hours or days, depending on the severity of the stimulus. Ultimately, resolution of the process depends largely

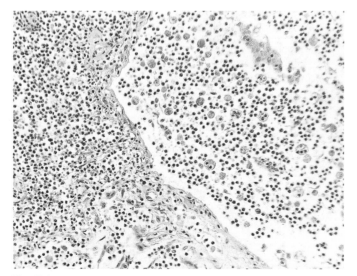

Fig. 5.14 Macrophages and neutrophils in inflamed bovine prostate. Neutrophils can be seen within macrophage phagosomes.

on the removal of the stimulus and tissue repair. Increased local blood flow and altered microvascular permeability subside, oedema is reversed by drainage of fluid and plasma proteins into the lymphatics. Fibrin deposits are broken down by plasmin and removed by the lymphatics. Neutrophils die locally and are replaced by macrophages, while discharged lysosomal contents are added to the inflammatory exudate and drain into the lymphatics. Macrophages ingest the majority of the cell debris and dead neutrophils (Fig. 5.14) and either leave in the lymphatics or remain in the tissue.

If the inflammatory stimulus persists or there are large areas of cell death then scar formation ensues. The area may be encapsulated within heavy fibrin deposits which may be too dense to be broken down by fibrinolytic enzymes. Mononuclear cells migrate into the fibrous tissue, followed by fibroblasts, vascularization of the tissue, and formation of a dense fibrous scar; this is discussed in the following sections.

5.2.6 Further reading

General

Charlesworth, E. N., Hood, A. F., Soter, N. A., *et al.* (1989). Cutaneous late-phase response to allergan. Mediator release and inflammatory cell infiltration. *Journal of Clinical Investigation* **83**, 1519–26.

Glynn, L. E., Houck, J. C., and Weissmann, G. (series eds). *The handbook of inflammation*, Vols 1–5. Elsevier, Amsterdam.

Henson, P. M. and Johnston, R. B. (1987). Tissue injury in inflammation. Oxidants, proteinases and cationic proteins. *Journal of Clinical Investigation* **79**, 669–74.

Willoughby, D. A. (ed.) (1987). *Inflammation—mediators and mechanisms*. *British Medical Bulletin*, Vol. 43, No. 2. Churchill Livingstone, London.

Cells

Anderson, D. C., Schmalsteig, M. J., Finegold, M. J., *et al.* (1985). The severe and moderate phenotypes of inheritable Mac-1, LFA-1 deficiency: their quantitative definition and relation to leukocyte dysfunction and clinical features. *Journal of Infectious Diseases* **152**, 668–89.

Johnston, R. B. (1988). Monocytes and macrophages. *New England Journal of Medicine* **318**, 747–52.

Hogg, J. C. (1987). Neutrophil kinetics and lung injury. *Physiology Review* **67**, 1249–95.

Malech, H. D. and Gallin, J. I. (1988). Neutrophils in human diseases. *New England Journal of Medicine* **37**, 687–94.

Savill, J. S., Wyllie, A. H., Henson, J. E., *et al.* (1989). Macrophage phagocytosis of aging neutrophils in inflammation. *Journal of Clinical Investigation* **83**, 865–76.

Schleiffman, B., Moser, R., Patarroyo, M., and Fehr, J. (1989). The cell surface glycoprotein Mac-1 (CD11b/CD18) mediates neutrophil adhesion and modulates degranulation independently of its quantitative cell surface expression. *Journal of Immunology* **142**, 3537–45.

Stevens, R. L. and Austen, K. F. (1989). Recent advances in the cellular and molecular biology of mast cells. *Immunology Today* **10**, 381–6.

Venge, P. (1990). What is the role of the eosinophil? *Thorax* **35**, 161–3.

Venge, P., Hakansson, L., and Peterson, G. B. (1987). Eosinophil activation in allergic disease. *International Archives in Allergy and Applied Immunology* **82**, 333–7.

Mediators

Barnes, P. J., Chung, K. F., and Page, C. P. (1988). Inflammatory mediators and asthma. *Pharmacological Review* **40**, 49–84.

Braquet, P., Touqui, L., Shen, T. Y., and Vargaftig, B. B. (1987). Perspectives in platelet-activating factor research. *Pharmacological Review* **39**, 97–145.

O'Flaherty, J. T. (1982). Lipid mediators of inflammation and allergy. *Laboratory Investigation* **47**, 314–29.

Mantovani, A. and Dejana, E. (1989). Cytokines as communication signals between leukocytes and endothelial cells. *Immunology Today* **10**, 371–5.

Pace-Asciak, C. and Granstrom, E. (eds) (1983). *Prostaglandins and related substances*. New Comprehensive Biochemistry, Vol. 5. Elsevier, Amsterdam.

Serafin, W. E. and Austen, K. F. (1987). Mediators of immediate hypersensitivity reactions. *New England Journal of Medicine* **317**, 30–4.

5.3 Repair and regenerative responses

M. R. Alison

In Section 5.2 we discussed the immediate responses of tissues to acute damage, be it trauma or mediated by one of the many agents that cause inflammation. In this section we survey the phenomena and mechanisms that ensue, leading to restitution of the injury.

5.3.1 Wound healing

Introduction

Man in general is subject to a wide range of injuries, both accidentally and deliberately inflicted, which are insufficient to cause death of the individual. *Healing*, a response to this injury, can comprise a number of processes including fibrosis and a partial or complete restitution of organ structure and function. Of course, inflammation is invariably associated with the healing response, although—only for convenience—the two processes are usually considered separately. It is customary to consider healing in two parts; *regeneration*, which is the replacement of lost cells by cells of the same type (usually applied to epithelial cells) and which can sometimes return the tissue to its pristine state, and *repair*, which involves the synthesis of connective tissue and its eventual maturation into scar tissue. In many cases, both processes contribute to the healing response and, for this reason, together with easy accessibility, the healing of linear skin wounds has been the subject of exhaustive investigation. While the regeneration and repair that follow skin wounding will serve as a prototype of the healing process, the discussion would not be complete without presenting the considerable information that is now available on healing processes in various internal organs. Local modifications of the general principles of healing can affect the degree of structural and functional reconstitution achieved in these organs. For example, vigorous healing responses can themselves on occasion generate new lesions of pathological significance: examples are the strictures and adhesions commonly found after irradiation of the gastrointestinal tract, and the portal hypertension that follows hepatic cirrhosis. Notwithstanding the vast array of toxic substances present in the environment to which man can be exposed through ingestion or inhalation, knowledge of organ-specific limitations in healing and the time parameters of such responses has accumulated through the introduction of intensive cytotoxic chemotherapy and wide-field irradiation in the treatment of neoplastic disease where there is a need to optimize the treatment modalities with maximum normal tissue-sparing effects.

The sequelae of biological events that result from injury to an organ and the acute inflammatory reaction which it elicits depend not only on the nature and magnitude of the injurious insult, but also on the ability of the various surviving cells to proliferate and repopulate the damaged area (see Fig. 5.15). *Static* cell populations (sometimes called permanent cells) show no cell proliferation in adult life; there are no epithelial cell populations in which all the cells are of this type, but neurones in the central nervous system (CNS) and cardiac muscle cells belong to this group. Healing in the CNS involves a response by

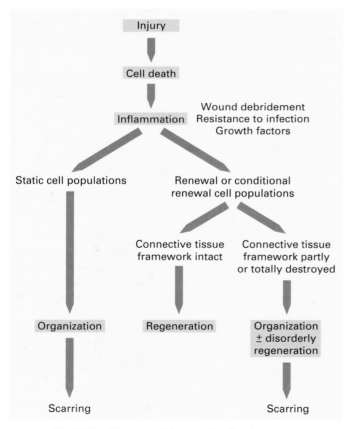

Fig. 5.15 The natural history of healing in organs.

the specialized supportive elements (*reactive gliosis*), whereas connective tissue repair follows the all-too-common myocardial infarction in man. This is basically the same process of healing that occurs in most non-osseous connective tissues, but the process is called *organization* when the connective tissue replaces dead tissue which cannot be reconstituted by the proliferation of like cells (see Section 5.3.3). Most other cell types are capable of rapid repopulation of damaged areas, and can be classified into one of two groups on the basis of their proliferative activity under normal physiological conditions. *Renewing* cell populations (labile cells), such as stratified squamous and gastro-intestinal epithelia, continue to proliferate throughout adult life because of the need for cell replacement due to persistent exfoliation of post-mitotic terminally differentiated cells from the surface (Wright and Alison 1984). Also included in this category are haemopoietic cells, where pluripotential stem cells, committed precursor cells, and maturing cells continue to proliferate to satisfy the large peripheral demand for mature cells. *Conditionally renewing* cell populations (stable cells) ordinarily exhibit a very low rate of cell proliferation, but they, too, are capable of rapid proliferation after loss of like cells because they retain the *potential* to replicate. Included in this category are the epithelial cells of virtually all glandular organs in the body, such as hepatocytes, renal tubular cells, and prostatic acinar cells; connective tissue cells (fibroblasts, chondrocytes, and osteocytes), vascular endothelial cells, and the smooth muscle cells present in the walls of viscera and blood vessels also belong to this group. The proliferative response of hepatocytes to partial hepatectomy is the classical example of healing in stable cells (see Section 5.3.2). There has been some controversy concerning the reparative ability of skeletal muscle fibres, but the fact that myogenic stem cells (satellite cells) divide in response to injury suggests that skeletal muscle is most correctly classified as that of a conditionally renewing population.

The restitution of normal structure and function within a damaged organ depends not only on the replicative ability of the surviving cells but also on the preservation of the supporting stroma to permit an orderly replacement. An intact basement membrane is probably critical in this respect, and provides the necessary scaffolding for the correct replacement of the lost parenchymal cells. When basement membranes are disrupted (Fig. 5.16), the epithelial cells may proliferate in a haphazard manner, forming disarranged masses of cells bearing no resemblance to the original structure. More severe conditions such as permanent ischaemia will result in no regenerative response whatsoever, and the gradual replacement of dead tissue by fibrotic tissue (scarring).

Healing of skin wounds

In the healing of a wound of the skin and subcutaneous tissue the formation of scar tissue is allied with epidermal regeneration; therefore almost by convention, this response is considered the archetype of wound healing; healing differences in other tissues being merely of degree rather than of kind (but see Section 5.3.2). It has become customary to consider the

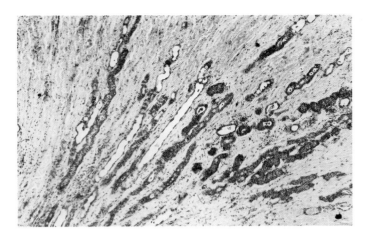

Fig. 5.16 Disorderly regeneration in the medulla of the rat kidney. Note the epithelial cells forming irregular cords, most of which are solid, within the infarcted area.

healing of a cleanly incised wound where the edges are in close apposition separately from those where there is a large tissue defect making it impossible for the edges to be stitched together. The healing of a clean surgical incision, where the edges are apposed by surgical sutures or tapes is the type of healing encountered in the vast majority of surgical wounds, and occurs without significant bacterial contamination and with a minimal loss of tissue; it is often referred to as *primary union*, or using the more archaic terminology *healing by first intention*. Likewise, healing of the more open type of wound is referred to as *secondary union* or *healing by second intention*. The formation of granulation tissue, fibrosis, and scarring are florid features of secondary rather than primary union, but the basic mechanism is the same for both; differences are thus quantitative not qualitative.

Healing of wounds with apposed edges (healing by first intention)

A simple incision causes the death of a small number of epidermal and connective tissue cells with or without minimal damage to adnexal structures in the dermis. The incision obviously severs many small blood vessels, causing haemorrhage, so the narrow incisional space is rapidly filled with clotted blood, rich in fibrin. *Fibronectin*, a homodimeric glycoprotein of molecular weight 440 000 Da, variously known as cold-insoluble globulin, opsonic protein, etc., is present in the extravasated plasma and can be cross-linked to fibrin, collagen, and other extracellular matrix components, to provide a provisional mechanical stabilization of the wound. Dehydration of the blood clot on the surface results in the formation of a *scab* which effectively seals the wound from the environment almost at once. During the first 24 h or so there is a mild inflammatory reaction at the wound edges with the exudation of fluid, deposition of further fibrin and migration of neutrophil polymorphs, monocytes, and lymphocytes. This acute inflammatory (exudative) phase in the response to injury heralds the phase of

demolition where the blood clot is digested by enzymes liberated from disintegrating neutrophil polymorphs. By the third day, neutrophils have largely disappeared from the scene and have been replaced by phagocytic macrophages which digest the remaining fibrin, damaged extracellular matrix, red cells, and cellular debris. The breakdown products from the injured cells, fibronectin, and released lysosomal enzymes from neutrophils all act as *chemoattractants* for these macrophages. Wound débridement (the excision of dead tissue) by the mononuclear phagocyte system during this inflammatory phase is probably aided by fibronectin, which opsonizes cell and tissue debris (Clark 1988).

Epithelial regeneration The response of the marginal epidermis involves *cell migration*, *cell proliferation*, and post-wounding *remodelling*. The onset of cell migration is one of the earliest signs of epithelial activity and occurs approximately 18–24 h after wounding in man. The stimulus for the initiation of cell movement is not entirely clear, but reasonably might be expected to be release from contact-inhibition by neighbouring cells; this naturally also provides a mechanism for the cessation of migration. Increased numbers of mitoses are found in marginal epidermis within 24–36 h of wounding, and soon tongues of epithelium, consisting of a sheet of flattened epithelial cells, can be seen 'dipping-down' from the margins, cleaving a path between the dead and living collagen fibres and thus displacing the remnants of the scab towards the surface. The cells only migrate over viable tissue, and are aided in this process both by the secretion of collagenase and plasminogen activators in order to dissect a pathway through the extracellular matrix (Grøndahl-Hansen *et al.* 1988) and by the presence of fibronectin which promotes the adhesion of cells to collagen and other substrates; in turn the trailing cells not only divide but secrete basement membrane components so that the continuity of the epidermal basement membrane is gradually restored. This epithelial response can be amazingly fast, so that within 48 h the whole epithelial defect can be covered by a continuous, though thin, epithelial layer (Fig. 5.17). The epithelial cells which participate in the proliferative response are both basal and

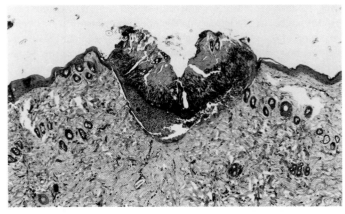

Fig. 5.17 Skin wound at 48 h after incision. Note the delicate sheet of epithelial cells more-or-less covering the wound floor, separating the viable collagen fibres from the overlying scab.

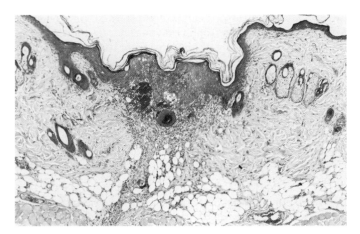

Fig. 5.18 Healed skin wound at 7 days after incision. The regenerated epidermis is markedly acanthotic and the track of the wound is delineated by the underlying cellular granulation tissue.

suprabasal cells, but the migrating cells which initially cover the wound are essentially *non-dividing*. Repeated observations on the proliferative activity in marginal epidermis of incised wounds in both man and experimental animals have shown that DNA synthesis and mitosis are extremely low or absent in the advancing epithelial tongue, and only become prominent at some distance away from the protruding tip. In a study of human volunteers, mitoses were never seen in the actively migrating tips and most were congregated some 15–20 cell diameters away from the tips, peak activity occurring between 2 and 5 days after wounding (Maibach and Rovee 1972); the cell-cycle time of the stimulus-responsive cells is much reduced compared with controls (Wright and Alison 1984).

As migration and proliferation appear to be two quite independent processes, it seems unlikely that indirect lateral pressure due to mitosis can be an important mechanism of migration. Some authors have described how advancing cells in the encroaching margin roll or slide over one another as in the movement of a caterpillar track, while others have maintained that epidermal cells move by amoeboid action mediated by pseudopodia. In pig epidermis the speed of migration has been recorded at 7 μm/h, and in general the epithelialization of the wound floor will occur more rapidly when occlusive or semi-occlusive dressings are used. These prevent excessive dehydration of the denuded dermis which would otherwise become incorporated into the scab, so causing the epithelial cells to move deeper, migrating as they must over a viable wound surface.

For epidermal wound healing to be complete, enhanced epithelial proliferation continues for a number of days, thickening the epidermal covering layer, with cell proliferation apparent in the wound floor epidermis from about day 3 onwards. A granular layer becomes apparent after about 4 days, and initially the 'healed' epidermis may be thicker than normal (acanthotic) due to an increased number of suprabasal cells (see Fig. 5.18); rete ridges are absent in the regenerated epidermis.

Repair of the dermis and subcutaneous tissue These tissues heal by proliferation of new blood vessels and fibroblasts to form *granulation tissue*. The term 'granulation tissue' derives from its pink, granular appearance on the surface of a large tissue defect, where the tiny granules correspond to loops of new capillaries which bleed easily. Vascular proliferation begins 2–3 days after injury with solid cords of endothelial cells growing out as buds or sprouts from the surviving capillaries at the wound edge, a process called *angiogenesis* or *neovascularization* (Fig. 5.19). At the tip of the elongating sprouts are migrating endothelial cells and, behind them, endothelial cells in mitosis.

The sprouts are solid at first but rapidly become canalized through the formation of a lumen in each endothelial cell in the sprout. Endothelial proliferation occurs just behind the growing tips which can advance at a rate of up to 0.6 mm/day, with the vascular sprouts exhibiting a strong disposition to anastomose with one another to form loops or arcades, well seen in the healing studies of Clark and Sandison using a transparent rabbit ear chamber (Florey 1970; Fig. 5.20).

The growth of new blood vessels also involves the local degradation of the parent capillary basement membrane at places where sprouts arise, and also changes to the extracellular matrix through which the capillaries must grow. Such changes are largely due to the generation of extracellular proteolytic activity by the endothelial cells themselves. Endothelial cells can produce two metalloproteinases, *collagenase*, which is capable of degrading the interstitial collagens, and *stromelysin*, which has a broad substrate-specificity including proteoglycans, fibronectin, laminin, and type IV collagen. Co-ordinated secretion of the connective tissue-degrading metalloproteinases and a *tissue inhibitor of metalloproteinase* (TIMP) may limit this degradation to the path of capillary endothelial cell migration during angiogenesis (Herron *et al.* 1986a,b). The conversion of the zymogen, plasminogen, to plasmin is another mechanism for generating extracellular proteolytic activity, and certainly cultured endothelial cells are capable of enhancing their production rate of plasminogen activators (serine proteases) in response to suitable stimuli. Likewise, this proteolytic activity can be limited by specific inhibitors; endothelial cells can produce a potent plasminogen activator inhibitor which has been called PAI-1 (Moscatelli and Rifkin 1988).

In the early stages the rudimentary new vessels have little basement membrane and behave as if acutely inflamed, being extremely leaky and allowing the passage of protein-rich fluid and red cells into the extravascular space; thus new granulation tissue is often oedematous. At its peak, granulation tissue is probably the most vascular tissue in the body, and, of course, provides an essential prerequisite for the rest of connective tissue healing, i.e. a blood supply. Within a few days some of the newly formed capillaries differentiate into arterioles or venules by the acquisition of smooth muscle cells, either by migration from pre-existing blood vessels, or possibly by differentiation from periadventitial cells (pericytes). With time, blood-vessels become less numerous in granulation tissue as some of them undergo thrombosis and degeneration and are resorbed.

Lymphatic channels are also found in granulation tissue and,

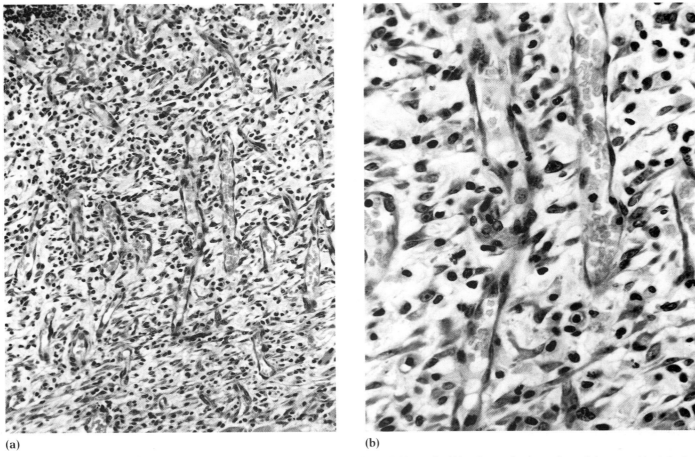

(a)

(b)

Fig. 5.19 A granulating wound showing the vertical orientation of newly formed thin-walled blood-vessels; the surface of the wound is at the top of the picture. (a) Low power; (b) high power.

like the blood circulation, the lymphatic circulation is re-established by similar process of budding and anastomosing.

In parallel with the process of neovascularization, the wounding of the connective tissue in the dermis also causes fibroblasts to migrate into the wound and undergo a brief period of intense mitotic activity. The origin of the fibroblasts is not entirely clear: they may be derived simply from resting fibroblasts but could conceivably also arise from the proliferation and differentiation of the mesenchymal stem cells. The chief function of the fibroblast with respect to wound healing is that of *secretion*, and by 4–5 days after injury these cells undergo a pronounced hypertrophy, acquiring increased amounts of rough endoplasmic reticulum and a prominent Golgi complex. These large, plump fibroblasts become active in the synthesis and secretion of extracellular matrix components, in particular the polysaccharide *glycosaminoglycans* (GAGs), which are usually covalently linked to protein to form *proteoglycans, fibronectin*, and *collagen types I and III* (see below). The concentrations of GAGs and proteoglycans in the wound area reaches a peak towards the end of the first week, and these molecules form a highly hydrated, gel-like 'ground substance' in which collagen fibres are embedded. The accumulation of fibronectin in the

wounded area follows a similar pattern to the proteoglycans, with normal levels of fibronectin re-attained after about 2 weeks.

The synthesis of collagen by fibroblasts begins within 24 h of wounding, but no significant collagen deposition in the tissue occurs before the third or fourth day; this corresponds with the first real increase in the breaking strength of the wound (Irvin 1981). Both type I and type III collagen are produced, although type III is the principal collagen synthesized in the wound, and the collagen fibres come to lie across the incision line and help to unite the cut edges from about the end of the first week after injury. At this time the rate of extracellular degradation of collagen at the healing site is greatly elevated, and this activity remains abnormally high for some months. Over this period a process of remodelling occurs; much of the type III collagen is replaced by type I collagen, and the new collagen fibres are orientated according to the new lines of mechanical stress. Collagen molecules are most likely degraded in a sequential fashion, initially by a collagenase which makes a single proteolytic cleavage at a specific site in each polypeptide chain, and then by a series of proteases which act on the reaction products to finally yield small peptides which are phagocytosed.

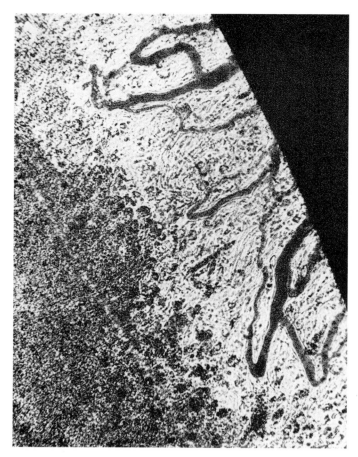

Fig. 5.20 Capillary loops growing into a blood clot situated in a transparent chamber embedded in a rabbit's ear. (From Florey 1970.)

Macrophages and fibroblasts are the major producers of collagenase in wound healing, although neutrophils and epithelial cells are also capable of producing the enzyme.

Although the collagen content of the wound reaches a maximum by about the third week, the development of the maximum tensile strength of the wound takes many months, and invariably never reaches the value for unwounded tissue. The tensile strength of the wound is usually gauged by simply measuring the load required to disrupt the wound, expressed as the *weight per unit cross-sectional area of scar tissue* (e.g. g/mm²). This slow acquisition of wound strength results from both the remodelling of the collagen, and the formation of stable intramolecular and intermolecular collagen cross-links within the collagen fibrils (see below). Thus the transition of newly produced granulation tissue into mature *scar* tissue is a protracted process featuring progressive devascularization, resorption of oedema fluid, remodelling of collagen, and the stabilization of the collagen molecules within the collagen fibrils. During maturation of the scar, type III collagen is gradually replaced by type I collagen and, eventually, the normal adult ratio (I:III, 85:15 per cent) of these collagen types is re-established. Other studies have demonstrated an appreciably higher type III colla-

gen content in embryonic or fetal tissues versus their adult counterparts; thus repair, in so far as collagen is concerned, involves a recapitulation of ontogeny.

Collagen synthesis The collagens are a family of highly characteristic fibrous proteins, which account for 25–30 per cent of the total body protein. The flexible fibres have a great resistance to pulling forces and, contrary to appearance, collagen is metabolically active and turnover rates of 5 per cent/day or more have been reported (Laurent 1987). At least 13 types of collagen have now been described (Miller and Gay 1987), but we only need concern ourselves with the stress-bearing *fibrillar collagens* (types I, II, and III) which contain a long stretch of hydrogen-bonded triple helix for most of the length of the mature molecule; these collagens account for over 95 per cent of the body's total collagen.

The central feature of all these three collagen types is the presence of a lengthy (300 nm) uninterrupted triple helix: three polypeptide chains of molecular weight 95 000 or greater, called α-*chains*, are wound around each other in a regular helix to generate a rope-like collagen molecule. In order to achieve this remarkable structure, the amino-acid sequence of each α-chain is most unusual; the most striking feature is the presence of *glycine* at every third residue which, because of its small size, can pack into the crowded interior of the collagen triple helix. So the amino-acid sequence of an α-chain helical domain can be written as $(Gly-X-Y)_n$ where $n = 338 \pm 2$ for all three fibrillar collagens. In addition, positions X and Y are often proline and hydroxyproline. The composition and distribution of the fibrillar collagens are summarized in Table 5.3.

Type I collagen is by far the most predominant collagen in vertebrate organisms, and the more common molecular species of type I is a heteropolymer of two α1(I) chains and one α2(I) chain; the Gly-X-Y triplets spanning a sequence of 1014 amino-acid residues. A homopolymer of three α1(I) chains is a minor type I collagen in some tissues.

Type II collagen is the major collagen in cartilage, and each molecule is a homopolymer of three α1(II) chains, with the fibrils into which these molecules aggregate being generally thinner than the type I collagen fibrils. Type III collagen is a homopolymer of three α1(III) chains and is generally found in association with large type I fibres in the more distensible connective tissues. It is abundant in embryonic tissues and is the first collagen deposited in wound healing.

The steps in the synthesis, secretion, and assembly into definitive extracellular structures of collagen are briefly summarized in Fig. 5.21. Individual polypeptide chains are synthesized on membrane-bound ribosomes, and, like other proteins destined for export, these pro-α-chains have a short sequence of amino acids at the N-terminal end which functions to direct the molecule into the cisternae of the endoplasmic reticulum; such *signal peptides* are cleaved shortly after translation. Pro-α-chains also have extra amino acids, called *extension peptides* or *propeptides*, at both the N- and C-terminal ends of the molecule, which do not intertwine to form a triple helix; neither do they contain long repeat triplets of Gly-X-Y form. Within the

Table 5.3 Characteristics of the major human fibrillar collagens (adapted from Sykes and Smith 1985)

Collagen type	Subunits	Known molecular configurations	Tissue distribution
I	$\alpha 1(I)$ $\alpha 2(I)$	$[\alpha 1(I)]_2 \alpha 2(I)$ and $[\alpha 1(I)]_3$	All tissues except cartilage and vitreous; very high concentrations in stress-bearing structures such as tendons, bone, dentine, ligaments, skin, blood-vessels
II	$\alpha 1(II)$	$[\alpha 1(II)]_3$	Cartilage, vitreous of the eye
III	$\alpha 1(III)$	$[\alpha 1(III)]_3$	Most tissues except bone and dentine; highest concentrations in pliable tissues such as skin, gut and blood-vessel walls, lung

Individual polypeptide chains are designated by the Greek letter α. The Arabic number after α characterizes the constituent chains of the trimer. Chains of different collagen types are distinguished by the Roman numeral of the corresponding type in parentheses.

various intracellular membranes (endoplasmic reticulum, Golgi and secretory vesicles), the nascent chains probably undergo more extensive post-translational modifications than any other group of proteins. In particular, there is no transfer RNA for hydroxyproline and hydroxylysine so many of the proline and lysine residues are hydroxylated in reactions involving specific enzymes (prolyl and lysyl hydroxylases), and these hydroxyl groups probably form inter-chain hydrogen bonds that help to stabilize the triple helix. Hydroxylation requires ascorbic acid (*vitamin C*), and the importance of the process is illustrated by the inadequate wound healing characteristic of vitamin C deficiency (scurvy). Two sugar residues, usually glucose and galactose, are covalently attached to the hydroxyl group of hydroxylysine, the degree of glycosylation varying greatly among different types of collagen. In a number of heritable disorders, such as osteogenesis imperfecta, Ehlers–Danlos syndrome, and Marfan's syndrome, which present as the mechanical failure of collagen-rich tissues, genetic deficiencies of various post-translational modifying enzymes have been described, as well as alterations in the amino-acid structure of the helical peptides (see Sykes and Smith 1985).

The assembly of the *procollagen* molecules involves each pro-α-chain, together with its extension peptides at both the N- and C-terminal ends, combining with two others to form a long stretch of hydrogen-bonded triple helix; extension peptides probably serve to guide triple-helix formation with the formation of inter-chain disulphide bonds between C-terminal peptides. The procollagen molecules are packaged into secretory vacuoles and eventually released into the extracellular matrix. Generally speaking, the extension peptides are removed by specific amino- and carboxy-proteases which act at protease-sensitive sites before fibril formation is instituted. This results in the triple-helix conformation existing for over 96 per cent of the total length (300 nm) of the *tropocollagen* molecule, with small non-helical regions (*telopeptides*) of 15–30 amino acids persisting at the end of each α-chain. This scheme may be an oversimplification, since collagen plus the carboxylpropeptide (pC-collagen) or collagen plus the aminopropeptide (pN-collagen) has been located on the surface of growing fibrils (Fleischmajer 1986). These intermediates may prevent premature polymerization of collagen molecules, with the remaining pN or pC domain being cleaved after the molecule has become resident within the fibrils; failure to cleave the propeptide could stop further growth of the fibril. Fibril formation involves the polymerization of collagen molecules in a staggered arrangement that gives the collagen fibrils their characteristic 67 nm periodicity, which not only maximizes the number of hydrogen bonds that can be formed, but also ensures that telopeptide domains are adjacent to triple-helical regions of neighbouring molecules. The development of the full tensile strength of the collagen fibrils essentially derives from the formation of covalent cross-links between the telopeptide segment of one molecule and the helical domain of an adjacent molecule. The extracellular copper-requiring enzyme *lysyl oxidase*, deaminates lysine and hydroxylysine residues to form highly reactive aldehyde groups which can react non-enzymatically with unmodified lysine and hydroxylysine residues in neighbouring molecules to form intermolecular covalent cross-links of the aldimine type (so-called Schiff bases); alternatively, two aldehyde groups can react together to form an aldol condensation product. Increasing the degree of cross-linking progressively renders the collagen fibrils insoluble. Certain substances are capable of preventing collagen cross-linking: β-aminopropionitrile (BAPN) contained in *Lathyrus odoratus*, the sweet pea, inhibits the oxidative deamination and aldehyde formation, and the affected collagen fibrils are quite unable to resist tensile forces. Apart from nitriles (*lathyrogens*) which chelate copper, other potentially anti-fibrotic drugs include colchicine, which affects protein secretion through its action on microtubules, and proline analogues which cannot be hydroxylated, thus reducing the stability of the triple helix.

Collagen fibrils can be quite long (10 μm or more) and vary in thickness from 10 to 200 nm, clearly visible in electron micrographs. Such fibrils are often grouped into larger bundles several or more μm in diameter, which are seen in the light microscope as collagen fibres.

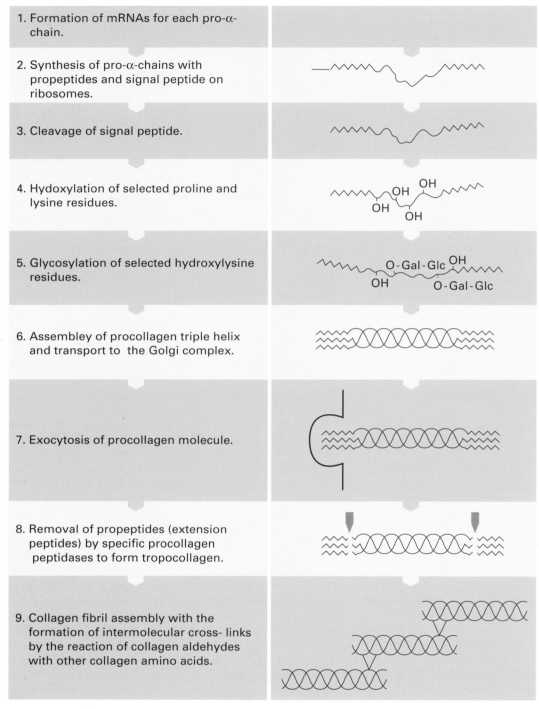

1. Formation of mRNAs for each pro-α-chain.

2. Synthesis of pro-α-chains with propeptides and signal peptide on ribosomes.

3. Cleavage of signal peptide.

4. Hydoxylation of selected proline and lysine residues.

5. Glycosylation of selected hydroxylysine residues.

6. Assembley of procollagen triple helix and transport to the Golgi complex.

7. Exocytosis of procollagen molecule.

8. Removal of propeptides (extension peptides) by specific procollagen peptidases to form tropocollagen.

9. Collagen fibril assembly with the formation of intermolecular cross- links by the reaction of collagen aldehydes with other collagen amino acids.

Fig. 5.21 Collagen biosynthesis: the intracellular and extracellular events.

Healing of wounds with separated edges (healing by second intention)

Where there is a more extensive loss of tissue to produce a wound with widely separated margins, then clearly the reparative response is slower than when the wound edges are closely apposed. In addition, the greater amounts of tissue and cellular debris provoke a more intense inflammatory response and, likewise, the production of granulation tissue is more exuberant leading to the possibility of large, deforming scars. The single most important feature which distinguishes healing by first intention from healing by second intention is the phenomenon of *wound contraction*, which assumes far greater significance in the healing of large excised wounds. Over a period of weeks, the area covered by a large surface wound can diminish by as much as 90 per cent or more, accompanied by equally dramatic changes in shape, transforming circular wounds into linear scars and square or rectangular wounds into stellate scars. Wound contraction is particularly well seen in lower animals where epithelialization may be regarded as a temporary repair, since, in the fully contracted wound, much of the migrated epithelium is ultimately lost. Wound contraction is not due to the shortening of collagen fibres, as it still occurs in scorbutic animals and in cases of lathyrism. It is most likely that the contraction of granulation tissue depends ultimately on the contraction of modified fibroblasts, termed *myofibroblasts*, which appear in granulation tissue. Myofibroblasts contain considerable amounts of contractile proteins, in particular, actin and myosin, whose similar distribution in the cytoplasm suggests that they interact to generate contraction (Rungger-Brandle and Gabbiani 1983). Thus strips of granulation tissue behave in a similar fashion as smooth muscle cells when exposed to substances which cause either muscle contraction (e.g. 5-hydroxytryptamine, vasopressin, and adrenalin) or relaxation (prostaglandins E_1 and E_2). In hollow visceral organs the contraction of granulation tissue in, for example, the base of an ulcer, can lead to symptoms of obstruction or at least the puckering of the overlying mucosa.

As in the incised wound, the production of a large tissue defect causes haemorrhage and the formation of a blood clot, rich in fibrin and fibronectin, to be followed by the immigration of neutrophil polymorphs and later, macrophages for the process of wound débridement. Epithelial migration is underway within 24 h if not before, but when there is a large tissue defect new epidermis is formed not only from the epidermis at the wound margins but also from the ducts of sweat glands and the outer root sheath of hair follicles (Fig. 5.22). Pinkus and Mehregan (1981) are of the opinion that these adnexal keratinocytes are modulated in wound healing, returning to a quasi-embryonic state before redifferentiating into epidermis. The scar tissue which replaces a large tissue defect is characterized by collagen bundles running a fairly straight course parallel to the skin surface; small blood-vessels extend perpendicularly between the epidermis and subcutis. Elastic fibres, which are either absent or very infrequent, run parallel to the collagen fibres. Moreover, dermal papillae and rete ridges are either

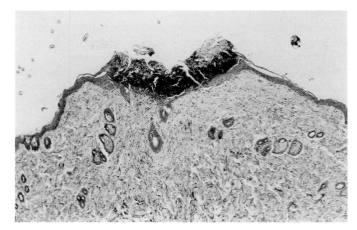

Fig. 5.22 A healing epidermal wound with re-epithelialization of the wound floor with new epidermis apparently arising from the outer root sheath of a hair follicle at the centre of the wound.

absent or poorly developed, and adnexal structures are apt to be absent in skin scars (Fig. 5.23).

Factors influencing wound healing

The factors which may adversely affect wound healing can be categorized into those which act locally (local factors) and those more general metabolic disturbances (systemic factors) which can interfere with the healing process.

Local factors

Adequacy of blood supply in an area of injury is a factor upon which the healing process ultimately depends; actively dividing fibroblasts are confined to regions where tissue oxgen tension is greater than 15 mmHg, and this is only found within 50–70 μm of the nearest functioning capillary. Any factors that

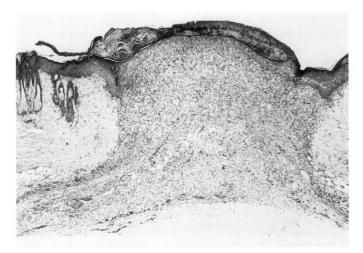

Fig. 5.23 Healing of a deep excised wound with exuberant granulation tissue and stratification of the regenerated epidermis. Note the absence of hair follicles and sebaceous glands amongst the granulation tissue.

limit blood flow (arterial disease, pressure) and venous abnormalities that retard drainage are well-known impairments to the healing of wounds. When the blood supply is compromised, quite trivial injuries may give rise to tissue damage out of all proportion to the injury. This is often seen in older patients with a poor blood supply to the lower limbs (atherosclerotic arterial insufficiency of the lower limb) where a minor injury leads to the formation of a large ulcer which heals very slowly.

Infection is the single most important local cause for delayed healing. In this context effective wound débridement is essential since dead tissue provides a portal of entry for micro-organisms. Infection delays epithelial regeneration and fibroblast proliferation, and promotes the production of greater amounts of granulation tissue due to more tissue destruction, with the resultant likelihood of larger, more deforming scars. Infection is a very common cause of death in burn injuries, and is a lethal complication in prosthetic implants in cardiovascular surgery.

Early *movement* causes mechanical stress of the wound and is clearly something to be avoided, no more so than in the healing of fractures where immobilization of the fracture and protection from mechanical stress are vital for a successful outcome. Following a laparotomy a sudden increase in mechanical stress brought about through coughing or vomiting is often the cause of abdominal wound disruption.

Extraneous *foreign material*, sutures, and dead and devitalized tissues can all impede the healing process through encouraging infection and/or exciting an inflammatory and macrophage foreign body-type reaction. Percutaneous sutures can afford micro-organisms a portal of entry, while the nature of the suture material has a strong bearing on the tissue reaction invoked. For example, absorbable plain catgut provokes a greater tissue reaction than non-absorbable braided polyester.

Ionizing radiation is, in general, deleterious to wound healing. Although the acute effects of irradiation can include a block in cell proliferation and cell death, these are generally of little consequence practically. More relevant are the late effects of irradiation seen in the healing of wounds in previously-irradiated tissues, where unstable granulation tissue and obliterative vascular changes make wounds prone to dehiscence. For these reasons, surgeons are advised against fashioning intestinal anastomoses from the immediately perilesional tissues following resection of locally irradiated malignant neoplasms.

Systemic factors

Without a great deal of evidence to support the notion, *ageing* is generally held to be associated with poorer qualities of healing. In many cases the so-called effects of ageing may have more to do with vascular insufficiency, malnutrition, or vitamin deficiency.

Metabolic status has a profound bearing on the healing of wounds, with protein deprivation having a particularly deleterious effect on the acquisition of wound strength through impairment of collagen and glycosaminoglycan synthesis. In rats, however, a loss of one-third of the total body weight had to occur before protein deprivation had a significant effect on the strength of incised skin wounds and colonic anastomoses (Irvin

1981); thus the wound site seems to enjoy a biological priority. Sulphydryl-containing amino acids, such as methionine, are essential for collagen and glycosaminoglycan synthesis, and it is claimed by some (but denied by others) that methionine supplementation can negate the adverse effects of protein deprivation. Of all the individual dietary factors that could affect healing, the most widely appreciated is ascorbic acid (vitamin C), the deficiency of which (scurvy) has been known to be associated with poor healing since the seventeenth century. Ascorbic acid is required in man for the activation of the enzymes prolyl and lysyl hydroxylase and probably also for the production of galactosamine, an essential component of chondroitin sulphate. Vitamin C deficiency results in the impaired synthesis of normal collagen, and the resultant underhydroxylated collagen is thermally unstable, poorly transported out of the cell, and is very susceptible to degradation. The collagen that is secreted fails to undergo normal fibrillogenesis and the condition recognized as *scurvy* develops. A deficiency of *zinc* has adverse effects on wound healing in man and experimental animals since the metal is a cofactor of several enzymes, including DNA and RNA polymerases. There is no evidence that zinc supplements are required after routine surgical operations, though patients with severe burns are likely to be zinc-deficient. Diabetics are more vulnerable to serious infections, which in turn impede healing responses. Likewise, other conditions that increase the susceptibility to bacterial infection (granulocytopenia, defects in leucocyte chemotaxis or phagocytosis) make wounds prone to slow healing.

Large doses of *corticosteroids* impair the healing response in experimental animals. Such steroids have been reported to have adverse effects on epithelial regeneration, the proliferation of fibroblasts, and the synthesis of the extracellular matrix. However, the fact that steroid therapy is only really effective when administered in the early postoperative period has led to the suspicion that the inhibitory effects on the healing response are exerted indirectly through a suppression of the inflammatory response. On the other hand, there has been a suggestion that cortisone stabilizes lysosomal membranes thus preventing tissue breakdown, which itself is important to the perpetuation of the reparative response.

Cytotoxic drugs used in immunosuppressive therapy or in the treatment of malignant disease could also, theoretically at least, inhibit various healing responses, since their mode of action is generally to interfere with macromolecular synthesis and have cytostatic or cytolethal effects on proliferating cells.

Complications of wound healing

The complications of wound healing are listed in Table 5.4, and are generally associated with the repair process. *Wound dehiscence* (bursting) is most likely to occur in the first few weeks after surgery before substantial completion of collagen cross-linking. Excessive wound tension, particularly sudden increases in mechanical stress, should be avoided, and systemic factors such as poor metabolic status (hypoproteinaemia, vitamin C deficiency) result in weak scars and thus an increased likelihood of

Table 5.4 Complications of wound healing

Wound dehiscence
Hypertrophic scars and keloids
Cicatrization
? Neoplasia
Miscellaneous (painful scars, weak scars, pigmentary changes,
    implantation cysts)

dehiscence. Hypertrophic scars and keloids result from post-traumatic tissue overproduction of connective tissue, leading to firm, raised flesh. Histologically the two conditions are very alike, often with thick hyalinized bands of collagen in whorls (Fig. 5.24); they occur most frequently on the face, neck, anterior chest, and shoulder. Hypertrophic scars flatten spontaneously over the course of one or two years, but keloids persist and may even extend beyond the site of the original injury. The aetiology of keloids is uncertain, but racial and familial factors are involved.

Wound contraction depends upon the action of myofibroblasts, and an exaggeration of this process is termed *contracture* or *cicatrization* and results in severe deformity at and around the wound site. It is often regions such as the palms and soles, which normally show minimal wound contraction, that are particularly prone to contractures. In the gastrointestinal tract, contracture can cause a narrowing of the bowel lumen and the associated problems of obstruction. There are several diseases that are characterized by contracture of superficial fascias, although there is no known precipitating injury; Dupuytren's contracture (palmoplantar fibromatosis) and Peyronie's disease (induratio penis plastica) are two such examples.

For a particular tissue, experimental studies strongly suggest that an enhancement in the rate of cell turnover increases the likelihood of tumour induction. Thus wound sites, with their elevated levels of cell proliferation, may be fertile grounds for such development and indeed the phenomenon of so-called 'suture-line cancers' is now well recognized.

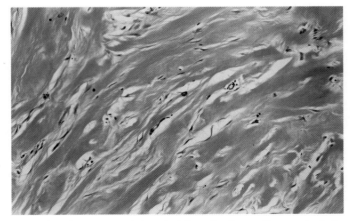

Fig. 5.24 Swollen, hyalinized bundles of collagen fibres typical of a keloid.

Control mechanisms in healing

Although the phenomenology of regenerative and repair processes in wound healing have been more than adequately described, information about the factors that control these various responses is only just emerging. Indeed, up until a few years ago the only general biological model of growth control was a chemical mechanism of self-inhibition, largely formulated from experiments on normal and wounded epidermis. This was the *chalone* hypothesis, which states that the rate of cell production in all tissues is under the control of a tissue-specific (but not species-specific) freely diffusible chemical agent, the chalone, produced locally by the functional cells of a tissue, which acts to inhibit cell proliferation. This concept can explain many growth phenomena after wounding: loss of differentiated epidermal tissue decreases the local chalone concentration, allowing cells to divide, and with the production of new functional cells which synthesize chalone, the local chalone concentration increases, and inhibits cell proliferation again; thus the initiation and curtailment of the proliferative response to wounding is explained. There is a certain amount of experimental evidence favouring this self-inhibition or negative-feedback hypothesis. For example, the amount of skin regenerated after abrasion can describe a series of damping oscillations about the control value with time after wounding, a situation characteristic of a negative-feedback loop. On the other hand, progress in elucidating the chemical composition of the effector molecule of such inhibition in any tissue has been so painfully slow or non-existent as to relegate further investigation from the mainstream of current biological thought. However, some progress has been made as far as the epidermis is concerned, with Elgjo *et al.* (1986) isolating and sequencing a mitosis-inhibiting pentapeptide from hairless mouse skin. Another mechanism of self-inhibition is that which follows cell contact during growth *in vitro*, but the importance of this in *in vivo* tissue systems is difficult to assess, although such extremely local inhibition could conceivably play a part in the curtailment of epidermal growth after wounding. The role of such *contact inhibition* in, say, the regenerative response after partial hepatectomy is more problematical.

Finally, in this discussion of controlling mechanisms we must, of necessity, consider the role of endogenous stimulators of cellular processes in regulating the healing process. Leaving aside the undoubted trophic effects of established hormones like androgens and oestrogens on their respective target tissues, there is now a growing list of *polypeptide growth factors* with pleiotropic biological effects, including the recruitment of new cells, the stimulation of extracellular matrix synthesis, and the promotion of neovascularization. These peptides appear to play a key role in the reparative process, acting in a paracrine fashion following release from injured cells, platelets, macrophages, and lymphocytes; common enough bedfellows at the wound site.

One of the most ubiquitous of these factors is platelet-derived growth factor (PDGF), a cationic glycoprotein first isolated from platelets, thus leaving little doubt as to its relevance in wound

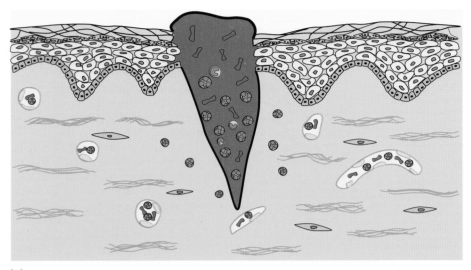

(a)

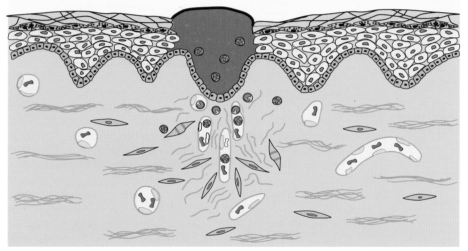

(b)

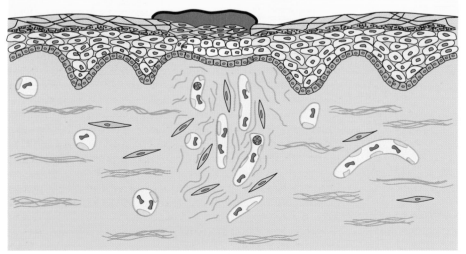

(c)

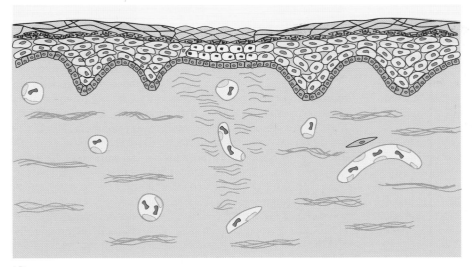

(d)

Fig. 5.25 A summary of skin healing. (a) In the exudative phase a fibrin-rich clot is formed and the immigration of neutrophils is soon followed by an influx of monocytes and lymphocytes. (b) Two or three days after injury, phagocytic cells are active in demolishing the clot (scab), and re-epithelialization of the wound floor is more-or-less complete through the migration of epithelial cells from the wound margin and proliferation of other basal and suprabasal cells some distance back from the pushing epithelial 'tongue'. Simultaneously, endothelial cells proliferate and neovascularization begins, while fibroblasts and myofibroblasts accumulate at the wound site. (c) Four or five days after injury, stratification of the regenerated epidermis is readily apparent as the scab is displaced towards the surface. The dermal injury is filled by very vascular granulation tissue and fibroblasts are highly active in the synthesis and secretion of the extracellular matrix components. (d) Much later, the once highly vascular granulation tissue has been replaced by relatively avascular scar tissue, with type I rather than type III being the principal fibrillar collagen. The overlying epidermis is of normal thickness but lacks rete ridges.

repair. PDGF is present in platelet α-granules, is released from the granules upon platelet aggregation and activation at sites of injury, and binds with high affinity to receptors on the surface of connective tissue cells. PDGF from human platelets is a disulphide-linked heterodimeric protein with a molecular weight of approximately 30 000, comprising one A (non-*sis*) and one B (*sis*) polypeptide chain. The B-chain is structurally and functionally almost identical to part of the protein product (p28 *sis*) of the v-*sis* oncogene, the transforming gene of simian sarcoma virus. In certain instances PDGF exists in A-chain or B-chain homodimeric forms (Ross *et al*. 1986), and additional sources of PDGF or PDGF-like molecules include monocytes, endothelial cells, and a variety of transformed cell lines. PDGF is a powerful chemoattractant for connective tissue cells (fibroblasts and smooth muscle cells) as well as inflammatory cells (monocytes and neutrophils), serving to direct cells to the site of tissue damage. Furthermore, PDGF is a mitogen for mesenchymal cells, e.g. fibroblasts, glial cells, and smooth muscle cells, and has been implicated in both the synthesis and remodelling of the extracellular matrix.

PDGF accounts for about half of the platelet-derived mitogenic activity of human serum as assayed on certain connective tissue cells; much of the remaining activity is derived from another polypeptide growth factor stored in the α-granules,

transforming growth factor-β (TGF-β). TGF-β is a homodimeric peptide, composed of two identical polypeptide chains each of molecular weight 12 500, which has been found in a variety of tissues since its original purification from platelets (see Sporn *et al*. 1987). The name of the peptide is derived from the functional assay for the originally purified TGF-β, namely the stimulation of anchorage-independent growth of normal fibroblasts. In various cell culture systems TGF-β has been found to be a mitogen for a variety of mesenchymal cells, but it appears to be a growth inhibitor for epithelial cells; indeed, TGF-β may serve to counteract the positive effects of other growth factors. TGF-β also has biological effects unrelated to proliferation, including the stimulation of wound contraction, and it appears to be intimately involved in the formation and conservation of the extracellular matrix through the combined actions of promoting collagen synthesis, inhibiting the secretion of proteases such as plasminogen activator and stromelysin, and increasing the secretion of protease inhibitors (TIMP and PAI-1).

Basic and acidic fibroblast growth factors (bFGF and aFGF) are single-chain peptides of 146 and 140 amino acids respectively, both characterized by a high affinity for heparin, and produced by a wide variety of mesoderm- and neuroectoderm-derived cells. Both growth factors have a wide spectrum of biological activities related to wound healing (Gospodarowicz *et al*.

1987), the most notable being the ability to promote neovascularization *in vivo* by being mitogens for endothelial cells. Acidic fibroblast growth factor has a 53 per cent sequence homology to bFGF, seems to bind to the same receptor, but is much less potent than bFGF in terms of stimulating endothelial cell proliferation; in the presence of heparin, aFGF is equipotent with bFGF. FGFs may also aid angiogenesis by stimulating plasminogen activator and latent collagenase production by endothelial cells.

Mononuclear leucocytes, which are invariably found in healing wounds, are responsible for producing a host of polypeptides and other factors which increase the number and activity of fibroblasts. These factors include interleukin-1 (IL-1) and tumour necrosis factor (TNF, formerly called cachectin), although cytokines such as TNF also have other biological effects related to healing, including being potent angiogenic factors.

Epidermal growth factor (EGF) is a well-characterized polypeptide which stimulates the proliferation of a large variety of cells *in vitro*. EGF is widely distributed among various organs and tissues, although it is notably concentrated in the submaxillary glands of male mice and in Brunner's glands in man. In man the polypeptide resembles β-urogastrone, and it has similar chemical (37 out of 53 amino-acid residues are common to both) and physiological properties to rat and mouse EGF (Cohen 1986). In organ culture EGF directly stimulates the proliferation of epidermal cells of chick embryo skin, but its role *in vivo* is still uncertain. EGF administration enhances epidermal growth and keratinization in new-born rats, and its topical application accelerates corneal re-epithelialization in rabbits with wounded corneas. In the gastrointestinal tract rendered hypoplastic by the absence of luminal nutrition, Goodlad *et al.* (1987) have found that EGF stimulates cell proliferation in a dose-dependent fashion, which together with its ability to inhibit gastric acid secretion suggests a possible role for EGF in the management of peptic ulcer disease. EGF can also act as an angiogenic factor through its mitogenic action on endothelial cells, a property it shares with transforming growth factor-α (TGF-α). TGF-α and EGF share only 35 per cent sequence homology but they bind to the same receptors, seemingly due to the identical positioning of the three disulphide bonds giving the molecules a similar conformation. Likewise, both EGF and TGF-α have proved useful, when administered topically, in promoting the re-epithelialization of cutaneous wounds.

Summary of wound healing

We can broadly summarize the process of wound healing using the healing of a linear skin wound as a prototype. With any wound the initial event at the site of injury is haemorrhage and the formation of a fibrin-rich clot (Fig. 5.25a, p. 376). Fibronectin stabilizes the clot before dehydration takes place and a scab is formed. Macrophages soon follow neutrophils to the site of tissue injury and wound débridement is aided by the opsonization of tissue debris by fibronectin. The epidermal response to wounding is initiated very rapidly and within a day or so 'tongues' of epidermal cells can be seen cleaving a path between the scab and the viable collagenous tissue underneath; two or three days after injury the wound floor is covered by a sheet of regenerated epidermal cells (Fig. 5.25b, p. 376). The formation of granulation tissue begins at about the same time with an influx and proliferation of fibroblasts and the beginnings of new capillary formation. Four to five days after wounding stratification of the wound-floor epidermis is readily apparent, fibroblasts are highly active in the manufacture and secretion of extracellular matrix compounds (principally GAGs and type III collagen) and the process of neovascularization is in full swing (Fig. 5.25c, p. 376). To achieve this invasive process endothelial cells must secrete a battery of proteinases (e.g. type IV collagenase, interstitial collagenase, elastase, stromelysin, and plasminogen activators) to degrade the basement membrane and the diverse components of the extracellular matrix. In time, the full thickness of the epidermis is restored without the reformation of rete ridges, much of the type III collagen which was initially laid down is replaced by type I collagen fibres, orientated parallel to lines of mechanical stress (collagen remodelling), and the once highly vascular granulation tissue undergoes a protracted process of devascularization as it matures into relatively avascular scar tissue (Fig. 5.25d, p. 376).

5.3.2   Tissue differences in healing

Gastrointestinal tract (GI tract)

Healing (both epithelial regeneration and connective tissue repair) in the GI tract is important from a number of standpoints of clinical significance: the rate of repair of the connective tissue largely determines the strength of gastrointestinal anastomoses, while the ability of the epithelium to regenerate is vital for both the reconstitution of the mucosa when areas of the bowel wall have been denuded as part of an ulcerative process, and for the repopulation of crypts and glands partly damaged by cytotoxic chemotherapeutic drugs and ionizing radiation. Indeed, gastrointestinal side-effects can be a limiting factor in the use of such treatment modalities in the treatment of neoplastic disease.

The management of anastomoses at various levels in the GI tract is a major aspect of a surgeon's workload since, for example, 60 per cent of patients with large bowel cancer are amenable to 'curative resection', i.e. complete removal of the macroscopic tumour. The biochemical, cellular, and mechanical aspects of the reparative process conform to primary wound healing, with the mechanical strength of the union usually assessed, experimentally at least, by the wound-bursting pressure—literally the lumen is inflated with air or filled with fluid and the intraluminal pressure at the moment of leakage is recorded. In rats with the colon transected and anastomosed, re-epithelialization is complete within 12 weeks and the anastomotic site can only be identified by the interruption in the muscularis propria where scar tissue replaces the smooth muscle (Roe *et al.* 1987). An elevated level of cell proliferation persists in the perilesional crypts for some 8–12 weeks post-operatively, and is presumably the reason why many more tumours than expected develop at the site of union when these rats are exposed to the carcinogen azoxymethane during the healing period: the 'suture line' may also be a fertile field for the development of large bowel cancer in man (Umpleby and Williamson 1987).

It is probably not uncommon for the gastric mucosa to be subjected to minor insults caused by agents such as aspirin and alcohol. Such perturbations can result in the desquamation of just a few surface cells, or more deeper losses which, however, do not involve the full thickness of the mucosa. The healing of these so-called *erosions* can be very rapid: Silen and Ito (1985) noted the complete re-epithelialization of totally desquamated surfaces within 1 h by migration of epithelial cells from neighbouring pits, a process termed *restitution* (the re-establishment of epithelial continuity before cell proliferation and inflammation). Circumscribed lesions involving loss of the full thickness of the mucosa with a variable degree of penetration into the underlying muscle coats are termed *ulcers*, and certainly peptic ulcer disease is a major cause of human morbidity. Simply stated, ulcers arise from the breakdown of the mucosal defence mechanisms (mucus gel formation and bicarbonate secretion) to the endogenous aggressors, acid and pepsin. At the present time the so-called anti-ulcer drugs do not directly stimulate the reparative process, but rather they alter the local environment so that healing can take place. The most effective medical therapy is to reduce acid secretion by blocking the promoting action of histamine on the acid-secreting parietal cells: in 1987 the H_2-receptor antagonists ranitidine (Zantac[R]) and cimetidine (Tagamet[R]) were first and second, respectively, in the league table of the world's top drugs, with combined sales worth £1590 million. In the normal situation the presence of food in the lumen stimulates the release of gastrin from the G-cells in the pyloric antrum; this in turn promotes acid secretion by the parietal cells and acid acts to limit gastrin release. Thus H_2-receptor antagonists can cause hypergastrinaemia and, in experimental animals at least, this is associated with an increased incidence of enterochromaffin cell (ECL cell) hyper-plasias and gastric ECL cell tumours.

In man, most ulcers occur in pyloric-type mucosa, and the consensus view is that healing does occur, but the regenerated glands are more irregular and fewer in number. McMinn (1969) studied the healing of experimentally induced ulcers in the gastric mucosa of rats and found that the cells migrating as a sheet across the ulcer floor were also able to divide. These migrating cells had the morphology of mucous neck cells, and within two weeks lesions of ~ 0.5 cm^2 had been re-epithelialized, with tubular invaginations readily apparent in the epithelial sheet; differentiation of these mucous neck-like cells into parietal and chief cells began to occur after about 1 month. Healing of ulcerative lesions can occur throughout the GI tract, and the general picture is that of an ability to reconstitute the mucosa with the reformation of specialized structures, be it gastric glands, crypts, or villi. EGF has been

shown to enhance the healing rate of both gastric and duodenal ulcerations in rats and, moreover, this has been attributed to a direct mitogenic effect of EGF on the epithelial cells rather than through an indirect action such as inhibiting acid secretion or stimulating gastrin release (Konturek *et al.* 1988). The relevance of such studies to the healing of gastrointestinal tissues is apparent from the discovery of an EGF-secreting cell lineage which is invariably present adjacent to areas of chronic ulceration (Wright *et al.* 1990). This lineage initially appears as a bud from the base of intestinal crypts; it grows locally to form a small gland and ultimately communicates with the lumen via a newly-formed duct. The lineage produces neutral mucin (Fig. 5.26) and secretes immunoreactive EGF, which is then available to assist in ulcer healing. If regeneration is complete, then the only trace of injury will be the collagenous scar tissue underneath. Like granulation tissue elsewhere, the fibrous base

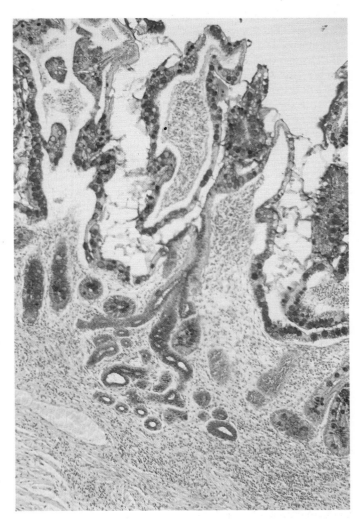

Fig. 5.26 The EGF-secreting lineage in the ileum from a patient with Crohn's disease, stained with Alcian blue/diastase periodic acid-Schiff (PAS) method. The lineage is well shown by its neutral mucin content, staining magenta with PAS but not Alcian blue. The deeper glandular portion has communicated with the villus epithelium by way of a duct.

of an ulcer can contract; in the pyloric canal this can result in stenosis sufficient to interfere with normal emptying. The base of an unhealed ulcer has four recognizable layers (Fig. 5.27): on the luminal aspect there is a narrow zone of fibrino-purulent exudate, underlying this is a layer of acidophilic necrotic tissue, then a zone of vascular granulation tissue which blends with the deepest layer of more dense scar tissue.

Ionizing radiation damages cells, and after a single large dose there is a rapid, but temporary, dose-dependent decline in the number of proliferating cells. Within a matter of hours cell death is seen in the lower regions of the crypt where proliferative cells are normally found, and if the dose has been sufficiently high whole crypts may disappear completely. The fraction of crypts surviving is measured by plotting a crypt survival curve after graded doses of irradiation (Fig. 5.28a; and see Potten *et al.* 1983). Above a dose of about 10 Gy there appears to be an exponential decline in crypt survival, suggesting that one further cell death in a crypt results in the loss of that crypt, i.e. the surviving crypts after such high doses originate from a single surviving repopulating or clonogenic cell. The fact that all possible cell lineages will be present in the newly regenerated crypts (e.g. Paneth, enteroendocrine, goblet, and columnar cells in the small intestine) argues strongly in favour of the existence of a multipotential stem cell capable of giving rise to all the various cell types present. After high doses of irradiation which ablate whole crypts, reduce the cellularity of others, and so cause a reduction in villus size, the survival of the animal as a whole depends on the regenerative capacity of the crypts to overcome the cellular depopulation before its consequences are fully felt. These include symptoms of the GI radiation syndrome such as haemorrhage, bacterial infection, and fluid loss. At 3–4 days after irradiation the process of re-

epithelialization has begun, with foci of regeneration present as discrete crypt-like structures called *microcolonies* (Fig. 5.28b). These structures continue to grow rapidly and very soon the crypt cellularity overshoots the normal value (Fig. 5.28c), but this excess cellularity is eliminated at a later time. If whole crypts have been lost, the crypt density will be increased by the surviving crypts undergoing crypt fission and initiating a 'budding' type of growth.

Most cytotoxic chemotherapeutic drugs are designed to cause the death of proliferative cells; consequently GI side-effects can be a limiting factor with such a treatment modality. In the small intestinal crypts of animals and man the cells towards the base of the crypts are known to divide very slowly compared with those in the remainder of the crypt. However, if rats are treated with hydroxyurea, a drug which kills cells in DNA synthesis, repopulation is initiated by a large increase in the rate of proliferation of basally sited crypt cells (Wright 1978). These cells are slowly cycling in normal circumstances, but could constitute a reserve pool, which, because they are dividing slowly, are relatively insensitive to such cell cycle phase-specific insult. Cytosine arabinoside (ara-C) also kills DNA-synthesizing cells (Fig. 5.29) and a suitably fractionated dosage schedule can reduce the cellularity of mouse small intestinal crypts by as much as 80 per cent (Wright and Al-Nafussi 1982). This in turn leads to a severe depletion in villus size, and then crypt repopulation, which results in the crypt cellularity considerably overshooting normal values and then describing a series of damping oscillations about this value. This pattern of response is suggestive of a loss in negative-feedback information (? caused by the reduction in the differentiated compartment size), but as yet there is no consistent message about the nature of an inhibitory molecule.

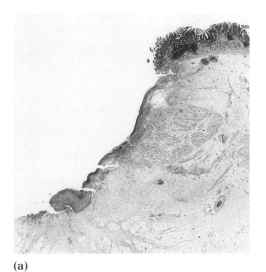

(a)

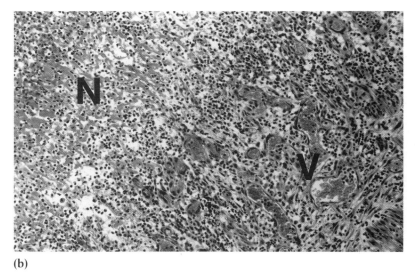

(b)

Fig. 5.27   (a) Low-power photomicrograph of a deep ulcer crater in the pyloric stomach, a layer of fibrino-purulent exudate covers the surface. (b) Beneath the exudate is a layer of necrotic (N) granulation tissue which overlies the highly cellular and richly vascular viable (V) granulation tissue.

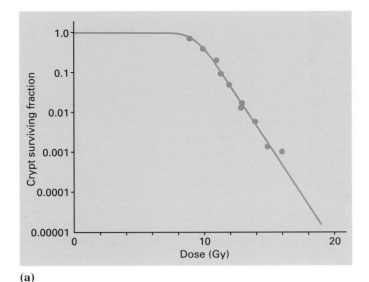

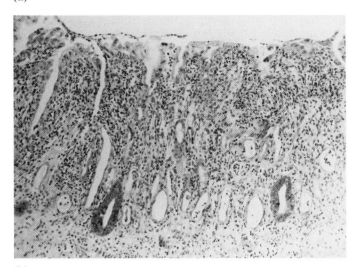

(a)

(b)

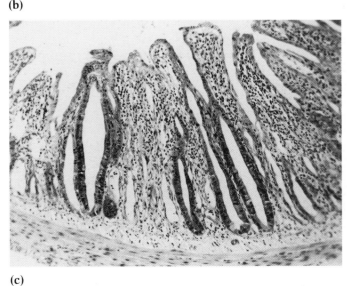

(c)

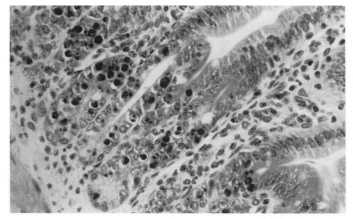

Fig. 5.29 Widespread occurrence of apoptotic cell death in the rat small intestine shortly after exposure to cytosine arabinoside. Recovery (regeneration) from this amount of intestinal death is readily accomplished.

Liver

The liver is often considered the model for regeneration *par excellence*. Most studies have been conducted on the rat liver after a two-thirds partial hepatectomy, a relatively simple surgical procedure involving removal of the anterior liver lobes. Strictly speaking, the proliferative response which is evoked by this operation is a *compensatory hyperplasia* since the remaining lobes are not actually damaged, while the remnants of the resected lobes do not regenerate but undergo infarction because of the necessary ligatures around the afferent and efferent blood vessels at the hilum. Nevertheless, the partial hepatectomy model of regeneration is widely adopted for the reasons of:

1. *reproducibility*: removal of anterior liver lobes inflicts the same degree of damage (loss) on each animal;

2. *completeness*: since hepatocytes have to be ejected from the G_0 phase they probably have to pass through all the necessary stages of biochemical preparation for DNA synthesis and mitosis;

3. *rapidity*: the response is essentially complete within 7–10 days (see Fig. 5.30); and

4. *simplicity*: the reparative response is largely one of regeneration uncomplicated by significant connective tissue healing.

Having said this, it is worth remembering that connective tissue

Fig. 5.28 (a) A crypt survival curve for the mouse small intestine in which the number of regenerative foci (microcolonies) per unit length present on the third or fourth day after irradiation is expressed as a fraction of the number of crypts normally present in such a length. (b) Two discrete regenerative foci (microcolonies) present near the muscularis mucosa in an area of rat small intestine otherwise devoid of gut epithelia; 3.5 days after 12 Gy X-irradiation. (c) Two or three days later the microcolonies have increased enormously in cellularity and begun to resemble normal crypts; the crypts are, in fact, hypercellular and no definitive villi are yet seen.

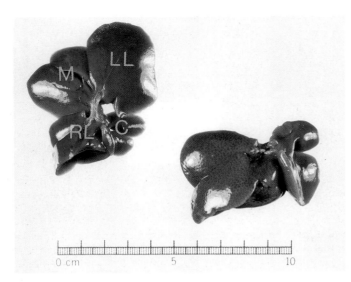

Fig. 5.30 A two-thirds partial hepatectomy in the rat involves removal of the median (M) and left lateral (LL) lobes. Ten days later hyperplasia in the right lateral (RL) and caudate (C) lobes has restored the liver to its pre-operative weight.

production in the liver in response to injury is a vital and beneficial component of the reparative process. However, when the process of fibrogenesis is prolonged the normal liver structure is seriously perturbed with the deposition of abnormal amounts of connective tissue leading to end-stage liver disease—*cirrhosis*, with catastrophic consequences for the individual. Cirrhosis seems to develop in response to the continual infliction of liver cell damage; in man, chronic alcohol abuse and hepatitis B

virus infection seem to be the most important aetiological factors, and similar lesions can be generated in experimental animals by chronic intermittent exposure to hepatotoxins such as carbon tetrachloride. Most cell types in the liver are able to produce the interstitial collagens but it seems that the fat-storing cells (called *Ito cells* or *lipocytes*) are the principal facultative fibroblasts of the liver. On the other hand, a single exposure to carbon tetrachloride does not lead to the development of cirrhosis, although up to 50 per cent of the parenchymal mass may be destroyed. Instead, a regenerative response is rapidly initiated by the unaffected hepatocytes in the periportal areas, which restores the liver to its normal appearance.

Following a two-thirds partial hepatectomy in the rat, very rapid and seemingly crucial accumulations of cAMP and polyamines precede a stimulation of DNA synthesis at about 15 h post-operatively (Fig. 5.31); at 24 h over one-third of all hepatocyte nuclei are in the phase of DNA synthesis at the same time, and some nuclei are already at the stage of mitosis. The response is distinctly ephemeral and the intensity of the proliferative response gradually subsides as the deficit in tissue mass is reduced and eventually totally replaced (Fig. 5.30). During the first 24 h or so of this hyperplastic response there is a distinct spatial distribution of proliferating cells, with most [³H]thymidine-labelled cells (DNA-synthesizing cells) being located in the outer third of the lobule (Fig. 5.32), in zone 1 of the hepatic acinus. From 48 h post-operatively, proliferating hepatocytes are randomly distributed within the liver, and while many of the periportally orientated hepatocytes may undergo two or three rounds of cell division, most of the more slowly responding centrilobular cells probably divide only once

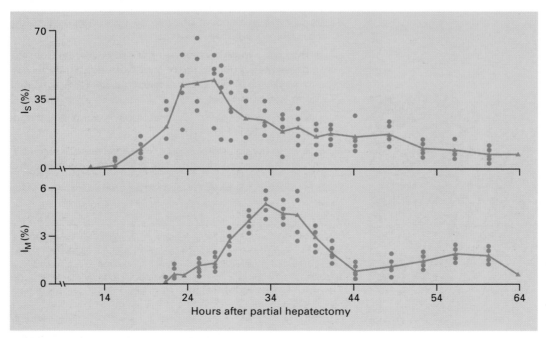

Fig. 5.31 Tritiated thymidine labelling index (I_S) and mitotic index (I_M) in the right lateral lobe of the rat liver following a two-thirds partial hepatectomy. (●) values from individual animals; (▲) mean values.

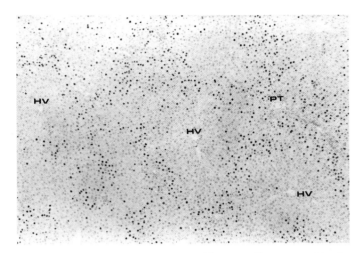

Fig. 5.32 An autoradiograph prepared from a rat liver exposed *in vivo* to tritiated thymidine shortly before the death of the animal at 24 h after partial hepatectomy. The labelled (DNA-synthesizing) nuclei appear black, and are congregated around the points of entry of the afferent blood supply, the small portal tracts (PT). Note the absence of labelled nuclei around the draining hepatic veins (HV).

(Wright and Alison 1984). Since all hepatocytes in the regenerating liver divide at least once it is distinctly unlikely that a stem cell compartment exists amongst the normal population of differentiated hepatocytes. On the other hand, when normal liver cells are prevented from responding to resection by a mito-inhibitory environment created by carcinogen exposure, then nondescript small cells found in the portal space (called *oval cells*) can proliferate and differentiate into hepatocytes and may deserve the appellation of *potential stem cells*. In addition to hepatocytes, all other cell types present in the liver (e.g. bile duct cells and sinusoidal-lining cells) respond to resection with a burst of cell proliferation, although invariably these responses lag a few hours behind those of hepatocytes. In man, extensive liver resection is also compatible with survival and a return to full health; almost complete restoration within 10 days has been reported following a right hepatic lobectomy in previously fit young individuals (Karran and McLaren 1985). Other studies in which individuals underwent right lobectomy (∼60 per cent resection) because of the presence of carcinoma have reported complete restoration of the remaining normal liver within 3 months (Nagasue *et al.* 1987).

The factors that control the regenerative response are not well understood; nutritional and hormonal status can have a modifying influence on the response, while in primary cultures of freshly isolated hepatocytes EGF and insulin appear to act in a synergistic manner to promote DNA synthesis. The reduction in liver size seems to be associated with a decrease in the concentration of a hepatic growth inhibitor and/or the production of a trophic factor which is also of hepatic origin (Alison 1986). The characteristics and amino acid sequence of these hepatic growth factors, the so-called *hepatopoietins*, are now described (Michalopoulos 1990).

Kidney and urinary bladder

The ability of the kidney to functionally compensate for a loss in renal mass is widely appreciated, and this adaptive response has been most extensively investigated in the rat following a unilateral nephrectomy. Over a period of 1 month the weight of the remaining contralateral kidney may increase by 50 per cent above its pre-operative value, and increases in the ratios of RNA/DNA and protein/DNA support the morphological observations that the bulk of this kidney enlargement is due to cellular *hypertrophy*. There is also a hyperplastic component in this response, principally confined to the cortical tubule cells, but which only increases the kidney DNA content by something less than 10 per cent: at the peak of the hyperplastic response the proportion of cortical tubule cells in DNA synthesis is less than 2 per cent (cf. the liver after partial hepatectomy, Fig. 5.31). The proximal segments of the nephron exhibit the most prominent growth reaction, with proximal convoluted tubules increasing by 35 per cent in length and 14 per cent in outside diameter, while distal convoluted tubules increase by 17 per cent in length and 10 per cent in outside diameter (see Wright and Alison 1984). The glomeruli also enlarge by hyperplasia and hypertrophy. In man and experimental animals the glomerular filtration rate (GFR) in the remaining kidney increases by 40–60 per cent above its pre-operative value (Harris *et al.* 1986), so that the total GFR is about 75 per cent of normal when the response is complete. This increase is all due to a rise in the single nephron glomerular filtration rate (SNGFR) as *no new nephrons are formed after renal ablation in adulthood*. The most vigorous compensatory growth reaction occurs in very young animals (< 1 month old), and likewise unilateral nephrectomy in early childhood results in the GFR in the solitary kidney equalling the total GFR in individuals with two kidneys.

In the short term at least, rats can also withstand severe reductions in renal mass involving losses of up to five-sixths of renal tissue. However, such sub-totally nephrectomized animals invariably progress to end-stage renal failure because of the process of sclerosis occurring in the glomeruli of the residual nephrons. Glomerular damage is thought to be initiated by the twin effects of hyperperfusion and hyperfiltration and can be hastened by feeding a high-protein diet. The low proliferative capability of the remnant kidney after unilateral nephrectomy in fact belies very efficient powers of regeneration, observed for instance after short periods of ischaemia or exposure to nephrotoxic chemicals. Heavy metals such as mercury, in particular mercuric chloride ($HgCl_2$), first cause damage to the *pars recta* (straight portion) of the proximal nephron (Fig. 5.33) but, provided the connective tissue framework remains intact, a vigorous regenerative response will repopulate the denuded basement membrane, returning the kidney to its pristine state.

The factors that control compensatory growth in the kidney are not fully elucidated, though earlier hypotheses based on so-called 'work hypertrophy' (e.g. increased urea excretion or increased sodium reabsorption) are now largely discounted. Experiments involving animals in parabiotic union support the existence of a humoral factor (Austin *et al.* 1981), and recent

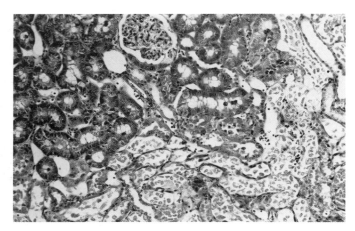

Fig. 5.33 Widespread tubular damage in the corticomedullary region of the rat kidney induced by mercuric chloride. The connective tissue framework is left intact so regeneration will restore the kidney to its normal state.

evidence suggests that this factor (renotropin) is normally present in the serum and urine and acts to inhibit growth (Snow *et al.* 1987).

Ulcerative lesions of the urinary bladder heal in much the same way as peptic ulcers: McMinn (1969) removed areas of mucosa of up to 1 cm² from the cat bladder and found epithelial cells spreading across the wound floor within 24 h, and by 48 h mitotic activity was seen not only in the perilesional mucosa but also in the migrating cells.

Adrenal gland

Each adrenal gland consists of an inner medulla, which is concerned with the production of sympathetic amines, and an outer cortex. There are three well-defined zones in the adrenal cortex: the outer *zona glomerulosa* is associated with electrolyte status and aldosterone secretion, while the *zona fasciculata* and the innermost cortical zone, the *zona reticularis*, are under the control of pituitary ACTH and secrete mainly glucocorticoids. Hypophysectomy or dexamethasone treatment sufficient to suppress ACTH secretion will cause atrophy of the rat adrenal gland, and likewise chronic ACTH treatment will cause both hypertrophy and hyperplasia in the normal gland (Dallman 1985).

The regenerative capabilities of the adrenal gland are well seen in the response to enucleation, a procedure in which the medulla and most of the cortex are 'shelled out' from under the capsule leaving behind a fibrous capsule with an irregular lining of glomerulosa cells. Following enucleation in the rat, cords of cells begin to grow inwards and can be 30 cells in length within a week, with the normal cortical structure restored after about 1 month. There is, of course, no regeneration of the medulla. Following bilateral enucleation, plasma ACTH levels rapidly become grossly elevated (up to 600 per cent of the levels in sham-operated controls) but remain so only for about 1 week (Dallman 1985). Hypophysectomy or treatment with corticosteroids will inhibit the regenerative response, suggesting that

ACTH or an ACTH-related peptide is required for the regenerative process. Even after many months the weight of the regenerated cortex does not exceed 80 per cent of normal.

A rapid compensatory growth response can also be induced in the adrenal by removal of the contralateral gland. Weight increases of 30 per cent and DNA content increases of 70 per cent have been registered just 1 day after unilateral adrenalectomy in the rat, with most of the DNA synthesis confined to the zona glomerulosa and outer zona fasciculata cells. Dexamethasone treatment does not inhibit this growth response, and likewise the response still occurs in hypophysectomized animals, although in both cases it is superimposed on a rapidly atrophying gland. These observations support the contention that adrenal growth is not simply due to a rise in ACTH levels resulting from a fall in corticosterone production, and in any case such changes are of an extremely transient nature after unilateral adrenalectomy (Engeland *et al.* 1975). Lowry *et al.* (1983) believe that a 74 amino acid fragment from the N-terminal fragment of the ACTH precursor, termed N-terminal proopiomelanocortin [N-POMC(1–74)], is involved in adrenal mitogenesis, and that cell proliferation results from a neurally mediated local cleavage of this molecule to generate a mitogenic factor N-POMC(1–48) not containing the γ-MSH sequence. Following bilateral enucleation it is believed that a change in the processing of POMC occurs in the pituitary itself, causing the preferential synthesis of the smaller mitogenically active N-POMC peptides (Estivariz *et al.* 1988).

Thyroid

Despite the prodigious growth potential of the thyroid, which can be seen when gland hormone production is impaired and overproduction of TSH occurs, regenerative capabilities are distinctly modest. Hemithyroidectomy in the rat causes an increase in the RNA/DNA ratio (hypertrophy) but little in the way of hyperplasia, and the gland is only 70 per cent of the preoperative weight once the response is curtailed. The response can be blocked by hypophysectomy or thyroxine therapy, suggesting that the overproduction of TSH is causally related. On the other hand, a very local mitotic response occurs in the follicular epithelia upon the infliction of a small incised wound. The thyroid is particularly susceptible to ionizing radiation, both by virtue of its ability to concentrate radioiodide, and because of its anatomical position. Though conventionally regarded as radioresistant, ionizing radiation can cause a very significant impairment of reproductive capacity in the follicular cells. If rats are treated with aminotriazole (a compound that blocks thyroid hormone synthesis and thus causes overproduction of TSH), the gland weight increases about threefold over a period of 1 month, but prior irradiation depresses this weight gain in a dose-dependent fashion (Table 5.5).

Salivary glands

Like the liver, kidney, and glandular organs discussed above, the salivary glands display little proliferative activity in adulthood. Nevertheless, major glands such as the submaxillary and

Table 5.5 Effects of prior irradiation on thyroid weight gain in rats treated with aminotriazole

Dose of X-irradiation (Gy)	Thyroid weight (mg)
0	76
0.5	72
2.5	66
5.0	54
7.5	47
10.0	37
15.0	28

Rats were administered aminotriazole for 4 weeks, starting 2 weeks after irradiation. The thyroid weighed about 25 mg in rats not challenged with aminotriazole. (Adapted from Gibson and Doniach 1967.)

parotid glands can undergo a prominent growth response to chronic treatment with β-sympathomimetic agents such as isoproterenol. This causes hypertrophy and hyperplasia in secretory acinar cells, and within 2–3 weeks gland weights and DNA content can be increased fivefold (Wright and Alison 1984). The response of these paired glands to unilateral extirpation is much more modest, and can in fact be completely abolished if the activity of the autonomic innervation to the residual gland is reduced by, say, switching the animals to a liquid diet. Thus functional demand seems to play a pivotal role in regenerative growth. The cell division that does occur seems to be localized to the intercalated duct region, and cells migrate distally to the acini and proximally to the ducts of increasing calibre.

Sex hormone-dependent tissues

In the male, accessory sex glands (prostate, seminal vesicles, etc.) are almost wholly dependent upon androgenic stimulation for the maintenance of normal function. If androgen levels are severely depleted, then these tissues undergo a profound atrophy, but tissue loss *per se* is not sufficient to elicit a compensatory response. However, if such atrophic tissues are presented with a functional demand in the shape of resumed androgenic stimulation, then all the regressive changes can be reversed by a wave of hypertrophy and hyperplasia (Alison and Wright 1979).

During the first half of the menstrual cycle the endometrial glands are in a state of active proliferation in response to a rising level of oestradiol in the plasma. Following ovulation these epithelial glands cease proliferation and enter the secretory phase, before ultimately most of the newly formed epithelial cells are shed at the end of the cycle, having undergone ischaemic cell death. Thus the oestradiol-induced wave of proliferation which starts anew at the beginning of each cycle is a regenerative response emanating from residual glandular elements at the base of the endometrium.

Lung

Lung tissue can undergo a compensatory growth response to partial excision (pneumonectomy) or regeneration in response to damage within the conducting airways or alveoli. Unilateral excision can result in the remaining lung achieving the same weight, volume, cell, and alveolar number as control animals. The response is probably more complete in young animals and begins with the proliferation of mesothelial and peripheral alveolar cells at 24 h after excision, and by 1 week there is diffuse pulmonary proliferation. The result of this increased cell proliferation is a large increase in the gas-exchanging surface area, although it is not entirely clear if this involves alveolar multiplication (Thurlbeck 1983). At least part of the stimulus for cell proliferation appears to be the increased ability of the remaining lung to expand, since *plombage* (packing the pleural cavity with inert material) on the pneumonectomized side delays the proliferative response.

Local wounds of the trachea heal by the migration of cells across the wound floor, with increased proliferation of marginal cells. Agents such as NO_2 cause the destruction of bronchiolar epithelium and alveolar lining cells, eliciting a regenerative response from Clara cells and type 2 pneumocytes, respectively. Bleomycin, an antitumour antibiotic, also causes the proliferation of type 2 pneumocytes (the supposed stem cells of the alveoli) by causing diffuse alveolar damage.

Nervous tissue

Neurones in the CNS are very sensitive to insults such as hypoxia, and in the postnatal human brain they are irreplaceable, although some limited regrowth of neuronal processes is possible. If axons in the CNS are severed, the cut ends swell due to continued axonal transport to form so-called *axon balloons* or *axon torpedos*. It is from these swellings at the distal ends of the proximal stumps that regeneration of fibres occurs, much more so in the peripheral nervous system than in the CNS. The cell body of the severed axon rapidly switches from a functional mode to one of attempted regeneration with accompanying morphological changes referred to as *chromatolysis* (Weller *et al.* 1983). There are overall reductions in the synthesis of transmitter-related enzymes, but significant increases in membrane protein synthesis. In response to CNS injury, astrocytes go through a phase of hypertrophy and hyperplasia (Takamiya *et al.* 1988), helping to absorb oedema and promoting neovascularization through the production of laminin. These so-called 'reactive' astrocytes also show a large increase in their content of *glial fibrillary acidic protein* (GFAP) (Fig. 5.34) and when these cells subsequently atrophy they leave behind a fibrous-like scar of glial filaments: failure of axonal regeneration may, in part, be due to an inability of the axon to penetrate this gliotic scar.

It could be argued that the failure of axonal regeneration in the CNS is beneficial since it lessens the likelihood of improper anatomical connections through local synaptogenesis in a tissue where the specificity of connections is vital for proper function. Certainly axonal regeneration is more successful in the peripheral nervous system where the demands for specific neuronal connections are less exacting. Here severing of the axon leads to degeneration of the distal portion and proliferation of the Schwann cells (Fig. 5.35) even while they are scavenging

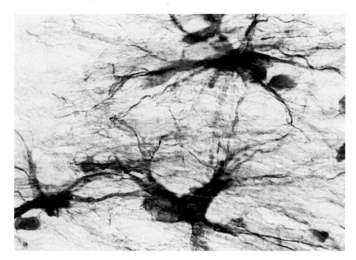

Fig. 5.34 Reactive astrocytes in the rat brain immunostained by the streptavidin-biotin technique for glial fibrillary acidic protein.

the axon and myelin debris (Fig. 5.35b). Within 3–4 days of transection regenerative features are seen (Fig. 5.35c). Chromatolysis of the neuronal cell body occurs and a number of axonal sprouts (neurites) can be seen growing out from the axon balloon. As the cluster of neurites grows down the line of Schwann cells, myelination occurs and finally one or more of the processes may make contact with an end organ such as muscle (Fig. 5.35d). Regenerated fibres can often be identified by their short (fetal-like) internode length.

Skeletal muscle

The replicative ability of skeletal muscle is due to the presence of

reserve (potential) myogenic stem cells called *satellite* cells (Mauro 1979). These small mononucleated cells are found between the external (basal) lamina and the plasma membrane of the muscle fibre, and probably account for only 1–2 per cent of all the muscle fibre nuclei. Satellite cells divide in response to injury, and the cells can fuse to form new multinucleated muscle fibres (*myotubes*). In cases of compensatory hypertrophy due to the incapacitation of synergistic muscles, newly formed cells can be incorporated into fibres (Schiaffino *et al.* 1976).

Arteries

Injury and repair of arteries are of considerable importance to the understanding of atherogenesis. Many studies have been made of endothelial and smooth muscle cell proliferation following dilatation injuries inflicted by balloon catheter. Endothelial regeneration in denuded arteries is strictly limited; proliferative rates are raised in the endothelial cells at the wound margin for 1–3 weeks, but cells migrate a distance of only 3–4 mm over the denuded surface in the first 3 months (Reidy 1988). Extensive endothelial denudaton can also cause smooth muscle accumulation in the arterial intima by the migration of both dividing and non-dividing cells from the tunica media (Clowes and Schwartz 1985). This migration and proliferation of smooth muscle cells is thought to be at least partly due to the adhesion of platelets to the exposed subendothelial collagen and the subsequent release of growth factors, including PDGF. The healing response at anastomotic sites follows a predictable course, with endothelial migration and mitoses and a prominent granulation tissue response; it is likely that the scar in the vessel wall remains a permanently inelastic structure. In most cases the newly formed connective tissue is not sufficiently strong to withstand the persistent mechanical stress or tension

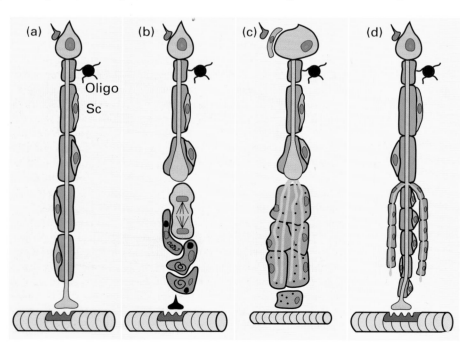

Fig. 5.35 Peripheral nerve regeneration. (a) Normal nerve and muscle; Schwann cell and myelin sheath (Sc), oligodendrocyte (ol). (b) Severing of the axon leads to the distal portion degenerating, Schwann cell proliferation, and axon ballooning. (c) Regeneration occurs through the formation of neurites from the axon balloon; the neuronal cell body undergoes chromatolysis and the denervated muscle atrophies. (d) Re-innervation of the end organ. (Drawn after Weller *et al.* 1983, with permission.)

in the normal arterial wall, in which case the permanent support of non-absorbable sutures is required.

Mesothelium

The pleural, pericardial, and peritoneal cavities are all lined by a monolayer of specialized cells, termed the mesothelium. The initial response to damage seems to be one of macrophage adherence to the wound surface, which may serve to prevent adhesions between visceral and parietal surfaces; macrophages may supply plasminogen activators as well as phagocytosing fibrin and cell debris. Within 24 h very high levels of cell proliferation are found in the mesothelial cells at the wound edge, and over the next few days mesothelial cells migrate centripetally to cover the denuded serosa (Whitaker and Papadimitriou 1985). In addition to their role in wound débridement, the adherent macrophages may also be a potent source of mitogenic factors for the mesothelial cells (Fotev et al. 1987).

5.3.3 Organization

Organization means the replacement, by granulation tissue, of solid, inanimate material such as necrotic tissue, inflammatory exudate, thrombus, or blood clot. Necrotic tissue is organized when, for example, the connective tissue framework of an organ is more or less destroyed permitting little in the way of regeneration (see Fig. 5.16). More often, organization occurs when tissue that has no inherent capability for self-renewal is partly destroyed, an all-too-common example being infarcted heart muscle.

Inflammatory exudates become organized when they persist and fail to resolve. In lobar pneumonia, for example, the conspicuous intra-alveolar exudate (Fig. 5.36) would normally be cleared by the combined actions of neutrophil polymorphs and macrophages returning the inflamed tissue to its pristine state (resolution), but occasionally resolution fails to occur and the exudate becomes organized leading to permanent fibrosis. This involves the ingrowth of fibroblasts and capillaries from the alveolar septae, converting the incompletely lysed fibrin into collagenous vascularized connective tissue (Fig. 5.36). Thus the affected alveoli are solid rather than spongy and aerated. Fibrinous exudates in serous cavities such as the pericardial and pleural cavities can be converted to fibrous adhesions which partly or totally obliterate the spaces. In some cases of pleurisy the thick layers of fibrin on both visceral and parietal pleura can be simultaneously organized, leading to the lung being firmly bound to the chest wall by fibrous tissue.

Like the inflammatory exudate, a thrombus may also resolve; that is, disappear leaving little or no trace of its presence. On the other hand, if the thrombus is too large to resolve, it may organize, transforming the thrombus into vascular connective tissue (Fig. 5.37). This begins with fibroblasts and capillaries proliferating and entering the thrombus from its points of attachment to the underlying vessel wall. At the same time, endothelium grows over the thrombus from its edges, and also lines any accessible clefts and spaces in an occluding thrombus. As organization proceeds the capillary channels may anastomose to produce thoroughfares that traverse the thrombus which have the function of restoring blood flow, a process known as recanalization. Mural thrombi tend to become less organized than occluding thrombi, probably because the high intra-luminal pressure prevents capillary ingrowth from the vasa vasorum. Recanalization of occlusive thrombi is also thought to occur more readily in veins than in arteries, though the re-establishment of an adequate blood flow is a slow process and may take several years. Other obliterative lesions in blood vessels can also be organized: Fig. 5.38 illustrates an atheromatous plaque which has embolized to the kidney and become partly organized.

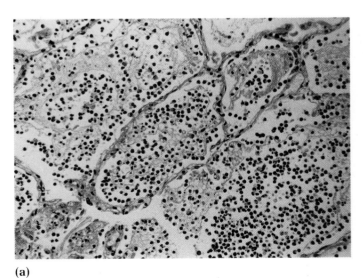

(a)

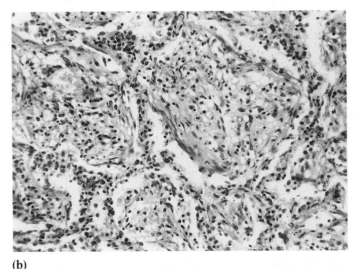

(b)

Fig. 5.36 (a) An example of lobar pneumonia with a conspicuous intra-alveolar exudate composed of fibrin and neutrophils. (b) Failure of the exudate to resolve has led to organization with the air spaces filled with connective tissue.

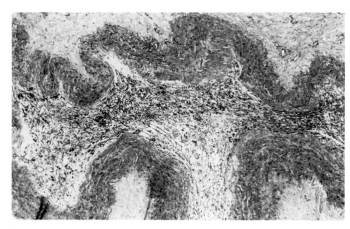

Fig. 5.37 In this pulmonary artery an occlusive thrombus has been completely organized, having been replaced by vascularized connective tissue.

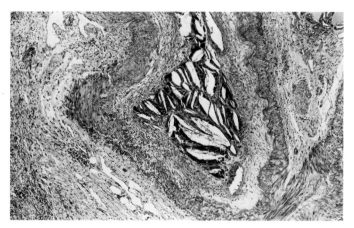

Fig. 5.38 Organization of an atheromatous embolus in a renal artery.

5.3.4   Bibliography

General

Clark, R. A. F. (1988). Potential roles of fibronectin in cutaneous wound repair. *Archives of Dermatology* **124**, 201–6.

Florey, H. (1970). *General pathology* (4th edn). Lloyd Luke, London.

Grøndahl-Hansen, J., Lund, L. R., Ralfkiaer, E., Ottevanger, V., and Danø, K. (1988). Urokinase and tissue-type plasminogen activators in keratinocytes during wound re-epithelialization *in vivo*. *Journal of Investigative Dermatology* **90**, 790–5.

Herron, G. S., Werb, Z., Dwyer, K., and Banda, M. J. (1986a). Secretion of metalloproteinases by stimulated capillary endothelial cells. [I]. Production of procollagenase and prostromelysin exceeds expression of proteolytic activity. *Journal of Biological Chemistry* **261**, 2810–13.

Herron, G. S., Banda, M. J., Clark, E. J., Gavrilovic, J., and Werb, Z. (1986b). Secretion of metalloproteinases by stimulated capillary endothelial cells. [II]. Expression of collagenase and stromelysin activities is regulated by endogenous inhibitors. *Journal of Biological Chemistry* **261**, 2814–18.

Irvin, T. T. (1981). *Wound healing. Principles and practice.* Chapman and Hall, London.

Moscatelli, D. and Rifkin, D. B. (1988). Membrane and matrix localization of proteinases: a common theme in tumour cell invasion and angiogenesis. *Biochimica et Biophysica Acta* **948**, 67–85.

Rungger-Brandle, E. and Gabbiani, G. (1983). The role of cytoskeletal and cytocontractile elements in pathological processes. *American Journal of Pathology* **110**, 361–92.

Wright, N. A. and Alison, M. R. (1984). *The biology of epithelial cell populations*, Vols 1 and 2. Clarendon Press, Oxford.

Collagen synthesis

Fleischmajer, R. (1986). Collagen fibrillogenesis: a mechanism of structural biology. *Journal of Investigative Dermatology* **87**, 553–4.

Laurent, G. J. (1987). Dynamic state of collagen: pathways of collagen degradation *in vivo* and their possible role in regulation of collagen mass. *American Journal of Physiology* **252** (*Cell Physiology* 21), C1–C9.

Miller, E. J. and Gay, S. (1987). The collagens: an overview and update. In *Methods in enzymology*, Vol. 144, *Structural and contractile proteins* (ed. L. W. Cunningham), pp. 3–41. Academic Press, New York.

Sykes, B. and Smith, R. (1985). Collagen and collagen gene disorders. *Quarterly Journal of Medicine, New Series* **56** (221), 533–47.

Control mechanisms

Cohen, S. (1986). Epidermal growth factor. *Bioscience Reports* **6**, 1017–27.

Goodlad, R. A., Wilson, T. J. G., Lenton, W., Gregory, H., McCullagh, K. G., and Wright, N. A. (1987). Intravenous but not intragastric urogastrone—EGF is trophic to the intestine of parenterally fed rats. *Gut* **28**, 573–82.

Gospodarowicz, D., Neufeld, G., and Schweigerer, L. (1987). Fibroblast growth factor: structural and biological properties. *Journal of Cellular Physiology*, Suppl. 5, 15–26.

Ross, R., Raines, E. W., and Bowen-Pope, D. F. (1986). The biology of platelet-derived growth factor. *Cell* **46**, 155–69.

Sporn, M. B., Roberts, A. B., Wakefield, L. M., and de Crombrugghe, B. (1987). Some recent advances in the chemistry and biology of transforming growth factor-beta. *Journal of Cell Biology* **105**, 1039–45.

Skin

Elgjo, K., Reichelt, K. L., Hennings, H., Michael, D., and Yuspa, S. H. (1986). Purified epidermal pentapeptide inhibits proliferation and enhances terminal differentiation in mouse epidermal cells. *Journal of Investigative Dermatology* **87**, 555–8.

Maibach, H. I. and Rovee, D. T. (1972). *Epidermal wound healing.* Year Book Medical Publishers, Chicago.

Pinkus, H. and Mehregan, A. H. (1981). *A guide to dermato-histopathology* (3rd edn). Appleton-Century-Crofts, New York.

Gastrointestinal tract

Konturek, S. J., Dembinski, A., Warzecha, Z., Bizozowski, T., and Gregory, H. (1988). Role of epidermal growth factor in healing of gastro duodenal ulcers in rats. *Gastroenterology* **94**, 1300–7.

McMinn, R. M. H. (1969). *Tissue repair.* Academic Press, New York.

Potten, C. S., Hendry, J. H., Moore, J. V., and Chwalinski, S. (1983). Cytotoxic effects in gastrointestinal epithelium (as exemplified by small intestine). In *Cytotoxic insult to tissue* (ed. C. S. Potten and J. H. Hendry), pp. 105–52. Churchill Livingstone, Edinburgh.

Roe, R., Fermor, B., and Williamson, R. C. N. (1987). Proliferative instability and experimental carcinogenesis at colonic anastomoses. *Gut* **28**, 808–15.

Silen, W. and Ito, S. (1985). Mechanisms for rapid re-epithelialization of the gastric mucosal surface. *Annual Reviews of Physiology* **47**, 217–29.

Umpleby, H. C. and Williamson, R. C. N. (1987). Anastomotic recurrence in large bowel cancer. *British Journal of Surgery* **74**, 873–8.

Wright, N. A. (1978). The cell population kinetics of repopulating cells in the intestine. In *Stem cells and tissue homeostasis* (ed. B. I. Lord, C. S. Potten, and R. J. Cole), pp. 335–58. Cambridge University Press, Cambridge.

Wright, N. A. and Al-Nafussi, A. (1982). The kinetics of villus cell populations in the mouse small intestine. *Cell and Tissue Kinetics* **15**, 611–21.

Wright, N. A., Pike, C., and Elia, G. (1990). Induction of a novel epidermal growth factor secreting cell lineage by mucosal ulceration in human gastrointestinal stem cells. *Nature* **343**, 82–5.

Liver

Alison, M. R. (1986). Regulation of hepatic growth. *Physiological Reviews* **66**, 499–541.

Karran, S. and McLaren, M. (1985). Physical aspects of hepatic regeneration. In *Liver and biliary disease* (2nd edn), (ed. R. Wright, G. H. Millward-Sadler, K. G. M. M. Alberti, and S. Karran), pp. 233–50. Baillière Tindall, London.

Michalopoulos, G. K. (1990). Liver regeneration: molecular mechanisms of growth control. *FASEB Journal* **4**, 176–87.

Nagasue, N., Yukaya, H., Ogawa, Y., Kohno, H., and Nakamura, T. (1987). Human liver regeneration after major hepatic resection. *Annals of Surgery* **206**, 30–9.

Kidney

Austin, H., Goldin, H., and Preuss, H. G. (1981). Humoral regulation of renal growth. *Nephron* **27**, 163–70.

Harris, R. C., Meyer, T. W., and Brenner, B. M. (1986). Nephron adaptation to renal injury. In *The kidney* (3rd edn) (ed. B. M. Brenner and F. C. Rector), pp. 1553–85. W. B. Saunders, Philadelphia.

Snow, B. W., Tarry, W. F., and Duckett, J. W. (1987). Compensatory renal growth: interactions of nephrectomy serum and urine antisera leading to a new theory of renal growth regulation. *Urological Research* **15**, 1–4.

Adrenal

Dallman, M. F. (1985). Control of adrenocortical growth *in vivo*. *Endocrine Research* **10**, 213–42.

Engeland, W. C., Shinsako, J., and Dallman, M. F. (1975). Corticosteroids and ACTH are not required for compensatory adrenal growth. *American Journal of Physiology* **229**, 1461–4.

Estivariz, F. E., Morano, M. I., Carino, M., Jackson, S., and Lowry, P. J. (1988). Adrenal regeneration in the rat is mediated by mitogenic N-terminal pro-opiomelanocortin peptides generated by changes in precursor processing in the anterior pituitary. *Journal of Endocrinology* **116**, 207–16.

Lowry, P. J., Silas, L., McLean, C., Linton, E. A., and Estivariz, F. E. (1983). Pro-γ-melanocyte-stimulating hormone cleavage in adrenal gland undergoing compensatory growth. *Nature* **306**, 70–3.

Thyroid

Gibson, J. M. and Doniach, I. (1967). Correlation of dose of X-radiation to the rat thyroid gland with degree of subsequent impairment of response to goitrogenic stimulus. *British Journal of Cancer* **21**, 524–30.

Accessory sex glands

Alison, M. R. and Wright, N. A. (1979). Testosterone induced cell proliferation in the accessory sex glands of mice at various times after castration. *Cell and Tissue Kinetics* **12**, 461–75.

Lung

Thurlbeck, W. M. (1983). Postpneumonectomy compensatory lung growth. *American Reviews of Respiratory Disease* **128**, 965–7.

Nervous tissue

Takamiya, Y., Kohsaka, S., Toya, S., Otani, M., and Tsukada, Y. (1988). Immunohistochemical studies on the proliferation of reactive astrocytes and the expression of cytochemical proteins following brain injury in rats. *Developmental Brain Research* **38**, 201–10.

Weller, R. O., Swash, M., McLellan, D. L., and Scholtz, C. L. (1983). *Clinical neuropathology*. Springer-Verlag, Berlin.

Skeletal muscle

Mauro, A. (1979). *Muscle regeneration*. Raven Press, New York.

Schiaffino, S., Pierobon Bormioli, S., and Aloisi, M. (1976). The fate of newly formed satellite cells during compensatory muscle hypertrophy. *Virchows Archives B—Cell Pathology* **21**, 113–18.

Arteries

Clowes, A. W. and Schwartz, S. M. (1985). Significance of quiescent smooth muscle migration in the injured rat carotid artery. *Circulation Research* **56**, 139–45.

Reidy, M. A. (1988). Endothelial regeneration. VIII. Interaction of smooth muscle muscle cells with endothelial regrowth. *Laboratory Investigation* **59**, 36–43.

Mesothelia

Fotev, Z., Whitaker, D., and Papadimitriou, J. M. (1987). Role of macrophages in mesothelial healing. *Journal of Pathology* **151**, 209–19.

Whitaker, D. and Papadimitriou, J. M. (1985). Mesothelial healing: morphological and kinetic investigations. *Journal of Pathology* **145**, 159–75.

5.4 Chronic inflammation

A. M. Flanagan and T. J. Chambers

5.4.1 Introduction

Injury evokes a sequence of events in living tissue, in which inflammation (a process by which tissue becomes hyperaemic and swollen due to exudation of white cells, plasma proteins, and fluid) is followed by demolition of injured tissue, and healing, either by resolution, regeneration, or repair. If the injurious agent acts briefly (burns, infarction) or is rapidly overcome (some infections), then inflammation will be of short duration (acute). If injury is prolonged, however, then the inflammatory response will be similarly prolonged, and will thus continue after the initiation of attempts at healing. Clinically, chronic inflammation is loosely defined as inflammation that has been present for weeks or months. Histologically, chronic inflammation is defined as inflammation that occurs simultaneously with attempted healing: processes that are sequential in acute inflammation (Fig. 5.39) occur simultaneously in chronic inflammation.

Although a clear distinction cannot always be made, especially clinically, between acute and chronic inflammation, prolongation of injury has consequences of its own: a transient injury may be followed by resolution even if the inflammation is intense (e.g. lobar pneumonia), but a prolonged injury will induce scar-tissue formation which makes resolution impossible when the injury subsides. Similarly, regeneration (defined in pathology as restoration of a normal number of specialized cells, not necessarily accompanied by restoration of normal tissue architecture) will occur with replacement of epithelial cells but not at the site of inflammation where the continuing injury prevents this, but in adjacent tissue. The regenerated tissue is generally hyperplastic and its normal architecture is disrupted (e.g. cirrhosis).

Chronic inflammation can arise in two ways: as persistence of any of the inflammatory stimuli that induce acute inflammation, or as a process that is distinctive from the outset. In the latter, there is minimal acute inflammation but rather an accumulation of cells of the mononuclear phagocyte system (macrophages), lymphocytes, and plasma cells. A primary chronic inflammatory reaction such as this occurs in two settings: first (a *granulomatous reaction*), in response to material that is difficult to digest, which also may be inherently toxic (e.g. silica) or becomes so when it evokes an immunological reaction (e.g. *Mycobacterium tuberculosis*). Secondly, there is a distinct group of diseases, which are characterized by a primary chronic inflammatory reaction (without preceding acute

inflammation), in which no obvious agent can be held responsible. This is considered to be the result of the immune response being inappropriately directed against an individual's own tissue (auto-immunity).

5.4.2   Persistence of acute inflammation

All forms of chronic inflammation caused by persistence of an injurious agent show in common exudative inflammation, with polymorphs and fluid exudate; macrophages, the cells of demolition; organization, as evidenced by new vessel formation, fibroblasts, and collagen deposition (i.e. granulation tissue); and regeneration in competent tissues (Fig. 5.40). Injury is usually difficult to identify directly, but may be recognized as loss of normal tissue components. Other cell types, such as plasma cells, lymphocytes, and eosinophils, are also present, depending upon the particular immunological properties of the inciting agent.

An important and distinctive subgroup of chronic inflammation that follows acute inflammation is *chronic suppurative inflammation*.

Chronic suppurative inflammation

Suppurative inflammation is characterized by the formation of an abscess cavity, consisting of an area of liquified tissue containing large numbers of living and dead polymorphonuclear leucocytes (*pus*). Fluid exudate in the inflammatory lesion maintains a high tissue tension, and the pus tends to track, under pressure, along lines of low tissue resistance. This may result in discharge of the pus on to a free surface, a process that enables discharge from the tissues of the inciting agent together with the liquefied tissue. This both assists host resistance and reduces the volume of tissue and exudate that requires organization and therefore the lesion is capable of healing more rapidly and with less fibrosis. Suppurative inflammation may persist, to become *chronic suppurative inflammation*, in which

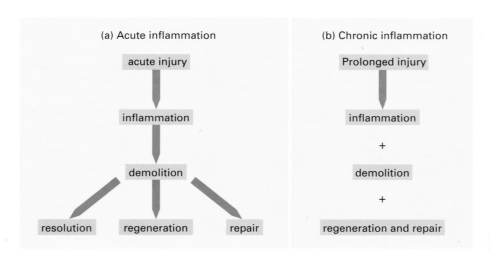

Fig. 5.39 (a) The sequelae of the acute inflammatory reaction; (b) the events of chronic inflammation.

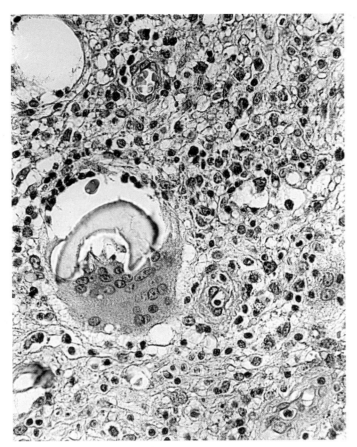

Fig. 5.40 The presence of part of a hair shaft in a sinus tract elicits a persistent inflammatory reaction with associated new blood-vessel formation: mononuclear phagocytes fuse in an attempt to engulf the foreign material which is resistant to degradation.

attempts at organization are seen in the wall of the abscess cavity while suppurative exudation is still occurring, in several circumstances.

Delay in evacuation

If the abscess cannot, for anatomical reasons, drain to an external surface, the inciting agent, rather than being evacuated, is more likely to persist in the abscess cavity, where it is relatively protected from host defences. The abscess cavity is avascular and structureless: this prevents the establishment of gradients for chemotaxis; polymorphs also have a longer distance to travel from vessels to reach organisms, and lack a solid substratum over which to migrate. Granulation tissue begins to form in the wall of the abscess cavity. The abscess cavity becomes lined with new, thin-walled, vascular sprouts, from which polymorphs continue to pour in large numbers from the 'pyogenic membrane' beneath which fibroblastic tissue proliferates and lays down collagen. This attempt at healing has the beneficial effect of walling off the abscess cavity from adjacent viable tissue, and thus localizing the infection, but also has the deleterious effect of making the abscess wall rigid. Thus even if the pus does eventually escape to an external surface, either naturally or through surgical intervention, the abscess will no longer collapse when tissue tension falls, and the inciting agent cannot be completely evacuated. Moreover, healing must then occur by infilling of the abscess cavity by granulation tissue, a prolonged process that will, at best, produce much scar tissue. Delay in evacuation is generally associated with intermittent discharge of pus at the external surface. Discharge of pus temporarily relieves tissue tension within the abscess cavity. The drainage track may then close, and drainage cease until tissue tension becomes sufficient to re-open the track once more.

Presence of necrotic or extraneous materials

Tissue or extraneous material that resists liquefaction during suppuration acts as a refuge within which organisms survive and proliferate relatively protected from host defences. Organisms may persist in crevices too small for access by polymorphs, or deep within necrotic tissue or material through which polymorph migration is difficult and prolonged. The best example of this is the necrotic bone that delays healing in *acute osteomyelitis*. Pyogenic infection within bone, especially cancellous bone, produces an area of suppurative inflammation within which organisms may be protected from engulfment by polymorphs in crevices and canaliculi on the bony trabeculae. There is, moreover, little opportunity for spontaneous evacuation of such an infection, and chronicity is the usual outcome. Viable bone trabeculae around the area of initial infection react with new bone formation, to surround the focus with dense, sclerotic new bone associated with the cells of acute (polymorphs) and chronic infection (macrophages, plasma cells, lymphocytes)—*chronic osteomyelitis*. If the initial inflammation is more intense, then the tissue tension within the unyielding confines of the bone rises and compromises the vascular supply, and leads to extensive infarction of bone and marrow. The pus tends to track under the periosteum, and the lifting of the periosteum from the bony cortex still further compromises the blood supply and may lead to more necrosis. Intraosseous pus may rupture through the periosteum and track into surrounding tissues and eventually reach the skin surface through a number of sinuses. The periosteum responds to the inflammatory process by producing reactive new bone, which surrounds the dead cortex in a sleeve-like fashion. The new bone is known as the *involucrum* (Fig. 5.41). Within the involucrum lies the dead bone, bathed in pus, which acts as a large foreign body within which microorganisms find sanctuary from host defences.

Chronic osteomyelitis is an archetypal example of an acute inflammatory reaction becoming chronic through inadequacy of drainage and the presence of a foreign body, in this case endogenous. A similar predisposition to chronicity is caused when extraneous material, such as dirt, wood, cloth, etc., is introduced into a wound, or surgical materials are erroneously left behind during surgical procedures.

Defective leucocyte function

Defective leucocyte function is also an important cause of chronic suppurative disease. The accummulation of neutrophil

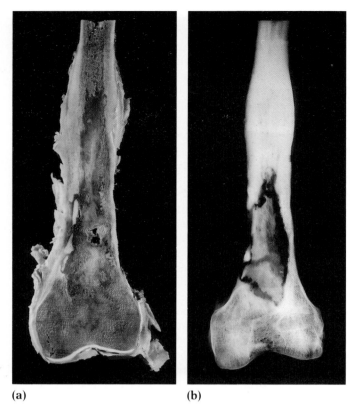

(a)   **(b)**

Fig. 5.41 A photograph (a) of chronic osteomyelitis of the tibia. There is thickened reactive periosteum and new bone formation, i.e. *involucrum*, surrounding a central area of necrosis. The corresponding X-ray (b) demonstrates dead bone (*sequestrum*) within the central cavity. (Courtesy of the Morbid Anatomy Department, Institute of Orthopaedics, Royal National Orthopaedic Hospital, Stanmore.)

polymorphs at a site of injury is dependent on normal chemotaxis and adherence of cell receptors to the substratum. On arrival at the site of injury, effective phagocytosis and degradation of the ingested materials is requisite for a brisk inflammatory reaction. If either of these latter functions are impaired, protracted injury of tissue by persistence of the inciting agent, tissue loss, and the accumulation of large numbers of functionally incompetent, although morphologically normal, neutrophil polymorphs occurs. The disease process in such individuals is manifested by increased susceptibility to infection and they commonly develop microabscesses as a result of only minor infections.

Examples of defects in phagocytosis by neutrophil polymorphs are seen in two important, although somewhat rare, genetically determined diseases: *C3 deficiency* and *X-linked Bruton's agammaglobulinaemia* (Pearl *et al.* 1978). In these diseases there is absence or deficiency of C3 and immunoglobulin respectively: both of these are well-characterized serum proteins which act as opsonins, coating foreign material, and are necessary for efficient attachment and phagocytosis by neutrophil polymorphs. Their absence results in the inefficient ingestion of material that occurs in the presence of large numbers of

acute inflammatory cells, which gives rise to chronic suppurative lesions.

Besides abnormalities of ingestion, derangement of enzymatic degradation may also occur. Microbicidal activity is largely dependent on the production of toxic oxygen metabolites by neutrophil polymorphs. In particular, the release of hydrogen peroxide (H_2O_2) in conjunction with myeloperoxidase is the principal means of killing organisms. *Chronic granulomatous disease of childhood* is characterized by an inherited enzymatic defect that results in the failure of production of H_2O_2 during phagocytosis (Babior 1978). This leads to inefficient killing of bacteria and fungi and results in individuals having a marked propensity for frequent chronic suppurative infections. Diabetes mellitus, a more common disease, is complicated frequently by chronic infections, e.g. carbuncles, pyelonephritis. Neutrophil polymorphs show impairment of phagocytosis and degradation, although the defective mechanism is less clearly defined than in Bruton's agammaglobulinaemia or in chronic granulomatous disease of childhood.

Non-specific chronic inflammation

Most examples of chronic inflammation are not associated with the formation of the pus typical of chronic suppurative inflammation. Lesser forms of injury do not produce liquefaction of tissue, but can nevertheless go on to chronic inflammation if the injury persists. This produces a typical histological pattern, in which there may be evidence of fluid exudate (fibrin deposition, oedema) and polymorphonuclear leucocytes, induced in response to injury. Superimposed on these are the responses seen in tissue that is attempting to heal: granulation tissue, fibrosis, the cells of demolition (macrophages), lymphocytes, and plasma cells. This histological pattern is seen as a response common to chronic injury in a wide variety of agents, and is frequently referred to as 'non-specific chronic inflammation'.

The injurious stimulus involved in non-specific chronic inflammatory reactions is usually of a low-grade nature and the severity of the tissue damage is largely dependent on the persistence of the injury, which is accompanied by inflammation and fibrosis. The particular site involved is also of major importance in determining the consequences of the chronic inflammation.

The presence of ill-fitting dentures results in continuous mucosal irritation inducing ulceration; an inflammatory infiltrate of acute and chronic inflammatory cells accumulates along with new blood-vessel formation and fibrosis. However, there is little or no serious functional loss as a result of injury at this site. In contrast, however, there are serious consequences following non-specific chronic inflammation as illustrated in chronic alcoholic liver disease. Ethanol and, more importantly, its metabolites acetaldehyde and acetate, are hepatotoxic, and ingestion of alcohol over a long period of time results in extensive hepatocyte injury and cell death. Chronic damage is followed by the usual sequence of events as described in Fig. 5.39b. Inflammatory cells, including neutrophil polymorphs, macrophages, and lymphocytes, are recruited to the site of injury. The neutrophil polymorphs characteristically cluster around dead hepatocytes within the parenchyma: this histological feature is termed

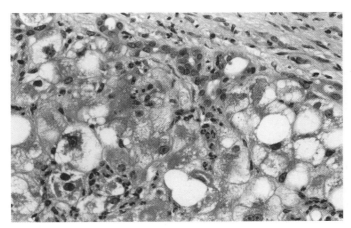

Fig. 5.42 Alcoholic liver disease: the photomicrograph shows fatty change and ballooning degeneration of hepatocytes. There is a predominantly neutrophil polymorph reaction to damaged hepatocytes.

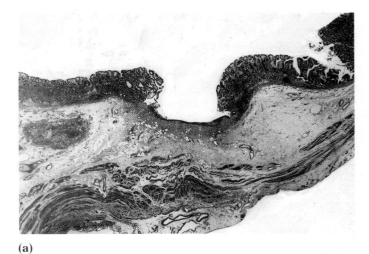

(a)

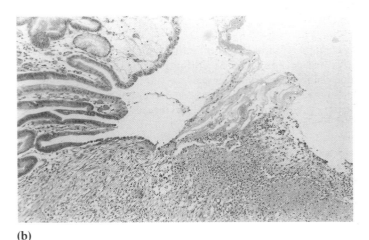

(b)

Fig. 5.44 A peptic ulcer (a) showing loss of the surface epithelium and replacement by granulation tissue. The high-power view (b) shows the necrotic slough and pus exuding from the ulcerated surface.

acute alcoholic hepatitis (Fig. 5.42). Chronic tissue loss is accompanied by attempted healing, manifested by regeneration of hepatocytes and fibrosis. This eventually leads to replacement of the normal lobular architecture by hyperplastic nodules of liver cells surrounded by thick bands of collagen: the histological picture recognized as *cirrhosis* (Fig. 5.43).

Another common disease where features of non-specific chronic inflammation are seen as a result of prolonged tissue damage is chronic peptic ulceration. This is believed to result from an imbalance between factors which protect the mucosa, such as mucus, blood flow, and bicarbonate, against those which are potentially injurious to mucosal cells; these include gastric acid, pepsinogen, bile, and ingested agents, e.g. alcohol and aspirin. In peptic ulceration, dead cells are sloughed from the mucosal surface (Fig. 5.44) and large numbers of acute and

chronic inflammatory cells are recruited to the site of tissue injury. A layer of granulation tissue is formed beneath the necrotic debris and fibroblasts proliferate, laying down collagen deep to the granulation tissue in an attempt at healing. The amount of fibrosis is related to the size and chronicity of the injury. If the inciting stimulus (acid) is removed, re-epithelialization may occur (as described in Section 5.3), but the fibrosis is irreversible and, if extensive, results in stenosis of the bowel wall (see also Section 5.3.2).

5.4.3 Primary chronic inflammation

Chronic inflammation does not always follow persistence of agents that cause acute inflammation, but can also arise as a process that is distinct from the outset. In this type of inflammation, also called chronic *de novo*, there is an absence of, or only

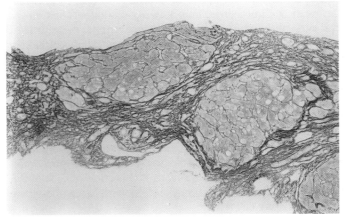

Fig. 5.43 A photomicrograph of a cirrhotic liver. The hyperplastic hepatic nodules are surrounded by thick bands of collagen, resulting in loss of the normal vascular relations, i.e. loss of the normal liver architecture.

an insignificant, phase of acute inflammation. From the beginning the cellular infiltrate is predominantly mononuclear, consisting of mononuclear phagocytes and lymphocytes, with few or no polymorphs. There are two main categories: those disorders in which the immune system itself is responsible for most of the injury, when tissue cells are recognized as foreign, and those disorders in which mononuclear phagocytes dominate the histological appearance. The latter, *granulomatous inflammation*, is a common response to many agents that are normally ingested by mononuclear phagocytes, but that resist degradation; these may cause injury to the engulfing macrophage either directly, due to inherent toxicity (e.g. silica), or indirectly through antigenicity (e.g. *Mycobacterium tuberculosis*). This pattern of inflammation will be described in Section 5.4.4. In the former category, lymphocytes are generally the dominant cell type, and local tissue cells show degenerative changes. There are associated attempts at healing, with regeneration and fibrosis as evidence of chronicity. Several important diseases fall into this category, amongst which *chronic active hepatitis* is perhaps the best example.

Hepatitis B viral (HBV) infection is a major cause of chronic liver disease and cirrhosis. Although the virus is hepatotropic and replicates within liver cells, it is not intrinsically cytotoxic (in contrast to alcohol). This is demonstrated by the absence of hepatocyte injury, death, and the paucity of an inflammatory reaction in the liver of infected individuals who are immunosuppressed. In contrast, HBV infection in immunocompetent individuals results in cell death brought about by cell-mediated immunity considered to be directed against the liver cell membrane altered by HBV (Scheuer 1986). The histological appearance of HBV-infected liver is that of predominantly periportal liver cell death in association with a dense chronic inflammatory infiltrate, mainly lymphocytes, and is referred to as *piecemeal necrosis* (Fig. 5.45). Chronic hepatocyte loss and inflammation, together with regeneration and fibrosis, leads to irreversible loss of the normal lobular architecture and the development of cirrhosis (Fig. 5.43).

Primary chronic inflammation is also seen in a group of diseases in which the immune response is directed against self antigens. The first described (and archetypal example) of such an organ-specific auto-immune disease is *Hashimoto's thyroiditis*; other examples include Graves' disease, Goodpasture's disease, and juvenile insulin-dependent diabetes. The aetiology of such diseases is not known, but they are seen more commonly in individuals of certain HLA groups, and HLA type seems to predispose individuals to auto-immune disorders (Bodmer 1987). In the case of Hashimoto's disease, the major defect is considered to be an abnormality of suppressor T-cell function, which is possibly generated by the immune-response genes of the HLA DR3 genotype, resulting in an unchallenged attack on the follicular cells by cytotoxic T-cells. There is also aberrant expression of MHC class II antigens on thyrocytes, an abnormality which is likely to be involved in the presentation of self antigens to the activated T-lymphocytes. However, the initiating factor precipitating such a sequence of events is not known.

Hashimoto's thyroiditis is characterized by a diffuse intense

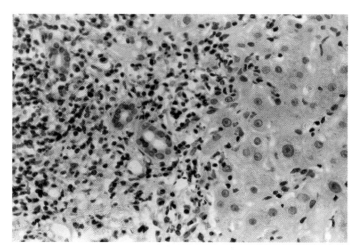

Fig. 5.45 A liver biopsy showing the features of chronic active hepatitis. The periportal predominantly lymphocytic infiltrate surrounds individual hepatocytes, causing hepatocyte degeneration.

infiltrate of lymphocytes and plasma cells throughout the thyroid parenchyma, associated with atrophic follicles and damaged follicular cells which appear strongly eosinophilic (Hürthle cells) (Fig. 5.46) and which are functionally inactive, leaving the individual in a hypothyroid state.

5.4.4   Granulomatous diseases

J. L. Turk

The term *granuloma* was introduced by Virchow in 1865 to describe certain well-circumscribed swellings, which he considered at the time to consist of 'granulation tissue', found in a number of chronic infectious diseases including tuberculosis, leprosy, syphilis, and leishmaniasis. Later authors distinguished large swollen epithelial-like cells, which they called 'epithelioid cells', from the lymphoid elements in these lesions. Metchnikoff in 1891 formally recognized that these cells were related to the new type of cell that he called the macrophage. The relation between these granulomatous diseases and allergic reactions of the delayed hypersensitivity type was recognized by Von Pirquet when he invented the term 'allergy'. This was the first indication that cell-mediated immune processes might be involved in the development of these reactions. A granuloma may be defined in modern terms as a collection of cells of the 'mononuclear phagocyte series' (MPS) with or without the addition of other cell types.

Mononuclear phagocytes, or macrophages, have both a phagocytic and a secretory function. Depending on the pathological state of the granuloma, these cells may take on a more phagocytic (Fig. 5.47) or a more secretory role (Fig. 5.48a,b). In

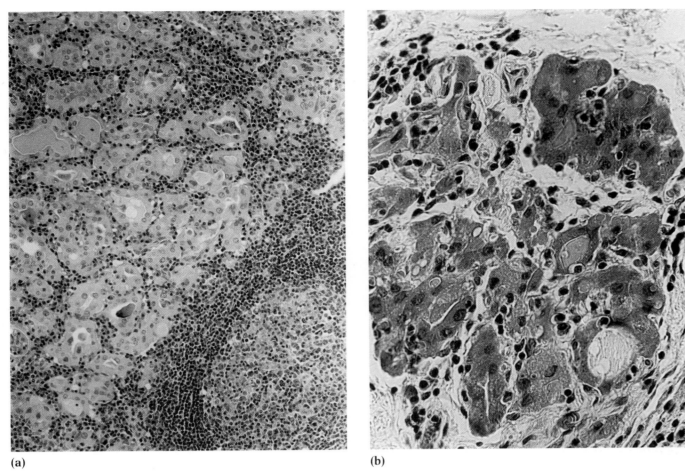

(a) (b)

Fig. 5.46 Hashimoto's thyroiditis: (a) note the diffuse lymphoid infiltrate and the presence of a lymphoid follicle with a germinal centre. The high-power photomicrograph (b) demonstrates the atrophic acini, the cells of which are large and contain abundant eosinophilic cytoplasm. Focal nuclear atypia is also a feature.

addition to a wide range of lysosomal enzymes, many of which are hydrolytic and particularly proteolytic, macrophages secrete prostaglandins, interleukin-1, interferons, and fibroblast activating factors. In its purest form, as a tissue reaction against a non-immunogenic foreign body, for example colloidal iron, a granuloma may contain only cells of the MPS; although such reactions may produce striking X-ray changes in the lungs, they do not lead to fibrotic changes, and there may be little change in the patient's vital capacity. One may, therefore, divide granulomatous changes into those which have an immunological association and those which are non-immunological (Table 5.6). The place of silicosis in this classification and its relation to other granulomas associated with fibrosis is of considerable interest and will be discussed separately. Metals such as beryllium and zirconium induce *immunological-type granulomatous reactions* associated with delayed-type hypersensitivity. The reaction to other metals such as aluminium are those of *non-immunological granulomas*. The granulomas in infectious diseases such as tuberculosis, associated with delayed hypersensitivity reactions, are characterized particularly by the

Table 5.6 Classification of granulomas

Immunological
  Tuberculosis
  Tuberculoid leprosy
  Syphilis
  Schistosomiasis
  Sarcoidosis
  Zirconium
  Beryllium

Non-immunological
  Non-toxic
    e.g. Plastic beads
        Carbon particles
        Non-toxic metals, Fe
  Toxic
    e.g. Silica
        Talc
        Asbestos
  Activation of C3
    e.g. Carageenan
        Kaolin
        Aluminium hydroxide

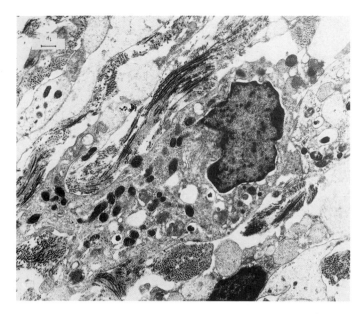

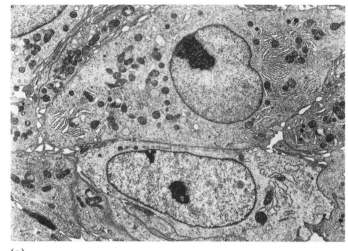

(a)

Fig. 5.47 Phagocytic macrophage: lepromatous leprosy granuloma containing large numbers of bacilli.

presence of fibroblast proliferation and fibrosis. Immunological granulomas also contain considerable numbers of lymphocytes. These may be T-lymphocytes or B-lymphocytes, many of which will have transformed into plasma cells. Eosinophils are a particular feature of granulomas caused by helminths, such as those around schistosome eggs. Granulocytes are found especially where there is tissue necrosis. In addition, the cells of the MPS take on the special appearance of 'epithelioid cells'. Although this term was originally used to describe all cells of the MPS in granulomas, the term *epithelioid cell* now has a special meaning to describe a particular class of cells of the MPS found mainly in immunological granulomas. These cells have a pale cytoplasm with a round or slightly oval nucleus with finely marginated chromatin and prominent nucleoli. Ultrastructurally, these cells are frequently characterized by the presence of a rough endoplasmic reticulum (Fig. 5.48a,b) and they are often poorly phagocytic. The ultrastructural appearance of rough endoplasmic reticulum associated with minimal or absent phagocytosis has been described in the granulomas of sarcoidosis, tuberculoid leprosy and beryllium and zirconium granulomas (Wanstrup and Christensen 1966; Elias and Epstein 1968). These cells have been described as *plasmacytoid* epithelioid cells because of their superficial resemblance to plasma cells. Plasmacytoid secretory epithelioid cells transform into vesicular epithelioid cells (Fig. 5.48c) containing numerous cytoplasmic membrane-bound vesicles. Such cells do not contain any endocytosed material (Williams 1982). Epithelioid cells carry the

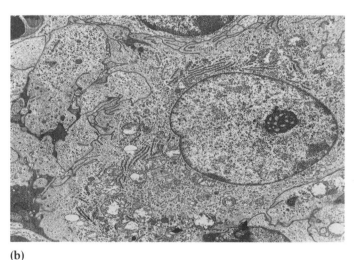

(b)

Fig. 5.48 Electron micrographs of epithelioid cells: (a) secretory—borderline tuberculoid leprosy; (b) secretory—BCG granuloma, note rough endoplasmic reticulum; (c) vesicular—borderline tuberculoid leprosy.

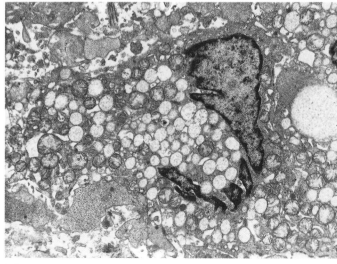

(c)

same specific cell-surface antigenic marker as other cells, but may express class II MHC antigens poorly as compared with phagocytosing macrophages. Epithelioid cell granulomas are well demarcated from the surrounding tissues by fibroblasts and evidence of recent collagen synthesis in the periphery (Fig. 5.49). They are also frequently but not inevitably associated with the presence of 'Langhans-type' giant cells in which the nuclei usually form a peripheral 'horseshoe' pattern (Fig. 5.50). It is the increased collagen synthesis, which is an inevitable part of these granulomas, that gives rise to such clinically important conditions as pulmonary fibrosis in tuberculosis, berylliosis, silicosis, and sarcoidosis, and the course periportal cirrhosis of schistosomiasis.

The increased collagen synthesis associated with epithelioid cell formation has given rise to the suggestion that the rough endoplasmic reticulum in these cells is associated with the increased secretion of fibroblast-activating factors (Table 5.6). Macrophages are known to secrete fibroblast chemotactic factors and fibroblast-activating factors. Interleukin-1 of macrophage origin also causes increased fibroblast proliferation. However, there are also factors that increase fibroblast proliferation and collagen synthesis secreted by lymphocytes. Schistosome granulomas have been found to give rise to factors that increase fibroblast proliferation.

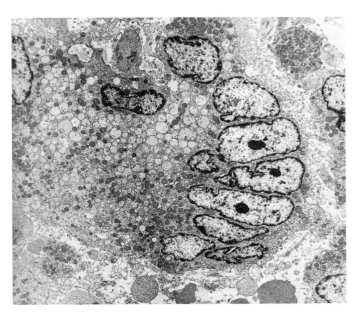

Fig. 5.50 Langhans-type giant cell, borderline tuberculoid leprosy.

Tissue destruction leading to caseation and cavitation is a particular feature of tuberculosis and is rarely, if at all, found in other immunological and non-immunological granulomas. One of the agents that has been postulated as a cause of caseation is *tumour necrosis factor* (TNF), which is released from cells of the MPS particularly by the action of endotoxin and can lead to vascular endothelial damage and fibrin deposition. It could be that there is increased release of TNF by cells of the MPS in patients with tuberculosis in the presence of certain components of *Mycobacterium tuberculosis* and this might account for the regular occurrence of *caseation*, the characteristic 'cheese-like' necrosis, in this disease. Caseation is also a feature of the epithelioid cell granulomas of tertiary syphilis known as *gummas* and, at the other end of the spectrum, absence of caseation is a diagnostic feature of the epithelioid cell granulomas of sarcoidosis. These differences could be explained on the basis of differences in local production of TNF.

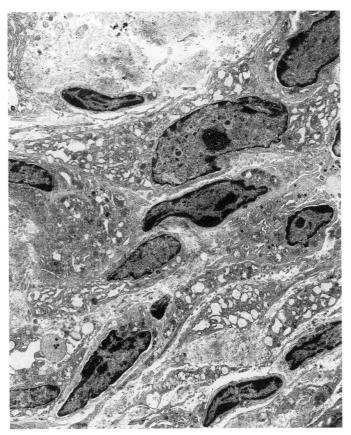

Fig. 5.49 Fibroblasts—zirconium granuloma.

Table 5.7 Factors affecting fibroblast growth and function

Macrophage origin
  Fibroblast chemotactic factor
  Fibroblast activating factor
    (increased [³H]thymidine uptake)
  Interleukin-1 →fibroblast proliferation

Lymphocyte origin
  Fibroblast proliferative activity
    (increased [³H]thymidine uptake)
  Increased protein synthesis
    collagen
    non-collagen proteins

Granuloma origin (schistosome)
  Fibroblast proliferation
    (increased [³H]thymidine uptake)

The association between epithelioid cell granuloma formation and delayed hypersensitivity in a number of diseases would explain the large number of T-lymphocytes found in the periphery of these lesions. Experimentally, it has been shown by transfer studies that such granulomas, particularly in schistosomiasis in the mouse, are T-lymphocyte mediated. However, the presence of plasma cells and eosinophils as well as epithelioid cells and lymphocytes in many granulomas of helminthic origin, including schistosomiasis, would indicate that B-lymphocytes might play an important role in their formation. The 'Hoeppli' phenomenon, in which eosinophilic and Schiff-positive fibrinoid material deposits, shown to contain immunoglobulin and complement, accumulate in granulomas around the eggs of *Schistosoma japonicum* would be consistent with this view.

The ovum showing the Hoeppli phenomenon (Smith and Lichtenburg 1967) is surrounded by an area of necrosis and infiltration with epithelioid cells, plasma cells, and lymphocytes, with eosinophils present in varying proportions. In most severe reactions there may be an eosinophil abscess. With the death of the ovum the epithelioid cells increase in number and fibrosis occurs. The lesions which also contain giant cells are referred to as *pseudo-tubercles*. The fibrosis and calcification in the liver may give rise to coarse portal cirrhosis and portal hypertension. Similar fibrosis and calcification occur in the wall of the urinary bladder in *S. haematobium* infection. Other sites of granuloma formation include the rectal mucosa. Schistosomiasis, like a number of other granulomatous diseases, is associated with circulating immune complexes which, in this case, can lead to the development of glomerulonephritis.

The role of the allergic reaction and particularly granuloma formation in resistance to infection has been a controversial subject throughout the past 100 years. Early workers in the field of tuberculosis considered that granulomas acted to wall off the infection and thus protect the individual from widespread disease. A less mechanistic view is that resistance to infection with mycobacteria is due to the strength of the T-cell-mediated immune response directed against the invading organism. The fibrotic reaction associated with the granuloma is more damaging to the patient and appears to play no role in protection. As will be discussed later, there has been a revolution in attitudes towards the pathogenesis and mechanisms of granulomatous disease in the past 25 years as workers have placed more emphasis on the study of the immunology of leprosy rather than tuberculosis by drawing analogies with changes seen across the clinical spectrum of leprosy.

The term 'foreign body' granuloma is used to cover the localized response to a range of substances that enter the body from the exterior. Granulomatous reactions may occur around thorns or other sharp objects that penetrate the skin. Many of these reactions are immunological responses against foreign antigens either as part of the object or on micro-organisms carried in by the object. Thus the lesions are frequently epithelioid granulomas with giant cells and there is also fibroblast proliferation. Frequently these lesions resolve by fibrosis. The lesions produced by talc are similar. Although talc is not anti-genic the reaction is one caused by its silica content and thus the lesion is related to those of silicosis which will be discussed later.

Mycobacterial diseases—leprosy and tuberculosis

Mycobacterial infections may take a low- or high-resistance course clinically with a broad spectrum of clinical and pathological positions in-between (Ridley and Jopling 1966). Polar low-resistance forms of the disease are *disseminated miliary tuberculosis* and *lepromatous leprosy* (LL). The polar high-resistance forms are the self-healing single pulmonary lesions (the *Ghon focus* with hilar lymphoadenopathy) of tuberculosis and the self-healing nerve and skin lesions of polar tuberculoid leprosy (TT). Between the two polar forms is a wider spectrum of disease in leprosy, the manifestations of which are referred to as *borderline tuberculoid*, *borderline*, or *borderline lepromatous leprosy* (BT, BB, or BL), or in tuberculosis are represented by the forms of *cavitating fibro-caseous tuberculosis* of varying severity, prognosis, and response to therapy. High-resistance forms of disease are associated with the presence of small numbers of infecting organisms, whereas in the low-resistance forms the tissues are teeming with micro-organisms. High resistance is associated with marked lymphocytic infiltration of the tissues as part of the granuloma, low resistance with the presence of few lymphocytes (Tables 5.8 and 5.9).

Low resistance in lepromatous leprosy is due to a failure of T-lymphocyte function which is specific to *Mycobacterium leprae*. There appears to be no single cause. Among the interacting factors suggested are suppressor T-lymphocytes, suppressor monocytes, specific depression of T-cell clones by high levels of antigen (immunological tolerance), poor response of T-cells to interleukin-2, and defective processing of antigen by macrophages leading to a failure of presentation of antigen by macrophages to lymphocytes.

In high-resistance disease the granuloma is of the epithelioid cell type and in low-resistance forms granulomas may contain few epithelioid cells and the cells are almost all phagocytosing macrophages. Fibroblast proliferation, increased collagen synthesis and fibrosis are features of high resistance rather than low resistance forms of the disease. Such a spectrum of clinical and pathological features leads to a realization that the different forms of mycobacterial disease occur as a result of a spectrum of immunological reactions. Immunological reactions are involved at two levels: one is in the resistance of the individual to the infecting organism; the other is in the type of granuloma that is produced. Granulomatous reactions, as discussed above, may be immunological or non-immunological. High-resistance forms of disease are usually associated with the development of immunological epithelioid cell granulomas, and low-resistance forms of the disease with non-immunological granulomas containing phagocytosing macrophages. Immunological granulomas in mycobacterial infections are T-cell mediated. T-cell-mediated reactions in the skin to soluble antigens such as tuberculin are delayed-hypersensitivity reactions, maximal at 48–72 h and resolving by 7 days. Granulomatous reactions to particulate mycobacterial organisms or their products occur

Table 5.8 Summary of the clinical, histological, bacteriological, and immunological findings of the five groups of the leprosy spectrum

Characteristics	TT	BT	BB	BL	LL
Skin lesions					
Numbers	1 to 3	Very few to moderate	Moderate	Moderate to many	Very many
Symmetry	Very symmetrical	Asymmetrical	Asymmetrical	Slightly asymmetrical	Symmetrical
Anaesthesia	Very marked	Marked	Marked to moderate	Slight to nil	Nil
Nerve enlargement					
Cutaneous sensory	Common	Occasional	0	0	0
Peripheral*	0 to 1	Common, asymmetrical	Common, asymmetrical	Moderately asymmetrical	Symmetrical
Skin histology					
Granuloma cell	Epithelioid	Epithelioid	Epithelioid	Histiocyte	Foamy histiocyte
Lymphocytes	+++	+++	+	± or ++	±
Dermal nerves	Destroyed	Mostly destroyed	Some visible	Visible	Easily visible
No. of bacilli (routine examinaton)	0	0, +, or ++	+, ++, or +++	++++	+++++
Lymph nodes					
Paracortical infiltrate	Nil, immunoblasts	Sarcoid-like	Diffuse epithelioid	Diffuse histiocytes	Massive infiltrate with foamy histiocytes and Virchow cells
Germinal centres	Normal	Normal	Normal	Some hypertrophy	Gross hypertrophy
Lepromin test	+++	++	± or 0	0	0
Reactions					
ENL†	0	0	0	Rare	Very common
Reversal (lepra)	?	Common	Very common	Very common	(Rare)‡

* Nerves of predilection, i.e. ulnar, median, lateral popliteal, facial, great auriclar, and posterior tibial.
† Erythema nodosum leprosum.
‡ Lepra reactions are occasionally seen in treated LL patients who have developed from borderline (BT, BB, or BL) in the absence of treatment.

Table 5.9 The spectrum of human tuberculosis, as defined on the basis of clinical, bacteriological, histological, and immunological data (Lenzini *et al.* 1977)

	Reactive (RR)	Reactive intermediate (RI)	Unreactive intermediate (UI)	Unreactive (UU)
Skin test to PPD*:				
Typical delayed reaction (%)	100	30	5	—
Early reaction (%)	—	13	15	—
Mixed reaction (%)	—	57	80	—
Leucocyte migration inhibition	+++	++−	±−−	−−−
Humoral anti-PPD antibodies (%)	5	70	98	100
Mycobacteria:				
In sputum	−−−	−−−	++−	+++
In the tissue	−−−	+−−	+++	+++
Immunologic change in lymph node:				
Germinal centres and plasma cells	−−+	−−+	+++	−−+
Paracortical area	+++	++−	+−−	−−−
Response to antimycobacterial treatment (%)	100	90	33	0

* Protein purified derivative of tuberculin.

maximally at 14–21 days with a nodular response after intradermal injection, as with the *Mitsuda lepromin reaction*, which when biopsied shows a typical epithelioid cell granuloma. The lepromin reaction (Mitsuda) is negative in the low-resistance (lepromatous) forms of the disease, whereas it is positive in the high-resistance forms of the disease (tuberculoid) that are associated with epithelioid cell granuloma development.

There has been considerable controversy as to whether the same T-cell line is involved in allergic reaction and resistance in mycobacterial infections. This goes back to a more mechanistic approach as to whether resistance to infection was due to the site of infection being actually walled off by the granuloma itself. Currently, evidence is more in favour of a dissociation between allergy and resistance. This is of more than theoretical importance, since when vaccines are developed for use in protection from mycobacterial infection it is crucial to be sure that the vaccine is not stimulating allergic reactivity alone. BCG vaccine, used in the protection of populations from tuberculosis for many decades now, generally stimulates both resistance to infection and tuberculin reactivity. However, in a proportion of cases individuals vaccinated may be tuberculin-negative and still protected. Conversely, it is well known that many individuals with progressive spreading tuberculosis may be strongly tuberculin positive throughout their disease.

BCG vaccination has been shown to be highly effective in the control of tuberculosis in the United Kingdom. The percentage efficacy shown in the Medical Research Council trial in an analysis of the ten-year incidence of the disease was 80 per cent. However, immunity conferred by the vaccine did not depend on the degree of tuberculin sensitivity induced in the individual. The annual incidence of tuberculosis per 1000 participants was found to be between 0.26 and 0.64 whether the subjects were tuberculin positive or negative. This would indicate that tuberculin testing has little value in assessing the efficacy of the vaccine. There are currently a number of trials of BCG vaccine with or without the addition of killed *M. leprae* in the prevention of leprosy in leprosy-endemic areas. BCG vaccine appears to be more effective in Africa where the incidence of tuberculoid leprosy is much higher than that of the lepromatous form of the disease. However, results of 'immunotherapy' of lepromatous patients, in which these vaccines are given to patients already with this disease, need to be studied more closely before any strong conclusions can be drawn as to the efficacy of this approach.

In addition to the actual granulomas, mycobacterial infections may be associated with other pathological features which are of allergic origin. These include pleural effusions and the condition of the skin known as *erythema nodosum*. This shows mainly a lymphocytic infiltration and is probably T-lymphocyte mediated. Acute reactions in tuberculoid leprosy or reversal reactions from borderline to tuberculoid leprosy are also T-lymphocyte mediated and have many of the features of acute delayed-hypersensitivity reactions. However, *erythema nodosum leprosum* which occurs at the lepromatous end of the leprosy spectrum is a necrotizing vasculitis associated with a polymorphonuclear leucocyte infiltration and is often associated with arthritis. This condition has all the features of immune-complex pathology. The local lesions are probably due to local formation of these complexes in the skin, whereas systemic features are due to circulating immune complexes depositing on the basement membrane of blood-vessels or on the synovial membrane.

Patients who would normally have a high resistance to mycobacterial infection or have disease at the tuberculoid end of the spectrum, whereby they would form epithelioid cell granulomas in which micro-organisms might be difficult to find, may have their disease modified by factors that suppress the immune response. This may occur as a result of malnutrition in childhood or the presence of an intercurrent viral infection. In 1907 Von Pirquet was the first to discover that during measles tubercular children lose the capacity to react to tuberculin for about one week. This is frequently associated with a spread of the tubercular disease process. Treatment of a patient who had a past history of healed leprosy with immunosuppressive drugs to control graft rejection following a renal transplant caused the development of lepromatous leprosy with extensive erythema nodosum leprosum. Recently it has been found that infection with the human immunodeficiency virus (HIV) will so depress the immune response that patients will develop rapidly spreading disseminated infection with the *Mycobacterium avium intracellulare* group or *Mycobacterium tuberculosis* itself. In these cases the lesions contain confluent macrophages full of mycobacteria, as in lepromatous leprosy, and the spread of the disease resembles the most severe form of miliary tuberculosis. Despite this, the patients may show little increase in constitutional upset as they are incapable of developing a hypersensitivity reaction.

Whereas disease due to *M. leprae* is mainly confined to the skin and nerves, *M. tuberculosis* causes granuloma formation throughout the body. The main sites are the lungs, lymphoid tissues (including the Peyer's patches of the intestines), bones, kidney, epididymis, testis, and brain. High-resistance disease may result in *tuberculoma* (a mass of tuberculous granulation tissue with caseation) formation in the brain, whereas low-resistance miliary tuberculosis may be accompanied by a tuberculous meningitis. Despite the large amount of literature on tuberculosis, an immunological spectrum similar to that for leprosy was only defined 10 years ago (Lenzini *et al.* 1977). Four points of the spectrum have been defined equivalent to TT, BT, BL, and LL. These are described as follows:

RR reactive; micronodular localized tuberculosis;

RI reactive intermediate; nodular or micronodular localized tuberculosis with cavitation; unilateral or bilateral lymphadenopathy; tubercular serositis;

UI unreactive intermediate; nodular or micronodular chronic diffuse tuberculosis with cavitation and fibrosis; tubercular lymphadenopathy complicated by fistula formation;

UU unreactive; acute miliary tuberculosis.

The definition of localized micronodular tuberculosis was based on the size and discrete quality of the lesion on X-ray, and their limitation to one or two segments of the lung. Nodular lesions were larger in size but still localized in their distribution. The lesions of nodular or micronodular chronic diffuse tuberculosis were characterized by one or more cavities and a prolonged course of disease and relative resistance to therapy.

The cell-mediated immune reactivity of the patients was assessed by tuberculin skin testing in which three types of reactivity were found:

1. typical delayed-hypersensitivity reaction present at 24 h peaking at 48 h with strong induration, and persisting up to 72 and 96 h;

2. early reactions with rapid development persisting until 24 h, chiefly with erythema and oedema gradually decreasing and disappearing at 48 h;

3. biphasic reactions with an early phase visible from 3 to 24 h with erythema and oedema, gradually decreasing at 48 h.

In addition, cell-mediated immune reactivity was assessed by the *leucocyte migration inhibition test* (LMT) using tuberculin as antigen. Typical delayed hypersensitivity skin reactions were found in 100 per cent of patients with RR, 30 per cent with RI, and 5 per cent with UI. UU patients showed no response to tuberculin. Reactivity assessed by LMT followed a similar pattern (Table 5.9). The presence of mycobacteria in the sputum and tissues was inversely proportional to cell-mediated immunity as assessed by these parameters. Humoral antibody levels were also inversely proportional to the parameters of cell-mediated immunity. The ability to respond to antimycobacterial therapy paralleled the strength of cell-mediated immune reactivity. Host resistance in tuberculosis, as in leprosy, could be genetically controlled and it will be of interest to find out whether a linkage with MHC haplotypes exists.

Allergic granulomas caused by the metals beryllium and zirconium

Granulomas to beryllium and zirconium develop on the background of delayed hypersensitivity to these metals, and are allergic granulomas mediated through a T-lymphocyte reaction. In both cases the lesions are typical epithelioid cell reactions with Langhans-type giant cells. These reactions may show little central necrosis, and in many ways resemble the lesions of sarcoidosis. Inhalation of beryllium results in the development of pulmonary berylliosis which leads to fibrosis in the lungs and fatal respiratory failure in at least 36 per cent of cases. In other cases of pulmonary berylliosis there may be a more widespread disseminated cellular infiltrate with little evidence of typical epithelioid cell granuloma formation. Local epithelioid cell granuloma formation in the skin, with central caseation, can occur from the entrance of beryllium into the skin after a cut from a fluorescent light tube coated with a mixture of zinc-beryllium silicate.

Epithelioid cell granulomas can also occur in the skin following the entrance of sodium-zirconium lactate used as an antiperspirant. These lesions are epithelioid cell granulomas with Langhans-type giant cells (Figs 5.51, 5.52). However, no caseation occurs in zirconium granulomas. Fibroblast proliferation and increased collagen synthesis are features of both beryllium and zirconium granulomas.

Sarcoidosis

Sarcoidosis is a generalized systemic disease in which epithelioid cell granulomas are widely distributed throughout the body. The main sites of distribution are the lungs, lymph nodes, and other areas of lymphoid tissues, including the spleen. A characteristic feature is bronchial hilar lymphadenopathy, and diffuse infiltration of the lungs is an important cause of severe pulmonary fibrosis. The lesions are typical circumscribed epithelioid cell granulomas incorporating giant cells, some of which enclose calcium-containing *asteroid* inclusion bodies (*Schaumann bodies*). The lesions are characterized also by fibroblast proliferation and increased collagen synthesis. Although characteristically not associated with caseation, the lesions of sarcoidosis may have a slight degree of 'coagulation' necrosis. Typical sarcoid granulomas may occur in the skin but there also may be lesions of erythema nodosum with a mainly lymphocytic infiltrate in the dermis. Patients may also present evidence suggesting circulating immune-complex disease such as migrating polyarthritis and acute iritis.

The *Kveim test* for sarcoidosis is the intradermal injection of a heat-sterilized suspension of sarcoid tissue from spleen or lymph nodes. A nodular granuloma appears at the site of injection in 80–90 per cent of sarcoid patients, 6–8 weeks after injection.

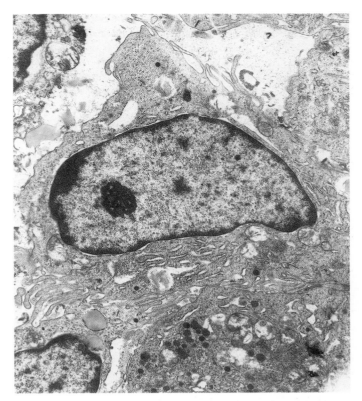

Fig. 5.51 Zirconium granuloma, epithelioid cell.

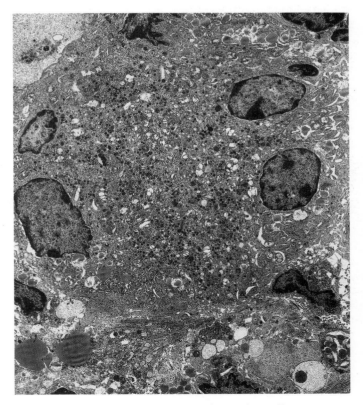

Fig. 5.52 Zirconium granuloma, giant cell.

Histologically, the lesion is a typical sarcoid granuloma. Another feature is the increased levels of *angiotensin converting enzyme* (ACE) in the serum in active disease, which may be twice that in control subjects.

Most patients with sarcoidosis fail to give a positive tuberculin reaction. However, if the tuberculin is combined with corticosteroids, the reaction is positive. This suggests that there is local suppression of the skin reaction by suppressor lymphocytes. Some authors have reported an excess of suppressor T-lymphocytes in the peripheral blood in sarcoidosis. However, there is no general agreement on the subject. Others have observed a normal helper:suppressor lymphocyte ratio but have suggested suppressor monocytes as a cause of reduced delayed hypersensitivity.

In contrast to the peripheral hyporesponsiveness, T-cell activity may be increased in broncho-alveolar lavages from the lung in active sarcoidosis. These T-cells are predominantly helper T-cells (CD4) and show evidence of activation by the expression of the IL-2 (Tac) receptor and the release of IL-2. Sarcoid alveolar macrophages can activate B-cells to secrete immunoglobulin. They also release IL-1 and γ-interferon spontaneously and they have an enhanced capacity to present antigen. This is associated with a diminished prostaglandin secretion and reduction in the regulation of the immune response.

No single aetiological agent has been found to underly sarcoidosis. The pathological features of the disease suggest a tissue response similar to that of tuberculoid leprosy, a high-resistance infectious disease in which the infectious agent is often difficult to demonstrate. Although the granulomatous features are consistent with T-cell-mediated reactions, there is also a suggestion of circulating immune-complex disease. In this connection it is of interest that the disease is frequently associated with a hypergammaglobulinaemia and over 50 per cent of patients with sarcoidosis have been reported to have circulating immune complexes. In view of the strong hypersensitivity gra-

nulomatous Kveim reaction, it is unlikely that the depression of the tuberculin reaction is related to the basic aetiology and pathogenesis of the disease. Whereas depressed tuberculin reactivity in measles is associated with spread of a tubercular infection, there is an interesting inverse relationship between sarcoidosis, with its depressed tuberculin reactivity, and tuberculosis. Sarcoidosis and tuberculosis are not seen in the same patient. The incidence of sarcoidosis in the population increases as that of tuberculosis drops. This has led to one hypothesis that sarcoidosis is a variant of tuberculosis itself.

Other granulomatous diseases

Syphilis

The explosive appearance of syphilis in Europe at the Siege of Naples in 1495 has many parallels with the rapid spread of AIDS in modern times. The metamorphosis from an acute lethal disease to the more chronic appearance seen in the pre-antibiotic era could be due to both a build-up in herd resistance as well as a change in the virulence of the organism, which might show parallels with AIDS in the future. There is a suggestion from studies of children born with congenital syphilis that the treponeme itself has some immunodepressive properties. It appears likely that syphilis was introduced into a population with a poor state of resistance to the organism, possibly from the 'New World' where treponemal infections were not uncommon, and lack of resistance was due to a lack of experience of many of the antigens carried by the organism.

Treponema pallidum is another organism that causes a chronic infection with a wide range of clinical manifestations (Table 5.10). Whereas in the case of leprosy and tuberculosis, patients can move from side to side across a spectrum, depending on the strength of host resistance, in syphilis there is a preditable progression from low resistance to high resistance during the course of disease. Initially resistance is low, so that the organism rapidly speads throughout the tissues. This is fol-

Table 5.10   Syphilis

	T-cell function				Presence of T. pallidum	B-cell function		
	Luetin skin test	LTT*		PHA†		Antibody	Immune complexes	Vasculitis
		T. pallidum						
		UK	Ethiopia					
Primary								
sero −ve	−	−	−	±	++	+		+
sero +ve		+	−	±	++	+		+
Secondary								
macular	−	−	−	±	+++	+++	++	?
papular	++	+	−	±	++	+		−
Latent	+ or −	+	±	+	−	+		−
Tertiary								
gumma	+++	+			+	+		++
neurosyphilis	±				+++	+++		++

* Lymphocyte transformation test.
† Phytohaemagglutinin.

lowed by a gradual increase in resistance sufficient to control the spread of the organism without actually eliminating it completely. This balance is, however, unstable and in a proportion of individuals it can be so disturbed as to result in the tertiary manifestations of the disease. These may take on either a high-resistance tuberculoid form (*gummatous*) or a low-resistance form (*cerebral*).

T. pallidum can enter cells in the same way as mycobacteria, and thus escape the action of circulating antibody (Sykes and Miller 1971). Antibody alone confers only partial resistance in experimental models. Moreover, diffuse spread of the organism can be otained in models in which cell-mediated immunity is reduced and antibody production remains normal. In addition, *T. pallidum* appears to have a natural ability to suppress the immune response of the host. When injected into new-born rabbits, the organism produces a runt-like syndrome associated with depletion of splenic lymphoid tissue, and babies born with congenital syphilis have depletion of the T-cell areas of the spleen.

Infection with *T. pallidum* runs a progressive and relentless course in many infected patients. This has been traditionally divided into four phases: *primary, secondary, latent,* and *tertiary* disease. The organism spreads rapidly throughout the body before the primary lesion has developed, and both the primary and secondary forms of the disease are characterized by a low state of host resistance. During the later phases of the secondary form of the disease, when the skin lesions may be papular rather than macular, resistance begins to improve and the patients begin to strike a balance with the organism which is all but eliminated. Then at a later date something happens, resistance fails and the patient goes into the tertiary form of the disease. This may take the form of localized gummatous lesions or the more diffuse proliferation of the organism characteristic of the neurological forms of the disease. if has been known for many years that whereas positive delayed hypersensitivity tests with treponemal antigens were found in late secondary and latent syphilis, they were almost universally negative in primary and early secondary syphilis. Moreover, in cerebrospinal syphilis the reaction is negative in 50 per cent of patients, whereas in the other tertiary forms of the disease it is positive in 95 per cent of patients. Recently it has been suggested that the immuno-deficiency associated with HIV infection can predispose to the development of neurosyphilis.

Lymphocyte transformation and proliferation of lymphocytes cultured with specific antigen *in vitro* (lymphocyte transformation test, LTT) has been used to investigate the spectrum of cellular immunity in syphilis (Friedmann and Turk 1975, 1978). These studies were made in England, and also in Ethiopia, where the course of the disease was somewhat different in that the secondary lesions were more of the papular type, and it was possible also to collect a series of patients with a cardiovascular tertiary form of the disease. In England, patients with sero-negative primary syphilis were universally negative in the LTT. Half the patients with sero-positive primary syphilis reacted to *T. pallidum* whereas cells from most patients with macular secondary syphilis were unresponsive. After 4–8 days of antibiotic therapy, patients even in the macular secondary stage of the disease showed a dramatic increase in lymphocyte reactivity. A similar increased skin-test reactivity to *T. pallidum* had also been described by Noguchi in 1911 in patients with secondary syphilis following treatment. In Ethiopian patients with early syphilis, regardless of clinical type, there was a complete failure of responsiveness to *T. pallidum*. This absence of reactivity in the LTT was found in forms of the disease in which many patients in the UK were antibody positive, e.g. sero-positive primary syphilis. Strong reactivity was found, however, in patients with latent and cardiovascular syphilis. Increased reactivity was found in only half the patients with early syphilis following treatment.

The consistent absence of specific reactivity in certain forms of early syphilis would, therefore, appear to be due to positive immunosuppression. There is accumulated evidence that this is to some extent non-specific. Thus it can be shown that there is a parallel depression of lymphocyte responsiveness to phyto-haemagglutinin (PHA) and tuberculin (purified protein derivative, PPD). In addition, a factor can be demonstrated in the plasma of these patients which inhibits the response of lymphocytes from normal individuals to PHA and PPD. This factor could be related to the release of antilymphocytic factors by *T. pallidum* or the presence of antigen–antibody complexes which, if formed in antibody excess, can specifically inhibit lymphocyte transformation to the homologous antigen, and, if complexed with IgM antibody, can non-specifically depress stimulation by mitogen. These inhibitory plasma factors may, however, be evidence of a deeper upset in immunological control mechanisms caused by the presence of excessive amounts of antigen in the tissues, and may parallel the presence of a population of immunologically specific suppressor cells. A similar phenomenon has been described in leprosy: it has been found that patients with borderline leprosy do not respond to *M. leprae* in the LT test and that plasma from these patients inhibits lymphocyte responsiveness to PHA. Some of these patients develop 'reversal reactions' in which their lesions become inflamed, probably as a result of delayed hypersensitivity. During the 'reaction' the patient's lymphocytes become reactive to *M. leprae* in the LT test and their plasma loses its inhibitory capacity.

Evidence is now beginning to accumulate which suggests that the lymphocyte transformation reaction correlates in both leprosy and syphilis with delayed hypersensitivity. However, the correlation between these two reactions and protective immunity is not as strong as might be expected. Patients with tuberculoid (TT) leprosy in whom protective immunity is highest do not show such strong lymphocyte reactivity to *M. leprae* as those with BT in whom protective immunity is weaker. Patients in England with syphilis re-infection clearly lack protective immunity. However, they frequently show strong reactivity to *T. pallidum* in the LTT. It would also appear from a number of studies that the clinical appearance of the lesion is related to delayed hypersensitivity rather than to immunity. The gummatous form of the disease is particularly associated with strong hypersensitivity reactions.

It is likely that immune-complex disease as well as cellular hypersensitivity may also contribute to the clinical manifestations of syphilis. Antibodies against *T. pallidum* occur early in the disease; during the time when the primary lesion is present the antibodies are initially IgM but later are IgG. The contribution of immune complexes to the clinical manifestations of the early (secondary macular) stages of the disease are suggested by the occasional occurrence of iridocyclitis, arthritis, and proteinuria. In addition, there may be a fully developed nephrotic syndrome with electron-microscopic evidence of immune-complex deposition on the glomerular basement membrane.

It is clear from a number of studies that patients who are infected with *T. pallidum* do not necessarily go through the whole spectrum of the disease. It is well documented, for instance, that only one-third of patients who have passed into the latent stage will develop tertiary stigmata. In a number of these it used to be considered that one-third developed neurosyphilis, one-third gummatous disease, and one-third cardiovascular disease. However, in a more recent survey in Ethiopia 10 years ago the only tertiary form of the disease discovered was the cardiovascular form. In addition, it is clear that not all patients will develop papular lesions in the secondary form of the disease. Thus the clinical manifestations that develop will depend, first, on the strength of protective immunity, which if developed sufficiently can terminate the infection at any stage. Secondly, the clinical manifestations developed will depend on the relative strengths of both cellular and humoral hypersensitivity reactions. Thus the clinical manifestations of secondary disease may be relatively weak or inapparent. Moreover, two-thirds of patients passing into the latent stage of the disease, in which the patient reaches a balance between protective immunity and the infecting organism, fail to pass into the tertiary phase of the disease. It could be that tertiary stigmata only develop if this balance between the host and the infecting organism is upset by external events. This could be the result of a temporary depression of protective immunity that might develop as a result of, for example, malnutrition or intercurrent infection.

Wegener's granulomatosis

This condition is a necrotizing granulomatous disease, principally of the nose and upper nasal sinuses and nasopharynx. It may also affect the lung and bronchial tree and be associated with a focal glomerulonephritis. The distinctive pathological feature that differentiates it from other granulomatous diseases is the presence of a necrotizing vasculitis and plasma cell infiltration. Epithelioid cells may be few or absent. Multinucleate giant cells are, however, common. Lesions may also occur in the orbit, skin, gastrointestinal tract, and peripheral and central nervous systems. The disease is associated in many cases with hypergammaglobulinaemia and the presence of rheumatoid factor in the serum, which with the primary vascular lesions suggests an immune-complex rather than a T-lymphocyte pathogenesis. The lesions of Wegener's granulomatosis respond to treatment with immunosuppressive therapy. Without such treatment patients invariably die from renal failure.

Granulomatous diseases of protozoal and fungal origin

Other infectious diseases with granulomatous features present aspects similar to those found in leprosy, tuberculosis, and syphilis (Turk and Bryceson 1971). This type of immunological spectrum with clear polar forms is found in cutaneous leishmaniasis (Table 5.11). *Diffuse cutaneous leishmaniasis* has a parasitized-macrophage-type granuloma with a negative

Table 5.11 The histological spectrum of cutaneous leishmaniasis

Designation	Histological features	
(MM) Macrophage	Thin intact epidermis, clear subdermal zone; dermal infiltration with macrophages, often vacuolated, full of parasites; histiocytes, many vessels containing monocytes, absence of lymphocytes	
(MI) Macrophage/intermediate	MM together with scanty lymphocytes scattered throughout or grouped deeply beneath the lesion	DCL* before treatment
(II) Intermediate	Epidermis thickened, intact early, may ulcerate later; no clear zone; lymphocyte intimately mixed with large fleshy histiocytes, moderate numbers of parasites or MM areas alongside IT or TT areas	
(IT) Intermediate/tuberculoid	Epidermis ulcerated; where intact shows reduplication of the layers, nuclear damage, and hyperkeratosis; lymphocytes predominate, early arrangement into tubercles around clumps of epithelioid cells, parasites scanty	Oriental sore and DCL in relapse
(TT) Tuberculoid	Epidermis ulcerated; tubercle formation, often with giant cells; parasites rare or invisible	Lupoid leishmaniasis; all types healing
(TF) Tuberculoid fibrosis	Tubercles being destroyed by fibrosis; re-epithelialization	
(F) Fibrosis		
(R) 'Resolving'	Patchy perivascular infiltration with lymphocytes and histiocytes; absence of tubercle formation and of parasites	DCL healing without immunological shift

* Diffuse cutaneous leishmaniasis.

delayed hypersensitivity reaction to leishmanin. In *lupoid*, or *recidiva*, leishmaniasis the lesions are epithelioid-type granulomas, often with giant cells from which parasites cannot be isolated, and the delayed hypersensitivity reaction to leishmanin is strongly positive. The more common *oriental sore* takes on a 'borderline' position on the spectrum. As in leprosy, patients within the 'borderline' region can move towards either polar positions. *Visceral leishmaniasis* due to *Leishmania donovani* is found only in the low-resistance form in which delayed hypersensitivity is absent and the granulomas consist only of parasitized macrophages, which are found in the spleen, liver, and blood. It is not known whether cell-mediated immunity fails to develop or whether it has become suppressed as the infection progresses. However, there is no failure of B-lymphocyte function, as antibodies against the parasite develop normally and the disease is characterized by high levels of IgG and IgM.

Low-resistance forms of the chronic mycoses are also well documented. *Chronic mucocutaneous candidiasis* develops in all conditions where there is a non-specific failure of T-lymphocyte function. This may be due to a failure of thymus development in fetal life or to a failure of the production of soluble mediators of cell-mediated immunity (CMI). It occurs in AIDS or when CMI is suppressed by immunosuppressive drugs, following defects of endocrine function, and in neoplastic disorders of lymphoid tissue such as Hodgkin's disease. Low-resistance macrophage-type granulomas occur in the systemic mycoses, such as *South American blastomycosis and histoplasmosis*. The lesions are generally systemic but in South American blastomycosis there is a diffuse cutaneous form of the disease. In the localized form of South American blastomycosis there is a delayed hypersensitivity to paracoccidioidin, a low level of complement-fixing antibodies to the polysaccharide antigen of *Paracoccidioides brasiliensis*, and a good response to treatment with sulphonamides. The disseminated cutaneous or systemic forms of the disease are associated with negative skin reactivity to paracoccidioidin and a high level of circulating antibodies against antigens derived from the infecting organism. These low-resistance forms respond poorly to treatment and have frequent relapses.

Silicosis

Silicosis is a granulomatous disease that does not fit easily into the simple classification of immunological/epithelioid cell granulomas leading to fibrosis and non-immunological/phagocytosing macrophage granulomas without fibrosis. Silicosis is recognized chiefly by the highly fibrogenic nature of the pathological processes observed. The granulomatous aspect of the disease has only been studied in any depth in experimental models. Following an intradermal injection of silica, three-quarters of the draining lymph nodes may be taken up by macrophage granuloma between the sixth and ninth day (Gaafar and Turk 1970). Many giant cells are seen, with strong lysosomal enzyme activity (Figs 5.53, 5.54). After inhalation of silica-containing material such as quartz, the initial inflammatory response is of polymorphonuclear leucocytes; this is followed by a rapid influx of macrophages, which become the

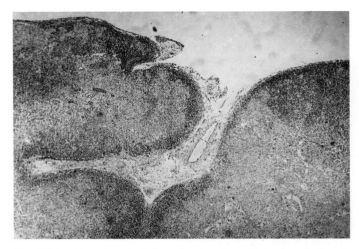

Fig. 5.53 A lymph node 6 days after intradermal injection of silica. A granuloma is infiltrating three-quarters of the node.

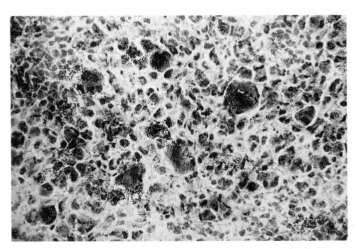

Fig. 5.54 A lymph node 9 days after intradermal injection of silica. Macrophages and giant cells in the granuloma. (Acid phosphatase.)

predominant cell in the infiltrate by 3 days. These macrophages may contain silica particles within phagosomes and also have a rough endoplasmic reticulum (Bowden and Adamson 1984). By the fifth day fibroblasts appear and become progressively an increasingly important part of the granuloma, persisting for up to 28 days after a single bolus of the silica-containing substance. In granulomas of six months of age, multinucleate giant cells have been seen in or around the granulomas. The fibrogenic action of silica has been attributed to a direct toxic action of silicic acid release from silica particles on cell membranes and the release of fibroblast-stimulating factors by macrophages. It has been suggested that the injury is mainly to lysosomal membranes. Experiments *in vitro* have demonstrated that phagocytosis of silica particles by macrophages results in a release of lysosomal enzymes into the surrounding medium. This is unlikely to be the whole story since aluminium hydroxide at the same concentration will release similar amounts of these enzymes and, indeed, produces localized granulomas without added fibroblast activation (Badenoch-Jones *et al.* 1978). Thus the specific fibrogenic activity of silica has not as yet been identified, and the results suggested by *in vitro* experiments in no way explain the pathological features that may be observed. There is no doubt, however, that silica has a strong *in vivo* fibroblast-proliferating effect that is not shown by a range of other minerals capable of inducing granulomas. This appears to be independent of any immunological mechanism found with similar granulomas associated with a high degree of fibroblast activation and increased collagen synthesis.

5.4.5 Bibliography

Chronic inflammation

Babior, B. (1978). Oxygen-dependent microbial killing by phagocytes. *New England Journal of Medicine* **298**, 659–68, 721–5.
Bodmer, W. F. (1987). The HLA system, structure and function. *Journal of Clinical Pathology* **40**, 948–58.
Pearl, E. R., *et al.* (1978). Lymphocyte precursors in human marrow: An analysis of normal individuals and patients with antibody deficiency states. *Journal of Immunology* **120**, 1169.
Scheuer, P. J. (1986). A review: changing views on chronic hepatitis. *Histopathology* **10**, 1–4.

Granulomatous diseases

Badenoch-Jones, P., Turk, J. L., and Parker, D. (1978). The effects of some aluminium and zirconium compounds on guinea pig peritoneal macrophages and skin fibroblasts in culture. *Journal of Pathology* **124**, 51–62.
Bowden, D. H. and Adamson, I. Y. R. (1984). The role of cell injury and the continuing inflammatory response in the generation of silicotic pulmonary fibrosis. *Journal of Pathology* **144**, 149–61.
Elias, P. M. and Epstein, W. L. (1968). Ultrastructural observations on experimentally induced foreign body and organised epithelioid-cell granulomas in man. *American Journal of Pathology* **52**, 1207–23.
Friedmann, P. S. and Turk, J. L. (1975). A spectrum of lymphocyte responsiveness in human syphilis. *Clinical and Experimental Immunology* **21**, 59–64.
Friedmann, P. S. and Turk, J. L. (1978). The role of cell-mediated immune mechanisms in syphilis in Ethiopia. *Clinical and Experimental Immunology* **31**, 59–65.
Gaafar, S. M. and Turk, J. L. (1970). Granuloma formation in lymph nodes. *Journal of Pathology* **100**, 9–20.
Lenzini, L., Rotolli, P., and Rotolli, L. (1977). The spectrum of human tuberculosis. *Clinical and Experimental Immunology* **27**, 230–7.
Ridley, D. S. and Jopling, W. H. (1966). A classification of leprosy according to immunity. A five group system. *International Journal of Leprosy* **34**, 255–73.
Smith, J. H. and Lichtenburg, F. von (1967). The Hoeppli phenomenon in schistosomiasis. II. Histochemistry. *American Journal of Tropical Pathology* **50**, 993–1007.
Sykes, J. A. and Miller, J. N. (1971). Intracellular location of *Treponema pallidum* (Nichols strain) in the rabbit testis. *Infection and Immunity* **4**, 307–14.
Turk, J. L. and Bryceson, A. D. M. (1971). Immunological phenomena in leprosy and related diseases. *Advances in Immunology* **13**, 209–66.
Wanstrup, J. and Christensen, H. E. (1966). Sarcoidosis. I. Ultrastructural investigations on epithelioid cell granulomas. *Acta Pathologica et Microbiologica Scandinavica* **66**, 169–85.
Williams, G. T. (1982). Isolated epithelioid cells from disaggregated BCG granulomas—an ultrastructural study. *Journal of Pathology* **136**, 1–13.

5.5 Amyloidosis

J. Bridger and Nicholas A. Wright

5.5.1 Introduction

Amyloid is the term used for a group of pathological extracellular proteinaceous substances that share common morphological characteristics and appear in a diverse number of clinical settings. When whole tissues or organs are stained by iodine followed by dilute sulphuric acid, amyloid shows a blue colour which is a staining characteristic shared by starch and led Virchov to suggest the term 'amyloid'. The main constituents of amyloid are protein fibrils whose protein subunits vary in the different forms of the disease and the chemical nature of which form the basis of classification. Amyloid may be localized or systemic in distribution. When localized it may only be an incidental finding at autopsy but in a more systemic form can cause serious morbidity or mortality. Amyloid rarely regresses, and causes its pathological effects by progressive accumulation which leads to atrophy of tissues. Diagnosis may be made by biopsy of the specifically affected tissues or by rectal biopsy, which demonstrates amyloid in 90 per cent of systemic cases provided adequate submucosal tissue is included. By light microscopy amyloid stains as hyaline, extracellular, eosinophilic material (Fig. 5.55a). With the *Congo red stain* it shows green birefringence when viewed under polarized light and this is pathognomonic of amyloid (Fig. 5.55c).

5.5.2 General features

Staining characteristics

Macroscopically, amyloid can be demonstrated by painting the cut surfaces of affected organs with iodine solution; amyloid is stained yellow–red which is transformed into blue or violet following application of dilute sulphuric acid. Microscopically, with routine sections stained with haematoxylin and eosin, amyloid appears as extracellular, amorphous, eosinophilic, hyaline material and a variety of special stains are available to differentiate it from other hyaline-appearing deposits.

Tinctorial methods

1. By definition, amyloid stains pink with Congo red and shows green birefringence when viewed under polarized light. Treatment of the sections with potassium permanganate before staining decolorizes *reactive systemic amyloid* (AA) and

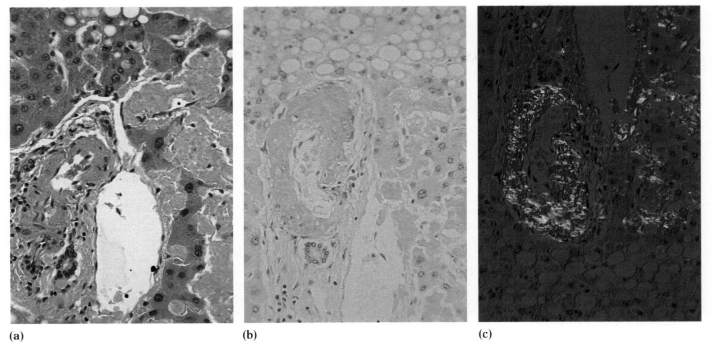

(a)   **(b)**   **(c)**

Fig. 5.55 Amyloidosis of the liver. (a) Haematoxylin and eosin stain; (b) Congo red stain with normal illumination; (c) Congo red stain with polarized light showing characteristic birefringence.

this may be used to discriminate it from that which occurs in immunocyte dyscrasias.

2. Amyloid shows metachromatic staining with methyl violet.

Fluorescent stains

Thioflavine-T, although not specific, causes amyloid to fluoresce when viewed under ultraviolet light.

Immunohistochemical stains

Isolation of various amyloid proteins has led to the preparation of both monoclonal and polyclonal antibodies to the various specific proteins and AP component (see below).

Nature of amyloid

Amyloid is composed of three main constituents.

1. About 90 per cent of amyloid is composed of fibrils, the nature of which varies with the underlying disease and which forms the basis for classification.

2. The remainder is predominantly *amyloid P component*, which appears ultrastructurally as pentagonal rings, maximum diameter 8.3 nm, and which may form linear arrays.

3. Glycosaminoglycans are a small but constant component.

Nearly all amyloids have a similar ultrastructural appearance: rigid, twisting, non-branching fibrils of indeterminate length, which are 10–15 nm in diameter. Each fibril appears to be formed of two filaments. In contrast, the intracerebral amyloid fibrils, particularly the paired helical filaments of *neurofibrillary*

tangles, which have distinctive biochemical properties different from those of all other types of amyloid, also have a slightly different morphology.

By definition, all amyloid stains positively with Congo red stain and shows red–green birefringence when viewed under polarized light. Previously, amyloid was considered to show an extensive β-pleated sheet arrangement in which the polypeptide chains are arranged in a plane perpendicular to the axis of the fibre (Fig. 5.56); furthermore the binding of Congo red dye to

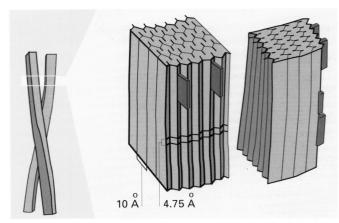

10 Å   4.75 Å

Fig. 5.56 Twisted β-pleated sheet antiparallel configuration of paired filaments of an amyloid fibril in acquired systemic amyloidosis. (Drawn after Glenner 1980, with permission.) The sites of binding of the planar Congo red dye are shown by the red blocks.

such a linear structure was invoked to explain the phenomenon of birefringence. However, recent work does not support this universal model, and a new structure for AA fibrils has been proposed, in which the fibrils are composed of a stack of globular subunits, each of which contains only some beta structure.

5.5.3 General classification and nomenclature

Recent advances in biochemical and aetiological information of amyloid have led to major changes in the classification of amyloidosis. Previous clinicopathological classifications have divided amyloid into different categories and the commonest of these is based on clinical presentation:

1. *Primary amyloidosis*, where there is absence of preceding disease and a predilection to nodular deposition with involvement of mesenchymal organs such as the heart. Amyloid associated with myeloma has a pattern of involvement similar to primary amyloid but was usually given a separate category.

2. *Secondary amyloidosis*, which appears as a complication of pre-existing disease, usually inflammatory or infectious, and was associated with amyloid deposits in parenchymal organs such as the spleen.

3. *Familial amyloidosis*, in which the different forms exhibit their own patterns of organ involvement.

4. *Isolated amyloidosis*, which may also be called *organ limited*. This was believed to be related to the primary form. It has been described in lung, heart, and joints and in association with endocrine tumours. It is most commonly found in the brain of patients with Alzheimer's disease.

However, isolation and characterization of many of the fibril proteins in the different forms of amyloid had led to a reclassification based on fibril type, and related clinical syndromes may now be recognized. This has rendered obsolete such ambiguous terms as primary and secondary amyloidosis.

5.5.4 Chemical nature of fibril proteins

AA amyloid

AA amyloid fibril protein has a molecular weight of about 8000 and consists of 76 amino acid residues. In contrast to AL amyloid, the amino-acid sequence is identical in all patients. The amino-acid sequence is identical to the amino-terminal sequence of *serum amyloid-associated protein* (SAA), suggesting that there is a precursor–product relationship between the two proteins. SAA is synthesized in the liver; it is an acute-phase protein whose concentration increases rapidly (500–1000-fold) during any inflammatory process. Native SAA has a molecular weight of 18 000 and in the serum it is associated with high-density lipoprotein.

AL amyloid

AL amyloid fibril protein consists of the whole, or fragments of, the variable region of monoclonal immunoglobulin light chains. The light chain of the circulating urinary or serum paraprotein is either identical to, or a precursor of, AL amyloid isolated from the individual deposits.

Prealbumin

Variant prealbumin has been identified as the major fibril subunit protein in several hereditary forms of systemic amyloidosis, including familial amyloid polyneuropathy types I and II. In these cases it has been shown that a single amino-acid residue change in the plasma prealbumin molecule, determined by a single base change of genomic DNA, makes the variant prealbumin amyloidogenic. Prealbumin is also the fibril subunit protein of *senile systemic amyloidosis* and there is evidence that these patients also have circulating variant prealbumin.

Endocrine amyloidosis

Endocrine tumours may be associated with isolated amyloid. The amyloid of medullary carcinoma of the thyroid seems to be derived from a calcitonin precursor molecule. Amyloid deposits associated with other endocrine tumours are thought to be related to their specific hormone products.

γ-trace protein (cystatin C)

The amyloid of *hereditary cerebral haemorrhage with amyloidosis* appears to be derived from cleavage of γ-trace protein, a peptide normally present in plasma and cerebrospinal fluid.

Haemodialysis-associated β_2-microglobulin

β_2-microglobulin is a polypeptide which is non-covalently associated with class I MHC molecules and catabolized in the kidney after glomerular filtration. However, it is poorly cleared by haemodialysis membranes.

β- (or A4) protein

This forms the *cerebral amyloid* in Alzheimer's disease, Down's syndrome, and in senile brains. β-protein has a molecular weight of 4200 Da and is a fragment of a very much larger protein which is probably a transmembrane cell-surface receptor. It is encoded by a gene on chromosome 21 located close to the locus associated with familial Alzheimer's disease. The pathogenesis may include:

(a) overproduction of the precursor in trisomy 21 or possible gene reduplication or abnormalities of expression in some Alzheimer's patients;

(b) possible variant forms of precursor; or

(c) possible proteolytic processing to produce β-protein itself.

Intraneuronal paired helical filaments, or *neurofibrillary tangles* are more specific for Alzheimer's than cortical plaques and cardiovascular amyloid, both of which are composed of β-protein. However, although they stain with Congo red and give green birefringence, they are not composed of β-protein and also differ from all other forms of amyloid by being intracellular.

Glycosaminoglycans

Glycosaminoglycans are a constant but small component of amyloid, along with the fibrils and P component. They appear to be synthesized by the cells at or near the amyloid deposits and may be involved in binding P component.

Amyloid P component

Amyloid P component (AP) is identical to serum amyloid P component and is a member of the *pentraxin* group of plasma proteins. It is present in all forms of amyloid except the intracortical plaques of Alzheimer's and senile brains. It comprises about 10–15 per cent of the mass of amyloid. A protein immunochemically indistinguishable from SAP is an integral constituent of glomerular basement membranes and is also found in association with elastic fibres throughout the body.

5.5.5 Clinical amyloidosis syndromes

Systemic amyloidosis

Reactive systemic (AA) amyloidosis

AA amyloid arises in association with chronic inflammatory or infectious disease and malignancy, in which the fibrils (AA) are thought to be derived from the acute-phase protein SAA. Before effective therapy existed, the commonest predisposing conditions were tuberculosis, bronchiectasis, and osteomyelitis, but now it most commonly complicates chronic rheumatic and connective tissue disease and inflammatory bowel disease. Amyloid occurs in 5–20 per cent of cases of rheumatoid arthritis but, in contrast, involvement in systemic lupus erythematosus (SLE) is rare. Similar differences exist in inflammatory bowel disease where amyloidosis has been reported in 1–8 per cent of cases of ulcerative colitis but rarely in Crohn's disease.

Among malignancies, Hodgkin's disease and renal carcinoma are most commonly associated with AA amyloid.

AA amyloid involves parenchymal organs and may be asymptomatic although widely distributed. The commonest presentation is proteinuria, often sufficient to cause nephrotic syndrome. Chronic renal failure is the cause of death in 40–60 per cent of cases. The next most common presentation is with organomegaly, e.g. hepato-splenomegaly or thyroid enlargement. Although deposition in the heart (50–60 per cent of cases) and gastrointestinal tract is common, it generally causes less functional impairment of affected organs than does AL amyloid.

Table 5.12 Clinical amyloidosis syndromes (adapted from Pepys 1988)

Distribution of deposits	Clinical syndromes	Fibril proteins and precursors
Systemic amyloidosis	Associated with immunocyte dyscrasia: myeloma, monoclonal gammopathy, occult dyscrasia	AL fibrils derived from monoclonal immunoglobulin light chains
	Associated with chronic active diseases: reactive systemic amyloidosis	AA fibrils derived from serum amyloid A protein (SAA)
	Hereditary syndromes:	
	Predominantly neuropathic forms (several types)	Prealbumin fibrils, genetic variant of plasma prealbumin
	Predominantly nephropathic forms include that associated with familial Mediterranean fever (autosomal recessive), typical AA amyloidosis	AA fibrils derived from serum amyloid A (SAA)
	Predominantly cardiomyopathic forms include	
	Senile systemic amyloidosis (formerly called senile cardiac amyloidosis)	Prealbumin fibrils derived from variant of plasma prealbumin
	Associated with chronic haemodialysis	β_2-microglobulin derived from high plasma levels
Localized amyloidosis	Senile amyloidosis (heart, brain, joints, seminal vesicles)	Atrial natriuretic peptide-related fibrils in isolated atrial amyloid, otherwise not known; different in different organs
	Cerebral amyloid angiopathy and cortical plaques in Alzheimer's disease, senile dementia, and Down's syndrome	β-protein fibrils, precursor encoded on chromosome 21
	Periarticular, bony, and renal amyloid in chronic haemodialysis patients	β_2-microglobulin derived from high plasma levels
	Endocrine amyloidosis	Precalcitonin-related fibrils in medullary carcinoma of thyroid; calcitonin gene-related peptide fibrils in islets of Langerhans; ? other peptide hormones
	Isolated massive nodular deposits (skin, lung, urogenital tract)	AL fibrils derived from monoclonal immunoglobulin light chains
	Primary localized cutaneous amyloid (macular, papular)	? Keratin-derived
	Hereditary syndromes:	
	Hereditary cerebral haemorrhage with amyloidosis Icelandic type	Cystatin C (γ-trace) fibrils, Glu58 genetic variant of cystatin C
	Dutch type	β-protein
	Cutaneous deposits (bullous, papular, poikilodermal)	Not known
	Ocular deposits (corneal, conjunctival)	Not known

Amyloidosis associated with immunocyte dyscrasias, AL amyloid

Because it is derived from free light chains, AL amyloid may occur in any dyscrasias of the B-lymphocyte lineage, such as multiple myeloma, Waldenstrom's macroglobulinaemia, solitary plasmocytomas, malignant lymphomas, and 'benign' monoclonal gammopathies. Of these conditions, multiple myeloma is the commonest cause, but still only accounts for about 20 per cent of cases of AL amyloid; conversely AL amyloid complicates 6–15 per cent of cases of multiple myeloma. The incidence in 'benign' monoclonal gammopathies is unknown but is probably about 5–10 per cent; here the gammopathy is not really benign because of the poor prognosis of the associated amyloidosis.

As AL amyloid is derived from free light chains, it should be possible to detect either a monoclonal paraprotein or free light chain in the serum or urine of all cases. However, this is not always possible with standard techniques. Sometimes the paraprotein manifests itself after the diagnosis of amyloid, and in other cases there may be other clues to the aetiology, such as low polyclonal immunoglobulins (reflecting immunosuppressive effects of a proliferating immunocyte clone) or increased numbers of marrow plasma cells.

AL amyloidosis predominantly affects the mesenchymal tissues to produce effects such as neuropathies, carpal tunnel syndrome and macroglossia, restrictive cardiomyopathy, and arthropathies of large joints. But organs such as the kidney and gastrointestinal tract may also be affected and, as with AA amyloid, any tissue may be involved. This marked overlap between AA and AL amyloid emphasizes the inaccuracy of the designations of primary and secondary amyloidosis.

AL amyloid, with or without myeloma, is commoner in men than women, and usually occurs in patients over 40 years old. Fatigue and weight loss are the commonest presenting symptoms. Although AL amyloid is said to involve the heart, tongue, gastrointestinal tract, nerves, and skin (as compared to AA amyloid, said to involve mainly liver, kidneys, and spleen), no consistent difference has been demonstrated between AL and AA amyloid either by organ distribution or by electron microscropy.

The heart is affected in 90 per cent of cases of AA amyloidosis, with cardiac dysfunction the presenting feature in 30 per cent and the cause of death in up to 50 per cent. It may lead to a restrictive cardiomyopathy or involve the conducting system, with development of arrhythmias. The gastrointestinal tract may be involved at any level, leading to macroglossia (seen only in AL amyloidosis), mobility disturbance (often due to autonomic dysfunction), malabsorption, haemorrhage, perforation, or obstruction. Neurological complications include peripheral and autonomic neuropathy and carpal tunnel syndrome. Skin involvement is either with plaques or nodules of amyloid or purpura due to infiltration of dermal vessels.

Heredo-familial systemic amyloidosis

Predominantly neuropathic, nephropathic, and cardiopathic type I. They occur predominantly in limited geographical areas. The only fibril types identified so far are variant forms of prealbumin. *Familial Mediterranean fever* is an autosomal recessive disease of unknown aetiology characterized by acute, self-limiting attacks of fever and inflammation of serosal membranes, leading to peritonitis, pleuritis, and synovitis. Erythematous skin rashes occur. Amyloidosis is a frequent and serious complication, and is an example of AA amyloid complicating an acute inflammatory process.

Senile systemic amyloidosis

Amyloid deposition invariably accompanies ageing, and autopsies in individuals over the age of 80 show amyloid in all cases. The amyloid may be localized and composed of different fibrils in the different sites. However, in up to 25 per cent of cases the fibrils are derived from prealbumin. The heart is the main organ affected (indeed it was previously called *senile cardiac amyloidosis*), but deposits are also found elsewhere, such as in the lungs. Major differences from other systemic amyloidoses are the few deposits found in the spleen and absence of renal glomerular involvement. Unless cardiac deposits are massive, it is generally accepted to have a minimal effect on cardiac function.

Localized amyloidosis

In the absence of systemic senile amyloidosis, amyloid deposits may be localized to particular organs or tissues, or distributed focally within one or more tissues and occur in various forms. The deposits may produce clinically obvious masses or be evident only on microscopic examination.

1. Related to extramedullary plasmocytomas. AL amyloid deposits, ranging from microscopic to massive, may be found associated with extramedullary plasmocytomas and often affects the larynx, genito-urinary tract, and skin. Sometimes there is predominance of amyloid over plasma cells in the lesion.

2. Amyloidosis may occur in a localized form as a part of the ageing process. The commonest form is part of senile systemic amyloidosis; amyloid is deposited in the myocardium of atria and ventricles. Isolated atrial amyloidosis has been reported in 78 per cent of patients over the age of 80 years. The amyloid fibrils contain immunoreactive human atrial natriuretic peptide. The amyloid occurs as fine deposits in or adjacent to the sarcolemma of muscle cells and affected small vessels. Intracellular deposits may occur, as in endocrine tumours. In the elderly population it has been suggested that atrial fibrillation is more common in patients with isolated atrial amyloidosis.

3. Cutaneous amyloidosis. *Nodular cutaneous amyloid* is derived from AL amyloid. Macular and papular forms also occur and it is suggested, although not proven, that they are derived from epidermal keratins.

4. Deposits are present in the seminal vesicles of 21 per cent of men over the age of 75 years. The fibril protein is not

known, although it may be the same as the focal amyloid deposits, corpora amylacea, which occur in the prostate.

5. Microscopic deposits may be found in tumours and tissues of the endocrine system. The commonest example is amyloid in medullary carcinoma, where it is derived from precalcitonin. In the pancreas, amyloid occurs in the islets of the ageing pancreas and in the islets of patients with diabetes mellitus. In type II diabetes the fibrils are immunochemically cross-reactive with insulin β-chains.

6. Cerebral amyloid. Cerebral amyoid occurs in three forms:

   (a) *cerebral amyloid angiopathy*, in which it is deposited within and around blood vessels;

   (b) as the core of senile and neuritic plaques; and

   (c) as neurofibrillary tangles within neuronal cell bodies and processes.

   In all these three forms they share the characteristic ultra-structural and staining features of amyloid. The plaques, seen in senile dementia and Alzheimer's disease, and the neurofibrillary tangles are the only forms of amyloid that do not contain amyloid P component. Interestingly, AP is present in the plaques of the spongiform encephalopathies. The amyloid fibril protein found in the plaques and cerebro-vascular amyloid of patients with Alzheimer's, senile dementia of Alzheimer type, and Down's syndrome is com-posed of β-protein.

7. *Cerebral amyloid angiopathy* is present in almost 100 per cent of brains from patients with Alzheimer's disease, as well as in a significant proportion of brains from mentally normal, elderly people. It is a rare cause of cerebral haemorrhage in the at-risk group. One other form is *heredi-tary cerebral haemorrhage with amyloidosis*, an autosomal dominant condition leading to fatal cerebral haemorrhage in middle age; the fibrils are closely related to γ-trace pro-tein. It is not known whether the cerebrovascular amyloid in non-demented patients without plaques or tangles is related.

8. Alzheimer's disease is characterized by neuritic plaques, neurofibrillary tangles, and cerebral amyloid angiopathy. The pathogenesis of the plaques and tangles is unknown. Senile dementia of Alzheimer's type has similar pathology but may not share the same aetiology and pathogenesis. The cerebral pathology found in Down's syndrome patients who develop dementia is also identical.

9. Plaques closely resembling senile neuritic plaques occur in the transmissible encephalopathies Kuru, Creutzfeldt–Jacob disease, and Gerstmann–Strausler syndrome. Ex-perimental purification of scrapie prions has shown the preparations to contain numerous rod-shaped particles; arrays of these prion rods ultrastructurally resemble amyl-oid and show green birefringence. It has been suggested that amyloid plaques in the transmissible encephalopathies may consist of prions.

10. Articular and peri-articular amyloid, usually affecting the carpal tunnel, is a complication of haemodialysis. Amyloid is also present in most osteoarthritic joints, usually associ-ated with chondrocalcinosis; the fibril protein is unknown.

5.5.6 Organ involvement in amyloidosis

Amyloidosis may be inapparent or organs may be atrophied or enlarged and firm with a waxy appearance. Amyloid is depos-ited along stromal networks, between cells, and often initially closely related to basement membranes. Progressive accumu-lation may lead to organ enlargement but, conversely, atrophy may occur due to vascular deposits causing circulatory impair-ment and also because of the compressive effects of the deposits themselves.

Liver

The liver is commonly involved in amyloidosis. Estimates range from 56 per cent, where it is reported as the next most common after spleen and kidney involvement, to 100 per cent. Symp-toms of liver disease are rare, although hepatomegaly is relatively common; jaundice is an uncommon sign and a poor prognostic feature. Macroscopically the liver is usually enlarged, smooth, pale, and of waxy or rubbery consistency. Amyloid is first deposited in the space of Disse between endo-thelial and parenchymal cells. Progressive accumulation leads to atrophy of hepatocytes through ischaemia or compression. There may be a zonal distribution with a tendency for peri-venular areas to be affected first. Amyloid around central veins and within portal tracts is common; however, as was pre-viously suggested, the distribution pattern cannot be used to discriminate between the different forms. Accompanying fea-tures include portal tract fibrosis, inflammation, and, rarely, cirrhosis.

Kidney

Proteinuria is present in most patients with amyloidosis; it is usually poorly selective and may contain a paraprotein. There is a great deal of overlap in the patterns and clinical pictures between the different forms. The glomeruli are nearly always involved in AA amyloid but in only about one-third of AL amyl-oid. Thrombosis of intrarenal veins may develop and precipitate acute renal failure. Renal amyloid is the commonest cause of death in familial Mediterranean fever. Macroscopically the kid-neys are usually large and pale. However, if there has been prolonged hypertension, they may show contraction with granular cortical surfaces. Microscopically, glomeruli are pre-dominantly involved but tubules, interstitial tissues, and blood-vessels are also affected. Progressive involvement of glomeruli, tubules, interstitial tissue, and vessels leads to tubular atrophy and interstitial fibrosis. Tubules may contain casts, and the overall appearance resembles the changes seen in chronic pyelonephritis; the casts may be laminated and may stain for amyloid in cases of multiple myeloma.

Localized amyloid may be present in the form of isolated deposits in the renal pelvis and/or ureters.

Heart

The heart may show the features of constrictive cardiomyopathy. Macroscopically the heart may be enlarged, heavy, and show ventricular dilatation. The endocardial surface may be granular, a feature characteristically seen in the left atrium. Microscopically, amyloid may be deposited between and compress myocardial fibres. Vascular involvement is common, infiltrating small and large vessels. Deposits within valves are common and the conducting system is frequently involved.

Spleen

The spleen may be of normal size or enlarged. Two forms of deposition are seen; the nodular form involves splenic follicles whereas the diffuse form infiltrates the red pulp. Parenchymal amyloidosis is usually accompanied by involvement of the vasculature; however, vessels alone may be affected.

Other organs

Amyloid is often found in the pancreatic islets of patients with non-insulin-dependent diabetes mellitus and to a lesser extent in islets from elderly patients without diabetes. It is found very rarely in islets of patients with diabetes of juvenile-onset type. Amyloid is also found associated with insulinomas and growth-hormone-producing tumours of the adenohypophysis.

5.5.7 Pathogenesis

One of the most important processes in amyloid formation is proteolytic cleavage of a precursor protein. This is the generally accepted mechanism for formation of AL and AA amyloid, but under other circumstances this view has to be modified because whole variant prealbumin molecules can polymerize to fibrils in some familial forms of amyloidosis, and the amyloid of haemodialysis consists of whole, unprocessed β_2-microglobulin.

It is generally believed that AA amyloid is produced by proteolytic cleavage of SAA. SAA is an acute-phase reactant whose concentration rises in response to tissue injury, infection, or inflammation. SAA has a molecular weight of 180 000 and is an apoprotein of high-density lipoprotein. Denaturation of the lipoprotein releases apo-SAA, which has a molecular weight of 12 000–14 000. Release of apo-SAA from hepatocytes is stimulated by interleukin-1 produced by macrophages. This apo-SAA consists of 104 residues, the first 76 of which, from the N-terminal end, are identical with AA amyloid from tissue deposits. The risk of developing AA amyloidosis is greater when the systemic response and acute protein response is higher. The overall rate of accumulation of SAA may also be an important factor—a low rate in SLE and ulcerative colitis (with a low incidence of amyloidosis), and a high rate in rheumatoid arthritis and Crohn's disease (with a higher incidence of amyloidosis). Experiments in mice have demonstrated an 'amyloid enhancing factor' in which injection of amyloidotic tissue leads to development of amyloid in only 1–2 days, but its significance in man is as yet unknown. Although six isotypes of apo-SAA have been identified in man, there is no conclusive evidence that any form of differential expression is related to development of AA amyloidosis.

AL amyloid formation is thought to be produced by proteolytic cleavage of monoclonal light chains. There is evidence that the AL proteins have unique amino-acid replacements or insertions compared to non-amyloid monoclonal proteins and this finding, together with the fact that AL amyloid is more commonly derived from λ light chains, suggests that some proteins are more amyloidogenic than others.

Proteolysis is not involved in the pathogenesis of some amyloidoses, notably in familial amyloidotic polyneuropathy.

The part that AP plays in the pathogenesis of amyloid is not known: it may be an epiphenomenon, its binding to amyloid fibrils a reflection of a shared ligand, or it may contribute to the formation and persistence of amyloid.

5.5.8 Bibliography

Glenner, G. G. (1980). Amyloid deposits and amyloidosis—the beta fibrilloses 1. *New England Journal of Medicine* **302**, 1283–92.

Pepys, M. B. (1988). Amyloidosis. In *Immunological disease* (4th edn) (ed. M. Samter *et al.*). Little, Brown and Co., Boston.

6

Pathophysiology of infection

6
Pathophysiology of infection

6.1 Microbial infection and host–parasite relationships

Heather M. Dick

6.1.1 Introduction

This chapter aims to illustrate selected important principles in the study of the pathophysiology of infection. It is not intended to be a comprehensive survey of the subject, for which readers are referred to some of the major texts on microbiology and immunology (see Chapter 4). Particular emphasis has been laid on the mechanisms of virulence and the means by which micro-organisms actually produce disease. Some seem to have a predilection for particular tissues, and some are particularly effective at spreading through the community. Readers should consult the relevant sections of this book for further details of specific infections of various organs and tissues, and are referred to specialized texts on microbiology for details of the methods used to isolate and identify micro-organisms and the treatment of infections (see Further reading).

Man comes into close contact with numerous micro-organisms at almost every stage of life, from the fetus *in utero*, throughout childhood, and as an adult. Many micro-organisms live in a close relationship with man, on skin, mucous membranes, in the gut, in food and water, and seldom give rise to infectious problems. Some constitute what is described as the 'normal flora' of sites such as the upper respiratory tract, the skin, the lower intestinal tract, and the genital tract, where they are not disease producers but are an integral part of the environment of these sites. These include staphylococci, some streptococci, lactobacilli, and many others. Infectious lesions as such are relatively rare and are usually the result of contact with a highly infectious and virulent organism or of a breakdown in the protective immunological defence mechanisms. There are also organisms that are seldom or never found in healthy individuals and, when they do occur, are closely associated with the presence of disease. These include some viruses and protozoan parasites as well as certain bacteria and fungi,

for example smallpox virus, malaria, rabies, and tuberculosis. Other organisms, commonly found in the environment, in animals, or in the soil, water, or food can be harmful to man if a sufficient dose is acquired, as in *Salmonella* food poisoning, or where tissue damage or spillage of gut contents occurs, as for example with gas gangrene, tetanus, and peritonitis.

Genetic differences exist in susceptibility to some infections and there may be widely differing degrees of resistance or susceptibility between species as well as between individuals within a species. Some of the differences in response are attributable to the influence of immune response genes, which are associated with resistance or susceptibility to particular diseases and influence both the type and magnitude of response; many of these genes are found on one of the autosomal chromosomes in close linkage with the genes which code for the major histocompatibility antigens, forming part of the region known as the major histocompatibility complex (MHC) in man and other mammals. The other important genes in this region code for the HLA antigens. Using highly inbred strains of mice to simplify the genetic mixture, it is possible to demonstrate that genes of the MHC determine not only resistance or susceptibility to some infectious agents, particularly viruses, but also code for many of the molecules that are essential to antigen recognition and cellular co-operation in the immune system. The MHC system is fully discussed in Chapter 4.

6.1.2 Infection and immunity

Non-specific immunity

Intact defence mechanisms will generally prevent or, at the least, hinder the attack of all but the most invasive organisms. The first-line non-specific defences are so called because they are not directed against any one individual virus or bacterial species, but rather act in a general way to prevent colonization and invasion (see Sections 4.2 and 6.2.1). The non-specific defences include the skin and mucous membranes, the cornea, the cilia of the respiratory tract, and numerous products of the tissues, including enzymes, such as lysozyme (found in tears), and the acids and lipids produced by the gut and the skin, respectively, as well as cell products such as the interferons, which are effective against viruses. These defences can prevent the access of micro-organisms to the deeper tissues, either by acting as a physical barrier or by their physiological activity—in wafting particles out of the respiratory tract as the ciliated epithelium does, or by slowing the growth rate of organisms, especially bacteria, as do lysozyme and the fatty acids in sebum, or by lethal effects as exemplified by the high-acid content of the stomach. Such responses, which are concentrated at the likely points of access for disease-producing micro-organisms, do not increase in magnitude with repeated exposure to the same organism but are, nevertheless, extremely effective in preventing infections as long as they remain intact. The phagocytic activities of neutrophils and cells of the macrophage series are also very important first-line defences, especially against bacteria. The additional effect of serum complement as an adjunct to the killing process after phagocytosis has taken place should not be underestimated, especially in the presence of specific antibodies, when they begin to appear, with the development of the specific response to infection.

Specific immunity

This specific second line of defence, the product of many cells, tissues, and organs, collectively, if ungrammatically referred to as 'the immune system', is dealt with in detail elsewhere (Chapter 4). Suffice it to say that the rapidly responsive and highly efficient mechanisms which form this 'system' include both cells and cellular products, the most important of which are antibodies and lymphocytes, together with their soluble products. Specific immunity is capable of increasing both in magnitude and in effectiveness on repeated exposure to the same organism. The importance of specific immunity was recognized in the earliest work of bacteriologists, particularly Pasteur, Koch, Ehrlich, and their colleagues, and formed the basis of their efforts to prepare vaccines to prevent or ameliorate infectious processes. They were a little better informed than Jenner, the first practitioner to use vaccination in the eighteenth century, because they at least were able to identify the bacterial cause of many conditions, but neither they nor Jenner understood the exact way in which the vaccination process produced the state of immunity. That understanding was to come, slowly at first and with increasing speed, in the past 20 years. We can now recognize not only which cells (lymphocytes, macrophages, and many others) and by what routes they achieve their purpose of eliminating or minimizing the spread of infection, and we are also aware of the many ways in which the processes can break down or become ineffective (Lydyard and Grossi, 1989; Lewis and McGee, 1992).

Virulence

The dose and disease-producing capabilities of the offending organism are also of great importance in determining whether an infection becomes established. Some bacteria are capable of producing infection after an initial dose of only a few bacilli, e.g. typhoid, and the same is true for some viruses, such as rabies. In other cases, quite large doses, probably of the order of tens of millions rather than hundreds, are needed before the bacteria can multiply successfully in the tissues, as with salmonella producing food-poisoning. In addition, many bacteria and parasites produce a wide range of cell-associated products, including organelles such as flagella, fimbriae, spores, enzymes, and chemical toxins (see Section 6.2), which assist them in their efforts to invade the tissues and to become established where they can multiply freely, avoiding the defence mechanisms, both specific and non-specific. The general term 'virulence mechanisms' is now applied to such factors.

Opportunistic infections

Some widely distributed organisms are usually of little significance as producers of infectious disease because they lack means to produce active infection, especially in healthy tissues, i.e. they are not highly virulent. However, given the correct set of circumstances, these opportunistic organisms can seize the chance to become established, leading to infection—hence, 'opportunists'. A breach in the normal defence mechanisms, such as trauma, a surgical wound, the insertion site of a needle or cannula, the implantation of a foreign body, such as an artificial hip joint, may offer a starting point for infections produced by organisms of low virulence. Serious defects which diminish the body's ability to make specific antibodies or to produce an effective T-lymphocyte response can also predispose to infection. For example, human immunodeficiency virus type 1 (HIV-1) in acquired immunodeficiency syndrome (AIDS) actually destroys those lymphocytes which are essential to both T- and B-lymphocyte responses to micro-organisms. The patient with AIDS is thus open to a wide range of infections from both exogenous and endogenous organisms. Existing foci of infection, for example with *Mycobacterium tuberculosis*, or herpes virus type 1, which were previously kept in check by the immune system or were in a latent state, may 'light-up' after HIV-1 infection because of the destruction by the HIV of the body's specific defences. Similar, but less dramatic (or perhaps less well publicized) problems occur with other patients who have had their immune system compromised by disease or treatment. The extent to which a patient is 'immunologically compromised' can vary widely, depending both on the original disease and the type and duration of treatment. Any one or several parts of their defences may be ineffective or diminished and it is often difficult to determine the precise nature of the defects and which particular functions are affected. The problems of such infections are dealt with in Section 6.7.

6.1.3 Further reading

Collee, J. G., Duguid, J. P., Fraser, A. G., and Marmion, B. P. (eds) (1989). *Mackie and McCartney practical medical microbiology* (13th edn). Churchill Livingstone, Edinburgh.

Klein, J. (1986). *The natural history of the major histocompatibility complex*. Wiley, New York.

Lewis, C. L. and McGee, J. O'D. (1992). *The natural immune system: the macrophage*. Oxford University Press.

Lewis, C. L. and McGee, J. O'D. (1992). *The natural immune system: the natural killer cell*. Oxford University Press.

Lydyard, P. and Grossi, C. (1989). Cells involved in the immune response. In *Immunology* (ed. I. M. Roitt, J. Brostoff and D. Male), (2nd edn), ch. 2. Churchill Livingstone, Edinburgh.

Mims, C. A. (1987). *The pathogenesis of infectious disease* (3rd edn). Academic Press, London.

Shanson, D. C. (1989). *Microbiology in clinical practice* (2nd edn). Wright, London.

Wilson, G. S., Miles, A. A., and Parker, M. T. (ed.) (1991). *Topley and Wilson's principles of bacteriology, virology and immunity* (8th edn). Arnold, London.

6.2 Virulence mechanisms

6.2.1 Adhesion, penetration, and colonization

David C. Old

Many bacterial infections in man and animals are initiated by colonization of the mucous membranes of the respiratory, genito-urinary and gastrointestinal tracts. These environments are notoriously hostile to bacteria which, furthermore, are challenged by the mechanical turmoil resulting from the upward movement of the mucus on ciliated mucosal surfaces, or the cleansing action of urine flow or the constant churning movements of intestinal contents. Bacteria attempting to survive in such difficult conditions must include among their armoury of survival attributes mechanisms whereby they can withstand the onslaught of the host defences.

Infections on mucosal surfaces involve a number of stages, including the attachment of bacteria to epithelial cells, followed thereafter by an increase in bacterial numbers that leads eventually to colonization. Regardless of their ultimate relationship with the host, many bacteria have been forced to develop mechanisms whereby they can attach to mucosal surfaces, and this phenomenon of attachment, designed as it is to prevent the forceable removal of bacteria from their favoured niches, is likely, when present, to provide considerable survival advantage over that of bacteria without attachment potential. The attachment to mucosae is likely to be equally as important to commensal as pathogenic bacteria because, for all of them, attachment aids survival.

Adhesion

For most bacteria the earliest stage of colonization occurs through a series of specific lock-and-key interactions between structures present at the bacterial surface and complementary sequences on the host substratum. In 1959 Duguid first coined the term adhesins to describe the bacterial structures involved in this attachment process; the term has remained popular ever since and, as far as medical microbiologists are concerned, its usage indicates the binding of bacteria to mammalian cells. The term receptor describes the complementary sequences recognized by the adhesins in their specific act of recognition. For some pathogenic bacteria, adhesion and subsequent colonization may be strictly localized and directed mainly towards the efficient delivery of bacterial toxins or other extracellular products that effect damage to the host tissues. For other bacteria, attachment is only the first of a series of complex interactions between bacterium and host leading either to penetration (invasion) and dissemination of bacteria through the host's tissues or even to a state of intracellular parasitism. That the process of recognition between bacterium and host receptor is highly selective is the fundamental aspect of adhesion. Tissue tropism, i.e. the predilection shown by some microbes for particular tissues or organs, was perhaps the first realization by medical microbiologists that tissue specificity and, indeed, host adaptations were acts of specific recognition.

The realization that adhesins are important virulence factors has stimulated much detailed study of the mechanisms whereby bacteria, particularly pathogenic ones, adhere to host cells. The apparatus of adhesion is as diverse as the microbes themselves, but each is essentially a surface macromolecule presented either as a structural organelle, or as a diffusible product. Among the surface materials known to have adhesion potential are: slime, capsule, other high molecular weight polysaccharides, cell-wall products such as lipoteichoic acids, glycocalyx, outer-membrane proteins, flagella, fibrillae, and fimbriae. The chemical nature of the macromolecules themselves is equally diverse.

Fimbrial adhesins

Escherichia coli is perhaps the most versatile pathogen in the family Enterobacteriaceae and certainly one that has amassed a vast array of virulence determinants, each suited for colonization of particular niches in the host. Information about the adhesins of *E. coli* has accumulated at an exciting, if daunting, pace over the past two decades. The demonstration by electron microscopy that many adhesive strains formed hair-like filaments, called fimbriae, the possession and expression of which correlated with the adhesive properties of a culture, led to the idea that the fimbriae themselves were the adhesins essential for attachment (Fig. 6.1).

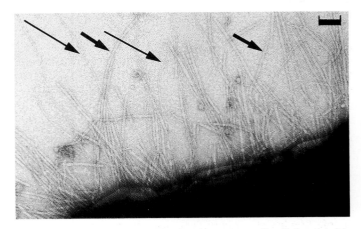

Fig. 6.1 Electron micrograph showing structurally distinguishable fimbriae present on an adhesive strain of Enterobacteriaceae. Fimbriae are: thin (≤4 nm diameter) and non-channelled (⟶), or thick (≥8 nm diameter) and channelled (➡). The bar marker represents 100 nm.

There was, indeed, good evidence for the role of fimbriae as specific organelles of attachment. An important breakthrough came in the 1960s when veterinary microbiologists, in particular Williams Smith and his colleagues, demonstrated that a major attribute of enteropathogenic strains of *E. coli* responsible for diarrhoeal illnesses in different species of domestic animals (including calves, lambs, and piglets) was their ability to attach to the epithelial cells of the small intestine of these animals. Proliferation in the small intestine of the host ensured accurate delivery of the bacterial enterotoxins to the very target cells in which hypersecretion would be induced, and affords a splendid example of localization and bacterial-cell economy. Strains of *E. coli* that lacked the capacity for localized colonization did not cause diarrhoea even if they could produce enterotoxin. Specific colonization antigens were first recognized serologically and, because they were thought to be capsular antigens, were designated as having new capsular antigens such as K88 and K99. The presence at the bacterial-cell surface of hair-like appendages that were clearly not capsules was subsequently established by electron microscopy. The name 'fimbriae' had first been proposed for the hair-like appendages of *E. coli* by Duguid in 1955 and this term, which will have priority, will be used rather than the synonym (pilus) introduced some years later.

It was of interest, and indeed was critical to the success of the genetic experiments of Williams Smith, that many of the adhesins (and enterotoxins) involved in diarrhoeal illnesses of animals were encoded by genes present on plasmids (accessory, extrachromosomal pieces of DNA). Loss or gain of adhesin-determining plasmids correlated well with the inability or ability to produce fimbriae and, hence, with the colonization of the epithelial cells of the small intestine. Somewhat later, similar fimbrial structures were described in enterotoxigenic strains of *E. coli* responsible for diarrhoeal illness in man. It should be noted, however, that some of the latter adhesins were not plasmid-determined.

Specificity Different strains of *E. coli* can be recognized for epidemiological purposes by serological identification of the surface antigens of their cell walls (o-somatic antigens), their capsules (κ-antigens), their flagella (h-antigens), and now their fimbriae (f-antigens). Strains of *E. coli* of particular serotypes are host-species specific. Thus, enterotoxigenic strains of *E. coli* that colonized the small intestine of, say, pigs belonged to serotypes that were different from those of strains that colonized the human intestine. Furthermore, it was also apparent that strains of *E. coli* causing diarrhoeal illness in man belonged to serotypes different from those responsible for urinary-tract infection (UTI).

Receptor recognition Perhaps the best studied example of receptor definition is that found among the 10 or so major serotypes of *E. coli* responsible for UTI in man. Among uropathogenic strains of *E. coli* the virulence determinants that are thought to be important are: haemolysin, capsule, type-1 fimbriae, and other adhesins. Considering the likely importance of adhesion to uro-epithelial cells, it was of interest that among strains of *E. coli* involved in the first episodes of non-obstructive pyelonephri-

tis (i.e. in which the upper urinary tract was involved) in women, more than 90 per cent of the strains produce a particular kind of adhesin associated with fimbriae called P fimbriae, so named because they bind specifically to receptor sites for α-D-galactosyl-β-D-galactoside (Gal–Gal). This receptor sequence is part of the P blood-group antigens on human red cells (which are, therefore, specifically agglutinated by P-fimbriated strains of *E. coli*) and is also found on uro-epithelial cells. The finding that glycolipids extracted from whole kidney and the upper ureters of man are rich in Gal–Gal residues of various complexities might explain why the P fimbriae-associated adhesin is the dominant one in uropathogenic strains of *E. coli*. Small saccharides containing Gal–Gal sequences inhibit adhesion of P-fimbriated bacteria to uro-epithelial cells and to human red cells of P-types, a useful confirmation of their receptor identity. Other urinary adhesins recognizing other diverse receptors have been described but occur less frequently than P fimbriae.

Fimbrial phase variation There are two further important observations that must now be made about the fimbrial adhesins of *E. coli*. First, genetic evidence has established unequivocally that expression of fimbriae is separable from that of adhesiveness. Thus, the actual adhesin molecule is encoded by a gene that is independent of those encoding the polypeptides (fimbrillins) which are assembled to form the structures we recognize as fimbriae. The adhesin is a minor component of the assembled organelle and the fimbriae should be regarded, therefore, as an effective architectural device whereby the adhesin, located at the tip of the fimbria, can be projected beyond the cell-wall paraphernalia and carried to wherever the adhesin's target receptor is to be found. Secondly, the expression of adhesin-bearing fimbriae can be switched on or off by a process of phase variation which occurs independently for each of the different classes of fimbriae possessed by an adhesive bacterium.

Non-fimbrial adhesins Many adhesive bacteria apparently do not form fimbriae and two important groups of non-fimbrial adhesins are known. In *E. coli* the best studied of them is the 'man-only' haemagglutinin (so called because it haemagglutinates human red cells only) associated with a hydrophobic surface protein presenting as a 'fuzzy' aggregate of very fine fimbrillae ($\leqslant 2$ nm in diameter) which are extremely difficult to observe by electron microscopy (Fig. 6.2). Other naturally occurring non-fimbrial adhesins seem to be associated with outer-membrane proteins.

Fimbrial antigenic variation

A common adhesin, e.g. the Gal–Gal-recognizing adhesin of *E. coli*, may be carried by any one of a variety of P fimbriae which are antigenically distinguishable and show little cross-reactivity. How then is a pathogenic bacterium able to switch so readily from the manufacture of one kind of fimbria to another that is antigenically, but not functionally or structurally, distinct?

The problem of antigenically variable fimbriae has been particularly well studied with *N. gonorrhoeae*. This species usually

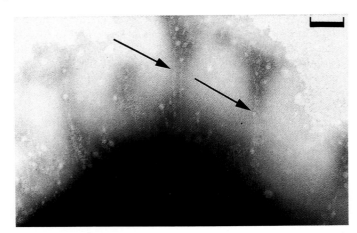

Fig. 6.2 Electron-micrograph of a non-fimbriate, adhesive strain of *Escherichia coli* bearing thin (⩽2 nm diameter) fibrillae. The bar marker repesents 100 nm. (Courtesy of Mr D. Yakubu.)

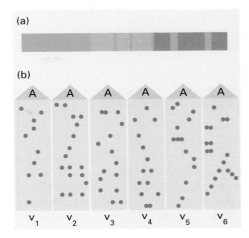

Fig. 6.3 Schematic representations of (a) fimbrillin polypeptide showing regions of the molecule that are highly conserved (green); variable (orange); or hypervariable (purple); (b) structurally identical fimbriae carrying at their tips the same kind of adhesin (A), but antigenically distinct (v_1–v_6) because of amino-acid sequences (red dots) in the variable and hypervariable regions of their fimbrillins that are unique and immunodominant.

colonizes the mucosal surfaces of the human urogenital tract but many other body sites are equally susceptible to infection. Its pathogenicity is very much associated with the ability to produce surface antigens that include fimbriae (often called pili in this species) and an outer-membrane protein PII (the opacity protein). Clinical isolates of gonococci have been shown to form fimbriae of many different antigenic types. Indeed, one strain of gonococcus isolated either from different cohorts in an epidemiologically related incident, or even from different body sites of one patient, may show considerable antigenic diversity of its fimbriae.

Comparison of the antigenically variant forms of gonococcal fimbriae shows that some regions of the fimbrillin polypeptides are highly conserved, whereas other regions are variable or hypervariable (Fig. 6.3). Conserved regions, in which changes are rarely tolerated, are probably those essential for correct assembly of the fimbrillin proteins to fimbriae and for the further assimilation of ancillary minor proteins into the intact fimbriae; the variable regions, where changes are tolerated without affecting correct assembly, represent the antigenically variable parts of the assembled fimbriae.

The gonococcus possesses several gene loci for the synthesis of fimbrillin, the major protein of its fimbriae. At any time, one of these loci will be expressed while the other loci remain 'silent'. By this mechanism the gonococcus can switch quickly from the synthesis of one antigenic kind of fimbriae to another. It is also able to generate new varieties of fimbrillin after transformation with exogenous DNA from lysed gonococci. Thus, the gonococcus has limitless potential for the generation of new antigenic forms of fimbriae, a process which has been demonstrated

1. in *in vitro* experiments;
2. after intra-urethral injection of human volunteers; and
3. in the course of natural epidemic spread.

By a combination of phase variation and antigenic variation, the gonococcus can display any of a multitude of attachment phenotypes; this flexibility helps the gonococcus to evade the attention of the host's immune system and to colonize different tissues and organs. A similar explanation seems equally valid for P and other fimbriae. The existence of antigenically variant adhesins may also help explain, at least in part, why some patients are subject to repeated episodes of gonorrhoea or UTI.

Anti-adhesin vaccines

The idea that it might be possible to neutralize the earliest, critical step of colonization in infectious diseases by the use of anti-adhesin vaccines is an attractive one. Without doubt, that hope has motivated much of the research and generated the excitement of adhesion in the past two decades. But, in fact, how practical an option does it now seem?

There have been many experimental demonstrations of the efficacy of fimbrial vaccines. For example, veterinary studies have shown that antibodies directed against the adhesins of enterotoxigenic strains of *E. coli* prevented diarrhoea in domestic animals. It is not certain, however, that this success can be attributed solely to the production of secretory immunoglobulins and interruption of attachment. The elimination from the herd environment of plasmid-carrying strains and their replacement by plasmidless strains was probably induced by the presence of circulating anti-adhesin antibodies in these animals. In both experimental models and in primates, there have been several demonstrations of the protection afforded by purified fimbriae against UTI by P-fimbriate *E. coli* and against gonorrhoea by gonococci.

As it emerged that there was antigenic drift even within a single class of functionally equivalent fimbriae, interest has shifted somewhat from the use of whole fimbriae to the search for short oligopeptide sequences that are immunogenic and common to all members of any class of fimbriae. But in the case of the gonococcus, for example, early hopes for the identification of conserved regions have subsequently been dashed. The variability of the fimbrial (and other) adhesin vectors thus far examined makes it difficult to see how a fimbrial vaccine (whole or fragment-based) is to be achieved:

Penetration

In their interaction with the host, many pathogenic bacteria exert their damage by penetration (invasion) of the cells of the host. Nevertheless, it is difficult to offer an all-embracing definition of this phenomenon because the synonyms penetration/invasion cover such a broad range of host–bacterium responses. The invasive process may be superficial as, for example, when it is associated with pathogenic bacteria ordinarily thought of as being non-invasive. Thus, for example, *Corynebacterium diphtheriae*, the agent of diphtheria, and *Bordetella pertussis*, the agent of whooping cough, are good examples of bacteria generally considered to be virulent by virtue of their production of powerful exotoxins. In both cases, an early stage of adhesion to the epithelial cells of the respiratory tract ensures localized proliferation at the site of attachment. There is inevitably some superficial invasion of the cells resulting from that colonization process, although the damage arising from that invasion contributes little to the overall virulence of the bacteria.

Invasion: Shigellae and enteroinvasive E. coli

For other pathogenic bacteria, however, the principal expression of their virulence is invasiveness. Among the Enterobacteriaceae there are many examples of invasive bacteria, including species of *Escherichia, Salmonella, Shigella,* and *Yersinia*. Illustration of this other extreme of penetration will be made by reference to the shigellae and their close relatives, the enteroinvasive *E. coli* (EIEC), which have been particularly well studied. These highly specialized pathogens cause a dysenteric syndrome in man (and a few primates) and are responsible for up to 20 per cent of all diarrhoeal illnesses world-wide. Shigellosis is illustrative of a highly localized invasion involving the epithelial cells of the colonic mucosae. By being invasive, shigellae escape from the highly competitive environment of the gut lumen to a more secluded niche within the colonic epithelial cells where they gain ready access to nutrients present in the blood system of the host. After penetration of the epithelial cells, and rapid proliferation in that protected intracellular environment, shigellae are released, kill the epithelial cells, and spread to other adjacent cells; that cycle of events leads eventually to death of the epithelium. The resultant dissemination of shigellae in the lamina propria provokes an inflammatory response which kills some of the shigellae but also causes mucosal damage that ranges from a mild inflammation to gross ulceration of the colon and produces the typical symptoms of shigellosis (dysentery).

Role of plasmids Laboratory models for the assay of invasiveness include the abilities to produce keratoconjunctivitis on instillation of shigellae to the guinea-pig eye and to invade tissue-culture cells such as HeLa cells. These two properties are associated with the presence of large plasmids. Although there are marked differences in the virulence of different serotypes of *Shigella* and in the severity of the illnesses they cause, it is of interest to note that there is sufficient homology in the sequences of the different large plasmids present in strains of different serotypes of shigellae and EIEC to suggest that they have a common ancestry and that essential genes have been conserved in all of them. These plasmids of shigellae must be critical for invasion because their loss leads to non-invasiveness and their introduction into non-pathogenic laboratory strains of *E. coli* renders the latter invasive.

Intracellular multiplication and killing In their transition from the lumen of the gut to inside the epithelial cell, the shigellae must cross the membrane barrier of the host cell. The active participation of the shigellae in this process is demonstrated by the finding that treatment of the shigellae with ultraviolet light or antibiotics interferes with their uptake. Shigellae probably induce their own phagocytic uptake by the epithelial cells by release of extracellular, heat-labile products of low molecular weight, that produce limited disaggregation (and immediate repair) of the plasma membrane of the epithelial cell. After multiplication within the vacuole, shigellae are released from it, when the same lytic product that initially induced their uptake damages the membrane of the vacuole, causing it to burst. Thereupon, the shigellae pass into the cytoplasm of the epithelial cell, an environment apparently suitable for expression of other virulence genes required for growth and survival. Little is known, however, about these latter products.

In *in vitro* experiments of phagocytes infected with shigellae, Sansonetti has shown that many dramatic events occur, including changes in the levels of intracellular ATP, severe impairment of respiration, and blockage of fermentation. The resultant killing is rapid; it probably reflects interference with the energy metabolism of host cells. The shiga toxin, produced by many shigellae and a known powerful inhibitor of protein synthesis, was previously believed to be responsible for host-cell death. But, if the shiga toxin is another virulence determinant of shigellae, it is more likely that it functions as an enterotoxin responsible for hypersecretion in the small intestine; diarrhoea is, of course, a frequent symptom in the early stages of shigellosis. As well as plasmid-determined genes carried on large plasmids, the virulence of shigellae also requires the participation of some chromosomal genes involved with, among other things, the structure of the repeat units of the lipopolysaccharide of its o-somatic antigen.

Invasion: other Enterobacteriaceae

The invasive process of *Salmonella* has little in common with that of shigellae. Thus, unlike shigellae, invasive salmonellae usually penetrate the epithelial cells of the ileum, do not proliferate there, invade the tissues more deeply, and ultimately are disseminated via the lymphatics and blood. That sequence of events is the usual outcome with serotypes such as *S. typhi* but may also occur, though less commonly, with the food-poisoning salmonellae. In some serotypes of *Salmonella*, invasiveness is associated with the carriage of large plasmids, the role of which is not well understood.

Some yersiniae, including *Y. pestis*, *Y. pseudotuberculosis*, and *Y. enterocolitica*, cause highly invasive infections in man and other mammals. The virulence determinants of yersiniae include adherence factors, outer-membrane proteins, fibrillae, serum resistance, and VW antigens, some of which are required for diarrhoeal illness, others for systemic involvement. Some of these virulence factors are determined by Vwa plasmids but the relationships among the different Vwa plasmids, and even among the different structures themselves, are complex and not fully understood at this time. It is clear, however, that the mechanics of invasiveness may be quite different even among closely related bacteria. For a more detailed discussion of these topics, the reader is directed to the excellent text of Mims (1987).

Colonization

The terms adhesion and colonization, though related, are not synonymous. Colonization, at least to this author, means not only that the stringent requirements of attachment have been satisfied but also that the bacteria survive, increase in numbers, and establish infection. Survival implies an ability to withstand the physical and chemical antibacterial devices of the host environment. Multiplication demands that the host environment then provides a sufficiency of the nutrients required for proliferation. Thus, colonization encompasses attachment, multiplication, and establishment of infection.

Our knowledge of the distribution of different growth factors and metabolites in the different tissues and cells of different host species is sparse, but an understanding of substrate availability sometimes explains different bacterial responses in different hosts. For example, in those animals that are susceptible to infectious abortion by brucellae, the bacteria show preferential colonization of the genital organs and the uterus of pregnant animals which, it transpires, are body sites rich in the growth-enhancing substrate, erythritol.

Again, we may be surprised when a pathogenic bacterium, apparently fully equipped with the virulence determinants of its species, is nevertheless not pathogenic for a particular host species. Thus, most strains of *Y. pestis* are pathogenic for both guinea-pigs and mice, but some naturally occurring strains that require asparagine for growth retain their virulence for mice but are avirulent in guinea-pigs. The activity of an asparaginase in the blood of the latter species prevents the growth of these asparagine-dependent strains. There have been many similar demonstrations of reductions in the virulence of other pathogens by mutations rendering them unable to grow because a required metabolite is absent, or present in low concentrations only, in the tissues or cells of the host. The recent development of attenuated vaccine strains of *Salmonella* provides an interesting twist to this story. Stable, non-reverting aromatic-dependent mutant strains of *S. dublin* and *S. typhimurium* and thymine- or purine-dependent *S. choleraesuis* have been constructed which cannot obtain sufficient required metabolite *in vivo*. Although of much reduced virulence, they can be used successfully as live attenuated vaccine strains in animals (and human volunteers), in whom they still elicit a cellular immune response.

The rapid progress made in this difficult area can be seen by reference to the need for iron for bacterial growth. Although present in host animals, it is often in a form not readily available to bacteria, which have, therefore, devised many means of scavenging host tissues for the iron required for enzyme function and for expression of virulence. Thus, many bacteria involved in extra-intestinal infections produce haemolysins that disrupt red cells to liberate the important source of bound iron. Many other bacteria excrete iron-chelating agents, or siderophores, such as aerobactin, enterobactin, ferrichrome, and rhodotorulic acid, which specifically sequester iron found in tissues and transport it via specific uptake systems. Further discussion of this aspect of colonization may be found in the texts of Sussman (1985) and Stocker and Mäkelä (1986).

Conclusions

The examples illustrating adhesion, penetration, and colonization were chosen to describe three aspects of baterial virulence that should be thought of as being related and interdependent. Emphasis was placed on the mechanisms of pathogenic bacteria, and rightly so, because so much is known about the virulence determinants that influence their interaction with the host. But we should not be surprised if eventually we learn that much of that holds equally true for commensals in their more 'friendly' interaction with the host. We should also remember that commensals will adopt the mantle of pathogenicity when the circumstances are right. Thus, the ability of, say, coagulase-negative staphylococci to colonize intravascular devices or prostheses depends, we might suggest, on determinants of opportunistic pathogenicity. Again, in those cases where members of the normal flora spill-over from their established state of commensalism to cause disease, e.g. the colonization of mucous membranes by *Clostridium difficile* in the gut, of *Candida* in the vagina, or haemophili in the respiratory tract, they do so presumably because they are better equipped than other bacteria that colonize these same tracts. Infrequent glimpses as to how such infections arise reveal an unsuspected skill in opportunism. For example, it seems that those secondary invaders of mucosal surfaces after primary damage by *B. pertussis* use an adhesin secreted by the whooping-cough bacillus itself, a phenomenon aptly named by Tuomanen as 'piracy of adhesins', a prototype of virulence determination probably more widespread than yet realized. The increasing application of the techniques of molecular biology to bacterial virulence promises to provide at the molecular level answers to many of our currently unanswered questions. The next few years should be an exciting time.

6.2.2 Toxins

J. P. Arbuthnott

In Section 6.2.1 it has been made clear that adhesion, penetration, and colonization are involved in the establishment of a pathogen on or in the tissues of the infected host and that, at the molecular level, the mechanisms involved include interactions between reactive surface determinants of the pathogen and receptors on the surface of host cells. The pathophysiological changes accompanying infection frequently also involve the action of another important class of microbial virulence determinants, namely toxins, which are, in effect, potent cell-damaging agents produced by micro-organisms. There are two main categories of toxins: exotoxins and endotoxins.

Exotoxins are diffusible toxic polypeptides secreted from the infecting organism into the surrounding tissue. These highly active agents include some of the most poisonous agents known to man and are capable of eliciting tissue damage either close to, or at a considerable distance from, the primary focus of infection.

Endotoxins, in contrast, comprise the lipopolysaccharide (LPS) component of the outer membrane of the Gram-negative bacterial envelope which, when released during lysis of the bacterial cell, triggers a complex cascade of pathophysiological changes that may culminate in endotoxic shock.

The principal general properties of exotoxins and endotoxins are summarized in Table 6.1.

Table 6.1 Comparison of exotoxins and endotoxins

Exotoxins	Endotoxins
Polypeptide in nature	Lipopolysaccharide in nature
Secreted from the bacterial cell	Located in outer membrane of Gram-negative bacteria
Diffusible in host tissue	Released in the form of vesicles on autolysis or disruption of bacterial cells
Most are thermolabile	Thermostable
Several can be converted to *toxoids* that have lost toxicity but retain antigenicity	Antigenicity resides in the polysaccharide region of the molecule
	Toxicity resides in Lipid A
	Cannot form *toxoids*

Exotoxins

Exotoxins are a diverse group of extracellular bacterial polypeptides, ranging in molecular weight from 3000 to 500 000. They were first discovered in the 'golden age' of microbiology, between 1880 and 1900. It is easy to imagine the scientific excitement and clinical interest that surrounded the observations that culture filtrates of three important pathogens, *Corynebacterium diphtheriae*, *Clostridium tetani*, and *Clostridium botulinum*, when injected into experimental animals, in the

absence of live organisms, were able to cause the specific symptoms of clinical disease. The agent responsible in each case proved to be a single antigenic protein against which protective neutralizing antibody could be raised in animals and in man. This discovery laid the foundations of protective immunization. Indeed, diphtheria and tetanus toxoid vaccine remain among the most effective bacterial vaccines in use today. Although the list of toxins now known is extensive, relatively few have proved to be highly effective as protective antigens. Though this is disappointing from the point of view of vaccine development, there is a ready explanation. Research over a number of years has established that mechanisms of bacterial pathogenesis are multifactorial, involving the interplay of several cell-associated extracellular components (Section 6.2.1) including exotoxins. Thus it is not surprising to observe that immunity to a single determinant is not always protective against challenge with the whole organism. It is accepted that vaccines of the future in many cases will consist of a mixture of cell-associated and toxic antigens. Indeed, just such a subunit vaccine is being developed as a second-generation vaccine against the whooping-cough organism, *Bordetella pertussis*.

The main purpose of this section is to describe the toxins that have been clearly implicated in pathogenesis, and to summarize what is known about their biological modes of action. It is important to bear in mind that bacterial protein exotoxins are synthesized and secreted in the same manner as other bacterial exoproteins. The genes that encode for toxins may be located on the chromosome, on a plasmid, or on a lysogenic bacteriophage; in few instances *tox* genes are located on transposons. Several such toxin genes have now been cloned and sequenced using standard molecular biological techniques. In addition, many toxins have been obtained in high purity and the study of their structure, mode of action, and role in pathogenesis has been greatly aided by the application of modern biochemical and molecular genetic analysis.

Toxicity of exotoxins

Bacterial exotoxins can be defined as a group of bacterial products whose principal common feature is that they are harmful to a variety of sensitive hosts when administered in relatively small doses. It is difficult to offer a more precise definition because exotoxins vary widely in potency and in the nature of the lesion or harmful effect produced. The main toxic effects of exotoxins include the following: lethal action in susceptible animals; skin effects; effects on the gastrointestinal tract; cytotoxic effects on individual cell types (e.g. cells in tissue culture or host-derived cells such as erythrocytes, polymorphonuclear leucocytes, monocytes, or lymphocytes); systemic effects, such as pyrogenic response. Examples of such toxic effects, which also form the basis of assays for toxins, are given in Table 6.2. Certain toxins are extraordinarily potent, e.g. botulinum toxin (lethal dose 2.5×10^{-14} g) and tetanus toxin (lethal dose 4×10^{-14} g). It is notable that several of the bacterial exotoxins exert their effects in several test systems. Quantitative measurements of biological potency are expressed in terms of effective doses. The effective dose is an indicator effect, e.g. death,

Table 6.2 Examples of toxic effects of bacterial exotoxins

Toxic effect	Examples
Lethal action	Botulinum toxin A: acts on neuromuscular junctions causing flaccid paralysis
	Tetanus toxin causes spastic paralysis of voluntary muscles
	Diphtheria toxin causes damage to heart, lungs, kidneys, liver
Pyrogenic effect (increase in body temperature by +1.5°C)	Pyrogenic exotoxins of *S. aureus* and *Strep. pyogenes*; staphylococcal toxic shock syndrome toxin-1
Toxic action on gastrointestinal tract	
Secretion of water and electrolyte in small intestine causing watery diarrhoea	Cholera enterotoxin, *E. coli* LT (heat-labile toxin)
	E. coli ST_a (heat-stable toxin)
	E. coli ST_b (heat-stable toxin)
Pseudomembranous colitis	*Cl. difficile* toxins A and B
Shigellosis—bloody diarrhoea	Shigella toxin
Vomiting	Staphylococcal enterotoxins A–E
Toxic action on skin	
Necrosis	Several clostridial toxins
	Staphylococcal α-toxin
Erythema	Diphtheria toxin
	Streptococcal erythrogenic toxin
Permeability of skin capillaries	Cholera enterotoxin, *E. coli* LT
Nikolsky sign (i.e. separation of epidermis from dermis)	Staphylococcal epidermolytic toxin
Cytolytic (membrane-damaging effects)	
Lysis of blood cells (erythrocytes and/or leucocytes)	Numerous membrane-damaging toxins including:
	Stephylococcal α-, β-, γ-, and δ-lysins, leucocidin
	Streptolysin O and S
	Cl. perfringens α-toxin, θ-toxin
Death or lysis of cells in tissue culture	*E. coli* α-haemolysin
	Vibrio parahaemolyticus direct haemolysin
Leakage of labelled markers	*Aeromonas hydrophila* aerolysin
Inhibition of metabolic activity, e.g. protein synthesis	Diphtheria toxin, shiga toxin
Change of cell shape	Cholera enterotoxin, *E. coli* LT

necrosis, or cell lysis, produced in a certain proportion of animals or tissue cells tested. It is desirable that the end-point should lie on the steepest part of the dose–response curve and if, for example, death is taken as the indicator, then the unit employed is usually the LD_{50}, i.e. the amount of toxin that kills 50 per cent of the animals tested. Variation between different animals must be taken into account in any bioassay.

Such tests in animals are now restricted for ethical reasons and for reasons of cost: experimental animals are very expensive to maintain. More emphasis is now placed on *in vitro* toxicity tests and serological methods of detection and assay. The latter make use of specific polyclonal or monoclonal antibodies raised against purified toxins and employ a variety of assay procedures [immunodiffusion, enzyme-linked immunosorbent assay (ELISA), or latex agglutination tests]. In serological tests, unknown toxin preparations can be compared with a reference sample, but it is important to note that such tests can only

detect antigenically active toxin. From time to time it may be necessary to confirm the toxicity of a toxin preparation in one of the bioassays listed in Table 6.2.

Molecular mode of action of exotoxins

With advances in protein biochemistry and molecular biology, knowledge of the molecular structure of bacterial protein exotoxins has increased. In several cases, the amino-acid sequence of the toxin has been determined both by peptide sequencing of the purified toxin and by sequencing the DNA of the structural gene encoding for toxin production. In a few fascinating instances not only is the structure of the toxin molecule known but the complexities of mode of action of the toxin at the molecular level have been unravelled and a fairly full picture exists of structure/function relationships. However, it must be remembered that not all toxins have been so well characterized. This is true particularly for toxins that have been discovered only recently, those that have been known for some time but have attracted little research interest, and yet others that have proved extremely difficult to characterize.

Bacterial exotoxins are of two main types:

1. cytolytic toxins that perturb the normal permeability properties of cell membranes;

2. bipartite (A–B) toxins that bind to a specific receptor by means of the binding or B region of the toxin molecule, and, after entering the cytoplasm, release the toxic A region which is responsible for cell damage within the target cell. The A and B components of such bipartite toxins may reside in different regions of a single polypeptide chain (e.g. diphtheria toxin) or in distinct subunits of a multimeric toxin (e.g. cholera toxin).

Cytolytic toxins The result of the exposure of susceptible cells to such membrane-damaging toxins depends on the concentration of toxin. At high concentrations, damage may be extensive, resulting in gross disturbance of ion and water fluxes and leakage of intracellular contents: cell death (cytotoxicity) usually ensues. At low toxin concentrations, such as may occur in lesions *in vitro*, the effect is likely to be much more subtle. Instead of cell death, an alteration of specific cell function occurs, such as impairment of the ability of polymorphs and macrophages to respond to a chemotactic stimulus. Thus cytolytic toxins may contribute to pathogenesis by causing tissue damage or by impairment of host defences. Cytolytic toxins are produced by many pathogenic bacteria, notably, *Staphylococcus aureus* (α-, β-, γ-, and δ-lysins and leucocidin), *Streptococcus pyogenes* (streptolysin O and streptolysin S), *Clostridium perfringens* (α- and θ-toxins), and *E. coli* (α-haemolysin). These toxins, often referred to as lysins or haemolysins, because of their ability to cause lysis of erythrocytes, form a diverse group of polypeptides differing widely in molecular weight and mode of action.

Mechanisms of membrane damage by cytolytic toxins. Membrane damage may result from enzymatic degradation of membrane phospholipids, as in the case of *Cl. perfringens* α-toxin, the first toxin to have its mode of action established unequivocally. It is a phospholipase C that hydrolyses phosphatidyl choline, sphingomyelin and, to a lesser extent, other membrane phospholipids.

Cl. perfringens α-toxin

$$\text{phosphatidyl choline} \underset{Ca^{2+}}{\rightleftharpoons} \text{diacylglycerol} + \text{phosphoryl choline}$$

The β-lysin of *Staph. aureus* also acts as a phospholipase but has a greater degree of substrate specificity in that it has a striking preference for sphingomyelin and preferentially lyses cells rich in membrane sphingomyelin.

Staph. aureus β-lysin

$$\text{sphingomyelin} \underset{Mg^{2+}}{\rightleftharpoons} \text{N-acylsphingosine} + \text{phosphoryl choline}$$

Another group of cytolytic toxins act not by enzymatic degradation but by causing physical derangement of the lipid bilayer either by detergent-like action of the toxin (staphylococcal δ-lysin) or by insertion of toxin molecules into the membrane, with the formation of discrete transmembrane pores (staphylococcal α-lysin, streptolysin O). Staphylococcal δ-lysin is a small molecular weight (M_r 3000) peptide consisting of 26 amino acids. Like the bee-venom toxin (melittin), the sequence of 20 amino acids from the N-terminus is rich in hydrophobic amino acids, whereas the C-terminal hexapeptide is rich in lysine and is therefore positively charged. Accordingly, the δ-lysin molecule exhibits both hydrophobic and charged hydrophilic properties. The biological activity of δ-lysin is typical of a surface-active agent, in that it induces almost instant disruption of a wide variety of membrane systems, resulting in non-selective release of large and small molecular weight from substances affected cells.

By contrast, pore-forming toxins, of which staphylococcal α-lysin is an example, act by initially binding to the target membrane, followed by polymerization (oligomerization) of monomeric subunits into ring-shaped structures that penetrate the hydrophobic region of the membrane to form transmembrane pores. In the case of staphylococcal α-lysin, these pores consist of hexameric oligomers and, from leakage studies performed with markers of differing molecular weight, the functional pore has been estimated to have a diameter of 2–3 nm. Much larger pores (15 nm) are formed by streptolysin O. Such pores allow free diffusion of ions and small molecules across the membrane.

Most cytolytic toxins that are not phosphilipases are likely to act as pore-formers or as surface-active agents. However, few have been studied in detail in terms of membrane/toxin interaction. It should be noted that in a few instances cytolytic toxins consist of two polypeptides that act synergistically to induce membrane damage. For example, staphylococcal γ-lysin consists of two components, γ_1 and γ_2, and staphylococcal leucocidin requires both its F and S components in optimal proportions for full biological activity.

Mode of action of bipartite (A–B) toxins Several major bacterial protein exotoxins have now been shown to be bipartite (A–B) toxins. Structure–function studies have revealed much about the specific recognition mechanism responsible for binding of the toxin to susceptible cells through the B region as well as details of the toxic action of the A region. It is most interesting to note that in five cases (diphtheria toxin, pseudomonas exotoxin A, cholera enterotoxin, *E. coli* enterotoxin, and pertussis toxin) the toxicity of the A region is due to enzymatic cleavage of NAD coupled with ADP-ribosylation of a key regulatory protein within the target cell. The main features of the structure and activity of these toxins are summarized in Table 6.3.

Exotoxins in disease

In classic bacterial toxinoses, such as diphtheria, tetanus, and botulism, the exotoxin produced by the causative organism is the principal determinant in the pathogenesis of disease. The main features of these diseases are summarized in Table 6.4. More commonly, pathogenesis depends on interactions involving cell-associated colonization factors and extracellular enzymes, as well as bacterial exotoxins. Despite this complexity, the contribution of certain exotoxins to the disease process is now clearly established for a number of infectious diseases. In some cases convincing evidence implicating toxin involvement has been obtained only recently by the application of modern molecular genetic approaches. Particular use has been made of the method of site-directed mutagenesis, in which the structural gene for the toxin under investigation is specifically modified such that active toxin is no longer expressed. Comparison of such site-directed mutants with fully toxigenic wild-type organisms in a suitable model system will show whether or not the toxin has a role in pathogenesis. Such studies have been crucial in establishing the importance of several toxins, including staphylococcal α-toxin and staphylococcal toxic shock syndrome toxin-1.

The site of toxin-mediated damage within the host depends on the degree of invasiveness of the bacterial pathogen, the degree of tissue tropism exhibited by the toxin, and whether its target tissue is superficial or is located in an internal organ (Fig. 6.4). It is also important to note that certain toxins induce abnormal function without causing tissue necrosis.

Action of enterotoxins on the intestine Cholera toxin and the heat-labile (LT) and heat-stable (ST) toxins of enterotoxigenic *E. coli* strains induce profuse watery diarrhoea without inducing inflammation or cytotoxic damage. These toxins are released on colonization of the small intestine by the relevant organism and act on membrane-associated adenylate cyclase of enterocytes. In contrast, some enteric pathogens do affect the structural integrity of intestinal epithelial cells, leading to local inflammation and cytotoxic damage. This can arise:

1. as a result of direct toxin-mediated cytotoxicity (*Cl. difficile*, *Cl. perfringens* type A, and *B. cereus*);

2. as a result of intimate contact between pathogen and brush border membranes [enteropathogenic *E. coli* (EPEC)]; or

3. from cell damage following invasion of intestinal epithelial cells and reproduction of shiga or shiga-like toxin [*Shigella dysenteriae* and enteroinvasive *E. coli* (EIEC)].

Table 6.3 Structure and mode of action of bipartite toxins that cause ADP-ribosylation

Toxin	Structure	Mode of action
Diphtheria toxin	Single polypeptide chain ($M_r = 58\,300$) activated by proteolytic nicking and thiol reduction to yield two fragments A ($M_r = 21\,100$) and B ($M_r = 37\,200$)	Binding of B region to membrane receptor followed by nicking leads to entry of the A fragment which causes ADP-ribosylation of elongation factor 2 (EF2) and consequent inhibition of protein synthesis
Intact toxin		$NAD + EF2 \rightleftharpoons ADP\text{-ribosyl-}EF2 + nicotinamide$ Diphtheria toxin
Proteolysis		
Thiol reduction		
Pseudomonas exotoxin A	Single polypeptide chain ($M_r\ 66\,600$) activated by conformational change. Limited evidence for proteolytic nicking	Binding to the membrane through two binding domains allows translocation and entry into the cytoplasm. Mode of action similar to diphtheria toxin $NAD + EF2 \rightleftharpoons ADP\text{-ribosyl-}EF2 + nicotinamide$ Pseudomonas exotoxin A This reaction results in inhibition of protein synthesis
Cholera enterotoxin	Consists of two types of subunits (A and B) The A ($M_r\ 27\,200$) subunit consists of two peptides, A_1 ($M_r\ 21\,800$) and A_2 ($M_r\ 5400$) linked by a disulphide bond. There are five B subunits each of $M_r\ 11\,700$ arranged as a pentamer. Thus the structure is A:5B. 	The toxin binds to susceptible cells by high-affinity binding of the B subunits to a membrane receptor (ganglioside GM-1). This results in translocation of the A_1 peptide which catalyses the ADP-ribosylation of the membrane-associated stimulatory G subunit of adenylate cyclase Cholera toxin $NAD + G\ subunit \rightleftharpoons ADP\text{-ribosyl-}Gs + nicotinamide$
5B subunits Subunit A_2 Subunit A_1		In turn this leads to overproduction and disturbance of ion and fluid balance in cells lining the small intestine: profuse diarrhoea results
E. coli LT toxin	Almost identical in structure to cholera enterotoxin	Virtually identical to cholera enterotoxin. Also causes ADP-ribosylation of the stimulatory G subunit of adenylate cyclase
Pertussis toxin	Has a complex subunit structure in which the A subunit (S_1) combines with two dimers ($S_2 : S_4$) and ($S_3 : S_4$) that fulfil the B function. The M_r values of S_1, S_2, S_3, S_4, and S_5 are $26\,200$, $22\,000$, $22\,000$, $12\,000$, and $11\,000$. The structure of the toxin is 	After internalization, the S_1 subunit catalyses the transfer of ADP-ribose from NAD to the regulatory protein, Ni, of the inhibitory arm of the adenylate cyclase complex. This removes the cyclase from inhibitory control and has the net effect of increasing the level of cAMP. The toxic effect depends on the target cell. Systemic effects include fever, lymphocytosis, leucocytosis, and impaired regulation of blood glucose $NAD + NI\ subunit \rightleftharpoons ADP\text{-ribosyl Ni} + nicotinamide$ Pertussis toxin

Toxins causing subepithelial or systemic damage When a focus of infection develops in subepithelial tissue as a result of multiplication of common pathogens such as *Staph. aureus*, *Str. pyogenes*, and *Cl. perfringens*, the release of cytolytic toxins can affect the host in several ways:

1. by impairing the response of phagocytic cells;
2. by release of soluble mediators from leucocytes; and
3. by causing necrosis and tissue damage.

An extreme example is gas gangrene in which the α-toxin of *Cl. perfringens* is probably the major factor responsible for the extensive necrosis and oedema that results from spreading damage to connective tissue, blood vessels, and muscle tissue.

Systemic effects can also arise from the ability of certain toxins, such as pertussis toxin and toxic shock syndrome toxin-1 (TSST-1), to release potent mediators that, in turn, initiate a cascade effect that leads to multisystem involvement, including activation of complement and/or coagulation.

Damage to particular organs and tissues In some diseases, toxin absorbed across an epithelial surface or diffusing out from a focus of infection spreads in the bloodstream, through lymphatic vessels or via neurones, to attack particular organs or tissues at distant sites. Examples of this sort of damage include the classic toxinoses diphtheria, tetanus, and botulism (Fig. 6.4). In diphtheria, elaboration of toxin in pharyngeal

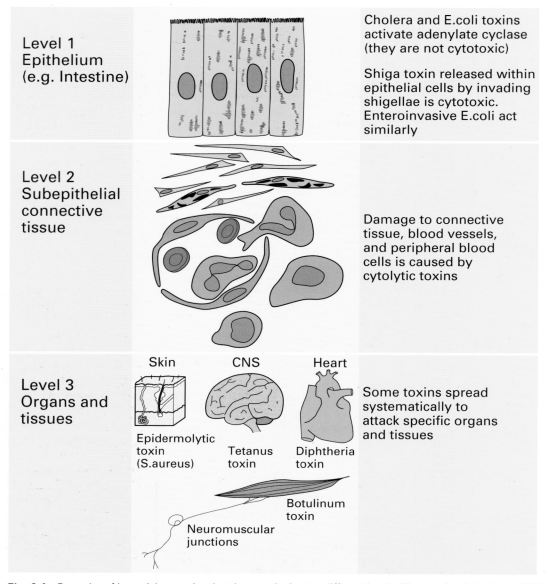

Level 1
Epithelium
(e.g. Intestine)

Cholera and E.coli toxins
activate adenylate cyclase
(they are not cytotoxic)

Shiga toxin released within
epithelial cells by invading
shigellae is cytotoxic.
Enteroinvasive E.coli act
similarly

Level 2
Subepithelial
connective
tissue

Damage to connective
tissue, blood vessels,
and peripheral blood
cells is caused by
cytolytic toxins

Level 3
Organs and
tissues

Skin   CNS   Heart

Epidermolytic
toxin
(S.aureus)   Tetanus   Diphtheria
                toxin   toxin

Some toxins spread
systematically to
attack specific organs
and tissues

Botulinum
toxin

Neuromuscular
junctions

Fig. 6.4 Examples of bacterial exotoxins that damage the host at different levels. (Drawn after Arbuthnott 1983, with permission.)

tissues by toxigenic diphtheria bacilli leads to formation of a pseudomembrane consisting of a tough fibrinous sheet containing fibrin, necrotic epithelial tissue, lymphocytes, leucocytes, and erythrocytes. Underlying the pseudomembrane is a necrotic haemorrhagic lesion. The local lesion can be fatal due to occlusion of the airways but death can also result from systemic spread of the toxin and damage to internal organs such as the heart, lungs, liver, kidneys, and nervous system. Unlike the toxin, the diphtheria bacilli remain at the site of infection.

In tetanus, toxin elaborated at a focus such as a wound containing sporing tetanus bacilli spreads to the CNS via nerve axons. The convulsive spasms of voluntary muscles, typical of tetanus, are a result of continuous excitation of motor neurones of the central reflex apparatus in the spinal cord. Tetanus toxin

exerts this action by preventing the release of inhibitory neurotransmitters. In botulism, preformed toxin ingested in contaminated food absorbed across the intestine, circulates systemically and acts on peripheral nerve endings to induce fatal flaccid paralysis by preventing release of acetylcholine.

Endotoxins

Unlike bacterial protein exotoxins, endotoxins are lipopolysaccharide (LPS) in nature. The LPS present in the outer membrane of Gram-negative bacteria is an important virulence factor and exerts a number of harmful effects. The toxicity of LPS resides in the lipid A region of the molecule (Fig. 6.5) which chemically consists of a $\beta 1,6$ glucosaminyl-glucosamine disaccharide substituted with phosphate groups and fatty acids.

Table 6.4 Features of some toxin-mediated diseases

Disease and Organism	Clinical features	Bacteriological comments	Mode of transmission	Treatment and prevention
Diphtheria (*Corynebacterium diphtheriae*)	Local inflammation of nasopharynx resulting in pseudomembrane formation, cervical adenopathy, and dysphagia. Systemic toxicity: all tissues affected but principal clinical manifestations are myocarditis and neurological toxicity—palatal paresis, cranial neuropathies, demyelinating peripheral neuritis, paralysis. Death due to asphyxia or cardiac failure. Cutaneous diphtheria. Indolent ulcers with grey membrane rarely associated with signs of intoxication. Skin lesions serve as a reservoir of *C. diphtheriae* and produce immunity.	Systemic effects due to diphtheria toxin. Exotoxin production by *C. diphtheriae* depends on presence of lysogenic β-phage which carries genes encoding for toxin (tox$^+$); tox$^-$ strains can cause localized diphtheria-like disease but do not produce systemic toxicity.	Airborne respiratory droplets. Direct contact with infected respiratory secretions or skin lesions.	*Treatment* Diphtheria antitoxin with supportive care and antibiotics. Penicillin or erythromycin have no effect on toxin but (1) kill bacteria preventing further toxin formation, (2) alleviate local symptoms, (3) prevent transmission of infection. *Prevention* Immunize with alum-adsorbed toxoid.
Tetanus (*Clostridium tetani*)	Local wound infection (may be trivial). Systemic toxicity due to absorption of neurotoxin tetanospasmin. Local or generalized stiffness. Increasing muscle rigidity resulting in trismus (lockjaw) and reflex spasms, tonic contractions, e.g. opisthotonus, risus sardonicus, laryngospasm. Autonomic dysfunction (see Section 6.5.3).	Anaerobic environment necessary for proliferation of organism and production of tetanospasmin.	Spores ubiquitous in soil. Any major or minor wound or closed infected area can act as nidus of infection.	*Treatment* Intensive monitoring including respiratory and cardiac support. Human tetanus immune globulin (HTIG); benzodiazepines (sedation anti-convulsant and muscle relaxant properties); antibiotics (penicillin or metronidazole) to kill vegetative organisms and prevent further toxin production. *Prevention* Immunize with alum-adsorbed toxoid.
Botulism (*Clostridium botulinum*)	Intoxication following consumption of contaminated food. Vomiting, constipation, weakness, lassitude, dry mouth. Cranial nerve pareses—diplopia, blurred vision, dysphonia, dysphagia. Weakness of respiratory and peripheral muscles. Death usually due to asphyxia. Infant botulism: *Cl. botulinum* from environmental sources colonizes the gastrointestinal tract and toxin production occurs *in vivo*. The baby becomes hypotonic, fails to thrive, flaccid paralysis of varying degree. Wound botulinism: rare condition in which *Cl. botulinum* intoxication results from wound infection (see Section 6.5.3).	Seven toxigenic serotypes. Serotypes A, B, E mainly responsible for human disease. Spores of *Cl. botulinum* very heat-resistant, can withstand 100°C for 22 h. Toxin destroyed by boiling for 10 min or 80°C for 30 min. Many factors determine survival, multiplication, and toxin production of *Cl. botulinum* in food, e.g. heavy contamination with spores, insufficient heating, alkaline pH, low salt, anaerobic conditions.	Spores ubiquitous in soil. Types A + B often associated with home preserved food. Type E usually associated with fish. Food which has been inadequately salted, smoked, dried, or pickled is the usual source. Honey implicated in some cases of infant botulism.	*Treatment* Intensive respiratory and supportive care. Antitoxin—polyvalent for types A, B, E, or monovalent if toxin type known. *Prevention* Ensure methods of food production are adequate to prevent proliferation of *Cl. botulinum* and its toxin in food.

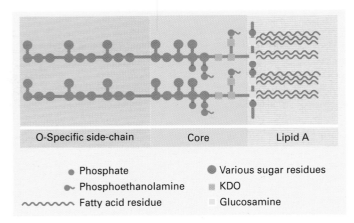

Fig. 6.5 Diagram of the structure of LPS. (Drawn after Reitschel *et al.* 1975, with permission.)

The biological properties of LPS are diverse and include the following:

1. pyrogenicity for man and rabbits;
2. lethal effect in animals;
3. activation of complement;
4. activation of clotting mechanisms;
5. B-cell mitogenicity;
6. induction of cytokines (TNF, IL-1);
7. Clotting of *Limulus* amoebocyte lysate.

The release of LPS from Gram-negative bacteria during Gram-negative septicaemia may lead to the symptoms of endotoxic shock (Fig. 6.6).

6.2.3   Antimicrobial resistance

Mary P. E. Slack

Introduction

The introduction of a new antimicrobial agent is almost inevitably followed by the appearance of strains of micro-organisms resistant to the drug. In some instances resistant strains have flourished to such an extent as to seriously limit the therapeutic value of a drug. For example, when penicillin was first used clinically in 1941 less than 1 per cent of strains of *Staphylococcus aureus* were penicillin resistant. Within a few years about 8 per cent of *Staph. aureus* isolates were resistant and now about 90 per cent of strains of *Staph. aureus* are resistant to penicillin. In this instance the selective pressure applied by penicillin usage has facilitated the growth and spread of a minority of the staphylococcal population which were already resistant to penicillin. Throughout this period the Group A streptococcus has remained uniformly sensitive to penicillin.

Since the early days of clinical trials of penicillin in Oxford, many hundreds of different β-lactams have been introduced for

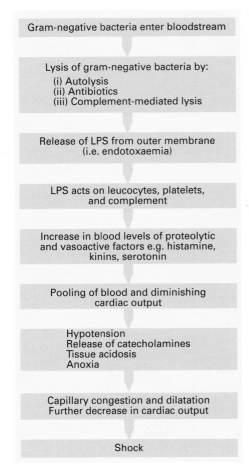

Fig. 6.6 Summary of the role of LPS in endotoxic shock.

clinical use. Many of the penicillin derivatives were produced in response to specific needs and represented major therapeutic advances. Thus, there was a clear need for penicillins resistant to staphylococcal penicillinase, such as methicillin and the isoxazolyl penicillins, cloxacillin and flucloxacillin.

Since the end of the 1970s there have been an increasing number of reports of severe infections due to methicillin-resistant *Staph. aureus* (MRSA). Outbreaks of MRSA are now encountered at differing frequencies in the United Kingdom, Europe, the United States, and Australia. Many of these strains have, in addition, exhibited varying degrees of resistance to the aminoglycosides.

The cephalosporins were introduced for clinical use in 1964 and have proliferated to an even greater extent than the penicillins. One of the most important developments in these compounds has been the production of agents with marked stability to Gram-negative β-lactamases.

For many years the gonococcus (*Neisseria gonorrhoeae*) remained susceptible to penicillin, although there was a gradual trend towards a decrease in susceptibility to this drug, necessitating the use of larger doses to effect a clinical cure. Within the past 15 years some strains of *N. gonorrhoeae* have acquired a plasmid-mediated β-lactamase which confers high-level resistance to penicillin. Penicillin resistance is now widespread amongst gonococci. Meningococci (*N. meningitidis*) have, in general, remained susceptible to penicillin, but there has been one report of a plasmid-mediated β-lactamase in a meningococcal strain in which the plasmid appeared identical to that of the 'Asian-type' plasmid found in penicillinase-producing *N. gonorrhoeae*. β-lactamase-mediated ampicillin resistance in *Haemophilus influenzae* and penicillin resistance in pneumococci have also appeared in the past 15 years, and it is now mandatory to screen for β-lactamase production and test for penicillin sensitivity, respectively, in these organisms.

Most hospitals harbour multiply-resistant Gram-negative bacteria of the Enterobacteriaceae (*Escherichia coli*, *Citrobacter* spp., *Enterobacter* spp., *Klebsiella* spp., *Serratia* spp.). These resistances are largely determined by conjugative plasmids. The prevalence of multiply-resistant Enterobacteriaceae varies considerably between countries and even between different hospitals. The overall trend is, however, towards resistance to an increasing number of antimicrobial drugs.

An organism is generally considered to be susceptible to a given antimicrobial if it is inhibited or killed *in vitro* by a concentration of the drug that would normally be therapeutically achieved. Bacterial resistance is thus the failure to be inhibited or killed *in vitro* by a concentration of the antimicrobial equal to or higher than that concentration which inhibits or kills susceptible strains. It must be emphasized that bacterial resistance or susceptibility is only one factor in the complex interactions between the host defence mechanisms (see Section 6.2.4), the particular type and site of the infection (e.g. intracellular or inaccessible foci), and the drug's pharmacokinetics which determine the clinical outcome in any individual. However, *in vitro* susceptibility testing gives a useful guide to the likely outcome of using a drug to treat an infection.

Mode of origin of antimicrobial resistance

Two forms of antimicrobial resistance are recognized: intrinsic and acquired resistance. Some bacterial species are naturally resistant to an antimicrobial agent (intrinsic resistance). For example, Group A streptococci are always resistant to gentamicin. *Pseudomonas aeruginosa* is resistant to penicillin by virtue of an inducible chromosomal β-lactamase. The mechanisms of intrinsic resistance include lack of a suitable target in the cell; inability to penetrate the cell wall; and the presence of naturally produced drug-destroying enzymes.

Most forms of antimicrobial resistance result from the acquisition of new or altered genetic material (acquired resistance). Acquired resistance may develop through chromosomal mutation or by the transfer of genes between micro-organisms, usually via extrachromosomal genetic elements, such as plasmids, transposons, or bacteriophages.

Mutational resistance

Random, spontaneous mutations generally occur at a frequency of 10^{-5}–10^{-10} cell divisions. In any large population of bacteria a small number of individual cells will be resistant to an antimicrobial. In the absence of the drug this will provide no selective advantage for survival but when the antimicrobial is administered it will act as a selective agent favouring the survival and multiplication of the resistant mutants. A well-known example of this is found in the treatment of tuberculosis. There are such large numbers of tubercle bacilli present within tuberculous lesions that spontaneous mutants resistant to antituberculous drugs will inevitably appear and flourish if a single agent is used in its treatment. The use of a combination of two drugs will markedly reduce the likelihood of spontaneous mutations to resistance to two drugs to about 10^{-15} cell divisions. Hence the use of more than one therapeutic agent in tuberculosis.

Transferable resistance (genetic exchange)

Genetic information conferring antibiotic resistance resides both in the bacterial chromosome and in extrachromosomal genetic elements (plasmids). Bacteria rarely exchange their chromosomal genes but plasmids are readily exchanged. Genes controlling resistance can pass readily from one cell to another by: (1) conjugation; (2) transduction; (3) transformation. These transfers occur *in vitro* and *in vivo*. Again, it must be stressed that a resistance appearing in a sensitive strain or population will only become widespread under the selective influence of antimicrobial chemotherapy.

Plasmids are extrachromosomal genetic elements composed of circular double-stranded DNA, and range in size from 10 to 400 kilobase pairs. Most bacterial cells carrying plasmids will only contain a single copy or a few copies of any given plasmid. Different plasmids may be found in a given cell but related plasmids often cannot co-exist in the same cell. This incompatibility of related plasmids is the basis of a classification scheme of plasmids (incompatibility groups).

Plasmids may determine a wide range of functions, including virulence, antimicrobial resistance, toxin production, bacteriocin production, metabolic activity, and immunity to some bacteriophages.

Plasmids are subdivided into two groups:

1. conjugative;
2. non-conjugative.

Conjugative plasmids are self-transmissible from one cell to another and possess a region which controls conjugation and the synthesis of thin protein structures—sex pili. Conjugation is the adherence of sex pili formed by one bacterial cell to specific receptor sites on another and the transfer of DNA from the donor cell to the recipient cell, possibly through the core of the sex pilus. Plasmids which transfer antimicrobial resistance by conjugation are referred to as 'R-factors' or resistance transfer factors. R-factor-mediated antimicrobial resistance is especially important in Gram-negative bacilli. It was first recognized in 1957 by Watanabe, who noted simultaneous resistance to chloramphenicol, streptomycin, sulphanilamide, and tetracycline developing during an outbreak of *Shigella dysenteriae* dysentery. This particular strain harboured a plasmid specifying all four resistances and the same R-plasmid was found in strains of *E. coli* isolated from these patients, implying that these plasmids could spread between bacterial genera. Multiple drug resistance of this type is now widely disseminated in Gram-negative bacteria throughout the world.

R-factors can spread from one bacterial strain to another or between species. This transfer can occur within the bowel, in burns, or in peritoneal dialysis fluid. There is clear evidence that antimicrobial resistances can spread in this way from members of the commensal flora to potentially pathogenic species. Genes conferring resistance to several unrelated antimicrobial agents can become linked together in a single plasmid and be transferred together from one cell to another. Treatment with one antibiotic may simultaneously select for multiple drug-resistance traits when they are carried on a single R-plasmid.

Non-conjugative plasmids are incapable of self-transfer and do not encode for a sex pilus. They are smaller than conjugative plasmids and do not usually encode for more than one or two antimicrobial resistances. Their transfer is mediated by co-resident conjugative plasmids or via transduction or transformation.

Transposons It is now recognized that some genes determining resistance can be transposed from one plasmid to another or from a plasmid to the bacterial chromosome. These highly promiscuous elements are called transposons and are capable of extensive dissemination. Transposons are small pieces of DNA in which resistance genes are flanked by an inverted terminal repeat sequence. They cannot replicate independently but must exist as part of a self-replicating element, either a plasmid or the chromosome. The inverted repeat sequences of DNA provide recognition sites for restriction endonucleases which catalyse the insertion of the transposon from one replicon to another. Transposons can move from plasmid to chromosome resulting in stable integration of the genes and conservation of the resistance genes in bacterial species in which plasmids are unstable. Conversely, transposons can move from chromosome to plasmid and from plasmid to plasmid, facilitating the increased dissemination of resistance. For example, the resistance genes can spread from a non-transmissible to a conjugative plasmid and become linked with other resistances or with virulence factors. Tn4 is the transposon which determines the production of a β-lactamase (TEM-1 β-lactamase) which is now very widespread amongst the Enterobacteriaceae. This transposon has also conferred β-lactamase activity on strains of *H. influenzae* and *N. gonorrhoeae*.

A special class of transposons confers antibiotic resistance in streptococci. These conjugative transposons induce conjugation between two cells and the transposon is transferred from the donor chromosome to that of the recipient. These conjugative transposons are of considerable importance in determining antibiotic resistance in streptococci. Most of them carry a determinant for tetracycline resistance, but some carry additional resistance determinants. Conjugative transposons of this type have also been detected in *Clostridium difficile* and *Bacteroides fragilis*.

Bacteriophages In staphylococci, bacteriophages are closely involved in the expression and spread of antimicrobial resistance. Bacteriophages mediate the transfer of antimicrobial resistance determinants by transduction or by 'phage-mediated conjugation'. Transduction is the transfer of bacterial DNA from one cell to another by means of a bacteriophage vector. β-lactamase production in *Staph. aureus* is usually determined by relatively small plasmids which are spread between cells by transduction. Aminoglycoside-resistance plasmids in *Staph. aureus* may be spread by a conjugative mechanism independent of bacteriophages.

Antibiotic resistance determinants can also be transferred between bacteria by transformation; that is the uptake and assimilation of naked DNA. Although this certainly happens *in vitro*, it has not been clearly demonstrated *in vivo*.

Biochemical mechanisms of antimicrobial resistance

In order to inhibit or kill susceptible bacteria an antimicrobial agent must enter the cell and inactivate its target. A knowledge of the mode of action of antimicrobial agents (Table 6.5) is an essential prerequisite to any consideration of the mechanisms of drug resistance.

There are four main mechanisms by which resistance may arise (Table 6.6).

Enzyme inactivation of the drug

This type of resistance is the most important mechanism encountered in clinical isolates. It is the principle mechanism of resistance to the β-lactam antibiotics (penicillins and cephalosporins), the aminoglycosides, and chloramphenicol.

β-Lactamases Resistance to β-lactam antibiotics is usually due to the production of β-lactamases, enzymes that catalyse the hydrolysis of the β-lactam bond which results in inactivation of the drug (Fig. 6.7). The primary function of β-lactamases is not to protect bacteria from the effect of β-lactam antibiotics, but to break bonds in a β-lactam structure which is a transitory intermediate in normal bacterial cell wall synthesis. It is therefore not surprising that β-lactamases have been detected in almost all Gram-positive and Gram-negative bacteria.

A β-lactamase may be an inducible or a constitutive enzyme. The β-lactamases of Gram-positive bacteria are usually inducible, i.e. only low levels of the enzyme are normally present, but considerably greater amounts of the enzyme are produced in the presence of an inducing substance. Staphylococcal β-lactamase may be induced by drugs, such as penicillin, which are hydrolysed by the enzyme, or by cephalosporins (e.g. cephaloridine) or isoxazolyl penicillins (e.g. cloxacillin), which are resistant to the staphylococcal β-lactamase. The β-lactamases of Gram-negative bacterial species are typically constitutive and are synthesized at the same rate both in the presence and absence of a β-lactam antibiotic. β-lactamases vary in their ability to hydrolyse individual penicillin and cephalosporin antibiotics. Determination of the substrate profile is one method used to classify β-lactamases. Other means of classification that have been employed include determining their isoelectric point

Table 6.5 Mode of action of some antimicrobial drugs

Site of action	Drug	Mode of action
Cell wall	β-lactams (penicillins and cephalosporins)	Interfere with cross-linkage of peptidoglycan strands
	Vancomycin ⎫ Teichoplanin ⎭	Inhibits polymerization of peptidoglycan by complexing with terminal D-alanyl-D-alanine precursor
	D-Cycloserine	Structural analogue of D-alanine
Cytoplasmic membrane	Polymyxins	Act as cationic detergents, disrupting membranes
	Polyenes (amphotericin B and nystatin)	Bind to sterols in fungal cell membrane creating pores
	Imidazoles (clotrimazole, fluconazole, ketoconazole)	Interfere with biosynthesis of ergosterol, causing leakage of fungal cell contents
Ribosomes	Aminoglycosides (gentamicin, netilmicin)	Interfere with m-RNA attachment to ribosome, and cause misreading of m-RNA
	Erythromycin ⎫ Clindamycin ⎪ Lincomycin ⎬ Sodium fusidate ⎭	Interfere with translocation/transpeptidation
	Tetracyclines	Interfere with binding of amino-acyl t-RNAs to acceptor site
	Chloramphenicol	Inhibits peptidyl transferase
Nucleic acid synthesis	Sulphonamides	Competitive inhibition of para-amino benzoic acid (paba)
	Trimethoprim	Inhibits dihydrofolate reductase
	Fluoroquinolones (ciprofloxacin, norfloxacin)	Inhibit DNA-gyrase
	Metronidazole	Intracellular reductive activation releases intermediate compounds which damage DNA
	Rifampicin	Inhibits DNA-dependent RNA-polymerase
	5-Fluorocytosine	Pyrimidine analogue, incorporated into fungal DNA causing synthesis of abnormal proteins
	Acyclovir (ACV)	Activated by viral thymidine-kinase to form ACV-triphosphate which inhibits viral DNA-polymerase
	Vidarabine (ara A)	Purine nucleoside analogue inhibits viral DNA-polymerase
	Zidovudine (AZT)	Inhibits viral RNA-dependent DNA-polymerase (reverse transcriptase)

Table 6.6 Mechanisms of antimicrobial resistance

Mechanism	Antimicrobial	Bacteria
Enzyme inactivation β-Lactamases	Penicillins, cephalosporins	Staph. aureus H. influenzae N. gonorrhoeae Enterobacteriaceae Pseudomonas spp.
Chloramphenicol acetyltransferase (CAT)	Chloramphenicol	H. influenzae Staph. aureus Enterobacteriaceae

Aminoglycoside-modifying enzymes
  adenylases
  acetylases
  phosphotransferases
	Aminoglycosides	Staph. aureus
		Enterobacteriaceae
		Pseudomonas spp.

Altered permeability Reduced active transport into cell	Aminoglycosides	Enterobacteriaceae Pseudomonas spp.
	Chloramphenicol	Staph. aureus Enterobacteriaceae
Increased active removal of drug from cell	Tetracyclines	Enterobacteriaceae
Alteration of target Penicillin-binding proteins	Penicillins	N. gonorrhoeae Str. pneumoniae Staph. aureus Enterobacteriaceae
DNA-gyrase	Fluoroquinolones	P. aeruginosa Staph. aureus
RNA-polymerase	Rifampicin	Enterobacteriaceae
Metabolic bypass Altered dihydropteroate synthetase	Sulphonamides	Staph. aureus Enterobacteriaceae
Altered dihydrofolate reductase	Trimethoprim	Enterobacteriaceae

(a)

Penicillin → Penicilloic acid

(b)

Cephalosporin → Cephalosporanic acid (unstable) → Mixed fragmentation products

Fig. 6.7 β-Lactamase hydrolysis of (a) a penicillin, to form penicilloic acid, which is antibacterially inactive; (b) a cephalosporin, to form cephalosporanic acid, which is usually unstable and disintegrates into smaller fragments. Chemical alterations of penicillins or cephalosporins at either the R_1 or R_2 position may significantly alter the capacity of β-lactamase to hydrolyse the β-lactam ring.

(pI) by isoelectric focusing; determining their susceptibility to β-lactamase inhibitors (clavulanic acid, sulbactam, p-chloromercuribenzoate, cloxacillin, and carbenicillin); determining their molecular weight; and determining their serological relatedness. Several different classification schemes have been proposed.

Numerous β-lactamases exist encoded either by chromosomal genes or by transferable genes carried on plasmids or transposons. The β-lactamases of Gram-positive bacteria are usually plasmid-mediated and preferentially hydrolyse penicillin. Most are inducible and the enzyme is excreted extracellularly. β-lactamases have been found in *Staph. aureus*, *Staph. epidermidis*, *Enterococcus faecalis*, and *Bacillus* spp. Gram-negative bacteria produce a plethora of chromosomal and plasmid-mediated β-lactamases with varying degrees of activity against pencillins and cephalosporins. Over 30 different plasmid-mediated β-lactamases have been described. All are produced constitutively. The enzyme remains bound to cells and destroys β-lactams as they pass through the cell envelope. The plasmid-mediated β-lactamases have been divided into three broad groups:

1. broad-spectrum enzymes that hydrolyse pencillins and cephalosporins at similar rates;

2. oxacillinases that rapidly hydrolyse oxacillin and related penicillins; and

3. carbenicillinases.

The most important β-lactamase in clinical practice is TEM-1,

which has a broad range of activity and is carried on a transposon (Tn4) which explains its very wide distribution.

Virtually all Gram-negative bacteria produce inducible chromosomal β-lactamases which preferentially hydrolyse cephalosporins, including the third-generation cephalosporins which are resistant to hydrolysis by the plasmid-determined enzymes. Normally the activity of these enzymes is low but in the presence of many of the newer β-lactam drugs, selection of stably derepressed mutants may occur which produce high levels of the β-lactamase, resulting in clinical resistance. The resistance is not due to temporary induction of the β-lactamase by the β-lactam. This form of resistance is well recognized, notably with *Enterobacter* spp. and *Pseudomonas* spp.

In some instances β-lactam resistance is due exclusively to the action of a β-lactamase, for example penicillin resistance in staphylococci. Resistance to penicillins and cephalosporins may also be due to alterations in the target site (penicillin-binding proteins, PBPs), which is the mechanism found in methicillin-resistant *Staph. aureus* or penicillin-resistant pneumococci. In Gram-negative bacteria, β-lactam resistance is often complex and results from a combination of β-lactamase activity, decreased permeability, and altered PBPs.

Aminoglycoside-modifying enzymes Resistance to the aminoglycosides is usually due to the production of modifying enzymes. The genes determining these modifying enzymes are carried on plasmids or on the bacterial chromosome. Several have been found on transposons. There are three main classes of enzymes, each of which catalyses a different type of modification:

1. adenylation of aminoglycoside hydroxyl groups;
2. phosphorylation of hydroxyl groups; or
3. acetylation of amino groups.

Within each class of enzymes there are different subclasses that modify a particular range of substrate aminoglycosides (Table 6.7). The nomenclature specifies the type of enzyme and the molecular site of modification (Fig. 6.8). The primary effect of the modifying enzymes is to interfere with the transport of the drug into the bacterial cell.

Table 6.7 Examples of aminoglycoside-modifying enzymes

Enzyme	Drugs modified	Bacterial distribution
Acetyl transferases		
AAC (2')	G,Neo.,Net.,S,T	*Providencia/Proteus*
AAC (3)	G,K,Neo.,S,T	Enterobacteriaceae *Pseudomonas*
AAC (6')	A,G,K,Neo.,Net.,S,T	*Staphylococcus* Enterobacteriaceae *Pseudomonas*
Adenyl transferases		
AAD (2″)	G,K,S,T	Enterobacteriaceae *Pseudomonas*
AAD (3″) (9)	Spect., Strep.	Enterobacteriaceae
ADD (4′) (4″)	A,K,Neo.,T	Staphylococci
AAD (9)	Spect.	Staphylococci
Phosphotransferases		
APH (2″)	G,K,T	Staphylococci
APH (3′)	K,Neo.	Staphylococci Enterobacteriaceae *Pseudomonas*
APH (3″)	Strep.	Staphylococci Enterobacteriaceae *Pseudomonas*
APH (6)	Strep.	*Pseudomonas*

A, amikacin; G, gentamicin; K, kanamycin; Neo., neomycin; Net., netilmicin; S, sissomicin; Spect., spectinomycin; Strep., streptomycin; T, tobramycin.

Aminoglycoside-modifying enzymes have been detected in many Gram-negative bacterial species and in a few Gram-positive species (*Staph. aureus, Staph. epidermidis, Enterococcus faecalis,* and *Enterococcus faecium*). In Gram-negative bacteria the enzyme remains within the periplasmic space and, by modifying small amounts of incoming aminoglycoside, can interfere with active uptake mechanisms and effectively block transport of the drug into the cell. There are two factors determining resistance to a given aminoglycoside: the rate of uptake of the drug by the cell and the affinity of the modifying enzyme for that drug. The presence of one enzyme can confer resistance to a number of aminoglycosides (cross-resistance). The prevalence of these modifying enzymes in clinical isolates varies from one geographical area to another. It is therefore essential to tailor one's choice of appropriate aminoglycoside therapy according to local susceptibility patterns.

Chloramphenicol acetyltransferase Resistance to chloramphenicol in both Gram-positive and Gram-negative bacteria is usually due to acetylation of the drug by an inactivating enzyme, a chloramphenicol acetyltransferase. The acetylated form of the drug cannot bind to the bacterial ribosome. The enzyme may be chromosomally or plasmid encoded. Many different chloramphenicol acetyltransferases have been described. This is the usual mechanism of chloramphenicol resistance in *Haemophilus influenzae*.

Erythromycin esterase Resistance to erythromycin is usually due to an altered target (see below) but an inactivating enzyme, erythromycin esterase, has recently been described in *Escherichia coli*. This enzyme is plasmid mediated, constitutive, and results in high-level resistance to erythromycin.

Altered permeability to antimicrobials

Alterations in cell permeability to antimicrobial drugs may result from changes in specific receptors, non-specific changes in permeability, or alterations in active transport mechanisms.

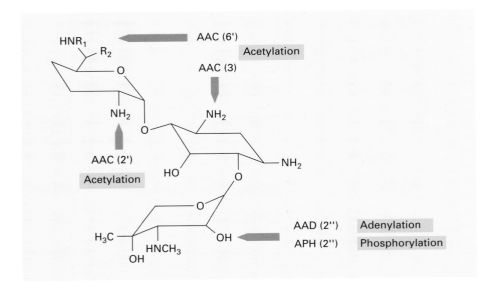

Fig. 6.8 Structure of gentamicin, showing sites of attack by modifying enzymes.

Hydrophilic antimicrobials traverse the outer membrane of the Gram-negative bacterial cell wall via porins. These porins are proteins which are so arranged as to form water-filled channels through which drugs may diffuse. In *E. coli* there are larger (OmpF) and smaller (OmpC) porin proteins. The rate of diffusion of a drug into a bacterial cell will be determined by the number and type of porin channels and by the physiochemical properties of the antimicrobial. Mutations resulting in loss of specific porins can occur in clinical isolates, resulting in increased resistance to β-lactam antibiotics. For example, a clinical isolate of *Salmonella typhimurium* which became resistant to a number of cephalosporins following cephalexin therapy was found to contain only OmpF protein while the parent strain produced both OmpF and OmpC strains. These strains also display reduced susceptibility to other antimicrobials that utilize these hydrophilic pathways, such as chloramphenicol and nalidixic acid.

Aminoglycosides are actively transported into bacteria. Some strains of *Pseudomonas aeruginosa* and other Gram-negative bacteria are resistant to the aminoglycosides because of a transport defect. This type of resistance, unlike that due to modifying enzymes, results in generalized cross-resistance to all the aminoglycosides, although the level of resistance may be low.

The uptake of tetracycline into cells also involves active transport. The major mechanism of tetracycline resistance in Gram-negative bacteria is due to the synthesis of a new protein which results in an increased efflux of the drug from the cell. Tetracycline entering the cell is simultaneously removed and the concentration of the drug remains subinhibitory. An active efflux system for removing fluoroquinolones from *E. coli* has also been described.

Alteration of the bacterial target

This type of resistance has been described for many antimicrobials. Resistance may result from alterations in the ribosomal binding sites. This has been described for erythromycin, clindamycin, fusidic acid, chloramphenicol, rifampicin, tetracycline, and streptomycin. The resistance arises from selection of rare pre-existing mutants. It is the principal form of resistance to erythromycin among Gram-positive organisms and is due to methylation of the 23S ribosomal RNA of the 50S ribosomal subunit by an inducible plasmid-mediated enzyme. Methylation of the ribosomal RNA renders the bacteria resistant to other macrolides and lincosamides (lincomycin and clindamycin). However, erythromycin is a specific inducer of the methylase and therefore bacteria carrying the plasmid are only resistant to these other drugs in the presence of erythromycin, so-called dissociated resistance.

Streptomycin binds to the S12 protein of the 30S subunit of the ribosome. A single mutation of one amino acid in S12 can interfere with streptomycin binding to the ribosome and result in high-level streptomycin resistance. Ribosomal resistance to other aminoglycosides, such as gentamicin and amikacin is rare and this is probably because these agents bind to several sites on the 30S and 50S subunits and resistance therefore requires multiple mutations.

Rifampicin-resistant mutants have an RNA polymerase with an altered β-subunit. It is inadvisable to use fusidic acid or rifampicin as monotherapy in staphylococcal infections since resistance of this type may readily emerge and result in treatment failure. The use of combinations of agents overcomes this problem.

Alterations in the penicillin-binding proteins (PBPs) may lead to β-lactam resistance. Methicillin-resistant *Staph. aureus* (MRSA) produce large amounts of a novel PBP (PBP-2′) which has a very low affinity for methicillin. Methicillin resistance in *Staph. aureus* also confers resistance to oxacillin, cloxacillin, flucloxacillin, and to cephalosporins. The majority of MRSA strains are also β-lactamase producers. Another class of MRSA has been described recently (Tomasz *et al.* 1989): these strains lack PBP-2′ and contain the normal PBPs with decreased penicillin-binding capacities. Penicillin-resistant pneumococci have several changes in their PBPs, including decreased affinity of some of the PBPs, new PBPs not present in sensitive strains, and deletion of other PBPs. Non-β-lactamase-producing strains of *N. gonorrhoeae* and *H. influenzae* may be resistant to penicillin and ampicillin by virtue of altered penicillin-binding proteins or by loss of outer membrane proteins.

Nalidixic acid and the newer fluoroquinolones act by inhibiting DNA gyrase, an enzyme that maintains superhelical twists in bacterial DNA. The enzyme contains four subunits: two A subunits encoded by the *gyr A* gene and two B subunits encoded by the *gyr B* gene. Several different mutations resulting in the production of a drug-resistant enzyme have been described in a variety of chromosomal loci. A second type of resistance is due to alteration in the outer membrane proteins (see above).

Metabolic bypass

Resistance to the sulphonamides may be mutational or plasmid mediated. The major cause of significant sulphonamide resistance is the plasmid-mediated production of an altered dihydropteroate synthetase with a 1000-fold lower affinity for the drug. Similarly, trimethoprim resistance is usually due to a plasmid-mediated dihydrofolate reductase that is several thousand times more resistant to the effects of trimethoprim than normal.

The emergence of resistance is, to some extent, an inevitable consequence of antimicrobial therapy. However, a rational approach to the use of antimicrobials and an understanding of the mechanisms by which resistance may occur can minimize the problem of antimicrobial resistance.

6.2.4 Host factors

Mary P. E. Slack

Introduction

Man is continuously being exposed to a wide variety of potentially pathogenic micro-organisms. The outcome of these encounters depends on a complex and dynamic web of interactions between the parasite and the host. The virulence factors of the micro-organism and the size of the infecting dose are weighed against a wide range of non-specific and specific host defence mechanisms which limit or eliminate any possible infection. Thus, the capacity of an organism to evade basic host defences is balanced against the host's ability to mobilize an inflammatory response augmented by specific immunological mechanisms.

Some bacteria possess specific properties which may render them pathogenic to normal hosts, and may be regarded as primary pathogens. The term 'pathogenicity' is defined as the ability to cause disease. However, we are increasingly aware of the consequences of impaired host defences rendering individuals susceptible to infection by micro-organisms not normally regarded as pathogens. This is termed 'opportunistic infection'. A wide range of diseases and therapeutic interventions can interfere with the normal host defence mechanisms and render the individual susceptible to opportunistic infections. In this context the classic view of an immunocompromised host is a rather narrow one. Indeed, every patient with an infection is to some extent a compromised host. There is a wide spectrum of impairment of host defences (Table 6.8) which increases the likelihood of such infections. It is probably true to say that many patients develop infections as a result of current clinical practice. For example, trauma to the skin or mucous membranes may introduce organisms to normally sterile tissues. This trauma may be due to the surgeon's knife, intravascular lines, tracheostomies, or in-dwelling urinary catheters. The body's microbial flora can be profoundly altered by the use of broad-spectrum antimicrobial therapy. The non-specific immune response may be markedly depressed by a variety of therapeutic agents.

Opportunistic pathogens are generally of low virulence. Virulence is defined as the degree of pathogenicity. A bacterial species may be of generally high or low virulence for a particular host, or a particular strain of that bacterial species may be relatively avirulent if it has lost an important virulence determinant. An example of this would be *Corynebacterium diphtheriae*, the cause of diphtheria, the pathogenic effects of which are wholly due to the production of an exotoxin. Non-toxigenic strains of *C. diphtheriae* are avirulent.

Bacterial virulence and resistance mechanisms have already been considered (see Sections 6.2.1–3). In this section we turn our attention to the defence mechanisms of the host. A complex array of non-specific (constitutive) and specific (immune) mechanisms, both at the surface and within the tissues, interact to defend the host from microbial assault (Table 6.9).

Non-specific surface defence mechanisms

These defences interfere with the colonization of body surfaces by potentially pathogenic organisms and prevent their access into the deeper tissues of the body. Such encounters are continually occurring and these defences are of vital importance in maintaining health.

Normal commensal flora

Under normal conditions the skin and much of the mucosal surface of the body are colonized with a rich and varied flora of micro-organisms. The skin and mucous membranes of the mouth, nose, conjunctivae, intestinal tract, and lower genital tract each have their own characteristic indigenous flora (Table 6.10). This microbial flora can be divided into two groups: the normal resident flora that is almost invariably present and which, if disturbed, will promptly become re-established; and a transient flora which may colonize the host for short periods but tends to be eliminated by competition from the resident flora or by the host's defence mechanisms. The transient flora may contain potentially pathogenic organisms, for example meningococci may be transiently carried in the nasopharynx of healthy individuals.

The exact pattern of colonization is influenced by microbial factors, host factors, and exogenous factors. One important microbial factor is adhesion to epithelial or mucosal cells (see Section 6.2.1). Some bacteria show a distinct affinity or tropism for particular types of epithelial cells. The normal flora may interfere with potential pathogens by competing with them for cell-surface receptors (Table 6.11). Both *Staphylococcus aureus* and Group A streptococci adhere to fibronectin on epithelial cell surfaces. The commensal flora may interfere with pathogenic organisms by producing bacteriocins, substances inhibitory to other bacteria (usually of the same species), or by competing for

Table 6.8 The spectrum of impaired host defences with some examples

Condition	Results
Trauma to skin or mucosa, e.g. intravascular cannula, surgical incision	Admits organisms to normally sterile tissues
Local lesion, e.g. furuncle, carbuncle	Multiplication of organisms; facilitates deeper invasion
Impaired non-specific (constitutive) defences white cell defects, e.g. chronic granulomatous disease	Recurrent pyogenic infections, e.g. *Staphylococcus aureus, Serratia marcescens*
complement component defects, e.g. C2 deficiency	Pneumococcal septicaemia + meningitis in children
C3 deficiency	Recurrent infections—*H. influenzae, Str. pneumoniae*
C5678 deficiency	Disseminated meningococcal and gonococcal infections
Impaired specific (immune) defects B-cell defects, e.g. hypogammaglobulinaemia	Recurrent respiratory infections, *Staph. aureus, Str. pneumoniae, H. influenzae*
T-cell defects, e.g. Di George syndrome	*Pneumocystis carinii* pneumonia, chronic mucocutaneous candidiasis

Table 6.9　Host defence mechanisms

	Non-specific (constitutive)	Specific (immune)
Surface defences (skin, mucous membranes)	Commensal microbial flora Colonization resistance Mechanical barrier Secretions: lysozyme 　　　　　　 lactoferrin 　　　　　　 gastric acid Directional flow: cilia 　　　　　　　 blinking 　　　　　　　 peristalsis 　　　　　　　 urination	Secretory IgA
Deeper defences Humoral	Lysozyme, lactoferrin Inflammation Acute phase reaction: cytokines Complement Fibronectin Interferons	B-lymphocytes Immunoglobulins
Cellular	Polymorphonuclear phagocytes Mononuclear phagocytes NK-cells	T-lymphocytes

Table 6.10　Predominant micro-organisms colonizing various body sites in health

Skin, external auditory canal
　Staphylococci (*Staph. epidermidis* and *Staph. aureus*)
　Propionobacterium acnes
　Corynebacterium spp. (coryneforms)
　Candida spp.

Oropharynx
　Viridans streptococci
　Neisseria spp.
　Branhamella catarrhalis
　Staphylococci
　Bacteroides spp.
　Fusobacterium spp.
　Anaerobic cocci

Nasopharynx
　Staphylococci
　Streptococci including *Str. pneumoniae*
　Haemophilus spp.
　Neisseria spp.

Conjunctiva
　Staphylococci
　Haemophilus spp.
　Diphtheroids

Large intestine
　Bacteroides spp.
　Clostridium spp.
　Fusobacterium spp.
　Escherichia coli
　Klebsiella spp.
　Staphylococci
　Yeasts

Lower genitourinary tract
　Staphylococci
　Streptococci
　Anaerobic cocci
　Corynebacterium spp.
　Lactobacilli (vagina)

Table 6.11　Mechanisms by which normal commensal flora inhibits potential pathogens

Competition for nutrients
Competition for cell-surface receptors
Production of bacteriocins
Stimulation of cross-reacting (natural) antibodies
Stimulation of clearance mechanisms

nutrients. Thus *Streptococcus mutans*, which is normally present in the oropharynx, can produce a bacteriocin (so-called viridicin) which is inhibitory to group A streptococci.

In these ways the normal flora forms an effective barrier limiting the opportunities for pathogens to colonize the surfaces of the host. This phenomenon has been called 'colonization resistance'. Upsetting the ecological balance of the flora can lead to serious problems. Broad-spectrum antimicrobial chemotherapy will deplete all the susceptible types of commensal bacteria from the gastrointestinal flora. Colonization resistance is impaired and potentially lethal pathogens can colonize the surface. When the treatment is stopped the resident flora will re-establish itself, but the more rapidly growing aerobic Gram-negative bacteria will reappear before the slower-growing anaerobic Gram-negative bacteria which normally comprise about 99 per cent of the commensal flora. In immunocompromised patients this distortion may result in a Gram-negative bacteraemia. Other consequences of suppressing the normal flora with broad-spectrum antimicrobials may be an overgrowth of yeasts, giving rise to thrush, or an overgrowth of the relatively antibiotic-resistant, anaerobic, toxigenic Gram-positive bacillus, *Clostridium difficile*, which causes a spectrum of problems ranging from antibiotic-associated diarrhoea to antibiotic-associated (pseudo-membranous) colitis.

Host factors that affect the normal flora include nutrition, age, hormones, and underlying diseases, including diabetes mellitus and malignancy. For example, bifidobacteria predominate in the relatively acid stools of breast-fed babies, whereas the less acidic stools of bottle-fed babies have a colonic flora more similar to that of older children and adults. The vaginal flora is under hormonal influence. The prepubertal and postmenopausal flora is scanty and consists of skin and colonic organisms. During the child-bearing years acidophilic lactobacilli predominate. Oestrogen stimulates the deposition of glycogen in vaginal epithelial cells. Lactobacilli can metabolize glycogen to lactic acid, producing an acid milieu (pH 4–5) which is inhibitory to many organisms but optimal for lactobacilli. The normal flora is beneficial in interfering with colonization by potential pathogens. It also gives rise to the production of cross-reacting or 'natural' antibodies. These antibodies are produced in response to antigenic stimuli provided by organisms colonizing the oropharynx or intestinal tract, which share cross-reacting antigens with potential pathogens. For example, in children colonization with *Neisseria lactamica* may be associated with an increased incidence of bactericidal antibodies to *N. meningitidis*. Certain strains of *Escherichia coli* stimulate the production of bactericidal antibodies to *N. meningitidis* or *Haemophilus influenzae* type b. It should be noted that these cross-reacting antibodies are not always beneficial. There is some evidence that IgA antibodies produced in response to commensal organisms that cross-react antigenically with meningococci may actually increase the patient's susceptibility to invasive meningococcal disease. These IgA-blocking antibodies compete with bactericidal IgG and IgM antibodies for binding sites on the surface of the meningococcus.

Mechanical barriers

Normal skin and mucous membranes provide effective barriers to the access of potentially pathogenic micro-organisms into the body. Most infectious agents cannot penetrate intact skin. Breeches in the skin following injury, insect bites, surgical incisions, or intravascular lines admit organisms to normally sterile tissues and are a major risk factor in the development of infection. Only a few organisms, for example the wart virus (papilloma virus), can penetrate intact skin.

Normal skin is inhospitable to many micro-organisms. It is relatively dry and acid (pH 5–6) due to the breakdown of triglycerides in sebum to free fatty acids and the lactic acid found in sweat. Higher bacterial counts are found on inflamed or moist skin, for example under occlusive dressings. Organisms on the skin surface are constantly being lost as skin scales desquamate. Hair follicles and sweat glands are chinks in the armour and may become colonized with *Staphylococcus aureus*, leading to furuncles, carbuncles, or abscesses. Damage to the biological activity of the skin, for example following burns, may lead to opportunistic infections, particularly with *Pseudomonas aeruginosa*. Similarly, cytotoxic drugs and irradiation cause thinning of the mucosal surface of the gastrointestinal tract, with patchy sloughing, which may lead to systemic invasion by the gut flora.

Surface secretions

Mucosal surfaces are bathed in secretions that contain a number of antimicrobial substances, the most important of which are lysozyme and lactoferrin. Lysozyme cleaves the linkage between *N*-acetyl muramic acid and *N*-acetyl glucosamine

in the bacterial cell wall, causing bacterial lysis, especially in Gram-positive bacteria. Lactoferrin interferes with bacterial iron metabolism. Local secretions also contain immunoglobulins, especially secretory IgA (sIgA), which, by coating micro-organisms, prevents their adherence to host cells. sIgA also inhibits bacterial motility, neutralizes toxins, and may agglutinate bacteria. It does not opsonize or mediate complement-dependent killing. It has been shown to be an important defence mechanism preventing infections by *Vibrio cholerae*, *Giardia lamblia*, and some respiratory viruses where primary attachment to mucosal surfaces is a vital stage in pathogenesis.

Gastric acid provides an effective barrier to most ingested micro-organisms, although some, such as *Mycobacterium tuberculosis* and enteroviruses, are indifferent to its effects. Achlorhydria is associated with colonization of the stomach and small bowel with Gram-negative bacteria. The use of H_2-antagonists similarly causes a rise in gastric pH. The infecting dose of cholera vibrios (ID_{50}) in healthy volunteers is about 10^8 organisms but this is reduced to about 10^6 organisms in patients with achlorhydria or following antacid ingestion. Unconjugated bile has antibacterial activity and probably inhibits the growth of bacteria in the small intestine. Intestinal peristalsis tends to prevent the bacterial overgrowth that occurs in blind loops of bowel.

Directional flow

The respiratory tract has a great array of antimicrobial defences. The air we breathe contains large numbers of suspended micro-organisms in droplets, droplet nuclei, or in dust particles. Particles $> 5 \, \mu m$ are trapped in the mucus layer coating the mucosal surface of the upper respiratory tract and are swept upwards by the directional ciliary motion to the back of the throat, where they are expectorated or swallowed. Smaller particles ($< 5 \, \mu m$) can penetrate to the alveoli where they are usually ingested by alveolar macrophages. The respiratory defence mechanisms are impaired by air pollutants, such as cigarette smoke, or by intercurrent infections. Thus influenza or pertussis may impair ciliary activity and predispose the patient to a secondary bacterial pneumonia. Intubation and tracheostomy bypass the normal defences of the upper airway and facilitate infection of the lower respiratory tract. In cystic fibrosis excessive quantities of abnormally viscid mucus are produced. In addition, ciliary clearance is poor and this results in recurrent pulmonary infections with *Staphylococcus aureus*, *Haemophilus influenzae*, and *Pseudomonas aeruginosa*.

The outer surfaces of the eyes are protected by blinking and the tears which dilute and wash away foreign material, including micro-organisms, via the nasolacrimal duct into the nasopharynx. Tears contain large amounts of lysozyme. When the nasolacrimal duct is blocked this defence mechanism is impaired and conjunctivitis often occurs.

Urine is an excellent bacterial culture medium and organisms introduced into the bladder will readily reach high numbers ($\geq 10^5$/ml). Regular voiding of urine is the principal defence mechanism. The relatively low pH of urine is inhibitory to many bacteria. The length of the male urethra protects against ascending infection, which is much more common in women because of the shortness of the female urethra. This defence mechanism is bypassed by urinary catheterization. Stasis due to prostatic hypertrophy, posterior urethral valves, or calculi also encourages infection.

During the child-bearing years the vaginal epithelium presents an acid environment, which is inimicable to many pathogens (see above).

The assorted surface defence mechanisms are extremely effective in preventing invasion of the body by potential pathogens. However, if the skin or mucosal surfaces are breached, allowing organisms to gain access, a local lesion may develop and organisms can multiply to a level at which deeper or progressive invasion can occur. A number of non-specific responses endeavour to limit this invasion.

Non-specific deeper defence mechanisms

These non-specific (constitutive) humoral and cellular mechanisms interact and augment one another to a great extent.

Non-specific humoral defence mechanisms As soon as micro-organisms gain access to subepithelial tissues they encounter intercellular fluids which contain a number of antimicrobial factors. Lysozyme is found in many body fluids (except cerebrospinal fluid, urine, and sweat) in sufficient concentration to lyse the cell wall of some Gram-positive bacteria. Lysozyme is unable to attack Gram-negative bacteria in the absence of antibody and complement. It also enhances the activity of complement.

Lactoferrin is an iron-binding protein that chelates iron, depriving micro-organisms of the free iron that the majority require for growth. Lysozyme and lactoferrin are also found in the secondary (specific) granules of neutrophils.

Inflammatory response The presence of multiplying bacteria within the tissues and the cell damage that they produce generally excites an inflammatory response (see Sections 4.4 and 5.2 for a full description). Capillaries in the vicinity dilate and become more permeable, allowing the extravasation of fluid containing proteins, immunoglobulins, and complement components. Leucocytes migrate from the capillaries into the tissues. Vasoactive substances such as histamine, bradykinin, prostaglandins, and leukotrienes modulate the inflammatory response. The effect of the inflammatory response is to limit the spread of the local lesion and prevent the dissemination of the invading micro-organisms.

Cytokines are peptides produced during the initial response to an invading micro-organism and have a number of important functions, including modulation of the immune system. They are produced by a number of cells, the principal sources being macrophages and activated lymphocytes. They are non-antigen specific. A large number of cytokines have now been identified,

the most important being interleukin-1, tumour necrosis factor-α (cachectin), α-, β-, and γ-interferon, and colony-stimulating factors (CSF). In response to foreign material a cascade of cytokine production occurs, increasing the host's non-specific resistance to infection. In this way cytokines form an effective defence mechanism prior to the onset of specific immunity.

Acute phase response The presence of microbial products, such as endotoxin, or trauma often leads to a marked rise in the circulating levels of a number of serum proteins, including:

1. complement;
2. coagulation proteins;
3. transport proteins (e.g. haptoglobin, caeruloplasmin), which compete with the pathogens for nutrients;
4. protease inhibitors, which limit tissue damage; and
5. adherence proteins (e.g. C-reactive protein), which bind to bacteria activating complement, enhance phagocytosis, and induce leucocyte migration.

This non-specific phenomenon is known as the acute phase response. A number of substances are known to induce the acute phase response, including prostaglandin PGE_1, interleukin-1, and tumour necrosis factor. Interleukin-1 stimulates the synthesis of C-reactive protein (CRP) by the liver. The concentration of CRP rises within a few hours of acute inflammation, increasing a thousandfold after 24–48 hours. CRP forms calcium-dependent complexes with the somatic C-polysaccharide of the pneumococcus and other polysaccharides present in a wide range of bacteria and fungi. Measurement of plasma concentrations of CRP has been advocated as an indicator of infection, especially in patients with underlying malignancy or where bacteriological results are equivocal. However, CRP levels are also elevated in non-infective inflammatory states such as rheumatoid arthritis, acute pancreatitis, and Crohn's disease.

Other features of the acute phase response include fever, which is a response of the action of cytokines (particularly interleukin-1, tumour necrosis factor, and α-interferon) on the hypothalamic thermoregulatory centre. The benefit to the host of fever is not completely clear. Serum iron and zinc levels fall. The virulence of many micro-organisms is diminished in iron-deficiency. This non-specific response is quite effective in the early stages of infection and is then augmented by the onset of specific immunological responses.

Complement The complement system (see Section 4.7) consists of at least 19 plasma proteins that mediate several aspects of the inflammatory process. Activation of the complement cascade may occur via immune complexes (the classical pathway) or via bacterial products (the alternative pathway) in the absence of specific antibody. Complement has a wide range of antimicrobial properties. Factors C5a, C5b67, and to a lesser extent C3a, are chemotactic for leucocytes and possibly monocytes. Factor C3b acts as an opsonin, and the complex C5b

C789 is able to penetrate cell membranes leading to the lysis of micro-organisms. Thus complement provides an effective defence system against micro-organisms, causing bacteriolysis and augmenting the antimicrobial activity of polymorphs and macrophages that can operate via the alternative pathway before a specific immune response has developed.

Fibronectin is a large molecular weight glycoprotein present on cell surfaces and in plasma. It is reported to opsonize and to interact with complement components. In experimental animals plasma fibronectin promotes the non-specific clearance of bacteria and other particles, such as cell debris and damaged platelets. Cell-surface-associated fibronectin is important in cell adhesion and cellular interactions. Patients undergoing cardiac surgery or in intensive therapy units lose fibronectin from their throats, resulting in depletion of the normal streptococcal flora and allowing coliforms to colonize the oropharynx.

Interferons (IFNs) The interferons (IFNs) are a family of relatively low molecular weight proteins, some of which are glycoproteins. Three main types are now recognized α-interferon (α-IFN), β-interferon (β-IFN) and γ-interferon (γ-IFN). The production of α-IFN and β-IFN is stimulated by any virus in any type of cell. α-IFN and β-IFN act mainly as antiviral agents, whereas the major function of γ-IFN is as an immune modulator. The antiviral efects of interferon are not virus-specific, though they do show host-species specificity. Interferons do not enter target cells but act via cell-surface receptors, inducing the synthesis of antiviral effector molecules which inhibit the translation of viral mRNA significantly more than host mRNA. Antiviral activity is also mediated by stimulation of host-defence mechanisms, especially natural killer (NK) cells and macrophages. γ-IFN is a major cytokine produced mainly by lymphocytes following antigen or mitogen stimulation.

Interferons are formed within hours of the onset of infection.

Non-specific cellular defence mechanisms

Phagocytic cells are the cells of the granulocytic series (neutrophil polymorphs and eosinophil polymorphs) and the mononuclear phagocytes (macrophages). They play a key role in the antimicrobial defence mechanisms of the host.

During acute inflammation an increased number of neutrophils, and sometimes eosinophils, appear in the area of inflammation, followed by an increasing number of macrophages. Actively growing bacteria release chemotactic factors, for example the tripeptide formyl-methionyl-leucyl-phenylalanine (FMLP), into the culture medium. Neutrophils have a specific membrane receptor for FMLP.

The exact nature of the cellular response varies both with time and with the type of invading micro-organism. Neutrophils are most effective against extracellular bacteria, whereas eosinophils are important in certain parasitic infections. Macrophages play a key role in the body's defences against intracellular pathogens such as mycobacteria and fungi. Lymphocytes provide the major cellular defence against viral attack.

Phagocytosis is the attachment and engulfment of particulate matter (>1 μm) by the cell. Some micro-organisms may be ingested in the absence of serum factors but the efficiency of phagocytosis is greatly enhanced if the particle is first coated with specific IgG, IgG3, or complement component C3b (opsonins). Some capsulated bacteria can only be effectively phagocytosed if they are trapped against a mechanical barrier such as occurs in the spleen. For this reason pneumococcal and *Haemophilus* infections are more severe following splenectomy.

The way in which polymorphs ingest and destroy microorganisms is described fully in Section 4.5.

During the process of phagocytosis and intracellular killing the neutrophils usually die and are ingested by macrophages, which have a greater ability to survive and can enzymically digest the phagocytosed material.

Mononuclear phagocytes (see Section 4.5) include circulating monocytes and fixed tissue macrophages. They have similar surface receptors for Fcγ and C3b to those found on neutrophils and are able to phagocytose opsonized micro-organisms. They contain cytoplasmic granules and lysosomes and can inhibit or kill phagocytosed organisms in a similar way to neutrophils. However, they are not able to kill a number of micro-organisms, including mycobacteria, *Listeria monocytogenes*, *Brucella* spp., *Legionella* spp., *Cryptococcus neoformans*, *Toxoplasma gondii*, and *Pneumocystis carinii*, which can survive and even multiply within the macrophages of a non-immune host. When T-cell immunity develops, activated T-helper cells produce a number of cytokines, the most important of which is γ-IFN. γ-IFN activates macrophages, and activated macrophages are able to kill some, but not all, of these intracellular pathogens.

When appropriately stimulated by microbial products, macrophages secrete a variety of cytokines, including interleukin-1 and tumour necrosis factor α, which mediate inflammation and interact with other cell types.

Natural killer cells (see Section 4.5) are a subpopulation of mononuclear cells which are able to kill certain virus-infected cells in the absence of prior sensitization. They are not phagocytic. NK cells recognize virally infected cells and produce perforin, which inserts into the cell membrane of such cells. After insertion perforin polymerizes, producing a transmembrane pore which leads to osmotic lysis of the infected cell. Phenotypically they are large granular lymphocytes. Their exact role is not known but there is a correlation between NK cell activity and susceptibility to herpes viruses and cytomegalovirus. There is a marked deficiency of NK cell activity in AIDS patients. The killing capacity of NK cells is markedly enhanced by interferon.

There is thus a complex array of non-specific humoral and cellular mechanisms which interact in many ways to produce a rapidly responding defence against microbial attack.

Specific immune defence mechanisms

The specific immune response follows the specific recognition of foreign antigens and involves T- and B-lymphocytes and cells of the macrophage–monocyte series. B-lymphocytes are involved in immunoglobulin production, whereas T-lymphocytes are the basis of cell-mediated immunity and interact with the B-lymphocytes in immunoglobulin production. Many interactions occur between the different cellular components of the specific immune response. Thus, macrophages stimulated by antigen secrete interleukin-1 which stimulates the activation and proliferation of T-lymphocytes. In turn, activated T-helper cells secrete several soluble factors (cytokines), including γ-interferon, macrophage chemotactic factor, migration inhibition factor, macrophage activation factor, and interleukin-2. These factors enhance the killing ability of macrophages. Interleukin-2 is responsible for the generation of cytotoxic T-cells, which can kill infected host cells. The overall effect of T-cell activation is to enhance the host's immunity to organisms sequestered within cells. Lymphokines from activated T-cells enhance the ability of macrophages to kill intracellular pathogens, and cytotoxic T-cells are generated which can kill infected host cells. A distinct group of cells with a cytotoxic function are K-cells, which are non-phagocytic mononuclear cells. They carry Fc receptors and can bind and kill material which is coated with IgG, such as bacteria, fungi, and parasites.

Antibody responses to most antigens depends on both T- and B-lymphocytes. The T-lymphocytes recognize antigens on the cell surface of the accessory cells (macrophages, monocytes) in association with HLA class II molecules and stimulate the proliferation of B-lymphocytes specific for the foreign antigen.

These B-lymphocytes differentiate into immunoglobulin-producing plasma cells.

For a full description of the immune responses see Section 4.2.

Factors affecting the quality of host defence mechanisms

The host defence mechanisms may be disturbed in a wide range of diseases and by an increasing number of therapeutic agents and iatrogenic procedures (Table 6.12). A number of constitutional factors influence the host's susceptibility to infection. There is also some evidence of genetic control of the quality of host defences. Congenital defects in the host's immune system are considered in Chapter 4.

Age The very young and the elderly are more susceptible to infection than other age groups. Neonates may be regarded as compromised hosts. The raw umbilicus provides an easy route of entry for micro-organisms, an ineffective blood–brain barrier allows organisms to enter readily the cerebrospinal fluid, and many of their host-defence mechanisms are immature. The antibody response to polysaccharide antigens is poor in young children, complement levels are low, and their phagocytic cells function poorly. Neonatal monocytes show defective killing of Group B streptococci and *Staph. aureus*, both important neonatal pathogens.

In the elderly the skin is atrophic, inelastic, and more easily

Table 6.12 Some examples of conditions which may impair host-defence mechanisms

Impaired surface defences		Impaired non-specific defences		Impaired specific (immune) defences	
Congenital	Acquired	Congenital	Acquired	Congenital	Acquired
Cystic fibrosis	Intravascular lines	Chronic granulatomous disease	Extremes of life (neonates + elderly)	Defects in antibody production	Myeloma
Kartagener syndrome	Surgical incisions	Complement deficiencies (C2, C3, C5678)	Malnutrition	X-linked hypogamma-globulinaemia	Sarcoidosis
	Drug abuse		Alcoholism + liver failure	Selective IgM deficiency	Hodgkin's disease
	Burns, pressure sores, ulcers	Chediak-Higashi syndrome	Renal failure	Selective IgA deficiency	Lymphoma
	Endoscopy	Cyclical neutropenia, etc	Diabetes mellitus		Leukaemia
	Loss of colonization resistance		Infection, e.g. influenza	Defects of cell-mediated immunity	Total-body irradiation
	Endotracheal intubation		Splenectomy	Di George syndrome	AIDS
	Urinary catheterization		Drugs—antibiotics	Severe combined immunodeficiency	Drugs
			Non-steroidal anti-inflammatory drugs		cytotoxics
			Auto-immune diseases		corticosteroids
			Rheumatoid arthritis		cyclosporin A
			Systemic lupus erythematosus		
			Non-haemopoietic malignancy		
			Trauma		

damaged, and there is a functional decline in cell-mediated immunity. Serum IgM levels are reduced. The elderly may also be dehydrated, malnourished, and have underlying diseases which impair host defences.

Nutritional state Severe protein energy malnutrition is a major problem in the developing countries but is also seen in patients with severe underlying diseases, such as malignancies. This severe malnutrition has marked effects on many aspects of host defence and may lead to infectious complications. Thus the skin and mucosal surfaces will become thin with decreased levels of secretory IgA and lysozyme. Complement levels are depressed and microbial killing by polymorphs is impaired. T-lymphocytes, especially helper T-cells are diminished and NK-cell activity is reduced. Many infections are more common in severe malnutrition, including tuberculosis, bacterial diarrhoea, measles, herpes simplex, pneumocystis pneumonia, candidiasis, and aspergillosis.

A shortage of some vitamins may affect cell-mediated immunity. Vitamin A deficiency predisposes to infection at epithelial surfaces such as the cornea. In experimental animals zinc deficiency impairs wound healing, produces disturbances of T-cell function, and increases susceptibility to listeriosis. Zinc deficiency has been reported during total parenteral nutrition. Iron deficiency has not been shown to be associated with an increased risk of infection. Indeed, replenishing iron stores in these patients can increase the risk of certain infections, such as tuberculosis. *Yersinia enterocolitica* septicaemia is more common in conditions of iron overload, such as haemachromatosis and thalassaemia.

Genetic factors There are some microbial diseases in which genetic factors clearly affect host susceptibility. For example, family studies suggest that although no one HLA antigen is associated with altered susceptibility or resistance to leprosy, HLA-type does seem to determine which type of leprosy the patient will develop (tuberculoid or lepromatous). Similarly, family and twin studies provide evidence of a genetic factor in host susceptibility to tuberculosis. Twin studies show an increased concordance for the disease in monozygotic rather than dizygotic twins. Possession of the HLA-B27 antigen increases the likelihood of reactive arthritis following gastrointestinal infections with *Salmonella* spp., *Shigella* spp., *Yersinia* spp., or *Campylobacter jejuni*. The likelihood of chronic liver disease developing after hepatitis B infection is HLA-related. An increased frequency of the B-cell alloantigen HLA-DR2 is seen in patients with the severe, chronic form of Lyme disease (caused by *Borrelia burgdorferi*).

Some infections are more frequently seen in patients of certain blood groups. For example, giardiasis is more common in people of blood group A than in other ABO blood groups.

Underlying diseases affecting host defences

A number of disease states are associated with alterations in the host defence mechanisms leading to an increased risk of infection, of which the following are only a limited example.

Diabetes mellitus In diabetes mellitus the skin is breeched by injections, and peripheral vacular disease and neuropathy increase the likelihood of injury. Keto-acidosis impairs neutrophil function. The reasons for the association between diabetes and unusual infections, such as rhinocerebral mucormycosis and malignant *Pseudomonas aeruginosa* otitis externa, are not known.

Alcoholism Minor trauma and aspiration of stomach contents into the lung are frequent problems in alcoholics which increase the likelihood of infection. These patients may have multiple vitamin deficiencies and protein-energy malnutrition. In alcoholic cirrhosis, cell-mediated immunity is depressed and circulating T-lymphocytes are depleted.

Chronic renal failure does not appear to impair humoral defence mechanisms. The major threat to the patient is during haemodialysis or peritoneal dialysis, where the integument is breached. Fluid overload predisposes the lungs to infection.

Malignant disease Immune responsiveness is impaired with disseminated malignancy and these patients often suffer opportunistic infections caused by low-grade pathogens. This is particularly seen in patients with leukaemias and lymphomas. Many factors contribute to the risk of infection, including granulocytopenia, mucosal damage due to cytotoxic therapy or irradiation, and intravascular lines breaching the skin.

Infections Many viral and parasitic infections *per se* produce an immunosuppressed state in the host and predispose the patient to secondary bacterial or fungal infections. For example, influenza virus impairs the defences of the respiratory mucosa and depresses polymorph function and results in an increased susceptibility to staphylococcal pneumonia. Measles results in impairment of both humoral and cell-mediated immunity, and bacterial pneumonias or gastroenteritis may supervene. HIV infection results in depletion of helper T-cells and is characterized by recurrent infections with low-grade pathogens, notably *Pneumocystis carinii* and *Toxoplasma gondii*.

Drugs Many drugs impair the host defences against infection, including corticosteroids and other immunosuppressive drugs, cytotoxics, and some antibiotics. Antibiotic therapy can alter the commensal flora, interfering with colonization resistance. A number of antibiotics may impair other aspects of the host's non-specific and specific defence mechanisms.

Conclusion

A system of complex defence mechanisms has been evolved to protect man from the myriad of potentially pathogenic organisms present in his environment. In normal hosts these defences are extremely effective, but a wide range of diseases and therapeutic interventions can interfere with one or more of these mechanisms, increasing the patient's risk of developing an infection. When two or more of these disorders occur together the patient may be severely immunocompromised.

6.2.5   Further reading

Adhesion, penetration, and colonization

Kapperud, G., Namork, E., Skurnik, M., and Nesbakken, T. (1987). Plasmid-mediated surface fibrillae of *Yersinia pseudotuberculosis* and *Yersinia enterocolitica*: relationship to the outer membrane protein YOP1 and possible importance for pathogenesis. *Infection and Immunity* **55**, 2247–54.

Lindberg, F., Lund, B., Johansson, L., and Normark, S. (1987). Localization of the receptor-binding protein adhesin at the tip of the bacterial pilus. *Nature* (London) **328**, 84–7.

Mims, C. A. (1987). *The pathogenesis of infectious diseases* (3rd edn). Academic Press, London.

Reid, G. and Sobel, J. D. (1987). Bacterial adherence in the pathogenesis of urinary tract infection. *Reviews of Infectious Diseases* **9**, 470–87.

Sansonetti, P. J. and Mounier, J. (1987). Metabolic events mediating early killing of host cells infected by *Shigella flexneri*. *Microbial Pathogenesis* **3**, 53–61.

Sparling, P. F., Cannon, J. G., and So, M. (1985). Phase and antigenic variation of pili and outer membrane protein II of *Neisseria gonorrhoeae*. *Journal of Infectious Diseases* **153**, 196–201.

Stocker, B. A. D. and Mäkelä, P. H. (1986). Genetic determination of bacterial virulence, with special reference to *Salmonella*. *Current Topics in Microbiology and Immunology* **124**, 149–72.

Sussman, M. (ed.) (1985). *The virulence of* Escherichia coli. Academic Press, London.

van Die, I., Hoekstra, W., and Bergmans, H. (1987). Analysis of the primary structure of P-fimbrillins of uropathogenic *Escherichia coli*. *Microbial Pathogenesis* **3**, 149–54.

Toxins, general

Dorner, F. and Drews, J. (eds) (1986). *Pharmacology of bacterial toxins*. Pergamon Books, Oxford.

Hardegree, M. C. and Tu, A. T. (eds) (1988). *Bacterial toxins*. Marcel Dekker, New York.

Harshman, S. (ed.) (1988). *Methods in enzymology*, Vol. 165, *Microbial toxins: tools in enzymology*. Academic Press, New York.

Toxins in pathogenesis

Arbuthnott, J. P. (1983). Host damage from bacterial toxins. In *The determinants of bacterial and viral pathogenicity* (ed. H. Smith, J. P. Arbuthnott, and C. A. Mims). The Royal Society, London.

Arbuthnott, J. P. (1988). Extracellular toxins: their role in virulence. In *Immunochemical and molecular genetic analysis of bacterial pathogens* (ed. P. Owen and T. J. Foster). Elsevier, Amsterdam.

Poxton, I. R. and Arbuthnott, J. P. (1991). Determinants of bacterial virulence. In *Topley and Wilson's principles of bacteriology, virology and immunity* (8th edn), Vol. 1 (ed. A. H. Linton and H. M. Dick). Edward Arnold, London, in press.

Toxins, specific reviews

Eidels, L. and Draper, R. K. (1988). Diphtheria toxin. In *Bacterial toxins* (ed. M. C. Hardegree and A. T. Tu). Marcel Dekker, New York.

Finkelstein, R. A. (1988). Structure of the cholera enterotoxin (choleragen) and the immunologically related ADP-ribosylating heatlabile enterotoxins. In *Bacterial toxins* (ed. M. C. Hardegree and A. T. Tu). Marcel Dekker, New York.

Reitschel, E. T., Galanos, C., and Luderitz, O. (1975). Structure, endotoxicity and immunogenicity of the lipid A component of bacterial lipopolysaccharides. In *Microbiology* (ed. D. Schlessinger). American Society for Microbiology, Washington.

Antimicrobial resistance

Appelbaum, P. C. (1987). World-wide development of antibiotic resistance in pneumococci. *European Journal of Clinical Microbiology* **6**, 367–77.

Hackbarth, C. J. and Chambers, H. F. (1989). Methicillin-resistant staphylococci: genetics and mechanisms of resistance. *Antimicrobial Agents and Chemotherapy* **33**, 991–4.

Huovinen, P. (1987). Trimethoprim resistance. *Antimicrobial Agents and Chemotherapy* **31**, 1451–6.

Livermore, D. M. (1987). Clinical significance of beta-lactamase induction and stable derepression in Gram-negative rods. *European Journal of Clinical Microbiology* **6**, 439–45.

Malouin, F. and Bryan, L. E. (1986). Modification of penicillin-binding proteins as mechanisms of β-lactam resistance. *Antimicrobial Agents and Chemotherapy* **30**, 1–5.

Nikaido, H. (1989). Outer membrane barrier as a mechanism of antimicrobial resistance. *Antimicrobial Agents and Chemotherapy* **33**, 1831–6.

Phillips, I. and Shannon, K. (1984). Aminoglycoside resistance. *British Medical Bulletin* **40**, 28–35.

Reynolds, P. E. (1984). Resistance of the antibiotic target site. *British Medical Bulletin* **40**, 3–10.

Tomasz, A., Drugeon, H. B., de Lencastre, H. M., Jabes, D., McDougall, L., and Bille, J. (1989). New mechanisms for methicillin resistance in *Staphylococcus aureus*: clinical isolates that lack the PBP2a gene and contain normal penicillin-binding proteins with modified penicillin-binding capacity. *Antimicrobial Agents and Chemotherapy* **33**, 1869–74.

Wolfson, J. S. (1989). Quinolone antimicrobial agents: adverse effects and bacterial resistance. *European Journal of Clinical Microbiology* **8**, 1080–92.

Host factors

Balkwill, F. R. (1989). Interferons. *Lancet* i, 1060–3.

Cooper, N. R. (1988). Complement and infectious agents. *Reviews of Infectious Diseases* **10** (Suppl. 2), 447–9.

Dhur, A., Galan, P., and Hercberg, S. (1989). Iron status, immune capacity and resistance to infections. *Comparative Biochemistry and Physiology* **94A**, 11–19.

Gardner, I. D. (1980). The effect of aging on susceptibility to infection. *Reviews of Infectious Diseases* **2**, 801–10.

Gluckman, S. J., Dvorak, V. C., and MacGregor, R. R. (1977). Host defences during prolonged alcohol consumption in a controlled environment. *Archives of Internal Medicine* **137**, 1539–43.

O'Garra, A. (1989). Peptide regulatory factors: interleukins and the immune system. *Lancet* i, 943–6; 1003–5.

O'Grady, F. (1985). Antibiotics and host defences. In *The scientific basis of antimicrobial chemotherapy*, (ed. D. Greenwood and F. O'Grady), pp. 341–64, 38th Symposium of the Society for General Microbiology. Cambridge University Press, Cambridge.

Pepys, M. B. (1981). C-reactive protein fifty years on. *Lancet* i, 653.

Proctor, R. A. (1987). Fibronectin: a brief overview of its structure, function and physiology. *Reviews of Infectious Diseases* **9** (Suppl. 4), 317–21.

Rager Zyman, B. and Bloom, B. R. (1985). Interferons and natural killer cells. *British Medical Bulletin* **41**, 22–7.

Sugarman, B. (1983). Zinc and infection. *Reviews of Infectious Diseases* **5**, 137–47.

Tracey, K. J., Vlassava, H., and Cerami, A. (1989). Cachectin/tumour necrosis factor. *Lancet* i, 1122–5.

6.3 Pathogenesis of viral infections

J. S. Porterfield

6.3.1 Introduction

Viruses are obligate subcellular microparasites which are capable of replicating only within susceptible cells. The cells may be of animal, plant, or bacterial origin, and viruses are subdivided according to which of these three types of host they infect. The distinction between viral infection, a cellular event which may or may not result in the death of the infected cell, and viral disease, which affects the entire host and is therefore applicable only to animals and plants, is an important one. In multicellular hosts, viral infection usually progresses through a series of replication cycles involving many cells, some of which may be killed. Viral disease is recognized when the functions of organs or tissues are affected, or when the life of the host is threatened. Some manifestations of viral disease in animals and man are not directly attributable to the effects of the virus, but are examples of immunopathology resulting from the killing of virus-infected cells by the immune system of the host.

Many viral infections are completely silent, being recognized only retrospectively by the detection of antiviral antibodies. The same virus can give rise to a silent infection in one individual, but may cause severe disease or death in another. The outcome of any viral infection is determined by the balance between two competing processes, the first involving the replication of the virus, and the second the mobilization of host immune defences which restrict viral replication. This balance can be affected by viral factors, such as dose, strain, and virulence; by host factors, such as immune status, age, nutrition, and genetic susceptibility; and by environmental factors, which may include the effects of drugs, antiviral chemotherapy, radiation, and other infectious agents, such as bacteria and parasites. We are now beginning to understand something of the molecular basis of viral pathogenicity, but much of this knowledge is fragmentary and is based upon model systems in cell cultures or in laboratory animals rather than on direct evidence from viral disease in man.

Viruses are divided into families, the names of which end in the suffix . . . viridae; some families are further divided into subfamilies, (ending . . . virinae). Within families there are genera, (ending . . . *virus*), and within genera there are individual viruses or species. All viruses in the same family share basic structural and biochemical features, but there may be major differences in pathogenicity between viruses within the same family or genus, or even between strains of the same virus. As a further complication, similar clinical disease syndromes may be associated with viruses in a number of different families.

6.3.2 Infection at the cellular level

Extracellular virus particles, or virions, occur in a variety of different structural forms. The simplest virions contain only the viral genome of either DNA or RNA (but not both) complexed with coat or capsid proteins to form a nucleocapsid. In more complex viruses there may be a double capsid shell, or the nucleocapsid may be surrounded by an envelope comprising other proteins, glycoproteins, or glycolipids. Extracellular virions are incapable of independent replication but have the potential to reproduce themselves if the viral genome is introduced inside susceptible host cells, genome replication following in the cytoplasm or in the nucleus with different viruses. For this to occur, the genome must somehow pass through two barriers, the first being the protective layers of the virus (capsid and/or envelope), and the second the plasma membrane of the host cell. The initial step in this sequence of events involves the attachment of the virion to the surface of the host cell.

A small amount of virus may adhere to the surface of a host cell through non-specific effects, such as those due to electrostatic charge, but most viral entry follows a specific interaction between a viral attachment protein on the surface of the virion and cellular surface receptors of appropriate specificity. The presence or absence of these specific surface receptors largely determines the host range and tissue tropism for animal viruses. For many enveloped viruses, the viral attachment protein is a glycoprotein, whereas in non-enveloped viruses it is one of the capsid proteins (usually non-glycosylated) that takes over this function. While much is known about the viral attachment proteins of several viruses, the precise nature of host cell receptors to which viruses attach is known for relatively few. Although the human immunodeficiency virus (HIV, Retroviridae) has been recognized only recently, its primary receptor is known to be the CD4 antigen expressed on human T-lymphocytes. Only cells which carry that receptor are therefore susceptible to infection with HIV. However, although the presence of the CD4 antigen is necessary for HIV infection, it is not sufficient. Thus, although HIV will not replicate in human cells of the HeLa line nor in mouse L-cells, the virus will replicate in HeLa cells that have been genetically manipulated to express CD4 antigen at their surface, but not in L-cells expressing the same antigen. Similarly, poliovirus receptors are present on cells in the human gastrointestinal tract that serve as entry points for polioviruses (Picornaviridae), but there are no such receptors on human kidney cells *in vivo*. However, if human or monkey kidney cells are cultured *in vitro*, receptors for poliovirus appear, and such cells are then susceptible to poliovirus infection. Chicken cells are insusceptible to polioviruses because they lack these receptors, but they are not non-permissive to poliovirus replication, because if poliovirus RNA is artificially introduced inside chicken cells, a single cycle of viral replication will follow, but there will be no further cell-to-cell spread.

Several enveloped viruses, notably the myxoviruses, bind to determinants containing sialic acid residues, which are often found at the end of the sugar chains of glycoproteins and glycolipids of common cell-surface proteins. However, different viruses within the same family or genus may use different receptors, and a single receptor can bind unrelated viruses.

Viral entry mechanisms

Living cells can take up nutrients and some foreign proteins either by pinocytosis or by receptor-mediated endocytosis (RME). In pinocytosis, a portion of the plasma membrane surrounds the nutrient or foreign material, internalizing it non-specifically inside a minute vesicle. In RME the binding of a ligand to its specific membrane receptor triggers the enclosure of the ligand in clathrin-coated vesicles which are drawn into the cell and delivered to endosomes. The internal pH of endosomes is maintained at pH 5.0–5.5 by proton-translocating ATPases. The low pH tends to dissociate ligands from the receptors; the ligands are absorbed into the cytosol or delivered to lysosomes and the receptors are returned to the cell surface or are degraded.

In the past, a distinction was drawn between the entry pathways of non-enveloped and enveloped viruses. The former were believed to enter by pinocytosis and the latter by receptor-mediated endocytosis (Fig. 6.9). Recent studies with non-enveloped polioviruses shows that, like many enveloped viruses, these too enter cells by the endocytic route. Since much is known about the entry of influenza viruses (Orthomyxoviridae) into host cells, this process will be described in some detail, comparing and contrasting this with the entry pathway for Paramyxoviridae and some other enveloped viruses.

Entry of enveloped viruses

The family Orthomyxoviridae contains two major pathogens, influenza A viruses (which infect birds, horses, seals, and swine, as well as man) and influenza B viruses (which are exclusively pathogens of man); there is also a third minor human pathogen, influenza C virus. Virions are spherical, or sometimes filamentous, and contain helical nucleocapsids enclosed within a matrix protein, outside which is the lipid envelope acquired as the virus buds through the cytoplasmic membrane. The genome comprises eight segments of single-stranded, negative-sense RNA (seven segments in influenza C viruses), and there is an associated viral transcriptase.

Viruses in the family Paramyxoviridae are roughly similar in size to influenza viruses, but have an entirely different internal structure. Their genome consists of a single molecule of linear, single-stranded, negative-sense RNA associated with a transcriptase. The family is divided into three genera; the genus *Paramyxovirus*, which contains several respiratory-tract pathogens (infecting man and wild and domestic animals, including birds) and mumps virus; the genus *Morbillivirus*, which contains measles virus and the related distemper and rinderpest viruses of animals; and the genus *Pneumovirus*, which includes the

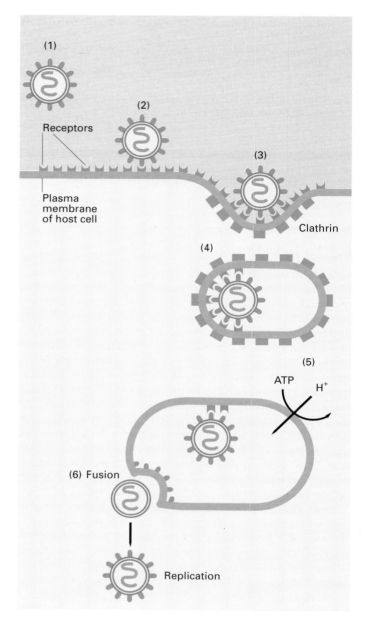

Fig. 6.9 Viral entry at the level of the cell by receptor-mediated endocytosis. (1) Extracellular enveloped virion; (2) glycoprotein on the viral surface binds to a receptor on the plasma membrane of the host cell; (3) attachment progresses through engulfment of the virion in a clathrin-coated pit; (4) endocytosis continues with closure of the plasma membrane and formation of a coated vesicle; (5) the coated vesicle loses its clathrin and fuses with an endosome; (6) the vesicle is acidified by proton-translocating ATPases. The viral envelope membrane fuses with the membrane of the endosome, liberating the viral nucleocapsid into the cytosol, where the replication process commences.

agent of respiratory syncytial disease and related animal pathogens.

Both ortho- and paramyxoviruses have two surface glycoproteins. In the former these are the haemagglutinin (HA), which also has fusogenic properties, and the neuraminidase (N). The haemagglutinin is so called because it attaches to red blood cells and causes them to clump, but more importantly it is the structure by which viruses attach to host cells prior to entry. In orthomyxoviruses the HA and N are separate structures, but in paramyxoviruses the two molecules occur as a single HN protein and there is a separate fusion protein F, which is also found in morbilliviruses and in pneumoviruses, which lack a neuraminidase.

The HA of influenza viruses has been studied intensively at the chemical, structural, and functional levels. The haemagglutinin is a trimeric protein which projects from the lipid envelope of the virus to which it is anchored by a tail composed of hydrophobic amino acids. Each monomer consists of a globular head (HA1) which carries the viral attachment site and neutralization epitopes linked by disulphide bonds to the stalk protein, HA2. HA1 and HA2 are derived by proteolytic cleavage from a single precursor polypeptide. Both the HA and N molecules of influenza A and B viruses are subject to antigenic drift, and a single amino-acid sequence change can alter reactivity with monoclonal antibodies.

The mechanism by which low pH induces fusion has been studied in detail with influenza virus. The N-terminal amino acids of HA2 are hydrophobic and are highly homologous to a portion of the fusion protein of paramyxoviruses. This 'fusion peptide' is buried within the trimeric stalk structure of HA at neutral pH, but upon exposure to pH values of 6.0 or below, the HA trimer undergoes a conformational change to reveal the fusion peptide, which is then free to insert into the endosomal membrane.

Several other enveloped viruses, including Semliki Forest virus (Togaviridae), West Nile virus (Flaviviridae), and many Bunyaviridae also enter cells by fusion with endosomal membranes at mildly acidic pH. After genome replication, progeny virus particles are assembled and are released by budding through the cell membrane with togaviruses, but into intracytoplasmic vesicles with flaviviruses and bunyaviruses.

The presence or absence of host cell proteases may determine whether or not a virus is pathogenic to a particular host. This effect is most clearly seen with viruses in the families Orthomyxoviridae and Paramyxoviridae, much of the evidence having come from laboratory studies with Sendai virus, a member of the second family. Like all other paramyxoviruses, Sendai virus has two surface glycoproteins, HN which has haemagglutinating (surface-binding) and neuraminidase activities, and F which is the fusion protein. After a single cycle of replication, Sendai virions are formed which contain the fusion protein in the form of a biologically inactive precursor, F_0. Such virions are non-infectious, but become infectious when F_0 is cleaved by proteases present in certain cells to the biologically active forms, F_1 and F_2 (see Fig. 6.10). Mutants of Sendai virus require different proteases, and thus have specificities for different cells. This requirement for F-protein cleavage is not simply a laboratory phenomenon, but explains the differences in virulence of field isolates of another paramyxovirus, Newcastle disease virus of chickens.

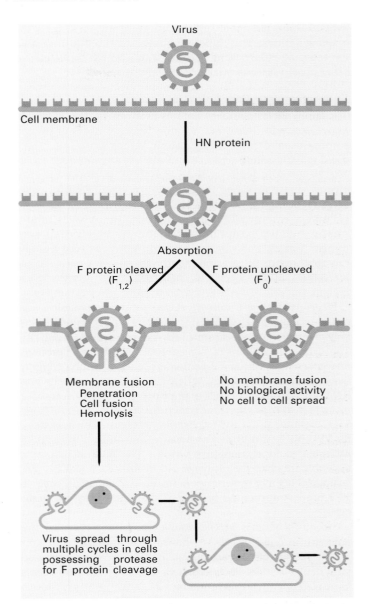

Fig. 6.10 Viral entry at the level of the cell: role of host proteases in the replication of Sendai virus. Virions first attach to the host cell by the binding of viral surface glycoprotein HN to receptors on the plasma membrane. If the host cell possesses the appropriate protease, there is cleavage of biologically inactive F_0 to F_1 and F_2, fusion occurs, penetration takes place, and further replication cycles follow. In cells lacking an appropriate protease, F_0 remains uncleaved, there is no fusion, and no further replication occurs. (Drawn after Choppin and Scheid 1980, with permission.)

Influenza viruses also rely upon a host cell protease for infectivity, and this partly determines the cells in which these viruses will replicate. Severe cases of influenzal pneumonia are not infrequently complicated by the presence of bacteria in the lungs. These were generally thought to be opportunistic organisms, but recent studies have shown that certain strains of *Staphylococcus aureus* secrete a serine protease that is able to activate some, but not all, influenza A viruses by cleavage of the haemagglutinin. This synergism may explain the increased mortality of influenza in persons with chronic bronchitis or other upper respiratory tract bacterial infections.

Entry of non-enveloped viruses

The family Picornaviridae contains four genera, two of which, *Enterovirus* and *Rhinovirus*, contain large numbers of human pathogens, and two further genera, *Aphthovirus* and *Cardiovirus*, contain smaller numbers of (mainly) animal pathogens. The *Enterovirus* genus includes the three serotypes of polioviruses that can cause the crippling or fatal disease, poliomyelitis; also some 30 coxsackie A and B viruses; 72 serotypes of human enteroviruses, including hepatitis A virus; and a smaller number of distinct enterovirus types affecting non-human species. Polioviruses, human rhinovirus type 14, and the aphthovirus of foot-and-mouth disease have been studied intensively at the chemical, structural, and genetic levels, making this one of the best characterized of all viral families.

Picornaviridae are non-enveloped viruses comprising four capsid proteins VP1, VP2, VP3, and VP4, and a protein-linked polyadenylated, single-stranded RNA of positive-sense polarity. The virus coat contains 60 copies of each of the capsid proteins, and is assembled from 12 pentamers, each of which contains five copies of each protein. When virus infects a cell, the viral RNA directs the synthesis of a single polyprotein which is subsequently cleaved to give three structural proteins, VP0, VP1, and VP3, and non-structural (replication) proteins. The next step is for VP0, VP1, and VP3 to associate in pentameric form and to assemble to form immature virions. The final step in viral assembly involves the cleavage of VP0 to VP2 and VP4. VP4 remains hidden in the interior of the virion, and all 60 copies of VP4 are lost during the process of viral entry into susceptible cells.

Structural studies at the atomic level have revealed that polioviruses and rhinoviruses have four immunogenic regions on the surface of the capsid proteins that are concerned with viral neutralization. Each icosahedral face of the virion bears a large cleft or canyon surrounding VP1, which contains the site of the attachment protein that binds to host cells; this site is inaccessible to immunoglobulins, whereas neutralizing antibodies readily reach neutralization sites located around the edge of the cleft. Coxsackie virus A2 and human rhinovirus 14 share the same receptor, and coxsackie virus B3 and adenovirus 2 (Adenoviridae) share another receptor; the cellular receptors for polioviruses are distinct from those of all other Picornaviridae.

Poliomyelitis can be prevented by vaccines prepared either from live, attenuated virus or from inactivated virus. Attenuated variants of the three virulent poliovirus prototypes were derived by serial passage through a variety of cell cultures, followed by virulence testing in monkeys. Analysis of the nucleotide sequences of the parental and attenuated viruses has now established how the vaccine strains differ from their wild-type parents. In the case of poliovirus type 1, a total of 55 nucleotide substitutions were found over the whole length of the genome,

representing 21 amino-acid replacements, seven in VP1, two in VP2, two in VP3, and one in VP4, with the remainder in the non-structural proteins. Similar studies have been carried out with type 3 polioviruses, which revealed only ten point mutations, representing only three amino-acid replacements between the wild type and the vaccine strains. Specific mutations have been introduced into the genome of type 3 poliovirus in order to determine which region is relevant for attenuation. The most important of these has been located in the non-translated region of the RNA, and the next most important mutation is that affecting that portion of the VP1 protein that is responsible for temperature sensitivity of the virus.

Although these sequence differences between wild type and vaccine strains are now established, the molecular basis of neuropathogenicity is still poorly understood. Attenuated virus binds to neural cells as well as does the wild-type virus, showing that there is no defect in adsorption with the vaccine strains. It is presumed that the block occurs at the level of replication, which may involve changes in the non-structural (replication) proteins rather than in the capsid proteins. Studies using genetically engineered cDNA recombinant clones strongly suggest that numerous mutations, and not one or a few, contribute to the attenuated phenotype of poliovirus type 1. Although attenuated poliovirus vaccines have a very good safety record, some reversion towards the virulent phenotype does occur. Sequence studies carried out on polioviruses recovered from the faeces of infants who had received vaccine showed that changes were detectable within four days.

The family Reoviridae contains members that are capable of replicating in a wide range of hosts, including vertebrates and invertebrates, plants and fungi. Analysis of the model system of reovirus infection in the mouse has provided valuable pointers to the pathogenesis of respiratory and gastrointestinal disease in children due to other members of this family. Reoviruses are non-enveloped viruses having ten segments of genomic, double-stranded RNA contained in a core which is enclosed within a second protein shell. Each genomic segment encodes a unique messenger RNA that is translated into a polypeptide. The ten segments are divided on the basis of molecular weight into three large segments (L1, L2, and L3), three medium-sized segments (M1, M2, and M3), and four small segments (S1, S2, S3, and S4), and the proteins are divided on the same basis into $\lambda 1$, $\lambda 2$, and $\lambda 3$ from the large segments, $\mu 1$, $\mu 2$, and $\mu 3$ from the medium segments, and $\sigma 1$, $\sigma 2$, $\sigma 3$, and $\sigma 4$ from the small segments. The viral RNAs and the locations of the viral proteins are presented in Table 6.13. The outer capsid contains three proteins, $\sigma 1$, $\sigma 3$, and $\mu 1C$, the last being derived from $\mu 1$ by proteolytic cleavage; these three proteins play distinct roles in determining the pathogenicity of reoviruses. Reoviruses types 1 and 3 differ with respect to the sensitivity of their capsid proteins to intestinal proteases. By preparing reassorted viruses that contain genome segments derived from different parents, it is possible to assign specific biological functions to distinct viral genes. The S1 gene segment has been found to code for the $\sigma 1$ protein that is responsible for the binding of virions to specific receptors present on host cells. The M2 gene segment codes for

Table 6.13 Relationship between viral RNA and proteins in Reoviridae (adapted from Sharpe and Fields 1985)

Genome segment	Genome M_r	Polypeptide	Polypeptide M_r	Location in virus
L1	2.8×10^6	$\lambda 3$	150 000	Core
L2	2.8×10^6	$\lambda 2$	140 000	Core
L3	2.8×10^6	$\lambda 1$	125 000	Core
M1	1.4×10^6	$\mu 2$	70 000	Core
M2	1.4×10^6	$\mu 1, \mu 1C$	80 000, 72 000	Outer capsid
M3	1.4×10^6	μNS	75 000	Non-structural
S1	0.7×10^6	$\sigma 1$	42 000	Outer capsid
S2	0.7×10^6	$\sigma 2$	38 000	Core
S3	0.7×10^6	σNS	36 000	Non-structural
S4	0.7×10^6	$\sigma 3$	34 000	Outer capsid

the $\mu 1C$ protein that determines whether or not the virus will be inactivated by proteases present in digestive juices in the intestinal tract, and thus controls susceptibility to infection by the alimentary route. The third capsid protein, $\sigma 3$, is responsible for controlling the inhibition of protein synthesis in the host cell, and it also plays a role in establishing persistent, rather than lytic, viral infections.

Polarized cells

Certain cell lines in culture exhibit polarization shown by epithelial tissues *in vivo*. Epithelial cells possess tight junctions which divide the cell membrane into an apical domain and a basal lateral domain. Diffusion of outer leaflet membrane molecules such as gangliosides, phospholipids, and glycoproteins is restricted between these two regions. In addition, such cells show the ability to target some newly synthesized proteins to the apical surface, and others to the basal lateral membrane. Enveloped viruses have been used to define the polarizing signals within the secreted proteins. Thus, vesicular stomatitis virus (Rhabdoviridae), and some herpes viruses and retroviruses bud only from the basal lateral membrane, whereas influenza virus buds only from the apical surface of polarized epithelial cells. These functional differences affect virus spread, and may therefore affect the localization of disease. The pathogenicity of respiratory syncytial virus (*Pneumovirus*, Paramyxoviridae) may be associated with the secretion of virus-induced surface filaments which block airways in the lungs of small children.

6.3.3 Infection at the level of the host

The skin is an effective barrier against most viruses, but it can be penetrated by biting arthropods which can introduce into the capillaries or subcutaneous tissues arthropod-borne viruses such as yellow fever, tick-borne encephalitis, and many other viruses. The skin can also be penetrated by needles, which may introduce hepatitis B virus or the human immunodeficiency virus (HIV). Both of these viruses, together with non-A, non-B hepatitis viruses (hepatitis C virus), and cytomegalovirus (Herpesviridae), may be present in contaminated blood given by transfusion. In Africa, Ebola virus (Filoviridae) caused many severe and fatal infections during an outbreak in which syringe transmission was prominent. The bite of a rabid dog, bat, or other reservoir host may introduce rabies virus into the tissues of a leg or other site, and the bite of a monkey silently infected with herpes virus simiae may result in fatal encephalitis in man. Wart viruses (Papovaviridae) and herpes simplex viruses can spread from person to person, and are able to infect through the skin, possibly through minor abrasions; cowpox, Orf, and the rarer monkeypox viruses (Poxviridae) can also infect man in this way (see Fig. 6.11).

Although much smaller in area in relation to the skin, the conjunctivae are probably more important as entry points for viruses. Measles and rubella viruses, and some adenoviruses, can enter that way, as can certain enteroviruses, notably human enterovirus type 70, an important cause of epidemic conjunctivitis.

Very many viruses enter the body via the respiratory and gastrointestinal tracts, members of some viral families such as the Orthomyxoviridae, Paramyxoviridae, and Coronaviridae entering almost exclusively by the former, whereas Adenoviridae and Picornaviridae are capable of infecting through either route. Reoviridae are principally enteric pathogens, but some can enter by the respiratory tract. Caliciviridae probably enter only through the gut.

Viruses in several families are capable of entering via the urogenital route. These include some members of the Herpesviridae, notably herpes simplex virus type 2 and cytomegalovirus, and certain Papovaviridae. Lassa fever and Junin fever viruses (Arenaviridae) have both been shown to be capable of transmission by sexual intercourse, and HIV is certainly capable of transmission by this route.

All the examples so far mentioned have been of horizontal transmission, but vertical transmission through the placenta is also possible. Rubella virus (Togaviridae), cytomegalovirus (Herpesviridae), and the human immunodeficiency virus (HIV, Retroviridae) are all capable of crossing the placenta barrier and infecting the developing fetus, as can other viruses such as Japanese encephalitis virus (Flaviviridae) and certain Picornaviridae, although rarely.

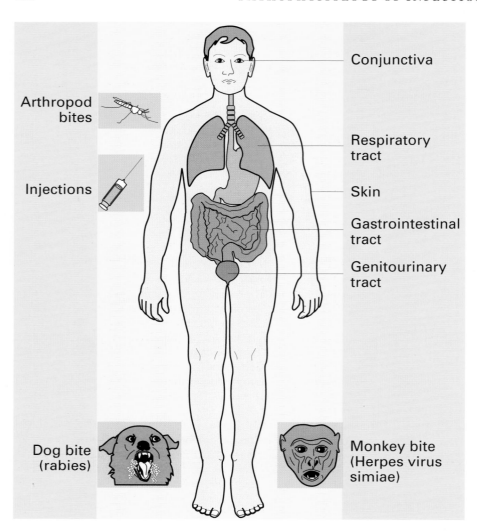

Arthropod bites

Injections

Dog bite (rabies)

Conjunctiva

Respiratory tract

Skin

Gastrointestinal tract

Genitourinary tract

Monkey bite (Herpes virus simiae)

Fig. 6.11 Viral entry at the level of the host. Conjunctiva: measles, rubella, some adenovirus and enterovirus types. Respiratory tract: rhinoviruses, coronaviruses, orthomyxoviruses, paramyxoviruses, adenoviruses, and herpes viruses. Gastrointestinal tract: picornaviruses, caliciviruses, reoviruses, and adenoviruses. Genitourinary tract: herpes viruses, papilloma viruses, retroviruses, and arenaviruses; trans-placental infection (rubella, cytomegalovirus). Skin: abrasions (poxviruses, herpes viruses), bites (rabies virus, arboviruses, B virus), and injections (hepatitis viruses, cytomegalovirus, human immunodeficiency virus).

6.3.4 Cell-to-cell spread

Once a virus has undergone a complete cycle of replication and has been released, either by cell lysis, or by budding, progeny virus particles can spread to neighbouring cells to initiate further replication cycles. Extracellular virus, however, may encounter antiviral antibody and cellular host defence mechanisms which can render it non-infectious. Some viruses, such as most Paramyxoviridae, are able to bring about the fusion of the plasma membranes of adjacent cells and, when this happens, virus spreads freely from cell to cell unrestrained by host defences. Rabies virus (genus *Lyssavirus*, Rhabdoviridae) is unusual in its ability to infect nerve cells. Members of this family have bullet-shaped virions with a genome of negative-stranded RNA. The genome codes for five proteins, an external glycoprotein (G) which functions as the attachment protein, a nucleocapsid protein (N), two membrane proteins (M1 and M2), and a large protein (L). The nature of the cellular receptor for rabies virus is still uncertain. There is some evidence that the nicotinic acetylcholine receptor functions as a viral receptor, but other

studies point to phospholipids or glycolipids. Whatever the precise mode of entry into nerve cells, transport therein is by retrograde axonal flow, and the incubation time for the onset of clinical disease reflects the distance to be travelled from the point of entry to the axon and subsequent further spread within the central nervous system. A number of mutants of the G protein of rabies virus show differences in neuropathogenicity, but to date the molecular basis of rabies virus virulence is still uncertain.

6.3.5 Spread to target organs

Some viruses produce their effects locally at the site of entry, while others cause disease by affecting internal tissues or organs distant from the initial point of viral entry. Where the effects are produced locally, as in a common cold, the incubation period (the time between first exposure to virus and the onset of clinical signs or symptoms of disease) is normally short. When an organ such as the liver or the brain is involved the incubation time is usually longer, because the virus has to undergo a series of cycles of replication before it reaches and damages the particular target organ (Fig. 6.12). After entry into the body through a peripheral route, such as the skin or mucous membranes, many viruses are carried to regional lymph nodes where they may be degraded. Some viruses, however, undergo a phase of multiplication in regional lymph nodes and are then released into the bloodstream where they give rise to a transient viraemia, or they may be transported in the lymph to distant sites. Other viruses may be transported to distant sites within monocytes which then lodge elsewhere in the body, releasing virus which can then invade other cells. Many viruses have tropisms for particular tissues. The body can tolerate the death of cells in non-critical tissues such as skin, muscle, or lining of the intestinal tract, whereas the death of cells in the brain, heart, liver, or pancreas can have more serious consequences.

In terms of disease severity, the brain is probably the most critical target for viral infection, and viruses in many different families are capable of replicating within the central nervous system. As already mentioned, rabies virus reaches the brain by travelling along nerve axons, but this is an unusual mode of entry. Most neurotropic viruses enter the brain from the bloodstream, although the precise mechanism by which virus crosses

the blood–brain barrier is not known. In certain cases, infection occurs via the brain capillaries, possibly by the migration of virus-infected monocytes, and in other instances infection enters through the choroid plexus. Viral encephalitis can be due to a variety of different enterovirus and coxsackie virus types, polioviruses, herpes viruses and mumps virus, several alphaviruses, flaviviruses, bunyaviruses, and orbiviruses (Reoviridae), and certain retroviruses; the target cells being neurones in different parts of the brain. Lymphocytic choriomeningitis (LCM) virus (Arenaviridae) differs from most other neurotropic virus in that it provokes an intense cellular infiltration spreading in from the meninges. As discussed in the section on immunopathology, the disease manifestations of LCM virus infection are a consequence of the vigorous cellular immune reaction of the host, and they are prevented if the host is immunosuppressed (see Section 6.3.9). Immunosuppression can, however, provoke disease due to latent viruses, as is discussed in Section 6.6.2 on chronic infections.

The intact skin provides an effective barrier against most viruses. Human wart virus (Papovaviridae) is capable of multiplying in the epidermal tissues, producing local proliferative lesions from which virus may spread to different skin areas. Herpes simplex virus produces its effects locally at the site of viral entry, but most viruses which produce skin lesions, such as chicken-pox (varicella virus, Herpesviridae), measles virus (rubeola virus, Paramyxoviridae), and rubella virus (rubivirus, Togaviridae) do not normally enter through the skin, but gain entrance through the upper respiratory tract or conjunctiva, spreading through the bloodstream to produce local effects in the skin. The rash that develops is caused by local capillary damage augmented by a cellular infiltration which causes a variable amount of swelling and local irritation. Several tropical diseases, such as dengue, sandfly, Chikungunya, and O'nyong-nyong fevers are associated with erythematous rashes caused by infection with different arthropod-borne viruses.

The upper respiratory tract provides a portal of entry for viruses in a number of different families. The clinical syndrome which is recognized as the common cold may be due to a rhinovirus, a coronavirus (Coronaviridae), an adenovirus, a parainfluenza virus, a classical influenza virus, a reovirus, or possibly other viruses. Irrespective of the virus, the sequence of events is likely to be similar. Virus shed in droplets from an infected individual is carried through the air until it impinges upon the upper respiratory tract of another person. Non-specific defence mechanisms, such as a layer of mucus, may prevent the infection of susceptible cells and the virus may be removed before it can do any harm. In other circumstances, virus may attach to receptors on susceptible epithelial cells, these cells are entered, virus replicates therein, producing cell death and the liberation of more infectious virus. The dead epithelial cells, mixed with inflammatory cells and fluid, are shed from the surface of the respiratory tract, producing the nasal secretion which is characteristic of the common cold, while the general constitutional effects, congestion and sometimes fever, result from the inflammatory response mediated by a variety of chemical substances, including interleukin-1 and γ-interferon,

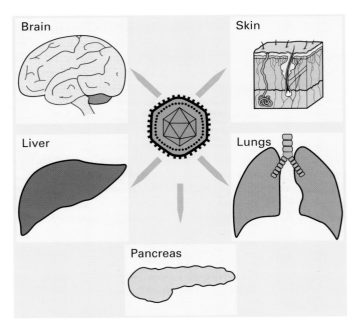

Fig. 6.12 Target organs for viruses. Following entry and initial replication at peripheral sites, viruses may spread, usually via the bloodstream, to target organs where they replicate and produce disease. The brain may be a target organ for poliovirus and other picornaviruses, for herpes, mumps, and measles viruses, several flaviviruses and togaviruses, and for rabies virus. The liver may be a target organ for hepatitis A, B, C, D, and E viruses and for yellow fever virus. The pancreas may be a target organ for certain coxsackie and cardiovirus serotypes, and also rubella, mumps, and reoviruses. The skin may be a target organ for herpes viruses, poxviruses, and papilloma viruses. The lungs, although usually infected via the respiratory tract, may be a target organ for blood-borne spread of measles, mumps, and cytomegaloviruses.

that accompany the specific cell-killing effects. In a severe rhinovirus infection much of the epithelial surface of the lining of the nose may be shed, but over the course of a few days a new epithelial layer regenerates and the subject recovers from his or her cold.

Several viruses, including coxsackie virus B4, encephalomyocarditis (EMC) virus, and reovirus 3 have been shown to have tropism for the β-cells of the pancreas and induce a diabetes-like syndrome in mice. There is evidence that coxsackie viruses and mumps virus may be responsible for some cases of juvenile-onset diabetes in children, the risk being higher with certain HLA types (DR3 and DR4).

6.3.6   Fetal and neonatal infections

The cells of the developing fetus are highly sensitive to infection with several viruses. Rubella virus (Togaviridae) is probably the best known viral cause of fetal death and congenital malformations in man, and *pestiviruses* (also Togaviridae) are responsible for very similar effects in cattle, sheep, and pigs. Cytomegaloviruses (Herpesviridae) are another important cause of neonatal disease in man. While the evidence that viruses in the family Parvoviridae are significant causes of teratogenic effects in man is fragmentary at present, there is substantial evidence that autonomous parvoviruses cause severe fetal and neonatal disease in several animal species. Parvoviruses enter cells through a receptor which contains sialic acid residues, and replicate only in actively dividing cells; hence their affinity for fetal tissues. When inoculated into neonatal hamsters, parvoviruses give rise to runting, 'mongoloid-like' deformities, and cerebellar dysplasia. Adult tissues, which have fewer dividing cells, are relatively resistant to parvovirus infection, but feline panleukopenia virus, mink enteritis virus, and canine parvovirus are closely related exceptions in which virus replicates well in the epithelial cells of the gastrointestinal tract, producing severe disease in animals. The human parvovirus B19 infects a subset of erythroid progenitor cells which are in active division, causing a juvenile erythematous fever, erythema infectiosum, or 'fifth disease', in otherwise healthy children, and precipitating aplastic crises in persons with hereditary haemolytic anaemia. Parvovirus B19 also causes hydrops fetalis *in utero* due to infection of fetal erythroid cells with the production of haemolytic anaemia and cardiac failure.

6.3.7   Viral cytopathology

The term 'viral cytopathology' is usually applied to describe the changes induced in cultured cells following viral infection. These may be gross, resulting in cell death, or they may be more subtle, causing structural and functional changes in cells that may be detected by a variety of different methods. A viral cytopathic effect (cpe) usually implies that viral replication has taken place, but ultraviolet irradiated virus in high doses may produce a cpe, and certain viral proteins, such as the fibre protein of adenoviruses, may be directly cytopathic without the

need for infectious virus. Since viruses differ widely in their replication strategies, it is not surprising that there is no single basis for viral cytopathology. The same virus may be cytopathic in one cell type but non-cytopathic in another. Thus, alphaviruses, flaviviruses, and bunyaviruses, which are capable of replicating in both vertebrate and invertebrate cells, are usually cytopathic in the former, but are normally non-cytopathic in the latter. There is no consistent link between the ability of a virus to produce a cpe *in vitro* and its pathogenicity *in vivo*, but cell-culture systems have provided valuable insights into the mechanisms of disease production in man and in animals.

Viral cytopathology may arise because the infecting virus represses host cell macromolecular synthesis, preventing the transcription and translation of host messenger RNA (mRNA). Eukaryotic protein synthesis is a complex multistage process, and viruses are capable of maximizing the expression of their own genes at the expense of the synthesis of host proteins by interfering with the normal events of eukaryotic gene expression. Viruses in several different families, such as picornaviruses, adenoviruses, and poxviruses, are known to be capable of bringing about a selective suppression of translation of host mRNA.

All eukaryotic cells have a 'cap' structure present at the 5' end of cytoplasmic (non-organelle) mRNA. The cap structure is concerned with the formation of stable complexes between 40S ribosomal subunits and mRNA that are needed for the initiation of translation. Several different initiation factors contribute to this process, acting through different cap binding proteins (CBP). Many viral RNAs possess a similar cap structure, but polioviruses and some plant viruses are different in that their RNA is uncapped. Poliovirus infection does not lead to the degradation of host mRNA, nor does it change the patterns of host cell mRNA capping, methylation, or polyadenylation. The specific block induced by poliovirus replication occurs at the level of translation of host cell protein synthesis, and appears to involve the specific inactivation by a virus-dependent protease of a p200 component of a CBP complex that is required for normal host cell protein synthesis. Since poliovirus mRNA is translated by a cap-independent mechanism, the synthesis of viral proteins proceeds unhindered. The precise mechanism by which proteolytic cleavage of the CBP complex results in functional loss is still controversial. Within the Picornaviridae, polioviruses and cardioviruses switch off protein synthesis by different blocks, and viruses in other families may achieve a similar functional loss by quite different pathways.

6.3.8   Host reactions

The consequences of viral infection are determined by the type of cell or cells infected; their number and location; the immune status of the host at the time of infection; and upon the speed and magnitude of the host's immune response. Intracellular virus is not normally accessible to the immune defences of the host, but if a cell expresses viral antigens at its surface, that cell is recognized as foreign and becomes subject to immune surveillance. Viral infection triggers a complex sequence of cellular responses which tend to limit the further spread of the virus.

The various branches of the immune response have different, but overlapping, roles in the defence of the host against viral infection. The earliest cellular response is the secretion of interferon, which reaches its peak within 1 or 2 days of infection. Interferon induces an antiviral state in cells adjacent to those initially infected, thus limiting spread. Natural killer cells contribute in the early stages but lack specificity for the virus. Cytotoxic T-lymphocytes play an important role in the termination of a viral infection and also contribute to the production of an immune state. The antibody response is relatively late in the course of an infection, but is important in protecting the host from re-infection with the same virus. Patients with agammaglobulinaemia, who cannot mount a satisfactory antibody response, nevertheless recover well from most viral infections, whereas patients with Di George syndrome, who are deficient in T-lymphocytes, are highly susceptible to viral diseases.

Following early non-specific host reactions are a series of virus-specific effects, involving antigen-presenting cells which include macrophages and dendritic cells; these process viral proteins, and present antigenic fragments to T- and B-lymphocytes. In the case of helper T-lymphocytes (which usually express CD4/T4), viral antigens are presented at the surface of macrophages or dendritic cells in association with class II antigens of the major histocompatibility (MHC) locus, whereas cytotoxic T-lymphocytes (CTL, which usually express CD8/T8) bind to viral antigens presented by infected macrophages in association with class I MHC antigens. Macrophages also secrete interleukin-1 (IL-1), which contributes to the activation of helper (T4) cells. In their turn, helper (T4) cells secrete interleukin-2 (IL-2); this stimulates cytotoxic (T8) cells that have recognized an antigen (together with MHC class I antigen) to divide, thus increasing the number of specific cytotoxic T-cells. Other CD8$^+$ cells later function as suppressor cells, switching off the proliferative response when this is no longer needed.

Activated T-helper cells also secrete a number of other molecules, including IL-4 and IL-5, which stimulate B-cells to mature, divide, and later differentiate either into plasma cells which secrete specific antiviral antibody, or into memory cells. Thus, for most viral antigens, B-cell maturation is dependent upon T4-helper-cell activation. The antibody produced by plasma cells can bind to free virus particles, neutralizing their infectivity. Antibody may neutralize virus by preventing viral attachment to cells, by preventing acid-mediated fusion in endosomes, or by restricting replication in later stages of the infection pathway. After virus has been eliminated, memory cells persist, and can be speedily reactivated upon further exposure to the same viral antigen.

Cytotoxic T-lymphocytes inactivate virus indirectly, by killing the cells in which virus is replicating. If a CTL of appropriate antigenic specificity makes contact with an infected cell, it attaches to the cell by its antigen receptors and it then secretes perforin (a protein which forms large holes in the target cell plasma membrane) and serine esterases into the cleft between two cells, thereby killing the infected cell.

6.3.9 Viral immunopathology

Host immune defences contribute to the recovery from the majority of viral infections, but with certain viral infections disease is directly attributable to the harmful effects of host immune responses. Lymphocytic choriomeningitis (LCM) virus (Arenaviridae) provides the clearest example of viral immunopathology. LCM virus, like other members of the same family, such as Lassa fever virus and Junin (or Argentinian haemorrhagic fever virus), infects wild rodents in nature and frequently causes persistent infections in its natural host, the house mouse, *Mus musculus*. If inoculated into new-born mice, LCM virus produces no overt disease, although the virus multiplies in the mice, producing a persistent, tolerant infection, and there may be late disease after several months. In adult mice, LCM virus produces severe meningoencephalitis and death after intracerebral inoculation, but no disease develops if the mice are immunosuppressed. If T-lymphocytes are prepared from the spleen removed from a non-immunosuppressed adult mouse which has been recovering from LCM virus infection and these are inoculated into a mouse with a persistent, tolerant infection, disease develops within a few days, due to the killing of virus-infected cells by immune T-cells. This T-cell response is histocompatibility restricted, being seen only when the T-cells are of the same MHC type as those of the mouse with the tolerant infection.

Macrophages, as has been noted, are one of the first of the cellular immune defences mounted against a virus. However, some viruses are able to replicate inside macrophages or monocytes, and antiviral antibodies at defined concentrations and of appropriate specificity may paradoxically increase viral entry into macrophages and enhance the yield of infectious virus released by these cells. Dengue haemorrhagic fever, an important cause of sickness and death affecting children, mainly in South-East Asia, is believed to be an example of antibody-dependent enhancement of viral infectivity in human peripheral blood mononuclear cells. There are four different dengue virus serotypes, each of which is capable of producing classical dengue fever, after which the subject is solidly immune against reinfection with the same serotype, but remains susceptible to infection with any of the other three serotypes. There is little or no cross-protection, and secondary infections with heterotypic dengue viruses can cause dengue haemorrhagic fever and/or the dengue shock syndrome, which can be fatal. A dramatic example of viral immunopathology was seen in Cuba in 1981 when there were more than 10 000 cases of severe dengue on the island, and 158 deaths, mainly in children, but some in adults. Severe disease was attributable to type 2 virus infection in 1981, following four years after an extensive, but benign, epidemic of classical dengue fever due to type 1 virus in 1978/79.

6.3.10 Viral persistence

This is considered in detail in Section 6.6.2.

6.3.11   Viral transformation and oncogenesis

Although the association between viruses and malignant tumours in animals and birds has been established for many years, the role of viruses in the causation of human cancer has been questioned until recently. Now, however, there can be no doubt that viruses are important causes of naturally occurring malignant tumours in man as well as in animals. Experimental studies on viral carcinogenesis have revealed the interplay between host genes and viral genes, and the recognition of viral and cellular oncogenes has 'transformed' our views on the causation of cancer.

Among the DNA viruses, Adenoviridae, Hepadnaviridae, Herpesviridae, and Papovaviridae have all been shown to be oncogenic. At least three adenovirus serotypes are oncogenic in the laboratory, but none has been clearly associated with naturally occurring human tumours. The association between hepatitis B virus and hepatocellular carcinoma is now beyond doubt. Epstein–Barr virus is causally linked with Burkitt's lymphoma in children, mainly in Africa, and with nasopharyngeal carcinoma in China; two other herpesviruses are less firmly associated with human malignancies, cytomegalovirus with Kaposi sarcoma and herpes simplex with carcinoma of the cervix. Human papilloma viruses cause benign tumours (warts) and some genotypes are causally linked to malignant tumours of the skin while others are becoming increasingly linked to cervical carcinoma.

Among the genes of certain DNA viruses which are the first to be expressed in infected cells are some which modify 'global' gene expression so as to facilitate the expression of later viral genes concerned with replication and assembly. Some of these early viral genes are capable of inducing excessive expression of host cell genes responsible for growth regulation as well as assisting later viral genes, and this activation of cellular genes may be one of the steps that allows a normal cell to transform into a malignant cell. For example, one of the immediate early genes of Epstein–Barr virus is responsible for the immortalization of B-lymphocytes *in vitro*.

The most compelling evidence for a link between viruses and cancer comes from studies on RNA viruses in the family Retroviridae which have a DNA phase in their replication, enabling them to be integrated into the genome of host cells as a provirus. Much of our understanding of oncogenes came from early studies on Rous sarcoma virus in chickens and on a variety of leukaemia viruses found in laboratory mice. These viruses have incorporated a copy of a cellular gene into their own genome, and are capable of producing tumours in their animal hosts with high frequency. The viral oncogene, *src*, and its cellular counterpart, the proto-oncogene, are capable of influencing the growth-factor-mediated control of cellular proliferation. The viral oncogene produces its effect either because it is expressed from the viral promoter in excessive amounts or because it has acquired mutations which alter its activity.

The majority of animal retroviruses take longer to produce tumours than is the case with Rous sarcoma virus, and these produce their effects by integrating into the host cell chromosome close to a proto-oncogene, thereby activating it. The retroviral promoter directs transcription 'outwards' from the retroviral genome and into flanking cellular genes.

Another retrovirus, the human T-cell leukaemia virus, HTLV-I, possesses a *trans*-acting activating gene, *tax*, which is capable of enhancing the expression of other viral genes. The regulatory sequences with which the Tax protein interacts are also found in the genes for interleukin-2 and its receptor. Since IL-2 is the T-cell growth factor, infection of T-cells with HTLV-I results in an autocrine stimulation of cellular proliferation.

It is now widely accepted that carcinogenesis is multifactorial in its aetiology, involving genetic and environmental elements, which include viruses. Viral genes may provide the transformation genes of DNA tumour viruses. Cellular oncogenes are involved in the control of cell growth, through growth factors, receptors for growth factors, and through the expression of genes acting in the nucleus or activating DNA synthesis. Different oncogenes may act synergistically, the end-result of a multi-stage progression being malignancy. This is discussed fully in Chapter 9.

6.3.12   Recovery from viral infections

Relatively few viral infections result in the death of the host; the majority are followed by recovery and a degree of protection against reinfection with the same virus that may be transient or lifelong. As has been stated earlier, viral infection provokes both non-specific and specific host responses, which involve both the cellular and humoral arms of the immune response. Since these two arms are intimately interwoven, it is difficult to analyse with certainty the respective contributions of each to the recovery process.

6.3.13   Further reading

Viral entry mechanisms

Helenius, A., *et al.* (1980). On the entry of Semliki Forest virus into BHK-21 cells. *Journal of Cell Biology* **84**, 404–20.

Marsh, M. (1984). The entry of enveloped viruses into cells by endocytosis. *Biochemical Journal* **218**, 1–10.

Viral receptors

Choppin, P. W. and Scheid, A. (1980). The role of viral glycoproteins in adsorption, penetration, and pathogenicity of viruses. *Reviews of Infectious Diseases* **2**, 40–61.

Co, M. S., Field, B. N., and Greene, M. I. (1986). Viral receptors serving host functions. In *Concepts in viral pathogenesis*, *II* (ed. A. L. Notkins and M. B. A. Oldstone), pp. 126–31. Springer-Verlag, New York.

Paulson, J. C. (1985). Interaction of animal viruses with cell surface receptors. In *The Receptors*, Vol. 2 (ed. P. M. Conn), pp. 131–219. Academic Press, New York.

Simons, K. and Fuller, S. D. (1986). Cell surface polarity in epithelia. *Annual Review of Cell Biology* **1**, 243–88.

Cytopathic effects

Klenk, H. D. and Rott, R. (1987). Synergistic role of staphylococcal proteases in the induction of influenza virus infection. *Virology* **157**, 421–30.

Wagner, R. R. (1984). Cytopathic effects of viruses: a general survey. In *Comprehensive virology*, Vol. 19 (ed. F. Fraenkel-Conrat and R. R. Wagner), pp. 1–63. Plenum Press, New York.

Pathogenesis (general)

Notkins, A. L. and Yoon, J.-L. (1984). Virus induced diabetes mellitus. In *Concepts in viral pathogenesis* (ed. A. L. Notkins and M. B. A. Oldstone), pp. 244–7. Springer-Verlag, New York.

Sharpe, A. H. and Fields, B. N. (1985). Pathogenesis of viral infections. Basic concepts derived from the reovirus model. *New England Journal of Medicine* **312**, 486–97.

Specific viruses

Air, G. M. and Laver, W. G. (1986). The molecular basis of antigenic variation in influenza virus. *Advances in Virus Research* **31**, 53–102.

Cotmore, S. F. and Tattersall, P. (1987). Autonomous parvoviruses. *Advances in Virus Research* **33**, 91–174.

Kawaoka, Y. and Webster, R. G. (1988). Molecular mechanism of acquisition of virulence in influenza virus in nature. *Microbial Pathogenesis* **5**, 311–18.

Sonenberg, N. (1987). Regulation of translation of poliovirus. *Advances in Virus Research* **33**, 175–204.

Wimmer, E., Emini, E. O., and Diamond, D. D. (1986). Mapping neutralization domains of viruses. In *Concepts in viral pathogenesis, II*, (ed. A. L. Notkins and M. B. A. Oldstone), pp. 159–73. Springer-Verlag, New York.

Viral transformation and oncogenesis

Weiss, R. A. (1985). Unravelling the complexities of carcinogenesis. In *Viruses and cancer* (ed. P. W. J. Rigby and N. M. Wilkie), Society for General Microbiology Symposium 37, pp. 1–21. Cambridge University Press, Cambridge.

6.4 Spread of infection

6.4.1 Mechanisms of spread

Heather M. Dick

Introduction

The ubiquity of micro-organisms and the ease with which some produce disease in man or other species, both in individuals and in groups of individuals in the community or within social groups, point to the existence of effective methods of spread for many micro-organisms, as well as to their possession of a variety of means by which they can invade the tissues—often referred to collectively as virulence mechanisms. For some organisms which are wholly parasitic and dependent on the host's cells for nutrition and even DNA, successful invasion and replication is a prerequisite to survival. Such is the case for most viruses, some bacteria that grow intracellularly, and even some parasites. Sometimes, more than one host is required to sustain the full life cycle, as with malaria, where both man and the mosquito are required to permit this protozoan parasite to go through both sexual and asexual phases of growth and multiplication. Spread may occur from either exogenous sources, originating outside the infected animal, or from endogenous sources, from pre-existing sites in the body, such as the skin or gut, as is frequently the case with infections in immunosuppressed patients. Many micro-organisms occur as part of the normal flora of some body sites, including the mouth and throat, the gut, and the vagina (see Section 6.2.4) and are rarely, if ever, the cause of clinical infection, whereas others, possessed of a particularly effective set of virulence factors, are almost always the cause of disease if an individual is exposed to them. Examples of the latter include the smallpox virus and typhoid bacillus. In individuals whose defence mechanisms are less than optimal, even organisms of relatively low virulence may gain a foothold and go on to multiply and cause disease, either localized or disseminated (see Section 6.2.4). There are organisms which are primarily infectious for animals and which rarely, if ever, cause disease in man. Occasionally close proximity or occupational exposure leads to the transfer of infection from the primary animal host, such as birds, goats and cattle, or dogs, as occurs with psittacosis, brucellosis, ringworm, and rabies, respectively.

Routes of infection
Airborne

The recognized routes and vehicles for the spread of micro-organisms are given in Table 6.14. It is relatively easy to identify the more obvious routes, such as inhalation or ingestion. Airborne transmission, particularly by droplets of moisture or saliva is a very common route by which infection can be acquired. Upper respiratory tract infections are probably the most rapidly spreading infectious conditions in the community, testifying to the ease and effectiveness of this route of spread, for viruses such as the common cold viruses, influenza, and glandular fever (Epstein–Barr virus) and for bacterial infections,

---

Table 6.14 Routes of spread and acquisition of organisms

Routes of spread
  Ingestion
  Inhalation
  Injection (including bites)
  Intra-uterine and perinatal

Vehicles for the spread of micro-organisms
  Food, milk, water, etc.
  Blood and injected fluids
  Animals, including man
  Insect and animal bites
  Inert objects—'fomites'
  Air, dust, soil

ranging from streptococcal sore throat to tuberculosis. Some fungal infections may also be acquired by this route. Similarly, most of the infectious diseases of childhood, such as measles, mumps, and whooping cough, are spread by the airborne (aerosol) route.

Ingestion

Ingestion of contaminated food, milk, or water is the route of infection for many bacteria and viruses which preferentially choose the gut for their primary site of multiplication, including the many types of salmonellae and other bacteria which cause food-poisoning, poliovirus and many of the enteroviruses (so named because of their predilection for gut tissues), the cholera vibrios, and many protozoal and worm (helminth) infections, such as amoebic dysentery, cryptosporidium, and tapeworms of several species.

Faecal–oral

At times, infection by the alimentary route occurs by transference from contaminated hands or objects, rather than directly by swallowing the affected food or liquid. Spread of infection in these cases is by the faecal–oral route, the infecting organism coming from the faeces of another infected case and transferred to another individual because of the handling of objects with hands which have not been properly washed or where hygiene is difficult to maintain. Examples might include those related to very young children; institutionalized severely handicapped patients; overcrowded conditions, for example in refugee camps; under combat conditions; or after natural disasters, where adequate facilities may not be available to minimize the risk of transfer, and clean water supplies are not plentiful.

Injection and bites

Infection may also be spread by those procedures which breach the intact skin, sometimes referred to as the 'injection' route, but since many of these mainly bacterial infections follow after surgical or other invasive procedures, the route of infection may not strictly be limited to sites of injection. The increased use of invasive procedures, such as intravenous therapy, obviously increases the risk of acquiring infection for many patients. Blood and blood products are also implicated in occasional infections, both of patients who may receive blood transfusions, platelet transfusions, or injections of blood products as part of their treatment, and of staff who receive accidental needle stick injuries or who are exposed to large amounts of freshly spilled blood or body fluids. Hepatitis B and non-A, non-B hepatitis (recently rechristened hepatitis C virus) and the human immunodeficiency virus (HIV-1) may all be transmitted by these materials, as can malaria, and, on very rare occasions, syphilis. This potential hazard emphasizes the value of a good screening programme, both for donors and for the blood itself, such as is available in the Western world, but not always in countries with fewer resources and health care facilities. Some agricultural methods seem designed to ensure the continued spread of parasites, such as schistosomes, which have a life cycle involving an aquatic snail, where the infection of man occurs from penetration of the skin by the free-swimming stage of the parasite, which is acquired as a result of standing or bathing in rivers or irrigation channels. Similarly, leptospirosis in man is often the sequel to immersion in water contaminated by the urine of rats, for example in sewage workers, rice planters, or after accidental immersion. Insect bites are the route of transmission of many infections, including malaria, yellow fever, and dengue. Occasionally animal bites or scratches, often from domestic pets, can give rise to sepsis, mainly because of the presence of anaerobic bacteria in the mouths of cats or dogs.

Sexual route

Infectious organisms may also be acquired by the sexual route: for some viruses and a few bacteria, this may be the commonest route of acquisition, presumably because the organism has evolved optimal survival mechanisms suited particularly to the conditions prevailing in the genital tract and to the close contact between the individuals. *Treponema pallidum* and *Neisseria gonorrhoeae* together with some viruses, including herpes type 2, are generally acquired by the sexual route, which is now also recognized as an important route for the transmission of both HIV-1 and hepatitis B. Infections may also be acquired *in utero* or at the time of birth, including rubella, hepatitis B, and cytomegalovirus.

'Multiple' routes

It should be recognized that some organisms may use different routes on separate occasions to gain access to the tissues, as with staphylococci and many streptococci. Others, particularly the viruses, tend to be acquired by a single main route, e.g. measles by the upper respiratory tract and rabies from the bite of a rabid animal. Sometimes the route of acquisition is critical in determining the type of infection which subsequently develops: thus, *Yersinia pestis* which enters via the bite of the rat flea will take the form of bubonic plague, with systemic manifestations due to infection carried via the bloodstream to many organs, including the liver and lymph nodes throughout the body; whereas the infection acquired by the respiratory route (generally in the course of nursing a case of plague) will often manifest itself as pneumonic plague in the first instance.

The importance of the hands as the means of transfer of infection cannot be overemphasized and does not only apply to intestinal infection. The transference of organisms, known as cross-infection, between staff and patients in hospital or in any nursing situation is all too common. Such hospital-acquired infections are a major problem in terms of morbidity and cost (see Section 6.7). The causative organisms can be of almost any species and the risk of subsequent infection will depend on the virulence of the species involved and on the severity of illness or susceptibility of the patient.

Factors affecting spread

It is possible to identify several factors which may influence spread, or which may be critical for the subsequent development of an infection. Where infection is acquired from exogenous sources, many variables in the environmental conditions or in the vehicle of spread can affect the likelihood of successful spread—that is, success for the micro-organism in reaching a new and susceptible host. Hostile features which may diminish the chances of viable organisms reaching another host include the size of the dose required to produce an infection, the presence of suitably sized dust particles to act as carriers, the distance to be travelled to reach a new host, sunlight, dehydration, and the presence of effective concentrations of disinfectant. Numerous examples can be cited. Tubercle bacilli will survive for months in dust which is not exposed to ultraviolet irradiation, anthrax bacilli in soil or dust can develop into the spore form, when they are highly resistant to adverse conditions, such as lack of nutrients and moisture, and many fungi are able to survive in a non-replicating state when conditions are unsuitable for growth, reverting to their vegetative form when better times arrive. Viruses are relatively more dependent on suitable environmental conditions, relying as they do on the presence of the biochemical systems of other cells for their survival and replication. However, they too have devised strategies to ensure survival and transfer, including the ability to become latent within the genetic material of another cell and, in a few instances, some capacity to resist adverse environmental conditions such as dehydration although, in most cases, probably not for as long as some bacteria and fungi. However, in the presence of proteinaceous material, such as dried blood or body fluids, some viruses can survive for hours, days, and even weeks.

Inert objects may also be the vehicles of transfer. The term 'fomites' is often used to describe the whole range of such objects, although its Latin derivation, from *foveo*, to keep warm (itself derived from the Latin for tinder), was originally applied only to clothing which might carry contagion such as the plague. Modern usage has widened the application and often refers to any object which might harbour micro-organisms, such as toilet seats, taps, cutlery, crockery, books, toys, etc. In fact, the risk of acquiring infection from such sources is probably minimal, given the likely dose, unless the object is grossly contaminated with dried blood or body fluids. Cleanliness is vitally important in this context, especially in hospital, but the use of detergent and hot water must be encouraged, rather than the indiscriminate use of disinfectants which are short lived in their action.

6.4.2 Epidemic infections

N. R. Grist

The term 'epidemic' refers to an increase in the incidence of cases (in this case of infections) which is clearly above that expected from previous experience in the community or region concerned. Incidence (the rate at which new cases arise, increasing to a peak in an epidemic before falling back again) should be clearly distinguished from prevalence (a static con-

cept—the total number of cases existing at a defined time or period in a specified population). Epidemics of infection can arise only when the infectious agent exists together with susceptible hosts and when there is effective means of transmission between them. An epidemic is provoked when one or more of these elements is created or, more usually, enhanced. An epidemic which involves most of the population of most of the world is termed a 'pandemic'. Currently the world is in the late stages of the seventh pandemic of cholera (Fig. 6.13) and the early stages of the pandemic of HIV-1 causing AIDS. Some examples of epidemics and the factors that cause them are described below.

Introduction of a new agent, new antigenic variant, or new source of infection

Measles brought by visiting ships to isolated island communities where it did not previously exist has caused devastating epidemics. It killed about a quarter of the population of Fiji in 1875 and affected almost the whole population of Tristan da Cunha in 1959. The previously unknown enterovirus type 30 caused epidemics of acute haemorrhagic conjunctivitis in most parts of the world after 1969. HIV-1 (the AIDS virus) is apparently new to our species and is now spreading widely.

Antigenic variation of influenza virus determines periodic epidemics, especially when major 'antigenic shift' of influenza A introduces antigens to which all or most of the population has no immunity, as in the pandemics of 1918–19, of 'Asian flu' in 1957 (Fig. 6.14), and 'Hong Kong flu' in 1968.

Introduction of new susceptible hosts into an area where the infectious agent already exists

International travellers often meet unfamiliar infections to which they are not immune. 'Travellers' diarrhoea', hepatitis A, poliomyelitis, and malaria are examples of diseases that impaired the health and effectiveness of troops deployed from Europe into Asia and Africa in wartime and which have caused outbreaks among holidaymakers.

Immigrants from isolated communities are often susceptible to serious illnesses caused by infection with agents, such as cold viruses, which are relatively innocuous in the largely immune population of the recipient area. Thus, the inhabitants of Tristan da Cunha suffered severe respiratory infections after their evacuation to Britain in 1961 to escape volcanic eruption.

Enhancement of transmission and creation of new routes of spread

Breakdown of preventive public health arrangements to avoid contamination of food or water by faecal organisms can cause epidemics of dysentery, salmonellosis, hepatitis A, and other such infections. Breakdowns of milk pasteurization plants have caused outbreaks of salmonellosis and *Campylobacter* infection. Lapses in food hygiene in group catering establishments are a common cause of outbreaks of food-borne infection, especially when the food has spent sufficient time at unchilled temperature for contaminants to multiply within it and provide a big

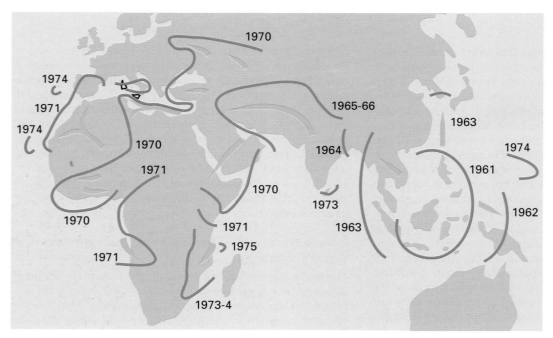

Fig. 6.13 The global spread of cholera, 1961–74 (after Velimirovic *et al.* 1984). Since 1974 cholera has spread more slowly to reach most of Africa, many countries of Asia and the Arabian peninsula, and the American continent (mainly around the Gulf of Mexico; and Peru in 1991), and with imported and secondary cases in Europe.

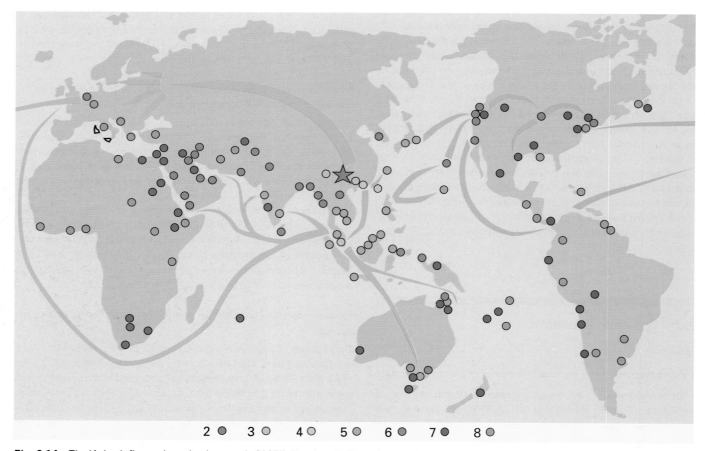

2 ●   3 ○   4 ○   5 ○   6 ●   7 ●   8 ○

Fig. 6.14 The 'Asian influenza' pandemic spread of 1957. Numbers indicate the month when the first epidemic cases were noted; the star indicates the probable origin of the epidemic. (Drawn after Stuart-Harris and Schild 1976, by permission of the World Health Organization.)

effective dose and/or substantial quantity of toxin for its consumers.

Technical innovations may cause unforseen new methods of spreading organisms. Thus, bacteria causing legionnaire's disease can spread to persons in hospitals or hotels by mechanical ventilation systems which have entrained infected water droplets derived from contaminated cooling plants. Whirlpool baths can propagate and spread Gram-negative bacteria and cause outbreaks of skin infection among members of spa clubs.

Crowding, especially of susceptible young, old, or ill persons (as in hospitals) increases the close contacts and opportunities for infections to spread, particularly in overcrowded urban communities, slums and Third World shanty towns. Diarrhoeal, respiratory, and skin infections are highly prevalent in slum conditions, with periodic epidemics especially affecting young children. Outbreaks of 'nosocomial' (hospital-acquired) infection are a serious threat requiring constant vigilance and careful technique from staff: the commonest means of spreading infection in hospitals and clinics is via the contaminated hands of staff. Both fingers and inadequately cleaned instruments have spread adenovirus type 8 from eye to eye, sometimes causing large epidemics of keratoconjunctivitis in eye hospitals and among industrial workers attending busy clinics because of eye injuries.

Seasonal variations in incidence often result from effects on crowding. The early upsurge of colds partly reflects the bringing together of susceptible young children in schools as new sessions begin. These children carry their infections home to infect their families. The winter peaks of respiratory infections also reflect the spending of more time together indoors by persons of all age-groups at this colder season. Seasonal epidemics may also reflect seasonal variations in the prevalence of vectors. Thus, malaria is transmitted by mosquitoes largely during the rainy seasons of the tropics, and the raised spring–summer incidence of tick-borne encephalitis in Europe reflects the increased activity of ixodid ticks in the warmer season.

Inadvertent use of infected blood or blood products has caused epidemics of viral hepatitis and AIDS in haemophiliacs and recipients of transfusions; these same infections are currently spreading among intravenous drug misusers who share equipment.

More 'permissive' attitudes to sexual intercourse and promiscuity have caused epidemics of both classical 'venereal diseases' and other sexually transmitted diseases such as viral hepatitis and AIDS, spread heterosexually and homosexually by oral, genital, orogenital, anogenital, and oro-anal routes.

Enhancement of susceptibility

The AIDS epidemic was first noticed in the USA because of the unusual increase in pneumocystis pneumonia caused by immune depression by HIV; this effect has now apparently also reversed the decline of tuberculosis in the USA and caused a dramatic increase of tuberculosis in Africa.

Decline of 'herd immunity' (immunity as a result of previous infection or immunization of members of the population) can allow renewed epidemic spread. This can happen because new

births have added new susceptibles to the population, as seen with annual epidemics of infant bronchiolitis caused by respiratory syncytial virus (Fig. 6.15) or the biennial epidemics of measles and four-yearly epidemics of poliomyelitis seen in Britain before immunization by vaccines. It was also shown by the

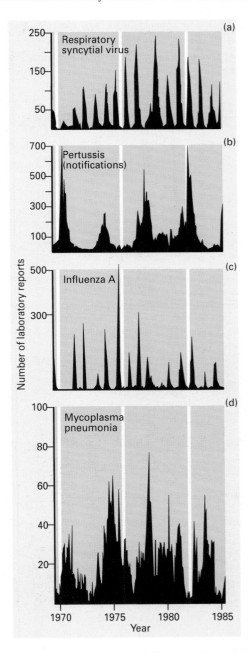

Fig. 6.15 Incidence of some common infections of the respiratory tract (based on Scottish reports, courtesy of the Communicable Diseases (Scotland) Unit). (a) Respiratory syncytial virus, annual winter epidemics; the increase in early years reflects the growing use of specific diagnostic tests. (b) Pertussis, four-yearly epidemics (because fewer children were immunized since 1972). (c) Influenza A, epidemics in most winters; (d) *Mycoplasma pneumoniae*, epidemics at intervals of 4–5 years. (Drawn after Grist *et al.* 1987, with permission.)

resurgence of pertussis after fears of 'vaccine damage' reduced uptake of that vaccine in Britain in the 1970s.

Patterns of epidemics

As mentioned above, many infections which are established in the host population show fairly regular epidemic fluctuations, either seasonal or at intervals of a few years (see Fig. 6.15). Other epidemics may occur sporadically as a result of changes, often temporary, in one or more of the determining factors described above.

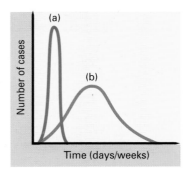

Fig. 6.16 Epidemic curves. (a) Abrupt rise, peak, and fall of incidence in an outbreak from a common point source. (b) Gradual rise, prolonged course, and slow decline of an epidemic from case-to-case transmission of infections. (Drawn after Grist *et al.* 1987, with permission.)

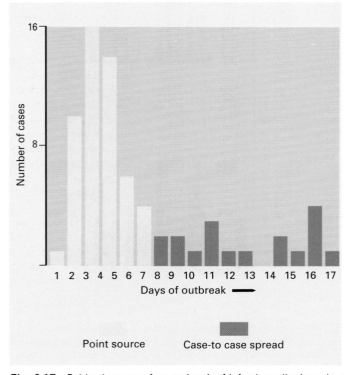

Fig. 6.17 Epidemic curve of an outbreak of infectious diarrhoea in a nursing home (courtesy of the Communicable Diseases (Scotland) Unit). Initial point source outbreak with subsequent case-to-case spread of infection. (Drawn after Grist *et al.* 1987, with permission.)

Epidemic curves

The time-course of an epidemic may give a useful guide to its probable source. The typically abrupt rise and fall in incidence of a 'point source epidemic' (Fig. 6.16) suggests a single episode of exposure to one common source of infection, e.g. consumption of contaminated food by a wedding party or conference group, or of milk distributed after a temporary breakdown of pasteurization. The decline of the outbreak may be relatively slow when there is also person-to-person spread of infection after the original episode (e.g. secondary cases of salmonellosis after a 'food-poisoning' episode) (Fig. 6.17). These patterns contrast with the smooth, prolonged course of an epidemic which is spread from person to person (Fig. 6.16), slowing as a growing proportion of the population gains resistance from post-infective active immunity, and eventually ending as this immune proportion becomes too high for the infection to maintain itself by reaching new susceptibles.

6.4.3   Further reading

Mechanisms of spread

Burnet, M. and White, D. O. (1972). *Natural history of infectious disease* (4th edn). Cambridge University Press, Cambridge.

Miles, A. (1983). Herd immunity. In *Topley and Wilson's principles of bacteriology, virology and immunity* (7th edn) (ed. G. S. Wilson and H. M. Dick), pp. 413–28. Edward Arnold, London.

Mims, C. A. (1987). *The pathogenesis of infectious disease* (3rd edn). Academic Press, London.

Zinsser, H. (1934). *Rats, lice and history*. Little, Brown and Co., USA. [Paperback edition (1985) Macmillan, London.]

Epidemic infections

Grist, N. R., Ho-Yen, D. O., Walker, E., and Williams, G. R. (1987). *Diseases of infection*. Oxford University Press, Oxford.

Stuart-Harris, C. H. and Schild, G. C. (1976). *Influenza—the viruses and the disease*. Edward Arnold, London.

Velimirovic, B., et al. (1984). Infectious disease in Europe: a fresh look. World Health Organization, Copenhagen.

6.5   Acute bacterial infections

6.5.1   Gram-positive aerobic infections

Mary P. E. Slack

The aerobic Gram-positive bacteria include cocci and rod-shaped organisms (Table 6.15). The Gram-positive cocci are the commonest cause of pyogenic infections in man (see Section 6.5.2). In contrast the aerobic Gram-positive rod shaped bacteria are predominantly commensals and the rare pathogenic species produce highly individual infections with diverse presentations. Examples of some of the more important infections

Table 6.15 The major Gram-positive aerobic pathogens and the diseases they cause

Organism	Diseases
Staphylococci	
Staph. aureus	Skin sepsis, bacteraemia, endocarditis, pneumonia, toxic shock syndrome, food poisoning
Staph. epidermidis and other coagulase negative staphylococci	Urinary tract infection, osteomyelitis, endocarditis, endophthalmitis, infection of indwelling lines, prostheses, etc.
Streptococci	
Str. pyogenes (Group A streptococcus)	Pharyngitis, scarlet fever, erysipelas, pyoderma, [Rheumatic fever or acute glomerulonephritis are non-suppurative sequelae of Str. pyogenes infection]
Str. agalactiae (group B streptococcus)	Neonatal sepsis and meningitis
Pneumococcus	Pneumonia, meningitis
Corynebacterium diphtheriae	Diphtheria
other "coryneforms"	Bacteraemia in immunocompromised, prosthetic valve endocarditis
Listeria monocytogenes	Listeriosis
Erysipelothrix rhusiopathiae	Erysipeloid
Bacillus anthracis	Anthrax
B. cereus	Food poisoning, endophthalmitis, bacteraemia in immunocompromised

caused by Gram-positive aerobic bacilli will be considered in this section.

Diphtheria

Diphtheria is a classic example of an infectious disease in which pathogenesis depends almost wholly on the production of an exotoxin by the infecting organism *Corynebacterium diphtheriae*. The primary site of infection is typically an area of mucosa on the tonsils or posterior pharyngeal wall. The bacteria remain confined to the superficial layers of the respiratory tract mucosa where they multiply and secrete diphtheria toxin. This exotoxin produces marked local inflammation and necrosis which results in the formation of a dense coagulum of fibrin, erythrocytes, polymorphs, necrotic cellular debris, and bacilli. This material forms a grey or brown 'pseudomembrane' over the infected area which reveals pinpoint bleeding of the underlying mucosa if it is removed. Diphtheria toxin is absorbed into the bloodstream resulting in toxaemia and the characteristic systemic effects of diphtheria. Diphtheria toxin can affect any tissues in the body since all human cells carry the membrane receptors for the toxin. However the major clinical manifestations are due to myocardial and neurological toxicity (see Table 6.4).

Pathogenesis

Diphtheria toxin is a bipartite (A–B) toxin which acts by inhibiting protein synthesis in mammalian cells but not in bacteria. In the laboratory, toxin production by strains of *C. diphtheriae* can be demonstrated by the *in vitro* immunodiffusion technique of Elek. The B segment binds to cell membrane receptors. Following proteolytic cleavage of the bound molecule the active A segment enters the cell where it catalyses the ADP-ribosylation of transfer RNA translocase (elongation factor 2 (EF2)) which is present in eukaryotic cells but not in bacteria. This inhibits protein synthesis (see Table 6.3). It is an extremely potent toxin, less than 1 μg being the lethal dose for a child. Toxin production by *C. diphtheriae* depends on the presence of a lysogenic bacteriophage, the β-phage. The genes encoding for diphtheria toxin (tox) are part of the phage genome. In its lysogenic state the phage genome becomes incorporated into the host bacterial chromosome and 'tox' gene is expressed. Strains of *C. diphtheriae* lacking the β-phage do not produce diphtheria toxin, but they can be converted to toxigenicity *in vitro* by infection with the lysogenic tox$^+$ phage. There is some evidence that this can also occur *in vivo* between toxigenic and non-toxigenic strains of *C. diphtheriae*. Because diphtheria remains endemic in many developing countries there is a theoretical risk that the non-toxigenic strains of *C. diphtheriae* normally carried in the respiratory tract in developed countries could become lysogenized by the tox$^+$ phage carried by an imported toxigenic strain. This underlines the importance of maintaining universal immunization against diphtheria in developed countries, despite the low incidence of diphtheria in these parts of the world.

The tox$^+$ phage from *C. diphtheriae* can also lysogenize *C. ulcerans* and *C. pseudotuberculosis* causing these organisms to secrete diphtheria toxin. Rarely these organisms have been associated with a diphtheria-like illness. Non-toxigenic (tox$^-$) strains of *C. diphtheriae* can produce a localized diphtheria-like pseudomembrane in the nasopharynx but they do not produce any systemic toxaemia.

Apart from causing classical faucial diphtheria, *C. diphtheriae* can infect skin and other mucous membranes. Cutaneous diphtheria occurs mainly in the tropics and results in indolent, punched-out ulcers with a grey membrane. They are rarely associated with any symptoms of intoxication but they can act as a reservoir of *C. diphtheriae* and may produce immunity.

The major toxic manifestations of diphtheria can be prevented by active immunization with inactivated diphtheria toxin or toxoid. In the United Kingdom alum-adsorbed diphtheria toxoid is routinely offered to all infants as part of the triple vaccine (diphtheria, tetanus, pertussis).

Other coryneform bacteria are frequently isolated from clinical material as several species are components of the normal skin flora. They can occasionally act as opportunistic pathogens (see Lipsky *et al.* 1982). Group JK coryneform bacteria are an important cause of bacteraemia and other infections in immunocompromised patients with haematological malignancies.

Listeriosis

Introduction

Listeria monocytogenes is a Gram-positive, non-spore-forming rod or coccobacillus which produces β-haemolysis on a range of blood agars, exhibits tumbling motility at room temperature, and which readily grows at 4 °C. *L. monocytogenes* is widespread in nature and is responsible for a variety of infections in animals and man; it may be carried in the gut of animals and man. In man the reported rates of faecal and genital tract carriage vary from 1 to 70 per cent per cent but generally the reported rate is 5–10 per cent. Some of the older studies of carriage rates are, however, misleading since listeriae were reclassified in 1985. Prior to that time the term *L. monocytogenes* was loosely applied to a number of species of listeria (*L. monocytogenes sensu lato*). The name *L. monocytogenes* is now restricted to a single species (*L. monocytogenes sensu stricto*) which is the major pathogen for man. It is not clear whether faecal carriage is transient or long-term nor is it certain whether infection develops from organisms colonizing the gut at a time when host immunity is depressed, for example, during pregnancy. *L. monocytogenes* is an opportunistic pathogen in man and causes infection relatively infrequently, usually in patients with impaired immunity. The main clinical syndromes in man are shown in Table 6.16.

L. monocytogenes is well known for its predilection for infecting pregnant women and immunocompromised hosts. Infection during pregnancy can carry risks for the fetus, resulting in abortion, premature labour, or intrauterine sepsis with a high risk of stillbirth or early neonatal mortality. The mother usually suffers only a mild flu-like, febrile illness. Damage to the fetus depends on the gestational age at the time of infection. Congenital listeriosis presents soon after birth as a pneumonia and septicaemia. Micro-abscesses and granulomata are found throughout the body, particularly in the spleen, liver, lungs,

brain, kidneys, and adrenals. This condition is known as *granulomatosis infantiseptica* and has a high mortality rate of 35–55 per cent. Many of the surviving infants have serious handicaps. Transmission of infection to the fetus does not always occur and it may be possible to treat the fetus *in utero* by the administration of parenteral antimicrobial therapy. The alleged link between listeriosis and habitual abortion is not proven. In contrast to congenital infection, neonatal infection, acquired during delivery from the maternal genital tract or later by cross-infection, can result in septicaemia or meningitis days or weeks after birth.

Pathogenesis

Listeriosis in adults can present in a number of ways. The most common manifestations are meningitis or meningo-encephalitis or bacteraemic infections but many other focal infections, such as osteomyelitis, endocarditis, and cholecystitis have been described (see review by Lamont *et al.* 1988). Approximately 70 per cent of non-pregnant adult patients have an underlying predisposing condition. These include lymphoid malignancies, immunosuppressive and steroid therapy, alcoholic liver disease, diabetes mellitus, and old age. A common factor in these groups is depressed cellular immunity.

It is clear from studies in experimental animals and man that T-lymphocytes and macrophages are of prime importance in the host defence against *L. monocytogenes*. Immune globulins and complement are also important. *L. monocytogenes* can act as a facultative intracellular parasite and may persist and grow within macrophages in the presence of active immune defences and effective antibodies. It was thought that *L. monocytogenes* persists as an intracellular L-form but this is now in doubt and the mechanism of the intracellular persistence is thought to be due to secreted bacterial products, in particular haemolysin (see below).

It is of interest that there have been few cases of listeriosis in patients infected with HIV where T cell-mediated immunity is impaired. Several hypotheses have been put forward to explain this finding, including the possibility that a T-cell subset other than CD4+ cells is of importance in immunity to listeria (see Berenguer *et al.* 1991).

L. monocytogenes produces one or more haemolysins *in vitro*, including α listeriolysin, a thiol-activated cytotoxin, which has similarities with streptolysin O, tetanolysin α, and β-listeriolysin. These enzymes damage erythrocytes, platelets, and phagocytes. They also disrupt the membranes of lysosomes and phagosomes and may help the bacteria to survive within macrophages by allowing them to escape from the phagolysosome into the cytoplasm. Non-haemolytic variants produced by transposon mutagenesis have greatly reduced virulence.

Virulence probably depends on other factors as well as haemolysin. *L. monocytogenes* produces superoxide and hydrogen peroxide, both of which are potentially cytotoxic. The bacterium also produces the enzymes superoxide dismutase and catalase which will tend to protect it from the toxic effects of superoxide and hydrogen peroxide. The cell wall almost cer-

Table 6.16 Listeriosis in Man

Clinical syndrome	Comments
Infections in pregnancy	Severity can vary from unapparent infection or mild flu-like illness to severe bacteraemic infection. Fetus may be unaffected or infection can result in abortion, stillbirth, premature labour, intrauterine sepsis, and early or late perinatal sepsis.
Congenital infection (Granulomatosis infantiseptica)	Pneumonia and septicaemia shortly after birth. Miliary micro abscesses and granulomata in liver, spleen, adrenals, lungs, kidney, brain. Mortality 35–55%.
Neonatal infection	Acquired during delivery (from maternal genital tract or later by cross-infection). Bacteraemia and meningitis days or weeks after birth.
Infections in adults	Central nervous system infections (meningitis, meningo-encephalitis) and primary bacteraemia are commonest manifestations; less frequently pneumonia, endocarditis, osteomyelitis, etc. 70% of adults have underlying illness predisposing to infection which depresses cell-mediated immunity (e.g. lymphoma, immuno-suppressive and steroid therapy, diabetes mellitus, alcoholic liver disease, old age).

tainly plays some part in virulence since rough strains that produce haemolysin are less virulent than wild-type smooth strains. A cell-wall extract has immunosuppressive and monocytosis-producing activity (MPA).

The epidemiology of listeriosis and man is poorly understood. The recent increase in the incidence of listeriosis, particularly cases which appear to be food-related has aroused considerable media concern. Supermarkets now sell a range of ready-prepared meals, stored for many days in chilled cabinets. *L. monocytogenes* can grow and even multiply at 4 °C. Indeed this property is exploited in the laboratory by the use of cold enrichment techniques to recover listeria from contaminated material. *L. monocytogenes* may be isolated from many foodstuffs including chicken, paté, cooked meats, and prepacked salads such as coleslaw. Whilst it is clear that many types of food may be contaminated with *L. monocytogenes* only in a small proportion of cases does exposure to the organism actually lead to disease. Much more work needs to be done to elucidate the epidemiology and pathogenicity of listeriosis.

Anthrax

Anthrax is caused by *Bacillus anthracis*, a Gram-positive sporing rod. Farmers, veterinary surgeons, butchers, slaughtermen, and pathologists who are in contact with infected animals may develop skin anthrax (malignant pustule) which is often self-limiting. Industrial cases occur in workers who process hides, leather, wool, or bones. These workers may contract cutaneous anthrax but there is a higher risk of pulmonary anthrax due to inhalation of anthrax spores (wool sorter's disease) which has a high mortality (see Chapter 13). In developing countries ingestion of contaminated meat from animals that have anthrax can result in an intestinal form of the disease. Anthrax spores persist for long periods in the environment. The soil of the Scottish island of Gruinard was still heavily contaminated with spores more than 40 years after bombs containing anthrax spores were detonated there in 1942. In 1986 the island was successfully decontaminated by the application of 50 litres/m^2 of 5 per cent formaldehyde in sea water (Manchee *et al.* 1990).

Pathogenesis

B. anthracis has a three-component exotoxin and an antiphagocytic poly-D-glutamic acid capsule. The toxin and the capsule are encoded in two large, distinct plasmids. The toxin consists of factor I or oedema factor (EF), factor II or protective antigen (PA), and factor III or lethal factor (LF). PA appears to bind to specific receptors on the host cell surface and produces a secondary binding site that is recognized by both EF and LF. EF is a calmodulin-dependent adenylate cyclase. The mode of action of LF is unknown. Antibodies to PA but not to LF and EF are necessary for protection. In fatal cases of anthrax there is a terminal bacteraemia. However, death appears to be due to the effects of the toxin rather than the bacteraemia. Antibiotic therapy at this stage will generally fail to prevent death. A human vaccine is available and should be administered to those whose occupations put them at risk of anthrax.

B. cereus is a well-known cause of food poisoning. It has also been associated with bacteraemia, endocarditis, pneumonia, and wound infection. The patient is often immunocompromised. *B. cereus* endopathalmitis may occur in intravenous drug abusers or following penetrating eye injuries. Other *Bacillus* species are opportunistic pathogens and have been implicated in a wide variety of infections (see review by Logan 1988).

Bibliography

Berenguer, J., Solera, J., Diaz, M. D., *et al.* (1991). Listeriosis in patients infected with human immunodeficiency virus. *Reviews of Infectious Diseases* 13, 115–19.

Lamont, R. J., Postlethwaite, R., and MacGowan, A. P. (1988). *Listeria monocytogenes* and its role in human infection. *Journal of Infection* 17, 7–28.

Lipsky, B. A., Goldberger, A. C., Tompkins, L. S., *et al.* (1982). Infections caused by non-diphtheria corynebacteria. *Reviews of Infectious Diseases* 4, 1220–35.

Logan, N. A. (1988). *Bacillus* species of medical and veterinary importance. *Journal of Medical Microbiology* 25, 157–65.

Manchee, R. J., Broster, M. G., Stagg, A. J., Hibbs, S. E., and Patience, B. (1990). Out of Gruinard Island. Salisbury Medical Bulletin 68 (special Supplement on Anthrax), 17–18.

Turnbull, P. C. B. (1990). *Anthrax. Topley & Wilson's principles of bacteriology, virology and immunity*, Vol 3. *Bacterial diseases* (eds G. R. Smith and C. S. F. Easmon), pp. 366–79. Edward Arnold, London.

6.5.2 Pyogenic infections

J. B. Selkon

Although many bacteria which infect man can produce pus, the most important pyogenic organisms are the Gram-positive cocci; in particular, the streptococcus, pneumococcus, and staphylococcus. The physical factors that protect them from phagocytosis and lysis, and the numerous enzymes and toxins they produce, present a fascinating picture of the wide and complex range of the biochemical determinants of microbial pathogenicity. There are certain similarities between these bacteria and even more interesting differences. They will therefore be considered separately, but compared where possible.

Streptococci

The principal streptococci responsible for pyogenic infections in man are the β-haemolytic streptococci which carry the Lancefield's Group A polysaccharide antigen, also known as *Streptococcus pyogenes*. In addition, pyogenic infections in man may be produced by Lancefield's Group C, *Str. equisimilis*, and the large-colony Group G strains. The streptococcal biotype, *Str. milleri* may also be pyogenic. However, it is a heterogeneous group of organisms and its virulence factors, though in some instances similar to those of *Str. pyogenes*, are poorly defined and understood; therefore they will not be considered further. The factors responsible for the pathogenicity of streptococci are discussed.

Cell surface

In the early stages of growth the strains produce a capsule-like surface coating of hyaluronic acid which protects them from phagocytosis. In addition they have, extending through their surface, fine filamentous appendages from the cell wall, composed of M protein and lipoteichoic acid, which are responsible for the adherence of streptococci to erythrocytes, epithelial cells, and phagocytes, and have significant antiphagocytic activity.

The peptidoglycan component of the cell wall is toxic to leucocytes and, on injection, causes fever and lysis of platelets. It also has some immunoadjuvenant activity, leading to a localized Schwartzman reaction, and may produce diffuse cellular infiltration of the myocardium.

Extracellular products

At least 20 products are released from Group A, C, and G β-haemolytic streptococci, and many of these are involved in their pathogenicity.

Toxins

Streptolysin O (oxygen labile) These haemolysins produced by streptococci of Groups A, C, and G are immunologically identical. They are responsible for the haemolysis seen around colonies on blood agar plates. The O haemolysin is also a powerful cardiotoxin, producing death in animals within seconds of intravenous injection, and may contribute to the heart damage which occurs in rheumatic fever. It acts principally as a leucocidin, which destroys neutrophils as well as erythrocytes and platelets. When reduced it becomes attached to the cholesterol molecules of the cell membrane and liberates the intracellular contents of lysosomal granules, such as the hydrolytic enzymes, which rapidly leads to cell destruction. It also inhibits leucocyte chemotaxis.

Streptolysin S (oxygen stable) This haemolysin is also a leucocidin and is antichemotactic. It is lethal for mice and it is possibly the more important of the haemolysins since, being cell-bound, it is able to destroy polymorphs which have engulfed streptococci. It is a small polypeptide of only 28 amino acids, is not antigenic, and does not produce immunity against subsequent attacks.

Erythrogenic toxin This is produced only by Group A streptococci and is responsible for the rash of scarlet fever. The toxin exists in three antigenically distinct forms, A, B, or C, and is released as a complex with hyaluronic acid. Apart from the skin rash, its toxic manifestations include pyrogenicity, low lethality, and myocardial necrosis. It is relatively stable to heat and is antigenic. There is growing evidence that the rash is due to a hypersensitivity reaction to toxin localized in the skin and not to a direct toxic effect on blood vessels.

Pyrogenic exotoxin This is a heat-labile exotoxin which has the property, in addition to pyrogenicity, of enhancing the lethal properties of the endotoxin of Gram-negative bacilli and other streptococcal toxins, such as streptolysin O. It is of low lethality in rabbits and enhances local Arthus reactions.

Enzymes

Hyaluronidase is produced by most strains of streptococci *in vivo*, including Lancefield's Groups A, C, and G. That produced by Group A strains is antigenically distinct from those produced by Groups C and G. It attacks the hyaluronic acid of connective tissue and may be responsible for the characteristic ability of this organism to spread rapidly through tissue. The M protein is unaffected by it; therefore, despite destroying hyaluronic acid, one of the components of the bacterial cell's protective envelope, it exposes this more important antiphagocytic factor.

Streptokinase This enzyme catalyses the activation of plasminogen into the protease, plasmin, which in turn lyses fibrin clots. It may, in this way, assist bacterial spread. It is produced by most strains of Group A streptococci and by some C and G strains, but in varying and smaller amounts. Experiments in animals suggest that it enhances the severity of streptococcal lesions. It is chemotactic.

Nucleases of four distinct types, A–D, which act on both deoxyribonucleic acid and ribonucleic acid, are enzymes that may be responsible for dissolving viscid pus and so assisting the spread of bacteria. They are produced by Groups A, C, and G, but in smaller amounts in the latter two serogroups.

Nicotinamide adenine dinucleotidase (NADase) This is an enzyme which removes the nicotinamide from NAD. It is doubtful whether NADase itself plays any part in pathogenesis but its presence is especially associated with nephritogenic strains, such as type 12. It is also formed by some strains of Groups C and G.

Proteinase This enzyme attacks casein, fibrin, and gelatin, and destroys several proteins produced by the streptococcus itself, including the M protein, haemolysin O, and the enzymes streptokinase and hyaluronidase. It is only released between pH 5.5 and 6.5 and as an inactive precursor which becomes active under the reducing conditions of the streptococcal cell wall. It is both antigenic and cardiotoxic.

Diseases produced by streptococci

The pyogenic streptococci are therefore well-equipped pathogens, protected from phagocytosis by their hyaluronic acid capsule and an M surface protein which is, in addition, highly toxic to leucocytes. They produce toxins that are highly active against human cells and several enzymes that enhance their ability to spread through pus and tissues. This combination of virulence factors has made *Str. pyogenes* one of mankind's most effective foes.

Pharyngitis The commonest infection due to the pyogenic

streptococci (Groups A, C, and G) is pharyngitis, particularly in those under 15 years of age. In addition to the local features of inflammation, there may be generalized effects, such as pyrexia, headache, malaise, nausea, abdominal pain, and even vomiting. If the strain of streptococcus produces the appropriate erythrogenic toxin, the patient may develop, within 48–72 hours, a generalized rash and even more severe systemic effects, a syndrome known as scarlet fever. This is less likely to occur in the present antibiotic era, as are the other complications, in particular local spread from the tonsils to produce peritonsillar or retropharyngeal abscesses. Bacteraemia may occur but is rare. Other common infections of the upper respiratory tract are otitis media, mastoiditis, and sinusitis, and their rare complication of extension through the skull to produce meningitis, brain abscess, or thrombosis of the intracranial venous sinuses.

Skin sepsis The other major form of infection is local skin sepsis. This may be limited to the epidermis and dermis and is called streptococcal pyoderma or impetigo. It occurs mainly in infants and young children. Alternatively, the infection may occur after a small, even non-detectable, break in the skin and involve the whole thickness of skin, producing indolent ulcers or spreading rapidly with a very active, raised, red inflammatory reaction, extending from the initial lesion with a sharply demarcated but irregular edge, known as erysipilas. In contrast to erysipilas, spread may be through the deeper tissues as a non-palpable, rapidly extending, inflammatory process with a distinct border, which is known as cellulitis. Either form of the infection may, within 24 hours, lead to bacteraemia. Lymphangitis may accompany cellulitis or it may occur separately.

If the infection is deeper, as may result from trauma or occasionally following a bacteraemia, it may involve the fascial planes overlying the muscles, producing a most destructive process known as necrotizing fasciitis.

Apparently localized pyogenic streptococcal infections may occasionally result in a bacteraemia which then leads to infection of any organ of the body, for example producing arthritis, osteomyelitis, or meningitis. Pneumonia may occasionally occur after viral or mycoplasma infections.

In addition to these direct actions of pathogenicity and suppuration, the Group A streptococci are able to produce two other important diseases through non-suppurative mechanisms.

Rheumatic fever is a condition characterized by a combination of inflammation of the endocardium, myocardium, and the large joints (see also Chapter 12). It is occasionally also associated with involvement of the brain, producing Sydenham chorea, production of subcutaneous nodules and the development of a skin rash known as erythema marginatum (annulare). It occurs in children and young adults, 2–4 weeks after a streptococcal pharyngitis. The process does not involve live streptococci, but is probably due to an immunological reaction or over-reaction. There are antigens present in Group A streptococci which are similar to determinants on cardiac muscle and the endocardium, particularly heart valves. Cross-reactions have been demonstrated between the Group A carbohydrate and the structural glycoproteins on heart valves and between M-associated antigens and cardiac muscle. However, this is not the full explanation, since antibodies are not present in Aschoff bodies (the characteristic pathological feature seen in the myocardium) and in the pericardium, even in the presence of pericarditis. Furthermore, there is no association between rheumatic fever and any specific serotypes of Group A streptococci, suggesting that the antigen involved must be common and very widely present in streptococci but as yet undetected, and that it cannot stimulate a detectable antibody response. However, the very high levels of antibodies to streptococcal products in patients with rheumatic fever, manifest by high anti-streptococcal O haemolysin and anti-DNase titres, suggest that the host's excessive immunological reaction to streptococcal infection is in some way responsible. Perhaps the cardiotoxic properties of streptolysin O and protease are in some way the initiators. The arthritis probably results from the deposition of antigen–antibody complexes in the joints, but this does not explain the mechanism for the other 'connective tissue disorders'.

Acute glomerulonephritis A further complication of *Streptococcus pyogenes* infection is the development, 1–3 weeks after pharyngitis or skin infections, of an acute glomerulonephritis. As with rheumatic fever, there is no evidence that post-streptococcal acute glomerulonephritis is due to streptococcal infection of the kidney. Only a limited series of serotypes, such as M types 12, 49, 55, 57, and 60, the so-called nephritogenic strains, are associated with the disease and, in contrast to rheumatic fever, recurrent attacks very rarely occur because of the protection arising from the development of specific anti-M protein antibodies. It is assumed that an unknown type-specific M-protein-associated antigen is responsible, and the disease represents a Type III hypersensitivity reaction to the deposition of antigen–antibody complexes in the basement membrane of glomerulocapillary walls. This results in the activation of complement, the influx of neutrophils, and the liberation of tissue-damaging enzymes (see also Chapter 19).

Pneumococci

The pneumococci conform to the genus *Streptococcus* and are a distinct species which are correctly referred to as *Streptococcus pneumoniae*.

Cell surface

Capsule The pneumococci have a similar structure to other streptococci but their most characteristic feature is a prominent polysaccharide capsule which is antiphagocytic and blocks opsonizing antibodies. This is its most important virulence factor. There are at least 83 serological types of polysaccharide, and antibodies to these specific capsular antigens confer immunity to infection. The capsular polysaccharide is distinct from the hyaluronic acid layer of β-haemolytic streptococci.

Cell wall The cell wall contains a species-specific carbohydrate, designated as C substance, which appears in the blood during the acute phase of infection, but its pathogenic role is unknown. The cell wall also contains type-specific M antigens which are similar to those of Group A streptococci, but are not antiphagocytic as in Group A streptococci and do not appear to be virulence factors. Thus, only capsulated pneumococci can establish infection in man or animals, while their non-encapsulated mutants or trypsinized cells are non-pathogenic.

Extracellular products

Pneumococci produce an intracellular haemolysin which is liberated by autolysis. This pneumolysin is oxygen and heat labile. It is serologically related to streptolysin O, and to the haemolysins of *Cl. perfringens* and *Cl. tetani*. It has lethal and dermonecrotic properties in animals. A pneumococcal leucocidin and a neuraminidase are produced by freshly isolated strains and it has been proposed that they contribute to the pathogenesis of pneumococcal pneumonia. Pneumococci also produce a hyalurnidase, but it is not thought to contribute to their virulence.

Pneumococci cause not only pneumonia, as their name implies, but also a wide range of other infections. Pneumococcal meningitis or brain abscess is the most lethal, while otitis media and sinusitis are the most common. The pneumococcus is responsible for about 25 per cent of instances of mucopurulent exacerbations of chronc bronchitis. Occasionally· it may give rise to septicaemia, bacterial endocarditis, or peritonitis.

Staphylococci

The staphylococci which produce coagulase, heat-resistant deoxyribonuclease, and ferment mannitol are classified as *Staphylococcus aureus* and are characteristically pyogenic. The remaining so-called coagulase-negative strains, although able to set up infection under special conditions (such as in association with foreign bodies or in immunocompromised patients), are not, in the convential use of this term, pyogenic organisms. One exception is *Staph. saprophyticus*, which is capable of causing urinary-tract infection with pyuria.

Staph. aureus produces a wide range of virulence factors in the form of toxins and enzymes, which by their combined action are highly pathogenic for man and animals.

Cell surface

As with streptococci, the staphylococci are protected from phagocytosis to a considerable extent by the structure of their cell surface.

Capsule Only a small proportion (4–18 per cent) of staphylococci produce a clearly discernible polysaccharide capsule. There are at least eight different antigenic types. A larger proportion of strains may produce microcapsules. The presence of these capsules is associated with enhanced pathogenicity resulting from protection from phagocytosis. In addition, most strains

of *Staph. aureus* produce a slime layer which is chemically distinct from the capsular polysaccharides. It enhances the ability of staphylococci to colonize catheters and may also impair phagocytosis.

Cell wall The cell wall is a relatively thick homogeneous layer which consists mainly of peptidoglycan (50–60 per cent of the dry weight of the wall) and teichoic acid. There are also a number of proteins, of which protein A is the most important. The staphylococcal peptidoglycan has important toxic properties, being pyrogenic, inhibiting leucocyte migration, and activating complement. The staphylococcal protein A has a minor role in enhancing pathogenicity, probably through impairing opsonization by binding to the Fc portion of the IgG antibody. It appears on the surface and is readily released into the environment of the cells.

In addition, the cell wall contains a protein known as clumping factor or bound coagulase, which reacts with a serum factor, probably fibrinogen and not related to thrombin activity. This is the mechanism responsible for the 'slide coagulase' reaction. Clumping factor is thought to be cytotoxic.

Extracellular products

Staphylococcus aureus excretes at least 25 known extracellular proteins into the environment during growth, Of these, nine have been characterized as toxins, while the remaining are non-toxic enzymes or enzyme activators. A comparison of the modes of action of those responsible for the pathogenicity of *Staph. aureus* and *Streptococcus pyogenes* are set out in Table 6.17.

Toxins

α-Haemolysin (α-toxin), which is the major haemolytic toxin of human strains, is both a haemolysin and a leucocidin. Its mode of action is unclear but may involve enzymatic activity on membrane proteins. It is also lethal on injection due to the induction of spasm in smooth muscle.

β-Haemolysin This is mainly encountered in animal strains and is most active on sheep and bovine erythrocytes and much less active on rabbit and human cells. It acts through its enzymatic action as a sphingomyelinase and weakens cell membranes, including human epithelial cells, making them vulnerable to other lytic agents.

γ-Haemolysin is principally lytic for sheep, rabbit, and human erythrocytes. It also has a leucocyte-damaging action.

σ-Haemolysin This is produced by most human strains and acts on the red cells and leucocytes of most animal species. It lyses leucocytes rapidly by its action on cell membranes, and liberates lysosomal enzymes. Its main role in pathogenicity is its synergistic interaction with α-haemolysins so that lysis occurs at well below the minimal lytic threshold of each. It is a small molecule and a very weak antigen.

Panton–Valentine (PV·) leucocidin This is the main leucocidin and is specifically toxic to human neutrophils and macrophages. It is

Table 6.17 Comparison of the structural and soluble products involved in the pathogenicity of *Streptococcus pyogenes* and *Staphylococcus aureus*

		Streptococcus pyogenes	Mode of action	*Staphylococcus aureus*	Mode of action
Structural	Capsule	hyaluronic acid	antiphagocytic	polysaccharide	antiphagocytic
	Cell wall	M protein	antiphagocytic	peptidoglycan	antiphagocytic
				protein A	inhibits opsonization
				clumping protein	? cytotoxic
Soluble	Toxins	streptolysin S	leucocidic	haemolysin α	leucocidic
				β	weakens cell membranes
		streptolysin O	leucocidic	γ	leucocidic
				σ	leucocidic and enhancing
				PV leucocidin	leucocidic
		erythrogenic toxin	skin rash	exfoliatin	separation of stratum granulosum
			fever		scalded-skin syndrome
			scarlet fever	TSST	toxic shock syndrome
				Pyrogenic toxin	fever
				Enterotoxins A–E	food-poisoning
	Enzymes	streptokinase	dissolves fibrin	staphylokinase	dissolves fibrin
		DNase	liquified pus	DNase	liquifies pus
		hyaluronidase	assists spread	hyaluronidase	assists spread
		proteinase	cardiotoxic	proteinase	?
				lipase	assists bacterial metabolism in skin
				coagulase	impedes leucocytes and phagocytosis

non-haemolytic. It has two protein components, F (fast) and S (slow), separable by electrophoresis. These two components are inactive alone, but when both are present they act successively on the triphosphinositide of the leucocyte cell membrane, altering permeability and resulting in an influx of Ca^{2+} ions into the cell and a loss of K^+ ions. The increase in intracellular Ca^{2+} activates membrane enzymes via the calcium-activated regulator protein, calmodulin, and results in degranulation with discharge of lysosomal enzymes. PV leucocidin also stimulates other membrane enzymes, including adenylate cyclase.

Enterotoxins Staph. aureus is a major cause of food-poisoning and more than 40 per cent of human strains form one or more of the antigenically distinct enterotoxins, A, B, C_1, C_2, D, or E. Enterotoxin A is responsible for three-quarters of *Staph. aureus* food-poisoning outbreaks. All the enterotoxins are heat resistant, withstanding boiling for 30 min, and are resistant to proteolytic enzymes such as trypsin. Therefore they can persist in cooked food and survive passage through the stomach. The enterotoxins act in an unknown manner, but it is known that they bind directly to nerve endings in the intestine and generate a sensory stimulus which travels via the sympathetic and vagus nerves to the vomiting centre of the brain. Enterotoxin B is a relatively uncommon cause of food-poisoning and in the 1950s and 1960s was associated with post-antibiotic enterocolitis. Phage type 94/96 strains, which produce enterotoxin B, may be associated with a toxic shock-like syndrome.

Epidermolytic toxin (exfoliatin) This acts on the intercellular connections between cells of the stratum granulosum of the skin. This most frequently occurs in neonates and results in detach-

ment and peeling of large areas of the outermost layer of the epidermis, producing the staphylococcal scalded-skin syndrome (see Chapter 28). The toxin may act locally at the site of an infection, such as an impetigo, or may be spread by the bloodstream, thus producing a generalized epidermolysis from which staphylococci are not isolated. This toxin is usually produced by phage II strains (particularly phage type 71) in association with a plasmid which is also responsible for a bacteriocin. However, occasionally toxin production may be determined chromosomally.

Pyrogenic exotoxins These have similar properties to streptococcal pyrogenic exotoxins and have low molecular weights. In rabbits they are pyrogenic and enhance susceptibility to endotoxic shock. There are three antigenic types, A, B, and C. Types A and B are produced by most strains of *Staph. aureus*.

Toxic shock syndrome toxin (TSST) This was thought previously to be an enterotoxin and was known as enterotoxin F. However, it is now accepted as a distinct toxin and is mainly produced by strains of phage group I. It is pyrogenic, toxic to muscle, induces vomiting, hypotension, erythroderma, impairment of hepatic and renal function, and thrombocytopenia. This combination of symptomatology is characteristic of the toxic shock syndrome.

Enzymes

Coagulase causes plasma to clot by activating prothrombin, or a prothrombin-like substance (called coagulase reacting factor), which generates thrombin, which in turn converts fibrinogen to fibrin. This localizes the lesion and in this way may protect the organisms, at least in the early stages, from phagocytosis. Although coagulase is non-toxic, it is an absolute marker of potential pathogenicity, and strains from different animal species coagulate homologous plasma and only a limited range of other plasmas.

Staphylokinase This is an enzyme which, like streptokinase, dissolves fibrin through activating plasminogen. It has the potential role of a spreading factor but it is doubtful how relevant this is in human infection. This enzyme is heat stable and potent but is not an essential requirement for virulence.

Hyaluronidase (hyaluronate lyase) As its name implies, hyaluronidase dissolves hyaluronic acid, and this may assist as a spreading factor. This may be more important in mixed infections or late in the disease but, like staphylokinase, does not appear to be related to pathogenicity, since strains without these two enzymes show no diminution of virulence in experimental infections.

Lipases These are common in staphylococci and may be useful in enabling them to metabolize sebaceous secretions on the skin. Thus, they may be particularly important in infections starting in hair follicles or sebaceous glands. The range of activity of lipases of different staphylococci varies, but the presence of lipases that attack Tween 80 is an invariable characteristic of strains that produce boils.

Deoxyribonuclease (DNase) DNase that resists boiling is produced by nearly all strains of *Staph. aureus*. It is a very potent enzyme and possibly is associated with pathogenicity, but its mode of action in this respect, like that in streptococci, is unknown.

There are a number of other enzymes produced by *Staph. aureus*, such as proteases (gelatinase), phosphatases, and lysozyme, but their contribution to pathogenicity is even less well understood and not thought to be significant.

Diseases produced by Staph. aureus

Most strains of *Staph. aureus* form most of the toxins and enzymes described above, but the only products that are consistently associated with pathogenicity are coagulase and heat-stable deoxyribonuclease, which are in themselves not principal virulence factors. The main determinants of virulence are α-haemolysin and PV leucocidin. However, virulence is, in general, due to a combination of all the factors described above. The only toxins that are associated with specific diseases are the enterotoxins, in particular A, which produces food-poisoning; epidermolytic toxin, which produces the scalded-skin syndrome; and TSST-1, which produces staphylococcal toxic shock syndrome.

The commonest site of staphylococcal infection is the skin. It takes the form of small abscesses arising in the hair follicles, or breaks in the skin which may, on occasions, enlarge considerably to produce a cluster of larger abscesses, known as a furuncle or carbuncle. Common predisposing factors to infection are immune suppression, diabetes melitus, or following

surgery, particularly in the presence of foreign bodies such as sutures or implants. *Staph. aureus* remains the commonest cause of post-surgical wound sepsis.

More rarely, and particularly in the young, a staphylococcal bacteraemia may occur even in the absence of local sepsis as a source of entry, and may give rise to a severe osteomyelitis or endocarditis. Staphylococcal endocarditis is particularly likely to occur in drug addicts or after intravenous infusions, in which adequate sterility has not been maintained.

The staphylococcal scalded-skin syndrome (toxic epidermal necrosis) occurs characteristically in neonates and sometimes as epidemics in nurseries. It may start as a small staphylococcal impetiginous lesion around the mouth, but then rapidly spreads to affect large areas of superficial layers of the skin, which then desquamate, leaving a moist, red, glistening surface. It may be fatal. Rarely, a similar disease may be seen in older children or even adults.

Toxic shock syndrome is characterized by vomiting, diarrhoea, high fever, circulatory collapse, erythroderma with subsequent desquamation, liver damage, renal failure, and thrombocytopenia. It may occur in either sex following local infection, but large outbreaks have occurred following colonization of vaginal tampons, which may have been due to the stimulation of TSST production by the components of some tampons.

Bronchopneumonia may occur after influenza virus pneumonia, measles, or whooping cough, or in immunosuppressed patients. It frequently results in cavitation of the lung and empyema.

Food-poisoning due to the enterotoxins usually occurs within 1–6 hours after ingestion of the preformed toxin, and starts with abdominal cramps, nausea, and vomiting. A degree of shock may occur due to the violent vomiting and mild diarrhoea may ensue.

6.5.3 Gram-negative aerobic infections

Adam Fraise

The range of Gram-negative infections

Gram-negative aerobic organisms (Table 6.18) are a major cause of bacteraemic infections. The commonest of these organisms is *Escherichia coli*, which accounts for aproximately 22 per cent of all bacteraemias. Other members of the enterobacteriaceae, e.g. *Klebsiella*, *Enterobacter*, and *Proteus*, and members of the pseudomonadaceae, e.g. *Pseudomons aeruginosa*, cause a large proportion of the remainder.

These organisms are common causes of urinary-tract infection and may enter the blood subsequently. Direct invasion from the gut may occur in patients on continuous ambulatory peritoneal dialysis (CAPD), and invasion via a poorly functioning liver may occur in patients with hepatic impairment. In

Table 6.18 Some Gram-negative pathogens and the diseases they cause

Organism	Disease
Enterobacteria	
Escherichia coli	
Proteus sp.	urinary-tract infection; nosocomial
Klebsiella sp.	pneumonia; 'Gram-negative
Enterobacter sp.	shock'
Serratia sp.	
Salmonella typhi	enteric fever
Salmonella spp.	gastroenteritis
Shigella spp.	bacillary dysentery
Vibrios	
Vibrio cholerae	cholera
Vibrio parahaemolyticus	diarrhoea/food-poisoning
Vibrio alginolyticus/vulnificus	soft-tissue infections
Pseudomonads	
Pseudomonas aeruginosa	exacerbations of cystic fibrosis; nosocomial pneumonia
Pseudomonas cepacia	end-stage disease in cystic fibrosis
Legionella pneumophilia	Legionnaire's disease; Pontiac fever
Parvobacteria	
Haemophilus influenzae	exacerbations of chronic bronchitis; meningitis; conjunctivitis; osteomyelitis
Bordetella pertussis	whooping cough
Pasteurella multocida	dog-bite infections
Fastidious Gram-negative rods	
Kingella kingae	
Eikenella corrodens	endocarditis
Cardiobacterium hominis	
Gram-negative cocci	
Neisseria gonorrhoeae	gonorrhoea
Neisseria meningitidis	meningitis

severe cases the clinical picture is that of Gram-negative shock. Hypotension, pyrexia, hyperventilation, and organ failure (cyanosis, acidosis, oliguria, jaundice, or congestive cardiac failure) are the main manifestations.

Although Gram-negative organisms constitute the bulk of the normal faecal flora, some species are pathogenic at this site. Examples include *Salmonella* spp. (the cause of enteric fever and sallmonella food-poisoning), *Shigella* spp. (the cause of bacillary dysentery), and *Campylobacter jejuni* (a spiral organism which is the commonest bacterial cause of diarrhoea in the developed world). Even the normally innocuous commensal *E. coli* can be pathogenic if virulent strains, which produce various exotoxins (see below), are ingested.

Vibrios are a group of curved Gram-negative rods which cause a range of infections. The most notorious species within this genus is *Vibrio cholerae*, which causes the profuse watery diarrhoea known as cholera. In this condition the patient may produce volumes of fluid so large that death can occur within 2–3 hours, although the time from the first liquid stool to death is more usually 1–3 days without treatment. *V. parahaemolyticus* is a marine organism which cause a milder diarrhoea after the consumption of contaminated shellfish, while *V. alginolyticus* and *V. vulnificus* can both cause soft-tissue infections, particularly in people swimming in water containing the organisms.

Pseudomonas spp. are the predominant organisms isolated from patients with cystic fibrosis, and are believed to play a role in the continued destruction of lung tissue which takes place in this disease. *P. aeruginosa* colonizes relatively early in the course of the disease but is replaced by more resistant members of the pseudomonadaceae (e.g. *P. cepacia* and *P. maltophilia*) as repeated courses of antibiotics are prescribed and the disease worsens. The isolation of *P. cepacia* is usually associated with end-stage disease.

Pseudomonas spp. are also major caues of bacteraemia in neutropenic patients who have become colonized with these relatively resistant organisms as a result of previous antibiotic therapy. Similarly, *P. aeruginosa* and other resistant Gram-negative bacteria (such as *Enterobacter cloacae* and *Serratia marcescens*) are important causes of nosocomial pneumonia in patients who have been treated with broad-spectrum antibiotics.

While infections due to the enterobacteriaceae and pseudomonadaceae are the commonest Gram-negative infections, many other Gram-negative aerobic organisms may cause systemic disease with a quite different clinical picture.

Legionella pneumophila is a short Gram-negative rod which stains poorly with Gram's stain. It is a cause of pneumonia (Legionnaire's disease) or an acute febrile illness without pneumonia (Pontiac fever).

Haemophilus influenzae is a pleomorphic Gram-negative rod, which colonizes patients with chronic chest disease and may cause pneumonia in those individuals. In these cases the strain is usually non-capsulate; however, capsulate strains exist and cause more severe infections, such as meningitis in children (mainly under the age of five) and epiglottitis (also in children, but under the age of seven). The most prevalent capsular type is type b.

Other infections caused by *H. influenzae* include otitis media and purulent conjunctivitis. Although these conditions are less severe than meningitis and acute epiglottitis, they are more prevalent and are consequently a significant cause of morbidity.

The family of small Gram-negative rods (parvobacteria) includes:

1. *Bordetella pertussis*—the cause of whooping cough; and
2. *Pasteurella multocida*—part of the normal oral flora of dogs and cats and consequently a cause of wound sepsis following bites from domestic animals.

Gram-negative cocci are important causes of human disease and the most significant of these are *Neisseria gonorrhoeae* and *N. meningitidis*.

N. gonorrhoeae is the cause of gonorrhoea, one of the major public health problems world-wide. In 1988, 22 884 infections were notified in England alone. Gonorrhoea is proving a particularly difficult problem to overcome as the organism has developed resistance to most of the commonly used drugs. Fortunately these resistant strains are rare, with the exception of penicillin-resistant strains in South-East Asia.

N. meningitidis, the causative agent of meningococcal meningitis, continues to be a problem. A recent outbreak in Britain has underlined the fulminating nature of this infection. It is unfortunate that the commonest serotype, type B, is poorly immunogenic and thus no effective vaccine is available.

Other aerobic Gram-negative rods may cause infections infrequently and tend to excite microbiologists but baffle clinicians. These include *Eikenella corrodens*, *Kingella kingae*, and *Cardiobacterium hominis*. These organisms and other similar pathogens may cause an indolent endocarditis which can take weeks to diagnose.

Epidemiology of Gram-negative aerobic infection

The human gastrointestinal tract is a huge reservoir of bacteria; faeces contain up to 10^{11} organisms per gram. While most of these are anaerobes, many are aerobic and act as an important source for urinary-tract infections. Organisms on the perineum may migrate up the female urethra spontaneously or during intercourse, to cause lower urinary-tract infections or pyelonephritis. As explained earlier, the gastrointestinal reservoir of aerobic bacteria plays an important role in the pathogenesis of bacteraemia in liver disease. In addition, the frequent bacteraemic episodes during post-chemotherapy neutropenia are probably secondary to migration of organisms across the intestinal wall and subsequent failure of neutrophil phagocytosis.

The administration of broad-spectrum antimicrobial agents has a significant effect upon the ecology of the bowel flora. Replacement of the normally sensitive *E. coli* (the most abundant aerobic Gram-negative rod in the normal host's intestinal flora) by more resistant organisms, such as *Pseudomonas aeruginosa* and *Enterobacter cloacae*, occurs quite quickly after implementation of broad-spectrum antimicrobial therapy. Consequently, these organisms frequently cause bacteraemia in neutropenic hosts who have been treated with these antibiotics.

The oropharynx in debilitated patients also acts as a reservoir for Gram-negative rods. The healthy host is not colonized with these organisms due to the protective effect of fibronectin (see Section 6.2.4); however, with general deterioration the fibronectin layer diminishes and allows colonization to take place. This oropharyngeal reservoir acts as a significant source of systemic invasion by Gram-negative organisms, and particularly as a precursor to nosocomial pneumonias caused by these bacteria. Gram-negative nosocomial pneumonia has also occurred following the use of poorly decontaminated respiratory equipment, such as ventilators and ventilator tubing.

Intravenous cannulae, monitoring devices, and pacemaker wires frequently become colonized with Gram-negative organisms, especially in hospitalized patients who have been exposed to antimicrobial agents. Secondary bacteraemias are not uncommon and may be life threatening. Other invasive devices, such as chest drains, abdominal drains, and urinary catheters, may also become colonized with Gram-negative organisms, and thus may be a source of systemic sepsis.

The natural habitat of legionellae is water and the organisms can colonize cooling towers and hot and cold water distribution systems. It is thought that aerosols of contaminated water are the usual source of infection.

Haemophilus influenzae is part of the normal pharyngeal flora and is spread from person to person by aerosols. Strains colonizing asymptomatic individuals are normally non-capsulate but capsulate strains are occasionally isolated. Following acquisition of a capsulate strain, invasion may take place. Invasion seems to be mediated by the type b capsule and results in bacteraemia and meningitis, predominantly in children under the age of five. Septic arthritis and epiglottis may also follow invasion.

Neisseria meningitidis, the causative agent of meningococcal meningitis, may also be carried in the nasopharynx of asymptomatic individuals. Transmission is probably mediated via respiratory secretions and the incidence of invasive disease, e.g. meningitis, is proportional to the rate of acquisition of the organism. It is believed that asymptomatic carriage is the means by which immunity is developed. Carriage of non-pathogenic *Neisseria* spp. may also stimulate the development of immunity to *N. meningitidis*.

The Gram-negative cell wall

The cell wall of Gram-negative bacteria consists of three layers: outer membrane, rigid peptidoglycan, and the inner cytoplasmic (or plasma) membrane (Fig. 6.18). The outer membrane consists of protein, lipid, and carbohydrate. The polysaccharide portion of the outer membrane is antigenic and is the 'O' or somatic antigen expressed by *Salmonella*, *E. coli*, and other enteric bacteria. Deeper within the outer membrane is the 'core' structure. The structure of the core region has been studied by analysing mutants of *Salmonella* spp. which have progressively less of the core structure attached to the lipid A (so called 'rough' mutants *Ra–Re*). The deepest rough mutants (*Re*) merely have 2-keto-3-deoxyoctonate (KDO) attached to the lipid A, while progressively less deep mutants (*Rd–Ra*) have heptose, galactose, glucose, and *N*-acetyl glucosamine attached sequentially.

Some workers have attempted to exploit the similarity between the core structures of different Gram-negative bacteria, and raise antibodies which will cross-react with various species. Infection with strains possessing the 'O' side-chain induces immunity only to that 'O' serotype, whereas the above approach avoids the problems of antigenic variation between

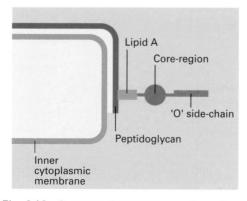

Fig. 6.18 Structure of the Gram-negative cell wall.

different species and, indeed, different strains of the same species. Early results were conflicting but recent advances with monoclonal antibodies have been promising (see below).

The peptidoglycan portion of the cell wall is a rigid structure containing *N*-acetyl glucosamine and *N*-acetyl muramic acid alternating in a chain. There are also peptide cross-linkages between these chains; this rigid structure protects the organism against osmotic rupture and is the site of action of *β*-lactam antibiotics.

The inner cytoplasmic (or plasma) membrane is a lipid bilayer pierced by proteins and phospholipids. These proteins are involved in various metabolic activities and in transport of nutrients and ions, synthesis of lipids, and electron transport.

Mechanisms of virulence

In order to exhibit virulence (Table 6.19) a micro-organism must first attach to the host, a phenomenon known as adherence. Following invasion, the micro-organism must be resistant to the antibacterial effects of serum and to killing by phagocytes. Irrespective of the invasive nature of the organism, toxins may be produced, many of which have no known function. However, some of these help the organism to survive and multiply and many have a deleterious effect on the host.

Table 6.19 Mechanisms of virulence

Adherence
Serum resistance
Anti-phagocytic properties
Toxins

Adherence

Most Gram-negative organisms possess specific adherence organelles called fimbriae (or pili) on their surface. These organelles are sometimes called adhesins because of their functional role; they adhere to specific receptors on host cells. The receptors may be oligosaccharides, glycoproteins, or glycolipids. Fimbriae play an important role in the pathogenesis of urinary-tract infections by attaching to the urothelium to avoid the flushing effect of urinary flow. Antibodies to fimbriae have been described in acute pyelonephritis, although their protective effect is unknown.

Adherence is also of fundamental importance in gonococcal infection. The gonococcus avoids antibody-mediated inhibition of adherence by variation of the antigenic type of the fimbriae. Many different fimbrial antigenic types may be expressed by different descendants of a single strain of *N. gonorrheae*, thus immunity to the original infecting organisms does not prevent adhesion of subsequent populations. Adhesins are discussed in Section 6.2.1.

Serum resistance

Gram-negative organisms vary in their susceptibility to complement-mediated lysis. The majority of strains causing bacteraemia are resistant to this bactericidal effect of serum, while a much lower percentage of isolates from faeces are resistant to serum killing. Furthermore, isolates of *Pseudomonas aeruginosa* from patients with cystic fibrosis are usually serum sensitive and rarely cause bacteraemias. This contrasts with isolates from patients with pseudomonas pneumonia (a complication of severe debilitation and prolonged intensive care), which are usually serum resistant. It has been suggested, therefore, that resistance to the bactericidal effect of serum is an important virulence factor for Gram-negative bacteria.

Antiphagocytic properties

Many organisms possess capsules which are functionally antiphagocytic. This capsule is usually polysaccharide in nature but some organisms possess protein components in their capsule, which also act to inhibit phagocytosis. Mutants of *E. coli* with capsules deficient in polysaccharide have been shown to be less virulent than the parent strain that possesses a complete capsule. This decrease in virulence was associated with an increase in the ability of the host's neutrophils to phagocytose the organisms.

The mechanism behind this inhibition of phagocytosis is unclear but seems to be related to the ease with which the C3 component of complement can bind to the organism. Capsulate strains bind less C3 than non-capsulate strains and are thus less susceptible to neutrophil phagocytosis.

Some organisms are effectively ingested by the phagocyte but manage to avoid intracellular killing. An example of this is in *Salmonella typhi* infection during which virulent strains are ingested by neutrophils. Normally, ingestion of a micro-organism is followed by a burst of metabolic activity which is essential for intracellular killing. While the oxidative burst takes place after ingestion of a virulent strain of *S. typhi*, the magnitude of this burst (as measured by oxygen consumption) is markedly reduced compared with that following ingestion of avirulent strains.

Survival of intracellular killing is thus an integral part of the pathogenesis of typhoid fever and is essential for the establishment of chronic intracellular infections, such as brucellosis.

Toxins

Toxins can be divided into two broad groups: endotoxins and exotoxins.

Endotoxins These are an integral part of the bacterial cell wall and are composed of lipopolysaccharide (a covalently linked complex of polysaccharides and lipid). They are involved in the pathogenesis of fever, inflammation, and related events.

Man is exquisitely sensitive to the effects of endotoxin; minute doses cause fever which is more marked than in animals. The fever commences 90–120 min after an injection of endotoxin and continues for 3–4 hours. This effect is probably mediated via the production of tumour necrosis factor (TNF) which is produced in large quantities when rabbits are injected with lethal doses of endotoxin and is also produced in human volunteers following injection of pure endotoxin. TNF, when injected alone, causes fever, a metabolic acidosis, adrenal haemorrhage, and acute renal tubular necrosis.

The effects of endotoxin are presumably not entirely detrimental and are possibly part of the body's non-specific defences. TNF has been shown to be viricidal and has been reported to increase neutrophil activity. The exact importance of these effects is still unclear.

Exotoxins These are released by bacteria during growth and are protein in nature. They are toxic to target cells and generally have a dual subunit structure. The first subunit, designated the 'A' portion, is enzymatic and responsible for the activity of the toxin. The second, or 'B', subunit mediates binding to target cells. Both subunits are necessary for the biological effect of toxins and toxins lacking one or other subunit are not biologically active (see Section 6.2.2).

There are many different toxins produced by Gram-negative bacteria and only two main examples are discussed here. For more detail see Section 6.2.2. Cholera and *E. coli* heat-labile toxin are similar in structure and function. They bind to intestinal cells and cause an increase in cyclic AMP (cAMP). This results in an outpouring of isotonic secretion, resulting in profuse watery diarrhoea (Fig. 6.19).

Shigella dysenteriae type 1 produces a toxin called shiga toxin which inactivates ribisomes and causes cytotoxicity and neurotoxicity in experimental animals. Its clinical effect in humans is to produce a severe bloody diarrhoea. Related toxins are produced by enteropathogenic *E. coli* (a cause of infantile diarrhoea) and by verotoxin-producing *E. coli* (VTEC), the causative agent of haemorrhagic colitis and haemolytic uraemic syndrome.

Pathophysiology of Gram-negative septicaemia

Gram-negative septicaemia has a characteristic clinical presentation which includes fever, hypotension, acidosis, and renal and respiratory failure. While this clinical picture is called 'Gram-negative shock' it is important to realize that Gram-positive organisms can cause an identical syndrome. Endotoxin

triggers the activation of a number of mediators, the most important of which is TNF (see above). Other cytokines activated by endotoxin include interleukin-1 (previously known as endogenous pyrogen), γ-interferon, and a group of colony stimulating factors.

As mentioned earlier, endotoxin, when injected into volunteers, results in an increase in the plasma concentration of TNF. Furthermore, injection of pure recombinant TNF into human volunteers results in many of the clinical and laboratory features of Gram-negative shock. These manifestations can be eliminated in animals by prior administration of anti-TNF antibodies.

Endotoxin also activates Hageman factor (factor XII of the clotting cascade) which, in turn, activates the intrinsic clotting cascade, resulting in the conversion of fibrinogen to fibrin and subsequent clot formation. Hageman factor also initiates the fibrinolytic cascade, resulting in conversion of plasminogen to plasmin. These two mechanisms (coagulation and fibrinolysis) acting together cause the syndrome of disseminated intravascular coagulation (see Chapter 7), which manifests as uncontrollable bleeding due to consumption of coagulation factors exacerbated by the dissolution of clot.

Conversion of pre-kallikrein to kallikrein, which in turn converts kininogen to bradykinin, also follows endotoxaemia and is reponsible for the hypotensive component of Gram-negative septicaemia.

The complement cascade is also activated by endotoxin, and both classical and alternate pathways are involved in the pathogenesis of Gram-negative septicaemia. Complement activity enhances phagocytosis and cause lysis of antibody-coated bacteria. It also has deleterious effects, such as inflammation and thrombocytopenia (see also Chapter 4).

Implications of the understanding of pathogenesis on treatment of Gram-negative septicaemia

The mainstay of treatment of Gram-negative sepsis is the use of antibiotics active against the infecting organism. However, recent progress in the understanding of the pathogenesis of Gram-negative sepsis has opened several new channels of investigation.

The initial causative role of endotoxin in the manifestations of Gram-negative septicaemia stimulated some workers to attempt treatment or prophylaxis of Gram-negative infection by serotherapy. Hyperimmune serum was raised by immunization with a killed suspension of a rough mutant of *E. coli* (designated J_5 and equivalent to the *Rc* mutant of *Salmonella* sp.) and was used in the treatment of bacteraemic patients. Patients treated with the hyperimmune serum had a lower mortality compared with those treated with placebo. These results have stimulated further work with animal and human monoclonal antibodies which protect against the effects of Gram-negative sepsis in animal models. Preliminary studies in humans have shown the mouse monoclonal antibody to be well tolerated, and results of clinical trials with both animal and human products are awaited.

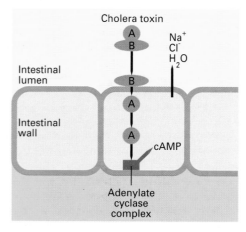

Fig. 6.19 The action of cholera toxin.

Since the elucidation of the central role of TNF in the pathogenesis of Gram-negative septicaemia, many workers have attempted to produce anti-TNF monoclonal antibodies. At present a multicentre trial of the efficacy of anti-TNF monoclonal antibodies in sepsis is being conducted. It may be that the reliance on antibiotics as the major treatment of Gram-negative sepsis could be significantly reduced as adjunctive forms of therapy become established.

6.5.4 Anaerobic and polymicrobial infections

H. R. Ingham and P. R. Sisson

Introduction

The concept of a particular disease being caused by a particular parasite is embodied in 'Koch's postulates', which state:

1. The organism should be found in all cases of the disease in question, and its distribution in the body should be in accordance with the lesions observed.

2. The organism should be cultivated outside the body of the host, in pure culture, for several generations.

3. The organism so isolated should reproduce the disease in other susceptible animals.

A subsequent caveat to the postulates is the demonstration of a specific immune response to the organism, evidenced by the presence of antibodies or hypersensitivity in an infected host.

Many disease-producing bacteria broadly fulfil Koch's criteria; however, it has been recognized that they cannot be applied *de rigueur*. The outcome of an encounter with a particular organism depends on the virulence of the latter and the susceptibility of the host. The ingestion of *Salmonella typhi* by non-immune individuals almost invariably produces systemic disease, whereas the body co-exists with *Staphylococcus aureus* until there is some local or general impairment of the defences. This spectrum of pathogenicity encompasses a whole range of organisms which individually may produce disease under appropriate conditions.

Historical perspective

In the past 25 years it has become apparent that many infections are caused by organisms which individually are relatively avirulent, but when acting in concert are highly pathogenic. The majority of these organisms form the normal flora of the alimentary tract, a complex ecosystem, the separate components of which act collectively in the metabolism of foodstuffs and their residues. These symbiotic relationships in which microorganisms conjointly produce results not achieved by individual bacteria acting alone fostered the term 'synergy', first used by Kammerer in 1924 to describe the conversion of bilirubin to urobilinogen by mixtures of bacteria in human faeces, an effect not achieved by individual organisms.

An early example of infective synergy was a report that *Clostridium tetani* and *Bacillus oedematiens* became virulent only when mixed with other organisms such as *Proteus vulgaris*. Bacterial synergy in the production of the commoner human infections was first referred to by Meleney in 1924, in his description of a spreading gangrenous infection of abdominal wounds associated with the combined presence of *Staph. aureus* and a microaerophilic streptococcus. These infections complicated surgical drainage of peritoneal sepsis in which the streptococcus was implicated, and were characterized by erythema, cellulitis, and subsequently gangrene around sutures. Culture of the latter additionally yielded staphylococci which had gained access to the wound from extrinsic sources. Both organisms were always present in these infections, termed synergistic gangrene, and were also required for the reproduction of the condition in animal models. Subsequent studies up to the late 1950s with anaerobic bacteria isolated from patients with appendicitis, infections of the female genital tract, and oral infections showed quite clearly that injection of mixtures of these organisms produced severe disease in experimental animals. By contrast, the lesions produced by pure cultures were smaller and resolved spontaneously (Figs 6.20, 6.21).

Causative organisms

The normal flora of the alimentary tract in health, located predominantly in the oropharynx, the gingival crevice and large bowel consists of a mixture of facultative and obligate anaerobes; similar organisms are encountered in the vagina.

Dental plaque, a normal constituent of the gingival crevice contains about 10^{10} bacteria per gram. About half of these are facultative anaerobes, mainly Gram-positive rods and cocci and there are equal numbers of obligate anaerobes, mainly non-spore-bearing. In the large bowel there are 10^{10-11} obligate anaerobes per gram of faeces; clostridia are present in addition to non-spore-bearing anaerobes and in total these outnumber facultative anaerobes by 100:1 (Table 6.20).

The facultative anaerobes of the gingival crevice include *Actinomyces* spp., diphtheroids, Gram-negative rods such as *Actinobacillus* and *Haemophilus* spp., and a wide variety of streptococci, one of which, *Streptococcus milleri*, is important in certain pyogenic infections. The anaerobic flora of the non-sporing anaerobes in the large bowel is distinguished from that of the gingival crevice by the species represented, the most important practical difference being the presence of large numbers of members of the *Bacteroides fragilis* group. In distinction to oral anaerobes the latter are always resistant to penicillin.

In certain circumstances there is a substantial increase in the bacterial load deriving from the normal flora, e.g. in patients with poor dental hygiene, Vincent's infection, and some tonsillar infections. Obstructive malignancies of the stomach may cause an increase in pH and mechanically impede passage, both of which favour overgrowth of oral bacteria. Likewise, obstruction to the large bowel results in faecal organisms colonizing the small bowel. The increase in total numbers of bacteria arising

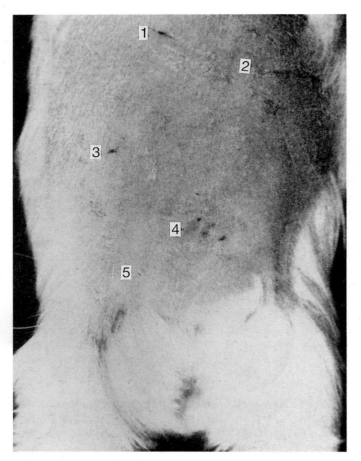

Fig. 6.20 Guinea-pig inoculated with five separate isolates from appendix infections. Note the minimal lesions. (Reproduced from Altemeier 1942, with permission.)

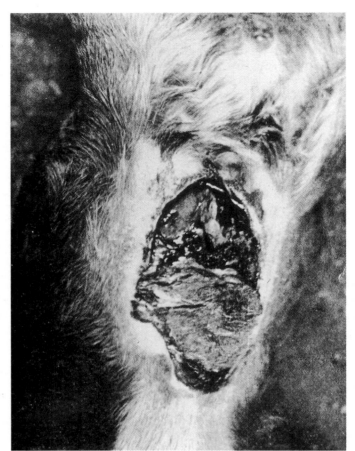

Fig. 6.21 Guinea-pig inoculated with a mixture containing the five isolates from appendicial infections shown in Fig. 6.20. Note the gross necrosis and sloughing. (Reproduced from Altemeier 1942, with permission.)

Table 6.20 The microbial flora of the gastrointestinal tract organisms/ml*

	Oesophagus	Stomach, duodenum, and upper small bowel	Large bowel
Aerobes			
Streptococci	$0-10^2$	$0-10^2$	10^{3-8}
Escherichia coli	$0-10^1$	$0-10^2$	10^7
Klebsiella	$0-10^1$	$0-10^1$	10^{5-6}
Faecal streptococci	$0-10^1$	$0-10^2$	10^{5-6}
Anaerobes			
Bacteroides fragilis	$0-10^1$	$0-10^1$	10^{6-9}
Bacteroides sp.	10^3-10^4	$0-10$	10^{10}
Non-sporing Gram-positive bacteria	10^3	$0-10^1$	10^{8-11}
Clostridia	0	0	10^{4-9}
Peptostrepto-cocci	$0-10^3$	$0-10^3$	10^{3-9}

*From Strachan and Wise (1979).

under these circumstances poses a greater challenge to the body defence mechanisms (see Section 6.2.4). In addition to the presence of adequate numbers of micro-organisms, certain precipitating events are necessary for the development of infections, illustrative examples of which will now be considered.

Common anaerobic and mixed infections
Acute ulcerative gingivitis

Acute ulcerative gingivitis (Vincent's infection) is predominantly associated with fusobacteria and spirochaetes. The aetiology of this condition is not entirely clear but poor dental hygiene appears to be a prerequisite, allowing accumulation of plaque which encroaches upon and elevates the gingival margin. Spirochaetes and fusobacteria, which form part of the flora of plaque, become more numerous and invade the adjacent gingival mucosa; however, attempts to reproduce the disease in volunteers with these two organisms alone have been unsuccessful. Evidence has been advanced for the additional participation of other oral anaerobes, such as *B. intermedius* in the pathogenesis of this condition.

Actinomycosis

A more insidious infection which may develop in relation to the oropharynx, chest, or abdomen, is actinomycosis. Classically the condition presents as a chronic indurated swelling, often associated with a persistent discharging sinus. *Actinomyces* are present in the oral cavity, especially where there is chronic inflammatory disease of the teeth, gingiva, or tonsils. In human infections associated with this organism the species commonly implicated is *Actinomyces israeli*. Actinomycotic lesions have a very characteristic histological appearance, with a central, almost amorphous area, in which branching Gram-positive rods may be present, and a peripheral zone consisting of radial clubs which some believe result from an interaction between host defences and the organism. Despite the predominance of actinomyces in such lesions, many studies have revealed the consistent presence of other oral bacteria, including obligate anaerobes. Attempts to reproduce the disease in experimental animals with pure cultures of actinomyces have been largely unsuccessful and it seems that actinomycosis may be yet another example of a mixed infection.

Acute dental infections

For many years it has been known that dental abscess, a term covering a variety of pyogenic conditions involving the teeth and adjacent tissues, respond to treatment with penicillin and appropriate surgery. Until relatively recently the only bacteria regularly isolated from these infections were comparatively non-pyogenic organisms such as *Str. viridans*, *Staph. albus*, diphtheroids, and occasionally *Staph. aureus*. Many of these organisms are sensitive to penicillin and were pragmatically incriminated in these conditions. Dental pus is characteristically malodorous, a distinguishing feature of anaerobic infections, and on microscopy is seen to contain numerous micro-organisms, both Gram-negative and Gram-positive. Latterly the isolation of large numbers of obligate anaerobes from such material, and the sensitivity of these organisms to penicillin strongly suggested their implication in this condition.

Demonstration of the efficacy of metronidazole in these infections finally delineated the role of obligate anaerobes, as this drug is without action against any of the facultative anaerobes commonly present. The recognition of the paramount importance of obligate anaerobes in dental infection has allowed a much clearer understanding of the bacterial aetiology of such diverse infections as human bites (Fig. 6.22), intracranial sepsis, and the pulmonary consequences of aspiration.

Tonsillar infections

Necrobacillosis The other site in the oropharynx where anaerobic infections occur is the tonsils. In the past a well-recognized form of tonsillar infection was due to *Fusobacterium necrophorum*, an organism causing a variety of infections in animals and which appears to be more virulent in humans than other non-sporing anaerobes. It is the sole pathogen in Lemierre syndrome, which is characterized by septicaemia with involvement of the lungs, liver, bones, brain, and meninges. The apparent decline in the incidence of this condition is perhaps attributable

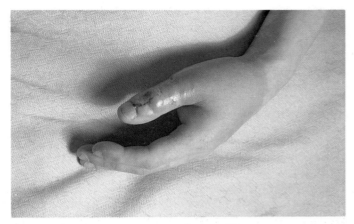

Fig. 6.22 Human bite. Pus from these lesions frequently contains oral anaerobes. Note the marked cellulitis and swelling.

to the widespread early use of antimicrobials, in particular penicillins, in patients with pharyngitis. Scattered recent reports of this condition are not accountable in terms of a reduction in sensitivity of these isolates to penicillin, but may reflect the destruction of the agent in the tonsillar bed by β-lactamase-producing anaerobes, whose presence in this site has been reported.

Acute bacterial tonsillitis The usual cause of acute bacterial tonsillitis, *Str. pyogenes*, is also commonly assumed to be responsible for peritonsillar abscess but there is growing evidence for the importance of oral anaerobes in this condition. The pus is typically malodorous, obligate anaerobes have been isolated from approximtely 75 per cent of abscesses in well-conducted studies, and Group A haemolytic streptococci from only 25 per cent.

Infected tonsils and teeth are primary foci for the spread of mixed infection to the compartments of the neck, the thorax, and intracranially. The deep structures of the neck are divided into a series of intercommunicating compartments by fascial layers which permit extension into the mediastinum anteriorally and into the posterior pharyngeal wall as far down as the psoas sheath. The lymph nodes in the retropharyngeal space, in addition to receiving drainage from nearby structures, also drain the nose, paranasal air sinuses, nasopharynx, pharynx, middle ears, and Eustachian tubes. Infections in any of these structures may give rise to retropharyngeal abscess.

Pulmonary infections

Mixed bacterial infections in the lungs and related structures are almost always the result of aspiration of material from the oral cavity. Such infections are uncommon in healthy individuals with normal respiratory mucosa and cough reflex but if the conscious level is impaired due to head injury, alcoholic stupor, poisoning, or anaesthesia, or there is interference with deglutition, infections due to aspiration are likely. Where there is poor oral hygiene much larger numbers of organisms are aspirated, increasing the likelihood of infective sequelae. These are most common in dependent parts of the lung and include acute pneumonitis, lung abscess, and empyema thoracis. Where aspiration is recurrent over a period of time, particularly in alcoholics, chronic destructive pneumonia results, with areas of fibrosis and granulation tissue co-existing with consolidation, pus formation, and cavitation.

Para-nasal air sinus infections

Although *Staph. aureus, H. influenzae,* and *Str. pneumoniae* are commonly responsible for infections of the para-nasal air sinus, mixtures of organisms derived from the oral flora may also be implicated. In the case of the maxillary antrum this is often a sequel to root canal infection in the associated teeth. One of the commonest organisms reported in pyogenic infections of the frontal air sinus, particularly where there are intracranial sequelae, is *Str. milleri* Lancefield Group F. It is often the sole organism isolated, but oral anaerobes may also be present.

Intracranial infections

Mixed infections involving teeth, tonsils, or sinuses may also extend intracranially, either directly through bony structures or via vascular channels. Extension by vascular routes is greatly facilitated by the rich venous plexuses in this region, which communicate with each other and the intracranial venous sinuses. Therefore, one of the infective complications which may ensue is thrombosis of the cavernous sinus. The high mortality associated with this condition is due in part to lack of early recognition, because of the obscure primary sources of these mixed infections. Thrombosis of the sagittal and lateral sinuses are less common. Spread of infection to the latter sinus is not from the oropharynx via the Eustachian tube, but from cholesteatoma (see Chapter 15) in the middle ear, associated with chronic suppurative otitis media.

Most cholesteatomas develop as a consequence of serous otitis media (glue ear) when the resultant drop in presssure consequent upon blockage of the Eustachian tube causes invagination of the upper part of the tympanic membrane. The resulting saccule accumulates dead squames, aural secretions, and bacteria. Gradual enlargement of the cholesteatoma causes erosion of the surrounding bony structures, allowing infection of the lateral venous sinus directly or via small venous channels. The commoner intracranial complication of cholesteatoma is a brain abscess, either in the cerebellum or the temporal lobe. The organisms that characterize otogenic brain abscess and that constitute the flora of cholesteatomas derive not from the oropharynx but from the large bowel, and include *E. coli, Proteus* spp., *Str. faecalis, Bacteroides* including *B. fragilis,* and anaerobic streptococci.

It is clear from the flora and mode of development of cholesteatoma that organisms are introduced via the external auditory meatus (see Chapter 15). This mixture of organisms is only rarely seen in other types of brain abscess due to direct spread from contiguous structures. Thus abscesses of the frontal lobe that are sinusitic in origin yield *Str. milleri* with or without oral anaerobes, which also characterize abscesses in this region of the brain secondary to a dental source. Likewise, subdural abs-

cess, which is almost always secondary to infections of the frontal air sinus, is commonly due to *Str. milleri,* although in some instances *Staph. aureus* is the causative organism. The presence of oral anaerobes in these abscesses should stimulate a search for communications between the sinuses and infected maxillary teeth.

Abdominal and pelvic infections

Abdominal and pelvic mixed infections of gastrointestinal origin arise spontaneously as a result of disease, or secondary to surgery or accidental trauma of the bowel. Because there are normally many more bacteria in the large than in the small bowel, endogenous infection is more likely following large bowel surgery or trauma. If the number of bacteria in the small bowel increases, for instance because of bacerial overgrowth or obstruction, the infective risks of operation rise. The likelihood of infection in operative procedures also relates directly to the degree of peritoneal soiling. In spontaneously occurring infections associated with perforation, the time elapsing before operation is obviously important in this context. Failure to secure haemostasis also greatly increases the likelihood of infection. The infections range from involvement of superficial wounds and localized intra-abdominal abscesses to generalized peritonitis, portal vein thrombosis, liver and subphrenic abscesses, and septicaemia.

In health the numerically dominant non-sporing anaerobes in the large bowel are members of the *B. fragilis* group, which are found in numbers of 10^{10}/g of faeces. This group comprises *B. fragilis, B. vulgatus, B. distasonis, B. thetaiotaomicron, B. uniformis, B. variabilis/eggerthii,* and *B. splanchnicus; B. fragilis* represents less than 10 per cent of these strains. However, in abdominal sepsis it is the dominant isolate. The latter observation strongly suggests that this species has particular virulence factors.

The recognition of the importance of non-sporing anaerobes in endogenous abdominal infections came with the use of metronidazole both in chemoprophylaxis and therapy in abdominal surgery. The dramatic reduction in infection rates were attributable to the effect on anaerobic bacteria of this agent, which is largely without action on facultative anaerobes.

Operations on, or disease of, the female pelvic organs may be associated with mixed infections. Studies of the healthy vaginal flora have revealed that anaerobes are present in as many as 65 per cent of individuals. The commonest organisms belong to the *B. melaninogenicus/oralis* group, members of the *B. fragilis* group are relatively uncommon. In symptomatic females attending departments of genital medicine, the number with vaginal anaerobes may reach 90 per cent, but the qualitative nature of the flora remains relatively constant and *B. fragilis* group is quite uncommon. By contrast, in deep-seated or surgical infections the *B. fragilis* group becomes more prevalent. Infections may simply involve superficial wounds or may extend to the uterus, tubo-ovarian abscess, pelvic vein thrombosis, and generalized peritonitis. As with abdominal infections due to non-sporing anaerobes, the introduction of metronidazole as a chemoprophylatic and therapeutic agent has markedly reduced the incidence and improved the outcome of these infections, leaving no doubt as to the pathogenic role of these organisms in this situation.

Clostridial infections

The examples of anaerobic and mixed infections thus far considered relate to organisms whose importance in the pathogenesis of human disease has been recognized only latterly, almost certainly because of the difficulties in establishing disease with pure cultures in animal models. By contrast, the association between the spore-bearing clostridia and their role in the pathogenesis of well-defined human infections has been long accepted. The diseases caused by clostridia are due to the effects of powerful exotoxins, but the intiation of the infective process is often dependent upon additional factors which result in multiplication of the organisms.

Tetanus

Tetanus results from the introduction of toxigenic strains of *Cl. tetani* into the body via injuries, raw surfaces or, more rarely, parenterally. In the developed countries most cases are seen in adults, often where the injury has occurred in an agricultural or horticultural setting; intravenous narcotic drug addicts present a further risk group. In the Third World about one-third of cases are neonatal tetanus and result from contamination of the umbilical stump.

The common clinical presentation is muscle rigidity with tonic reflex muscular spasm. In the commoner 'descending' form of the disease, toxin reaches the brain stem via the bloodstream and motor nerves; characteristically the masseters are involved at an early stage. In 'ascending' tetanus, in which the lower extremities are first affected, the toxin 'ascends' the motor nerves to the anterior horn cells. The injection of toxin-free spores of *Cl. tetani* into the guinea-pig is without effect, but disease results if there is injury at the injection site producing necrosis or bruising, or a second species of bacteria is present, or small quantities of ionizable calcium salts are included in the inoculum.

These various forms of tissue damage are thought to cause a fall in the oxidation–reduction potential to levels permitting germination of the spores. Growth of the vegetative form is accompanied by production of the potent neurotoxin which, reaching the central nervous system via the motor nerves and the bloodstream (see above), binds to a specific receptor, possibly a ganglioside. The mode of action of the toxin appears to be selective depression of impulses which normally act upon the motor neurones to prevent motor hyperactivity.

Gas gangrene

Gas gangrene is a clostridial myositis. The prerequisites for the development of the disease are similar to those operative in tetanus, although tissue damage is generally more severe. Characteristically, the condition complicates gross trauma such as war wounds, occasionally it follows elective surgery. Several species of clostridia may cause the disease, either alone, or in combination with each other, or with aerobic organisms. Anaerobic streptococci may, infrequently, cause a clinically similar condition. The three most important clostridia associated with gas gangrene are *Cl. perfringens*, *Cl. novyi*, and *Cl. septicum*. All three species elaborate exotoxins, those produced by *Cl. perfringens* include lecithinase, collagenase, hyaluronidase, deoxyribonuclease, and fibrinolysin. Inoculation of toxic amounts of culture filtrates of the organism into animals produces oedema, necrosis, capillary and venous thrombosis. Substances present in the culture filtrate are implicated in the initiation of the infection as well as producing the characteristic picture. Thus, washed bacilli are non-pathogenic when injected into guinea-pigs, but if a non-lethal dose of culture filtrate is added to such an inoculum it becomes extremely virulent. This effect appears in part to be due to the presence in culture filtrates of non-toxic substances which activate the infection by impeding phagocytic killing, permitting the growth of toxigenic bacilli.

Intestinal disease

Just as the aforementioned species cause gas gangrene by means of the exotoxins they elaborate, these and other toxigenic clostridia have also been associated with various intestinal diseases in man. Food-poisoning due to *Cl. perfringens* type A is usually associated with the consumption of meat that has been inadequately cooked, stored at a relatively high ambient temperature, and insufficiently reheated. Germination of the surviving heat-resistant spores produces large numbers of vegetative organisms which, on injection, germinate in the intestine, releasing enterotoxin. Oral administration of purified enterotoxin to appropriate laboratory animals and human volunteers produces diarrhoea. Related but much more severe, sometimes fatal, conditions are enteritis necrotans and pig-bel due to *Cl. perfringens* types F and C, respectively.

Botulism

Some species of clostridia produce toxins that are so powerful that their ingestion alone can produce disease. Thus botulism, characterized by vomiting, ocular and pharyngeal pareses, with a clear sensorium, may be regarded as an intoxication rather than an infection. Usually *Cl. botulinum* multiplies in contaminated food, producing soluble neural toxins which, on ingestion, are readily absorbed from the intestine and cause the disease by acting peripherally on both the efferent autonomic nerve supply to muscle and glands and somatic nerves to striped muscles. In rare instances multiplication of *Cl. botulinum* in the gut, with concomitant toxin production, has been suspected. Thus, infant botulism may arise not from the ingestion of pre-formed toxin in milk preparations, but from in-gut production by the bacteria. This hypothesis is supported by the finding of very large numbers of *Cl. botulinum* in the faeces of affected babies and the continued presence of toxin in the faeces long after resolution of the initial illness. Very rarely, botulism has been reported as a consequence of wound infection.

Pseudomembranous enterocolitis

Cl. difficile has been implicated as causing pseudomembranous enterocolitis, a disease that sometimes complicates broad-spectrum antimicrobial treatment in the seriously ill. Faeces from affected patients contain high titres of cytopathic toxin derived from antibiotic-resistant *Cl. difficile*. In addition, an enterotoxin of *Cl. difficile* has been demonstrated, which may be responsible for the observed colitis.

For further information on anaerobic infections readers are referred to the relevant chapters in Wilson *et al.* (1991).

Mixed infections due to extrinsic micro-organisms

Not all mixed infections encountered in man involve endogenous organisms. One of the commonest of such infections is tinea pedis (athletes' foot) in which the interdigital spaces of the toes are infected with a fungus, commonly *Trichophyton rubrum*, *T. interdigitalis*, or *Epidermophyton floccosum*, usually acquired in communal bathing facilities such as swimming or communal baths. This produces a low-grade scaly condition known as dermatophytosis simplex which, if unrelieved, may, through the concomitant multiplication of brevibacteria, progress to the development of painful soggy interspaces which characterize dermatophytosis complex. It has been demonstrated experimentally using antifungal and antibacterial agents alone or in combination that the more severe form of the disease is dependent upon the presence of both types of organisms. The reciprocal benefits of this association are not clear, but it has been suggested that antimicrobial substances produced by the fungi favour the overgrowth of the relatively antibiotic-resistant brevibacteria.

Having considered the source of bacteria in mixed and anaerobic infections and clinical examples of these we must now examine the pathogenic mechanisms employed by these organisms.

Pathogenetic mechanisms

Although Meleney's synergistic gangrene was one of the first examples of mixed infections to be described, little is known of the individual contributions made by *Staph. aureus* and the microaerophilic streptococcus that characterize this condition, other than that both are required to reproduce the disease in experimental animals. Studies of a variety of other mixed infections have cast more light on the means whereby the individual components contribute to the synergistic process.

Animal models

Appendicitis and gingival infections Studies in the 1940s by Altemeier of organisms recovered from peritoneal exudates in patients with acute appendicitis showed that subcutaneous (sc) or intraperitoneal (ip) inoculation of the individual strains into guinea-pigs usually failed to produce progressive disease. However, sc injection of mixtures of the strains resulted in extensive cellulitis which was often gangrenous. Similarly, fatal peritonitis frequently followed the ip injection of such mixtures. One of the organisms consistently present in these samples was *B.*

melaninogenicus, usually in conjunction with a non-haemolytic streptococcus, which was difficult to culture without the anaerobe.

Further light was shed on this observation in studies of the bacteriology of human gingival infections in which guinea-pigs were inoculated with material from the gingival and periodontal lesions of acute necrotizing ulcerative gingivitis. Of the 20 strains of bacteria isolated from the resulting abscesses, only four were essential for transmission of infection to further animals. These strains were *B. melaninogenicus*, two other strains of *Bacteroides*, and a facultative diphtheroid. The apparent function of the diphtheroid in this mixture appeared to be the provision of a growth factor for *B. melaninogenicus*, subsequently shown to be a napthaquinone, a precursor of vitamin K. Media supplemented with vitamin K derivatives such as menadione supported the growth of the strain of *B. melaninogenicus*. Strains of *B. melaninogenicus* that grew in the absence of menadione produced lesions in guinea-pigs in the presence of only one other strain of *Bacteroides*, indicating that menadione dependence resulted in a reduction of virulence.

The provision of essential growth factors by one bacterium for another is one of the mechanisms proposed to explain synergy. The difficulty in establishing single-organism experimental infections in animals, even with bacteria not requiring demonstrable growth factors, suggests that bacterial synergy must be a multifactorial process.

A further hypothesis advanced to explain the pathogenesis of these infections has been the provision by one part of the inoculum of factors that protect other component organisms against the defence mechanisms of the host. An example of this was demonstrated elegantly in a study of the bacteriology of foot-rot in sheep. This is a disease seen in flocks living in wet conditions, and represents progression of the normally self-limiting condition, ovine interdigital dermatitis, to a more destructive disease, which may eventually result in separation of the hoof. In experimental studies with sheep and guinea-pigs it was shown that in ovine interdigital dermatitis *F. necrophorum*, by means of the leucocidal action of its exotoxin, allowed the growth of *Corynebacterium pyogenes*, and the latter produced a filtrable agent that stimulated the growth of *F. necrophorum*. In foot-rot, further organisms are present that provide additional growth factors for *F. necrophorum* and maintain persistent infection in periods of relative quiescence between acute destructive episodes due to *F. necrophorum*.

Until recently (see below), efforts to establish an animal model of human infections with a single species of non-sporing anaerobes, with the exception of *F. necrophorum*, were not successful, except in the presence of inert factors in the inoculum such as agar, mucin, or barium sulphate. The latter substances presumably impede phagocytic activity, allowing the organisms to gain a foothold, very much in the manner of a foreign body in a naturally occurring infection.

Rat model of intra-abdominal sepsis In attempts to reproduce in experimental animals infections with organisms typical of the flora of abdominal sepsis, Weinstein (in the 1970s) inoculated rat caecal contents into the peritoneal cavity of Wistar rats. The inoculum was contained in gelatin capsules and essential components of this inoculum were found to be barium sulphate and autoclaved rat caecal contents.

A bimodel illness ensued in which there was an early, septicaemic phase caused by *E. coli* with a high mortality, followed by the development of intra-abdominal abscesses in the survivors. The abscesses contained most of the organisms in the original inoculum but when the work was repeated with individual components of the purified cultures, only *E. coli* and *B. fragilis* were found to be essential in this model.

Studies with antimicrobial agents, commenced 4 hours after insertion of the capsules, revealed that gentamicin, active only against *E. coli*, reduced the mortality from 37 to 4 per cent but had no effect on abscess formation in the survivors. Clindamycin, active against *B. fragilis* but not *E. coli*, had no effect on mortality but reduced abscess formation from 100 to 5 per cent. When both agents were given together both mortality and abscess formation were markedly reduced.

Unexpectedly, administration of metronidazole not only reduced abscess formation from 100 to 13 per cent but also mortality from 37 to 10 per cent. It thus appeared that, as metronidazole is extremely active against obligate anaerobes but has little or no action against facultative anaerobes, it might be exerting an effect on mortality indirectly by killing the anaerobic components of the inoculum and thus impairing the synergistic partnership. It soon became apparent that this explanation was unlikely as it was demonstrated that metronidazole, under appropriate conditions, was active against facultative anaerobes such as *E. coli* (Ingham *et al.* 1980) and also that the early septicaemia and mortality due to *E. coli* was purely a function of the number of these organisms in the initial inoculum. The synergy apparent in this model was, therefore, restricted to abscess formation.

Subsequent studies showed that the original strain of *B. fragilis* employed had been non-capsulate. The substitution of a capsulate strain of *B. fragilis* in this model obviated the need for *E. coli*, and it proved possible to produce abscesses with the purified capsular polysaccharide. Immunization of animals with capsular polysaccharide prevented these experimental abscesses when the homologous strain was employed as the inoculum, proving the importance of the capsule as a virulence factor. Further supportive evidence is seen in recent reports that encapsulated strains of *Bacteroides* sp. and anaerobic cocci cause abscesses in mice when injected alone. Moreover, non-encapsulated strains, when used as part of a mixed inoculum in such experiments, became heavily encapsulated during development of the abscesses and subsequently induced such lesions when injected alone. A clinical corollary to this is the report that, in contrast to strains of anaerobes isolated from the healthy throat or mouth, those present in patients with active infections in these areas are capsulate.

Capsular material is thought to enhance the virulence of bacteria by interfering with the opsonophagocytic process, either by preventing ingestion or subsequent intracellular killing. The importance of capsulation in the pathogenicity of non-sporing

anaerobes is underlined by the observation that *B. fragilis*, the most frequently encountered strain in abdominal and pelvic sepsis, is regularly encapsulated, in contrast to other members of the group. The ability of apparently non-capsulate strains of non-sporing anaerobes to develop these structures when they are present as part of a mixed infection suggests that in many such organisms this property is innate but not usually expressed. In such organisms, capsule formation may be regarded as a survival mechanism rather than, a priori, a virulence factor.

Encapsulation is not the sole virulence factor (see Section 6.2) in experimental infections, as judged by recent reports of another rat model of peritoneal sepsis in which *E. coli* and various species of bacteroides were inoculated ip in fibrin clots. In this model the mortality due to *E. coli* was genuinely enhanced by the bacteroides, some strains of which were non-capsulate.

In vitro studies

Effect of anaerobes on the phagocytic process Further information on the role of capsule in infections involving non-sporing anaerobes has emerged from studies of the interaction between these organisms and the polymorphonuclear leucocytes (PMNL) *in vitro*. In the 1970s Okuda and Takazoe showed that encapsulated strains of *B. melaninogenicus* were more resistant to phagocytic killing than non-capsulated varieties and that phagocytosis and phagocytic killing of *Staph. aureus* was inhibited when extracted capsular material from *B. melaninogenicus* was present in the test system. In 1977 Ingham and colleagues demonstrated that the ability to inhibit phagocytic killing was a property shared to a greater or lesser degree by all Gram-negative non-sporing anaerobes. The extent of this activity varied, being greatest with *B. fragilis* and *B. melaninogenicus* groups and least with *B. ruminicola* and *Veillonella*. The effect was associated with the bacterial cell, only seen with high inocula, and appeared to be specific to obligate anaerobes as it was not exhibited by equivalent numbers of aerobes and facultative anaerobes. It was further observed that not only did obligate anaerobes inhibit their own phagocytic killing but also that of facultative anaerobes included in the test system. The primary effect of anaerobes in this experimental system appeared to be inactivation of heat-labile and heat-stable serum components concerned with the opsonization of micro-organisms prior to ingestion. Ingestion *per se* did not appear to be inhibited as at the end of the experiment PMNL contained large numbers of viable bacteria, and it seems likely that the primary effect is directed against opsonic factors essential for intracellular killing.

Other workers have broadly confirmed these findings although suggesting that, at least in the early stages of phagocytosis, there is impairment of uptake of micro-organisms. The phagocytic process includes all events from the initial movement of PMNL towards the infected focus, to attachment, engulfment, and intracellular killing of micro-organisms. These apparently conflicting results have been partially reconciled by subsequent studies reporting the production of diffusible substances by non-sporing obligate anaerobes which, by direct action on PMNL, inhibit chemotaxis, degranulation, and cell membrane function. Chemotaxis is a process whereby polymorphs are positively attracted towards bacteria, usually under the influence of chemotaxins produced by the organisms or generated by an interaction between the bacteria and serum components. Degranulation is associated with the metabolic burst occurring in PMNL in relation to intracellular killing, and intact cell membrane function is essential for the intracellular transmission of signals generated by the binding of chemotactic factors. Impairment of any or all of these functions could thus retard the initial uptake of bacteria by polymorphs.

The factors in anaerobic bacteria responsible for the inhibitory effect on the phagocytic process have not been fully characterized. In non-sporing anaerobes they appear to be heat-stable substances intimately associated with the bacterial cell, and inhibition is optimally expressed by whole cells rather than extracts. Capsular polysaccharide extracted from these organisms is capable of inhibiting phagocytic killing, although not as efficiently as whole cells. Others have linked the inhibition of chemotaxis and phagocytic killing with the production by obligate anaerobes of short-chain fatty acids or other diffusible substances, but in both instances the inhibition is mediated through an effect on the white cells rather than a serum component.

In summary, *in vitro* studies indicate that non-sporing anaerobes inhibit chemotaxis and killing by PMNL of themselves and associated organisms directly and by interacting with serum factors. These effects are mediated by cell-associated components, including bacterial capsule, and diffusible substances.

Bacterial toxins

Endotoxins The success of micro-organisms as pathogens depends not only on their ability to gain a foothold at a particular locus in the body but also on the production of progressive disease. Mixed infections, if uncontrolled, may produce septicaemia with the development of metastatic foci but, unless Gram-negative facultative anaerobes are implicated, endotoxic shock is unusual. This has been attributed to the fact that the cell wall of non-sporing anaerobes is substantially different from that of Gram-negative facultative anaerobes, in particular in the structure of the lipopolysaccharide (LPS) that is responsible for endotoxicity. The latter is due to the lipid A fraction, which in experimental animals causes fever, leucopenia followed by leucocytosis, hyperglycemia, purpura, Shwartzman reaction, and, in larger doses, irreversible shock. The LPS of *B. fragilis* is only weakly endotoxic as measured by animal studies, and in the *Limulus* lysate test, an *in vitro* assay, a much higher concentration is required to produce a positive result compared with endotoxins from Gram-negative facultative anaerobes. These differences are attributed to the absence of 2-keto-3-deoxyoctonate (KDO) and heptose, which characterize LPS in Gram-negative facultative anaerobes. It is of interest that *F. necrophorum*, one of the few organisms capable of producing pure anaerobic infection in man, does exhibit some of these biological activities in experimental animals, and the cell wall contains small amounts of KDO.

Exotoxins The focal effects of mixed infections depend upon the location and size of lesions and involement of adjacent tissue. Although these may result from further embarrassment of local defence mechanisms, it is possible that tissue-active bacterial toxins are implicated. Non-sporing anaerobes produce a range of such enzymes, which include heparinase, collagenase, proteinases, fibrinolysin, hyaluronidase, and chondroitin sulphatase. However, studies to date have not shown a clear association between the production of these enzymes and the virulence of particular clinical isolates of non-sporing anaerobes. The rapid time-course and degree of swelling of cellulitis characteristic of some of these infections strongly suggests the involvement of such 'spreading' factors (Figs 6.23, 6.24). Likewise, there is a clear role for heparinase in the aetiology of the thromboembolic complications that characterize many of these infections.

Apart from obligate anaerobes and facultative Gram-negative anaerobes, the role of other organisms in mixed infections has, in general, been little studied and is poorly understood. An exception to this is seen in *Str. milleri*, which forms part of the normal flora of the gingival crevice, the large bowel, and the vagina, and is present in many mixed infections due to endogenous organisms. This organism may possess Lancefield antigens A, C, G, or F and strains carrying the latter are most commonly implicated in infective processes. The organism is reported most often in liver and brain abscesses, where it may be the sole isolate, and it seems likely that this organism was the microaerophilic streptococcus implicated in Meleney's gangrene.

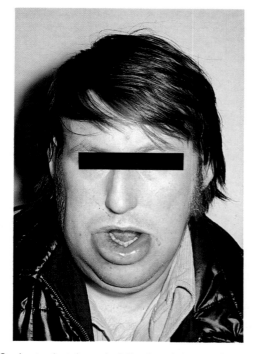

Fig. 6.23 Acute dental sepsis following the extraction of a lower molar. Note the gross swelling of the face and lower lip. (Reproduced from Ingham *et al.* 1977b, with permission.)

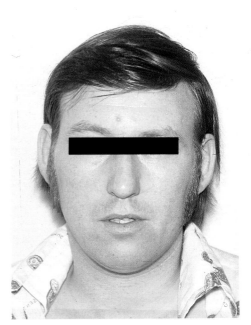

Fig. 6.24 The appearance of the patient shown in Fig. 6.23, after resolution of the infection. (Reproduced from Ingham *et al.* 1977b, with permission.)

Indirect pathogenicity

Another process that may contribute to the overall success of mixed infections in the clinical context is the production of enzymes that inactivate antimicrobial agents. Unquestionably, the most important example of this is cephalosporinase production which is a constant characteristic of members of the *B. fragilis* group, which are also inherently resistant to penicillin and many cephalosporins. This has the effect of rendering these organisms highly resistant to penicillins in general, as the inherent resistance permits multiplication of these organisms and the production of large amounts of drug-destroying enzymes. Latterly, similar cephalosporinases have been reported increasingly in normally penicillin-sensitive strains, such as members of the *B. melaninogenicus/oralis* group. The *B. fragilis* group also produces enzymes that inactivate chloramphenicol.

The production of these enzymes has profound implications for the management of mixed infections, as not only are the parent bacteria resistant to the particular antibiotics but any coexisting sensitive organisms in mixed infections are protected from their action, which has given rise to the term 'indirect pathogenicity'.

Conclusion

It will be apparent from the foregoing text that mixed infections constitute a prime example of microbial opportunism, whereby organisms forming the normal flora of various regions of the body conjointly exploit breaches in the defences. The initiating events in such infections are easily comprehended and should be revealed in most instances by a careful clinical history, particularly when this is supplemented by bacteriological data, which may provide a 'fingerprint' of the primary source. The more widespread recognition of these infections should stimulate the detailed studies required for a fuller comprehension of the pathogenic mechanisms employed.

6.5.5 Further reading

Pyogenic infections

Easmon, C. S. F. and Adlam, C. (1983). *Staphylococci and staphylococcal infections*, Vol. 2. *The organism* in vivo *and* in vitro. Academic Press, London.

Taussig, M. (1984). *Processes in pathology and microbiology* (2nd edn). Blackwell Scientific Publications, Oxford.

Wilson, G., Miles, A., and Parker, M. T. (1983). *Topley and Wilson's principles of bacteriology, virology and immunity* (7th edn), Vol. 2. *Systemic bacteriology*, chs 29 and 30. Edward Arnold, London.

Gram-negative anaerobic infections

General

Young, L. S. (1990). Gram-negative sepsis. In *Principles and practice of infectious diseases* (3rd edn) (ed. G. L. Mandell, R. G. Douglas Jr., and J. E. Bennett). Churchill Livingstone, New York.

Young, L. S., Martin, W. J., Meyer, R. D., Weinstein, R. J., and Anderson, R. T. (1977). Gram-negative rod bacteraemia: microbiologic, immunologic, and therapeutic considerations. *Annals of Internal Medicine* **86**, 456–71.

The gram-negative cell wall

Ingraham, J. L., Maaloe, O., and Neidhardt, F. C. (1983). Composition, organisation and structure of the bacterial cell. In *Growth of the bacterial cell*. Sinauer Associates, Inc., Sunderland, Massachusetts.

Mechanisms of virulence

Densen, P. and Mandell, G. L. (1980). Phagocyte strategy vs. microbial tactics. *Reviews of Infectious Diseases* **2** (5), 817–38.

Toxins

Wolff, S. M. (1973). Biological effects of endotoxins in man. *Journal of Infectious Disease* **128**, S259–S264.

Ziegler, E. J., *et al.* (1982). Treatment of Gram-negative bacteraemia and shock with human antiserum to a mutant *Escherichia coli*. *New England Journal of Medicine* **307** (20), 1225–30.

Anaerobic and polymicrobial infections

Altemeier, W. A. (1942) The pathogenicity of the bacteria of appendicitis and peritonitis. *Surgery* **11**, 375–6.

Brook, I. (1987). Role of encapsulated anaerobic bacteria in synergistic infections. *CRC Critical Reviews in Microbiology* **14**, 171–93.

Ingham, H. R. and Sisson, P. R. (1984). Pathogenic synergism. *Microbiological Sciences* **1**, 206–8.

Ingham, H. R., Sisson, P. R., Tharagonnet, D., Selkon, J. B., and Codd, A. A. (1977). Inhibition of phagocytosis *in vitro* by obligate anaerobes. *Lancet* **ii**, 1252–4.

Ingham, H. R., *et al.* (1977b). Metronidazole compared with penicillin in the treatment of acute dental infections. *British Journal of Oral Surgery* **14**, 266–72.

Ingham, H. R., Hall, C. J., Sisson, P. R., Tharagonnet, D., and Selkon, J. B. (1980). The activity of metronidazole against facultatively anaerobic bacteria. *Journal of Antimicrobial Chemotherapy* 6, 343–7.

Okuda, K. and Takazoe, I. (1973). Antiphagocytic effects of the capsular structure of a pathogenic strain of *Bacteroides melanogenicus*. *Bulletin of the Tokyo Dental College* 14, 99–104.

Rotstein, O. D., Pruett, T. L., and Simmons, R. L. (1985). Mechanisms of microbial synergy in polymicrobial surgical infections. *Reviews of Infectious Diseases* 7, 151–69.

Strachan, C. J. L. and Wise, R. (1979). *Surgical Sepsis*. Academic Press, London.

Wilson, G., Miles, A., Parker, M. T., and Smith, G. R. (eds) (1991). *Topley and Wilson's principles of bacteriology, virology and immunity*, Vol. 3 (8th edn). Edward Arnold, London.

6.6 Chronic infections

6.6.1 Chronic bacterial infections

Mary P. E. Slack

The majority of bacterial infections run an acute course. They provoke an acute inflammatory response which usually results in the elimination of the infecting organisms from the body. Less frequently, the host fails to mount an adequate response and the infection may then prove rapidly destructive, even fatal. There is, however, an intermediate group of infections in which the bacteria are not eliminated from the body, but persist for months or years. These chronic infections may represent a failure of host defences, or some special adaptation of the pathogen which permits its survival.

Chronic infections cannot, by definition, be acutely lethal to the host, and usually the infecting organism is of low pathogenicity, permitting the survival of the host despite the persistent infection. The pathological changes characteristic of the chronic infection are not necessarily due to the toxic properties of the bacterial pathogen, but may be a result of immune mechanisms, for example antibody- or immune complex-related phenomena or the effects of cell-mediated immunity.

There are several reasons why infections show chronicity (Table 6.21). Almost all bacteria that cause acute infections can cause infections with some degree of chronicity, but some bacterial species are particularly associated with chronic infections. *Mycobaterium tuberculosis*, *M. leprae*, and *Treponema pallidum* often cause chronic infections.

This section will first discuss the ways in which chronic infections arise and then the pathogenesis of some chronic bacterial infections will be considered in more detail.

Evasion of immune response
Intracellular sequestration
A feature common to many of the bacteria associated with

Table 6.21 Pathogenic mechanisms of chronic infections

Mechanism	Examples
Evasion of immune mechanisms	
Intracellular sequestration	*Mycobacterium tuberculosis*
	Mycobacterium leprae
	Listeria monocytogenes
	Salmonella typhi
	Treponema pallidum
	Brucella abortus
Antigenic variation	*Borrelia recurrentis*
	Borrelia burgdorferi
Protected sites of infection	
Foreign bodies	
prosthetic heart valve	*Staphylococcus epidermidis* endocarditis
necrotic sequestrum of bone	*Staph. aureus* osteomyelitis
Relatively avascular sites	
damaged heart valve	*Viridans streptococcal* endocarditis
aqueous humour	Diphtheroid endophthalmitis
scarred gall bladder	*Salmonella typhi* carriage
Anatomical defects	
bladder diverticula in prostatic hypertrophy	*Escherichia coli* urinary-tract infection
bronchiectasis	Pneumococcus and *Haemophilus influenzae* infection
Defective immunity	
White cell defects	
chronic granulomatous disease	recurrent and chronic *Staphylococcus aureus* and *Serratia marcescens* infections
Antibody deficiency	
hypogammaglobulinaemia	recurrent respiratory infections leading to chronic disease
Complement deficiency	
C6, C7, C8 deficiency	chronic meningococcaemia chronic gonococcaemia
Cell-mediated immunity	lepromatous leprosy

chronic infections is that they are obligate or facultative intracellular parasites and thus are protected from the extracellular defence mechanisms of the host, in particular circulating antibodies. *Mycobacterium leprae* is an obligate intracellular parasite. Facultative intracellular parasites include *M. tuberculosis*, *M. bovis*, *M. avium*, *Listeria monocytogenes*, *Salmonella typhi*, *Brucella* spp., and *Treponema pallidum*. Typically, intracellular bacteria induce granulomata formation, whereas extracellular bacteria, when localized in tissues, produce abscesses (see Chapters 4 and 5). The immunity to intracellular bacteria is mediated by T-cells which activate macrophages by releasing soluble cytokines such as γ-interferon.

Antigenic variation
Individual antigens are controlled by individual genes and only one antigen encoded by a gene at a particular locus can be expressed at any one time. Some organisms possess the capacity to express a number of different antigenic types corresponding

to the genes present at that locus and can, under adverse conditions, switch gene activity and produce a different antigen. The presence of specific antibody is a trigger for this switch. This mechanism of evasion of host defences is especially common among parasitic infections such as trypanasomiasis. It is also the mechanism underlying the remissions and relapses which are characteristic of infection with *Borrelia recurrentis* (relapsing fever) and *B. burgdorferi* (Lyme disease).

Protected sites of infection

In some instances a bacterial infection may tend to become chronic because the site of the infection, for example the renal parenchyma or heart valves, affords considerable protection against the defence mechanisms of the host. For example, leptospires can persist in the renal tubules of the rat kidney for long periods of time, with chronic shedding of organisms into the urine. The bacteria responsible for infective endocarditis are, to a large extent, protected by being encased in vegetations of platelets and fibrin. The presence of a foreign body severely impairs the ability of the host to eliminate an infection. The introduction of low-grade pathogens into prosthetic material in a patient can result in an indolent, chronic infection which can be very difficult to eradicate. Examples of this type of infection include prosthetic valve endocarditis and prosthetic joint infections. Necrotic debris, such as a sequestrum of bone in chronic osteomyelitis (see Chapter 27), similarly provides shelter for pathogens from the action of the host defences.

In some cases of typhoid, *S. typhi* can persist for months or even years in the gall bladder or urinary bladder. Scarred, relatively avascular areas of the gall bladder or urinary bladder become colonized and the organisms are protected from the host defence mechanisms. *S. typhi* will be excreted intermittently via the bile into the faeces or from the bladder into the urine. Bacteria may also reside in anatomical defects such as bladder diverticula associated with prostatic hypertrophy, and provide a source of chronic urinary tract infection. Renal and biliary calculi may contain bacteria that are protected from host defences.

Defective immunity

Many of the congenital immunodeficiency syndromes are characterized by severe, recurrent episodes of infection which can result in chronic disease. Patients with phagocyte defects, such as chronic granulomatous disease, have recurrent pyogenic infections with *Staphylococcus aureus* and *Serratia marcescens* which result in cellulitis, abscesses, pneumonia, or osteomyelitis. Antibody-deficiency syndromes are also characterized by severe, recurrent, pyogenic bacterial infections. These patients almost invariably suffer recurrent respiratory infections, which include suppurative otitis media, mastoiditis, sinusitis, bronchitis, and pneumonia, which often result in bronchiectasis and chronic respiratory disease. They also suffer other systemic infections including osteomyelitis and meningitis. See Chapter 4 for a full discussion of these antibody and complement (see below) deficiency syndromes.

Congenital deficiencies in the complement system are often associated with infections similar to those observed in hypogammaglobulinaemia and include respiratory infections and meningitis. Patients with a congenital lack of the terminal complement components C6, C7, and C8 are prone to repeated episodes of disseminated chronic infections with *Neisseria meningitidis* and *N. gonorrhoeae*. These are cases of chronic meningococcaemia and chronic gonococcaemia rather than recurrent episodes of meningoccal meningitis or gonorrrhoea.

Infections with *M. leprae* form a spectrum ranging from localized disease (tuberculoid leprosy), to the widespread anergic form of the disease (lepromatous leprosy) (see Chapter 29 for a full discussion of leprosy). In lepromatous leprosy there is defective cell-mediated immunity, the underlying mechanism of which is still not clearly understood.

Other factors can affect host resistance and favour chronicity in a particular individual. These include nutritional state and intercurrent infections. There is also some evidence for a genetic predisposition to some forms of chronic infections. Individuals with the HLA-DR2 or HLA-DR3 haplotype or both may be predisposed to tuberculoid leprosy while DR2-DQWI may be associated with lepromatous leprosy.

Mycobacterial infections

Tuberculosis

Mycobacterium tuberculosis is still the most important chronic infectious disease in the world. *M. tuberculosis* produces neither exotoxins nor endotoxins and no single antigenic structure or mechanism can explain its virulence. However, there are a number of properties which are usually associated with the capacity of virulent strains of *M. tuberculosis* to cause disease. These include the possession of lipids such as the cord factor—a glycolipid, trehalose-6,6'-dimycolate—and sulphatides. In experimental animals cord factor inhibits polymorphonuclear leucocyte migration, induces granulomata formation, and inhibits mitochondrial oxidative phosphorylation. The sulphatides potentiate the toxicity of cord factor and *in vitro* they inhibit the fusion of secondary lysosomes with phagosomes to form phagolysosomes in macrophages. Because *M. tuberculosis* is an intracellular parasite, these virulence factors may promote survival by preventing exposure of the organisms to lysosomal hydrolases.

The response of an individual after exposure to virulent tubercle bacilli depends on the balance between acquired cell-mediated immunity and delayed hypersensitivity. Hypersensitivity to the proteins of the tubercle bacilli is the cause of the tissue destruction seen in tuberculosis. After the inhalation of virulent tubercle bacilli the organisms reach the alveoli where they are ingested by alveolar macrophages. The organisms multiply slowly, with a generation time of 15–20 hours, most other bacteria having a generation time of about 1 hour. Since these intracellular bacilli do not secrete any enzymes or toxins, they initially provoke little inflammatory response in the non-immune host. (Other extracellular organisms which do not produce toxins, such as the pneumococcus, provoke a marked inflammatory response during the early stages of infection.) By about 3 weeks there will be approximately 10^6 bacilli present in alveolar macrophages and in non-resident macrophages that have collected in the area. Macrophages, laden with mycobacteria, spread along the lymphatics to the hilar lymph nodes where at 6–8 weeks an immune response, dominated by T-helper cells, and tissue hypersensitivity develops. Tissue hypersensitivity is manifested by a positive tuberculin skin test and granulomata formation. Tissue hypersensitivity is enhanced by the potent adjuvant properties of mycobacterial lipids. The detailed pathology of tuberculosis is discussed in Chapter 13.

When helper T-cells encounter the macrophages which contain intracellular tubercle antigen they are activated, producing a variety of cytokines, including γ-interferon. These cytokines attract and activate macrophages at the site of the infection. Activated macrophages produce high concentrations of lytic enzymes which are mycobactericidal but which also cause tissue necrosis when released from the cells. Interleukin-1, secreted by the macrophages, causes fever. Tumour necrosis factor interferes with lipid metabolism and results in severe weight loss. Epithelioid cells, which are pathognomonic of tubercles, are highly stimulated macrophages. Activated macrophages secrete a fibroblast-stimulating substance which results in the formation of collagen and ultimately fibrosis. Langhans giant cells are fused macrophages lying around tubercle bacilli.

The majority of patients successfully contain the infection at this stage of a small primary lung lesion or tubercle which does not progress. If cell-mediated immunity is inadequate, the infection will extend to give progressive primary tuberculosis or disseminated disease. Healed and inactive granulomata contain small numbers of dormant but viable tubercle bacilli, and in about 3–5 per cent of cases these lesions can break down or reactivate to give post-primary or re-infection tuberculosis. Reactivation is primarily associated with old age, malnutrition, or immunosuppression, including HIV infection (AIDS). These persistent organisms also help to maintain a population of memory immune T-cells which can prevent exogenous re-infection.

In any given population a few patients are unable to mount an adequate immune response to *M. tuberculosis*. The infection spreads rapidly through the body to give a disseminated miliary form of the disease. Infection with *M. tuberculosis* stimulates the production of a number of antibodies but these seem to play no significant role in the pathogenesis or immunity to tuberculosis. Recent studies have indicated that host resistance to tuberculosis is to some extent genetically determined.

Disseminated infection with both *M. tuberculosis* and the opportunistic species *M. avium*, *M. intracellulare*, *M. kansasii*, *M. fortuitum*, *M. xenopi*, and *M. gordonae* is now a well-recognized problem in patients with AIDS (see Chapters 4 and 29). The source of these non-tuberculous species appears to be the environment, including contaminated drinking water.

Leprosy

Leprosy is a chronic infection, caused by *M. leprae*, which mainly involves the skin, peripheral nerves, and, in some cases, mucous membranes. The clinical features of the disease are due to bacterial proliferation, the immunological response of the host to the bacilli, and the resulting peripheral neuritis. *M. leprae* is of low infectivity and even in an endemic area most people resist infection. Indeed only about 1 in 200 people infected with *M. leprae* go on to develop overt clinical disease. The incubation period is about 2–4 years. The hallmarks of leprosy are skin lesions, skin anaesthesia, and enlarged peripheral nerves. Individuals who are unable to resist infection with *M. leprae* initially develop a few hypopigmented skin lesions with minimal sensory loss. This phase is called indeterminate leprosy. About three-quarters of cases spontaneously resolve at this stage. Some remain indeterminate for a long time, and the remainder will progress to one of the established forms of leprosy.

The spectrum of established leprosy has been well defined (Table 6.22). Cases are placed into one of five categories, which range from localized, self-healing, granulomatous disease with very few demonstrable bacilli and a marked immune response (polar tuberculoid leprosy) to a widespread, progressive, anergic form of the disease (polar lepromatous leprosy). The groups are no more than arbitrary points on a continuous spectrum. Patients in the borderline areas may develop immunity and move towards the tuberculoid end of the spectrum or lose resistance and drift towards lepromatous leprosy. Premature or abrupt cessation of treatment may result in loss of resistance. (For a full description of the types of leprosy, see Chapter 29.)

M. leprae is an obligate intracellular pathogen which cannot be cultured *in vitro*. It can be cultured in the mouse footpad or in the nine-banded armadillo. The organism multiples within mononuclear phagocytes, particularly histiocytes in the skin and Schwann cells of nerves. *M. leprae* is very slow-growing, with a generation time of about 12 days. Its virulence factors have still to be identified.

Leprosy is a disease in which there is a close correlation between the nature of the host response and the clinical forms of disease. In tuberculoid leprosy there is well-developed cell-mediated immunity, resulting in well-organized granulomata in the basal layer of the epidermis. These consist of epithelioid cells, multinucleated giant cells, and many lymphocytes. Acid-fast bacilli are scanty or absent. The organisms invade the nerves and multiply in Schwann cells. The nerves are swollen

Table 6.22 The spectrum of leprosy (Ridley–Jopling classification)

Abbreviation	Pathology	Resistance
T.T.	Polar tuberculoid	high
B.T.	Borderline tuberculoid	
B.B.	Borderline	
B.L.	Borderline lepromatous	
L.L.	Polar lepromatous	low

and destroyed by granulomata. The nerve damage is non-specific and is due to the cell-mediated response. Macrophages, activated by cytokines (γ-interferon) released from sensitized helper T-cells play a key role in epithelioid cell granuloma formation. Patients with tuberculoid leprosy exhibit a strong delayed hypersensitivity to lepromin, a heat-killed suspension of *M. leprae*.

The histopathology of lepromatous leprosy is strikingly different to that of tuberculoid leprosy. Epithelioid and giant cells are absent and only a few lymphocytes are found in the lesions. The inflammatory infiltrate contains many histiocytes, which have a foamy appearance due to the accumulation of a unique phenolic glycolipid (PGL-1). This compound possesses a trisaccharide that is specific for *M. leprae* and highly immunogenic.

As the pattern of disease moves across the spectrum towards lepromatous leprosy, there is a progressive loss of hypersensitivity and development of an anergic state. A loss of cell-mediated immunity parallels the decline in delayed hypersensitivity to *M. leprae* antigens. It must be stressed that patients with lepromatous leprosy do not have a general suppression of their cell-mediated immunity, rather they lack specific cell-mediated responses to *M. leprae* antigens. There is a deficiency of T-helper cells specific for *M. leprae* antigens at the lepromatous end of the spectrum but the reason for this is unclear. Other studies have demonstrated *M. leprae*-specific suppressor T-cells in the peripheral blood of lepromatous leprosy patients. It also seems likely that macrophage function is impaired in these patients.

Patients with lepromatous leprosy have high circulating levels of antibodies to *M. leprae* antigens and often show polyclonal hypergammaglobulinaemia. Patients with tuberculoid leprosy have only low levels of these antibodies. These antibodies are of no protective value, which is hardly surprising since *M. leprae* is an obligate intracellular parasite. Humoral antibodies do play a role in the pathogenesis of erythema nodosum leprosum which occurs in about 50 per cent of cases of lepromatous leprosy as a result of immune-complex deposition in the tissues.

Syphilis

Treponema pallidum is another bacterium that causes a slowly evolving chronic infection (Fig. 6.25). It principally infects vascular tissue and can involve almost every tissue of the body. In leprosy the disease state can move from one side of the clinical spectrum to the other, depending on the level of host resistance.

In syphilis there is a sequential progression from a state of low resistance during the early stages to high resistance in the later stages of the infection.

T. pallidum enters the body through mucous membranes or through intact skin, possibly via microscopic abrasions, and quickly spreads via blood and lymphatics throughout the body. Multiplication of organisms occurs at the site of entry, resulting in a single, painless papule, the primary chancre. *T. pallidum* has a generation time of about 30–33 hours. The primary chancre consists of an inflammatory response characterized by lymphocytes, plasma cells, monocytes, and some macrophages. Metachromatic acidic mucopolysaccharides accumulate, which gives the lesion its characteristic firmness. These mucopolysaccharides are in part derived from the capsules of the treponemes, and in part are host-tissue constituents. The mucopolysaccharides readily adhere to the surface of the treponemes and enable the organisms to avoid antibody recognition and also impair cellular immune responses to the spirochaete. *T. pallidum* also produces a mucopolysaccharidase that can degrade cell-surface mucopolysaccharides. This enzyme may degrade the mucopolysaccharides that join capillary endothelial cells. By cleaving these cells the treponemes can gain access to the perivascular area. Further degradation of mucopolysaccharides in blood vessels may account for the obliterative endarteritis characteristic of syphilis.

Chancres usually heal spontaneously in 2–8 weeks, but may persist for longer in immunocompromised individuals, such as AIDS patients. Healing probably depends on both humoral and cell-mediated immunity. Within lesions *T. pallidum* is essentially extracellular. These organisms are susceptible to antibodies and to phagocytosis by macrophages and polymorphonuclear leucocytes and by activated T-lymphocytes. A small number of treponemes are sequestered intracellularly. This intracellularity may explain the chronic, relapsing nature of syphilis.

Secondary or disseminated syphilis occurs 2–12 weeks after contact. Lesions that are histologically similar to the primary lesions can occur in many sites, including lymph nodes, liver, skin, genital tissue, heart, bone, joint, brain, meninges, or kidneys. It is remarkable that these lesions develop so soon after the host defences have brought the primary lesion under control. It has been suggested that secondary syphilis results from selective immunosuppression of the host defences. The treponemal capsular mucopolysaccharide may inactivate B-lymphocytes, T-lymphocytes, and macrophages. Intracellular treponemes

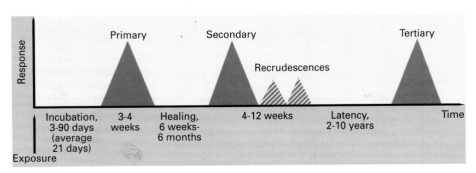

Fig. 6.25 The clinical course of untreated syphilis.

could then emerge from cells, multiplying extracellularly to produce secondary lesions. The cycle is then repeated, with both cell-mediated and humoral responses developing, which eventually lead to healing of the secondary lesions. Clearly, this hypothesis leaves many questions unanswered and does not fully explain latency and tertiary syphilis. *T. pallidum* may become sequestered in immunologically privileged sites, such as the brain or aqueous humour. Organisms in these areas are relatively protected from circulating antibodies and thus may be able to persist for long periods of time. The immune response is brisk during the secondary stage and an immune-complex glomerulonephritis may occur. After the secondary stage subsides the patient enters a latent period, during which there are no signs or symptoms of syphilis. Relapses of secondary syphilis can occur for up to 4 years in the early latent period. The subsequent latent period is known as the late latent stage. Tertiary syphilitic lesions may develop more than 2–10 years after the last evidence of secondary syphilis. About one-third of untreated patients will develop tertiary lesions. Most of these lesions are similar to primary and secondary lesions. An unusual feature of the tertiary stage is the occasional occurrence of gummata in the spleen, skin, liver, or bones. Few treponemes are present in these lesions and they may be due to hypersensitivity reactions.

It is clear that syphilis is a very complicated disease, both in terms of the pathogenicity of the organism and the host immune responses. Many questions about the pathogenesis of the disease remain, as yet, unanswered.

Chronic bacterial infections thus provide many fascinating examples of the complex realtionship between the pathogenicity of the organism and the strength and nature of the host's immune response.

6.6.2 Chronic viral infections

Paul Griffiths

The main aim in life of a virus is to survive. In order to do this, a virus that infects only humans must infect at least one further individual before the host immune response destroys it. Most viruses achieve this by replicating so quickly that they can spread to other humans before the immune system is fully mobilized (see Fig. 6.26a). This type of infection is termed productive because daughter viruses are produced in abundance. The tactics of the viruses are analogous to vast numbers of troops attempting to break through a heavily defended stronghold; there will be heavy losses but at least some of the 'soldiers' will succeed in escaping.

A rather more subtle tactic, analogous to guerilla warfare, is seen in persistent virus infection. Only low levels of daughter viruses are produced and they develop a variety of methods to

either avoid stimulating the host immune response or to suppress it.

Finally, viruses can act as 'moles' by lying latent within cells that appear to be normal. However, months or years after the latent infection was established, the latent virus can reactivate to a short-lived productive infection. Obviously, the immune system will recognize the productive infection and, being already primed immunologically, will respond rapidly to destroy the virus. It is as if latent viruses know this and so they choose to reactivate when the immune system is in some way temporarily debilitated, i.e. they act as opportunists.

The differences between productive, persistent, and latent infections are summarized in Table 6.23. Although different viruses have evolved to cause one of these distinct types of infection preferentially, it is important to note that infected cells of all three types have the potential to be productive of daughter viruses. This potential resides in the nucleic acid of the virus which encodes the genetic information required to produce and assemble daughter viruses. Viruses that have RNA as their nucleic acid cannot become truly latent except as retroviruses (RNA viruses containing a reverse transcriptase) which make DNA copies of their genomes which then act as repositories of genetic information in the cell.

Table 6.23 Characteristics of latent, persistent, and productive viral infection

Characteristic	Type of virus infection		
	Latent	Persistent	Productive
Detectable nucleic acid	+	+	+ +
Detectable early antigens	±	+	+ +
Detectable late antigens	−	+	+ +
Infectious virus usually produced	−	+	+ +
Infectious virus can be produced	+	+	+
Reported for DNA viruses	+	+	+
Reported for RNA viruses	− *	+	+

* Retroviruses can be + here once the DNA copy of the RNA virus has been integrated into host DNA.

Reactivation of latent viruses

Figure 6.26b shows schematically the reactivation of varicella-zoster virus. During primary infection, the virus grows centripetally along sensory nerves supplying the dermatome affected by chicken-pox. It then establishes latency in the dorsal root ganglion at that sensory level and remains there, unexpressed, for decades. With advancing age, the virus suddenly reactivates to grow back down the sensory nerve and erupt on the skin of that individual. Clearly the best chance of survival for that virus is to encounter an immunologically susceptible individual who can then become infected. This tactic of reactivating only once in a lifetime can be improved upon from the standpoint of virus transmission. Thus, herpes simplex virus (HSV) reactivates many times during the life of an individual and so has more opportunities of encountering other susceptibles (see Fig. 6.26c). However, reactivations of HSV have the disadvantage of

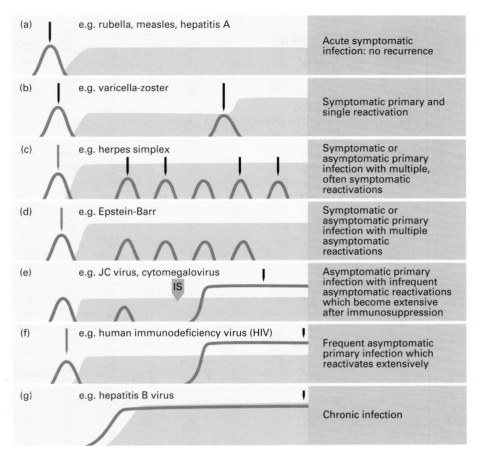

Fig. 6.26 Patterns of viral replication and clinical disease. Purple line = viral replication; the pink shaded area = humoral immune response; black arrows = symptoms produced; red arrows = symptoms may, or may not be produced; IS = immunosuppression.

often revealing themselves clinically; people are less inclined to kiss those who have obvious cold sores. This deficiency has been overcome by another herpes virus, Epstein–Barr virus (EBV) whose reactivations are entirely asymptomatic (see Fig. 6.26d). Susceptible contacts can thus enjoy the pleasure of oral–oral contact oblivious to the fact that they are acquiring EBV infection in the process.

The tendency for latently infected cells within the body to reactivate is held in check by cell-mediated immune (CMI) effector cells. This 'immune surveillance' usually stops the first signs of reactivation so that the virus rarely reaches the external surfaces of the body. However, if this otherwise efficient system is impaired by general stress or debilitation, or by the administration of immunosuppressive drugs, then viral reactivation can become florid and life threatening. Figure 6.26e shows examples where cytomegalovirus (CMV) can reactivate to cause fatal pneumonitis and where polyoma virus JC can reactivate to cause the fatal demyelinating brain disease, progressive multifocal leukoencephalopathy. Likewise, human immunodeficiency virus (HIV) can reactivate and cause extensive damage to CD4-positive lymphocytes (Fig. 6.26f). Since these cells are responsible for inducing cytotoxic T-lymphocytes (CD8$^+$) to recognize and destroy HIV-infected cells, this establishes a vicious circle which leads ultimately to profound loss of CMI effector cells.

Persistent virus infections

Some viruses establish persistent infections from the time of first virus replication. For example, some people who encounter hepatitis B virus (HBV) do not mount an effective CMI response which is required for virus eradication. The patients gain by not getting acute hepatitis, since this syndrome is caused by the CMI response rather than by the virus, yet they lose because they do not eradicate HBV. Although they may remain entirely asymptomatic for years, such individuals are at risk of chronic hepatitis, cirrhosis, and primary liver cancer due to chronic HBV infection (see Fig. 6.26g and Chapter 17).

Factors favouring viral persistence

There are many ways in which viruses have evolved to enable them to establish persistent infections. For example, as shown in Fig. 6.27, the virus may remain within its intracellular environment so that extracellular antibody molecules cannot react to it: also shown in Fig. 6.27 is a tactic used by CMV. Because the circulating antibodies are directed against surface proteins of the virus, CMV has evolved the ability to coat itself in a host protein (β_2 microglobulin) which protects the virus from neutralization. CMV can thus spread from cell to cell extracellularly despite the presence of a vast excess of antibody that can neutralize uncoated virions *in vitro*. This coating tactic is so elegantly simple that it might be expected to be employed by

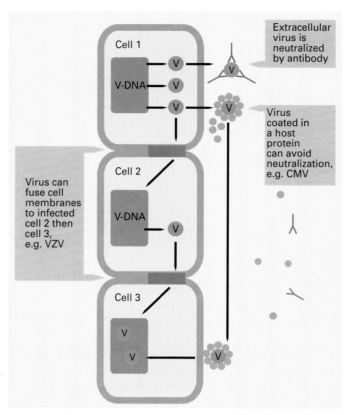

Fig. 6.27 Strategies used by viruses to avoid extracellular neutralizing antibody. In attempting to leave cell 1 and reach cell 3, viruses run the risk of being neutralized by extracellular antibody. They avoid this by remaining intracellular following fusion of membranes or by coating themselves in a host protein. V, virus; Y, neutralizing antibody; green ● host protein; V-DNA, viral DNA; VZV, varicella zoster virus.

other viruses. For example, the gene coding for the surface protein of scrapie agent is now known to be present in all normal hosts, so it is possible that this protein surrounds and protects a small nucleic acid molecule which has not yet been identified. This suggestion is speculative, but it could explain why such infections fail to stimulate host immune responses, since the coated agent would not be recognized as foreign.

Even those viruses that remain intracellular are potentially vulnerable because they express specific proteins at the surface of infected cells and so can be detected by cytotoxic T-lymphocytes (see Fig. 6.28). Papilloma viruses only produce such structural proteins once epithelial cells have differentiated to keratinocytes, by which time the cells are not readily accessible to immune surveillance cells from blood vessels in the dermis. Even when viruses do not display whole proteins at the cell surface, their proteins may well be cycled through the endosome/lysosome compartments so that their peptide breakdown products can be expressed at the cell surface. Specific epitopes of these peptides can be recognized by cytotoxic T-cells which react to destroy the infected cell, so that successful persistence may involve reduction of surface antigen expression. Since such cytotoxic T-cells recognize antigen in the context of class I MHC molecules, another tactic is for the virus to persist in cells, such as liver or brain, which express only low amounts of MHC antigens. Adenoviruses have evolved another strategy for reducing MHC display; they produce a cytoplasmic protein which binds MHC molecules and so hinders their transport to the cell membrane.

Clinical effects of persisting viruses

Whether or not a virus persisting within an individual cell induces disease must depend on the amount of cell damage incurred and the uniqueness of the function performed by that cell. For example, if a neural cell supplying the only efferent signals to a muscle is infected, this may lead to weakness or even paralysis, depending on the extent to which other neural cells can supply compensating signals to neighbouring muscle

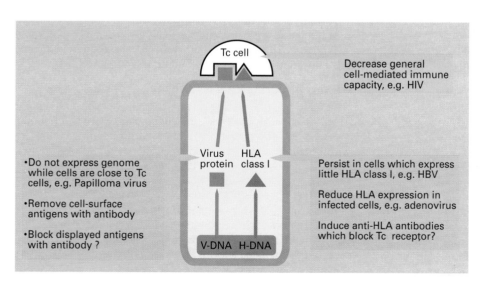

Fig. 6.28 Tactics used by viruses to decrease specific cytotoxic T-cell responses. The cytotoxic T-lymphocyte recognizes epitopes of virus proteins together with HLA class I molecules. A virus can therefore decrease the effectiveness of such cells by reducing display of either protein or by generally suppressing cell-mediated immunity. V-DNA, virus DNA; H-DNA, host DNA.

groups. In contrast, persistent infection of a single liver cell would not produce liver dysfunction because of the vast reserve of biochemical capacity present within that organ. If persistent infection of the liver is to produce disease, it follows that a large number of cells must be infected and damaged. As a corollary, we must consider the possibility that persistent infection is established in many apparently normal individuals but that it remains clinically silent because only a few cells are infected. Nevertheless, some patients do present with disease that is due to persistent viral infections, and several pathogenic mechanisms can be envisaged.

Immune-complex disease The chronic production of virus antigens by infected cells, coupled with the continuous production of virus-specific antibodies, would be expected to represent a perfect recipe for induction of immune-complex disease. In practice, most individuals with proven persistent virus infection do not develop chronic immune-complex disease, although symptoms such as arthralgia or rash may be present at certain times during the acute phase of their infections. Nevertheless, there are specific medical and veterinary examples where pathogenic immune complexes can be induced by known viruses. The major medical example is polyarteritis nodosa, where in many cases the immune complexes contain hepatitis B surface antigen. Thus, a patient can have asymptomatic HBV infection of the liver and present with systemic disease caused by the production of immune complexes.

Induction of cancer Chronic viral infection within cells of a particular organ may lead to induction of malignant tumours. The fine details of this induction process are only now becoming defined (see Chapter 9) but may be classified into those that act directly on the cellular DNA and those acting by indirect mechanisms.

Direct mechanisms Viruses in this group integrate their DNA (or DNA copies of their RNA genomes) into host DNA. This leads to perturbation of host oncogenes by a variety of mechanisms (see Chapter 9 for details) with subsequent excess production of the products of naturally occurring oncogenes. The products confer growth advantages on the infected cells and enable them to bypass the normal signals that control cell division. The result is a clone of cells replicating autonomously, which we label as 'cancer'. Several viruses are thought to act in this way: e.g. EBV and Burkitt's lymphoma; HBV and primary liver cell cancer; human papilloma viruses and carcinoma of the cervix; and human T-cell lymphotrophic virus (HTLV-1) and adult T-cell leukaemia.

Indirect mechanisms Here the virus DNA is not found in the tumour cells but the virus has acted on another cell to permit development of the tumour. An excellent example is HIV which induces immunosuppression and loss of immune surveillance. This, in turn, may allow clones of endothelium or lymphoid tissue to expand without control, leading to development of Kaposi's sarcoma or lymphoma, respectively. Although HIV does not infect these target cells directly, such tumours would not develop if the virus were not infecting and damaging the CD4$^+$ lymphocytes which are presumed to be responsible for inducing the cytotoxic T-lymphocytes to keep such micro-tumour production under control.

Progressive target organ damage Low-grade replication of viruses within cells of a target organ can lead to progressive loss of the function of that organ. For example, chronic HBV infection of hepatocytes leads to symptoms due to the failure of the secretory and/or excretory function of the liver. Regeneration of uninfected cells can lead to compensation of biochemical defects but may produce undesirable architectural or haemodynamic developments, which we label 'chronic hepatitis' or 'cirrhosis'. Thus, the 'disease' seen at death may seem to bear little relationship to the mild infection that precipitated the series of pathological processes culminating in disease.

A similar example concerns HIV. This infection is clinically mild in its acute phase yet can lead to progressive loss of function of CD4$^+$ lymphocytes or brain cells. The 'disease' experienced by the patient (see Chapter 4 for details) consists of opportunistic infections or tumours or intellectual impairment which superficially bear no relationship to the target cell attacked by the underlying virus infection.

Loss of luxury functions Until now we have considered that a virus produces symptoms by markedly deranging the whole functioning of a cell. However, we must consider the consequences if the virus allows the cell's synthetic and replicative machinery to function normally, and only inhibits the specialized functions of highly differentiated cells. The advantage to the virus would be that its intracellular home remains viable but the disadvantage to the host is that absence of the specialized functions can lead to debilitating disease. For example, in animal models of certain virus infections, loss of growth hormone secretory ability can produce impaired size. One wonders how many human patients with chronic debilitating illnesses of the nervous or endocrine systems might have underlying chronic low-grade viral infections of cells responsible for the provision of 'luxury' functions.

6.6.3 Fungal infections

M. D. Richardson

Introduction

Although there are 250 000–300 000 species of fungi widely distributed in all ecosystems, there is only a limited number of fungi known to be pathogenic for man and which have become well adapted to a parasitic mode of existence. The 80 genera of pathogenic fungi include more than 200 species. Diseases caused by fungi are known collectively as mycoses, and range from very common, mild, chronic infections affecting the skin, deep cutaneous, or subcutaneous infections, to acute and chronic infections of the viscera and deep tissues. Mammalian hosts are exposed to fungi from the moment of birth in one or more ways:

1. exposure due to true pathogenic fungi normally growing as saprophytes in geographical areas where these fungi are found;

2. when weakened or more susceptible because of intercurrent pathologies or iatrogenic factors—the fungi found in this setting are termed the opportunistic pathogens;

3. when individuals are exposed to infective propagules of pathogenic fungi, principally dermatophytes (ringworm fungi), which are very well adapted to parasitism and quite capable of invading the host.

Fungal adaptation

There are five broad groups of fungi, classified according to the degree of parasitic adaptation.

1. Those fungi that are common in man's surroundings whose spores are inhaled. These fungi are able to invade and develop in the healthy tissues of the host. The principal infections here are histoplasmosis, blastomycosis, coccidioidomycosis, and paracoccidioidomycosis.

2. Those fungi that are implanted into healthy tissue by trauma of the integument, e.g. chromomycosis and mycetoma.

3. Those fungi which are ubiquitous in man's environment and either invade through the mucous membranes (zygomycosis) or are inhaled (aspergillosis, cryptococcosis). These infections generally occur in weakened hosts.

4. Other than the infections caused by dermatophytes, infections by *Candida* outnumber all other mycoses. Members of the genus *Candida* are regarded as endogenous pathogens and can cause both superficial and deep-seated diseases which are world-wide in distribution. Of relatively low virulence when compared with bacteria and viruses, *Candida* species are generally classified as opportunistic pathogens, causing disease in hosts that are compromised by some underlying pathological process or deficiency state. They are prone to attack the new-born, debilitated, or pregnant, and the immunosuppressed as a consequence of certain malignant diseases, prominent amongst which is leukaemia. *Candida* also causes endocarditis, renal disease, and other visceral mycoses. Other yeasts cause various superficial diseases, for example, pityriasis versicolor, white piedra. Many of the yeasts that cause disease are commensals, exerting pathogenic effects only when the balance between the host and its indigenous flora is deranged. Opportunity for yeasts to invade tissues is afforded by many of the procedures of modern medicine, such as organ transplantation, open-heart surgery, prolonged intravenous hyperalimentation, and the use of cytotoxic and immunosuppressive drugs, as well as of antibiotics that suppress the normal bacterial flora. Deep-seated infections caused by these fungi are serious and life threatening, for all have an extremely grave prognosis if

not diagnosed or predicted promptly. It is also important to note, however, that certain species of *Candida* possess morphological and biochemical attributes that may enhance the ability to invade susceptible hosts. For instance, the high incidence of *C. albicans* isolated from cases of systemic infection, compared with other species of *Candida*, may be due to a number of virulence determinants not possessed by these other species.

5. The last major group of fungi is that comprised of the dermatophytes which cause superficial cutaneous infections which primarily involve keratinized tissues of the epidermis, pilosebaceous follicle, and nails.

Pathogenetic mechanisms

To be regarded as pathogenic, a fungus has to be able to complete a number of steps in order to initiate infection and counteract a range of non-specific and specific host defence mechanisms. For the majority of fungi, if these steps are not achieved the fungus is not regarded as a successful pathogen. There are many ways in which fungi can express determinants of virulence which enable the host to be invaded and the fungus to survive in the host's internal environment by, for example, perturbing or avoiding host defences. The attributes of a successful pathogen are:

1. adherence to the stratum corneum or mucous surfaces;

2. penetration of host tissues to facilitate access to target organs or body fluids;

3. the ability to multiply *in vivo*; this requires the fungus to be thermotolerant and to adapt to the physiochemical conditions of the host;

4. avoidance of host defence mechanisms;

5. even if the previous criteria have been fulfilled, a fungus is not regarded as being pathogenic if it has not been able to damage host tissue.

Each of these facets will be discussed in turn, with examples to illustrate the concepts presented.

Adherence

Adherence is necessary for saprophytic colonization and as a prelude to tissue penetration. Situations where the adherence of fungal propagules to host surfaces have been studied include the attachment of dermatophyte arthrospores to corneocytes of the stratum corneum, impaction of *Rhizopus* sporangiospores to the mucosal surfaces of the nasal sinuses, impaction of conidia of *Aspergillus fumigatus* to mucous surfaces of the respiratory tract, and attachment of blastospores of *Candida albicans* to corneocytes of the skin, epithelial cells of the oral cavity, vagina, urinary tract, gut mucosa, and endothelial cells of blood vessels (Fig. 6.29). It is considered that the superficial layers of the cell wall of *Candida* are responsible for the adherence of the cells to the host. Although the transition of *C. albicans* and other yeast species from saprophytism to parasitism remains largely unexplained, it is generally considered that the adherence or the

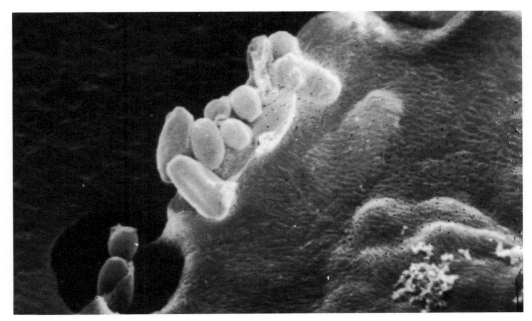

Fig. 6.29 Adherence of blastospores of *Candida albicans* to a buccal epithelial cell. The blastospores and epithelial cells have been mixed for 30 min and then filtered through a capillary pore polycarbonate filter. Note the blastospores adhering to a portion of an epithelial cell drawn into a pore of the membrane.

association of fungal cells to the host surfaces is an essential initial step. However, the adherence to mucosal surfaces is not necessary for fungal survival or growth. Adherence appears to be related to the production of an additional wall surface layer: a fibrogranular cell wall coat that is much less developed or not detectable in non-adhering forms. Adherence may also be influenced by various sugar compounds and by specific antibody to *C. albicans*. In the vagina, enhanced adherence is seen when a large proportion of intermediate epithelial cells are present.

Tissue invasion

Structures that enable fungi to penetrate host tissues are absent on most zooparasitic fungi, unlike the numerous examples seen in phytopathogenic fungi. However, a few human pathogens can undergo different types of dimorphism, generally expressed by the transition from a filamentous form to a yeast mode of growth, when they invade tissues. In contrast *Candida* species develop pseudohyphae and true mycelium when they act as pathogens.

The morphological changes expressed by pathogenic fungi due to adaptation to parasitism and tissue invasion can usually be observed as they develop in the host. The variety of tissue forms of pathogenic fungi can be seen using a range of staining techniques. In aspergillosis, conidia impacted on to respiratory mucous surfaces during inhalation swell and then germinate. The germlings develop into wide, branching aseptate hyphae. In the later stages of invasion the hyphae assume a more characteristic saprophytic appearance, which may suggest resistance to host defences (Fig. 6.30). In dermatophytosis, the

hyphal change little *in vivo*, although the hyphae of *Trichophyton rubrum* may appear thinner when invading the thin stratum corneum of the inguinal area compared to the broader appearance when growing in the much thicker stratum corneum of the sole of the foot. Dermatophyte fungi produce keratinase enzymes which appear to assist the penetration of the organisms between the individual corneocytes of the stratum corneum. The true pathogenic fungi (*Blastomyces dermatitidis, Histoplasma capsulatum, Coccidioides immitis,* and *Sporothrix shenckii*) exhibit dimorphism, which probably results from a metabolic alteration of the fungal cells provoked by confrontation with the tissues of the host which determines important modifications. The process appears to enable pathogenic fungi to adapt to a parasitic mode of existence when faced with selective pressures exerted by the tissues of the host. The acquisition of a yeast-like morphology is not, however, always linked to enhanced pathogenicity. The pathogenic potential of *C. albicans* appears to be linked to the formation of germ tubes and the development of pseudohyphae and true hyphae. Normally, however, all the various growth forms of *C. albicans* are seen in host tissues. Therefore, there appears to be no direct correlation between a filamentous form and pathogenicity, although the concept is an attractive one.

Multiplication within tissue

The morphological variations and dimorphism seen in pathogenic fungi are essentially phenotypic modifications that enable the fungi to survive the non-specific and specific defences of the host and to multiply in the tissues of the host. However, these changes in growth form, in general, do not constitute any

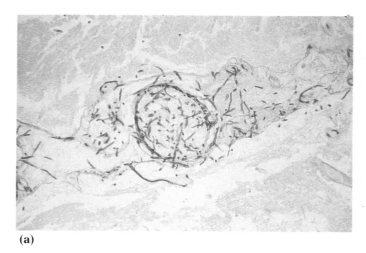

(a)

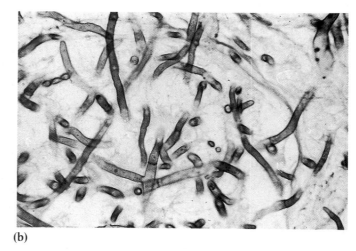

(b)

Fig. 6.30 (a) Section through lung which showed multiple confluent indurated nodules. Acutely branching hyphae of *Aspergillus flavus* can be seen. (b) Septation within the hyphae is also present.

morphological specializations to penetrate the cells of the host. Exceptions to this include the penetration of epithelial cells by *C. albicans* and corneocytes by dermatophyte hyphae. Having survived the non-specific defence mechanisms where a fungus makes initial contact with a human host, and having established a focal point of tissue invasion, the pathogen has to assure itself of a continued existence by multiplication and possible dissemination to target organs and specific tissues.

Factors considered essential to the growth of fungi in tissues include thermotolerance, expression of enzymes for particular substrates, utilization of nutrients, and competition with other micro-organisms for essential food materials. However, to penetrate the tissues of the host and develop there, pathogenic fungi have to possess certain mechanisms that enable them to resist the specific and non-specific host defences. Fungi appear to exploit and acquire a number of mechanisms that enable them to do this once they have become established. These attributes are directly connected to the morphological form assumed in tissue, the rate of growth, and the biochemical architecture of the fungal cell wall. These mechanisms include: fungal invasion of weakly protected tissues, for example the stratum corneum; the secretion of proteolytic enzymes or of efficient cytotoxins against immunocompetent cells; the secretion by pathogenic fungi of cortisone-like substances that 'stabilize' biological membranes, allowing the multiplication of fungi within pulmonary macrophages, for example *Histoplasma*; the morphological form of the fungus, e.g. true hyphae; the presence of a capsule or other cell wall material which could inhibit phagocytosis (Fig. 6.31); the massive release of antigenic material in tissue and body fluids which could produce immunotolerance; and, finally, the secretion of substances inhibiting the proliferation of T-lymphocytes, for example in histoplasmosis and candidosis.

Other ways in which fungi may be able to overcome host defence mechanisms include: immobilization of phagocytes; hindering contact with phagocytes; preventing ingestion by

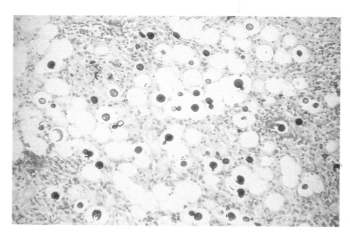

Fig. 6.31 Cryptococcal encephalitis in a mouse. Note numerous budding cells of *Cryptococcus neoformans* embedded in the brain parenchyma. The clear spaces surrounding the yeast cells are apparently due to shrinkage and loss of capsular material during processing.

phagocytes; and interfering with intracellular killing by phagocytes. Nevertheless, most fungal propagules are readily ingested by host effector cells (Fig. 6.32) and some that are too large to be engulfed by neutrophils or macrophages, for example the spherule of *Coccidioides immitis* or the hyphae of *Rhizopus* species, are killed extracellularly.

Tissue damage

The successful completion of the pathogenic process by fungi includes damage to tissue. This is often accompanied by a characteristic inflammatory response. For the fungus to survive once localized in a particular target organ, there must be a tissue environment suitable for continued existence and multiplication.

In general, fungi are indolent as inflammatory irritants compared with many bacteria. It is not clear that variations in

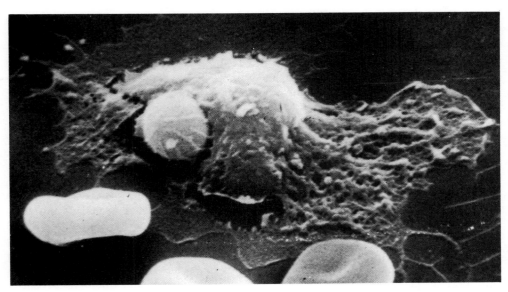

Fig. 6.32 Scanning electron micrograph of a glass adherent mouse neutrophil after 10 min incubation with *Candida albicans* blastospores. Phagocyte lamellipodia can be seen surrounding the yeast cell prior to making contact at the distal end of the organism and completing ingestion.

chemical composition of different organisms have much effect on basic immunological responses. No one tissue change seems to be entirely characteristic or pathognomonic of fungal diseases. The changes seen may include the degree of suppuration; the presence of macrophages and giant cells; and the presence of caseous necrosis and fibrosis. A number of general observations can be made.

1. A number of subcutaneous and deep infections, for example sporotrichosis and coccidioidomycosis, show all of these tissue changes.

2. Mycetoma and chromomycosis show all of these changes except caseous necrosis.

3. Zygomycosis, a spectrum of diseases caused by *Mucor*-like fungi and related fungi, can run an entire course with only infarction due to vascular thrombosis and with minimal acute inflammation.

4. Suppuration is absent or minimal in many lesions of histoplasmosis and cryptococcosis.

5. Superficial diseases often appear to have no inflammatory response, for example tinea capitis caused by *Trichophyton tonsurans*, but in cattle ringworm and other dermatophytoses caused by zoophilic dermatophytes all forms of acute and chronic inflammation can be seen.

Chronic suppuration with fibrosis is the most general tissue change in deep fungus infection and the neutrophil is usually the primary reacting cell. However, in some instances the macrophage or giant cell may be the primary effector cell. Factors responsible for the tissue changes seen in fungal infections include the following:

1. large and variable size of the organism, for example the spherules of *Coccidioides immitis*, some 400 μm in diameter, and the variable cell size and capsule width of *Cryptococcus neoformans*;

2. location of the fungus, whether it is superficial or in deep tissue;

3. the production of endotoxins and the chemical constitution of the organism;

4. development of hypersensitivity to the fungus;

5. chronicity of the process.

The host–parasite relationship in both superficial and systemic fungal disease is poorly understood. However, it is evident that the mechanism by which the fungus establishes itself and provokes tissue damage apparently does not depend directly on the toxic activity of some product of the fungi. It is possible that the persistence of the fungus in the host, regardless of the host's immune status, may be a result of a mechanism that permits evasion of the immune response. Many of these aspects provide interesting areas of research.

6.6.4 Further reading

Chronic bacterial infections

Collins, F. M. (1989). Mycobacterial disease, immunosuppression and acquired immunodeficiency syndrome. *Clinical Microbiology Reviews* **2**, 360–77.

Fitzgerald, T. J. (1981). Pathogenesis and immunology of *Treponema pallidum*. *Annual Review of Microbiology* **35**, 29–54.

Hastings, R. C., Gillis, T. P., Krahenbuhl, J. L., and Franzblau, S. G. (1988). Leprosy. *Clinical Microbiology Reviews* **1**, 330–48.

Hill, H. R. (1988). Infections complicating congenital immunodeficiency syndromes. In *Clinical approach to infection in the compromised host* (ed. R. H. Rubin and L. S. Young) (2nd edn), pp. 407–38. Plenum Medical, New York.

Meisler, D. M., *et al.* (1986). Chronic *Propionibacterium* endophthalmitis after extracapsular cataract extraction and intraocular lens implantation. *American Journal of Ophthalmology* **102**, 733–5.

Mims, C. A. (1987). *The pathogenesis of infectious disease* (3rd edn). Academic Press, London.

Ridley, D. S. and Jopling, W. B. (1966). Classification of leprosy according to immunity. A five group system. *International Journal of Leprosy* **34**, 255–73.

Scheld, W. M. (1984). Pathogenesis and pathophysiology of infective endocarditis. In *Endocarditis* (ed. M. A. Sande, D. Kaye, and R. K. Root). *Contemporary issues in infectious diseases*, Vol. 1, pp. 1–32. Churchill Livingstone, London.

Stoenner, H. G., Dodd, T., and Larsen, D. (1982). Antigenic variation of *Borrelia hermsii*. *Journal of Experimental Medicine* **156**, 1297–301.

Waldrogel, R., Medoff, G., and Swartz, M. (1970). Osteomyelitis: A review of clinical features, therapeutic considerations and unusual aspects. *New England Journal of Medicine* **282**, 198–206.

Wiegeshaus, E., Balasubramanian, V., and Smith, D. W. (1989). Immunity to tuberculosis from the perspective of pathogenesis. *Infection and Immunity* **57**, 3671–6.

Chronic viral infections

Southern, P. and Oldstone, M. B. A. (1986). Medical consequences of persistent viral infection. *New England Journal of Medicine* **314**, 359–67.

Fungal infections

Douglas, L. J. (1985). Adhesion of pathogenic *Candida* to host surfaces. *Microbiological Sciences* **2**, 243–7.

Evans, E. G. V. and Gentles, J. C. (1985). *Essentials of medical mycology*. Churchill Livingstone, Edinburgh.

Hay, R. J. (1988). Histopathology. In *Medical mycology, a practical approach* (ed. E. G. V. Evans and M. D. Richardson), pp. 261–81. IRL Press, Oxford.

Richardson, M. D. and Shankland, G. S. (1991). Pathogenesis of fungal infection in the non-compromised host. In *Fungal infection in the compromised patient* (2nd edn), pp. 1–22. John Wiley & Sons, Chichester.

Szaniszlo, P. J. (1985). *Fungal dimorphism*. Plenum Press, New York.

6.7   Hospital-acquired and opportunistic infections

Heather M. Dick

6.7.1   Hospital-acquired infections

Hospital-acquired infections are also known as nosocomial infections (from the Greek, *nosokomeian*—a hospital). Such infections are now recognized as a major problem in terms of morbidity, mortality, and cost, the latter including extra days in hospital, as well as the costs of treatment with antimicrobial agents. An international survey published in 1988 (Mayon-

White *et al.* 1988) and covering 47 hospitals in 14 countries on four continents, revealed that the prevalence of such infections ranged from 3 to 21 per cent with a mean of 8.4 per cent. The highest rates occurred in intensive care units, closely followed by surgical and orthopaedic units. Children under 1 year of age and adults over 64 years were most often affected. Up to 30 per cent of patients in the hospitals surveyed (which covered both general and specialized units, and both teaching and non-teaching hospitals) were receiving antimicrobials, including penicillin, ampicillin, amoxycillin, and gentamicin, and 50 per cent of these were receiving two or more antimicrobials. Urinary-tract infection featured high in the lists, especially in patients over 1 year of age, reaching nearly 5 per cent of all patients and over 30 per cent in catheterized patients, especially those with in-dwelling catheters but not sparing those who had had short-term catheterization, for example postoperatively (Carson 1988). Surgical wound infections were most prevalent in adults, with the reported values ranging from 13 per cent for 'clean' operations, i.e. those not involving traumatized tissue or the gastrointestinal tract, to 29 per cent in 'dirty' operations, involving contaminated sites. Many patients had intravenous lines, and infection rates for these sites were generally around 5–10 per cent, with higher rates for those with three-way taps and, presumably, more intervention by staff for administration of drugs and sampling of blood.

It is possible from the published data to identify many of the risk factors that predispose patients to become infected during their stay in hospital (Table 6.24), and to list the commonest microbial isolates from such patients (Table 6.25). Minor defects in the ability to respond to infection are very common in hospital patients and may account for the relative susceptibility of a wide variety of patients to infection. Many diseases are known to carry an increased risk of infection, e.g. rheumatic valvular disease. Sometimes it is possible to postulate the exact nature of the immunological problem, although in many instances additional risk factors may play an important role in predisposing the patient to infections, e.g. the vascular pathology of diabetes or the anaemia of end-stage renal failure. Anaethesia, surgery, blood transfusion, steroids, and even anti-

Table 6.24   Examples of factors predisposing to hospital-acquired infections

Invasive procedures, breaching skin
   Surgery
   Intravenous lines, superficial and deep
   Injections
Implanted devices
   Urinary catheters
   Assisted respiration
   Pacemakers
   Shunts and Spitz–Holtzer valves
   Joint replacements
   Artificial heart valves
Trauma
Advanced malignancy, especially involving haematopoietic tissues
Immunosuppressive therapy

Table 6.25 Main organisms involved in hospital-acquired infections

Organisms	Sites affected
Staphylococcus aureus and *Staph. epidermidis*	Skin
Streptococcus pneumoniae	Respiratory tract
Escherichia coli, *Klebsiella* sp., *Pseudomonas* sp., *Proteus* sp.	Urinary tract, wounds, respiratory tract
Bacteroides sp.	Peritoneal cavity, genital tract
Streptococcus pyogenes	Skin, genital tract
Candida albicans	Heart valves, systemic
Clostridium difficile	Gut

biotics may each contribute to a temporary state of relative immunodeficiency by reducing the population of circulating T-cells or even of specific subpopulations of T-cells, or, in the case of some antibiotics, by affecting phagocytosis and bacterial cell-killing.

Endogenous organisms

It should be recognized that nosocomial infections can arise from two sources. The organisms may spread from the patient's own flora, that is, from those anatomical sites with a 'normal' background of micro-organisms, i.e. sites such as the mouth, the gut, and the skin. Such infections with endogenous organisms are difficult to prevent entirely, especially in debilitated patients and at the extremes of age, where the normal defence mechanisms of the body are diminished. Prophylactic antibiotics can offer short-term, peri-operative cover but, although this may reduce the incidence of bacterial infection, it is not an ideal solution and may even contribute to the development of antibiotic resistance by selective pressure (Gugliemo and Brooks 1986). Attempts to use antimicrobials to sterilize the gut are never successful; partly because of the natural resistance of many bacterial species and of viruses and most fungi; but mainly because of the vast numbers of organisms that are present in the normal gut and on the skin, which means that only a shift in the flora can be hoped for, by reduction in the numbers of those species which are susceptible to the antibiotics chosen, and even that change is temporary. Claims for reduction in infection or colonization rates (two very different states, because an organism may be present at a site without causing an infective focus), for example in intensive care units, by the use of so-called 'decontamination regimes' of mixtures of antibiotics have come largely from units with previous high rates of infection and cross-infection in patients with multiple problems prior to admission to the units. Again, there may be temporary changes in the colonizing flora, especially of the upper respiratory tract, but the most concrete measure of success, a reduction in bacteraemia or septicaemia, is less often achieved. Although the speed with which new admissions become colonized with the prevailing strains may be slowed, there is little real evidence that colonization, with the consequent risk of infection, particularly with Gram-negative bacteria, is substantially altered in the long run. The problems of preventing infection where there are both endogenous and exogenous sources of micro-organisms are formidable.

Exogenous organisms

The second principal source of hospital-acquired infection is exogenous, i.e. from sources outside the patient. Such sources include the environment, medical and nursing staff, other patients, instrumentation, surgery, blood transfusion, food, water, visitors, etc. Scrupulous hygiene and the strict application of aseptic techniques in surgery, for dealing with intravascular lines (Elliot 1988), catheters, and other invasive procedures can help to reduce the likelihood of infection from such sources, but probably will never eliminate the risk. Much depends on the physiological state of the patient and the effective working of the normal defence mechanisms. The problem with hospital patients is that they are sick and are often receiving treatment which may interfere with these normal mechanisms, or the nature of their disease is such that they are unable to cope with even a minor load of an otherwise almost non-pathogenic organism, far less a major threat from a virulent virus, bacterium, or fungus. This is frequently the case in patients with leukaemia where the disease process may have replaced many of the cells (in the bone marrow and lymph nodes) required to fight infection, such as polymorphonuclear leucocytes and lymphocytes, and where anaemia may also have diminished the capacity to deal with infection. Aggressive chemotherapy and/or radiation, designed to eliminate the leukaemic cells, may further reduce the already depleted population of cells of the immune system. The use of isolation procedures, including reverse barrier nursing, sterilization of food, and laminar flow (where a curtain of filtered air is interposed between the patient and the environment) can provide temporary protection for highly susceptible patients, but cannot be sustained indefinitely if the defect cannot be corrected.

Other examples of patients whose immunological defence mechanisms are compromised (hence, the use of the term 'immunocompromised host') can be identified, ranging from the infant with physiologically immature responses to the very old, and other types of patient, such as those with end-stage renal disease, diabetes, auto-immune disorders, and now including those with the acquired immunodeficiency syndrome (AIDS), where the slow and inexorable destruction of T-lymphocytes is due to infection with human immunodeficiency virus type 1 (HIV-1).

Many micro-organisms, regarded in the past as of low virulence, with little capacity to produce infection in man, are increasingly being implicated in cases of hospital-acquired infection, where they now rank alongside the classical pathogens such as *Staphylococcus aureus* as a major cause of morbidity and mortality (McGowan and Acar 1984). It was previously the practice in some microbiological texts to deal with hospital-acquired infections due to recognized pathogens quite separately from the so-called opportunistic infections, but the change in the relative frequency of each group has made the differentiation somewhat artificial. Since the main sites of hospital-acquired infection, including skin, wound sites, and both superficial and deep infections, and infections of the respiratory tract and the gut are all equally prone to infections with both opportunists and recognized pathogens in the older sense, there seems little point in continuing the separation.

6.7.2   Opportunistic infections

True opportunistic infections are those caused by organisms which are either not commonly associated with infection in humans (e.g. some animal infections) or are of low virulence, especially in healthy individuals, and which can occur both inside and outside hospital. Predisposing factors include close contact, as in the case of some exogenously acquired infections, e.g. ringworm and some parasitic infections. These are often occupationally acquired as, for example, hydatid disease in shepherds or some skin infections in abattoir workers. Important features are that the organisms must gain access and that the conditions must be right for their multiplication, thus damaged skin, prolonged exposure to water, or close daily contact may be involved. However, by far the greatest clinical problem with opportunistic infections is created by those occurring in hospital patients who are immunocompromised by pre-existing disease or by treatment (see Section 6.1 and above). It may, however, be pertinent to comment on two points. Cross-infection, i.e. the transfer of infectious micro-organisms from one patient to another or to and from staff, can occur with opportunistic organisms as well as with the major pathogens. Organisms involved include such well-recognized pathogens as *Staph. aureus*, *E. coli*, *Streptococcus pyogenes*, together with several species previously regarded as of low virulence, such as *Candida*, *Staph. epidermidis*, *Pseudomonas aeruginosa*, and *Listeria monocytogenes*. The latter organism has been recognized as a cause of neo-natal infection, which may lead to meningitis or, if acquired *in utero*, to abortion, although maternal infection is often mild, with minimal symptoms. It has been suggested that *Listeria monocytogenes* may also be implicated in some cases of food poisoning, but the direct link between specific items of food and illness is poorly substantiated. It should also not be forgotten that viruses may be implicated in cross-infection, affecting both patients and staff. Two common examples are respiratory infections due to respiratory syncytial virus occurring in children's wards and rotavirus gastroenteritis affecting the very young and the elderly. The hazards of hepatitis B and HIV-1 must also be included, as should herpetic infections and rubella, particularly for nursing staff. Infections of the gut acquired in hospital may occasionally be classical infections such as salmonellosis, acquired from contaminated food or from other patients, but

also include conditions such as antibiotic-associated diarrhoea—due to *Clostridium difficile*—which is perhaps more truly 'opportunistic' in origin since the organism is found in the normal faeces in small numbers.

6.7.3   Infection in patients with congenital immunodeficiency

Rarely, congenital defects in one or more of the cell populations or organs can occur, exposing affected individuals to the risks of infection. Much has been learned about the precise role of individual cell populations by the careful study of these congenital conditions. The nature of the actual defect often determines the organisms to which the patient will succumb. Major defects often lead to serious, or even fatal, infections with recognized pathogens, such as staphylococci or herpes viruses, but these patients are also prone to infections by relatively minor pathogens or to chronic infections, especially with fungi. Lack of a normal thymus at birth leads to failure to develop normal T-lymphocytes, with consequent inability to cope with infections caused by viruses and fungi, as in di George's syndrome. B-lymphocyte defects also occur, for example in congenital or acquired hypogammaglobulinaemia, when bacterial infections may be life threatening because of the lack of specific antibodies. Many other forms of congenital immunodeficiency have been recognized, including lack of individual complement components, phagocytic and chemotactic defects, and those forms where more than one element of the immune system is absent or faulty (see Chapter 4). In some cases, where the defects are multiple and the infections life threatening, isolation in specially built rooms, etc. has been attempted, but without some way of correcting the defect, such as bone marrow transplantation, this can only be a temporary state for most patients with congenital defects.

6.7.4   Bibliography

Carson, C. C. (1988). Nosocomial urinary tract infections. *Surgical Clinics of North America* **68**, 1147–55.

Elliot, T. S. J. (1988). Intravascular device infections. *Journal of Medical Microbiology* **27**, 161–7.

Gugliemo, B. J. and Brooks, G. F. (1986). Surgical antibiotic prophylaxis. In *Medical microbiology* (ed. C. S. F. Easmon, J. Jeljaszewicz), Vol. 5, ch. 1. Academic Press, London.

McGowan, J. E. and Acar, J. A. (1984). Nosocomial infections. In *Infections: recognition, understanding, treatment* (ed. J.-C. Pechere *et al.*), ch. 34. Lea and Febiger, Philadelphia.

Mayon-White, R. T., Ducel, G., Keresilidze, T. and Tikomirov, E. (1988). An international survey of the prevalence of hospital-acquired infection. *Journal of Hospital Infection* **11**, Suppl A, 43–8.

7

Circulatory disorders

7

Circulatory disorders

In order to maintain normal function each cell in the body must be surrounded by, or have to access to, the body fluid. The composition of this fluid is carefully controlled and depends to a large extent on the maintenance of the normal circulation of the blood as well as other factors such as the chemical composition of the blood, renal function, and lymphatic drainage. Disturbances of these factors, loosely grouped together as 'disorders of the circulation' are responsible for a wide variety of disease states. The general principles of disorders of the circulation are discussed in this chapter.

7.1 Vessel wall

R. Ross

Introduction

All vessels in the circulatory system are lined by a continuous endothelium that rests on a basement membrane, which separates it from the underlying smooth muscle cells that make up the media of the vessel. The media is covered by a layer of connective tissue of varying density and thickness, termed the adventitia, which contains variable numbers of cells consisting of some smooth muscle cells and fibroblasts, and numerous capillaries and nerves. The thickness and content of the adventitia depends upon the size of the artery under consideration. In all cases in mammals, the media (or middle layer) appears to consist only of smooth muscle cells. The size of this layer determines the functional capacity of the artery and is reflected in its content of elastic fibres, collagen, and proteoglycan. Small and medium-sized arteries and veins contain variable numbers of smooth muscle cells in the media. These are separated from the endothelium by a relatively well-defined and continuous elastic lamina on the luminal aspect of the media, and from the adventitia by a less well defined and discontinuous elastic lamina on the outer aspect.

7.1.1 The endothelium

The endothelium provides a continuous non-interrupted monolayer of cells that, when viewed from the lumen, vary in shape from polygonal to rhomboid or ellipsoid. The rhomboidal or ellipsoidal cells generally have their long axes in the direction of blood flow, and the polygonal cells appear to be so shaped because they are located at sites such as branches and bifurcations, where blood flow is either discontinuous or where there may be eddy, or back currents, so that the cells are exposed to varying rheological forces (Fig. 7.1). The endothelial cells represent one of the groups of cells in the body that are probably truly 'contact inhibited'. These cells appear to be incapable, after injury, of crawling over one another to replace lost cells at a site distal to the injury. Apparently such cellular losses can be replaced only by cells at or near the margin of the missing cells, and thus require division of closely neighbouring cells together with their migration to fill any gaps that may have occurred. Such replacement properties may play a role in the process of atherogenesis (see Section 12.12). Each endothelial cell is attached to its neighbour by a series of junctional complexes that consist of both gap junctions and tight junctions. The gap junctions are sites of intercellular communication and the tight junctions provide seals of varying lengths that normally prevent passage of substances between the cells.

Permeability

The endothelial cells serve as a permeable barrier to the vessel and determine the nature and amount of substances that pass from the plasma in the arterial lumen into the surrounding tissues by processes of both active and passive transport. Such transport occurs via vesicles derived from the luminal surface that pass through the cells, fuse with the plasma membrane on the other surface, and release their contents. Transcellular channels have also been described. In the process of transcellular transport, endothelial cells have been demonstrated to be capable of modifying some of the substances that are transported, such as lipoproteins, which they can oxidize and variably modify. Endothelial cells also appear to bind lipoprotein lipase, which can act on lipoprotein particles in the plasma and

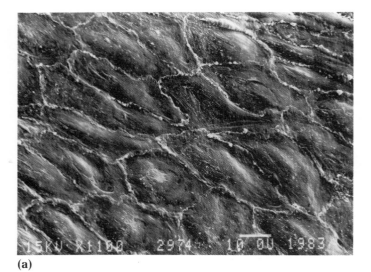

(a)

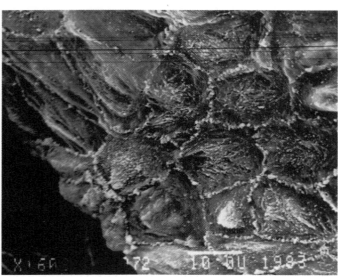

(b)

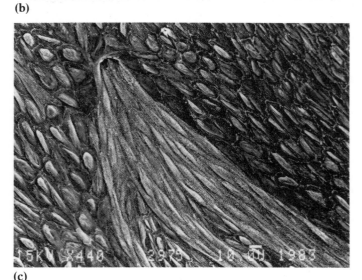

(c)

thus play a critical role in lipid transfer and in lipoprotein metabolism.

Interaction with blood cells

As discussed elsewhere (see Section 12.11), endothelial cells have the capacity, depending upon the cells with which they interact and the presence of appropriate molecules in the plasma, to form both procoagulant and antiogoagulant substances, as well as factors that can stimulate vasodilation (prostacyclin, PGI_2, and endothelial-derived releasing factor, EDRF) and vasoconstriction (angiotensin converting enzyme, ACE, and platelet-derived growth factor, PDGF). Normally as the blood flows by, depending upon the size of the vessel, white cells tend to roll along the perimeter and brush against the surface of the endothelium, whereas most red cells flow through the central part of the lumen where the flow is laminar. Alterations in the surface characteristics of the endothelium and/or the white blood cells may lead to changes that precede inflammatory responses of different types. These changes consist of margination of the leucocytes associated with increased adherence of the leucocytes to the endothelial cells followed by their migration between endothelial cells due to chemotactic attraction, so that the leucocytes become located subendothelially within the vessel wall. The factors responsible for these reactions can include altered cell-surface glycoproteins and chemotactic factors generated by the arterial cells as a result of the inflammatory response.

Synthetic properties

Recently it has been discovered that, like many other cells, endothelial cells can make growth factors. and cytokines. Among the factors that appropriately activated endothelial cells

Fig. 7.1 (a) This scanning electron micrograph presents an *en face* view of the surface of endothelial cells in the thoracic aorta of a normal individual. The border of each cell is clearly demarcated, and overlaps can be seen between the different endothelial cells. Raised areas representing the underlying nuclei of many cells are visible. These endothelial cells are generally ellipsoid in shape and suggest a diagonal flow of blood in the direction of the long axis of the ellipse. Such a view would be seen from a blood cell travelling in the circulation looking down upon the surface of the endothelium, and suggests the normal contours of endothelium within the arterial tree. (b) This scanning electron micrograph provides an *en face* view of endothelium that lies at the edge of an ostium of an intercostal artery in the thoracic aorta of a normal individual. The rhomboidal or ellipsoidal shape of the endothelial cells seen in (a) is not observed; instead, these cells appear more polygonal in shape, which is probably due to the change in the rheologic properties of the flow of blood in such a region. Contrast the cells in this figure with those in (a) and (c). (c) This scanning electron micrograph demonstrates an outflow track from a small ostium in the endothelial lining of the iliac artery of a normal individual. The change in direction, slenderness, and raised appearance of the endothelial cells in the track as compared to endothelial cells on both sides are probably due to the increase in rate of the flow of blood in the artery at this site, and demonstrate the effect of rheological forces on endothelial shape and direction.

can produce are: both A- and B-chains of PDGF, fibroblast growth factor (FGF), and interleukin-1 (IL-1). Endothelial cells respond to various injurious agents or other forms of 'injury' by expressing genes for these different factors, as determined by detection of the presence of mRNA for each factor using appropriate cDNA probes. This is done using Northern blot analysis (hybridization on a filter of a given cDNA with RNA extracts from endothelial cells), which demonstrates mRNA formation and thus gene expression for the different growth factors. Using this technique, it has been observed that exposure to thrombin, factor Xa, platelet releaseate, tumour necrosis factor-alpha (TNFα), or the stimulus derived from undergoing numerous rounds of division in cell culture, results in growth-factor gene expression. This is subsequently accompanied by synthesis and release of particular cytokines or mitogens. The release of IL-1 may also be related to the fact that endothelial cells are capable of presenting antigens and of expressing components of the major histocompatibility complex. As a consequence, they are undoubtedly major participants in immune responses as well.

In addition to the formation of cytokines, endothelial cells can be actively involved in the synthesis and secretion of connective tissue matrix macromolecules, including basement membrane collagen, elastic fibre proteins, and proteoglycans.

Thus endothelial cells serve at the interface between the blood and the tissue to line the blood container, act as a permeability barrier, serve as a non-thrombogenic surface, balance procoagulant versus anticoagulant activities, and synthesize and release cytokines that can affect cells as diverse as fibroblasts and smooth muscle as well as other endothelial cells and leucocytes. As a consequence, alterations of the environment in which the endothelial cells find themselves can have profound effects, not only upon the endothelial cells, but upon the underlying cells of the artery wall as well as the cells of the blood with which they come in contact.

Interaction with monocytes

Endothelial cells may carefully monitor the status of circulating blood cells, particularly lymphocytes and monocytes, and have an effect on the capacity of these cells to enter into the arterial wall, based upon surface constituents of the endothelial cells as well as changes in the surface of the white blood cells themselves. For example, when endothelial cells are pretreated with endotoxin, with IL-1, or with TNFα, increased adherence of polymorphonuclear neutrophilic leucocytes and/or monocytes may occur at the endothelial surface. This increased adherence may be due in part to the synthesis of new glycoproteins by the endothelial cells that interact with leucocyte cell-surface glycoproteins that are similar to the glycoprotein-IIb, IIIa complex on the surface of platelets. These glycoproteins are similar to the LFA-1/MAC-1/P150,95 glycoproteins described on the surface of leucocytes, which may be important for leucocyte adhesion. Leukotriene B4, a lipoxygenase product of granulocytes, can induce increased adhesion of other leucocytes, particularly monocytes, to endothelial cells at sites of disturbance, thus leading to inflammation. When endothelial cells migrate to regener-

ate a wound at a site of endothelial injury, they also appear to alter their cell-surface constituents so that monocytes may more readily adhere to the migrating and injured endothelial cells than to normal intact confluent endothelium.

Since monocytes represent a key cell type in the process of atherogenesis (see Section 12.12), understanding the factors important for monocyte–endothelial interaction may provide clues for prevention of this disease process as well as for altering the process of inflammation. Monocytes behave in many ways like neutrophils in terms of aggregation and margination at sites of inflammation, and apparently are chemotactically attracted into vessel walls in a similar fashion. Monocytes can secrete factors that may be cytotoxic or that may alter the function of endothelial cells and, in addition, can release phospholipases that can alter endothelial permeability. In turn, endothelial cells can oxidize lipoproteins by free-radical oxidation, and when they are exposed to plasma low-density lipoprotein (LDL), they can oxidize the LDL, which can become toxic to proliferating cells such as fibroblasts or smooth muscle. Such oxidized LDL can be taken up via the scavenger LDL receptor and by bulk-phase endocytosis, or phagocytosis, on the surface of macrophages. This may play a role in lipid accumulation and foam cell formation by macrophages. Thus endothelial–monocyte interactions in the presence of increased and/or altered lipoproteins may have profound effects in generating the early ubiquitous lesion of atherosclerosis, the fatty streak. Since endothelial cells can express class II (Ia) antigens of the major histocompatibility complex, and since T-lymphocyte activation requires that antigen be presented in the context of class II antigens, endothelial cells and macrophages may play important roles in antigen presentation and in subsequent T-cell proliferation and differentiation. It has been demonstrated that endothelial cells can serve as antigen-presenting cells and that T-cell products, such as gamma interferon, can in turn act upon endothelial cells and macrophages to augment class II antigen presentation. The capacity of both endothelial cells and macrophages to secrete IL-1 also puts them in a position to augment T-cell proliferation. Since T-cells have been observed in the advanced lesions of atherosclerosis (the fibrous plaque, or complicated lesion), this capacity of endothelium and macrophages to present antigen and to release appropriate cytokines could be significant in the development of the immune responses associated with atherosclerosis. Finally, endothelial cells have the capacity to bind and take up LDL as well as oxidized or modified LDL. They apparently do so via separate, specific, high-affinity receptors. As a consequence, in addition to the actions described above, the endothelial cells play a critical role in lipid entry into the artery wall.

7.1.2   Smooth muscle cells

As late as 1968, smooth muscle cells were considered to have the capacity to contract and thus provide a level of tonus to the vessel wall, but were not considered capable of other functions. Since that time and with the development of methodology to grow smooth muscle cells in conditions of culture in which they retain their differentiated phenotype, it has been shown that these cells are capable of numerous functional activities including synthesis and secretion of connective tissue matrix macromolecules, including collagen, elastic fibres, and proteoglycans. Under particular conditions, they are capable of forming growth factors (the A-chain of PDGF) and of presenting antigens in a fashion similar to endothelial cells.

Microanatomy

The smooth muscle cells in the media of each artery form a continuous interlocking spiral band of contractile cells that respond to agents such as angiotensin in maintaining tonus in the arteries. In the media of veins, the arrangement of the smooth muscle cells is not so highly developed, and thus may be less effective in this process. In addition, in the larger elastic arteries, the smooth muscle cells are attached by specific junctions to each other and thus form functionally continuous bundles of cells that are located between each elastic lamina. These elastic laminae consist of fenestrated sheets of elastic fibres that have sufficient numbers of relatively large fenestrations to allow substances to pass readily between the layers of smooth muscle cells. They do, however, offer a barrier for the passage of cells, requiring cells to find fenestrae or openings through which they can squeeze. The cells are capable of doing so if they are sufficiently attracted to migrate to a distant site. Smooth muscle cells surround themselves with various types of collagen and synthesize all of the protein components of the elastic fibre, as well as the numerous elements of proteoglycan that make up the matrix. Thus they belong to the family of connective tissue synthetic cells consisting of fibroblasts, osteoblasts, and chondroblasts.

When the fine structure of smooth muscle cells is examined by electron microscopy, actively synthetic cells are seen to contain an extensively developed rough endoplastic reticulum and Golgi complex. These organelles are associated with cells that are in the process of synthesizing secretory proteins such as connective tissue proteins. In general, when smooth muscle cells are in a contractile state they do not manifest these organelles, but rather their cytoplasm is rich in contractile actomyosin filaments (Fig. 7.2). There is data to suggest that the state of the cells reflects their capacity to respond to agonists, such as PDGF, and may be important in lesions of atherosclerosis (see Section 12.12).

Synthetic properties

Under special conditions, smooth muscle cells have been shown to be capable of forming growth factors, including PDGF A-chain and IL-1. Their capacity to form PDGF was first observed in new-born rat aortic smooth muscle cells grown in culture. In contrast to new-born rat smooth muscle, adult rat medial smooth muscle cells do not appear to be involved in growth-factor production. This capacity to form growth factors was also observed in smooth muscle cells derived from intimal proliferative lesions in the rat carotid artery that were induced by balloon catheter de-endothelialization. More recently it has

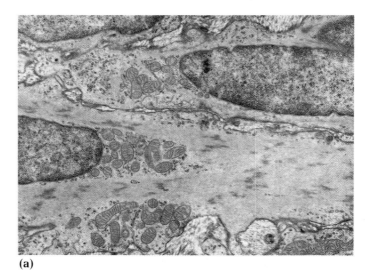

(a)

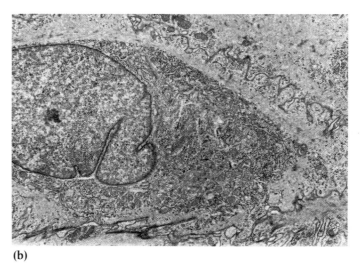

(b)

Fig. 7.2 (a) This is a transmission electron micrograph of a smooth muscle cell in a 'contractile' state in which the cytoplasm of the cell is rich in myofilaments and contains relatively few organelles, although a few perinuclear and peripheral mitochondria and small clusters of ribosomes can be seen within the cytoplasm. (b) This is the appearance of a smooth muscle cell in a synthetic state. In contrast to the cell seen in (a), this cell has an extensively developed rough endoplasmic reticulum and Golgi complex. The development of this secretory protein synthetic apparatus results in compression of the myofilaments to the periphery of the cell. These two states (contractile versus synthetic) represent the capacity of the smooth muscle cell to provide tonus to the artery wall in the relative absence of secretory protein synthesis versus a cell that can presumably synthesize secretory proteins such as collagen, elastic fibre proteins, and proteoglycans. It is not clear how heterogeneous or homogeneous the cells are in the media of most normal arteries.

been shown that smooth muscle cells derived from fibrous plaques of the human carotid artery express mRNA for PDGF A-chain *in situ*, and secrete PDGF when grown in culture. Thus, when appropriately activated, smooth muscle cells appear to be capable of expressing at least one PDGF gene and of playing potentially important roles in the generation of growth factors that could have profound effects upon neighbouring cells as well as upon the smooth muscle cells themselves, if they are able to respond in an autocrine fashion. Factors important in the control of genes that express these mitogens, circumstances that lead to repression of their expression in the normal artery, and induction of their expression in disease states, such as atherosclerosis, remain to be determined. Nevertheless, these observations have important ramifications in our understanding of the role of the smooth muscle cell in normal tissue homeostasis as well as in various pathologic states in which smooth muscle proliferation occurs. In addition, the capacity of the smooth muscle cell to make growth factors, to respond in an autocrine fashion to these factors and thus 'control its own destiny', is potentially important in situations such as embryogenesis and development.

Interaction with endothelium

Smooth muscle cells can interact with endothelium both via direct endothelial–smooth muscle cellular connections as well as via factors released by each of the two cell types. Specific junctional complexes have been observed between endothelial cells and smooth muscle cells *in vivo*, and when grown in co-culture, endothelial cells will reduce cholesterol ester hydrolysis by smooth muscle cells and increase the rate of incorporation of cholesterol oleate into the cells, resulting in increased accumulation of lipid within the smooth muscle. Smooth muscle cells have the capacity to take up LDL via specific high-affinity cell-surface receptors for LDL, as well as via low-affinity, bulk-phase endocytosis of these and other lipid particles. When exposed to mitogens such as PDGF, smooth muscle cells develop increased numbers of LDL receptors and take up increased lipid.

Role in atherosclerosis

The smooth muscle cells in the media probably act as a contractile unit when exposed to contractile agents, such as angiotensin or PDGF, or to relaxing agents, such as PGI$_2$ and EDRF. Although one of their chief functional roles is to maintain the tonus of the artery wall, smooth muscle cells can also migrate into the intima during formation of lesions of atherosclerosis. They can form new connective tissue matrix macromolecules, take up and modify lipids to become foam cells, and can secrete growth factors that may play a role in further lesion progression. These features will be further discussed in the section on atherogenesis (see Section 12.12).

7.1.3 Intimal thickening

Intimal thickening was originally thought to be the hallmark of atherosclerosis. However, Stary has recently studied a relatively large number of children who died during the first five years of life and has observed that the coronary arteries of the majority of these children had eccentric intimal thickening at bifurcations of the coronaries in the half of the artery opposite the flow divider. He suggests that the eccentric thickening may form as a response to intrinsic changes in the haemodynamic properties of the artery and thus represent a physiologic adaptation to rheologic forces as the vascular system develops.

In addition, a concentric, diffuse thickening of the intima is also present with increasing age. This contains relatively uniformly distributed smooth muscle and connective tissue (Fig. 7.3). This diffuse intimal thickening is regularly found throughout the arterial tree, and the extent of the thickness depends upon the artery and the age of the individual. The older the person, the greater the thickness of the artery.

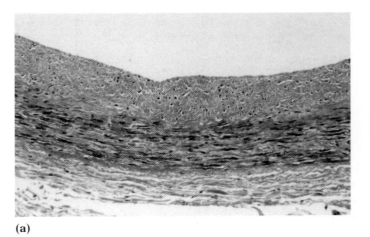

(a)

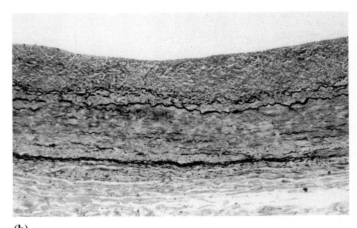

(b)

Fig. 7.3 (a) This light micrograph demonstrates a transverse section of a coronary artery, stained with haematoxylin and eosin, showing a concentric, uniform thickening of the intima that occurs gradually with increasing age. Although it cannot be seen in this micrograph, the thickened intima has not compromised the lumen of the artery to any severe degree. (b) This micrograph shows an adjacent section of the same artery as in (a), stained for connective tissue. The elastic fibres are dark and help to delineate the intima, medial, and adventitia.

If changes occur that predispose to the development of atherosclerosis, both these forms of intimal thickening, as well as regions of completely normal-appearing artery, may serve as sites where lesions of atherosclerosis may form. Sites of diffuse intimal thickening may serve as beds of intimal cells that can go on to proliferate further and develop into advanced lesions of atherosclerosis.

7.1.4   Further reading

DiCorleto, P. E. (1984). Cultured endothelial cells produce multiple growth factors for connective tissue cells. *Experimental Cell Research* **153**, 167–72.

DiCorleto, P. E. and de la Motte, C. A. (1985). Characterization of the adhesion of the human monocytic cell line U937 to cultured endothelial cells. *Journal of Clinical Investigation* **75**, 1153–61.

Hajjar, D. P., Falcone, D. J., Amberson, J. B., and Hefton, J. M. (1985). Interaction of arterial cells. I. Endothelial cells alter cholesterol metabolism in co-cultured smooth muscle cells. *Journal of Lipid Research* **26**, 1212–23.

Harlan, J. M. (1985). Leucocyte–endothelial interactions. *Blood* **65**, 513–25.

Montesano, R., Orci, L., and Vassalli, P. (1985). Human endothelial cell cultures: phenotypic modulation by leucocyte interleukins. *Journal of Cellular Physiology* **122**, 424–34.

Pohlman, T. H., Stanness, K. A., Beatty, P. G., Ochs, H. D., and Harlan, J. M. (1986). An endothelial cell surface factor(s) induced *in vitro* by lipopolysaccharide, interleukin 1, and tumor necrosis factor-α increases neutrophil adherence by a CDw18-dependent mechanism. *Journal of Immunology* **136**, 4548–53.

Stary, H. C. (1987). Macrophages, macrophage foam cells, and eccentric intimal thickening in the coronary arteries of young children. *Atherosclerosis* **64**, 91–108.

Walker, L. N. and Bowyer, D. E. (1984). Endothelial healing in the rabbit aorta and the effect of risk factors for atherosclerosis: hypercholesterolemia. *Arteriosclerosis* **4**, 479–88.

7.2   Haemostasis and blood coagulation

C. R. Rizza

7.2.1   Introduction

The evolution in higher animals of a complex vascular system with blood circulating under pressure through a network of tubes of different sizes and structures has entailed the development of a finely balanced mechanism which, on the one hand, is capable of preventing loss of blood from the body following injury but, on the other, must be delicately balanced so as not to block the system with unwanted clots. In many unicellular animals the primitive 'haemostatic' mechanism consists essentially of a surface precipitation reaction in the protoplasm as it flows from the damaged cell. In slightly less primitive creatures loss of body fluid following injury is prevented by aggregation of specialized cells and release of clottable protein from those cells at the site of injury and formation of a plug. In many primitive animals the haemostatic process serves as much to prevent ingress of foreign organisms as to prevent loss of body fluid. When one considers the vast area of the capillary bed (calculated as 6000 m² in human muscle alone) and how prone it is to

injury in everyday life, it is easy to see why an efficient haemostatic mechanism is of such great importance. In the majority of people this mechanism is so effective that it is taken for granted. Even quite large injuries, for example during major surgery, usually stop bleeding spontaneously in a short time. The importance of the haemostatic process is most clearly seen in individuals who suffer from inherited bleeding disorders and who may bleed to death from the most minor injuries unless steps are taken to correct the deficiency state. On the other hand, haemostasis must act only where and when it is needed, otherwise thrombosis may occur. Because of this there has to be a powerful inhibitor system to prevent the coagulation process spreading away from the site of injury and into the general circulation.

7.2.2   The mechanism of haemostasis

The mechanism of haemostasis in a wound is thought to consist of three separate but closely interlinked processes. The first of these is the reaction of the damaged blood vessels. The second is the adhesion and aggregation of platelets at the site of injury to form a platelet plug, and the third is the coagulation of the blood. The first two stages are referred to as the primary phase of haemostasis and are responsible for the initial staunching of blood flow from damaged capillaries. The blood coagulation phase of the reaction to injury is referred to as the secondary phase of haemostasis and results in the laying down of fibrin strands within and about the adherent platelet mass. In this way the platelet mass is consolidated and less likely to be washed away when full blood flow through the capillary is re-established. Failure of primary haemostasis, due either to a vascular defect or a platelet defect, results in a type of bleeding different from that seen when the clotting or secondary phase fails; failure of primary haemostasis leads to bleeding immediately after injury, whereas failure of secondary haemostasis usually results in bleeding that starts after a short delay or even as long as days after the injury. Thrombocytopenic purpura and haemophilia are well-known examples of failure of primary and secondary haemostasis, respectively (see Chapter 5).

The description above suggests a distinct sequence of events with the vascular, platelet, and coagulation components coming into play at different times. This is almost certainly not the case. It is more likely that the various components of the mechanism are brought into play simultaneously by injury and act upon each other from that moment.

The role of the blood vessels, platelets, and coagulation process will now be discussed in more detail.

Reaction of the blood vessels

The reaction of blood vessels to injury has been studied extensively in humans and in animals but we still know very little about the mechanisms involved. The response to injury of vessels depends on the size of the damaged vessel, the rate of blood flow through it, and the extent of the injury.

In the case of small vessels, observations made using the hamster cheek pouch and other animal systems show that injured and transected capillaries contract, or may seem to disappear completely, within a few seconds of the injury. Other vessels in the vicinity may also contract and others open up to provide shunts which allow blood to be diverted from the injured part.

The mechanism of these reactions is still not well understood, although there is some evidence that capillary contraction may be due to contraction of myofibrils within the endothelial cells. Also, endothelial cells at the site of injury may become sticky and adhere to each other causing obliteration of the lumen of the vessel. Furthermore, the capillaries may be acted upon by vaso-active substances such as serotonin (5-HT), adrenaline, and thromboxane A_2 released from platelets at the site of injury. Other substances, such as bradykinin, released following activation of the blood coagulation system via factor XII may also play a role by increasing capillary permeability and allowing water to pass out. As a consequence there is an increase of blood viscosity locally with slowing of flow and an increase of pressure on the capillaries from outside by the exuded fluid. All of this assists in reducing blood loss.

Following injury to arteries and veins, active constriction of these vessels is seen to take place and this, along with clot formation, is an important function in reducing blood loss from vessels of this size. Platelet aggregation probably plays a minor role in controlling bleeding from such large vessels, as the volume and pressure of blood flow are likely to wash away the platelet plugs. It is not known for certain how these large vessels contract after injury, but it is probably by a reflex nerve mechanism triggered by trauma.

Platelets in haemostasis

In 1882 Hayem observed that an incision in the jugular vein of a dog stopped bleeding because of the accumulation of 'haematoblasts' (platelets) at the site of the injury. This observation has been confirmed many times since and the underlying mechanism intensively investigated. Platelets are small, non-nucleated, round or oval cells 2–3 μm in size. Normal blood contains 200 000–400 000 platelets/μl. Electron microscopy studies of platelets show many subcellular granules (α-granules and dense bodies), a complex system of microtubules and filaments, as well as mitochondria. The dense bodies contain adenosine diphosphate (ADP), adenosine triphosphate (ATP), 5-HT, and calcium ions. The α-granules contain fibrinogen, β-thromboglobulin, von Willebrand's factor (vWF), platelet factor 4 (PF4), and other substances. Platelets also contain the contractile proteins actin and myosin, which are essential for the shape change that takes place during adhesion and aggregation. On their surface membranes they carry platelet factor 3 (PF3), a lipoprotein important for blood coagulation, also several glycoproteins that act as receptor sites for fibrinogen and von Willebrand's factor, which are important in the haemostatic process. Finally, platelets contain enzymes necessary for synthesis of fatty acids and phospholipids, and have mechanisms for breaking down lipids via arachidonic acid to produce thromboxane A2, a labile but potent platelet aggregating agent.

When blood vessels are damaged and subendothelial structures are exposed, the platelets, which until then have been circulating as discrete non-adherent cells, mainly in the non-axial plasma stream, suddenly change their behaviour and begin to adhere to the site of injury. The mechanisms of this important and very striking phenomenon is still not fully understood, although the trigger is thought to be a reaction between exposed collagen in the subendothelium and receptors on the surface of the platelets.

Platelet adhesion to damaged vessel wall is impaired in Bernard–Soulier syndrome in which there is a lack of glycoprotein Ib (GPIb) in the platelet membrane. Also, platelets fail to adhere to vessel walls in von Willebrand's disease in which there is a quantitative or qualitative deficiency of von Willebrand's factor (vWF).

vWF is a multimeric protein with a molecular weight sometimes as high as 20 million. Treatment with reducing agents such as dithiothreitol or mercaptoethanol results in a subunit species with a molecular weight of approximately 200 000 as measured by polyacrylamide gel electrophoresis. This is probably the basic subunit. Multimers are thought to be built up from these basic subunits linked by disulphide bonds. The larger multimers seem particularly important in the reaction with platelets and subendothelium. The smaller multimers seem to be less able to participate in the haemostatic reactions. This difficulty may be simply due to the fact that the larger multimers, by virtue of their repeating subunits, provide a high local concentration of binding sites.

Immunological and tissue-culture techniques have shown that vWF is synthesized by endothelial cells and megakaryocytes. Platelets also contain significant amounts of vWF. The gene for vWF has been partially cloned, and *in situ* hybridization techniques have localized the gene to chromosome 12.

The role of vWF in haemostasis is to bring about adhesion of platelets to exposed subendothelium and to each other with formation of a platelet plug. The mechanism of this reaction has been intensively studied *in vitro*, using perfusion chambers containing segments of animal or human veins and arteries from which the endothelium has been removed. From these experiments it appears that von Willebrand's factor first binds to subendothelium and probably undergoes some conformational change that then allows it to react with glycoproteins on the platelet membrane and to act as a bridge between endothelium and platelets and between platelets. It should be noted that von Willebrand's factor in plasma does not normally bind to resting or non-activated platelets. But in the presence of the antibiotic, ristocetin, aggregation takes place (Howard and Firkin 1971) and this reaction has been used as the basis of an assay for vWF (Macfarlane *et al.* 1975).

Once adhesion to subendothelium has taken place the attached platelets undergo complex biochemical and physical changes which have a profound effect on other platelets nearby. The most important of these changes is the release reaction, which entails the breakdown of ATP by ATPase and the release of ADP, 5-HT and other amines, thromboxane A_2, and PF3. ADP and thromboxane A_2 are powerful platelet-aggregating agents and cause more platelets to stick to the wound and to each other, and in this way the platelet plug is enlarged. PF3 is a platelet membrane phospholipid that plays an important part in the coagulation process by providing a surface for coagulation factor interactions. Following this stage of adhesion and cohesion the platelets begin to lose their surface membranes and they fuse to form an amorphous hyaline mass. At about the same time as fusion takes place strands of fibrin begin to appear in the platelet mass and so complete the formation of a compact strong haemostatic plug firmly adherent to the damaged vessel.

The role of blood coagulation in haemostasis

In normal people when blood escapes or is drawn from the body and allowed to come into contact with a foreign surface, it is transformed in a few minutes from a free-flowing fluid into a semi-solid gelatinous mass. This dramatic change has captured the imagination and curiosity of scientists and laymen over the centuries and has provoked much research, discussion, and argument as to its cause.

One of the earliest attempts to draw up a hypothesis of blood coagulation was made at the beginning of this century by Morawitz (1905). His hypothesis, which came to be known as the 'classical theory' (Fig. 7.4), stated that prothrombin, which circulates in an inactive state in the blood, is converted to an active enzyme, thrombin, by tissue thromboplastin released from damaged tissue, platelets, or white cells. This reaction required the presence of calcium ions. The thrombin formed then acted on the insoluble protein fibrinogen converting it into insoluble threads of fibrin to form a clot.

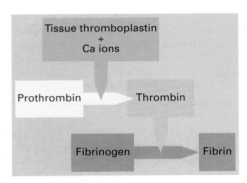

Fig. 7.4 Classical 'theory' of blood coagulation (Morawitz 1905).

This hypothesis of blood coagulation was accepted for nearly 40 years and proved to be a useful working hypothesis. But it failed to explain the nature of the coagulation defect in certain severe haemorrhagic disorders in humans and animals. In particular, it did not explain why it was that blood coagulation in haemophiliacs was abnormal despite the fact that their tissue thromboplastin, fibrinogen, and prothrombin had all been shown to be normal. As a consequence it became necessary to modify the classical theory over the years. The blood coagulation process is now envisaged as an enzyme cascade (Fig. 7.5) in each step of which an inactive precursor is converted to an active form which, in turn, activates the next enzyme in the

chain (Davie and Ratnoff 1964, Macfarlane 1964). Each of the proenzyme to enzyme transformations results in amplification of the 'signal' until, finally, large amounts of thrombin are formed, which act on fibrinogen to change it into fibrin clot. Several of the activated clotting factors, notably XIa, Xa, IXa, and thrombin (IIa) have been shown to have the amino acid serine at their active site and belong to the family of enzymes known as serine proteases. The primary structures of factors IXa, Xa, and thrombin show considerable sequence homology with other mammalian serine proteases, such as trypsin.

Blood has intrinsically all of the factors necessary for coagulation to take place but, in addition to the intrinsic system of blood coagulation, there is also an extrinsic mechanism involving exposure of blood to tissue juice (tissue thromboplastin) following injury, and consequent activation of the clotting cascade at several points in the chain. The concept of two systems of blood coagulation, an extrinsic system and an intrinsic system, is useful for descriptive purposes and also for interpreting the results of laboratory tests. It is clear, however, that there are several links between the two pathways, that they are complementary systems, and that both play important roles in the living animal.

Table 7.1 shows the various blood coagulation factors with their common names, roman numeral designation, and some of their properties.

The intrinsic blood coagulation pathway

The intrinsic pathway of blood coagulation is initiated by contact of blood with a foreign surface or substance (Margolis 1957, Nossel 1964). These include substances with negative surface charge such as kaolin, glass, celite, dextran sulphate, ellagic acid, or more biological substances such as fatty acids, skin, certain forms of collagen, urate crystals, and bacterial endotoxins. Collagen is particularly important as it is present in the subendothelium of vessels and, on exposure following injury, may activate the blood coagulation process as well as cause aggregation of platelets.

Four plasma factors are involved in the contact phase of blood coagulation, these are the Hageman factor (factor XII), factor XI, pre-kallikrein, and high molecular weight kininogen (HMWK). All four factors are strongly adsorbed on to the types of surface mentioned above, and are thereby enabled to react with each other more effectively. This stage of the reaction, unlike many later stages, does not require the presence of calcium ions. Also, it is now clear that the activation of the above factors by contact is important not only for the blood coagulation process but also for other components of the body's homeostatic and defence mechanisms, such as the activation of complement and fibrinolysis and the generation of kinins, which produce pain and increase vascular permeability.

The first stage of contact activation involves adsorption of factors XII, XI, plasma pre-kallikrein, and HMWK to the activating surface. Factor XII is a single polypeptide chain glycoprotein with a molecular weight of 90 000. As a result of adsorption to the foreign surface it is thought that factor XII undergoes a

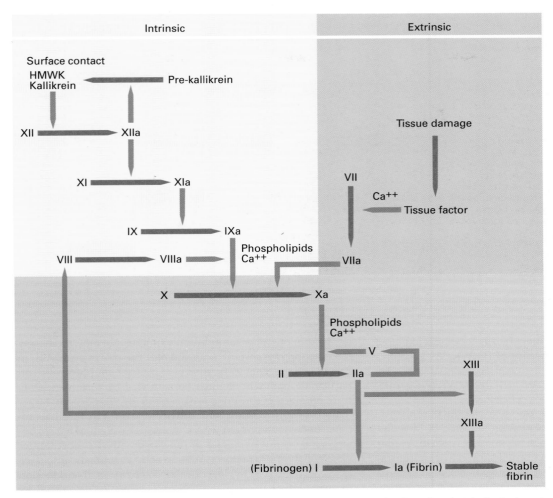

Fig. 7.5 A simplified schematic representation of the blood coagulation mechanism, showing the intrinsic and extrinsic pathways. Solid lines represent transformation from inactive to activated factors; activated factors are represented by 'a'; the purple arrows represent action on the next factor in the chain. All of the reaction stages, apart from that involving factor XII and factor XI, require calcium ions and probably take place on a phospholipid surface provided by tissue thromboplastin or platelet lipids.

conformational change that exposes active sites and thereby develops enzyme activity. The activated factor XII (XIIa) then acts on pre-kallikrein, changing it to kallikrein, which in turn acts back on factor XII to produce more XIIa. The kallikrein feedback stage results in proteolytic cleavage of factor XII and greatly accentuates the initial effects of contact. Factor XIIa next acts on factor XI in the presence of HMWK to produce activated factor XI (XIa) a powerful serine protease. Factor XI is a plasma protein with a molecular weight of approximately 160 000 and is made up of two polypeptide chains held together by disulphide bonds. Factor XIIa cleaves factor XI at two internal peptide bonds, producing two light chains, which contain the active sites, and two heavy chains.

Although it has been known for many years that plasma pre-kallikrein plays an important role in the kinin-forming system of plasma, its importance in blood coagulation *in vitro* was discovered only recently, from studies of patients deficient in the

factor (Fletcher trait). However, these patients do not bleed, and a role for pre-kallikrein in the *in vivo* haemostatic process has not been found so far. Pre-kallikrein is a single-chain polypeptide with a molecular weight of approximately 80 000, and it circulates in plasma as a complex with HMWK. It is present in plasma at a concentration of approximately 50 μg/ml. This complex is adsorbed on to the surface along with factor XII and the pre-kallikrein is converted to kallikrein in a reaction in which factor XIIa cleaves the chain to form a heavy chain and a light chain. The light chain carries the active site. As mentioned already, active kallikrein then acts back on factor XII. In addition it acts on HMWK, splitting off bradykinin, which has several important biological activities in the body's reaction to injury and in the inflammatory process.

High molecular weight kininogen is a plasma protein with a molecular weight of 120 000. It is a single-chain polypeptide which is thought to act as a carrier or co-factor for

Table 7.1 Some properties of factors involved in blood coagulation and haemostasis

Factor	Common name	Molecular weight	Approximate amount in 1 ml normal plasma	*In vivo* half-life
I	Fibrinogen	340 000	3–4 mg	3–4 days
II	Prothrombin	72 000	200 μg	72 hours
III	Tissue factor	220 000–300 000	0	
IV	Calcium ion	—	50 μg	
V	Proaccelerin	300 000	10 μg	15 hours
VII	Proconvertin	63 000	1 μg	4 hours
VIII	Antihaemophilic factor	280 000	50 ng	8–12 hours
IX	Christmas factor	55 000	4 μg	12–24 hours
X	Stuart–Power factor	55 000	6–8 μg	50 hours
XI	Plasma thromboplastin antecedent	160 000	8 μg	60 hours
XII	Hageman factor	90 000	40 μg	50 hours
XIII	Fibrin stabilizing factor	320 000	30 μg	4–7 days
Pre-kallikrein	(Fletcher factor)	80 000	30–40 μg	
High molecular weight kininogen	(HMWK; Fitzgerald, Flaujeac, or Williams factor)	120 000	80 μg	
	Protein C	62 000	5 μg	
	von Willebrand's factor	>1.5 million subunits 220 000	8 μg	24 hours

pre-kallikrein and factor XII, as these two factors show impaired adsorption to surface in the absence of HMWK. As with pre-kallikrein, the role of HMWK in blood coagulation was discovered from studies of patients deficient in HMWK (Fitzgerald, Flaujeac factor, or Williams factor deficiency).

Following contact activation, the next step in the intrinsic blood-clotting system involves activation of factor IX by factor XIa. Factor IX is a single-chain polypeptide and has a molecular weight of 55 000. It is present in normal plasma in a concentration of approximately 0.3 mg/100 ml and is deficient in patients suffering from haemophilia B (Christmas disease). It is synthesized in the liver and vitamin K is required for production of the biologically active protein. The complete amino-acid sequence of human factor IX has been elucidated and the molecule has been shown to be composed of 415 amino acids. Before release from the hepatocytes into the bloodstream, and in order to become biologically active, it undergoes several post-translational modifications, including carboxylation of glutamic acid residues under the influence of vitamin K and the addition of several carbohydrate residues. Synthesis of factor IX is regulated by a gene on the X chromosome. The gene is 34 kbp long, contains eight exons and six introns (Choo *et al.* 1982), and is situated near the end of the long arm of the X chromosome at the Xq 26-qter region.

During the process of coagulation, the inactive factor IX chain is cleaved in two proteolytic steps by factor XIa in the presence of calcium ions, to produce a two-chained activated form (factor IXa).

The next stage of the process brings about conversion of factor X to the active form, factor Xa, and involves a reaction between IXa, factor VIII, phospholipid, factor X, and calcium ions. Factors IXa and X bind to phospholipid molecules via their γ-carboxyglutamic acid residues and calcium ion bridges to form multimolecular complexes in which the reacting factors

are held in close proximity to one another, thereby increasing the reaction rate several thousandfold. The role of factor VIII in this reaction seems to be that of a cofactor and before it can participate optimally it must be activated by thrombin. Only trace amounts of thrombin are necesary for this purpose; larger amounts destroy factor VIII activity. Factor VIII (antihaemophilic factor) is a protein with a molecular weight of approximately 250 000. It circulates in the blood with the much larger von Willebrand's factor (vWF) which, as already discussed (p. 503), takes part in platelet-related activity such as adhesion to subendothelial collagen. The two molecules are linked by non-covalent bonds and can be dissociated easily *in vitro* by relatively simple procedures. The close association of factor VIII with vWF is important biologically as it presumably leads to a high concentration of procoagulant factor VIII at the site of injury by virtue of the binding of vWF to the damaged endothelium and to platelets. In addition, there is evidence that vWF acts as a stabilizer of factor VIII and when the two are separated factor VIII becomes unstable and loses activity rapidly. Some of the properties of factor VIII and vWF are shown in Table 7.2. Factor VIII is thought to be synthesized in the liver. Evidence for this comes from:

1. experiments in which normal dog livers were transplanted into haemophilic dogs with resultant increase of factor VIII activity in the recipients;

2. the finding of mRNA for factor VIII in the liver;

3. identification of factor VIII in hepatic sinusoidal endothelial cells using a monoclonal antibody acting against factor VIII coagulant activity.

The factor VIII gene has been cloned and the complete amino-acid sequence of the protein is now available (Gitschier *et al.* 1984). The gene, which is the largest gene clone so far, is situ-

Table 7.2 Some properties of factor VIII and von Willebrand's factor

	Factor VIII (VIII:C)	von Willebrand's factor (vWF)
Gene locus	Xq28	Chromosome 12
Site of synthesis	?Liver sinusoid cells ?Hepatocytes	Endothelial cells and megakaryocytes
Molecular weight	280 000	220 000–10 × 10^6 (multimers)
Functional assay	Based on ability to correct coagulation defect in haemophilic plasma	Based on ability to support platelet aggregation in presence of ristocetin (ristocetin–co-factor assay)
Antigen assay	VIII:C Ag assay by radioimmuno methods	vWF antigen by Laurell electroimmuno assay or immuno radiometric assay
Plasma concentration	5 ng/ml	10 μg/ml
Biological function	Co-factor for activation of factor X by IXa in the intrinsic system	(1) necessary for platelet adhesion (2) carrier of factor VIII

ated on the X chromosome in the Xq28 region and is 180 kbp long with 26 exons. Typically, factor VIII is deficient in the blood of haemophiliacs but the level of vWF and its associated activities are normal.

Factor X is centrally placed in the blood coagulation process and can be activated through the intrinsic or extrinsic system (see Fig. 7.5). It is a glycoprotein with a molecular weight of 52 000, is synthesized in the liver and is present in normal plasma at a concentration of approximately 1 mg/100 ml. It is made up of two chains, a heavy and a light chain, held together by disulphide bonds. During activation a peptide bond in the heavy chain is cleaved, releasing a small fragment and unmasking the active serine site which is situated in the heavy chain. The factor Xa (plasma thromboplastin, prothrombinase, 'tenase') thus produced then acts on prothrombin to yield the active enzyme thrombin.

The extrinsic blood coagulation pathway

Activation of factor X by the above process involves coagulation factors that are all circulating in the blood, but factor X can be activated by an extrinsic system of coagulation in a reaction involving factor VII, calcium ions, and a factor present in tissues.

Tissue factor (tissue thromboplastin) is a liproprotein found in all tissues. Brain, liver, and the placenta are the most commonly used for experimental work. Both the phospholipid and the protein portion of the complex are necessary for the reaction with factor VII and for development of coagulant activity. Factor VII is a plasma protein with a molecular weight of 60 000. It is produced in the liver, requires vitamin K for its production, and is present in plasma in very small amounts, approximately 0.05 mg/100 ml. It is a single polypeptide chain and, like all the other vitamin-K-dependent clotting factors, contains γ-carboxyglutamic acid residues which are essential for its biological function. When clotting takes place by the extrinsic system, factor VII forms a complex with calcium ions and the lipid component of tissue factor and is changed into a double-chain structure with enzymic activity that activates factor X, yielding factor Xa. In addition to the above activation pathways, fac-

factor X may be activated directly by trypsin or by Russell's viper venom. The nature of the reaction between Russell's viper venom and factor X has been intensively investigated by many research workers and the elucidation of the mechanism was an important stimulus to the formulation of the 'cascade' (Macfarlane 1964) or 'waterfall' (Davie and Ratnoff 1964) hypothesis of blood coagulation.

The common blood coagulation pathway

In this stage of the clotting process prothrombin is converted to the active enzyme, thrombin, by the action of factor Xa, the thrombin then acting on fibrinogen to produce the fibrin clot.

Prothrombin is a single-chain glycoprotein with a molecular weight of 70 000. It is produced in the liver under the influence of vitamin K and is present in normal plasma at a concentration of 10 mg/100 ml. During conversion of prothrombin to thrombin, two peptide bonds in the prothrombin molecule are split by factor Xa to release thrombin. Factor V, phospholipid, and calcium ions are necessary for this reaction to proceed at optimal rates. The phospholipid acts as a surface on to which prothrombin, factor V, factor Xa, and calcium ions are adsorbed, ensuring close proximity of the reactants. The formation of this factor V–Xa–phospholipid–Ca^{2+} is analogous to the complex of factor VIII–factor IXa–phospholipid–Ca^{2+} seen in an earlier reaction. Factor V is a plasma protein that is produced in the liver. Its molecular weight is 250 000–300 000 and it is present in normal plasma at a concentration of approximately 1 mg/100 ml. Like factor VIII, it seems to act as a co-factor in the clotting process and requires to be activated by trace amounts of thrombin before it can participate fully in the coagulation process, and it is destroyed by large amounts of thrombin.

The final stage of clot formation involves the conversion of the soluble protein, fibrinogen, to insoluble strands of fibrin. Fibrinogen is a plasma protein with a molecular weight of 340 000; it is synthesized in the liver and is present in normal plasma at a concentration of approximately 300 mg/100 ml. The fibrinogen molecule is a dimer, each half of the dimer being composed of three non-identical peptide chains designated as Aα, Bβ, and γ. The peptide chains are held together by

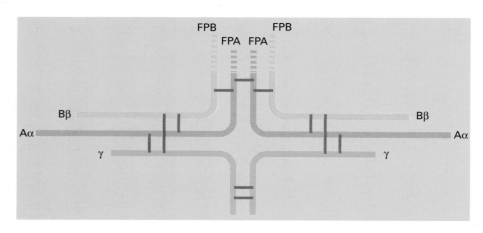

Fig. 7.6 Diagrammatic representation of the fibrinogen molecule showing the paired polypeptide chains. The disulphide bonds are represented by red lines; FPA, fibrinopeptide A; FPB, fibrinopeptide B.

sulphide bonds, as are the two halves of the dimer (Fig. 7.6). The conversion of fibrinogen to a stable fibrin clot occurs in three stages. During the first stage, thrombin acts on the amino-terminal ends of both $A\alpha$ and $B\beta$ chains, releasing two fibrino-peptides A and two fibrinopeptides B respectively. It is thought that these fibrinopeptides shield specific polymerization sites on the parent molecule and that their removal allows the remainder of the molecules (fibrin monomer) to aggregate spontaneously, aligning themselves side to side and end to end to form polymers of fibrin. The fibrin strands formed initially are not stable and can be broken down easily by fibrinolytic enzymes, as well as by non-physiological agents such as urea and monochloroacetic acid. The third stage of the reaction involves cross-linking of the fibrin polymer by covalent bonds. This requires the presence of factor XIII. Following activation by thrombin, factor XIII, which is a transamidating agent, catalyses the formation of γ-glutamyl–ϵ lysine bridges between the side-chains of fibrin molecules. In this way the fibrin clot is rendered more stable, more rigid, and more effective in haemostasis.

It has been estimated that the amount of thrombin generated from 1 ml of plasma is more than sufficient to clot all of the fibrinogen in the circulating blood. Clearly, therefore, there must be a system of inhibitors that limits the coagulation process to the site of injury, otherwise coagulation might spread throughout the general circulation with disastrous consequences. Mention has already been made of the fact that trace amounts of thrombin activate factors V and VIII and that large amounts generated during clotting then destroy these factors, thereby 'switching off' the reaction. In addition to this negative feedback process there are several inhibitors that act at various stages of the clotting cascade. The most closely studied and the best understood are antithrombin III (ATIII, heparin co-factor), α_1 antitrypsin, α_2 macroglobulin, and protein C.

Antithrombin III, as the name implies, is an inhibitor of thrombin. It is a single-chain polypeptide with a molecular weight of 65 000. It inhibits thrombin in a reaction in which an arginine residue in antithrombin III binds to the active serine site in thrombin. Heparin enhances this action greatly by binding to antithrombin III and bringing about a conformational

change in the ATIII molecule which is thought to expose the arginine site, making binding to the serine site in thrombin easier (Fig. 7.7). In addition to inhibiting thrombin, antithrombin III acts against XIIa, XIa, IXa, Xa, plasma kallikrein, and plasmin.

Inherited deficiency of ATIII to 50–60 per cent of the normal level results in repeated episodes of venous thrombosis and thromboembolism.

α_1 antitrypsin and α_2 macroglobulin seem to play a minor role in inhibiting thrombin. α_1 antitrypsin has some effect on thrombin, factor IXa, and plasmin; and α_2 macroglobulin inhibits

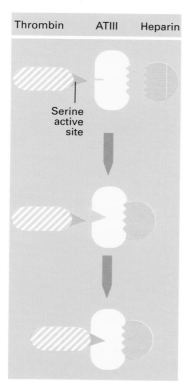

Fig. 7.7 Scheme to show how heparin is thought to act in enhancing the reaction between antithrombin III and thrombin.

thrombin, plasma kallikrein, and plasmin. Deficiencies of these two factors have not been associated with any thrombosing tendency.

Protein C is a vitamin-K-dependent plasma protein, synthesized in the liver. Following activation by thrombin, protein C inactivates both factors V and VIII in the presence of phospholipid and calcium ions. Protein C deficiency may predispose to thrombosis.

7.2.3   Bibliography

Choo, K. H., Gould, K. G., Rees, D. J. G., and Brownlee, G. G. (1982). Molecular cloning of the gene for human antihaemophilic factor IX. *Nature* **299**, 178–80.

Davie, E. W. and Ratnoff, O. D. (1964). Waterfall sequence for intrinsic blood clotting. *Science* **145**, 1310–12.

Gitschier, J., *et al.* (1984). Characterization of the human factor VIII gene. *Nature* **312**, 326–30.

Hayem, G. (1882). Sur le mécanisme de l'arrêt hémorrhagies. *Comptes Rendus hebdomadaires des Seances de l'Academie des Sciences* **95**, 18.

Heilbrunn, L. V. (1961). The evolution of the haemostatic mechanism. In *Functions of the blood* (ed. R. G. Macfarlane and A. H. T. Robb-Smith), p. 283. Academic Press, New York.

Howard, M. A. and Firkin, B. G. (1971). Ristocetin—a new tool in the investigation of platelet aggregation. *Thrombosis et Diathesis Haemorrhagica* **26**, 362–9.

Macfarlane, D. E., Stibbe, K., Kirby, E. P., Zucker, M. B., Grant, R. A., and McPherson, J. (1975). A method of assaying von Willebrand factor (ristocetin co-factor). *Thrombosis et Diathesis Haemorrhagica* **34**, 306–8.

Macfarlane, R. G. (1964). An enzyme cascade in the blood clotting mechanism and its function as a biochemical amplifier. *Nature (London)* **202**, 498–9.

Margolis, J. (1957). Initiation of blood coagulation by glass and related surfaces. *Journal of Physiology* **137**, 95–109.

Morawitz, P. (1905). Die Chemie der Blutgerinnung. In *Ergebnisse der Physiologie* **4**, 307–423.

Needham, A. E. (1970). Haemostatic mechanism in the invertebrata. In *The haemostatic mechanism in man and other animals* (ed. R. G. Macfarlane), p. 19. Published for the Zoological Society of London by Academic Press.

Nossel, H. L. (1964). *The contact phase of blood coagulation.* Blackwell, Oxford.

7.2.4   Further reading

Biggs, R. and Rizza, C. R. (eds) (1984). *Human blood coagulation haemostasis and thrombosis.* Blackwell Scientific, Oxford.

Bloom A. L. and Thomas, D. P. (eds) (1987). *Haemostasis and thrombosis* (2nd edn.). Churchill Livingstone, Edinburgh.

Brownlee, G. G. (1986). The molecular genetics of haemophilia A and B. *Journal of Cell Science, Suppl.* **4**, 445–58.

Macfarlane, R. G. (1961). The reaction of the blood to injury. In *Functions of the blood* (ed. R. G. Macfarlane and A. H. T. Robb-Smith), p. 303. Academic Press, New York.

Macfarlane, R. G. (ed.) (1970). *The haemostatic mechanism in man and other animals.* Symposia of the Zoological Society of London, No. 27. Academic Press, London.

7.3   Thrombosis

N. Woolf

7.3.1   Introduction

A thrombus was defined by Welch (1887) as a solid mass or plug formed within the heart, arteries, veins, or capillaries from the components of the streaming blood. It is a matter for regret that many speak of thrombosis as being more or less synonymous with clotting of blood, and important that the fundamental differences between the two processes should be appreciated. In *clotting* the initiation of a cascade system within the blood leads to the generation of thrombin and thus to the conversion of the soluble plasma protein fibrinogen to the insoluble fibrin polymer. Thrombosis, on the other hand, is characterized by a series of events which involve both the blood *platelets* and the coagulation system. Whether platelet activation or fibrin formation predominate in any single thrombus depends on the relative interactions of the three main factors believed to underlie the pathogenesis of thrombosis, these being:

1. changes in the vessel wall;
2. changes in the constituents of the blood; and
3. changes in the flow patterns of the blood.

7.3.2   Platelets, haemostasis, and thrombosis

Thrombosis may be viewed as an abnormal outcome of a set of normal mechanisms. The latter are those that must be activated when injury to blood vessels is followed by the formation of a haemostatic plug, and both platelet activation and the triggering of the clotting system contribute to haemostasis. It has been known for many years that *normal platelets in normal numbers are essential if bleeding from a damaged blood vessel is to be brought under control*; the mechanisms involved in the formation of a haemostatic plug and the formation of an arterial thrombus are essentially similar. Both haemostatic plugs and thrombi occurring in the arterial circulation and in the heart are composed largely of platelet aggregates that adhere at sites of injury to the endothelial surface. Strands of fibrin around the platelets serve to stabilize the platelet mass. Thus, a significant decline in the number of circulating platelets (thrombocytopenia) or some intrinsic abnormality, either in the platelets or in the endothelial cell (e.g. von Willebrand's disease), may be associated with abnormal bleeding.

Platelet activities in thrombus formation

In the course of thrombus formation, platelets first must adhere to sites of endothelial cell loss or areas where the endothelial cells are otherwise abnormal and, in the course of undergoing a shape change, release a number of very potent factors which lead to the *aggregation* of further platelets at the site of the initial adhesion, to the local formation of fibrin, to changes in vessel permeability, and to a stimulatory effect on the connective tissue cells in the underlying vessel wall (Fig. 7.8). As already stated, the mechanisms involved in thrombosis do not differ significantly from those that operate in the formation of a haemostatic plug, although local environment circumstances, such as the size of the vesels affected and the local blood flow characteristics modulate the end result.

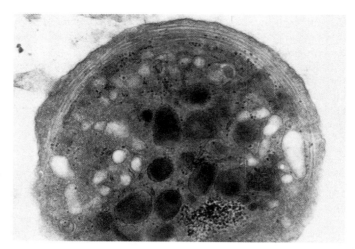

Fig. 7.9 A transmission electron micrograph of a non-activated, and hence disciform, platelet showing the arrangement of the cytoskeleton beneath the plasma membrane.

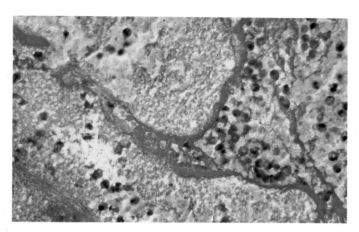

Fig. 7.8 Section of a three-day-old thrombus produced by direct endothelial injury and stained to differentiate between platelets (mauve), fibrin (red), and red cells (yellow). The bulk of the material can be seen to consist of aggregated platelets; there is relatively minor scaffolding of fibrin and some incorporated red cells. The appearance is of that seen in arterial thrombi formed under conditions of rapid flow (Picro-Mallory).

The complex series of changes undergone by platelets in the course of haemostatic plug or thrombus formation is mirrored in the microanatomy of these very small but remarkable cells. Some of the structure–function correlates that deserve our attention are, for instance, those which relate to:

1. the ability of the platelet, under normal circumstances, to circulate in the plasma in a completely non-active form;

2. the ability of the platelet to respond rapidly to signals generated from sites of vessel wall injury;

3. the ability of the platelet to contract after adhesion has taken place and thus release its store of pharmacologically active compounds—some of these contribute to aggregation, while others can produce striking proliferative changes in the underlying vessel wall.

The circulating platelet

Non-activated platelets circulate as flattened discs (Fig. 7.9). The maintenance of this shape depends on the activity of a peripheral band of microtubules, which are arranged in circumferential patterns, and on a system of microfilaments, which lie just beneath the unit membrane of the cell. The microtubules maintain a normal discoid shape; treatment of platelets with

compounds such as colchicine, which interferes with microtubule assembly, leads very rapidly to dissolution of the tubules and loss of the normal discoid shape (Figs 7.10, 7.11).

Signal reception

Of all the cells in the circulating blood the platelet is the most sensitive to a wide range of chemical and physical signals, and it is capable of localizing to submicroscopic areas of endothelial cell injury with exquisite precision.

This ability depends, in part, on the presence of a number of glycoprotein receptors located in the glycocalyx, and, in part, on the fact that for its volume the platelet has a very large surface area. This is due to the existence of a deeply ramifying series of canals running from the cell surface (the 'open canalicular system'). This enhances the chances of ligand–receptor binding and also provides a series of conduits for the active compounds secreted by the platelet as part of the 'release' phase that follows adhesion. Ligand–receptor binding may occur simply as a consequence of local release of a signal, such as von Willebrand's factor, or may depend on a prior conformational change in a receptor complex, such as is believed to occur in relation to the binding of fibrinogen to the platelet surface.

Platelet contraction

Platelet contraction, like other parts of the activation process, is mediated through changes in cytosolic calcium concentrations. This is largely dependent on a system of tubules known as the dense tubular system. This is made up of smooth endoplasmic reticulum derived from the parent megakaryocyte. In some areas within the cell the membranes of the dense tubular system and those of the open canalicular system are closely apposed, in a manner similar to the relationship between sarcotubules and transverse tubules in muscle cells.

The role of these membrane systems can be appreciated most easily if one looks upon the platelet as being in some respects

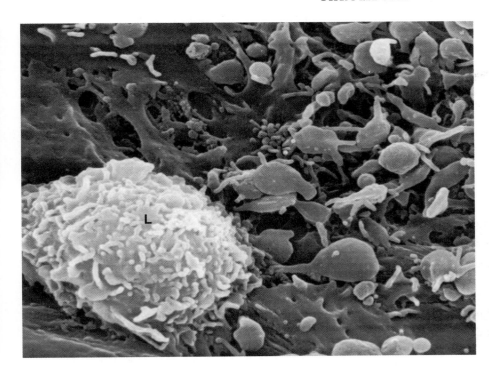

Fig. 7.10 Scanning electron micrograph of a damaged endothelial surface to which many platelets have adhered. Most of these have undergone a shape change and show the presence of blunt pseudopod-like processes. The size of the platelets can be compared with a leucocyte (L) which is also adhering to the vascular surface.

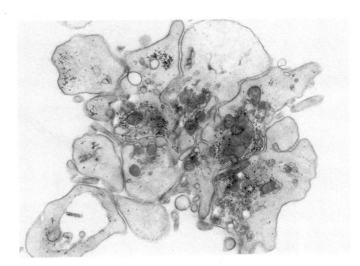

Fig. 7.11 Transmission electron micrograph showing aggregated platelets that have undergone shape change, this being associated with extensive degranulation.

rather like a muscle cell, in that both cells contract on stimulation. The contraction of platelet actomyosin, as in other situations, is modulated by calcium flux. In the platelet the dense tubular system is the site in which calcium is sequestered when the cell has not been activated. Signals reach the platelet interior via the open canalicular system, and the connections between this and the dense tubular system lead to the extrusion of calcium from the dense tubular system into the cytoplasm,

this being followed by contraction of actomyosin and shape change. When the platelet is not activated by a chemical signal, the cytoplasmic calcium is maintained at low levels by the operation of a calcium pump which transports cytoplasmic calcium into the dense tubular system, and which appears to be essential for maintaining the platelet in its resting, discoid form. If there is a rise in intracellular cAMP, the activity of the calcium pump is enhanced. It is not without interest that chemical agents appearing to inhibit platelet activity, such as the anti-aggregatory prostaglandins (E_1, D_2, and I_2), act by stimulating the platelet adenylate cyclase to produce a rise in intracellular cAMP. In addition to a role in modulating contractile functions, the dense tubular system also appears to be the site of prostaglandin synthesis within the platelet.

7.3.3 Factors promoting thrombosis

The very complexity of the interrelating processes involved in platelet adhesion, release, and aggregation that have been described in the preceding section suggests that a number of different circumstances may influence platelet/vessel wall behaviour. In the 1860s, when thrombosis was recognized (but not the existence of the platelet), Rudolf Virchow suggested that the factors likely to promote thrombus formation fell naturally into *three* major groups, which have been alluded to in the introduction. These:

1. changes in the pattern of blood flow;
2. changes in the intimal surface of the vessel;
3. changes in the constituents of the blood;

are known as *Virchow's triad*.

Changes in the pattern of blood flow

The important changes in blood flow pattern that are believed to increase the risk of thrombus formation are, first, changes in the *speed* of normal laminar flow and, secondly, actual *loss of the normal laminar pattern and its replacement by a turbulent pattern*. Slowing of the speed of blood flow without loss of the normal laminar pattern appears to be of particular significance in relation to the formation of thrombi in *veins*, while in the *heart and arteries* turbulence plays a more important haemodynamic role.

Reduced speed of flow

A reduction in the speed of blood flow may be either a general or a local phenomenon. The first of these may occur in patients with severe congestive cardiac failure, in whom the circulation time can be reduced significantly. The second tends to occur particularly in the veins of the leg under a number of different circumstances of which the most important are:

1. prolonged dependence of the limb;
2. reduced muscle pumping activity;
3. proximal occlusion of the venous drainage.

Venous thrombi are most frequently found to originate within the valve pockets, this anatomical site, under conditions of reduced flow, favouring local accumulation of activated clotting factors and increasing the chances of contact between platelets and the underlying vessel wall. These circumstances are most likely to arise in a patient immobilized in bed, especially after surgery. So far as the development of venous thrombosis is concerned, a hospital is a very high-risk area. Dissection of the deep veins of the calf has shown the presence of thrombi in more than 30 per cent of medical patients coming to necropsy and about 60 per cent of surgical patients. The clinical diagnosis of such thrombi is difficult and only perhaps 50 per cent are correctly diagnosed during life, by the presence of some swelling and tenderness in the affected calf and by pain in the calf being elicited on dorsiflexion of the foot (Homan's sign). Rational prevention related to minimizing changes in the pattern of blood flow, which is likely to be much more useful than treament of an established thrombus, should include routine physiotherapy with exercises emphasizing calf and thigh muscle contraction, early post-operative ambulation, and avoidance of prolonged dependency of lower limbs.

Stasis of blood can also occur in the heart and large vessels such as the aorta if either the cardiac chambers or a segment of a major artery are abnormally dilated. This is found in aortic and other arterial *aneurysms*, in the dilated chambers of the heart in a disorder of heart muscle known as *congestive or dilated cardiomyopathy* (Fig. 7.12), and in the dilated atria of patients with mitral valve disease, especially if there is associated atrial fibrillation. A situation rather similar to this occurs in patients in whom a large segment of the left ventricular wall has been rendered severely ischaemic following coronary artery occlusion (myocardial infarction). The dead heart muscle is replaced by scar tissue, which is non-contractile, and this can lead to local disturbances of flow during ventricular systole, and the formation of thrombi over the area of lost cardiac muscle.

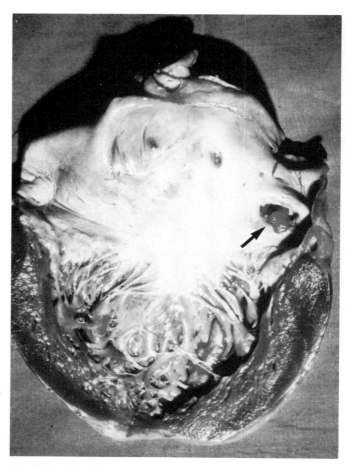

Fig. 7.12 Heart from patient dying with dilated cardiomyopathy. The thrombus has protruded from the left atrial appendage (arrow) and a thrombus is also present on the ventricular wall.

Turbulence

Turbulent flow is of particular importance in relation to points where arteries branch and to narrowed segments of arteries, such narrowing being due chiefly to atherosclerosis. The haemodynamic circumstances obtaining at points of branching are such that platelets tend to collect on the outer walls of branches. This has been demonstrated by introducing extracorporeal shunts, made either of glass or plastic, into the arterial system of animals, and then studying the sites at which platelets accumulate preferentially. In such a model system, the wall surface is uniform and thus the effect of flow can be studied in isolation (Figs 7.13, 7.14).

Changes in the vessel wall surface

Change in the surface of the vessel wall is recognized to be of major importance in the pathogenesis of arterial thrombi. The most important of these changes is *atherosclerosis*, the lesions of which are described in Chapter 12. However, injury (using the word in its broadest sense), inflammation, or neoplasms may also be associated with damage to the vessel wall. Of all the

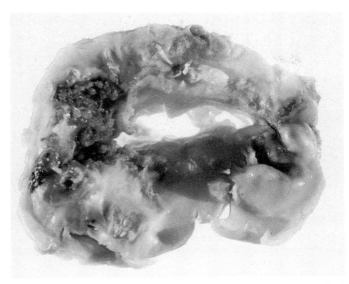

Fig. 7.13 Surgically removed mitral valve from a patient with mitral stenosis and incompetence. The abnormal regurgitant jut across the valve has resulted in the formation of thrombi as a result of haemo-dynamic injury.

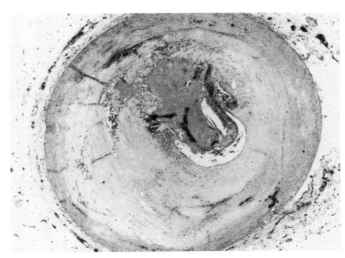

Fig. 7.15 An atherosclerotic plaque in which rupture of the connective tissue cap has occurred at one point with the rapid formation of thrombus, consisting almost entirely of platelets. The patient died suddenly.

structural elements of the vessel wall likely to undergo change as a 'pre-thrombotic' event, the one most likely to be implicated is the endothelial cell. In any situation where there is actual loss of endothelial cells with exposure of the subendothelial collagen, platelet adhesion is the inevitable sequel. This certainly happens in complicated atherosclerotic plaques when splitting of the connective tissue 'cap' of the plaque occurs (Fig. 7.15). Endothelial cell desquamation can also take place in the rare inherited metabolic disorder, homocystinaemia, in which lack of the enzyme cystathionine synthetase causes a block in the metabolic pathway from methionine to cystine. This leads to the accumulation of homocystine in the blood, which is associated with endothelial cell damage and widespread thrombosis involving both veins and arteries. It has also been claimed that desquamated endothelial cells can be identified in significant numbers in the plasma following cigarette smoking.

One of the dogmas of vascular pathology is that platelets do not adhere to intact endothelium. However, in some experimental models such adhesion has been seen. This has followed infusions of the enzyme, neuraminidase, which alters the proteoglycans in the luminal glycocalyx of the endothelial cell, and has also been noted in animals exposed to fresh cigarette smoke. A reduction in the amount of prostaglandin I_2 (prostacyclin) produced by aortic rings of rats exposed to fresh cigarette smoke has also been reported. These data, scanty as they are, suggest that certain factors may alter the structure and function of endothelium in such a way as to promote platelet–vessel wall interactions, without it being necessary for focal necrosis of endothelium to take place.

Trauma

Trauma to the endothelium of a sufficient degree to cause thrombosis can occur under a number of circumstances. At a rather extreme level, thrombosis can occur after burning or freezing (e.g. the capillary thrombosis seen in cases of 'frostbite'). Mechanical trauma to endothelium occurs in association with the presence of indwelling cannulae. Another type of much less easily provable endothelium trauma has been suggested as being one of the factors operating in the production of post-operative venous thrombi in the lower limb. During anaesthesia there is marked loss of the normal muscle tone, and the view has been put forward that the interaction between the dead weight of the limb and the hard surface of the operating table might be sufficient to cause trauma to the venous endothelium. There is no direct evidence for such trauma at the moment, although surgery certainly appears to be a very potent thrombogenic stimulus as far as the veins are concerned.

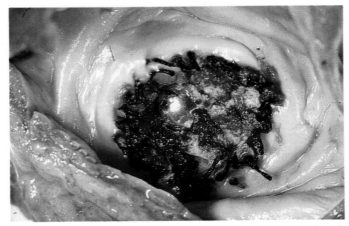

Fig. 7.14 A thrombosis occurring in relation to a Starr–Edwards prosthesis, which is virtually covered by the thrombotic mass.

Chemical trauma certainly exists and thrombosis may follow infusion of certain compounds into veins. This fact is made use of in certain treatments of both varicose veins and haemorrhoids, where sclerosing chemicals may be injected into the affected veins with the deliberate intention of causing thrombosis.

Inflammation

Thrombi occur frequently in situations where the vascular channels are involved in an inflammatory process. This may occur in the heart valves in patients with either rheumatic or infective endocarditis (Figs 7.16, 7.17). Arteries involved in an immune-complex-mediated inflammatory reaction, such as in *polyarteritis nodosa* or *temporal arteritis*, are often thrombosed, and both veins and capillaries passing through an inflamed area may be affected in the same way.

Neoplastic involvement

The invasion of small venules by malignant cells is often accompanied by thrombosis, and there is evidence to suggest that fibrin formed in relation to the tumour cells in the course of this process may enhance their chances of survival and, hence, of multiplying.

Changes in the constituents of the blood

Platelets

It seems obvious that changes in platelet behaviour should be considered in relation to the three main constituents of platelet function: adhesion, release, and aggregation.

In addition, their concentration within the blood should be

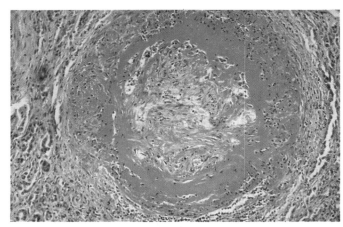

Fig. 7.17 A small artery in a patient with polyarteritis nodosa. The wall of the vessel shows fibrinoid necrosis and the lumen is occluded by partly organized thrombus.

determined since it is known that a low platelet count is associated with an abnormal bleeding tendency, and a high one with an increased likelihood of thrombosis.

In the laboratory it is common practice to measure the aggregatability of platelets to a given stimulus. ADP, collagen, or thrombin are added to a suspension of platelets in a cuvette and the turbidimetric changes resulting from aggregation measured. Platelet adhesiveness can also be measured. Here the suspension of platelets (of known concentration) is passed at a constant rate across glass beads and the drop in platelet numbers occurring as a result of this passage is determined. The release reaction can be monitored by measuring the changes in concentration of products derived from the α-granules: platelet factor 4 (an anti-heparin factor) and β-thromboglobulin. If sufficient care is taken in the sampling of the blood, a rise in the concentration of these compounds is prima-facie evidence of thrombosis having taken place. However, the half-lives of both platelet factor 4 and β-thromboglobulin in plasma are very short and thus the timing of sampling is critical.

Prostaglandins and platelets The results of epidemiological studies among the Eskimos of north-western Greenland suggest that alterations in the plasma concentrations of certain lipids may influence the balance between thromboxane A_2 and prostaglandin I_2. The incidence of ischaemic heart disease in this Eskimo community is very low. They have low levels of cholesterol and low-density lipoprotein in the blood and correspondingly high levels of high-density lipoprotein. This plasma lipid pattern is not genetic in origin but appears to be mediated by the diet. In addition, platelet aggregatability is lower than in age- and sex-matched Danes and the bleeding time is prolonged. One of the outstanding features of the Eskimo diet is a high intake of eicosapentaenoic acid (which is present in fish); Eskimos have high plasma concentrations of this fatty acid and low plasma concentrations of arachidonic acid. Eicosapentaenoic acid (EPA) is a starting point for the synthesis of prostaglandin I_3, which is anti-aggregatory, but the thromboxane derived from

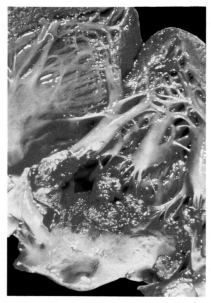

Fig. 7.16 The aortic valve of an intravenous drug abuser with acute bacterial endocarditis and a mass of infarcted thrombus on the aortic valve. (Courtesy of Professor M. J. Davies, St. George's Hospital Medical School, London.)

EPA is said not to be pro-aggregatory. Diets rich in cod-liver oil, which contains large amounts of EPA, have been shown to reduce the tendency to thrombosis in extra-corporeal shunts inserted into rat aortas.

Platelet aggregation and plasma lipid patterns Other evidence that plasma lipid concentrations and pattern may influence platelet behaviour is derived from patients with Type IIa hyperlipidaemia. Their platelets are many times more sensitive to doses of aggregating agents such as collagen, ADP, or thrombin than are those of normal subjects, though the lipid composition of the platelets themselves differs little, if at all. However, platelets from these hyperlipidaemics convert more arachidonic acid to thromboxane A_2 than to those from normal subjects.

In rabbits, feeding a diet high in saturated fat results in an increase in agggregatability of platelets in response to a standard dose of thrombin. This change takes place before any increase in the cholesterol concentration in the artery wall can be demonstrated. Similar data have been obtained from human studies.

Cigarette smoking and platelet function There is a strong positive correlation between heavy smoking (of cigarettes) and the risk of one of the major clinical manifestations of occlusive arterial disease. Cigarette smoking could operate as a risk factor in a number of ways and, clearly, the possibility of an effect on platelet behaviour is an area that requires investigation. Acute smoking experiments have yielded conflicting data on platelet aggregatability, but some studies suggest that smoking may have an effect on the adhesion of platelets to the underlying arterial wall.

7.3.4   Venous thrombosis

The process of thrombus formation in a non-inflamed vein is usually termed *phlebothrombosis*. When thrombosis occurs in a vein which is inflamed it is spoken of as *thrombophlebitis*. This is most commonly seen in superficial veins.

Understanding the pathogenesis of phlebothrombosis poses much greater problems than exist in the arterial counterpart. The site of initiation of the process is usually the valve pocket and if these areas are examined in sections of some, but by no means all, thrombosed veins, small clumps of platelets can be seen adhering to the luminal surface. It is a moot point whether this is preceded by damage to the endothelium in this area. Thus far no positive evidence that such damage is occurring has been presented, but the technical problems in carrying out such a study are daunting and it is, perhaps, too early to write off endothelial injury as being an important starting point for the process of venous thrombosis.

Any satisfactory hypothesis has to encompass a number of observed features:

1. the absence of significant damage to the venous endothelium in the valve pockets of thrombosed veins;
2. the marked tendency for phlebothrombosis to occur in the veins of the lower limbs, and pelvis;

3. the predilection for such thrombi to occur in subjects over 40 years of age, who have been kept at rest in bed, this being associated with recovery from surgery, attacks of myocardial ischaemia, and childbirth;
4. the observed decrease in risk which is brought about either by measures designed to reduce stasis in the veins of the lower limb or prophylactically to impair thrombin generation by the administration of anticoagulant drugs.

A possible role for leucocyte emigration induced by stasis

Some workers have noted the presence of leucocytes rather than platelets in these valve pockets, and it is possible that these cells could bring about changes in the endothelium sufficient to expose sub-endothelial collagen and thus cause platelet adhesion and aggregation. Certainly stasis alone does appear to be associated with increased adhesion of leucocytes to the endothelial surface.

The role of such leucocyte adhesion in relation to venous thrombosis was re-examined by Thomas *et al.* (1983) who compared the endothelial surfaces of blood containing segments of jugular vein ligated for 30–60 minutes with contralateral control segments. The ligated segments certainly showed the presence of leucocytes emigrating between adjacent endothelial cells and this was associated with some sub-endothelial oedema. However, there was no evidence in the ligated segments of either adhesion or aggregation of platelets.

The effect of thrombin and of activated coagulation factors

Wessler (1962) suggested that venous thrombi owed their origin to a combination of stasis in the venous circulation and local increases in thrombin concentrations, rather than to interactions between platelets and a damaged vein wall. Thrombin can cause signs of injury to cultured endothelial cells but there is no evidence that this occurs *in vivo*. Activated clotting factors are efficient in producing thrombi in stagnant columns of venous blood in animals and the further away such factors are from the actual process of fibrin formation, the smaller the dose that needs to be administered, a striking illustration of the importance of amplification in biological cascade systems. These experimental findings suggest that the formation of venous thrombi in humans occurs as a result of increased local generation (or decreased removal) of activated clotting factors at points of retarded venous blood flow, though why this should occur in some patients and not in others is not clear. The demonstration, referred to previously, that prophylactic treatment with low doses of thrombin-inhibiting compounds, such as heparin, prevents the formation of venous thrombi provides support for this view.

The evolution of venous thrombi

Once platelets are aggregated, clotting factors are activated locally and fibrin strands stabilize the platelet aggregate and help to anchor it to the underlying vein wall. When this has taken place a second phase begins in which a further batch of platelets is laid down over the initial aggregate. At this stage of the development of the thrombus, the platelets can be seen to have aggregated in the form of laminae that project from the surface of the initial aggregate and lie across the stream of blood (Fig. 7.18). As a result of the forces exerted by the streaming blood, these platelet laminae are bent in the direction of flow and form a somewhat coralline structure. Between the platelet laminae are large numbers of red cells, some fibrin strands, and a moderate number of leucocytes. The laminar arrangement of the platelets coupled with shortening of the fibrin strands between the laminae give rise to a curious 'rippled' appearance when the thrombi are viewed from above. The appearances are reminiscent of what one sees when a wind has blown across a beach and produced rippling of the sand. In both instances the 'ripples' lie concave to the direction of the force; in the case of the platelet laminae this having been the bloodstream. These elevated ridges on the surface of thrombi are known as *lines of Zahn* in commemoration of the pathologist who first described them. They are clearly visible with the naked eye but may be seen best with the aid of a hand lens. The more rapid the streaming of the blood in the segment of vessel where thrombosis has occurred, the more prominent are the lines of Zahn. They are most easily seen, therefore, in large arteries such as the aorta.

At this stage the process may come to an end. The thrombus will then become covered by new endothelial cells and be incorporated into the structure of the underlying vessel wall. However, if the deposition of platelets and fibrin continues, a third phase ensues and, as the coralline mass of platelets admixed with clotted blood continues to grow, the stream of blood through the affected segment slows still further and occlusion may occur ultimately. This phase is mediated predominantly by activation of coagulation pathways rather than by adhesion and aggregation.

Once a segment of vein is occluded in this way, the flow of blood cephalad to the occlusion stops. Thus a stagnant column of blood exists between the point of occlusion and the point cephalad to it where the next venous tributary enters. This stagnant column of blood coagulates and forms what is termed a 'consecutive clot' in continuity with the original thrombus.

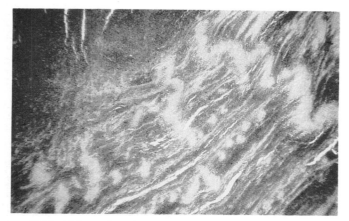

Fig. 7.18 This section shows a thrombus in a vein. Note the large numbers of darkly staining red cells and the pale staining lamina of the platelets.

This is the first step in a process known as *propagation* of the thrombus. There are two basic patterns in which this process may occur:

1. As mentioned above, consecutive clot forms between the original occlusion and the tributary immediately cephalad to it. At this point blood enters from the tributary and passes across the surface of the clot. Platelets then adhere to the fibrin meshwork and aggregation follows with the formation of another small platelet thrombus. If this, too, grows enough to occlude the lumen, propagation may occur again and another segment of vein filled with fresh clot. In effect, a long segment of the venous drainage of the limb can become occluded in a series of 'jumps' or episodes of clotting, each of which is triggered by the adhesion of platelets. On phlebography such thrombi appear as filling defects, which appear in marked contrast to the segments of vein that are filled by contrast medium. Such filling defects remain unchanged on screening. The mixed mass of platelet thrombi and consecutive clot is anchored to the underlying vein wall only at those sites where there has been adhesion of platelets.

2. If the venous return from the limb as a whole is slowed down, propagation by the formation of consecutive clot may occur on a massive scale. Cephalad to the original, occlusive platelet–fibrin thrombus, a long cord of clotted blood may form which fills the vein lumen and which is anchored only at its origin. With the eventual shortening of fibrin strands that takes place more or less inevitably after the formation of any clot, this mass of clotted blood comes to lie quite loosely within the lumen except at the point where the original thrombus is attached. If the thrombus becomes dislodged from its attachment point, then the whole mass is carried away in the systemic venous circulation until impaction takes place within the pulmonary arteries (pulmonary embolism).

7.3.5   The natural history of thrombi

Lysis

Some thrombi may undergo lysis through the action of plasmin and are completely removed. From the pragmatic point of view this is clearly the most desirable outcome, especially in relation to occlusive thrombosis within the arterial tree. It is not without interest that the plasminogen activator, plasmin, which converts plasminogen to the active form is present in greater concentrations within venous than within arterial intima.

Embolization

Thrombi may become detached from the underlying vascular wall, be it vein, artery, or heart. When this occurs the detached portion of thrombus travels at high speed in the systemic venous circulation (if its origin is a vein) or within the systemic arterial circulation (if the site of origin was an artery or the heart). At some point a vessel will be reached whose calibre is less than the diameter of the thrombotic material and impaction occurs. This can have serious structural and functional consequences which will be discussed in Section 7.4.

Organization

If the thrombus persists, the processes of organization, as described in Chapter 5, are triggered. Much will depend on whether the thrombus is occlusive, or whether it lies in a plaque-like fashion on the surface of the vessel wall without seriously impeding the flow of blood. Such a thrombus is called a *mural* thrombus.

The organization of occlusive thrombi

If a segment of a vessel remains plugged by thrombus, new vessels of granulation tissue capillary type grow out from the vasa vasorum in the adventitia, across the media, into and across the intima, and, ultimately, into the thrombus itself. At the same time, the removal of thrombotic material, largely through the action of macrophages, is proceeding. Eventually, at the worst, the occlusive thrombus may be replaced by a solid plug of collagenous tissue and all chance of re-establishing flow is lost.

Fortunately, however, the picture is not by any means always so gloomy. Quite early on after the formation of an occlusive thrombus, clefts may appear within the thrombotic material. These clefts often lie in the long axis of the occluded segment and hence, by implication, in the same axis as the blood flow. Not infrequently they link up with one another to form new channels which pass through the occluding plug of thrombus–granulation tissue from one patent segment of the vessel to another (Figs 7.19, 7.20). The clefts become lined within a few days by flattened cells of mesenchymal origin, which ultimately differentiate into endothelial cells. Occasionally some of the mesenchymal stem cells close to the new vascular channels differentiate into smooth muscle and arrange themselves round the clefts in a concentric fashion. The whole process by which a greater or lesser degree of blood flow through the occluded segment of vessel is re-established is known as *recanalization*.

The organization of mural thrombi

In this situation the pattern of organization is different because the pathophysiological circumstances differ so much from what obtains in an occluded segment of a vessel. Since flowing blood passes over the surface of the mural thrombus, the superficial portion of the thrombus is the seat of infiltration by oxygenated plasma, and granulation tissue type capillaries derived from the vasa grow only very slowly, if at all, into the thrombus. The lack of this feature may be mediated, in part at least, by the normal intramural tension within the affected part of the vessel.

Many of the platelets disaggregate and are either washed away by the passing stream of blood or are phagocytosed. In arteries this means that, within a short time, the major part of the remaining thrombus consists of a spongy mass of polymerized fibrin which tends to become packed down on to the surface of the underlying vessel wall. Within a few days the surface of the thrombus becomes partly covered by a layer of flattened cells. Originally it was thought that these were new endothelial cells, but there is some evidence to suggest that the cells making up the early neo-intima are smooth muscle cells (Fig. 7.21).

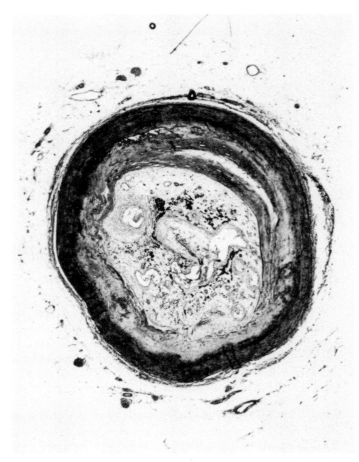

Fig. 7.19 Coronary artery, the lumen of which is completely occluded by a mass of organized and partly canalized connective tissue in which a few darkly staining thrombotic residua can be seen.

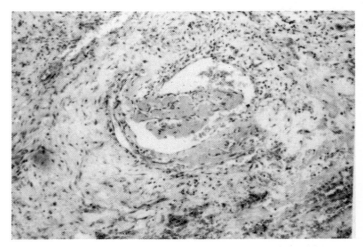

Fig. 7.20 A seven-day-old thrombus in a small vessel within the bed of the thyroid showing retraction of the thrombus and the formation of clefts within it that are lined by new endothelium.

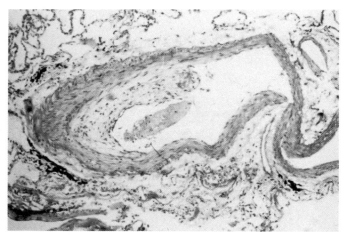

Fig. 7.21 A small artery within the lung, which was the seat of an embolus. Note the focal fibro-muscular hyperplasia on the intima in which a few plaques of persisting thrombus can be seen.

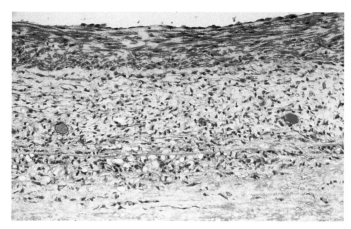

Fig. 7.22 Aortic intima at the seat of a previous post-traumatic thrombus. The intima is now many times as thick as normal and shows the presence of many red-staining new smooth muscle cells, some of which are arranged parallel to the intimal surface.

As in other situations where organization is taking place, the mass of fibrin and platelets becomes vascularized. An unusual feature, however, is the fact that the new vascular channels, which can be seen within a few days of the thrombus being formed, are derived from the main lumen of the vessel and grow down into the thrombus rather than upwards across the media from the vasa vasorum.

Intimal thickening with a striking degree of smooth muscle cell proliferation is a regular consequence of mural thrombosis. The major part of this proliferation of smooth muscle cells, and of the increase in extracellular connective tissue elements, such as collagen, which accompanies it, appears to take place on the lumenal aspect of the thrombus, so that the latter comes to lie deep within the thick new intima. This process is likely to be due to the interaction of platelet-derived growth factor with smooth muscle cells in the underlying vessel wall.

Platelet-derived growth factor (PDGF) is a basic protein with a molecular weight between 27 000 and 32 000. There are two distinct subunit chains, designated A and B, which are linked by disulphide bridges. There is considerable homology between these two chains. Of even greater interest is the 87 per cent homology that exists between the amino-acid sequence of the B-chain with a sequence of the transforming protein p28^{sis} of the simian sarcoma virus. It is now known that the human *c-sis* locus, which is found on chromosome 22, encodes the B-chain of PDGF. Like other proto-oncogenes, *sis* appears to have been highly conserved during evolution, and it seems likely that PDGF has a role in normal growth and development. Specific receptors for this growth factor have been identified on cultured human fibroblasts and on vascular smooth muscle cells, and these receptors appear to be quite distinct from those which bind other known growth factors. PDGF can also act as a chemotactic factor for fibroblasts, smooth muscle cells, neutrophils, and monocytes, and this activity is not lost when the molecule is split into its constituent chains, as is the case with its mitogenic function (Figs 7.22, 7.23, 7.24).

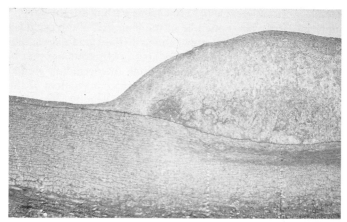

Fig. 7.23 Aortic intima 30 days after induction of a post-traumatic thrombus. A well-formed fibro-muscular plaque can be seen at the site.

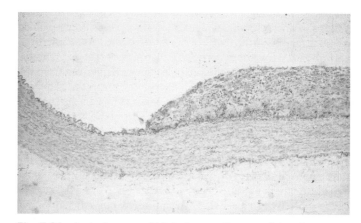

Fig. 7.24 Aorta from a rabbit fed on a diet containing 1 per cent cholesterol. The aorta was injured five weeks before killing and shows the presence of a well formed lipid-rich plaque of equal thickness to the underlying media.

7.3.6 Further reading

Thrombosis—general

Davies, M. I. and Thomas, A. (1984). Thrombosis and acute coronary artery lesions in the study of cardiac ischemic death. *New England Journal of Medicine* **310**, 1140.

Gordon, J. L. and Pearson, J. D. (1987). Biology of the vascular endothelium. In *Haemostasis and thrombosis* (ed. A. L. Bloom and D. P. Thomas), p. 303. Churchill Livingstone, Edinburgh and London.

Ross, R. and Glomset, J. A. (1976). Pathogenesis of atherosclerosis. *New England Journal of Medicine* **295**, 369.

Sixma, J. J. (1987). Role of blood vessels, plasma proteins and vessel wall in haemostasis. In *Haemostasis and thrombosis* (ed. A. L. Bloom and D. P. Thomas), p. 283. Churchill Livingstone, Edinburgh and London.

Virchow, R. (1866). *Cellular pathology*. John Churchill, London.

Wall, R. T. and Harker, L. A. (1980). Endothelium and thrombosis. *Annual Review of Medicine* **31**, 361.

Wessler, S. and Yiu, E. T. (1969). On the mechanism of thrombosis. *Progress in Haematology* **6**, 201.

Woolf, N. (1987). Thrombosis and atherosclerosis. In *Haemostasis and thrombosis* (ed. A. L. Bloom and D. P. Thomas), p. 651. Churchill Livingstone, Edinburgh and London.

Venous thrombosis

Sevitt, S. (1974). The structure and growth of valve pocket thrombi in femoral veins. *Journal of Clinical Pathology* **27**, 517.

Sixma, J. J. (1980). The thrombotic state. *British Journal of Haematology* **46**, 515.

Thomas, D. P. (1987). The pathogenesis of venous thrombosis. In *Haemostasis and thrombosis* (ed. A. L. Bloom and D. P. Thomas), p. 767. Churchill Livingstone, Edinburgh and London.

Wessler, S. (1962). Thrombosis in the presence of vascular studies. *American Journal of Medicine* **33**, 648.

7.3.7 Disseminated intravascular coagulation

J. S. Wainscoat

Disseminated intravascular coagulation (DIC) is a syndrome characterized by the activation of coagulation within the vascular system, resulting in a deposition of fibrin in small blood vessels and a consumption of coagulation factors and platelets. Many alternative terms have been used to describe this syndrome, including defibrination syndrome, consumption coagulopathy, and acquired hypofibrinogenaemia. Many cases of DIC result from tissue injury which causes the release of tissue factors into the circulation and activation of the extrinsic pathway, a good example is abruptio placentae in which placental tissue factors are released (Fig. 7.25). In addition to direct tissue injury by trauma there are several other causes of tissue-factor release, including dehydration, hypoxia, acidosis, and burns. DIC is often found in association with Gram-negative septicaemias and is caused, at least in part, by injury to the endothelium, exposure of the subendothelial collagen, and subsequent

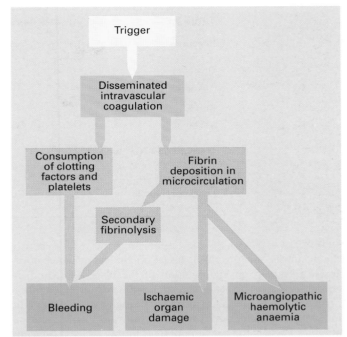

Fig. 7.25 Pathophysiology of disseminated intravascular coagulation.

activation of factor XII. The thrombin which is generated in DIC cleaves fibrinogen to fibrin, resulting in the formation of microthrombi, which are sieved off by the microvasculature of the organs through which they pass, giving rise to ischaemic organ damage. In addition, the thin fibrin strands that traverse the lumens of small vessels may cause mechanical damage to red cells, giving rise to a microangiopathic haemolytic anaemia.

Although DIC has been classified sometimes according to the mechanism of the activation of coagulation, in most clinical situations there are probably multiple precipitating factors. For example, in meningococcal disease, endothelial cell damage results in factor XII activation of the intrinsic system and endotoxin releases activators from leucocytes.

Clinical presentation

The best-known presentation of DIC is an acute bleeding tendency with incoagulable blood. Easy bruising and oozing from venepuncture sites may be followed rapidly by more significant bleeding from the gastrointestinal tract or into the central nervous system. Although bleeding is often the most dramatic clinical picture, there may also be severe organ dysfunction resulting from the generation of microvascular thrombi. Occasionally cases of low-grade DIC may be encountered; characteristically these are seen in association with mucin-secreting tumours. It seems that some tumour products are able to activate factor X directly. Table 7.3 lists some conditions that may be associated with DIC; it is inevitably incomplete since any condition with tissue injury may be complicated by DIC.

Table 7.3 Conditions which may be associated with DIC

Infections	Septicaemia
	Falciparum malaria
Obstetric	Amniotic fluid embolism
	Abruptio placentae
	Intrauterine death
Shock	
Malignancy	Disseminated cancer
	Leukaemia (in particular acute promyelocytic)
Mismatched ABO blood transfusion	
Snake bite	
Local consumption	Giant haemangioma
	Aortic aneurysm

Diagnosis

The diagnosis of acute DIC is based on clinical evidence of excessive bleeding, on examination of the blood film, and on laboratory tests. The blood film often shows distorted and fragmented red cells characteristic of microangiopathic haemolytic anaemia. The platelet count is almost always low and coagulation tests reflect the consumption of clotting factors. Typically the prothrombin time, partial thromboplastin time, and thrombin time are all prolonged. The fibrinogen concentration is not necessarily low since DIC may occur in a setting where the fibrinogen levels were previously high. In contrast, fibrinogen may be low in liver disease owing to decreased synthesis. Although levels of fibrin(ogen) degradation products (FDPs) are usually raised, such levels are not necessarily indicative of DIC. The widely available laboratory tests do not differentiate between degradation products of fibrin and fibrinogen; FDP levels are elevated in fibrinogenolysis unaccompanied by DIC. FDPs may also be spuriously elevated in inflammatory conditions.

The detection of fibrin monomer is a potentially important test in DIC because the monomer is produced from fibrinogen solely by the specific action of thrombin. One such test detects fibrinopeptide A, which is cleaved from fibrinogen when fibrin monomer is formed. However, the test is time consuming, expensive, and may be too sensitive for routine clinical application. Another recently introduced test detects the presence of a cross-linked fibrin degradation product, the D-dimer; its value in clinical practice remains to be determined.

Treatment

The treatment of DIC is first and foremost that of the underlying condition. In addition, fresh frozen plasma is used to correct the haemostatic defect, and platelet transfusions given when there is severe thrombocytopenia. There has been much controversy in relation to the treatment of DIC with heparin. However, there is no good evidence that heparin is beneficial in acute DIC and, indeed, may be very dangerous in patients already suffering from excessive bleeding. Occasionally heparin may prove useful in chronic DIC where the clinical picture is dominated by thrombosis rather than bleeding. The mortality of DIC is dependent on the underlying disorder; in shock and infection it may be as high as 90 per cent.

Pathology

The pathological diagnosis of DIC is based on the presence of fibrin thrombi in arterioles, capillaries, and venules, although there is no agreed definition as to the number of fibrin microthrombi which need to be observed before a diagnosis of DIC can be made. Very careful microscopic examination is necessary for the diagnosis since there is variation both between organs and within organs in relation to the presence of microthrombi. The organs frequently involved in DIC are brain, heart, lungs, and kidney.

In terms of clinicopathology, the cases may be divided into three groups:

1. clinical diagnosis of DIC with post-mortem examination showing characteristic intravascular thrombi;
2. clinical diagnosis of DIC with no evidence of thrombi on pathological examination;
3. patients not suspected as having DIC, but post-mortem examination demonstrating intravascular thrombi.

In Kims's study of 768 autopsies (Kim *et al.* 1976) there were three cases in group (1), nine cases in group (2), and 21 cases in group (3). In another study, Tanaka and Imamura reported 109 cases where DIC had already been diagnosed on clinical and laboratory grounds and found no evidence of microthrombi in 67 of them. These findings demonstrate the spectrum of DIC, from cases with a dramatic clinical picture of bleeding with no postmortem evidence of thrombi to cases with no clinical evidence suggestive of either bleeding or thrombosis but nevertheless with undoubted postmortem findings of widespread microthrombi. The rapid fibrinolysis which accompanies DIC may partly explain the poor correlation between clinical and pathological findings.

7.3.8 Further reading

Kim, H.-S., Suzuki, M., Lie, M. D., and Titus, J. L. (1976). Clinically unsuspected DIC—an autopsy survey. *American Journal of Clinical Pathology* **66**, 31.

Preston, F. E. (1982). Disseminated intravascular coagulation. *British Journal of Hospital Medicine* **28**, 129.

Tanaka, K. and Imamura, T. (1983). Incidence and clinicopathological significance of DIC in autopsy cases. In *Fibrogen degradation products* (ed. M. Vernstraete, J. Vermylen, and M. Donati), pp. 72–92. Munksgaard, Copenhagen.

Wilde, J. T., Roberts, K. M., Greaves, M., and Preston, F. E. (1988). Association between necropsy evidence of disseminated intravascular coagulation and coagulation variables before death in patients in intensive care units. *Journal of Clinical Pathology* **41**, 138.

7.4 Embolism

N. Woolf

An *embolus* is an abnormal mass of material, either solid or gaseous, which is transported in the bloodstream from one part of the circulation to another and which finally *impacts* in the lumen of vessels which are of too small a calibre to allow the embolus to pass.

Emboli may consist of:

- thrombus,
- mixed thrombus and blood clot,
- air,
- nitrogen,
- fat,
- small pieces of bone marrow,
- debris from the base of atherosclerotic plaques,
- groups of tumour cells (embolization constitutes an important means of tumour spread).

7.4.1 Origin of emboli

Roughly 99 per cent of emboli are derived from thrombus or from thrombus mixed with blood clot such as is found in the veins of the lower limb or, more rarely, in large pelvic veins. Amongst women, pregnancy and the taking of oral contraceptives constitute additional risk factors, and several cases of fatal pulmonary embolism have been reported in young women 'on the pill' who were thought to be in perfect health. The risk of this occuring appears to be enhanced by cigarette smoking.

The frequency with which venous thrombi in the lower limbs amongst patients with clinical evidence of embolism can be found at necropsy has been reported as being between 80 and 100 per cent although the clinical diagnosis of such thrombosis is established in only about 50 per cent of the cases.

When the origin of the embolus is a venous thrombus the end result, except in those very rare instances where the embolus passes through a septal defect to the left side of the heart, must be impaction in the pulmonary arterial tree. This is one of the commonest forms of embolization in man and also one of the most dangerous. Some 600 000 cases of pulmonary embolization occur each year in the United States and the number of patients reported as dying there in these circumstances ranges from 20 000 to 50 000 annually. In unselected necropsies, pulmonary emboli can be identified with the naked eye in about 10 per cent of cases. If the necropsy sample is a more selected one (patients who have had orthopaedic operations on the lower limb, or patients with severe burns or fractures), the frequency with which emboli can be identified rises steeply. The pathophysiological effects of pulmonary embolization depend on the interaction between two factors. These are:

1. the size of the embolus and hence the degree of mechanical obstruction that it causes;

2. the presence or absence of congestion in the pulmonary circulation at the time of impaction.

7.4.2 Pulmonary embolism

Massive pulmonary embolism

The logical correlate of massive pulmonary embolization is that the embolus has been derived from the thrombus *occluding a long segment of the venous drainage of the lower limb* (Figs 7.26, 7.27). In effect this means that the thrombotic process has involved the ilio-femoral part of the venous system. Even then it must be remembered that the calibre of the main pulmonary arteries exceeds that of the iliac or femoral veins, and in order for blocking of one of the major pulmonary vessels to occur, the length of mixed thrombus and clot must be loosely bundled together to form a mass of the appropriate dimensions. Massive pulmonary embolism usually presents with extreme suddenness. Often the symptoms appear when the patient is straining, as for example at stool. The affected patients may die suddenly or complain of chest pain, and experience shortness of breath.

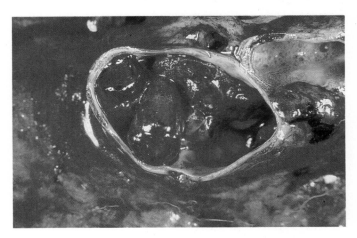

Fig. 7.26 This photograph shows a coiled-up embolus, derived from the ileal femoral veins, that has completely occluded one of the many pulmonary arteries.

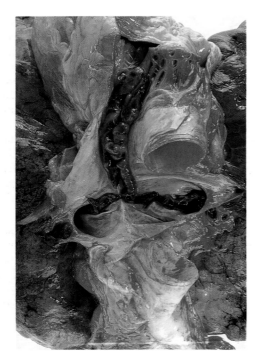

Fig. 7.27 This shows a 'saddle embolus' blocking both main pulmonary arteries.

The signs of circulatory collapse are usually present. It is humiliating to have to confess that the mechanisms involved in the production of the dramatic clinical picture are still not well understood. The factors that may be involved obviously include mechanical obstruction, and if more than 50 per cent of the pulmonary vascular bed is deprived of its blood supply then acute cor pulmonale and sudden death is the likely outcome. However, mechanical obstruction *per se* is unlikely to be the sole cause of this catastrophic syndrome, since it is possible to occlude one major pulmonary artery with an inflatable balloon in conscious normal subjects without producing any distress. While an embolus of this size would produce catastrophic effects, these subjects show no change in metabolic rate, total cardiac output, systemic arterial and left atrial blood pressures and heart rate. The ligation of the main pulmonary artery in the course of surgical resection of the lung for cancer is also without any obvious circulatory consequences. It is likely, therefore, that reflex neural and humoral mechanisms, such as those listed below, may play a part in the syndrome of massive pulmonary embolism.

Explanations that have been canvassed are:

1. a vagal reflex inducing spasm of the coronary and pulmonary arteries;
2. a reflex that produces marked peripheral vasodilatation;
3. a reflex producing cardiac arrest;
4. a massive release of platelet-derived thromboxane, which can provoke vasospasm in the pulmonary vasculature.

Support for the concept that humoral factors contribute to the haemodynamic and respiratory changes seen in massive pulmonary embolism comes from cross-circulation experiments in sheep. Pulmonary embolism induced in one animal simultaneously induced a rise in pulmonary artery pressure and a fall in lung compliance in both. Injection of barium sulphate, collagen, or thrombin into the pulmonary circulation of animals results, in addition to an increase in pulmonary vascular resistance, in constriction of the alveolar ducts and terminal bronchioles, with a marked decrease in lung compliance. It has been suggested that these compounds exert their effect through the medium of platelet activation, with a consequent release of both vaso-active and bronchiolar-constricting molecules.

Small pulmonary emboli

Small emboli are usually clinically 'silent' and are often multiple. Retraction of the thrombotic material from the wall of the vessel in which they are impacted frequently takes place, and the combination of such retraction with the organization described in Section 7.3.5 may leave small fibrous tissue cords, criss-crossing the lumen of the affected vessel in a web- or band-like fashion, as the only marker of the embolic episodes. In other cases the emboli retract so much that the thrombotic mass becomes packed down on to the vessel wall in the same way as occurs with a mural thrombus. These emboli then become covered by new endothelium and are incorporated into the vessel wall, this process of incorporation being accompanied by the proliferation of smooth muscle cells and the formation of a thicker than normal intimal layer. If this sequence of events is repeated many times, the increased thickness of the intima in the pulmonary arterial bed leads to a decrease in the compliance of the vessels, and ultimately to a rise in pulmonary artery pressure (pulmonary hypertension). In a few cases this may be of such magnitude as to result in a pulmonary artery pressure exceeding that in the systemic vascular bed, which can lead to reversal of 'left to right' shunts and thus to the appearance of central cyanosis.

Emboli of moderate size

Under certain circumstances, pulmonary emboli of moderate size (i.e. large enough to block secondary or tertiary branches of the pulmonary arteries) may reduce the perfusion of a segment of lung tissue sufficiently to produce a localized area of necrosis. Such areas of necrosis secondary to ischaemia are known as infarcts and occur in less than 10 per cent of cases of pulmonary embolism in humans. The lung infarcts less readily than many other tissues and this relative protection is due to its double blood supply. This was first shown by Virchow who found, in the course of some animal experiments, that ligation of the pulmonary artery on one side failed to produce any necrosis of lung tissue provided that the bronchial arteries (derived from the aorta) were normal. Experimental pulmonary artery ligation is followed by dilatation of the bronchial arteries and a very large increase in the flow of blood through these vessels. Indeed, left ventricular hypertrophy developed as a result of the increase in output from the left side of the heart. Pulmonary infarction is considered further in Section 7.5.

7.4.3 Systemic embolism

Most thrombotic, systemic emboli are derived from the left side of the heart. The thrombi may arise in the atrial appendages (this being particularly likely to occur in patients with dilated atria and/or those suffering from the arrhythmia—atrial fibrillation). Intraventricular thrombi may occur as a consequence of transmural myocardial infarction or in congestive cardio-myopathy, a muscle disorder in which the myocardium is flabby and the ventricles are dilated. There is a marked decrease in the systolic ejection fraction and thus a volume overload on the ventricular muscle. In life, the presence of these thrombi can be detected by echocardiography. Thrombi affecting the heart valves, of a size sufficient to give rise to significant emboli, are usually related to the presence of *infective endocarditis*, a disorder produced by the combination of haemodynamically induced endocardial injury and bacteraemia. The infected thrombi or *vegetations* as they are often called, may be bulky and friable. Portions of the vegetations can break off readily and travel in the systemic arterial circulation until they impact. This may, of course, occur in a very large number of situations but the brain, lower limbs, spleen, and kidneys are favoured sites. When an infected thrombus impacts, it may set up a localized inflammatory reaction leading to partial destruction of the wall of the vessel in which impaction has taken place. This leads to a dilatation of the affected arterial segment and rupture followed by haemorrhage may occur. Such a lesion is spoken of as being a *mycotic aneurysm*, a misleading term since fungi have nothing to do with the pathogenesis (*mycos*: mushroom).

Small *platelet thrombi* occur quite commonly in relation to atherosclerotic plaques at the point in the neck where the common carotid artery divides. Emboli derived from these platelet masses lodge in the cerebral circulation, often in small vessels, where they may give rise to permanent or transient neurological deficiencies.

Gaseous emboli

Air may be introduced into the systemic circulation under a number of circumstances. These include:

1. operations on the head and neck where a large vein is opened inadvertently;
2. mismanagement of blood transfusions where positive pressure is being used to speed up the flow of blood;
3. during haemodialysis for renal failure;
4. following on insufflation of air into the fallopian tubes in the course of investigation of sterility;
5. interference with the placental site during criminal abortion.

The air enters the right side of the heart where, in the right ventricle, it is whipped up into a frothy mass. It is this mass that can block the flow of blood through the pulmonary arteries, and the clinical picture that develops closely mimics that of massive pulmonary embolization by thrombus derived from the leg veins. In some cases the froth may gain access to the systemic arterial circulation and impact there. The most frequent site for this is the brain and cases have been reported also of embolization of vessels supplying the spinal cord. As little as 40 ml of air can have serious clinical results and 100 ml can be fatal, though there have been rare cases in which 200 ml have been tolerated. If air embolism is suspected as the cause of death, it is necessary to have the heart and pulmonary arteries under water, when they are opened, in order to detect the escape of the air bubbles from the blocked vessels.

Nitrogen embolization occurs in decompression sickness, also known as 'caisson disease'. It is found in persons whose occupation causes them to work at very high pressures and who may then be returned too quickly to normal atmospheric pressure (deep-sea divers, tunnellers, etc.).

At high pressures, inert gases, of which nitrogen is the most important, are dissolved in the plasma and in interstitial tissue, especially in adipose tissue. If the persons at risk return too quickly to normal atmospheric pressure, the gas comes out of solution and small bubbles are formed within the interstitial tissues and blood, platelets being often associated with gas bubbles in the latter situation. These bubbles may coalesce to form quite large masses and the clinical features are produced either by emboli in the circulating blood or by the presence of bubbles in the interstitial tissues, especially in relation to tendons, joints, and ligaments. When this happens the patients complain of excruciating pain (the syndrome being known as 'the bends'). The central nervous system may be affected and the sudden onset of respiratory distress has also been described. The symptoms may be relieved by placing the patient in a compression chamber and forcing the gases back into solution. Once this has been done, slow and careful decompression should avoid a recurrence. Occasionally the presence of nitrogen emboli in the systemic circulation is followed by ischaemic damage to the ends of long bones, this being associated with secondary damage to the articular cartilages and joints.

Fat embolism

Fat embolism is relatively common under certain circumstances but significant clinical consequences are, happily, quite rare. It has been most frequently associated with fractures of long bones, with severe burns, and with severe and extensive soft tissue trauma, but may also be found in patients with hyperlipidaemias and following ischaemic bone-marrow necrosis in patients with sickle-cell disease. The fact that the syndrome can occur in the absence of trauma suggests a multifactorial pathogenesis. In patients with fractures, especially multiple fractures, fat globules are thought to enter veins at the fracture site that are torn at the time of injury. These globules are then carried in the systemic venous circulation to the lungs where they may impact in small vessels and cause the sudden onset of respiratory distress some 24–72 hours following injury. In such patients it may be possible to identify droplets of fat in the sputum by staining sputum smears with fat-soluble dyes, such as Oil Red O. Despite the fact that the fat is said to enter the venous circulation, some patients present with predominant involvement of the central nervous system. They may become agitated at first and then lapse into coma; a high proportion of such patients die. At autopsy, if they have survived the onset of unconsciousness for a day or two, the brain shows oedema and *very many tiny haemorrhages*. These occur both in the grey and white matter but are more easily seen in the latter site. Frozen sections of brain stained with fat-soluble dyes show the presence of fat globules within the lumena of cerebral capillaries.

As mentioned above, fat emboli occur more frequently than does the *fat embolization syndrome*. When autopsies were carried out on Korean war battle casualties dying within four weeks of having been injured, evidence of fat embolization was found in the tissues in 90 per cent of cases. However, in only 1 per cent could any part of the clinical picture in these patients be attributed to the fat emboli.

The *pathogenesis* of fat embolism is a more complex matter than was previously thought. While one could accept the old simple hypothesis that it was due to the entry of fat into traumatized veins in patients with multiple fractures, this cannot account for the cases that occur in the absence of trauma. Other mechanisms that have been suggested include the possibility that under certain circumstances, particularly where there is a rise in endogenous catecholamine levels, chylomicrons much larger than usual are formed and that this arises from some instability of the normal emulsion represented by chylomicrons and plasma.

Bone-marrow emboli

Bone-marrow emboli are found, not infrequently, on histological examination of post-mortem samples of lung tissue from patients who have had episodes of cardiac arrest due to ventricular fibrillation, and in whom the attempts at resuscitation have included external cardiac massage. In middle-aged and elderly people, in whom the costal cartilages have long since become ossified, repeated pressure on the rib cage usually results in the fracture of several ribs and it is from these sites that the bone marrow is squeezed into the veins. What the clinical effects, if any, of such emboli are is simply unknown (Fig. 7.28).

Emboli derived from atheromatous debris

Atheromatous emboli obviously occur only in the systemic arterial tree and are derived from plaques that ulcerate and in which there is a massive basally situated pool of lipid and tissue debris, as described in Chapter 12. The emboli are usually found incidentally on histological examination of tissue and can be easily recognized since they consist of a mixture of thrombotic material and lipid-rich debris in which highly characteristic, cigar- or torpedo-shaped cholesterol crystals are present. While

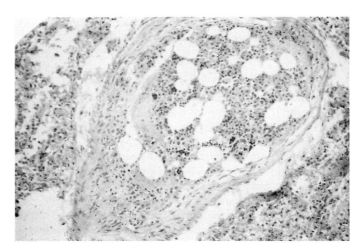

Fig. 7.28 This shows a small vessel in the lung occluded by a bone marrow embolus in which fatty spaces and haemopoietic cells can be seen.

for the most part such emboli, probably because they are usually small, do not cause significant damage in the tissues supplied by the vessels in which they have become impacted, they may occasionally be associated with ischaemic damage.

7.4.4 Further reading

Becker, D. M. (1986). Venous thrombi and embolism. Epidemiology, diagnosis and prevention. *Journal of General Internal Medicine* 1, 402.

Heath, D. and Smith, P. (1988). Disorders of the vascular system. In *The pathology of the lung* (ed. W. M. Thurlbeck), p. 687. Tiemer Medical Publishers Inc., Stuttgart and New York.

Kakkar, W. and Sasahara, A. A. (1987). Diagnosis of venous thrombosis and femoral embolism. In *Haemostasis and thrombosis* (ed. A. L. Bloom and D. P. Thomas), p. 779. Churchill Livingstone, Edinburgh and London.

7.5 Ischaemia and infarction

N. Woolf

Ischaemia may be defined as *the state existing when an organ or tissue has its perfusion lowered relative to its metabolic needs*. This definition is often broadened to include the functional changes that are produced by such a diminution of perfusion. An *infarct* is a *morphological* entity: a large, localized area of tissue necrosis that is brought about by *ischaemia*, although it must be realized that there is a wide range of structural changes short of infarction that can be brought about by ischaemia.

Ischaemia is most often caused by some local interference with the perfusion of the organ or tissue concerned. On some occasions, however, the ischaemic state may be generalized. This occurs only rarely and is associated with a fall in cardiac output. While acute reductions in cardiac output are by no means uncommon, they are not often expressed in the form of ischaemic changes in individual tissues. Rarely, gangrene of the extremities may be seen following either extensive myocardial infarction or the sudden onset of ventricular arrhythmia, both of which may be associated with a severe drop in cardiac output. Disorders of cardiac rhythm, including pathological changes in the conducting system, are not uncommon causes of cerebral ischaemia. An obvious and important example of this is *complete heart block* in which sudden periods of unconsciousness (Stokes–Adams attacks) occur. If adequate perfusion of the brain is not restored within 3–4 minutes, irreparable damage to the neurones occurs.

7.5.1　Local causes of ischaemia

The most important of the pathological bases of ischaemia have been described in the foregoing sections dealing with atherosclerosis, thrombosis, and embolism; and the arteritides, immune and non-immune, leading to luminal blockage have also been considered separately. In addition, arterial perfusion may be interfered with by spasm of the smooth muscle in the vessel wall or by pressure on the vessel from without. However, it is worth remembering that interruption of arterial blood flow is not the only way in which ischaemia may be produced; pathological changes affecting veins and capillaries can also lead to underperfusion of tissues.

7.5.2　Ischaemia caused by venous obstruction

The pathogenesis of *ischaemia due to venous occlusion* starts with blockage of local venous outflow, which leads to a rise in the hydrostatic pressure of the capillary bed drained by the blocked vein or veins. This, in turn, leads to transudation of fluid from the vascular to the extravascular compartment and a consequent increase in tissue tension within the extravascular compartment. This may be of such a degree as to impair the local arterial inflow and thus lead to ischaemia. It is clear that ischaemia on such a basis is likely to occur only in certain anatomical situations, where it may not be possible for the blood to bypass the obstruction via collateral drainage channels, and that, because of the local interuption to venous return, the affected tissues are likely to be *intensely congested and, possibly, even haemorrhagic*. The circumstances under which such *venous infarction* is likely to occur include:

1. extensive mesenteric venous thrombosis leading to infarction of the small intestine;

2. so-called strangulation of herniae, where entrapment of segments of bowel wall occurs, leading to oedema and pressure on the draining veins;

3. cavernous sinus thrombosis, which may lead in turn to thrombosis of the retinal vein and, ultimately, to blindness;

4. thrombosis of the superior longitudinal sinus within the dura—this can occur in children, severely dehydrated as a result of gastroenteritis, and leads to patchy haemorrhagic necrosis in the cerebral cortex;

5. a very rare variant of thrombosis in the ilio-femoral system, which may be followed by gangrenous changes in the lower limb.

7.5.3　Ischaemia caused by pathological changes in capillaries

Ischaemia due to capillary obstruction can occur as a consequence of physical damage to the capillaries, as in 'frostbite'. Rarely, capillaries may be occluded by parasites, as in cerebral malaria; by abnormal red cells, in sickle-cell disease or in certain auto-immune haemolytic anaemias; by fibrin, where disseminated intravascular coagulation has occurred; by antigen–antibody complexes; by fat or gas emboli, and by external pressure, as seen in 'bed sores'.

7.5.4　Ischaemia caused by arterial obstruction

Obstruction of arterial inflow may be followed by a spectrum of functional and/or structural events, which range from no detectable effect to extensive tissue necrosis. If neither functional nor structural changes can be observed, we can infer that the collateral arterial supply to the target area is good and that no significant reduction in perfusion has occurred.

Functional disturbances are usually noted when the collateral supply is only good enough to maintain adequate perfusion so long as the metabolic demands of the tissue are at a basal level. If these demands are increased, as for example in the heart or the muscle of the lower limb during exercise, then a state of ischaemia will be produced and the patient will experience either substernal pain (*angina pectoris*) or a cramp-like pain in the calf (*intermittent claudication*). Cessation of activity leads, in most instances, to disappearance of the pain.

The significant changes in the function of an organ or tissue that has been rendered ischaemic may result either from loss of cells or from abnormal or deficient behaviour on the part of surviving cells. In ischaemic myocardium there is a marked tendency for electrical disturbances to occur and these frequently give rise to fatal arrhythmias, such as ventricular fibrillation. Indeed, at least half the patients who die in the course of their first clinically apparent episode of myocardial ischaemia, die in this way. Similarly, the presence of ischaemic sensory nerve bundles may lead to qualitative abnormalities in the sensory patterns interpreted within the central nervous system, and it has been suggested that this mechanism may underlie the phenomenon of persistent pain sometimes seen in patients with limb ischaemia.

If the degree of ischaemia is greater than that described above, then structural damage to cells and tissues will occur. This may take the form, on the one hand, of patchy loss of parenchymal cells, such as is seen in the myocardium of patients with a long history of angina pectoris or, on the other, of massive necrosis. In either event, if the patient survives the ischaemic episode, the lost tissue is replaced, except in the case of the brain, by fibrous tissue in a manner identical with that described in Section 5.3. The degree of post-ischaemic necrosis is proportional to the degree of ischaemia, which, in turn, depends on the balance between the needs of an individual tissue and the degree to which arterial perfusion is compromised. When the ischaemia is slow in onset and chronic in nature the characteristic feature is the tendency for cell death to affect either individual cells or small groups of cells. Initially these may show the changes of intracellular oedema or fatty change but eventually they die and, for instance in the heart where no regeneration of muscle cells can take place, they are replaced by small foci of fibrous tissue. Such chronic myocardial ischaemia gives the heart muscle a curious flecked appearance because of the 'drop out' of small numbers of cells and their replacement by collagen fibres. In chronic lower limb ischaemia, the dermal papillae of the skin become flattened and both the epidermis and the dermis are thinned. Skin appendages, such as hair follicles, sweat glands, and sebaceous glands may also become atrophic and eventually disappear and, as a result of these changes, the skin appears shiny, hairless, and dry.

The degree of ischaemia is determined by a number of interacting variables. These include:

1. the metabolic needs of the underperfused tissue;
2. the speed of onset of arterial occlusion;
3. the completeness or otherwise of the arterial blocking;
4. the anatomy of the local blood supply;
5. the state of patency of the collateral blood supply.

Metabolic needs of the underperfused tissue

Tissues vary in their capacity to withstand a reduction in their arterial perfusion. The brain is the most sensitive in this respect, and deprivation of oxygen for more than 3–4 minutes will cause irreversible damage to the nerve cells. The myocardium, too, is very susceptible to damage following underperfusion. It is doubly unfortunate that both brain and heart should have, on the whole, rather poor collateral blood supplies and that neither heart muscle cells nor neurones are able to regenerate.

The speed of onset of underperfusion

If arterial occlusion takes place very rapidly as, for example, when an atherosclerotic coronary artery plaque ruptures, the effects of this are more severe than with slow narrowing of the same segment of artery, since there is little or no time for collateral vessels to open.

Completeness of the arterial blocking

Other things being equal, complete occlusion of an arterial lumen causes more extensive damage to the affected area than does severe stenosis. It must be equally obvious that the more proximally the occlusion is situated in a given arterial tree, the greater will be the area of tissue affected by ischaemia.

The anatomy of the local blood supply

Some organs or tissues have no collateral blood supply and the arteries that perfuse such parts are known as *end arteries*. The retina is an example of such a tissue. It is supplied by a single vessel, the central retinal artery, which only branches once it has reached the retina. If occlusion of the central retinal artery occurs and is not rapidly relieved, irreparable ischaemic damage will be produced within the retina. The smaller arteries within the cerebral cortex also function as end arteries. In contrast, some tissues, such as the lung, have a *double* arterial supply. Occlusion of one part of this blood supply need not lead to necrosis of the underperfused area since the supply from the other may be sufficient to maintain tissue viability.

Patency of the collateral blood supply

A good collateral supply, in the anatomical sense, can only compensate for blockage in the main arterial tree if the collateral vessels themselves are neither stenosed by atherosclerotic plaques nor in spasm.

7.5.5 General pathology of infarction

An infarct can be defined as a fairly large area of tissue necrosis (usually coagulative in type) that results from ischaemia. Blood may seep into the ischaemic area for some time, partly as a result of back flow from venules and escape of blood through the walls of vessels in the local microcirculation that have been damaged in the course of the ischaemic process. Thus many infarcts contain a good deal of blood in the early stages of their natural history. In spongy tissue such as the lung, the escape of red blood cells and fibrin is a conspicuous feature and the ischaemic lung tissue becomes firmer than normal. At necropsy, infarcts of this type can be appreciated as wedge-shaped lumps on the pleural aspect of the lung and, even when the lung is cut into, the infarcted area tends to bulge and to stand proud of the surrounding normal lung. This outpouring or 'stuffing' of blood into the devitalized areas is merely an epiphenomenon and not the core event in infarction. Failure of pathologists to appreciate this led to the introduction of the archaic and essentially unhelpful term *infarct* which is derived from the latin verb *infarcire*—to stuff.

With the passage of time the dying cells often swell. This tends to squeeze blood out of the interstitial tissue in the infarcted area and the infarct becomes much paler. In the heart, for example it takes 24–36 hours for this process to become complete. The pallor is a most useful marker for the macroscopic diagnosis of infarction at necropsy (Figs 7.29, 7.30). However, because this pallor takes a considerable time to develop, it may be difficult to make such a necropsy diagnosis in the early stages of the natural history of a myocardial infarct. The application of enzyme histochemical methods to this problem can be of great assistance in arriving at an accurate diagnosis on macroscopic examination of the heart (see p. 528), but even these techniques fail to identify necrotic muscle tissue unless the patient has survived for 6–9 hours after the cutting

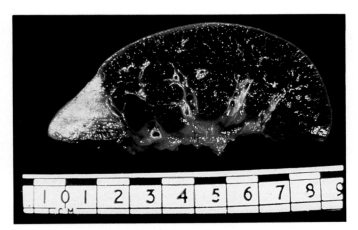

Fig. 7.29 This shows a large pale area of coagulative necrosis in the spleen, the result of systemic embolism in a patient with endocarditis. (Courtesy of Professor M. J. Davies, St George's Hospital Medical School, London.)

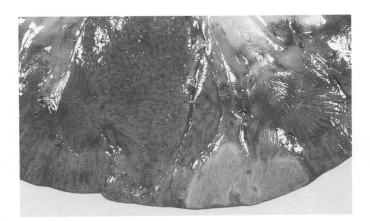

Fig. 7.30 This shows a pale wedge-shaped infarct, the result of systemic embolization in the kidney.

off of the blood supply to an area of the myocardium. The division of infarcts into 'pale' and 'red' varieties is pointless. Many infarcts start off as red and become pale as the blood is squeezed out of the infarcted area by swelling of the dying cells. Cerebral infarcts are usually pale *ab initio* (unless they are embolic in origin) and infarcts in the spongy lung tissue remain red and undergo repair while still at that stage.

The dead parenchymal cells in the infarcted area undergo autolysis and the diapedesed red cells haemolyse. At the same time a brisk inflammatory reaction occurs at the margins of the infarct and first neutrophils and then macrophages infiltrate the necrotic tissue. Breakdown products of haemoglobin, haematoidin (bile pigment), and haemosiderin (aggregated molecules of ferritin) may be seen in relation to the infarcted area and are ingested by macrophages. At this stage, usually about one week after the cutting off of the arterial supply, an infarct in a solid organ is usually firm in consistency and a dull yellow in colour, with a red zone of hyperaemia at the margins.

The presence of large numbers of macrophages corresponds with what is seen in the *demolition* phase in the case of an inflammatory reaction, and is of equal importance in the context of infarction. In some tissues, for example the *heart*, dead parenchymal cells are removed rapidly and there is an equally rapid replacement of these cells, first by granulation tissue and then by scar tissue. In other situations, such as the *kidney*, the infarcted area persists, sometimes for months, before being replaced by scar tissue. Histological examination of such an area shows the 'ghost outlines' of the architectural elements of the tissue, the tubules and glomeruli, although the constituent parenchymal cells are clearly dead. A slow but progressive ingrowth of connective tissue occurs even in these cases and, eventually, the infarct becomes converted to a fibrous scar in which some calcium salts may be deposited (dystrophic calcification).

The sequence of events described in the preceding paragraphs may be interrupted, at any time, by the death of the patient.

7.5.6 Ischaemia in specific sites

The central nervous system

The generalizations made above relating to the development of infarcts do not apply to the brain (Fig. 7.31). Here the processes involved, after the rendering of part of the brain ischaemic, are somewhat different. The type of necrosis is typically liquefactive

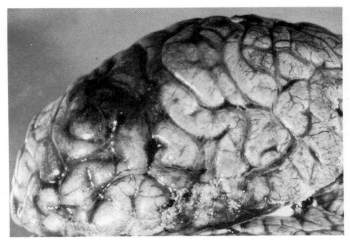

Fig. 7.31 This shows the brain from a patient having died from post-embolic cerebral infarction. Note the haemorrhagic appearances which are strongly suggestive of the lesion's embolic origin.

rather than coagulative and this may, in the long term, lead to the formation of a cavity. Histologically, the early stages of the development of a cerebral infarct are characterized by a transient neutrophil response, which is followed by a period of intense phagocytic activity by the *microglial* cells. These cells, which, in their resting phase, are normally small, cluster in the infarcted area and phagocytose the lipid that is liberated from degenerate myelin. The cytoplasm of the microglia, therefore, increases in bulk very markedly and appears foamy or granular in appearance. (Classically these swollen microglia are referred to as *compound granular corpuscles*.) Reactive astrocytes now gather at the margins of the infarcted area and synthesize new glial fibres which eventually replace part or all of the infarcted tissue.

The heart

Cardiac ischaemia is the single most important cause of death in Western communities. Approximately 150 000 adults in the United Kingdom die every year from ischaemic heart disease (about 25 per cent of all deaths). A decrease in the arterial perfusion of the myocardium may express itself in a number of ways, and it is important to realize that, while all occur against the background of myocardial ischaemia, the different clinical pictures may be brought about by different pathogenetic mechanisms. The patients may:

1. complain of angina on effort;
2. die suddenly;
3. develop acute myocardial necrosis (infarction of different patterns and with different pathogeneses;
4. develop failure of muscle pumping activity.

Angina pectoris

At autopsy on patients dying *with* rather than *from* angina pectoris, the myocardium may show no macroscopic abnormalities. In some instances there will have been ischaemic necrosis of small groups of heart muscle cells, and the marker of this having taken place is the presence of small flecks of fibrous tissue in the muscle wall of the left ventricle. The coronary arteries invariably show the presence of stenosing atherosclerotic lesions, which may affect one or more of the major coronary artery branches.

Sudden death

Sudden death may be defined as death occurring from myocardial ischaemia within one hour of the onset of acute symptoms. In practice many of these deaths occur within a few minutes. Sudden death is a major part of the overall problem of ischaemic heart disease, since at least 50 per cent of the deaths due to a first attack of ischaemia occur in this way, without the patient having the benefit of medical attention. Death is due to the onset of severe ventricular arrhythmias, most notably ventricular fibrillation, these being associated with loss of cardiac output. Of the patients who collapse with such severe arrhythmias and who are resuscitated, only 16 per cent develop a Q wave on electrocardiography (suggestive of myocardial necrosis involving most of the left ventricular wall thickness), and 45 per cent show elevations in the plasma concentrations of enzymes derived from heart muscle. Thus a majority of these living patients show no clinical or biochemical evidence of their arrhythmia being associated with acute myocardial necrosis. Post-mortem examination of patients dying suddenly in this way reveals evidence of acute, though not necessarily occlusive thrombosis in

a majority, though the prevalence of *occlusive* thrombi is lower than in patients dying with myocardial infarction. Narrowing of coronary artery lumena by 80 per cent or more is very frequent in these patients.

Acute myocardial necrosis

Acute myocardial necrosis occurs in two distinct patterns, although, from time to time, a combination of these may be seen. It is useful to be able to distinguish between these patterns since the pathogenesis of each differs considerably. Before being able to distinguish between the *patterns* of acute myocardial necrosis, it is necessary to be able to identify irreversibly damaged heart muscle. If the heart is examined some 18–36 hours after the onset of severe underperfusion there is no problem. The ischaemic heart muscle shows all the features of coagulative necrosis; macroscopically the necrotic area is a dull, yellowish, 'wash-leather'-like colour with a hyperaemic zone at the periphery. However, if the patient dies at an earlier stage of the natural history of myocardial necrosis the recognition of ischaemic damage is much more difficult. So long as the patient has survived for 6–9 hours after the onset of the acute ischaemia, the difficulty can be overcome by using a simple histochemical technique. This depends on the fact that a cell which is irreversibly damaged loses its intracellular content of water-soluble enzymes. The presence of respiratory enzymes, such as succinic dehydrogenase, in normal heart muscle can be shown by immersing a slice of unfixed heart muscle in a solution of the dye nitro-blue-tetrazolium. This is a yellow dye which acts as a hydrogen acceptor. In the presence of a cell with a normal content of dehydrogenase, the yellow dye turns a bluish-purple colour and is deposited on the tissue at the site where the reaction has taken place. Where a cell has been irreversibly damaged and has lost its intracellular dehydrogenases, no such colour reaction takes place and thus viable and non-viable muscle can be distinguished from each other with relative ease.

Regional myocardial infarction

The commonest pattern of acute ischaemic necrosis in the myocardium is so-called regional infarction. This occurs as a large single area of coagulative necrosis, measuring at least 3 cm along one of its axes and usually involving more than 50 per cent of the thickness of the ventricular wall. In more than 90 per cent of cases this pattern of necrosis is associated with occlusive thrombosis in the coronary artery segment supplying the affected area of muscle, and the majority of these thrombi occur in relation to breaks in the connective tissue caps of underlying atherosclerotic plaques.

Subendocardial necrosis

Subendocardial necrosis in its pure form is much less commonly seen at necropsy than regional infarction. Here the ischaemic necrosis is confined to the *inner half* of the left ventricular myocardium, a very thin layer of viable muscle immediately beneath the endocardium always being present. This type of necrosis may be segmental or can extend to involve the whole circumference of the left ventricle. Occlusive thrombi in the coronary arteries are found in only about 15 per cent of cases, though severe stenosing atherosclerosis is widespread within the coronary artery tree.

Subendocardial ischaemic necrosis is the morphological expression of a *generalized lowering* of myocardial perfusion and can occur in the absence of coronary artery disease in such situations as severe aortic stenosis or incompetence. Its pathogenesis can be understood most easily if one recalls two facts. These are that perfusion of the myocardium takes place during *diastole* and that the wall tension in the left ventricular myocardium is greater in the subendocardial zone than in the subepicardial region. In a person with normal coronary arteries, the *perfusion drive* can be represented as the difference between the diastolic pressure in the aortic root and the intracavity pressure in the left ventricle (LV). The total perfusion during any single cardiac cycle is determined by the time during which the *drive* is allowed to act and, hence by the length of diastole. Any circumstance that lessens the pressure difference between aortic root and LV intracavity pressure, or which shortens the diastolic interval, may reduce myocardial perfusion sufficiently to produce ischaemic necrosis.

Complications of myocardial infarction

Each stage of the natural history of myocardial infarction may hold dangers for the patient.

In the early stages the chief danger is the possible development of ventricular fibrillation leading to asystole and sudden death. As the coagulative necrosis develops and the dead muscle elicits a brisk acute inflammatory response, focal softening of necrotic muscle may occur. This can lead to rupture of the left ventricle either of the free wall into the pericardial cavity, death being due to the rapid accumulation of blood within the pericardial sac (*cardiac tamponade*), or of the septum, with the production of a defect in the interventricular septum. Similar softening can affect the papillary muscles and, if rupture of one or more of these occurs, the patient will develop a torrential regurgitant jet through the mitral valve. A somewhat less dramatic development of mitral valve incompetence may occur simply as a result of ischaemic necrosis and scarring of papillary muscles, and this is not uncommonly seen.

The abnormal haemodynamics that can obtain within the left ventricular cavity following infarction may lead to the formation of mural thrombi, and portions of these can break off and embolize the systemic circulation.

Healing of the infarcted muscle can also be associated with circumstances unfavourable to the patient. If there has been extensive loss of cardiac muscle in the process of infarction, correspondingly large amounts of fibrous tissue are formed during healing. This collagenous tissue lacks the power of recoil possessed by muscle and, due to the normal rise of intracavity pressure during ventricular systole, becomes gradually stretched and thinned. This may lead to a local dilatation or *ventricular aneurysm*, which can be a severe haemodynamic disadvantage to the patient. Extensive fibrosis following infarction of the anterior wall of the left ventricle may involve both bundle branches and lead to complete heart block.

The lung

Fewer than 10 per cent of pulmonary emboli cause infarction in the lung, a figure which emphasizes the importance of the state of the pulmonary circulation at the time when embolization occurs. Thus in young people, whose cardiac status is good, infarction is rare, this relative sparing is thought to be due, at least in part, to the double blood supply of the lung from the pulmonary and bronchial arteries.

Any rise in pressure in the pulmonary veins, as occurs in mitral stenosis or left ventricular failure, markedly increases the chances of infarction occurring if medium-sized branches of the pulmonary arteries become occluded. The vast majority of infarcts are due to emboli derived from thrombi in the leg veins; about 10 per cent are, however, derived from thrombi formed in the right side of the heart.

The infarcts are generally described as being wedge-shaped, with the base of the wedge situated towards the pleural aspect of the lung, and, in their early stages, are deep red in colour. At necropsy these infarcts are often more easily felt than seen. A fibrinous pleural reaction over the infarcted area is common and there may, on occasions, be small haemorrhagic effusions in the pleural cavity. Organization of pulmonary infarcts usually proceeds rapidly, perhaps because of the right vascular network in the surrounding lung tissue. The infarcts are converted into inconspicuous scars, which tend to be concealed by the surrounding lung tissue, which often shows compensatory overdistention.

The liver

True infarcts in the liver are rare, presumably because spontaneous occlusion of the hepatic artery is correspondingly rare, and because, like the lung, the liver has a double blood supply. However, accidental ligation of the hepatic artery in the course of surgery may produce true infarcts in the liver, and patchy hepatic infarction may also occur if hepatic artery branches within the liver are involved in immune-complex-mediated diseases, such as polyarteritis nodosa.

The intestine

The commonest cause of intestinal ischaemia are mechanical; hernial strangulation, volvulus (twisting of a segment of intestine), and intussusception. In the latter, excessive peristaltic contraction drives the affected segment of bowel forward so that the segment of bowel immediately distal lies in a sleeve-like manner over it. Some of the mesentery is included in the portion of bowel that is pushed forward, and the resulting local oedema leads to local ischaemia. Apart from such mechanical disasters, intestinal ischaemia can result from thrombotic or embolic occlusion of mesenteric arteries, or even from extensive mesenteric venous thrombosis. In this last instance, the interference with venous drainage leads to a very marked degree of congestion affecting the mucosal and submucosal vessels and the patient may pass fresh blood per rectum

The structural changes seen in ischaemic gut depend, as in other tissues, on the severity of the decrease in perfusion. In the most severe form of ischaemia (most commonly affecting the small intestine) the bowel wall shows *transmural* damage and is spoken of as being infarcted or gangrenous. If the reduction in blood flow has been less severe, then the ischaemic damage is confined either to the *mucosa* or to the *mucosa, submucosa, and the luminal aspect of the muscularis propria.*

Gangrene (transmural infarction)

When the degree of intestinal ischaemia is sufficient to cause infarction, the bowel wall feels stiffer than normal and is a dark plum colour. The serosal surface is the seat of a fibrinous inflammatory response so that instead of the normal shiny appearance of the serosa, it is dull and slightly roughened (Fig. 7.32). The necrotic bowel wall becomes colonized quite rapidly by the saprophytic organisms in the lumen and thus may show the putrefactive features characteristic of true gangrene. Factors that may contribute to the death of such patients include intestinal paralysis (ileus) with loss of fluid and electrolytes into the gut lumen, haemorrhage, perforation, which causes generalized peritonitis, and bacteriaemic shock.

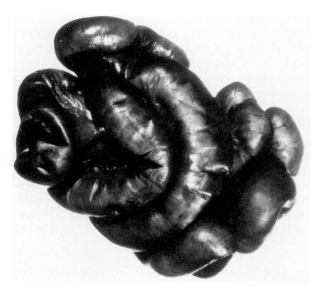

Fig. 7.32 This shows gangrenous bowel from a patient with volvulus. Note the deep discolouration of the bowel wall and rather matt serosal surface, which is due to the presence of a fibrinous exudate.

Mucosal and mural ischaemic damage

Ischaemia of the gut need not lead in all cases to such a dramatic conclusion. It is now well recognized that periods of lowered arterial perfusion, affecting particularly the region of the splenic flexure, may lead to localized mucosal ulceration. These lesions may be patchy and affect more than one segment of the bowel. Ischaemia is frequently associated with reductions in perfusion caused either by falls in the cardiac output, as seen in patients with severe cardiac failure, or by a combination of a decline in cardiac output and vasoconstriction of the splanchnic

vessels supplying the affected segment of gut. The mucosa shows the picture of coagulative necrosis often associated with haemorrhagic changes in both mucosa and submucosa and, in some instances, mimics the appearances seen in pseudomembranous enterocolitis caused by bacterial toxins. Healing of these ulcers is accompanied by a very considerable degree of scar-tissue formation, which may lead to localized narrowing of the gut lumen in the affected areas. During the healing phase these post-ischaemic ulcers show the presence of a broad band of granulation tissue extending into the submucosa, and the granulation tissue contains many macrophages laden with haemosiderin derived from broken-down red blood cells.

7.5.7   Further reading

Crawford, T. (1977). *Pathology of ischaemic heart disease*. Butterworth.

Davies, M. J. (1990). Morphology and natural history of atherosclerotic lesions in human coronary artery tree. In *Atheroma: atherosclerosis and ischaemic heart disease. Part 1: Th mechanisms* (ed. M. J. Davies and N. Woolf). Science Press Ltd.

Davies, M. J., Woolf, N., and Robertson, W. B. (1976). Pathology of acute myocardial infarction with particular reference to occlusive coronary thrombi. *British Heart Journal* **38**, 659.

Fuster, V. Barimol, L. Cohen, M., Ambrose, J. A., Badimon, J. J., and Cheseborough, J. (1988). Insights into the pathogenesis of acute ischaemic syndromes. *Circulation* **77**, 1213.

Reimer, K. A. and Deker, R. E. (1987). Myocardial ischemia and infarction: anatomic and biological substances in ischemic cell death and ventricular arrhythmias. *Human Pathology* **18**, 462.

Woolf, N. and Davies, M. J. (1980). Morphological variants and acute myocardial necrosis and their relationship to coronary artery thrombosis. *Acta Medica Scandinavia* (Suppl.), **642**, 92.

7.6   Oedema

J. D. Firth and J. G. G. Ledingham

Oedema is the term used to describe the swelling of tissues caused by an excess of fluid in the interstitial space. It may be localized, e.g. to a single organ or limb, or generalized. Generalized oedema, the hallmark of extracellular fluid volume expansion, is associated with renal sodium retention, except on rare occasions when it may be due to grossly excessive intake of salt and water, and may be accompanied by the formation of free fluid within the serous cavities (ascites, pleural effusion, pericardial effusion).

An understanding of the pathophysiology of the various processes that can lead to the development of oedema is dependent upon an appreciation of the normal mechanisms of control of extracellular fluid volume, and of the factors that determine the partition of extracellular fluid between the vascular and interstitial compartments. 'Inflammatory oedema', secondary to a local response to acute injury, will not be considered in this section (see Chapter 5).

7.6.1 Control of extracellular fluid volume

Extracellular fluid constitutes roughly 20 per cent of body weight; comprising interstitial fluid (16 per cent) and blood plasma (4 per cent). These values are normally maintained within narrow limits despite day-to-day variations (sometimes huge) in the dietary intake of salt and water. The physiological mechanisms that permit the regulation comprise:

1. sensors that detect changes in extracellular fluid volume relative to the capacitance of the vascular and interstitial compartments;
2. mechanisms—central, renal, or cardiac—capable of integrating the sensory inputs and modulating effector mechanisms; and
3. effector mechanisms that ultimately adjust the rate of renal sodium excretion to return the extracellular fluid volume towards a preset level.

This model should not be taken to imply that the capacitance of the vascular and interstitial compartments is fixed and that the control of extracellular fluid volume consists solely of means whereby the body maintains a constant fluid volume in a rigid system; the capacitance of the vascular and interstitial compartments are themselves modulated to an important degree by neural and humoral influences.

Afferent input: sensors of extracellular fluid volume

Volume detectors reside at several sites within the vascular bed and can be regarded as monitoring a particular characteristic of overall circulatory function, e.g. cardiac filling, renal perfusion. Table 7.4 lists the main receptor types, the stimuli to which each receptor responds, and the afferent pathways involved. Further information can be found in articles by Humphreys and Rector (1985) and by Seifter *et al.* (1986).

Efferent output: mechanisms controlling extracellular fluid volume

Although there are losses from the body of fluid and electrolytes in stools, sweating, and insensible losses, ultimate control over fluid and electrolyte excretion is exercised by the kidneys. Urine formation begins with the separation of an almost protein-free ultrafiltrate from plasma by the glomerular capillaries. In man roughly 1000 mmol of sodium are filtered each hour, of which approximately 990–995 mmol are reabsorbed by the tubules. It is clear from consideration of these facts that minute changes in either the filtered load of sodium or in the fraction reabsorbed by the tubules can exert an enormous influence on the quantity of sodium finally excreted, and hence on extracellular fluid volume. Many factors can influence renal handling of sodium, of which the most important are listed in Table 7.5. The articles by Humphreys and Rector (1985) and by Seifter *et al.* (1986) contain further details.

The brief description given above illustrates the many and varied means by which the body is able to monitor extracellular fluid volume and manipulate renal sodium excretion accordingly. No single mechanism operates in isolation, all are interrelated. When the system is working normally it can be difficult

Table 7.4 The major sensing mechanisms of extracellular fluid volume

Sensor type	Respond to	Afferent pathway
Intrathoracic (low pressure)		
type B atrial receptors	Atrial distention	Vagus
ventricular receptors	Increased diastolic filling	Vagus
juxtapulmonary capillary (J) receptors	Pulmonary interstitial volume	Vagus
atrial myocytes	Atrial distension	Atrial natriuretic peptide release
Arterial (high pressure)		
baroreceptors in carotid sinus and aortic arch	Rise in arterial pressure	Glossopharyngeal and vagus
volume receptors	'Filling of arterial tree'	Unknown
Renal		
juxtaglomerular apparatus	Reduction in delivery of filtrate to macula densa	Renin release*
Hepatic		
chemoreceptors	Sodium concentration in portal vein	Vagus
mechanoreceptors	Rise in pressure in vena cava	Anterior hepatic nerves*
Central		
chemoreceptors	Sodium concentration in carotid arterial plasma and CSF	

Activation of the afferent pathway leads to increased sodium excretion, except: * stimulation results in reduced sodium excretion.

Table 7.5 The major factors influencing renal sodium excretion (and hence extracellular fluid volume)

Glomerular filtration rate

Peritubular and luminal factors
    peritubular capillary Starling forces
    luminal composition
    medullary interstitial composition
    transtubular ion gradients

Humoral effector mechanisms
    renin–angiotensin–aldosterone system
    prostaglandins
    kallikrein–kinin system
    atrial natruiretic peptide
    other natriuretic hormone(s)

Renal nerves

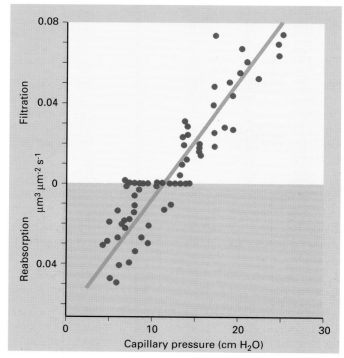

Fig. 7.33 Relationship between capillary pressure and initial rate of filtration or reabsorption of fluid after occlusion of frog mesentery capillaries. Each point represents a measurement from a single capillary. The slope of the regression line is the average hydraulic conductivity of the walls of mesenteric capillaries. (Drawn after Landis 1927, with permission.)

to ascribe greater or lesser importance to one mechanism than to another in any particular situation; similarly, when the system is deranged, it is often difficult to incriminate one aspect as being at fault rather than another.

7.6.2 Factors determining partition between vascular and interstitial compartments

The idea that interstitial fluid was formed by filtration of blood through capillary walls was first proposed by Ludwig, on the basis of studies that appeared to show that the chief factor determining the flow of lymph was the capillary blood pressure. An alternative theory, that lymph was the product of secretion by capillary endothelial cells, was finally overturned by Starling (1896) who suggested, on the basis of qualitative experiments, that the capillary wall behaved as a passive filter through which the exchange of fluid was governed by opposing hydrostatic and osmotic forces. Quantitative support for Starling's hypothesis came from Landis (1927) who measured capillary hydrostatic pressure in frog mesenteric vessels directly by micropuncture, temporarily occluded the vessel, and estimated fluid movement through the capillary wall by observing the motion of red blood cells relative to the point of occlusion. The relationship that he demonstrated between capillary pressure and initial filtration rate is shown in Fig. 7.33: net transcapillary fluid movement was zero when capillary pressure lay in the range from 7 to 14 cm H_2O, a value closely approximate to the plasma osmotic pressure of frogs from the same species. Evidence for Starling's hypothesis in mammalian capillary beds came from the work of Pappenheimer and Soto-Rivera (1948) on isolated hind limbs of cats and dogs.

The capillary hydrostatic pressure in human nailfold skin has been measured directly at 43.5 cm H_2O at the arteriolar end, falling to 16.5 cm H_2O at the venular end. Since the plasma colloid osmotic pressure is 28–38 cm H_2O, the balance of hydrostatic and oncotic forces favours filtration at the arteriolar end

and reabsorption at the venular end of the capillary. This suggests a continual recirculation of fluid between the vascular and interstitial compartments, any excess of filtration over reabsorption being returned to the circulation by the lymphatics. A comprehensive review of the literature concerning the movement of fluid across capillary walls has been written by Michel (1979).

One of the greatest difficulties in applying the Starling hypothesis to problems of fluid balance in man has been the absence of local oedema in the dependent parts of normal individuals. If the vessels of the foot behaved as rigid tubes, it is estimated that capillary hydrostatic pressure would reach 160 cm H_2O on quiet standing; if other determinants of filtration across the capillary wall remained constant, this would lead to an enormous excess of filtration over reabsorption and the rapid development of oedema. That this does not occur is due to precapillary vasoconstriction, which so slows capillary flow that local plasma oncotic pressure may rise as high as 60 cm H_2O after 60 minutes of quiet sitting.

The development of oedema in any circumstance means that the net amount of fluid filtered from the capillaries has exceeded that returned to the circulation via the lymphatics. Such an imbalance could theoretically be caused by:

1. an increase in capillary hydrostatic pressure;

2. a decrease in capillary oncotic pressure;

3. a fall in interstitial hydrostatic pressure (variation in the compliance of the interstitial space may exert important effects);

4. a rise in interstitial oncotic pressure;

5. an alteration in the capillary filtration coefficient (determined by the hydraulic conductivity of the capillary wall, see Fig. 7.33, and by its surface area), i.e. capillary permeability;

6. defective function of the precapillary vasoconstrictor mechanism; or

7. lymphatic insufficiency.

In some situations where oedema occurs, e.g. lymphatic blockage by tumour, it is clear that a single factor is dominant, but in other cases there may be contributions from a combination of the factors listed.

7.6.3 Localized oedema

Localized oedema, which is confined to a single part of the body or single organ, follows from a local imbalance in the forces determining the partition of fluid between the vascular and interstitial compartments.

Pulmonary oedema

An abnormal increase in the amount of interstitial fluid in the lung is described as pulmonary oedema. Experiments performed by Guyton and Lindsey (1959) demonstrated very elegantly that such an increase could be caused by either an increase in the hydrostatic pressure or a reduction in the oncotic pressure within lung capillaries, as predicted by Starling's hypothesis. An anaesthetized dog's left atrial pressure was elevated and then maintained constant by tightening and adjusting, as necessary, a clamp placed around the aorta; after 30 minutes the lungs were removed, drained of blood and weighed. The results can be seen in Fig. 7.34: when the plasma protein concentration was normal the critical left atrial pressure at which fluid began to transude into the lungs was 25 mm Hg, whereas when plasma protein concentration was reduced by about one-half the critical pressure was 11 mm Hg. Similarly, when lung capillary permeability is increased there is excessive flux from the capillary lumen to the interstitial space.

When fluid first begins to accumulate in the interstitial tissues it does so without a great change in tissue pressure in the loosely structured peribronchial connective tissue, where strongly anionic glycoproteins soak up water like a sponge. When the capacity of this sponge has been exceeded interstitial swelling spreads to the alveolar walls, causing impairment of gas exchange. Finally, fluid begins to accumulate in the alveoli themselves; initially this is confined to the alveolar angles but subsequently complete flooding of individual alveoli occurs. The lung lymphatic system provides an important defence against the development of oedema. Normally total lung lymph flow, propelled by active pulsation of the lymphatic channels and

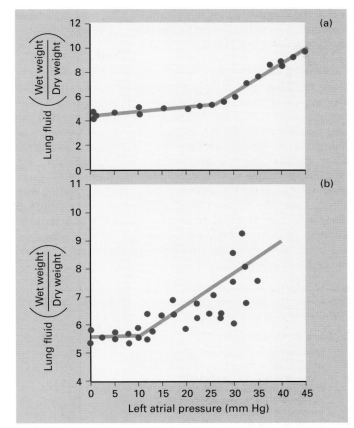

Fig. 7.34 (a) Ratio of lung wet weight to lung dry weight in 19 dogs exposed to various left atrial pressures for 30 minutes. (b) Ratio of wet to dry lung weight in 33 dogs exposed to various left atrial pressures for 30 minutes after reduction of plasma protein concentration to 47 per cent of normal by plasmaphoresis. (Drawn after Guyton and Lindsey 1959, with permission.)

lung movement acting in conjunction with endolymphatic valves, is less than 10 ml/hour. This rate can normally be increased at least tenfold, and in chronic pulmonary venous hypertension hypertrophy of lymphatics may increase the capacity still further.

The engorgement of the pulmonary veins and presence of increased interstitial fluid reduce lung compliance and increase the work needed to move air into and out of the chest. It is probably the disparity between the work needed and the benefit felt that leads patients to complain of breathlessness. The redistribution of blood between the systemic and pulmonary circulations that occurs on moving from the upright to the horizontal posture exacerbates matters, hence the common complaint of breathlessness on lying flat that is relieved by sitting up (orthopnoea).

The oedematous lung at post-mortem has a rubbery consistency. On sectioning there is a free escape of frothy, sanguinous fluid representing a mixture of air, blood, and oedema. On histological examination there is widening of septal walls due to capillary congestion and intraseptal interstitial oedema. Severe oedema is manifest by the presence of proteinaceous coagulate within the alveolar spaces. Such intra-alveolar fluid is prone to secondary infection, often with bacteria of low intrinsic virulence, producing hypostatic pneumonia.

Pulmonary oedema with normal capillary permeability

There are no pathological states causing a local reduction of plasma protein concentration in lung capillaries, but many circumstances in which the hydrostatic pressure is locally elevated. The most frequent of these is left ventricular failure, most commonly in Western societies a consequence of ischaemic heart disease (see Section 7.5.6) or hypertension (see Chapter 12), while in less 'developed' countries mitral valve disease would be the predominant cause (see Chapter 12). Any process that, directly or indirectly, compromises the pumping efficiency of the left side of the heart will tend to lead to a rise in left atrial pressure, pulmonary venous and capillary pressures, and hence pulmonary oedema: a more complete list of causes can be found in Table 7.6.

Table 7.6 Causes of pulmonary oedema with normal capillary permeability

Excessive capillary pressure
(1) with venous hypertension
         left ventricular failure
         mitral stenosis
         cardiomyopathies
         loculated–constricting pericarditis
         left atrial myxoma
         left atrial thrombus
         cor triatriatum
         pulmonary venous thromboses
(2) with acute pulmonary arterial hypertension*
         pulmonary emboli
         collagen diseases
         idiopathic pulmonary hypertension
         drugs (aminorex fumarate)
         secondary to reflex systemic vasoconstriction/release of
             catecholamines (acute intracranial lesions)

Reduced plasma colloid osmotic pressure†
         nephrotic syndrome
         hepatic failure
         malabsorption
         malnutrition
         overhydration (iatrogenic)

Failure of lymph clearance
         mediastinal obstruction
         carcinomatous lymphatic infiltration
         prolonged inadequate positive pressure ventilation

Unknown
         re-expansion of collapsed lung
         high altitude
         post-cardioversion
         post-anaesthesia
         post-cardiopulmonary bypass

 * Pulmonary arterial hypertension is rarely associated with pulmonary oedema: possible mechanisms include local overperfusion of relatively normal parts of the vascular bed and local alteration of capillary permeability.
 † It is not certain that reduced plasma colloid osmotic pressure is primarily responsible for pulmonary oedema. In some circumstances multiple factors may contribute to the development of oedema.

Pulmonary oedema with high capillary permeability

A wide variety of conditions can damage the integrity of the pulmonary capillary endothelium and lead to increased transudation of fluid into the interstitium. In addition to the movement of fluid there is also a transcapillary leak of protein; thus the oedema formed differs from that seen in the context of normal capillary permeability, which has a low protein content. This has a number of important consequences: the oncotic pressure of the interstitial fluid rises so that one of the major mechanisms for limiting the development of oedema is rendered impotent; fibrinogen enters the interstitium and alveoli and coagulates, stimulating interstitial fibrosis and impairing lymphatic drainage.

High-permeability oedema can be caused by mechanical or chemical insults directly damaging to the capillary endothelium or, more often, results from the seemingly inappropriate activation of the normal lung defence mechanisms, which produces a damaging inflammatory response similar to that seen following alveolar challenge with microbes. This condition is referred to clinically as the adult respiratory distress syndrome (ARDS) and is associated most commonly with major trauma, hypovolaemic shock, Gram-negative septicaemia, and severe pulmonary infection, but with an increasing recognition of other causative disorders. The onset of ARDS is unpredictable and the mechanism not clearly understood, although aggregation of granulocytes in lung capillaries, complement activation, and the generation of toxic free-oxygen radicals and liberation of proteases appear to be important factors. A list of the conditions reported as causing high-permeability pulmonary oedema is found in Table 7.7.

Cerebral oedema

In cerebral oedema there is an abnormal increase in the amount of interstitial fluid in the brain. Because the brain is enclosed by a rigid (in adults) skull vault only a relatively small increase in volume can be tolerated before intracranial pressure rises: this leads to symptoms of headache, vomiting, and drowsiness, progressing to visual failure and depression of consciousness before death, which is often caused by brain-stem compression following tentorial or tonsillar herniation. The pathological states that can lead to such a situation include primary and secondary brain tumours, abscesses, haemorrhage, and cerebral trauma. The mechanism involves an increase in capillary permeability, which is normally reduced in the brain compared to other organs (blood–brain barrier). There are no lymphatic channels in the brain to carry away any excess of interstitial fluid.

The definition of cerebral oedema given above, consistent with our general use of the term oedema to describe an abnormal accumulation of interstitial fluid, is more restrictive than that used in many textbooks, which would apply the term 'vasogenic oedema' to this situation and invoke 'cytotoxic oedema' to describe the swelling of brain cells. Such brain-cell swelling is a consequence of metabolic injury, that leads to accumulation of sodium and water within the cell and a reduction in extracellular fluid volume. The overall effect is nevertheless

Table 7.7 Causes of pulmonary oedema with high capillary permeability

Hypovolaemic shock

Infection
    pulmonary
    extrapulmonary (septicaemia)

Trauma

Embolism
    thrombus
    fat
    amniotic fluid
    tumour

Inhalation
    gas: smoke, nitric oxide, oxygen (high concentration)
    liquid: drowning, gastric contents

Haematological
    disseminated intravascular coagulation
    massive blood transfusion

Metabolic
    diabetic ketosis
    uraemia
    hepatic failure

Neurogenic
    cerebral oedema
    intracranial haemorrhage
    acute hydrocephalus
    post-ictal

Drugs/poisons
    heroin, aspirin, propoxyphene, barbiturates, paraquat, snake venom

Other
    pancreatitis
    high altitude

an increase in intracranial pressure with the potential consequences described above. The most common context in which brain-cell swelling occurs is following ischaemia, either focal or general, but it may also occur as a complication of many states, including water intoxication, treatment of hypernatraemia, hepatic failure, and rapid ascent to altitude (mountain sickness). In some of these circumstances the pathogenesis may be mixed, with both expansion of interstitial fluid volume and cell swelling.

Impaired venous drainage

Impairment of venous drainage lasting for days or longer may result in oedema of the part drained as a consequence of raised capillary hydrostatic pressure and probably an impairment of function of the precapillary vasoconstriction mechanism. Most commonly, such oedema is found in the leg as a consequence of deep vein thrombosis (see Section 7.3.4), incompetent venous valves in varicose veins (Section 12.3.3), or extrinsic compression of veins by tumours, surgical stockings, or plaster casts.

Impaired lymphatic drainage

The normal tendency for filtration across the capillary wall to slightly exceed reabsorption is accommodated by removal of the

excess through lymphatic channels. If these channels are deficient, then oedema may result. The deficiency may be due to congenital hypoplasia (Milroy's disease) or to structural damage as a consequence of neoplastic infiltration, scarring from trauma or irradiation, or of chronic lymphangitis from such infective agents as *Wucheria bancrofti* (filariasis), lymphogranuloma venereum, or recurrent streptococcal infection. Lymphatic oedema is often long-standing and becomes 'brawny' (firm and non-pitting). The skin itself may become considerably thickened and pigmented. Indolent ulcers tend to develop at sites of pressure.

Impaired neural control of vessels

One of the most important mechanisms in preventing rapid oedema formation when a limb is dependent is precapillary vasoconstriction. The normal working of this mechanism requires intact vasomotor innervation: if this is disrupted, e.g. following poliomyelitis affecting the innervation of a limb, oedema often results. This is exacerbated by the lack of action of the 'muscle pumps' which, on movement of a limb, intermittently compress veins and increase the return of blood to the heart. Both mechanisms may be involved in causing the characteristic oedema of paralysed limbs.

Localized oedema can be secondary to a local inflammatory response, which is often immunologically mediated. For details of these hypersensitivity reactions, including urticaria and hereditary angio-oedema, see Chapter 4.

7.6.4 Generalized oedema

Generalized oedema formation is a consequence of expansion of extracellular fluid volume. This can only occur as a result of a period of positive sodium balance during which renal excretion of salt and water has failed to keep pace with intake: once established, however, oedema can persist even though sodium intake and output might become equal through a decrease in intake or an increase in output. Why should the kidney retain sodium to such an extent that oedema, often massive, ensues? There are two broad possibilities; either there is an intrinsic abnormality of renal function, or the kidney is responding appropriately to signals that it is receiving—signals that are inappropriate to the extracellular fluid volume status, but perhaps essential to some other aspect of homeostasis. It can be exceedingly difficult to distinguish between these possibilities in the pathological states that cause oedema; the nature of the apparently errant signal(s) can be elusive.

Cardiac oedema

'Heart failure' is notoriously difficult to define. We use the term to indicate a primary abnormality of the heart leading to a situation in which the cardiac output is unable to satisfy the metabolic requirements of the body at rest and during reasonable exercise.

In established heart failure the kidney behaves in a manner that strikingly resembles its response to haemorrhage.

However, plasma volume is either normal or increased in patients with established heart failure and the reduced renal plasma flow and increased filtration fraction observed cannot be attributed to a diminished plasma volume. For this reason, the concept of a reduction in 'effective' blood volume has been invoked to try to explain renal behaviour. This concept refers to the possibility that the impaired pumping action of the heart could lead to a subtle disturbance of the perfusion of the arterial tree, perception by receptors of this inadequacy of perfusion as equivalent to a reduction in blood volume, and initiation of a renal response similar to that elicited when blood volume is indeed reduced. Such a mechanism has been termed the 'forward failure' hypothesis.

Despite uncertainty as to the nature of the arterial receptor(s) required by this hypothesis, although the baroreceptors in the carotid artery and aorta are obvious candidates, there is a great deal of evidence to support the contention that events in the arterial bed can initiate renal salt retention. In the model of heart failure in which a reduction in cardiac output is caused by vena caval constriction, positive sodium balance is mitigated by blood transfusion, which restores cardiac output to normal while causing further elevation of hepatic and renal venous pressures. In man the importance of blood flow in the arterial bed has been convincingly demonstrated by the renal response to the closure and reopening of an arteriovenous fistula: closure of the fistula results in a natriuresis, coinciding with a fall in atrial and pulmonary arterial pressure; reopening the fistula again reduces sodium excretion.

An alternative to the 'forward failure' hypothesis is that of 'backward failure'. This proposes that impairment of cardiac function causes an increase in venous pressure, leading to increased filtration and decreased reabsorption of fluid by the capillaries and hence oedema and a reduction in plasma volume, which serves as a stimulus for renal sodium retention. This simple analysis is unconvincing; at no stage in the development of various forms of experimental heart failure or of human heart failure has plasma volume been shown to be reduced. Furthermore, sodium retention has been seen to precede any rise in central venous pressure during the evolution of congestive heart failure in some patients. There are, however, reasons to believe that an elevation in venous pressure may contribute to the precipitation of cardiac oedema in some circumstances. In a study of patients with severe valvular heart disease, the only haemodynamic parameter measured that separated the oedematous from oedema-free patients was an elevation of right ventricular end-diastolic pressure. In the dog, chronic elevation of left ventricular end-diastolic pressure without elevation of right-sided pressures, caused by the creation of an anastomosis between the left subclavian artery and the left atrium, does not lead to sodium retention. This contrasts with the observation, discussed above, that sodium retention does occur when a fistula is created between an artery and a systemic vein, in which case a rise in right-sided pressures is observed. It must be stressed that these observations contradict expectations based on acute studies of the effects of elevation of central venous pressure, which tends to induce sodium excretion rather than retention (Table 7.4). It has been shown that chronic elevation of venous pressure decreases the sensitivity of atrial receptors to stretch: such impairment of the normal acute responses to an increase in venous pressure may contribute to the progressive fluid retention seen in patients with heart failure.

The effector mechanisms by which the kidney retains sodium and water in heart failure are haemodynamic, neurogenic, and hormonal; there is evidence that all three factors interact to determine the renal response.

In patients with heart failure and reduced cardiac output there is a striking and consistent reduction in renal plasma flow but because of an increase in filtration fraction the glomerular filtration rate (GFR) is relatively preserved. In patients with less severe heart failure, renal plasma flow and GFR may be within the normal range if measured at rest, but on minimal exercise there is a sharp reduction in renal plasma flow and a fall in GFR. Intrarenal haemodynamic changes have been examined in rats with ventricular dysfunction following myocardial infarction: glomerular plasma flow rate was markedly impaired, while the reduction in single-nephron GFR was proportionally less. These changes, mirroring those found in whole organ studies, were due to intense constriction of the efferent arterioles: the resulting decrease in peritubular hydraulic pressure and increase in peritubular oncotic pressure would be expected to lead to increased proximal tubular fluid reabsorption. The fact that these haemodynamic abnormalities are worsened by even minimal exercise may have bearing on two clinical observations. Firstly, the efficacy of bed rest as a treatment for severe cardiac failure. Secondly, the benefit of physical training in patients with milder forms of the condition.

The sympathetic nervous system may be a mediator of renal vasoconstriction in heart failure. Administration of sympatholytic agents to some patients with heart failure causes a diuresis, and infusion of an alpha-adrenergic blocking agent into the renal artery of a dog with heart failure due to experimental valvular disease resulted in an ipsilateral natriuresis and diuresis. However, the changes in electrolyte excretion produced by adrenergic blockade in patients with heart failure are generally small, and the characteristic picture of renal dysfunction in heart failure can be seen in transplanted and denervated kidneys. Thus, the role of the renal nerves in heart failure is variable, being critical in some instances and less important in others.

Many hormonal systems are abnormal in heart failure and these may be divided into two broad classes; those that induce vasoconstriction and promote sodium and water retention [renin–angiotensin–aldosterone, arginine vasopressin (AVP), adrenaline noradrenaline], and those that stimulate vasodilation and encourage natriuresis (prostaglandins, dopamine, atrial natriuretic factor). Renal behaviour represents an integrated response to the influence of these opposing factors, but the balance of effects favours vasoconstriction and sodium retention.

The changes in glomerular and proximal tubular function that characterize most models of heart failure are virtually identical to those that occur with the infusion of angiotensin II, which selectively constricts the glomerular efferent arteriole in addition to a direct action stimulating proximal tubule sodium reabsorption. Angiotensin blockade in patients and animals with heart failure may result in improvement in renal blood flow and sodium excretion. The predominant effect of the renin–angiotensin–aldosterone axis on distal nephron function is mediated by the action of aldosterone on the collecting duct, which causes increased net sodium reabsorption and decreased sodium backleak. The importance of these mechanisms in the genesis of cardiac oedema is, again, variable. Some studies have found a relationship between sodium retention and elevated levels of renin, angiotensin II, and aldosterone in heart failure; in other studies no consistent relationship could be established. Acute experimental impairment of cardiac function is associated with massive activation of the sympathetic nervous system, renin–angiotension–aldosterone system, and AVP release. These systems maintain systemic blood pressure and promote renal salt and water retention during the acute phase. In the chronic phase extracellular fluid volume is expanded, blood pressure is restored, and the plasma levels of the hormones return towards normal. Similar patterns occur in human cardiac failure and these stages of overt renal salt retention and return to salt balance must be considered when interpreting measurements of plasma renin, angiotensin II, and aldosterone.

At the same time as endogenous vasoconstrictor mechanisms are activated in heart failure, there is evidence that humoral vasodilator mechanisms are also activated. Studies in patients with heart failure demonstrate a linear relationship between the magnitude of systemic vasoconstrictor forces, as reflected by plasma renin activity and angiotensin II levels, and the magnitude of systemic vasodilator forces, as measured by circulating levels of prostaglandin E_2 and I_2 metabolites. In patients in heart failure with high levels of these prostaglandin metabolites indomethacin, a prostaglandin synthetase inhibitor, causes a reduction in cardiac output and a rise in arterial pressure: when prostaglandin levels are normal indomethacin has no such effect. Circulating plasma levels of dopamine are also elevated in heart failure: infusion of exogenous dopamine in heart failure may cause selective renal vasodilation and may initiate a diuresis, oral dopaminergic therapy may also have beneficial haemodynamic effects. Atrial natriuretic factor plasma levels are elevated in heart failure in proportion to the level of atrial pressure. The biological significance of these humoral vasodilators in heart failure is unknown, the renal response to them is blunted, either by hypotension or a combination of the factors tending to encourage sodium retention.

Elevation of venous pressure may contribute directly to the formation of oedema by impairing lymphatic drainage, causing resetting of pre- and post-capillary resistance vessels to favour an increase in capillary hydrostatic pressure, and perhaps by a direct action on renal sodium handling in some instances.

The mechanisms described are depicted in Fig. 7.35; it should be emphasized that the importance of each element can vary considerably from situation to situation and from time to time. Fuller discussion of the issues involved can be found in articles by Hollenberg and Schulman (1985) and Humphreys and Rector (1985).

Renal oedema

Reduced glomerular filtration

Profound reduction in the glomerular filtration rate (GFR), as occurs in advanced acute or chronic renal failure (Chapter 19), can lead to a situation in which the maximal rate of sodium excretion by the kidneys is less than the amount ingested. Positive sodium balance results. In chronic renal failure the fraction of filtered sodium that is excreted is much higher than normal, but this adaptive mechanism, perhaps involving circulating natriuretic substances, is ultimately unable to compensate fully for the degree of impairment of GFR. In acute renal failure secondary to pathological processes primarily affecting the glomerulus, e.g. acute glomerulonephritis (Chapter 19), there is sometimes avid renal tubular sodium reabsorption which, together with the fall in GFR, leads to a virtual cessation of sodium excretion. In acute renal failure resulting from tubular damage, 'acute tubular necrosis', fractional sodium excretion is elevated but GFR is drastically reduced by mechanisms that are complex and contentious (Chapter 19). In all of these situations a consequence of the primary renal sodium retention is expansion of the extracellular fluid and plasma volumes, leading to hypertension and/or oedema. It is characteristic of such oedema that it often occurs around the face and the eyelids.

Nephrotic syndrome

The traditional explanation for sodium retention in the nephrotic syndrome suggests that heavy urinary protein loss, occurring because of abnormal glomerular permeability, leads to hypoalbuminaemia and decreased plasma oncotic pressure. It is then supposed that the reduction in plasma oncotic pressure causes increased filtration and decreased reabsorption in tissue capillaries, leading to oedema and a contraction of plasma volume, which precipitates vigorous renal salt retention.

This explanation is superficially plausible; but close examination of experimental and human nephrosis has revealed, with the exception, perhaps, of most cases of nephrosis due to minimal change disease (Chapter 19) in children and some in adults, serious discrepancies between the observed facts and the requirements of the hypothesis. Early studies did suggest a reduction of plasma volume in nephrotic patients, but more recent work, paying scrupulous attention to methodological difficulties, has demonstrated that in adults with the nephrotic syndrome plasma volume is almost invariably normal or increased. There is no good evidence that the kidney is responding to a reduction in 'effective' blood volume; although plasma renin and aldosterone levels are increased in some nephrotic patients, in others they are reduced, and there is no association between such levels and the degree of sodium retention in the nephrotic syndrome; moreover captopril (an inhibitor of angiotension-converting enzyme) does not provoke natriuresis. Study of patients before and after steroid-induced remission has shown a fall in blood volume after remission, coupled with a rise

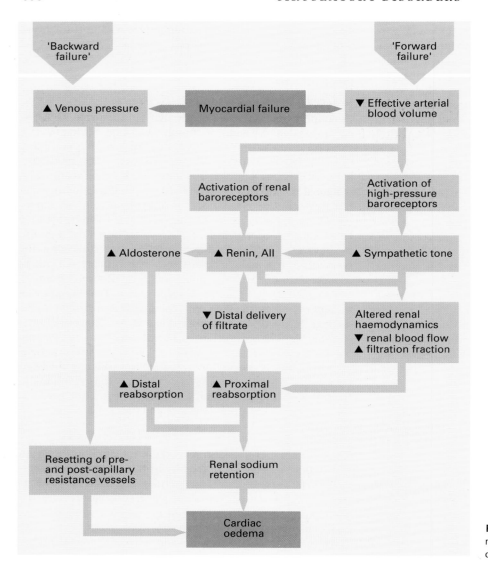

Fig. 7.35 Diagram showing the important mechanisms operating in the formation of cardiac oedema.

in plasma renin activity, contrary to the expectations of the traditional hypothesis. Further, the suggestion that a decrease in plasma oncotic pressure may disturb Starling's forces to produce oedema does not accommodate the observation that the oncotic pressure of the intestitial fluid is similarly reduced, such that there is very little change in the oncotic pressure gradient between the capillary lumen and the interstitial space. There is little or no correlation in nephrotic patients between the plasma albumin concentration and the presence or degree of fluid retention. Hypoalbuminaemia induced by plasmaphoresis does not lead to expansion of extracellular fluid volume unless accompanied by sodium loading; congenital analbuminaemia is not necessarily associated with the development of oedema.

These difficulties have led to increasing attention being paid to the possibility that sodium retention is due to an intrinsic renal abnormality. Ingenious experiments have demonstrated this may be the case, at least in the experimental model of nephrosis that follows administration of puromycin aminonucleoside

to rats. When only one kidney is exposed to the chemical, sodium retention is confined to that kidney; the contralateral kidney, which shares the same systemic milieu, is unaffected. The kidney removed from a rat rendered nephrotic by exposure to puromycin aminonucleoside fails to excrete sodium normally when perfused in isolation.

The weight of experimental evidence suggests that renal sodium retention in nephrosis is either a function of the distal tubule, or of some part of deep nephrons that are not accessible to study by micropuncture.

Hepatic oedema

As in the nephrotic syndrome, the traditional explanation of fluid retention in cirrhosis relates to the notion that hypoalbuminaemia is the cause of a postulated reduction in plasma volume. Indeed, there is good evidence that in cirrhosis—as in heart failure—the kidney behaves as if blood volume were reduced, but careful measurements show that it is usually elevated. Once again the concept of a reduction in 'effective' blood volume has been invoked to try and explain renal behaviour. Because cirrhosis is characterized by the development of multiple arteriovenous (AV) shunts in the pulmonary and systemic circulations it is reasonable to consider that the renal adjustments to fistulas in other circumstances, namely an increase in tubular sodium reabsorption coupled with an elevation in cardiac output and expansion of plasma volume, might also occur as AV shunts develop in the cirrhotic. The finding of increased plasma catecholamines, renin, aldosterone, and AVP in some, but not all, cirrhotic patients is consistent with the view that the circulation is perceived as being underfilled in certain cases.

There is experimental evidence to indicate that obstruction to hepatic venous outflow may also be fundamental. When hepatic venous outflow is selectively obstructed in the dog, either by intrahepatic histamine infusion or by surgical ligation, there is a dramatic fall in urinary sodium excretion. Pressure sensors responding specifically to elevation of hepatic venous pressure have been defined and section of the autonomic plexus around the hepatic artery eliminates the reflex increase in renal sympathetic activity that follows occlusion of the inferior vena cava at the diaphragm. An early rise in hepatic intrasinusoidal pressure has been documented in experimental cirrhosis associated with sodium retention. Furthermore, hepatic sinusoids, unlike capillaries elsewhere in the body, are highly permeable to plasma proteins. As a result, the partitioning of fluid between the vascular and interstitial compartments is largely determined by the hydrostatic pressure gradient, and a small rise in intrasinusoidal pressure augments filtration markedly. When filtration exceeds the capacity for lymph return fluid accumulates in the peritoneal space as ascites. A role for hepatic chemoreceptors is suggested by the observation that in cats, dogs, and rats intraportal infusion of hypertonic saline, but not equivalently hypertonic sucrose, results in a natriuresis which is abolished by vagotomy. This response is markedly reduced in cirrhotic rats.

As in established heart failure, renal blood flow is reduced and the filtration fraction is increased in established cirrhosis; as described in the section on cardiac oedema, this leads to an enhancement of proximal tubule sodium reabsorption. In circumstances where delivery from the proximal to distal tubule is preserved, increased distal reabsorption has been demonstrated. In some situations, action of the sympathetic nervous system, angiotensin, and aldosterone may contribute to sodium retention. Figure 7.36 shows schematically the mechanisms that may be involved, including the possibility that sodium retention in cirrhosis is due to a primary renal defect—although

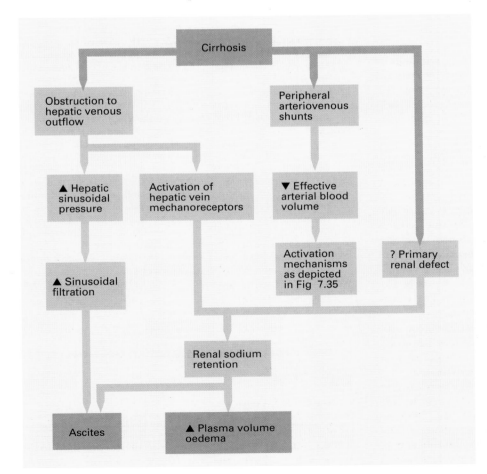

Fig. 7.36 Diagram showing the important mechanisms operating in the formation of cirrhotic oedema.

this seems unlikely in the model of cirrhosis produced in the rat by carbon tetrachloride administration, since the kidney handles sodium in a normal manner when perfused in isolation.

Pregnancy-associated oedema

Normal pregnancy

Normal pregnancy is associated with an average weight gain of about 12 kg; of this 1.25 kg is attributable to expansion of maternal blood volume and 1.7 kg to accumulation of interstitial fluid, which largely occurs between the 30th week of gestation and term. Many normal pregnant women develop generalized oedema, characterized by swelling of the fingers and face. Despite the marked rise in measured plasma volume, elevated levels of plasma renin and aldosterone would suggest that receptor mechanisms do not perceive blood volume to be increased. Renin and aldosterone levels respond appropriately to changes in sodium intake but 'reset' at a higher level. It may be that the uteroplacental circulation acts as an anteriovenous shunt in distorting perception of plasma volume. Physical factors can contribute to the control of sodium excretion during pregnancy: the antinatriuretic effects of standing upright are exaggerated and in late gestation turning from a supine to a lateral position promotes sodium excretion (for further discussion of this, and of the pathogenesis of other oedematous states, see Schrier 1988).

Pregnancy with hypertension

Pre-eclampsia is associated with generalized fluid retention in 85 per cent of cases; however, when oedema is present plasma volume is reduced as compared with normal pregnancy. The mechanism of sodium retention is uncertain, but involves early abnormalities of tubular function, with reduced uric acid clearance, and late impairment of GFR.

Other forms of generalized oedema

Idiopathic oedema of women is a condition in which episodic or more constant fluid retention occurs without obvious evidence of cardiac, renal, hepatic, or other disease known to cause oedema. Some women who appear to have idiopathic oedema abuse diuretics and suffer rebound oedema when these are stopped: this, however, is not a satisfactory explanation in all cases—there is evidence of an othostatic leak of plasma volume and plasma protein into the interstitial space, which may be due to abnormal function of the pre- and the post-capillary resistance vessels (Edwards and Bayliss 1976).

Generalized oedema is one of the cardinal features of kwashiorkor: gross expansion of the interstitial space may be associated with reduction of plasma volume. The cause of sodium retention is unknown and the 'standard' explanation that hypoalbuminaemia leads to oedema, as has been mentioned in the context of the nephrotic syndrome, is inadequate for the same reasons. During treatment of kwashiorkor oedema may be lost with no change in plasma albumin concentration. Equally puzzling is the observation that the sudden introduction of high-energy feeding to severely malnourished children or adults can sometimes precipitate oedema: the mechanism is unknown, but may be related to the response of leucocytes from such patients, which in vitro extrude sodium rapidly if provided with an energy supply. Very little work has been done in this area.

7.6.5   Bibliography

Edwards, O. M. and Bayliss, R. I. S. (1976). Idiopathic oedema of women. *Quarterly Journal of Medicine* **45**, 125.

Fisher, A. and Foex, P. (1987). Adult respiratory distress syndrome. In *Oxford textbook of medicine* (2nd edn) (ed. D. J. Weatherall, J. G. G. Ledingham, and D. A. Warrell), 15.161. Oxford University Press.

Guyton, A. C. and Lindsey, A. W. (1959). Effect of elevated left atrial pressure and decreased plasma protein concentration on the development of pulmonary oedema. *Circulation Research* **7**, 649.

Hollenberg, N. K. and Schulman, G. (1985). Renal perfusion and function in sodium-retaining states. In *The kidney: physiology and pathophysiology* (ed. D. W. Seldin and G. Giebisch), p. 1119. Raven Press, New York.

Humphreys, M. H. and Rector, F. C. (1985). Pathophysiology of edema formation. In *The kidney: physiology and pathophysiology* (ed. D. W. Seldin and G. Giebisch), p. 1163. Raven Press, New York.

Landis, E. M. (1927). Micro-injection studies of capillary permeability. II. The relation between capillary pressure and the rate at which fluid passes through the walls of single capillaries. *American Journal of Physiology* **82**, 217.

Michel, C. C. (1979). Fluid movements through capillary walls. In *Handbook of physiology—the cardiovascular system*, Vol. IV (2nd edn), p. 375. American Physiological Society, Washington.

Pappenheimer, J. R. and Soto-Rivera, A. (1948). Effective osmotic pressure of the plasma proteins and other quantities associated with the capillary circulation in the hind-limbs of cats and dogs. *American Journal of Physiology* **152**, 471.

Prichard, J. S. and Lee, G, de J. (1987). Pulmonary oedema. In *Oxford textbook of medicine* (2nd edn) (ed. D. J. Weatherall, J. G. G. Ledingham and D. A. Warrell), 13.334. Oxford University Press.

Schrier, R. W. (1988). Pathogenesis of sodium and water retention in high-output and low-output cardiac failure, nephrotic syndrome, cirrhosis and pregnancy. *New England Journal of Medicine* **319**, 1065 and 1127.

Seifter, J. L., Skorecki, K. L., Strivelman, J. C., Hanpert, G., and Brenner, B. M. (1986). Control of extracellular fluid volume and pathophysiology of edema formation. In *The kidney* (3rd edn) (ed. B. M. Brenner and F. C. Rector), p. 343. W. B. Saunders, Philadelphia.

Starling, E. H. (1896). On the absorption of fluids from connective tissue spaces. *Journal of Physiology (London)* **19**, 312.

Suki, W. N. and Eknoyan, G. (1981). *The kidney in systemic disease* (2nd edn). John Wiley & Sons, New York.

Wesson, L. G. (1969). *Physiology of the human kidney*. Grune and Stratton, New York.

7.7   Shock

T. Krausz and J. Cohen

A patient in severe shock is easy to recognize but hard to describe. More precisely, the term 'shock' is difficult to define in strict pathophysiological terms, since it is a loose description of the end result of a major acute circulatory disturbance, which may have many causes. Thus 'shock' cannot be measured, it has no single aetiology, and treatment depends on the particular circumstances. With these caveats, it is reasonable to think of shock as a state of prolonged tissue hypoperfusion. The principal causes are given in Table 7.8.

7.7.1 Pathogenesis

Adequate tissue perfusion is dependent upon a number of closely related factors—notably the systemic arterial pressure, the peripheral vascular resistance, and the patency of the tissue capillary bed—and most causes of shock can be explained by a disorder of one or more of these factors. As an example, arterial pressure is determined by the total vascular resistance and the cardiac output. Cardiac output is, in turn, a product of the heart rate and the stroke volume. Thus, after compensatory mechanisms are overwhelmed, a fall in stroke volume will cause hypotension and, ultimately, shock. Shock due to fall in stroke volume can therefore result equally from gastrointestinal haemorrhage (decreased filling pressure) or from myocarditis (decreased myocardial contractility).

It is convenient to consider the types of shock based on the main underlying cause, but in reality there is considerable overlap, as will become evident.

Hypovolaemia

An abrupt loss of intravascular volume will cause a fall in the stroke volume and, in turn, the cardiac output.

Haemorrhage

This may be external (as in major gastrointestinal bleeding or trauma) or internal, e.g. fracture of the femur with extensive blood loss into the soft tissue. A fall in stroke volume will lead to a compensatory tachycardia, but this can become self-defeating since an increased heart rate will shorten diastolic filling time and limit cardiac output. An acute drop in the cardiac output by 50 per cent or more will cause severe shock.

Excess fluid loss

Excess fluid loss, other than blood can also result in hypovolaemia. The severe vomiting which accompanies pyloric stenosis, or the catastrophic diarrhoea of cholera, are good examples. Decreased intravascular volume can also result from conditions such as diabetes insipidus or inappropriate diuretic therapy, although it is unusual for these patients to present in shock.

Burns

Burns represent a more complex situation. There is no doubt that extensive burns are associated with marked fluid loss (which must be replaced), but it is likely that some of the features of shock in burned patients are due to vaso-active mediators released from macrophages activated by thermal injury.

Vasodilatation

Vasodilatation causes peripheral pooling and relative hypovolaemia. Vascular smooth muscle tone is determined both by circulating vaso-active substances and neurogenically via the sympathetic nervous system. Arterial and ventricular baroreceptors respond to decreased systemic pressure by stimulating sympathetic efferent activity leading to peripheral vasoconstriction in an effort to 'protect' the cardiac output. Likewise, hypoxia (a common accompaniment to severe shock) activates the chemoreceptor reflex, which also increases sympathetic tone.

Several humoral factors play a part in regulating peripheral vascular resistance. Important amongst these are *renin*, which is released by the kidney in response to hypotension and which acts through *angiotensin*, resulting in peripheral vasoconstriction. *Bradykinin* and associated peptides, and *prostaglandins*,

---

Table 7.8 Causes of shock

Hypovolaemia	
haemorrhage	Includes external loss such as haematemesis, and internal loss, e.g. fractures
excess fluid loss	Vomiting, burns
vasodilatation	Hypovolaemia; neuropathic causes (e.g. spinal cord injury), anaesthesia, Addisonian crisis
Cardiac shock	
myocardial infarction	Cardiogenic shock
outflow obstruction	Tamponade, tension pneumothorax, major pulmonary embolus
valve rupture	Also septal and cardiac rupture
myocarditis	
arrhythmias	
Shock and infection	
bacterial infection	Gram-negative 'septic shock', and Gram-positive infections
non-bacterial infection	Viral, e.g. dengue; protozoal, e.g. malaria
Anaphylactic shock	

notably *prostacyclin* and *thromboxane* A_2, have potent vaso-active effects. The role of these mediators is discussed below.

Thus hypovolaemia due to vasodilatation is seen following autonomic blockade (for instance as a complication of anaes-thesia), after spinal injury, and perhaps more importantly, as one of the features of septic shock (see below).

Cardiac shock ('pump failure')

Myocardial infarction

The most obvious cause of pump failure is a massive myocardial infarction. Many such patients are hypotensive, but a propor-tion (approximately 10 per cent) develop a syndrome of low blood pressure, raised left ventricular filling pressure, peripheral vasoconstriction, and oliguria, which is called cardiogenic shock. This term is not used for patients with potentially revers-ible causes, such as arrythmias or hypovolaemia, and at a clini-cal level this distinction is probably worthwhile, since the prognosis for the patients in cardiogenic shock is extremely poor. Nevertheless, all these patients share a common physio-logical abnormality, i.e. a low cardiac output because of pump failure.

The main reason for the very poor outcome of cardiogenic shock is the extent of the lesion. If there is little remaining effect-ive myocardium, there will be an inevitable fall in the cardiac output. This, in turn, will lead to a fall in coronary perfusion pressure, and very soon there is a 'positive feedback loop' of increasing myocardial dysfunction. Eventually, arrhythmias and metabolic acidosis contribute to the mortality. Despite its attractive simplicity, this explanation may conceal the role of other contributory factors. For instance, the hypotension that occurs in septic shock (see below) is associated with a circulat-ing myocardial depressant factor, a protein which directly impairs myocardial cell activity in tissue culture. Since a myo-cardial infarction is known to induce a brisk and substantial acute phase response, it is plausible that some of the patho-physiological features of cardiogenic shock result from humoral factors released from activated macrophages.

Several other cardiac disorders can be associated with cardiac shock. *Rupture of the interventricular septum* or of the *papillary muscle*, and *cardiac rupture*, which is more common, can all present as acute haemodynamic collapse. *Arrythmias*, usually in the setting of an acute infarction, can, if persistent, cause prolonged hypotension and lead to shock. *Myocarditis* is always quoted as a potential cause of pump failure, but in our exper-ience it is an extremely uncommon cause of shock.

Outflow obstruction

A second group of conditions associated with cardiac shock can be thought of as due to outflow obstruction; principal amongst these is the shock associated with *acute massive pulmonary em-bolism*. The primary event is impaction of an embolus in the pulmonary arterial tree. If the extent of the occlusion is suffi-cient (generally, more than 50 per cent of the vascular bed), there will be a significant obstruction to the right ventricular

outflow, acute dilatation of the right ventricle, and *right vent-ricular failure*.

The second consequence of a major pulmonary embolism is a large area of the lung that is ventilated but no longer perfused, i.e. a *ventilation–perfusion mismatch*. Dyspnoea and hypoxia are almost always present, but the mechanism of these effects is not entirely clear. The simplest explanation is mechanical obstruc-tion to the pulmonary vascular bed leading to pulmonary hypertension, but there is also some evidence that humoral fac-tors (notably serotonin) are implicated.

Shock is the third component of this triad of haemodynamic features of acute pulmonary embolism. A fall in pulmonary venous return to the left heart leads to a fall in cardiac output which, if prolonged, leads to all the classical features of shock. It is important to distinguish shock associated with pulmonary embolism in which right ventricular failure predominates, from true cardiogenic shock, which is dominated by left heart failure.

Another cause of acute outflow obstruction is *cardiac tampon-ade*. In most cases inflammatory or infiltrative disorders cause a gradual accumulation of fluid in the pericardial space, but oc-casionally, e.g. following trauma, it develops very quickly. As pericardial pressure rises various compensatory mechanisms attempt to maintain the cardiac output. Right and left atrial pressures rise, a sinus tachycardia occurs and the peripheral vascular resistance increases. Ultimately these devices are insufficient, and the patient presents with low cardiac output shock. *Tension pneumothorax* is a further example of an extrinsic cause of cardiac compression that may lead to cardiovascular collapse.

Shock and infection

Very many infections can cause a shock-like state (Table 7.9). The term 'septic shock' is usually reserved for shock associated with Gram-negative septicaemia, but the same clinical syn-drome can occur as a complication of staphylococcal, strepto-coccal, or even candidal infections. The pathogenesis of shock in infection can be thought of in four stages:

1. microbial and host factors that lead to the establishment of infection;
2. tissue injury and/or toxin production;
3. generation of inflammatory/injurious mediators;
4. haemodynamic consequences.

For convenience, we will describe in turn shock associated with Gram-negative bacteria, Gram-positive bacteria, and then non-bacterial infections. It will become apparent that while there is considerable variation in the virulence factors that permit micro-organisms to establish infection and cause tissue damage, the later stages of the pathway, i.e. the mechanisms of injury and the haemodynamic effects, are remarkably similar, irrespective of the nature of the original infection.

Gram-negative bacteria: 'septic' or 'endotoxic' shock

A variety of bacterial properties contribute to their patho-genicity, i.e. their ability to cause infection. These properties

Table 7.9 Shock and infection

Gram-negative bacteria	'Coliforms', *Pseudomonas aeruginosa*, *Neisseria*. spp., cholera, typhoid, plague, brucellosis
Gram-positive bacteria	*Staphylococcus aureus*, *Clostridia*, haemolytic streptococci, *Streptococcus pneumoniae*, diphtheria, anthrax
Spirochaetes	Syphilis, relapsing fever, leptospirosis (Jarisch–Herxheimer reaction)
Rickettsia	Rocky Mountain Spotted Fever, louse-borne typhus
Viral	Haemorrhagic fevers; arenaviruses; dengue; Coxsackie B
Fungal	*Candida, Aspergillus*?
Parasitic	Malaria; trypasonomiasis?

include capsules, mobility, serum resistance, iron transport, and the presence of fimbriae or pili. In addition, certain bacteria produce toxins, and amongst Gram-negative bacteria *endotoxin* is the most important.

Endotoxin is a lipopolysaccharide situated in the outer part of the cell wall of most Gram-negative bacteria. It has three parts: the outermost is the 'O' side-chain, a series of sugars which are different in each bacterial strain. Deep to the 'O' chain is the core region, which is linked in turn to lipid A. It was found that the structure of the lipid A was the same in virtually all Gram-negative bacteria, and this was particularly interesting because isolation and purification of lipid A showed that it was responsible for all of the biological properties of intact endotoxin. This provided a clear explanation for the observation that the clinical and pathological features of Gram-negative septicaemia were always the same, irrespective of the causative organism.

Injection of purified endotoxin into animals—and even, cautiously, in man—confirmed that it could elicit virtually all the typical features of Gram-negative shock, including fever, hypotension, haematological and biochemical abnormalities. Indeed, so diverse are its properties that it seemed likely that it works by activating a series of cascades. This proved to be the case: included amongst the many systems involved are complement, the fibrinolytic pathway, endorphins, and phospholipase products such as platelet activating factor and the prostaglandins (Table 7.10). Although all these mediators certainly play some part in the syndrome of septic shock, none can alone reproduce all the features, and the precise mode of action of endotoxin was something of an enigma. However, it has

Table 7.10 Mediators of shock

Complement
Cytokines
'Myocardial depressant factor'
Fibrinolytic cascade
Endorphins
Platelet activating factor
Prostaglandins
Reactive oxygen intermediates
Kinins
Coagulation cascade

emerged recently that the toxicity of endotoxin is largely mediated through a substance called *tumour necrosis factor (TNF)*, also referred to as *cachectin*.

Tumour necrosis factor (TNF) is a lymphokine, or cytokine, a family of proteins which includes the interferons, interleukins, and colony-stimulating factors. They have a number of overlapping functions, generally concerned with immunoregulation, but TNF is unusual in that when present in excess it reproduces the effect of endotoxin. The evidence suggesting that TNF plays a major role in endotoxin-induced shock can be summarized as follows:

1. Administration of recombinant human TNF to mice induces pathophysiological effects typical of septic shock.

2. When healthy volunteers were challenged with intravenous endotoxin, clinical and biochemical responses were temporally associated with elevated circulating levels of TNF.

3. Mice and rabbits passively immunized with polyclonal anti-TNF antiserum were protected from the lethal action of endotoxin.

4. Baboons passively immunized with a monoclonal anti-TNF antibody were protected from shock and death after challenge with live *E. coli*.

5. Preliminary clinical data suggest that in meningococcal septicaemia high serum TNF levels are associated with a poor outcome.

Although it seems very likely that TNF is the principal mediator of endotoxicity, the details of its mode of action are not yet known. Nevertheless, it is particularly interesting that it appears to be responsible not just for the shock syndrome associated with Gram-negative septicaemia, but is also implicated in at least some cases of Gram-positive infection, thus providing for the first time an explanation for the well-known difficulty of distinguishing these two syndromes on clinical grounds.

Endotoxin release and TNF induction probably underlie almost all Gram-negative infections, including diseases such as typhoid, brucellosis, and meningococcal septicaemia. There are two exceptions, the most important being cholera. *Vibrio cholerae* produces a chromosomally encoded exotoxin—choleragen—which acts locally on intestinal epithelial cells to activate adenylate cyclase. The cells go into 'overdrive' and there is a massive loss of fluid into the bowel lumen, which continues until the cells are shed. It is this fluid loss which leads to hypovolaemia and shock. The other exception is *Pseudomonas aeruginosa*, which in addition to a classical endotoxin also possesses an exotoxin. Pseudomonas exotoxin A inhibits protein synthesis by inhibiting Elongation Factor 2, but not all strains produce the exotoxin and its clinical significance is questionable.

Gram-positive bacteria

Shock syndromes can be produced by several Gram-positive bacteria (Table 7.9), but the best example is provided by *Staphylococcus aureus*, which can cause shock through at least four different mechanisms.

S. aureus produces many *exotoxins*, amongst them haemolysins, exfoliatin (responsible for the scalded skin syndrome), and a group of six enterotoxins A–F. Ingestion of foods containing pre-formed enterotoxin causes acute staphylococcal food poisoning; occasionally the symptoms are so severe that hypovolaemic shock ensues.

Another familiar facet of staphylococcal disease is its *ability to invade tissue* and produce destructive, pyogenic lesions with a brisk inflammatory response. When this occurs in the region of the heart valves (typically as a complication of bacteraemias in intravenous drug abusers) the destruction proceeds rapidly. Unless treatment is given promptly the valve ruptures and the patient presents in cardiogenic shock. Staphylococci can also cause purulent pericarditis, and shock due to outflow obstruction.

A third mechanism of induction of shock mimics that seen due to *endotoxin* in Gram-negative bacteria. In the case of staphylococci it is the teichoic acid–peptidiglycan complex in the cell wall that activates complement and other vaso-active mediators, resulting eventually in a capillary leak syndrome. Not all patients with staphylococcal bacteraemia develop shock, in part because in most strains the techoic acid complex is hidden beneath an outer capsule.

The final, and most dramatic, effect of staphylococcal infection is the *toxic shock syndrome*. First recognized in association with tampon use in young women, patients developed high fever, profuse nausea and vomiting, conjunctivitis and rash, and finally hypotension and full-blown shock. The cause was traced to strains of *S. aureus* producing a toxin, called variously enterotoxin F, pyrogenic exotoxin C, and now, thankfully, toxic shock syndrome toxin 1. The toxin produces its damage both directly on tissues and also acts synergistically with endotoxin. The precise mechanism is unknown, although it is very likely that cytokines such as TNF play a part.

Non-bacterial infections

Table 7.9 provides an extensive list of other infections that are associated with shock. Often little is known of the underlying mechanisms, but there are some exceptions. *Spirochaetes*, for example, have cell walls that are similar in many respects to those of Gram-negative bacteria, and some of the clinical syndromes are clearly related to endotoxin-type effects. The *arenaviruses* cause many of the viral haemorrhagic fevers, such as Marburg and Ebola; the pathology is due in part to hypovolaemia and in part to reduced tissue perfusion due to disseminated intravascular coagulation. Very recently, TNF has been shown to play a central role in the pathogenesis of *cerebral malaria*. In rickettsial diseases such as *Rocky Mountain Spotted Fever* a capillary leak syndrome results from damage to the vascular endothelium.

Anaphylactic shock

In a small number of people, the injection of a foreign serum or protein, or sometimes an insect or snake bite, leads within a few minutes to a dramatic and life-threatening illness with profound hypotension, dyspnoea, and urticaria. The symptoms are caused by vaso-active mediators—histamine, serotonin, kinins—released from granules in mast cells triggered by the foreign antigen combining with cell-bound IgE. The role of the antibody is really just that of an intermediary, allowing the antigen to bind, and thus cross-link, IgE receptor molecules on the surface of the mast cell. This cross-linking brings about a conformational change in the cell membrane, which results in degranulation and mediator release.

Not all cases of 'anaphylactic shock' can be explained in this way. Mast cells can also be induced to degranulate by lectins or by complement components. Toxic reactions to drugs or venoms are often more complex, as in the case of collapse following the administration of radiological contrast media. These events are not IgE mediated, but are probably due to the consequences of intense complement activation.

7.7.2   Pathology of shock

General principles

Tissue hypoperfusion

Inadequate tissue perfusion is the main abnormality both in clinical and experimental shock. The defective tissue perfusion produces not only hypoxia but the accumulation of a variety of metabolites, the combined effect of which causes the lesions of shock. Interestingly, hypoxia alone does not produce these lesions. Unless the reduction in tissue perfusion is corrected in time, organ, tissue, and cell failure and, eventually, death occur. Most tissues and organs are affected to a lesser or greater extent. However, not all organ changes are manifest clinically and generally, organ dysfunction being difficult to assess because of the masking effect of the shock itself. Fatal shock lesions are present most commonly in the lung and the heart but occasionally injury of the other organs may contribute to a patient's death or even be the major cause.

Some organs are more at risk from ischaemia than others, the risk depending on such factors as anastomoses, watershed zones, and by the presence or absence of any vascular disease. In order of frequency the most commonly affected organs are the *lung, liver, heart, kidney, intestine, adrenals, brain, and pancreas*.

Basic pathology

The basic pathological changes in shock are *haemorrhages*, cell or tissue *necrosis*, and *fibrin thrombi* in capillaries, venules, and small veins. These changes are similar to the tissue manifestations of the Shwartzman reaction. The histological picture of shock-induced lesions varies from organ to organ; in some, necrosis, haemorrhage, and fibrin thrombi are all present, while in others there may be only haemorrhage or necrosis.

Microthrombi are almost always present in shock lesions of the intestine and brain, while in other organs their incidence varies from 0 to 20 per cent. The frequency of fibrin thrombi also depends on the time between the onset of shock and death. Remmele and Harms (1969) noted microthrombi in 50 per cent of patients dying within four hours of the onset of shock, and in almost all patients dying between 24 hours to 48 hours of the onset of shock. However, after 48 hours thrombi were difficult to find.

There is considerable debate as to whether the fibrin thrombi are the result of disseminated intravascular coagulation or merely the result of diminished perfusion. In support of the latter view is the fact that volvulus or incarceration of the intestine can lead to lesions identical to those seen in shock. However, it is also known that shock is frequently associated with DIC.

Necroses are frequent manifestations of the shock syndrome as a direct result of hypoperfusion. The site and extent of the necroses reflect the different vulnerability of different tissues, the time elapsed between the onset of the shock, and the state of the vasculature of the individual organs.

Haemorrhages in different organs, on mucocutaneous surfaces, and on serous membranes can occur in a number of diseases, one of which is the shock syndrome, where they are quite frequently found. The exact mechanism of the haemorrhages is not clear but the restricted, rather than generalized, distribution suggests that apart from thrombocytopenia, hypofibrinogenaemia, and fibrinolysis probably some local factors are also important in their pathogenesis.

The brain

Shock lesions in the brain are relatively rare, being present in 6.8 per cent of fatal shock cases, in comparison to the incidence of lesions in the lung, liver, heart, and kidneys. However, sometimes they may lead to the patient's death or, in case of recovery, serious neurological or psychological disturbances. The relative rarity of brain injury in shock could be attributed to the highly efficient autoregulatory mechanism that ensures a constant cerebral blood flow within an arterial pressure range from 65 to 140 mm Hg. The cerebral blood flow falls if arterial pressure goes below 65 mm Hg. The rate of blood flow also depends on the cerebrovascular resistance, which is determined by the intracranial pressure (normally 5 mm Hg), the tone of the smooth muscle in the vessel wall, and the viscosity of the blood. An increase of the intracranial pressure above 45 mm Hg leads to a decrease of the cerebral blood flow. In shock, when the systemic arterial pressure drops below the critical level, the compensatory autoregulatory mechanism of cerebral blood flow fails. This results in cerebral hypoperfusion, ischaemic hypoxia of the neural tissue, and the consequence is *hypoxic brain damage*. In severe cases this may be associated with 'cytotoxic' cerebral oedema which, through increased intracranial pressure, can reduce further the cerebral perfusion. The likelihood of developing shock-induced brain damage is greater in older patients with cerebrovascular atherosclerosis. The lesions of *hypoxic brain damage* characteristically occur in certain parts of the brain that are particularly vulnerable to ischaemia. Thus, lesions of hypoxic damage are usually found in the *border zones* (watershed zones) of major cerebral arterial territories (Fig. 7.37), in the *hippocampus*, in the *basal ganglia*, and in the *cerebellum*. The boundary zones are between the territories of the anterior and middle cerebral arteries, the posterior and middle cerebral arteries, the superior cerebellar and posterior inferior cerebellar arteries. The severity of the lesions varies from focal damage and *loss of neurones*, as seen microscopically, to frank *infarcts* visible at gross examination. In *infants* certain brain-stem nuclei may show increased susceptibility to hypoxia, and brain-stem necrosis has been described.

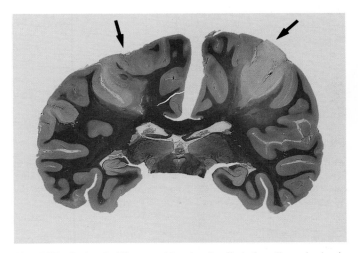

Fig. 7.37 Brain of a 52-year-old male who died of cardiogenic shock, illustrating bilateral watershed infarcts (arrows). Celloidin embedding, Luxol fast blue-cresyl violet. (Courtesy of Dr R. O. Barnard.)

Microscopical examination of the neurons in the Sommer's sector of the hippocampus (Fig. 7.38), the Purkinje cells of the cerebellum, and the neurones of the third and fourth cortical layers of the cerebral hemispheres reveals features of ischaemic injury. In the early stage following hypoxic damage there is cytoplasmic vacuolation, followed by shrinkage of the cytoplasm and nucleus. Eventually the cytoplasm becomes pale, homogenized, and karyopyknosis occurs. These changes can be observed between 2–18 hours following the hypoxic episode. After 24 hours reactive changes may be noticed in the astrocytes, microglia, and endothelial cells. Finally the necrotic neurones disappear and within a few days reactive changes become prominent. If the hypoperfusion is severe enough, then

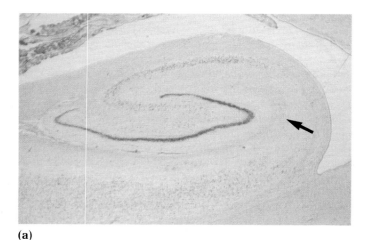

(a)

(b)

Fig. 7.38 (a) Hippocampus from a 16-year-old girl who died of septic shock, showing severe loss of neurons in the Sommer's sector (arrow). (b) Normal hippocampus, for comparison, with normal cellularity. (Courtesy of Dr R. O. Barnard.)

not only *selective neuronal necrosis* but *infarction*, where the necrosis affects not only the neurones but the glia and the blood vessels, occurs. Infarction can be noticed on *gross examination*. Anaemic infarcts become macroscopically visible only after 18–24 hours. The infarcted area in the cortex is usually confined to a few gyri but may extend into the white matter. Histological examination of the infarct reveals cell necrosis which is sometimes associated with haemorrhage and fibrin thrombi in some of the venules.

These lesions are not specific for shock. Similar lesions affecting the border zones may occur whenever the perfusion of these areas is compromised (e.g. following cardiac surgery, ligation of the common carotid artery, obstruction of the calcarine artery when it is compressed against the tentorium by tumour or cerebral oedema).

The heart

The heart is the principal organ affected in the development of

cardiogenic shock, as well as a frequent site of secondary shock lesions in all major types of shock. McGovern and Tiller (1980) found cardiac shock lesions in 204 (36.6 per cent) of 557 post-mortems in patients dying of shock other than cardiogenic shock. After the lung, the heart is the most common site where shock lesions can be found at post-mortem examination. Lesions in the heart are more common in patients with cardiogenic and hypovolaemic shock than in cases of septic shock. At post-mortem examination of patients dying of shock, the heart often shows petechial *haemorrhages* in the epicardium. Sub-endocardial haemorrhages may occur, most commonly in the left ventricle. Haemorrhage into the bundle of His is also well documented and could be responsible for the cardiac arrythmias and conduction blocks that often occur.

Necrosis of myocardial fibres or fibres of the conducting system is the other major type of lesion that can occur during shock. This is usually not a regional type infarct in the territory supplied by one major coronary artery but the diffuse form of necrosis due to the inadequate overall myocardial perfusion. The extent of the diffuse type of infarction can vary from microscopical foci of necrosis to extensive circumferential subendocardial infarction, especially if there is left ventricular hypertrophy (Fig. 7.39). In severe cases the right ventricular muscle may also be affected. Patients with coronary atherosclerosis are more susceptible than those without to the development of necrosis during shock. However, myocardial necrosis of a varying extent can occur as a result of shock in patients with no evidence of any coronary artery disease. The diffuse type of necrosis is not specific for shock, as has been observed in cases of high-grade coronary stenosis and in association with hyperkalaemia and high levels of circulating catecholamines. Depending on the extent and the age of the necrosis it may be seen on gross examination, but more frequently it becomes apparent only on histological study. The microscopical forms of the necrosis include myocytolysis, contraction band necrosis (Fig. 7.40), and coagulative necrosis.

In *cardiogenic shock* due to myocardial infarction additional

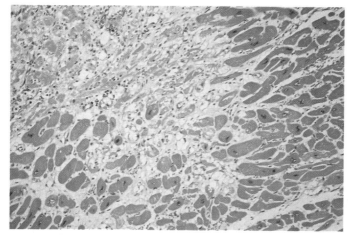

Fig. 7.39 Focal myocardial necrosis in a 48-year-old man who died of hypovolaemic shock.

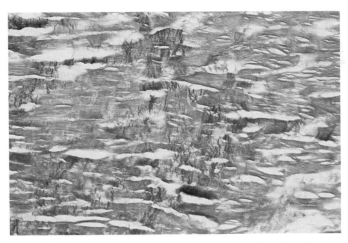

Fig. 7.40 Contraction band necrosis of the myocardium in a 38-year-old man who died of septic shock. Darkly staining vertical lines of hypercontracted segments are seen.

necrosis may develop as a consequence of reduced perfusion due to the initial shock episode, and the vicious circle of shock–necrosis–shock frequently leads to death. Histological examination of the heart in such cases reveals scattered additional foci of infarction varying in age and often at sites remote from the original infarct. Sometimes a regional transmural infarct causing shock can be followed by an extensive additional subendocardial infarct. Cardiogenic shock subsequent to cardiac surgery often results in foci of contraction band necrosis mainly in a subendocardial location. This type of necrosis can also be seen adjacent to coagulative necrosis of a massive regional infarct. In McGovern's series, 55.7 per cent of patients dying after elective cardiopulmonary bypass surgery had shock lesions in the heart, most frequently involving the interventricular septum and the conduction system.

In *hypovolaemic shock* the survival of the patients following blood loss depends on the volume of blood lost and the time which elapses before the blood volume is replaced. Patients who do not respond to restoration of blood volume are often in cardiogenic shock due to foci of myocardial necrosis resulting from the initial haemorrhagic shock. Shock lesions in the heart are present in the majority of the cases at necropsy in patients dying within 2–3 days after the onset of hypovolaemic shock.

In patients dying of *septic shock* cardiac lesions were present in only 17 per cent of the cases described by McGovern and Tiller (1980). However, dysrhythmias before death were much more frequent in these patients, indicating that the cardiac function had been disturbed.

The lungs

The development of *adult respiratory distress syndrome* (ARDS) is one of the most common (50.3 per cent in McGovern's series) and often fatal complications of shock. This was first recognized in war casualties and has been given various names, such as traumatic wet lung, Da Nang lung, post-traumatic pulmonary

insufficiency, congestive atelectasis, progressive pulmonary consolidation, and shock lung. (Later it became clear that shock is only one among the numerous other causes of ARDS (see Chapter 13).) ARDS can develop not only after traumatic shock but following hypovolaemic, septic, and cardiogenic shock as well. It is relatively common in septic shock and rare in pure hypovolaemic shock without trauma.

Most of the patients with ARDS require oxygen therapy; however, it is known, mainly from animal experiments, that oxygen can have a direct toxic effect on the lung and it is therefore difficult to distinguish changes that are due to oxygen from those that are the result of the initial injury.

Clinically ARDS is a form of acute respiratory failure characterized by severe refractory hypoxaemia and falling pulmonary compliance with an increasing shunt fraction, which leads to dyspnoea, tachypnoea, and cyanosis in a spontaneously breathing patient. Usually there are bilateral pulmonary infiltrates on chest X-ray.

Macroscopically the shock lung is bulky, moderately firm, almost rubbery in consistency and petechial haemorrhages are often present beneath the pleura. The weight of the lung is increased to 3 or 4 times normal, often 1000 g each. On sectioning, the lung is oedematous and the escaping fluid is blood-stained. There is lack of aeration but areas of collapse are distinctly uncommon.

Microscopically the findings are those of *diffuse alveolar damage* (DAD) the features of which are different in early, subacute, or late phase of the disease. In the initial stage of the development of alveolar damage the changes can be appreciated only at ultrastructural level unless there is direct traumatic lung injury, such as contusion of the chest wall or blast injury. Leucostasis with accumulation of polymorphonuclear leucocytes that show partial degranulation is seen in the capillary bed. The polymorphs also show a tendency to infiltrate the interstitium. The degranulation of polymorphs leads to liberation of proteolytic enzymes and oxygen free radicals, causing damage to the endothelial cells, which show cytoplasmic swelling and necrosis. All these changes are accompanied by interstitial oedema and defective development of surfactant in type 2 pneumocytes. Necrosis of membranous pneumocytes (type 1 pneumocytes) occurs later and subsequently the morphological alterations become clearly visible on light microscopical examination.

The first week of the lung injury is the *acute or exudative stage,* characterized by exudation, and interstitial and intra-alveolar oedema with haemorrhage and hyaline membrane formation. In the first three days, interstitial and intra-alveolar oedema and varying degrees of intra-alveolar haemorrhage with fibrin deposition dominate the histological picture. The oedema and haemorrhages are not confined to the dependent parts of the lung, as they occur on a non-cardiogenic basis. Pulmonary haemorrhages may be particularly severe in septic shock but are less common in hypovolaemic shock.

Hyaline membranes are formed from the first day but become most prominent 3–7 days following the injury (Fig. 7.41). This signifies the necrosis and sloughing of the membranous (type 1) pneumocytes with varying degrees of denudation of the

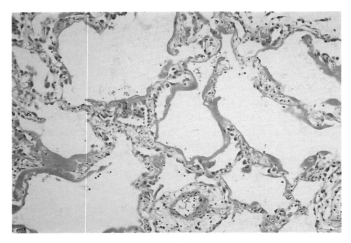

Fig. 7.41 Diffuse alveolar damage with hyaline membranes lining the alveolar spaces in a 50-year-old man who died of septic shock.

alveolar basement membrane. Microscopically, the hyaline membrane is a deeply eosinophilic, homogeneous material attached to the denuded alveolar wall. Ultrastructurally, it is composed of cell debris from necrotic type 1 cells mixed with fibrin and other proteinaceous material.

Fibrin thrombi may be seen in some of the alveolar capillaries and small pulmonary vessels. However, the incidence of microthrombi found in the lungs at autopsy varies greatly and they are not present in all the cases.

Alveolar lining cell hyperplasia develops 3–7 days following injury and persists throughout the organizing stage of DAD. This hyperplasia is the result of type 2 (granular) pneumocyte proliferation and appears as regularly spaced cuboidal cells along the alveolar wall. The proliferation of type 2 cells represents a reparative phenomenon, as they replace the sloughed type 1 cells and have the capacity to differentiate into type 1 cells in the recovery phase.

Interstitial inflammatory cell infiltrate, composed of lymphocytes, plasma cells, histiocytes, and a variable number of polymorphonuclear leucocytes, becomes prominent in the second week when organization develops.

The organizing stage of DAD is characterized by organization of hyaline membranes with associated interstitial and focal intraalveolar fibrosis. Phagocytosis of intra-alveolar debris and detached fragments of hyalin membrane by alveolar macrophages is common. The interstitial fibrosis, type 2 pneumocyte hyperplasia, and incorporation of organizing hyaline membrane into the alveolar septae result in varying degree of thickening of alveolar wall. Although local fibrosis has been observed as early as three days following pulmonary injury, the fibrosis becomes prominent after about one week. In addition to fibrosis in the alveolar wall, a small degree of peribronchial fibrosis may also be seen. In fatal cases, fibrosis may progress for several weeks, with restructuring of the lung parenchyma and formation of honeycomb lung. Animal experiments have shown that

the damage to the lung parenchyma will heal completely only as long as the basal membrane remains intact. However, in the majority of human cases damage to the basal membrane occurs, which explains why shock-induced pulmonary fibrosis cannot heal completely as far as the structure and the function of the lung is concerned. The mortality rate associated with DAD averages 50 per cent, with rates ranging from 10 to 90 per cent, depending on the severity and the cause of the lung injury.

The kidneys

Patients with shock frequently show evidence of *acute renal failure* (ARF), with a sudden deterioration of renal function characterized by rapid rise in blood urea and creatinine, with associated fluid overload, hyperkalaemia, and acidosis. In most cases there is oliguria and rarely anuria, although a nonoliguric variant of ARF has been recognized. The likely cause of ARF in shock is hypoperfusion (ischaemia) of the kidney, possibly with an additional toxic component in the cases of septic shock.

The main pathological changes in patients with ARF are in the renal tubules in the form of *tubular necrosis*. This was seen by McGovern and Tiller (1980) in 159 (21.1 per cent) of 754 autopsies on shock subjects. Rare types of shock lesions in the kidney include *cortical necrosis* and *microthrombi* in the glomerular capillaries.

On *gross examination* the kidneys may be enlarged, with a floppy consistency in cases of tubular necrosis. The dark, congested medulla is usually in a rather sharp contrast to the widened, pale cortex.

Microscopically, the glomeruli show no significant abnormality, though minor alterations, such as dilatation of the Bowman's space and tubularization of the Bowman's capsule epithelium, have been demonstrated. The most obvious changes of *tubular necrosis* occur in the distal convoluted tubules: the tubular lumen is dilated and lined by low epithelial cells showing regenerative features, including some mitotic figures (Fig. 7.42). Focal losses of tubular epithelial cells are also present, but frank coagulative necrosis of the tubular epithelium, as in heavy-metal poisoning, is not seen. Regenerative changes usually occur only after a few days. At an early stage, without the features of regeneration, the histological recognition of tubular necrosis can be difficult, especially in autolytic autopsy material. The presence of pigmented, granular, or hyaline casts in the tubular lumen is characteristic. The tubules also contain myoglobin in cases of crush syndrome.

Bilateral cortical necrosis is a very rare manifestation of shock. It is usually bilateral and it may be partial or complete. The extent of the necrosis can vary from minute lesions affecting a few glomeruli and tubules to gross cortical necrosis where the cortex is almost entirely necrotic with the exception of a narrow surviving area under the capsule. Histologically the extent of the necrosis may vary in different areas, affecting glomeruli, tubules, and blood vessels. *Microthrombi* composed of platelets and fibrin, as a result of intravascular coagulation, may be present in the glomerular capillaries, but their occurrence in shock is rare.

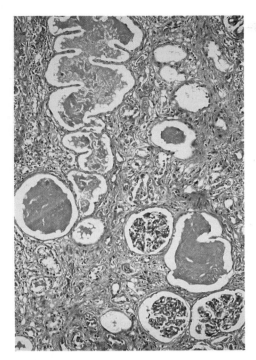

Fig. 7.42 Severe acute tubular necrosis of the kidney due to traumatic shock, showing markedly dilated tubules that are filled by casts. The tubular epithelium is flattened and focally damaged.

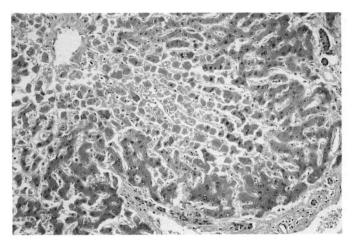

Fig. 7.43 Centrilobular necrosis of liver in a patient who died of cardiogenic shock. The periportal parenchyma is preserved.

The liver

Severe hypoperfusion of the liver during shock leads to alterations in the hepatocyte. In the early phase of shock there are no visible lesions in the liver on histological examination, nor are there clinical symptoms of liver injury. *Ultrastructural examination*, however, reveals significant changes in the liver cells, even in biopsies taken two hours after the primary injury. At this stage the cellular alterations are reversible and include clumping of the nuclear chromatin, dilatation of the endoplasmic reticulum, and condensation or swelling of mitochondria and hypoxic vacuoles at the cell periphery. If preventative measures are not introduced for three or four hours following the onset of shock, flocculant densities of the mitochondria, the hallmarks of irreversible injury, occur as a result of calcium accumulation.

Eventually severe hypoperfusion leads to hepatocellular death. At this stage *light microscopical examination* reveals *sinusoidal dilatation* and *congestion with zonal necroses*. The necrosis usually affects acinar zone 3 but sometimes it may extend to acinar zone 2, and occasionally it is limited to the latter zone. The necrosis usually provokes no inflammatory reaction, but occasionally neutrophils, mononuclear cells, and pigmented macrophages may be present in the affected areas. The necrosis is accompanied by condensation of the reticulin framework. The periportal areas remain normal (Fig. 7.43). In prolonged cases regenerative changes may occur in the residual parenchyma. The hepatic necrotic lesions of shock are usually asymmetrical in zone 3 regions, in contrast to the symmetrical lesions of congestive cardiac failure. In the series of McGovern and Tiller (1980) the incidence of liver cell necroses were 46.1 per cent in hypovolaemic shock, 56.3 per cent in cardiogenic shock, and 32 per cent in septic shock. Fatty change has also been observed in patients who survived more than 18 hours.

The likelihood of developing *liver failure* in shock depends not only on the extent of the necrosis but also whether there was any pre-existing liver disease, such as cirrhosis. The cirrhotic liver is particularly prone to anoxic necrosis when there is bleeding from oesophageal varices. The nodules of cirrhosis are probably poorly oxygenated as a result of abnormal vascular relations and shunting of the portal blood, and a fall in hepatic artery pressure during shock may lead to necrosis. Therefore patients with hepatic cirrhosis are more prone to develop liver failure in shock syndrome.

The pancreas

Shock lesions occur relatively rarely in the pancreas. McGovern and Tiller (1980) found pancreatitis in only 6.4 per cent of 754 autopsies for shock syndrome. However, hypoperfusion of the human pancreas may result in *necrosis* of the exocrine acinar cells. The extent of the necrosis varies from small *focal lesions* to extensive *haemorrhagic pancreatitis*. On one hand, acute haemorrhagic pancreatitis may be a manifestation of shock and, on the other, it may be the cause of it. The pathological picture is identical. Shock-related injury of the pancreatic islets of Langerhans has also been observed in newborn and young infants.

The gastrointestinal tract

Disorders of the alimentary system including oesophageal rupture, gastric and duodenal ulcers, pancreatitis, and necrosis of the intestine may cause hypovolaemic or septic shock. Conversely, shock of different aetiologies can cause lesions in the gastrointestinal tract. McGovern (1984) reported the incidence of shock lesions affecting the gastrointestinal tract as 8.8 per cent, 16.2 per cent, and 26 per cent at post-mortem examination in patients dying of hypovolaemic, cardiogenic, and septic shock, respectively. *Gastric and duodenal erosions* and *ischaemic bowel disease* are the most frequent complications of shock, but occasional cases of *acalculous cholecystitis* have also been described in association with shock. The pathogenesis of these lesions can be explained on the basis of hypoperfusion or direct endotoxin damage. In shock there is vasoconstriction of the splanchnic vessels and the low perfusion state may lead to ischaemic changes in the gastrointestinal tract. There is strong evidence that the splanchnic vasospastic response to shock is mediated by the renin–angiotensin axis. In the stomach and duodenum *petechial haemorrhages, erosions,* and *acute ulcers* may occur, but these are non-specific as similar lesions can occur in response to stress of other kinds or in association with Cushing's disease, therapeutic administration of adrenocorticosteroids, lesions of the hypothalamus, or the Curling's ulcers following extensive cutaneous burns, which are believed to result from stimulation of the pituitary–hypothalamic axis.

Ischaemic bowel disease may involve both the small and the large intestines in the form of ischaemic necrosis. The extent of the necrosis depends on the state of the blood vessels, anatomy of the blood supply, duration of the hypoxic episode, and the bacterial population in the lumen of the bowel. Diseases other than shock, such as occlusive atherosclerosis, thromboembolism, and vasculitis, can cause similar necrotizing lesions in the intestine. The jejunum, ileum, the splenic flexure, and the descending colon are most frequently affected but the whole large intestine, including the rectum, may also be involved. Severe cases present as surgical emergencies. Macroscopically the bowel is dilated, darkly congested with oedematous mucosa and friable wall. The lumen is usually filled by altered blood, and superficial or deep ulcerations of the mucosa, or even perforation of the wall, may occur. Histologically, *necrosis* can be seen, sometimes affecting only the superficial portion of the mucosa, while in severe cases the full thickness of the wall may be necrotic (Fig. 7.44). In this acute stage the mucosa shows disrupted, necrotic crypts and haemorrhage in the lamina propria, and only a sparse infiltrate of neutrophil polymorphs. *Fibrin thrombi* in the mucosal and submucosal capillaries are frequent. Later, polymorphs become more numerous and ulceration due to sloughing of the mucosa occur. Colonization of the mucosa and submucosa by bacteria can be observed, which can lead to septicaemia. Necrotizing lesions of the intestine are often responsible for the irreversibility of shock and for the death of the patient.

Limited forms of ischaemic lesions may be followed by a reparative phase with chronic inflammation and fibrosis, which often result in ischaemic *strictures* of the intestine.

The pituitary

Circulatory disturbances of shock may lead to *necrosis* or *haemorrhage* in the pituitary. Small foci of necrosis are not infrequent findings in unselected autopsies and have been observed

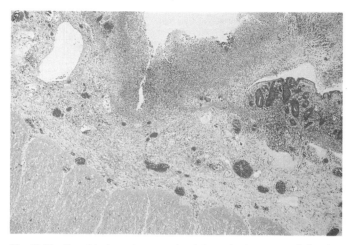

Fig. 7.44 Focal ischaemic necrosis of the colonic mucosa following hypovolaemic shock. The muscularis propria is not affected.

in 1–8 per cent of cases by both Kovacs (1969, 1972) and Plaut (1952). Sheehan and Davis (1968) noted that their occurrence in shock, especially in obstetric (post-partum) shock, is even more frequent. Haemorrhage of the pituitary or its extreme form, pituitary apoplexy, is extremely rare in shock, unless there is an associated head injury or a pituitary neoplasm. The pathogenesis of pituitary infarction is not entirely clear in shock; however, ischaemia, as a result of hypoperfusion, has a major role.

Microscopically, pituitary infarction is seen as coagulative necrosis, which may affect the entire or only a portion of the adenohypophysis. The stalk and the posterior lobe are less frequently involved.

Interestingly, destruction of the adenohypophysis does not produce clinical symptoms unless more than 90 per cent of the functional parenchyma is destroyed (Kovacs 1969). If the stalk and posterior lobe are affected, then diabetes insipidus might develop. Pituitary necrosis heals with fibrous scarring and, as cells of the adenohypophysis are not capable of significant regeneration, in cases of extensive damage permanent hypopituitarism may occur. Necrosis of the pituitary occurs not only in shock but has been observed following head injury, after the stalk of the pituitary has been transected, in cases of increased intracranial pressure, and in patients who required ventilation for a variety of diseases.

The adrenals

The adrenals may show morphological changes in all major types of shock. In McGovern and Tiller's (1980) post-mortem series of patients dying due to shock the frequency of adrenal lesions was 14.1 per cent. Interestingly, the plasma corticosteroid and adrenaline levels are usually elevated in shock in spite of the damage to the adrenal. The reason for this is that damage is usually focal, and even in fulminant cases of Waterhouse–Friderichsen syndrome the cause of death is septic shock rather than adrenal insufficiency.

The lesions of the adrenal that may be associated with shock are *lipid depletion*, *degenerative changes*, *haemorrhage*, *necrosis*, and *fibrin thrombi*. These lesions are not specific for shock and they have been observed in other conditions as well. In most cases the shock lesions are bilateral but occasionally only one gland is involved. Their distribution may differ in young children and adults.

Lipid depletion of the cortical cells is the most frequent but the least specific alteration, since it occurs with stress and trauma. Histologically, it is characterized by the presence of compact cells occupying the zona fasciculata at the expense of the lipid-filled clear cells. In adults the lipid depletion is focal and segmental, while in young children it is usually diffuse. Cytolytic *degenerative changes* of the zona fasciculata may be seen in addition to lipid depletion, which results in breaking up the outer portion of the zona fasciculata with the formation of spaces between the remaining cells' columns.

Adrenal haemorrhage can occur not only in the Waterhouse–Friderichsen syndrome due to meningococcal septicaemia but also in association with other infections or trauma, or as a complication of burns, pregnancy, leukaemia, and hypertension. *Necrosis* may be associated with the haemorrhage, but it sometimes occurs without haemorrhage.

In severe cases of haemorrhagic adrenal (adrenal apoplexy) the haemorrhage is centred on the reticular plexus and the medulla is pushed aside, with a varying extent of corticomedullary infarction.

Frequently, the haemorrhage ruptures through the adrenal cortex to form an extracapsular haematoma. In children younger than six months old, the haemorrhagic necrosis is mainly localized to the fetal cortex but extension into the definitive cortex may occur. In older children the focal haemorrhage and necrosis is most prominent in the zona fasciculata but may involve the full thickness of the cortex. Infiltration by polymorphonuclear leucocytes can also occur, especially adjacent to necrotic areas. In adults the pattern is similar to that found in older children, but corticomedullary infarcts and focal cortical infarcts with or without haemorrhage can also occur. *Thrombi* can be present in the central vein or in its branches.

The exact mechanism of adrenal haemorrhage and necrosis in shock is not clear, but diminished perfusion and endotoxin damage are likely to be the most important pathogenetic factors.

7.7.3 Bibliography

Ashbaugh, D., Bigelow, D., Petty, T., and Levine, B. (1967). Acute respiratory distress in adults. *Lancet* 1, 319–23.

Bailey, R. W., Bulkley, G. B., Hamilton, S. R., Morris, J. B., Haglund, U. H., and Meilahn, J. E. (1987). The fundamental hemodynamic mechanism underlying gastric 'stress ulceration' in cardiogenic shock. *Annals of Surgery* 205, 597–612.

Blaisdell, F. (1974). Pathophysiology of the respiratory distress syndrome. *Archives of Surgery* 108, 44–9.

Corrin, B. (1980). Lung pathology in septic shock. *Journal of Clinical Pathology* 33, 891–4.

Cowley, R. A., Hankins, J. R., Jones, R. T., and Trump, B. F. (1982). Pathology and pathophysiology of the liver. In *Pathophysiology of shock, anoxia and ischaemia* (ed. R. A. Cowley and B. Trump), pp. 285–301. Williams and Wilkins, Baltimore.

Fallat, R. J., Mielke, C. H., and Rodvien, R. (1980). Adult respiratory distress syndrome and Gram-negative sepsis: a deadly duo. *Archives of Internal Medicine (Chicago)* 140, 612–13.

Janzer, R. C. and Friede, R. L. (1980). Hypotensive brain stem necrosis or cardiac arrest encephalopathy? *Acta Neuropathologica (Berlin)* 50, 53–6.

Keren, A., Klein, J., and Stern, S. (1980). Adult respiratory distress syndrome in the course of acute myocardial infarction. *Chest* 77, 161–4.

Kovacs, K. (1969). Necrosis of anterior pituitary in humans I and II. *Neuroendocrinology* 4, 170–241.

Kovacs, K. (1972). Adenohypophysial necrosis in routine autopsies. *Endokrinologie* 60, 309–16.

Lawson, A. and Bihari, D. (1988). The clinical presentation and diagnosis of the adult respiratory distress syndrome. In *Shock and the adult respiratory distress syndrome* (ed. W. Kox and D. Bihari), pp. 225–34. Springer-Verlag, London.

Lefkowitch, J. H. and Mendez, L. (1986). Morphologic features of hepatic injury in cardiac disease and shock. *Journal of Hepatology (Amsterdam)* 2, 313–27.

McGovern, V. J. (1984). Shock revisited. *Pathology Annual* 19, 15–36.

McGovern, V. J. and Tiller, D. J. (1980). *Shock. A clinicopathological correlation*. Masson, New York.

Morrison, D. C. and Ryan, J. (1987). Endotoxin and disease mechanisms. *Annual Review of Medicine* 38, 417–32.

Page, D. L., Caulfield, J. B., Kastor, J. A., De Sanctis, R. B., and Sanders, C. A. (1971). Myocardial changes associated with cardiogenic shock. *New England Journal of Medicine* 285, 133–7.

Plaut, A. (1952). Pituitary necrosis in routine necropsies. *American Journal of Pathology (Philadelphia)* 28, 883–99.

Remmele, W. and Harms, D. (1969). Zur pathologischen Anatomie des Kreislaufshocks beim Menschen. I. Mikrothrombose der peripheren Blutgefasse. *Klinische Wochenschrift (Berlin)* 46, 352–7.

Schlag, G. and Redl, H. (1988). The morphology of adult respiratory distress syndrome. In *Shock and the adult respiratory distress syndrome* (ed. W. Kox and D. Bihari), pp. 21–31. Springer-Verlag, London.

Sheehan, H. L. (1965). The repair of post-partum necrosis of the anterior lobe of the pituitary gland. *Acta Endocrinologica (Copenhagen)* 48, 40–60.

Sheehan, H. L. and Davis, J. C. (1968). Pituitary necrosis. *British Medical Bulletin* 24, 59–70.

Todd, J. K. (1985). Staphylococcal toxin syndromes. *Annual Review of Medicine* 36, 337–47.

Tracey, K. J., Lowry, S. F., and Cerami, A. (1988). Cachectin: A hormone that triggers acute shock and chronic cachexia. *Journal of Infectious Diseases* 157, 413–20.

8

Cell growth, size, and differentiation

8

Cell growth, size, and differentiation

8.1 Introduction

Nicholas A. Wright

In this chapter we consider some aspects of the basic mechanisms by which cell population size is controlled, and then go on to discuss conditions where cells and cell populations react to altered circumstances by increasing or reducing their cell number, or by varying the size of individual cells. Most of the tissues of the body are plastic in this way, and these cellular events are pivotal in the understanding of the reasons underlying many pathological events.

8.2 The control of cell proliferation

Nicholas A. Wright

We have already, to some extent, considered the ways in which mammalian cells reproduce, their cell cycle, and the spatial and hierarchical organization of tissues in Section 1.1.5, and discussed pathways and mechanisms of differentiation in Section 1.1.4. However, the phenomenology of the cell cycle tells us little of how the rate of cell proliferation, and consequently the rate of cell production, is controlled.

If we refer to the familiar classical cell cycle model (Fig. 1.70), we will see that cells pass clockwise around the cycle; during the S-phase they synthesize DNA, and two new individuals are produced at mitosis. As far as control of this process goes, it is generally considered that, once committed to DNA synthesis, mammalian cells will in fact complete mitosis and contribute to cell production. There is little evidence for cells stopping or resting during DNA synthesis, and while there may be considerable variation in the rate at which cells traverse the G_2-phase, mammalian cells are again not generally considered to leave the cell cycle during this phase, unlike the position in plant cells.

It follows that any physiological control point should therefore be detected before the onset of DNA synthesis; Fig. 1.70 suggests that, during the G_1-phase, cells have to 'decide' upon three options—to re-enter the cell cycle (to *recycle*), to enter a quiescent phase of G_0, from which, if conditions are appropriate, they can return to the cell cycle, or to terminally differentiate and lose for ever the ability to reproduce. Why do we believe that this 'critical control point' is in the G_1-phase? Well, one good reason has already been mentioned, and is displayed in Fig. 5.31. When two-thirds of the liver is removed, for a short time there is no evidence of compensatory cell division; then we have the phenomenon of hepatocytes entering first DNA synthesis, as evidenced by a rise in the labelling index, and then proceeding through to mitosis, shown by the later rise in the mitotic index. Thus resting liver cells, a classical conditional renewal population as defined in Section 1.3, have been ejected from G_0 into the G_1-phase. Moreover, cells which terminally differentiate, such as suprabasal keratinocytes in the epidermis, and villus epithelial cells (called enterocytes) in the small intestine, differentiate with a G_1, or diploid DNA content, and so have left the cell cycle in the G_1-phase. Thus it is to G_1 that we should look for controlling mechanisms.

While we cannot yet explain in detail the molecular mechanisms responsible for the cells recycling or decycling, we are beginning to obtain a good idea. It is clear that cell cycle progression is genetically controlled: a set of genes can be identified, by differential cDNA hybridization, which are expressed during the G_0 to G_1 transition and which accumulate and decay rapidly after stimulation of quiescent cells. In late G_1, shortly before the onset of DNA synthesis, there is transcription of genes encoding DNA synthesizing enzymes, such as the DNA polymerases and thymidine kinase. As we shall see in Chapter 9, many of the cellular oncogenes described in recent years are transcribed during the cell cycle or as early events in the stimulation of conditional renewal systems such as the liver. It is becoming increasing clear that many oncogenes encode for growth factors or parts of growth factors, for growth factor receptors, or for nuclear transcription factors: the *sis* gene product is the β-chain of platelet-derived growth factor (PDGF) itself, and the *erb B* gene encodes for a truncated epidermal growth factor receptor molecule. The *fos* gene and the *jun* gene are activated by many peptide growth factors: *fos* probably acts as a third messenger, associating cytoplasmic signals with nuclear transcription events; it interacts with p39, the *jun* oncoprotein, to stimulate DNA transcription, and growth signals given to cells result in increased synthesis of *jun*- and *fos*-related proteins.

We have made the point that many tissues respond to pathological conditions by increasing or reducing cell production, so evidently cells can 'sense' the need to augment or decrease the proliferative rate. The ways in which cell populations do this are straightforward, and can be derived from Fig. 1.70; cells can be recruited from a resting G_0 pool, if such is available, as in the liver or kidney. However, in renewing populations, for example the epidermis or intestine, there are few or no G_0 cells, and increases in cell production are initiated in one of two ways— shortening the time taken to complete mitosis (a reduction in the cell-cycle time), or an increase in number of cells in the cell cycle, usually called the proliferating population. An illustrative example from human pathology is the epidermis in psoriasis (Fig. 8.1), a common skin disease. In normal human epidermis, cells divide about once every 200 h, but in psoriasis the cell-cycle time is reduced to less than 50 h. In addition, while proliferating cells in normal epidermis are confined to the basal layer, in psoriasis there may be as many as three or four layers of proliferating cells, as the proliferating population or compartment is expanded. Thus cell production is materially increased in this so-called 'proliferative skin disease'. A similar proliferative situation is seen in the hyperproliferative crypts of coeliac disease (Fig. 8.2). Conversely, when we consider hypoplasia,

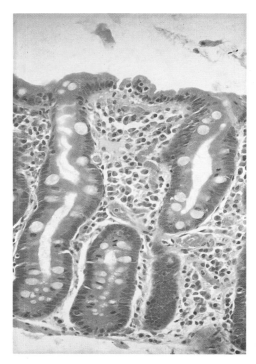

Fig. 8.2 Hyperplastic small intestinal crypts in coeliac disease. The crypts are markedly enlarged and show increased mitotic activity.

for example in the small intestine after intestinal bypass surgery, crypts are small, produced by a lengthening of the cell-cycle time and a reduction in the proliferating compartment.

Even in normal tissues, with normal cell production rates, there will be some constraints on the rates of cell proliferation and differentiation. Until comparatively recently, concepts of how this control was exerted were nebulous in the extreme. Now, however, it is clear that cells can not only receive signals to increase proliferation, or to stop proliferating and differentiate, but can also send such signals. These signals are small protein or polypeptide molecules called *growth factors*.

8.2.1 Growth factors

Figure 8.3 displays the now familiar diagrammatic representation, originated by Sporn and Todaro, of the three ways in which cells can co-ordinate signals for growth responses. Classical *endocrine secretion* is where cells secrete a hormone directly into a blood-vessel; the hormone then acts on target cells, usually at some distance from the source—a suitable example is where androgen or oestrogen from the gonads induce growth responses in the prostate/seminal vesicles or endometrium. However, the immune system can be regarded as a *mobile endocrine system*, targeted to specific sites as required, capable of producing whole families of *cytokines*, many of which induce or repress growth. *Paracrine secretion* occurs where an appropriate cell produces a peptide, while the receptors for the peptide are localized on other cells adjacent to the secreting cell. The usual examples given are several families of neuro-endocrine cells in

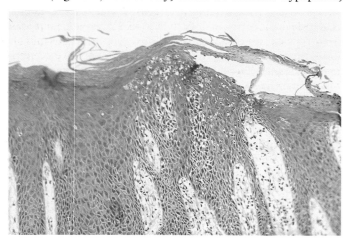

Fig. 8.1 The hyperplastic human epidermis in psoriasis. Note the elongation of the rete pegs.

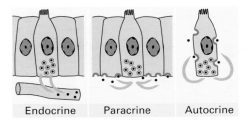

Endocrine   Paracrine   Autocrine

Fig. 8.3 A diagrammatic representation of autocrine, paracrine, and endocrine secretion. Growth factors are indicated as granules within the cells, and receptors are shown by semicircular areas on the cell membrane. (Drawn after Sporn and Roberts 1990, with permission.)

the gastrointestinal tract which produce multiple locally acting peptides, some of which undoubtedly influence growth. The third mechanism is the *autocrine loop*, where the same cell produces both a growth factor and has receptors for that growth factor, thus producing self-stimulation or inhibition. The archetypal example is where small cell ('oat cell') carcinoma cells secrete *bombesin*, and *themselves bear bombesin receptors*: it is possible to inhibit cell proliferation in these cells with monoclonal antibodies against bombesin, showing that the peptide is responsible for maintaining cell proliferation in this system. These well-established ideas may have to be modified in the light of recent work on the interactions of growth factors with classical hormones such as growth hormone, ACTH, and oestrogens. For example, the multifunctional polypeptide *transforming growth factor-β* (TGF-β) is induced by oestrogen, and can also regulate regular oestrogen synthesis in the ovary, and the interrelationships of these controlling factors have yet to be determined.

There are now several recognized growth factor families: Table 8.1 displays the major groups. It is quite fascinating that, in almost every case, the type of action exerted by the growth factor is far greater than suspected initially. For example, *epidermal growth factor* (EGF) was first detected by its action in advancing eyelid opening in neonatal mice, and is now known not only to be a major mitogen for many cell lineages, but also to induce differentiation and to have other non-related actions such as stimulating muscular contraction and inhibiting gastric-acid secretion. Further examples are the *interleukins* (IL): IL-1 produces effects on cells as diverse as keratinocytes, fibroblasts, astrocytes, and chondrocytes, while IL-6, in addition to controlling growth and differentiation in B-lymphocytes, regulates protein synthesis in hepatocytes and neurone-like chromaffin cells. Conversely, peptides such as TGF-β, isolated from non-immune cells, have immunoregulatory actions: TGF-β is 10 000 times more potent than cyclosporin A as a suppressor of T-lymphocyte function, while IL-6 itself is produced by fibroblasts, yet regulates immunoglobulin secretion by B-lymphocytes.

The effects of growth factors on cells are largely determined by the circumstances in question. TGF-β is inhibitory to fibroblast growth in the presence of EGF, but stimulates cell division when platelet-derived growth factor (PDGF) is present; TGF-β stimulates fibroblast growth in the early embryo, but inhibits

Table 8.1 The major growth factor families

EGF family
  EGF
  TGFα
  Pox virus growth factors
  Amphiregulin

Platelet-derived growth factor

Insulin-like growth factors
  IGFI
  IGFII

Fibroblast growth factors
  Basic FGF
  Acid FGF
  hst/kS3
  Int-2
  FGF-5

TGFβ family
  at lest 5 forms

Interleukin family
  Interleukin 1–6

Colony stimulating factor

Granulocyte colony stimulating factor

Granulocyte macrophage stimulating factor

Erythropoietin

Interferon family

Tumour necrosis factor family

Nerve growth factor

Bombesin family

the same cells later in development. Early lineage chondrocytes are stimulated to produce collagen II in the presence of TGF-β: later on in development, type II collagen synthesis is inhibited.

Growth factor effects can also be modulated by *extracellular matrix molecules* (ECM). It is now known that ECM themselves, *fibronectin* and *laminin*, can stimulate DNA synthesis in certain cells; collagen can switch it off. These ECM molecules interact with cells by combining with specific receptors called *integrins*. Many growth factors regulate the formation and destruction of ECM, controlling expression of ECM genes themselves, or of the several classes of integrins, or indeed of the enzymes that regulate the destruction of ECM. It is fairly clear that growth factors themselves have multiple and important roles to play in controlling tissue and organ growth.

And how do these growth factors exert their effects? We know that they combine with glycoprotein molecules, called *receptors*, on the cell surface. Isolated cDNA clones encoding numerous growth-factor receptors have allowed analysis of their amino-acid sequence and the development of antipeptide antibodies and molecular probes, and model systems have been developed in cultured cells to achieve high expression of receptor molecules.

The receptors for growth factors have a great deal in common. The basic architectural design is similar (Fig. 8.4). Each

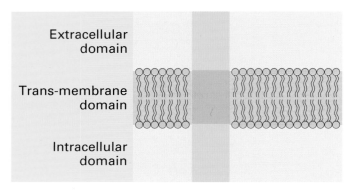

Fig. 8.4 A diagrammatic representation of a typical growth factor receptor. The cell membrane is indicated as a lipid bilayer.

receptor has a *single extracellular region* responsible for binding with the growth factor or ligand, attached to a single *hydrophobic peptide region*, which makes one pass through the lipid membrane bilayer and a single linear peptide sequence within the cytoplasmic domain, which possesses, though not in all cases, *tyrosine kinase activity*. Additionally, many receptors show extensive sequence homology, but show measurably different functional capabilities; for example the receptors for EGF and the oncogene product *HER-2/neu glycoprotein* show 50 per cent sequence homology, similar tyrosine kinase domains, but different ligand-binding properties—EGF does not bind HER-2/neu glycoprotein. However, receptor groups with divergent protein structures have the ability to bind similar peptide growth factors: receptors for *insulin-like growth factor I* (IGF-I) and IGF-II show no significant amino-acid homology, but both bind IGF-II with high affinity; moreover, EGF receptors bind TGF-α with equal or near equal affinity to EGF.

The *transmembrane domain* does not show much sequence homology between different receptors, indicating that precise sequence may not be required for receptor function and signal transduction. But a single point mutation in the transmembrane domain of the *neu* oncogene induces transforming activity, suggesting that the mutation stimulates the tyrosine kinase activity of the intracytoplasmic domain. However, similar mutations in the EGF receptor gene have no such effect, and any role of the transmembrane domain in activation is probably minor.

There are extensive amino-acid sequence homologies among the cytoplasmic domains of receptors with tyrosine kinase activity. The activation of receptor tyrosine kinase activity is the first cellular response to ligand–receptor binding. The mechanisms by which this activity induces the various cellular responses is not known; possibilities include the catalysis of exogenous substrates, or autophosphorylation of the receptor, changing its conformation so that interaction with effector molecules is possible. Thus a point mutation in the ATP-binding site of the tyrosine kinase of the insulin receptor inhibits tyrosine kinase activity and insulin response in affected cells; ATP-binding site mutations in the EGF receptor produce similar effects. Thus, whatever its role in receptor activation, tyrosine kinase activity is essential for receptor function. It should be remembered, however, that some of the growth factor receptors (e.g. IGF-II) lack tyrosine kinase activity; we do not know which regions are responsible for intracellular signalling, although it is currently thought that the intracytoplasmic part of these receptors associate with other membrane proteins that produce signal transduction.

Table 8.1 summarizes the more important growth factor families, and their activities. Many of the properties of growth factors can be seen in the example of the epidermal growth

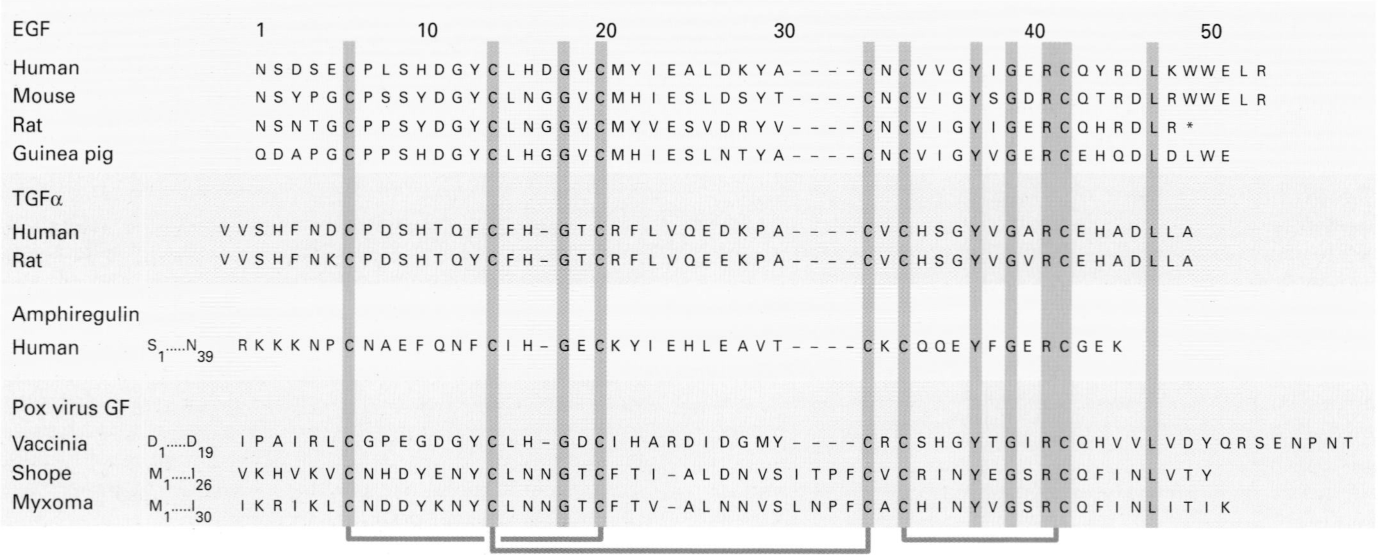

EGF	1	10	20	30	40	50
Human	N S D S E C P L S H D G Y C L H D G V C M Y I E A L D K Y A – – – – C N C V V G Y I G E R C Q Y R D L K W W E L R					
Mouse	N S Y P G C P S S Y D G Y C L N G G V C M H I E S L D S Y T – – – – C N C V I G Y S G D R C Q T R D L R W W E L R					
Rat	N S N T G C P P S Y D G Y C L N G G V C M Y V E S V D R Y V – – – – C N C V I G Y I G E R C Q H R D L R *					
Guinea pig	Q D A P G C P P S H D G Y C L H G G V C M H I E S L N T Y A – – – – C N C V I G Y V G E R C E H Q D L D L W E					
TGFα						
Human	V V S H F N D C P D S H T Q F C F H – G T C R F L V Q E D K P A – – – – C V C H S G Y V G A R C E H A D L L A					
Rat	V V S H F N K C P D S H T Q Y C F H – G T C R F L V Q E E K P A – – – – C V C H S G Y V G V R C E H A D L L A					
Amphiregulin						
Human	S_1.....N_{39} R K K K N P C N A E F Q N F C I H – G E C K Y I E H L E A V T – – – – C K C Q Q E Y F G E R C G E K					
Pox virus GF						
Vaccinia	D_1.....D_{19} I P A I R L C G P E G D G Y C L H – G D C I H A R D I D G M Y – – – – C R C S H G Y T G I R C Q H V V L V D Y Q R S E N P N T					
Shope	M_1.....I_{26} V K H V K V C N H D Y E N Y C L N N G T C F T I – A L D N V S I T P F C V C R I N Y E G S R C Q F I N L V T Y					
Myxoma	M_1.....I_{30} I K R I K L C N D D Y K N Y C L N N G T C F T V – A L N N V S L N P F C A C H I N Y V G S R C Q F I N L I T I K					

Fig. 8.5 Primary sequence for the EGF family of growth factors. The consensus sequences are indicated, and the solid lines connect the cysteine residues. (Drawn after Sporn and Roberts 1990, with permission.)

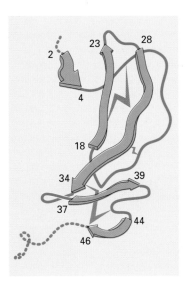

Fig. 8.6 Polypeptide backbone structure of mouse EGF. Arrowed ribbons indicate the position and direction of the β-sheets; disulphide bonds by lightning bolts. (Drawn after Sporn and Roberts 1990, with permission.)

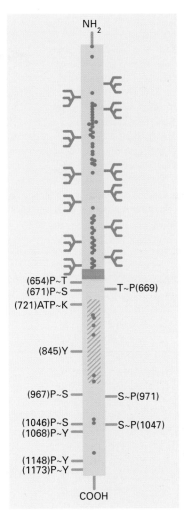

Fig. 8.7 The EGF receptor. The olive band shows the hydrophobic membrane anchor sequence, the branched structures indicate potential N-linked glycosylation sites in the extracellular domain, and the hatched area the tyrosine kinase domain. (Drawn after Sporn and Roberts 1990, with permission.)

factor family. EGF was discovered by Stanley Cohen in 1962, as a heat-stable protein from mouse submaxillary glands, which induced early eyelid opening and tooth eruption when injected into neonatal mice. EGF was later shown to increase epidermal thickening and keratinization. Transforming growth factor-α (TGF-α) was isolated as an EGF-like activity in sarcomas; pox virus genes encoding an EGF-like molecule were found, while *amphiregulin*, an EGF-like molecule, was isolated from tumour cells treated with phorbol esters.

The members of the EGF family share two properties: (1) they mimic EGF in biological activity, and (2) have an amino-acid sequence similar to EGF (Fig. 8.5). The primary structure of EGF has been known for some time, and recently the three-dimensional structure of EGF has been worked out (Fig. 8.6); EGF has no α-helical content, but contains about 22 per cent β-sheet structure. EGF is produced initially as a precursor molecule, and the genes encoding EGF are found on chromosome 4 in the q25–27 region in the human, and in the mouse on chromosome 3. The human TGF-α gene is on chromosome 3p11→13. It is now known that mouse EGF is highly homologous with the human polypeptide hormone *urogastrone* (URO), originally isolated from the urine of pregnant women, and now regarded as the human homologue of EGF.

The EGF/URO receptor conforms to our general remarks about growth factor receptors (Fig. 8.7), with an extracellular binding domain with several potential sites for N-linked glycosylation and a hydrophobic membrane anchor sequence. The intracytoplasmic component contains a tyrosine kinase domain, several autophosphorylation sites, and serine–threonine phosphorylation sites. After ligand–receptor binding, clustering of EGF-receptor complexes at coated pit areas on the plasma membrane occurs; the complexes are then internalized,

are sorted through intracytoplasmic compartments, eventually reaching the lysosomes where both receptor and ligand are degraded. Until the receptors are resynthesized, the cell may remain refractory to EGF stimulation: the receptors are then said to be *downregulated*. EGF binding induces rapid changes in the tyrosine kinase activity. The substrates for this activity include a variety of proteins, including the 35 kDa protein *lipocortin 1* which binds phospholipids in the presence of calcium, and possibly *phospholipase C*. However, the relationship between these activities and cellular activation is as yet unclear.

EGF is widely distributed in biological fluids. In man, mammary secretions, saliva, and duodenal juice are rich in EGF; the peptide is synthesized in breast, salivary glands, and Brunner's glands. TGF-α distribution in normal tissues is only now being worked out, but TGF-α mRNA and peptide has been found in villous enterocytes and suprabasal keratinocytes.

The physiological role of EGF has yet to be established, but the responses to exogenous EGF/URO are many and manifold, including stimulation of gastrointestinal, liver, kidney, mammary, and keratinocyte proliferation, but also multiple effects on differentiation and metabolism in multiple cell lineages, including mesenchymal cells such as endothelium. TGF-α actions are less well-studied, but its actions resemble EGF, although differences in potency in different systems do exist.

It is clear that the control of cell proliferation will eventually be understood as a complex interplay between the secretion of multiple growth factors and the synthesis of the appropriate receptors. The relationship between these two activities, and the cellular responses to ligand–receptor binding, remain problems for the immediate future.

8.3   Hyperplasia

Nicholas A. Wright

Hyperplasia is usually defined as an increase in the number of cells in a tissue or organ; it is usually associated with an increase in size. It should be remembered that hyperplasia can be relative, when a constituent cell or component of a tissue or organ becomes increased in number, but there is no overt increase in size. An example is the hyperplasia of gastric endocrine cells which accompany the elevation of serum gastrin in pernicious anaemia; the atrophic gastritis destroys the source of gastric acid (the parietal cells), and the G cells in the antrum respond by secreting *gastrin*, stimulating the *ECL cells (enterochromaffin-like cells)* in the fundus. However, the gastric mucosa itself is thinned.

There are several classifications of hyperplastic processes, most of which are artificial. For example, it is usual to distinguish *physiological hyperplasia*, such as growth of the adolescent breast at puberty or during pregnancy and lactation, from *pathological hyperplasia*, say the *endometrial hyperplasia* which occurs in perimenopausal women, leading to menstrual irregularities. But this distinction *is* artificial, since the cause of both these processes is an increase in the levels of circulating hormones, most importantly *oestrogens*. Thus it is better to call this *target-organ hyperplasia*. Similarly, we speak of *compensatory hyperplasia*, as when the liver regenerates after partial resection or, more appropriately, when a paired organ such as the kidney grows after unilateral resection. However, it is clear that, in the liver for example, growth factors are involved in the response, with *EGF*, *TGF-α*, and the specific *hepatotrophins* being involved. Thus this is also a form of target-organ hyperplasia. In the small intestine, resection of the jejunum leads to ileal hyperplasia— so-called *intestinal adaptation*; coeliac disease, produced by a sensitivity to the gluten component of cereals, induces loss of villi, 'villous atrophy' in the proximal small bowel: the ileum

responds by hyperplasia, 'compensating' for the loss of functioning absorptive cells proximally. Several gut hormones, especially gut glucagon, or *enteroglucagon*, have been incriminated in this response, again a target-organ effect.

Other instances of hyperplasia, which are less clear in respect of their causation, include psoriasis, a very common skin disease, in which there is unequivocal epidermal hyperplasia, and the lymphoid hyperplasia which accompanies common viral infections. Nevertheless, it is highly probable that these also will turn out to be target-organ effects: TGF-α is increased eighteen-fold in psoriatic epidermis, and the many cytokines released during virus infections are certainly mitogenic. So it is probable that all hyperplasias are, in the end, target-organ hyperplasias. Thus it is probably best to consider hyperplasia as an organ-specific process.

8.3.1   The dynamics of hyperplasia

Conceptually, it is easy to understand hyperplasia in an organ not usually given to self-renewal, the so-called 'conditional renewal systems', such as the thyroid gland. Excess levels of thyroid stimulating hormone (TSH) in iodine deficiency, or of thyroid auto-antibodies which act on the TSH receptor, lead to increases in cell production, and therefore net growth. But in renewing epithelia, such as the epidermis, the situation is more complex. Cells are produced in the basal layers; in most examples of epidermal hyperplasia, such as in the skin disease psoriasis, the progenitor cells in the basal layer are increased in number, increasing the proliferative population, as we have seen. While this increases the thickness of the epidermis, this is not the whole story, because merely increasing the rate of cell production in the basal layers will increase the rate of movement or transit through the above Malpighian layer. But we see that the Malpighian layer is itself increased in size in psoriasis (Fig. 8.1). Thus the rate of differentiation may also be a factor in this process; if it remained constant, we might expect an increase in Malpighian layer thickness as more cells enter from below. An increase in the rate of differentiation might maintain epidermal thickness at normal levels, and certainly hyperproliferative epidermis with normal Malpighian cell number is described—for example *lichen planus*, but here the individual cells are enlarged—'*pseudoacanthosis*'; cell proliferation is increased. Although methods are available to measure the differentiation rate, we know little about the processes that define it.

8.3.2   Hyperplasia in endocrine target organs

As mentioned above, this is a normal physiological event in the female breast at puberty, and during pregnancy and lactation, produced by an interplay between several different hormones. To a lesser extent, hyperplastic changes occur during each menstrual cycle, followed by regression. Both epithelial and connective tissue components contribute to this change; it is seen in exaggerated form in the condition called variously cystic disease, cystic hyperplasia, or even benign mammary dysplasia, a common benign proliferation of the breast where ducts and lobules show epithelial hyperplasia and metaplasia, and there is also stromal overgrowth (see Chapter 22). Exogenous oestrogens can cause breast hyperplasia in the male, but gynaecomastia can also occur during adolescence or in advanced liver disease.

The endometrial glands and stroma also go through a cyclical growth and regression process, under the influence of oestrogens and progestogens from the corpus luteum. Hyperplasia of the endometrium occurs in several instances: most cases are idiopathic, but are thought to be associated with increased levels of circulating oestrogens (see Chapter 21). Oestrogen-secreting tumours of the ovary, such as the *granulosa cell tumour*, also induce endometrial hyperplasia, and of course the common administration of oestrogens given during hormone replacement therapy causes a degree of endometrial hyperplasia.

In the male, hyperplasia of the prostate gland is a depressingly common manifestation of the aging process. There is epithelial, stromal, and smooth muscle hyperplasia, resulting in an increased size of the organ and consequent obstructive urinary symptoms. While generally felt to be associated with defective androgen metabolism, the details are by no means clear.

8.3.3   Hyperplasia in endocrine organs

These are excellent examples of hyperplasia: the diffuse hyperplasia of *Graves' disease in the thyroid*, the bilateral hyperplasia of the adrenals associated with an *ACTH-secreting pituitary adenoma* or with an *oat cell carcinoma secreting ACTH-like peptide fragments*, and *parathyroid hyperplasia*, which might be primary or secondary to the electrolyte disturbances of chronic renal failure. The details of these are discussed in Chapter 26.

8.3.4   Hyperplasia in surface epithelia

Epidermal hyperplasia is a very common manifestation of injury: after acute injury, such as stripping off the superficial layers of the epidermis with Scotch tape, or chronic injury, as seen in eczematous dermatitis ('lichen simplex chronicus circumscripta'). Other hyperplastic conditions are at present idiopathic, such as psoriasis (Fig. 8.1) and pityriasis rubra pilaris—the so-called *hyperproliferative dermatoses*.

In the gastrointestinal tract, hyperplasia is common—in the villous atrophy of coeliac disease the crypts undergo hyperplasia, presumably as a result of the reduction in the surface cell population (see Section 16.8.2); in ulcerative conditions of the stomach and intestine, the surrounding mucosa undergoes hyperplasia. In chronic ulcerative colitis the colonic crypts are large, hypercellular, and show active proliferation, often resulting in a reduction of specialized cells such as goblet cells (see Section 16.13.2).

8.3.5   Hyperplasia in bone marrow and lymphoid tissue

Any demand for increased blood cells is associated with bone marrow hyperplasia. After *haemorrhage,* or *haemolysis*, there is marked *erythroid hyperplasia* and, in the adult, the red or cellular marrow extends into the shafts of the long bones, which are usually filled with fatty yellow marrow. In *chronic haemolysis*, extramedullary haemopoiesis is seen, mainly in the liver and spleen. *Chronic hypoxia*, as in lung disease, *cyanotic heart disease*, or *high-altitude sickness*, is also associated with erythroid hyperplasia.

Hyperplasia of the myeloid series is seen in conditions where increased white blood cells are called for, as in pyogenic and other infections. *Lymphoid hyperplasias* commonly follow chronic infections, such as the spleen in malaria, etc.

8.3.6   Hyperplasia in paired organs and liver

The general manifestations of damage to the liver and after excision of paired organs such as the kidney have already been discussed (see Section 5.3.2). Here we should note, however, that some paired organs, such as the seminal vesicles and thyroid lobes, show little or no hyperplastic response to excision of one gland or lobe; why some paired organs show such growth responses and others do not, is at present unclear.

8.3.7   Hyperplasia—conclusions

It is fairly clear that most growth responses in mammalian organs result from a specific cause; in some instances we are beginning to understand this in terms of ligand–receptor binding. However, while the mechanisms of the initiation of hyperplasia are being intensively sought, there is, as yet, no unified hypothesis of how such mechanisms are set in motion. How does the kidney 'sense' the loss of its partner? Why do the intestinal crypts proliferate after damage to villus cells? Such phenomena were explained in the past by the *chalone hypothesis*, now *passé*, and a *negative feedback mechanism* operating on cell number. But despite the eclipse of the chalone hypothesis, there is substantial experimental evidence for a negative feedback mechanism in many growth situations, which will have to be explained.

8.3.8   Further reading

Sporn, M. B. and Roberts, A. B. (1990). *Peptide growth factors and their receptors*. Springer-Verlag, Berlin.
Wright, N. A. and Alison, M. R. (1984). *The biology of epithelial cell populations*, Vols 1 and 2. Clarendon Press, Oxford.

8.4   Hypoplasia

Nicholas A. Wright

This is a decrease in the size of an organ or tissue due to a reduction in cell number. Such hypoplasias can be *congenital*, or can be the result of a *physiological* or *pathological* change. Examples of congenital hypoplasias are seen in endocrine organs such as the thyroid, while physiological hypoplasia is seen in the intestine after prolonged bypass or parenteral feeding. Hypoplasia as part of a disease process is commonly seen in skin disorders, such as *lupus erythematosus* or *lichen sclerosus et atrophicus* (see Chapter 28). In these conditions the antithesis of growth stimulations obtains: cell production rates decline as a result of reduced stimulation or increased inhibition, which, with a normal rate of cell loss, leads to hypoplasia.

8.5　Atrophy

M. R. Alison

Atrophy is a reversible, adaptive response on the part of the cell to reduce its mass of functional cytoplasm. Causes of atrophy include:

1. *reduced functional activity*;
2. *loss of innervation*;
3. *reduced blood supply*;
4. *diminished nutrition*; and
5. *loss of hormonal or growth factor stimulation*.

Atrophic cells are smaller than their normal counterparts, thus atrophy can be readily detected microscopically by an increase in nuclear density, and is manifest biochemically by an increase in the concentration of DNA per unit of tissue weight. Some forms of atrophy are clearly *physiological*, such as the shrinkage of the endometrial glands after the fall in ovarian hormones following the menopause, while other forms are definitely *pathological*, like the atrophy of skeletal muscle following the destruction of anterior horn cells in the spinal cord by polioviruses. Whatever the cause, atrophy represents an attempt by the cell to survive (adjust) in the face of changes in the local environment. The term, *atrophy,* is also used in a wider sense to describe the involution of whole tissues or organs by processes which involve, not only individual cell shrinkage, but also cell destruction and lack of self-renewal. These include the well-known age-associated changes in the gonads and thymus gland; auto-immune diseases, which destroy the parenchymal tissue of the thyroid gland and adrenal cortex; and other conditions, such as coeliac disease (gluten-induced enteropathy) in which the small intestinal villi can be severely reduced in size (villus atrophy) (although the crypts are hyperplastic, see Section 8.3.4).

One of the commonest forms of atrophy results from *reduced functional activity*. This can be readily demonstrated by paralysing skeletal muscle through severing its nerve supply, and this so-called *disuse atrophy of muscle* is invariably seen in limbs immobilized in a cast as treatment for a bone fracture. The *muscular dystrophies* are a group of genetically determined disorders

characterized by progressive skeletal muscle weakness in which the main pathological change is an increased variability in the size of the muscle fibres due to atrophy of some of the fibres. *Duchenne muscular dystrophy* (DMD) is a relatively common X-linked disease affecting about 1 in 3500 male new-borns, and the disease is associated with the deficiency of a large ($\sim$ 400 kDa), low-abundance protein called *dystrophin*. Dystrophin is thought to be located on the inner surface of the muscle sarcolemma and may have a role in maintaining the elasticity of the muscle fibre; a mutant strain of mouse, the *mdx mouse*, in common with DMD patients, has no demonstrable dystrophin in skeletal muscle. The *neurogenic atrophies* closely mimic the clinical pattern of the muscular dystrophies but result from a denervating process. As one motor neurone supplies many fibres, denervation results in atrophic fibres randomly scattered in a biopsy specimen. The atrophic fibres are often clustered in groups, and the number of fibres per group increases with the severity of denervation. The presence of this 'small group' or 'large group' atrophy is, in fact, pathognomonic of denervation (Dubowitz 1985). Histographic analysis of fibre diameter in such cases often reveals a *bimodal distribution*, since not all motor neurons are simultaneously affected, and those fibres with an intact motor nerve may even hypertrophy as they try to compensate for the loss of function in the atrophic muscle fibres. *Spinal muscular atrophy* is one of the commonest neurogenic atrophies and large groups of atrophied fibres are often interspersed with fascicles of hypertrophied fibres (Fig. 8.8).

The integrity of all cells depends upon an adequate blood supply, and the atrophy of the brain in later life may be caused by hypoperfusion as arteriosclerosis narrows its blood supply. Inadequate nutrition associated with chronic disease leads to atrophy, particularly in skeletal muscle. In certain circumstances, the atrophy caused by *partial ischaemia* may, in fact, be due to a lack of nutrients. Depriving the liver of portal blood causes hepatocytes to atrophy, though this may have more to do with a reduced exposure to a high concentration of putative *hepatotrophic factors*, such as insulin and glucagon, than to a

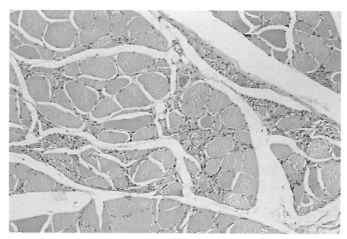

Fig. 8.8 Photomicrograph of a case of spinal muscular atrophy where large groups of atrophied skeletal muscle fibres (indicated by groups of closely packed nuclei) are interspersed with much larger fibres.

lack of nutrients. All cells are influenced by particular external signals (hormones, growth factors, or neurotransmitters) which act to regulate cellular processes such as mitosis and biosynthetic activity. Removal of the source of the trophic signal through, for example, ablation of an endocrine gland or denervation will invariably lead to atrophy of the target tissue. This is well illustrated in the sex-hormone-dependent tissues following withdrawal of hormonal stimulation. Endometrial glands become much smaller and scarcer after the fall in ovarian hormone levels following the menopause, while hypophysectomy or castration have dramatic effects on the male accessory sex glands (prostate, seminal vesicles, etc). If male rodents are castrated, the accessory sex glands lose more than half their mass within 1 week; the secretory epithelial cells dedifferentiate with a loss of rough endoplasmic reticulum, Golgi membranes, and secretory vacuoles so that normally tall columnar cells atrophy to cuboidal cells. The regression of the glands is also achieved by some of the secretory acinar cells undergoing *apoptosis,* with the net result that the acini are considerably shrunken in the atrophic gland and the supporting connective tissue stroma is much more prominent (Fig. 8.9).

Individual cell atrophy can also be the means by which excessively large organs return to normality. For example, thyroid follicular cells in a goitrous gland will atrophy if rats are switched back to a normal diet from an iodine-deficient diet, and likewise atrophy of hypertrophied hepatocytes occurs upon cessation of exposure to an enzyme-inducing compound (e.g. phenobarbital).

Atrophy involves a reduction in the structural components of the cell, such as discrete organelles and surplus enzymes, and in practice can be achieved by either enhanced protein degradation or reduced protein synthesis, or even both mechanisms. In eukaryotic cells, *lysosomes* form an important degradative system, each membrane-bound vacuole containing a rich selection of proteolytic enzymes (active in an acidic environment, pH 4.7–5.5) capable of the total breakdown of proteins. However, these acid hydrolases are not simply released into the cytoplasm to cause uncontrolled destruction, instead the organelles and/or cytosol destined for destruction are first compartmentalized in membrane-bound vacuoles termed *autophagosomes.* Substrates (organelles, etc.) and hydrolytic enzymes get together through membrane fusion, lysosomes and autophagosomes merging to form *autophagolysosomes.* Autophagosomes and autophagolysosomes are not readily distinguished from one another, the term *autophagic vacuole* (AV) encompasses both types of vacuole, and in many cases atrophy is associated with a marked increase in the number of AVs (Pfeifer 1987). The whole process of *autophagic degradation* is both active and rapid; inhibitors of protein synthesis block the further formation of AVs and cause a rapid decay in the volume fraction (proportion of cytoplasm occupied by AV-profiles) of AVs, suggesting a morphological half-life of something less than 10 mins.

8.5.1 Bibliography

Dubowitz, V. (1985). *Muscle biopsy. A practical approach.* Baillière Tindall, London.
Pfeifer, U. (1987). Functional morphology of lysosomes. In *Lysosomes: their role in protein degradation* (ed. H. Glaumann and F. J. Ballard), pp. 1–59. Academic Press, London.

8.6 Hypertrophy

M. R. Alison

A reversible increase in the size of a cell through an accumulation of more structural components is known as hypertrophy, and should not be confused with processes, such as cell and organelle oedema (formerly called 'hydropic degeneration'),

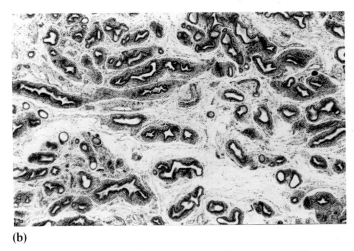

(a)

(b)

Fig. 8.9 (a) A prostate gland from a normal rat in which the secretory acini are almost back-to-back with little intervening stroma. (b) The same tissue 6 weeks after castration; all the acini are considerably shrunken due to cell loss and cell atrophy, with the result that the stroma is much more prominent in the atrophic gland.

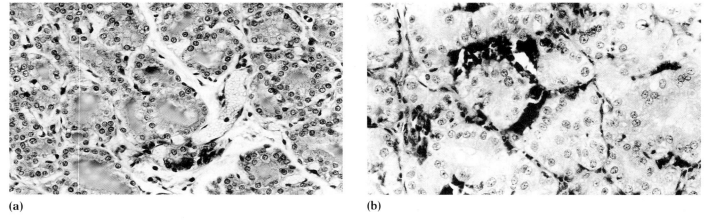

(a)   **(b)**

Fig. 8.10   (a) Follicles in a normal rat thyroid gland; (b) hypertrophied follicles in a goitrous thyroid gland.

which can also result in larger cells but is in fact a sublethal or prelethal event. *Thus, the purely hypertrophied organ has no new cells, just bigger ones.* As a consequence, the concentration of DNA per unit of tissue weight is less in hypertrophic tissue, and there is generally a sharp rise in the RNA/DNA ratio during the enlargement phase. Skeletal muscle hypertrophy induced by training has been traditionally taken as the prototype of such a process. Like atrophic responses, hypertrophic responses can be both physiological and pathological. *Physiological hypertrophy* can be effected by hormonal stimulation, one such example being the growth of the uterus during pregnancy: at the end of pregnancy in the guinea-pig the smooth muscle cells of the myometrium can be more than twice their normal size and be packed with greatly increased amounts of organelles (endoplasmic reticulum, Golgi complex, and mitochondria). Hypertrophy also occurs in response to abnormal levels of hormones. The activity of the thyroid gland is dependent on the production of TSH by the pituitary, but if there is insufficient iodine, or thyroid hormonogenesis is disrupted by some other means, then there is no feedback inhibition of TSH secretion and thyroid enlargement (goitre) occurs as a result of the overproduction of TSH. This enlargement is, in fact, due to both hyperplasia (an increase in cell number) and hypertrophy of the thyroid follicular cells (Fig. 8.10), demonstrating quite convincingly that these two adaptive responses are not mutually exclusive, a not uncommon finding. Anabolic steroids are taken by body-building athletes to increase their muscle mass through hypertrophy, although recent reports of seemingly associated liver tumours suggest the practice be abandoned.

Hypertrophy caused by *increased functional demand* is exemplified by the effects of exercise on skeletal muscle, in that under the stress of repetitive and sustained work muscle fibres will increase in size. Histographic analysis shows that there is usually a bell-shaped distribution curve of fibre diameters, and that, due to exercise, the curve is shifted to the right. But, on the other hand, if normal fibres hypertrophy to compensate for the loss of function in smaller atrophic fibres (induced by a denervating disease), then one might well see a twin-peaked distribution curve of fibre diameters. In exercise-induced hypertrophy of

skeletal muscle, there is also evidence that *satellite cells* (presumptive muscle stem cells) proliferate and become incorporated into the existing enlarging fibres (*myotubes*). The liver can be subjected to increased functional demand through exposure to compounds that are metabolized by the mixed-function oxidase system. Phenobarbital is one such substrate for this system, and its administration causes the rapid induction of cytochrome P_{450}-dependent enzymes with multiplication of smooth endoplasmic reticulum and thus hypertrophy of the responsive hepatocytes (Fig. 8.11). Likewise, hypolipidaemic agents, such as clofibrate, cause the hypertrophy of hepatocytes, although this is related to the multiplication of peroxisomes.

Perhaps the best example of adaptive hypertrophy occurs in the heart under pathological conditions, when it is called upon to increase its contractile force because of impedence with aortic outflow, or because of systemic hypertension. In the latter case, the heart may double in weight (Fig. 8.12), while the hearts of rats subjected to chronic exercise (6 h swimming/day for 14 days) will increase by over 25 per cent in weight. *Myocardial hypertrophy* can be induced experimentally by causing stenosis of either the ascending aorta (for left ventricular hypertrophy) or the pulmonary artery (for right ventricular hypertrophy).

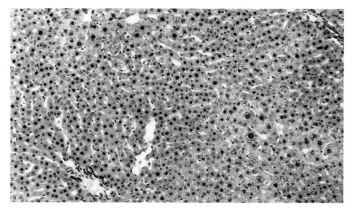

Fig. 8.11   Pronounced centrilobular hepatocyte hypertrophy in a rat exposed to phenobarbital.

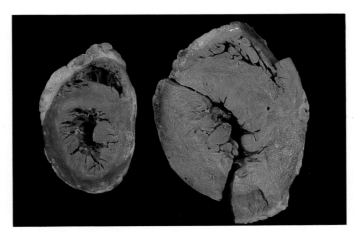

Fig. 8.12 Left ventricular hypertrophy in a hypertensive subject; by comparison the normal heart (left-hand side) weighs only half as much.

However, the acute pressure overload induced by this abrupt 'banding' can cause myocardial defects (focal necrosis, changes in mechanical performance and energy availability) not normally associated with hypertrophic myocardium where the onset of pressure overload has been more gradual. For this reason, hypertrophy induced by swimming or thyroxine administration are considered to be more appropriate models of human disease. As expected, hypertrophied myocytes contain more organelles than usual, in particular mitochondria, endoplasmic reticulum, and myofibrils. An increased functional demand may also be imposed upon an organ through the loss of some of the functional mass. This could possibly be the trigger for the growth response which ensues in the remaining kidney after a unilateral nephrectomy. Whatever the signal, removal of one kidney from the rat causes the weight of the contralateral kidney to increase by as much as 30 per cent within 5 days, with the bulk of the change due to hypertrophy of the renal tubular cells.

In many instances of hypertrophy there is no consistent message as to whether protein degradation is reduced or protein synthesis is enhanced during the growth phase. In fact, overloaded muscles can have elevated rates of degradation, but even greater increases in synthesis, enabling additional growth to be realized. In the growth of salivary glands induced by the β-sympathomimetic amine, *isoproterenol*, the initial response is one of an inhibition of cellular autophagy, as evidenced by a dramatic fall in the volume fraction of autophagic vacuoles.

8.7 Metaplasia

J. M. W. Slack

8.7.1 Differentiated cells

The normal events of embryonic development ensure the for-

mation of about 200 types of differentiated cell. From a cell kinetic viewpoint these fall into three classes: those, like neurones, which do not divide during adult life; those which are normally quiescent but which may proliferate under special conditions; and those which are continuously generated from populations of stem cells. In general, it is the connective tissues which make up the second class, and the epithelia which make up the third, although there are centres of continuous proliferation which are not epithelial, the bone marrow being the most obvious example. Within a particular renewal pathway, such as the progression from a basal layer epidermal cell to a terminal keratinocyte, there is a smooth gradation of cellular appearance. However, in the post-embryonic organism there are no graduations between the different lineages themselves; the boundaries between them are sharp, discrete, and persistent. This is particularly clearly seen at the junctions between different epithelia arising from a common embryonic cell sheet. For example the oesophageo-gastric junction shows an abrupt change from stratified squamous to columnar epithelium, and the same is true for the ecto-endocervical junction of the cervix uteri.

The molecular basis for the heritability of the differentiated state is still unclear, although three possible mechanisms have been suggested:

1. *positive feedback*, whereby genes are maintained in the active state by the presence of their own products;

2. *DNA methylation*, which can be maintained so long as one strand of the duplex is already methylated; and

3. *higher-order structures in DNA*, such as *supercoils*, which can be maintained through replication if the ends of DNA loops are anchored to other structures.

The extreme rarity of changes of cell lineage from one differentiated state to another gives such changes a special interest when they do occur. They are called 'metaplasia' from the Greek '*metaplasis*'—a moulding afresh. This section will consider what types of metaplasia occur in man, what normal mechanisms might be disturbed to bring about such changes, and what is their clinical significance.

8.7.2 Metaplasia in animals

First, however, it may of interest to mention a few of the more celebrated examples of metaplasia from the non-human world. Some workers have always been sceptical about the very existence of the phenomenon, but even they are silenced when confronted with Wolffian regeneration of the lens in newts. If the lens is removed, then over the next few weeks a region of the pigmented epithelium of the iris dedifferentiates to form a blastema which grows and differentiates into a new lens. The obvious requirement for dedifferentiation and growth in this example illustrates the first rule of metaplasia: *it is always associated with some abnormal stimulation of tissue growth, often wound healing or sometimes excessive hormonal stimulation of a responsive tissue.*

The Arthropoda provide many spectacular examples of metaplasia. In Crustacea the amputation of an appendage may be followed by the regeneration not of a copy of the original, but of an appendage which belongs elsewhere on the body (*heteromorphic regeneration*). For example, if an eye of the crayfish *Palinurus* is amputated near the base of its stalk then it will often regenerate not as an eye but as an antenna. In the fruit fly *Drosophila* similar transformations, called *transdeterminations*, occur when the larval *imaginal discs*, which normally form the different adult appendages, are extensively cultured. In these cases there is not necessarily a change of *histological cell type*, since the sorts of cells making up two appendages may be rather similar. However, their arrangement is different, and it is clear that what has changed is a label identifying higher-order subdivision of the developmental hierarchy. The genes that have this function of identifying regions of the embryo are known as *homoeotic genes*. Here then we have the second important rule of metaplasia: *the change responsible is not between two terminally differentiated cells themselves but between precursor cells whose commitment is to form a particular tissue, organ, or part of the body*.

The product of a metaplastic change may be a completely normal cell lineage which has arisen in an abnormal position but does not differ in any other way from its normal counterparts elsewhere in the body. This suggests that, unlike neoplasia, metaplasia does not necessarily involve a defect of a gene or molecule within the cell. It is true that there are also a number of types of metaplasia where the products are not normal, but the possibility of transformations between normal cell lineages establishes the third rule of metaplasia: *the changes represent changes in the normal sequence of logical decisions taken by cells during embryogenesis*. This means that metaplasias have a particular interest for those concerned with the mechanisms of embryonic development.

8.7.3 Epithelial metaplasias

Most or all epithelia are renewal tissues in which the cell population continuously turns over, being ultimately fed from a small proportion of stem cells. Many epithelia contain several different types of differentiated cell and, although the evidence is rarely conclusive, it is generally believed that for a given tissue all the types arise from a common stem cell. It is not known whether metaplasia arises initially from a single cell or a group of cells, but in either case it must arise within the stem-cell population in order to persist, since all the other cells of the tissue are destined to differentiate and die. It is also necessary, if the metaplasia is to expand from a small focus up to a visible patch, that the altered cells should have some selective advantage over the unaltered ones. This need not be large, for metaplasia is often occasioned by tissue damage and so the epithelium will be regenerating across areas of damage and both original and metaplastic regions may have an opportunity to expand.

Squamous metaplasia

A large group of epithelial metaplasias involve transformation from a mucinous to a stratified squamous type. In fact, almost any glandular epithelium may develop squamous metaplasia in response to continuous mechanical or toxic damage. One of the best-known examples is squamous metaplasia of the bronchus, which is commonly found among cigarette-smokers (see Chapter 9). This is of some clinical significance since although the metaplasia itself is relatively harmless, it is the parent tissue of squamous cell carcinoma: the most common type of lung cancer. By contrast, bronchial adenocarcinoma, which arises directly from the respiratory epithelium of small bronchioles, is much less common and its formation is promoted by smoking to a far lower extent. Another important example is squamous metaplasia in the urinary bladder, which is often occasioned by calculi or by parasitic infections such as schistosomiasis. In such cases, patches of squamous metaplasia may give rise to squamous cell carcinoma, although overall this is a less common type of cancer than transitional cell carcinoma arising from the parent tissue.

Glandular metaplasia

This group is of perhaps the greatest biological interest since glandular epithelia are usually characteristic of individual organs, and so changes between them are clear counterparts of the homoeotic transformations well known in arthropods.

A well-investigated case is *intestinal metaplasia* in the stomach, which is often associated with gastric ulcers. There are two types, called 'complete' and 'incomplete'. The complete type involves a total transformation of gastric glands to small intestinal crypts, with Paneth cells at the base and goblet and mucous cells on the villi. In incomplete metaplasia, Paneth cells are not found and there may be other histochemical differences, such as the presence of sulphomucins or the absence of certain enzymes such as trehalase. Gastric carcinoma of the 'intestinal' type is thought to originate within areas of incomplete metaplasia (see Section 16.3.2).

The converse situation of gastric tissue in the intestine is common in Crohn's disease. Here the ectopic tissue is usually of pyloric type, although there are a few cases in which body-type epithelium is found containing parietal and chief cells.

We have already mentioned squamous metaplasia of the urothelium. This tissue may also show glandular metaplasia in chronic cystitis or pyelitis. In these conditions 'von Brunn's nests' may sprout from the basal layer and the lining cells become oriented as glands. In the form known as *cystitis glandularis* these are intestinal in character and contain goblet and Paneth cells. Although adenocarcinoma of the bladder is rare, when it occurs it probably arises in such areas of metaplasia (see Section 19.3.5).

It may be significant that the three types of epithelium: gastric, intestinal and urothelial, arise from contiguous areas of the endoderm in the early embryo, and so it is possible that the three different precursor cell populations are distinguished from each neighbour by the state of activity of a single homoeotic gene. If in adult life this gene becomes turned on where it is normally off, or vice versa, either by mutation or an epigenetic event, then the commitment of the stem cell will become altered to that of the appropriate neighbouring tissue and a metaplasia will result.

Reproductive epithelia

Another important group of metaplasias occur between the various epithelia of the female reproductive tract. The most impressive potency is shown by the surface (so-called 'germinal') epithelium of the ovary. During the reproductive years this experiences repeated trauma as a result of ovulation, and may undergo hyperplasia. This damage can result in the formation of cysts lined with metaplastic epithelium of one of five different types. *Serous cystadenomas* resemble normal fallopian epithelium and often progress to *serous carcinomas*. *Mucinous cystadenomas* may either consist of columnar epithelium resembling the normal endocervix, or of a pseudostratified epithelium resembling the small intestine and containing absorptive, goblet, and argentaffin cells. Next, there is a group of neoplasms called *Brenner tumours*, which are arranged as cords and tunnels of tissue resembling urothelium. Finally, there are 'chocolate cysts' containing tissue resembling the endometrium, although in this case there must be some possibility of an implantational origin as is usually supposed to underlie peritoneal endometriosis.

The endometrium itself is, of course, in a situation of continual regeneration, and patches of ectopic tubal or endocervical epithelium are not uncommon. They became even more common in *endometrial hyperplasia,* associated with excessive oestrogen production and a suppression of ovulation.

Once again, the different levels of the female reproductive tract, from the ovaries to the proximal part of the vagina, arise from a contiguous zone of tissue, the so-called 'intermediate mesoderm' of the early embryo, and it is quite possible that the stem cells of each differ from their neighbours by the state of a single homoeotic gene.

8.7.4 Connective tissue metaplasias

A number of transformations are found between mesodermally derived tissues; and probably in all cases the precursor cells is the ubiquitous 'fibroblast'. Whether fibroblasts in different tissues or organs are actually identical to each other is not known, and it seems probable that one cell morphology may represent several cell types. However, fibroblasts in many parts of the body seem able to give rise to bone, with or without associated cartilage and marrow tissue. Such bony metaplasia may arise in surgical scars, sometimes long after the original operation. It may occur in muscle subjected to repeated mechanical trauma ('myositis ossificans'), in the walls of sclerotic calcified arteries, or in heart values calcified in chronic endocarditis. Small bony nodules may appear disseminated in the lungs in cases of mitral stenosis. In addition, bony deposits may arise in the stroma of a variety of tumours, presumably in response to factors secreted by the malignant epithelium. In view of the relative frequency of osseous metaplasia, it is of interest that two proteins have recently been purified that can induce local bone formation after subcutaneous implantation in rodents (*osteogenin* and *bone morphogenetic protein*).

Although the ectopic formation of bone and cartilage are by far the most common types of connective tissue metaplasia, there have also been described other transformations, such as the formation of adipose tissue in goitres or of striated muscle in mixed tumours of the endometrium.

8.7.5 Embryonic heterotopia

It is usual to distinguish sharply between heterotopia and metaplasia, mainly because metaplasia always arises in zones of tissue regeneration, whether provoked by mechanical damage, toxicity, infection, or abnormal hormonal stimulation. Whether or not a particular type of metaplasia makes cancer more likely, this sort of chronic tissue damage will also quite independently predispose to cancer and thus be a cause for concern. Heterotopic structures, on the other hand, have differentiated in the wrong place during embryogenesis, will not usually be associated with tissue damage, and may persist undetected throughout life. However from the point of view of the underlying biological mechanisms it seems probable that the homoeotic genes, whose states distinguish neighbouring tissues, are involved alike in the causation of metaplasia and heterotopia. It is never possible to prove that a given ectopic structure is a genuine heterotopia rather than a division, displacement, or abnormal migration of a normal structure, since the developmental history of an abnormal individual embryo cannot be observed as it occurs. However, heterotopic differentiation does seem the most likely cause for patches of gastric tissue found in the intestine or the vitellointestinal duct, for pancreas in the stomach or intestine, or for bone in the kidneys. These types of heterotopia may be compared to 'phenocopies' in the fruit fly *Drosophila,* in which patches of transformed tissue can develop after treatment of early embryos with ether. The transformations seen in phenocopies are very similar to those obtained by mutation of homoeotic genes.

8.7.6 Clinical significance of metaplasia

Few heterotopias or metaplasias cause much trouble in their own right. There are occasional problems from inappropriate secretions, such as HCl from heterotopic gastric tissue, but in most cases the ectopic tissue itself is harmless. More important is the question of to what extent and how these lesions can predispose to cancer, and here it is necessary to be careful about the different types of predisposition and causation.

As we have seen, metaplasias are associated with chronic tissue damage. So are many cancers; therefore the presence of metaplasia may simply be a warning of conditions that can also, independently, cause cancer. At the next level we may note that cancers often originate near junctions between epithelial tissues, such as the gastroduodenal junction or the ectoendocervical junction. This may again be because there is a small-scale 'ebb and flow' of the two tissues, with associated formation of new proliferation units. Metaplasia inevitably results in the creation of new boundaries with a sharp discontinuity of cell type, and so this may in itself increase the risk of cancer. Finally, there is the case where cancer probably arises from a cell within a patch of metaplasia, and resembles the metaplasia rather than the parent tissue. In some tissues these cancers are rarer than those arising directly from the parent tissue, but in others they are more common, and particularly important examples of this are squamous cell carcinoma of the bronchus arising from areas of squamous metaplasia, and 'intestinal type' carcinoma of the stomach arising from areas of incomplete intestinal metaplasia.

8.7.7 Summary

Metaplasias are patches of ectopic tissue. They arise in areas of abnormal growth by transformation of one type of precursor cell into another. Epithelial metaplasias may be glandular to squamous or glandular to glandular, the latter often being transformations between tissues which normally arise from adjacent areas of an embryonic epithelium. Connective tissue metaplasia usually involves the ectopic formation of bone. Some metaplasias predispose to the corresponding histological type of cancer.

8.7.8 Further reading

Nicholson, G. W. (1922). The heteromorphoses in the human body. *Guy's Hospital Reports* **72**, 75–127.

Schridde, H. (1909). Die ortsfremden Epithelgewebe des Menschen. *Sammlung anatomischer und physiologischer Vorträge und Aufsätze* **6**, 199–259.

Slack, J. M. W. (1985). Homoeotic transformations in Man: Implications for the mechanism of embryonic development and for the organization of epithelia. *Journal of Theoretical Biology* **114**, 463–90.

Taylor, A. L. (1927). The epithelial heterotopias of the alimentary tract. *Journal of Pathology and Bacteriology* **30**, 415–49.

Willis, R. A. (1962). *The borderland of embryology and pathology* (2nd edn). Butterworths, London.

9

Neoplasia

9

Neoplasia

9.1 Neoplasia

D. G. Harnden and James O'D. McGee

9.1.1 Introduction

Cancer, or related phenomena, occurs widely throughout both animal and plant kingdoms. We are aware of it as a common human disease and largely because of experimental cancer research work, we have all become familiar with the idea that cancer also occurs in inbred mice and other experimental animals. Similarly, cancers and other neoplasms occur in domestic animals and some are of considerable economic importance, for example, avian leucosis and bovine lymphomatosis.

The situation in wild animals is quite different. There is no record of a true cancer being found in a wild mouse in the United Kingdom and only a few cases have been recorded world-wide. This seems to pose a paradox. The explanation is almost certainly that the laboratory mouse may live for something like 2 years, whereas in the wild only a small proportion of mice live longer than 3 months; and since cancer is strongly age-correlated, wild mice simply do not live long enough to get cancer. Additionally, laboratory mice are highly inbred and, therefore, more genetically homogeneous.

True cancers are found occasionally in wild mammals and are particularly common in deer. There are also undoubted cancers in all the other classes of vertebrate animals; birds, reptiles, amphibians, and even fish. Growths do occur in invertebrate animals and while they are reported more commonly in the more advanced orders, the Mollusca and the Arthropoda, they have been reported in almost every group of animals without backbones. There is some debate as to whether these are true cancers, but that neoplasms occur (see below) is unquestioned.

There is ample evidence that cancer has not arisen recently. Paleopathologists have shown that cancer occurred in many animals long since extinct. 'Growths' have even been recognized in the remains of dinosaurs dating back over 100 000 000 years, but it is not possible to say whether or not these are true cancers. By these standards man is a relative newcomer on the scene and while there are growths in earlier hominid remains, the earliest true cancer is an osteogenic sarcoma in a fragment of mandible found in East Africa, dating from the lower Pleistocene era about 100 000 years ago. Some ancient Egyptian mummies show clear evidence of both sarcomas and carcinomas; descriptions of conditions which could well be cancer are recorded in some Egyptian papyri, particularly the Papyrus Ebbers, dating from the IVth dynasty. The number of firmly diagnosed cases is small. The suggestion has been made, therefore, that although cancer did exist in these times the incidence was very low and that the high incidence in modern man is an indication of a dramatic increase. However, in various early human populations the majority of the population died before they reached the age when cancer becomes common. A cross-section of present-day human populations of comparable age would probably give the same low incidence of malignant disease.

The ancient Greeks were familiar with the main features of cancer. They had treatments which, in some cases, do not differ greatly in principle from some of the radical procedures employed today. The Greeks were aware of the poor prognosis associated with cancer and were the first to compare cancer and the crab. The original analogy is usually attributed to Galen 'As a crab is furnished with claws on both sides of the body so in this disease the veins which extend from the tumour represent with it a figure much like that of a crab'.

9.1.2 Definitions of cancer *in vivo*

Cancer is a group of diseases which share common features. Cancer may affect any organ or tissue in the body, and the characteristics of the disease may differ from organ to organ. The aetiology is complex. Any one cancer may have many different causes. Equally, a single causal factor may be associated with many different cancer types. Some cancers, e.g. basal cell carcinoma of skin, are easily curable whereas others, e.g. carcinoma of the bronchus, have low cure rates. In this chapter these issues will be considered in detail, but first some of the terms used in defining cancer *in vivo* and *in vitro* will be introduced.

A *neoplasm* is literally a new growth of cells. A *tumour* is a neoplasm which can be recognized as a distinct lump or lesion. The generic term neoplasm, however, includes new growth of cells which may not form a distinct local lesion (e.g. haemopoietic cells, leukaemia). In clinical practice, neoplasm and tumour are used interchangeably.

Benign neoplasms

Neoplasms are of two principal kinds, benign and malignant. A *benign neoplasm* is localized and does not usually infiltrate normal tissue. Often it is circumscribed by a layer of fibrous tissue or compressed normal tissue. It will cause serious harm only when, in a confined space, it compresses or occludes normal tissues. The benign nature of a tumour is often (but not always) denoted by the suffix '-oma' as in *leiomyoma*, a benign neoplasm of smooth muscle; or *adenoma*, a benign neoplasm of glandular tissue. This is not an invariable rule (see below).

Malignant neoplasms

Nomenclature

A *malignant* neoplasm, i.e. cancer, exhibits the properties of:

1. *invasion* when its cells infiltrate the surrounding normal tissue; and

2. *metastasis*, the capacity of cancer cells to spread and grow at sites distant from the origin of the neoplasm.

Distant spread may occur early in the development of a cancer but in some cases the original *primary cancer* may grow to a substantial size before metastasis occurs. Metastatic deposits are also referred to as *secondary cancer* or *secondaries* (see Section 9.5).

The malignant nature of a neoplasm is often indicated by the term *carcinoma*, which literally means a cancer of an epithelial tissue. Carcinoma is used as a collective term for all epithelial tumours. It is also used as a suffix for particular kinds of carcinoma, as in *adenocarcinoma*—a cancer of glandular epithelium.

Similarly, a *sarcoma* is a malignant tumour of connective tissue or mesenchymal origin. As a suffix, '-sarcoma', identifies cancers of specific mesenchymal origin as in *fibrosarcoma*, a cancer of fibroblastic origin.

Malignant tumours of embryonic origin are usually named after the cell of origin with the suffix '-blastoma', e.g. *retinoblastoma*, a cancer of the neural retina; *neuroblastoma*, a cancer of ganglion cells of the peripheral nervous system. Corresponding benign tumours are *retinoma* and *ganglioneuroma*. Tumours of the central nervous system are again usually named after the cell type. *Astrocytoma* is a cancer derived from astrocytes. This is a deviation from the general meaning of the suffix '-oma'; most astrocytomas have a malignant outcome.

Neoplasms of blood-forming cells are of two types. *Leukaemias*, where the cell of origin is in the bone marrow and their neoplastic cells are present in the peripheral blood. *Lymphomas* have their origin in lymph nodes, or other lymphoid organs. Initially, they may be confined to the site of origin and present as a clinical lump; they are sometimes associated with 'leukaemic' cells in blood. Lymphoma is synonymous with malignant lymphoma.

Tumour spread

When tumour cells invade normal tissues, they do so by infiltrating directly into adjacent normal tissues or spread along natural routes such as nerve sheaths (*local spread*). They may also be transported by blood (*haematogenous spread*) or via lymphatic vessels (*lymphatic spread*) to distant sites. They may also exfoliate into body cavities (e.g. *transcoelomic spread*) where they continue to grow and provoke fluid accumulation.

Microscopic features of cancer

Invasion The single most important histopathological characteristic of cancer is that the lesion does not have a clearly marked boundary. The cells spread into adjacent normal tissue. Groups of cells or single cells may be seen at some distance from the main mass. By contrast, benign lesions are usually sharply delineated. The degree of invasion varies from a few wandering cells having broken through a basement membrane, to massive incursions into, and replacement of, normal tissue. Some lesions with many of the cellular characteristics of cancer that remain confined within a mucosal surface, without breach of the underlying basement membrane, are referred to as carcinoma *in situ* (see Section 9.3).

Terminology Hyperplasia (see Chapter 8) is a limited and sometimes reversible process, where in response to a stimulus, normal cells are produced in excessive numbers. The tissue essentially retains the normal pattern of differentiation for that organ. If, however, the tissue and or cellular architecture is distorted or deficient the tissue is *dysplastic*. Where one cell type is replaced by another (e.g. columnar by squamous epithelium) the tissue is said to be *metaplastic*. While these two latter features may occur in cancer, they are not diagnostic of cancer. When the normal tissue architecture is disrupted, the individual cells are abnormal in shape and size and particularly if nuclear shape and size are abnormal and variable, and binucleate or multinucleate cells are present the tissue is said to be *pleomorphic*. If this process has continued to the point where the original differentiated state can no longer be recognized, the lesion is said to be *anaplastic*. This is characteristic of many cancers. Not all cancers display anaplasia throughout the whole lesion and may retain obvious signs of the differentiated tissues within which the cancer arose—a *well-differentiated* cancer. Such cancers may be less aggressive in their behaviour. A *poorly differentiated* anaplastic cancer is likely to be more aggressive and associated with a relatively poor prognosis.

Nucleocytoplasmic ratio Many cancer cells have a relatively large nucleus in relation to the amount of cytoplasm. This feature varies very considerably from one cancer to another and within constituent cells of the tumour. Some lymphomas have a very high *nucleocytoplasmic ratio* whereas clear cell carcinoma of the kidney may have cells with relatively large amounts of cytoplasm.

Mitotic index Many cancers show large numbers of cells in division. It is not unusual for these mitotic figures to be abnormal, e.g. the cell may have three or more polar bodies instead of two to give a *tripolar mitosis* or *multipolar mitosis*. The mitotic index of a tumour is defined as the number of mitoses per unit of microscopic area. It is important to note, however, that not all cancers have a high mitotic index.

Necrosis The presence of a tumour stimulates the growth of blood vessels which serve the tumour—*angiogenesis*. As the tumour increases in size, the blood supply may become inadequate. This leads to areas of cell death, *necrosis*, which may be extensive, usually in the centre of large tumours. Associated with this, the tumour cells may thrive in the areas immediately around the blood vessels to form *tumour chords*. Damage to blood vessels may cause extensive areas of *haemorrhage*.

Tumour infiltration by normal cells Many tumours are infiltrated by large numbers of *macrophages* which, in some tumours, may constitute as much as 50 per cent of the total cell content of the tumour mass. Extensive infiltration by *lymphocytes* suggests an immune response to the tumour. In certain cases, there is some correlation between the presence of large numbers of lymphocytes and good prognosis. Medullary carcinoma of the breast with heavy lymphocytic infiltration has a good prognosis, while lymphocyte-depleted Hodgkin disease tends to do badly.

Cellular differentiation This varies from perfect recapitulation of the differentiation programme of the normal cells of the organ from which the tumour derives to complete lack of differentiation typical of the normal cell counterpart (see Sections 9.2 and 9.4 for a detailed discussion of the methodology for assessing tumour differentiation).

9.1.3 *In vitro* criteria of malignancy

Cancer is defined by the pathologist in terms of the material available, namely gross morphology of the biopsy or organ, together with the structure and ultrastructure of sectioned material or whole mounts treated in a variety of ways with stains, antibodies (etc.) and viewed with a whole range of microscopic techniques.

Cancer cells can be cultured *in vitro*, thus permitting study of their structure and behaviour in a way which is not possible *in vivo*. By a variety of techniques normal cells may be altered or 'transformed' *in vitro* so that they acquire some of the characteristics of cancer cells *in vivo*.

A cancer, however, is not a cellularly homogeneous structure. It contains many different kinds of cells including stromal cells (fibroblasts and endothelial cells) and infiltrating normal cells, such as macrophages and lymphocytes, and, of course, tumour cells *per se*. Not all tumour cells have the capacity for unlimited growth. The current concept is that tumour growth is maintained by a subset of *clonogenic cells* which do have the capacity for unlimited proliferation. These cells are sometimes referred to as *stem cells*, but this term is better reserved for the normal cells in proliferating tissues which have the dual capacity of self-renewal and the production of differentiating cell lineages. A tumour-cell *clone*, on the other hand, is a group of cells which are the progeny of a single cell. This does not imply a capacity for maintaining the cell of origin and, of course, cells within a clone may evolve to differ from each other. Thus, when cancer cells are cultured, one must be careful to determine which components are being grown and studied.

Tumourigenicity testing

The ultimate test of whether a cell derived by *in vitro* techniques is cancerous is to determine whether or not it will produce a tumour on inoculation into a compatible host animal. For animal tumours the host can be either of two types.

1. A *syngeneic* animal, i.e. an animal of the same species and the same histocompatibility type. The necessity for immunological compatibility has led to the development of *inbred strains* of animals. These animals are genetically identical and accept reciprocal tissue grafts. In some instances, tumours, or more frequently transformed cells, have acquired new cell-surface antigens which makes growth in the syngeneic host difficult.

2. An *immunodeficient host* animal of the same or different species may be used for tumour grafts. Genetically immunodeficient mice such as the athymic or *nude mouse* are frequently used. These mice lack the T-cell component of the cell-mediated immune response and accept grafts not only from mice of a different strain but also from other species, including humans. By carrying out neonatal thymectomy and administering appropriate sublethal doses of ionizing radiation, normal mice can be made to accept tissue from immunologically incompatible donors. Similar procedures can be carried out with rats but tumourigenicity testing in other species is difficult because of the absence of inbred strains.

Tumours grown in immune suppressed animals and derived from a different species are known as *xenografts*. For example, many human tumours can be grown in mice as xenografts; this procedure can be useful for maintaining tumour cell lines; for ascertaining the tumourigenic potential of human cells transformed *in vitro*; and for certain experimental procedures, such as drug testing. It is vitally important, when such procedures are used, to check that any nodule formed is of donor origin and not reactive host tissue. When tumour cells are inoculated, they provoke a host response which provides the stroma, including the vasculature, which supports the growing tumour of foreign origin.

Tumour cell inoculation may be carried out at a variety of different sites, subcutaneous, intradermal, intramuscular, intracranial, intraperitoneal, or intravenous. Not all tumours or transformed cells will grow as xenografts. This does not mean that these cells are not fully transformed (see below).

Tumour cells in culture

General considerations

Cells from tumours are not always easy to grow in culture. There are many reasons. Tumours are composed of both normal and malignant cells so that, when tumour tissue is grown in culture either as solid explants or as dissociated cells, normal cells, usually fibroblasts, tend to outgrow the tumour cells. Many early reports of cultured tumours are invalid because the investigators failed to check that the cells growing were of tumour and not of stromal origin.

All cells in culture require a number of specific *growth factors*.

These are normally supplied by a complex growth medium containing serum which is rich in growth factors. For the growth of particular cells, it may be necessary to supply specific growth factors, e.g. some haemopoietic cells require specific growth factors, such as *interleukin-3*, which are involved in the normal control of haemopoiesis. If a medium is deficient in specific factors, attempts at culture may fail. Some cells produce growth factors that stimulate their own growth (*autocrine* stimulation) and those of adjacent cells (*paracrine* stimulation).

Types of cell culture

Explant culture A small piece of tumour is anchored in a culture dish in some way and cells permitted to grow out. While this method is used to initiate cultures, it is rarely used experimentally, except in studies where two types of tissue are grown in juxtaposition to study cellular interactions as cells grow out and intermingle.

Monolayer culture This is growth of cells on a solid substratum, which may be glass or plastic. In practice, tumour cells often grow several layers deep and this characteristic, together with a disordered pattern of growth, may be useful in discriminating tumour cells from normal cells. This is referred to as lack of contact inhibition of cell growth.

Suspension cultures In liquid media, some tumour cell types can be grown in suspension by agitation, e.g. by means of a magnetic stirrer. It is unusual for cells from solid tumours to grow easily in this way but cells may be adapted by selection for growth in suspension. The exceptions are leukaemic or lymphoma cells, which can be frequently maintained in suspension culture.

Agar culture Growth in suspension in agar, or methylcellulose-containing culture medium, is possible for some tumour and some transformed cells. Normal cells do not grow under such conditions.

Spheroids Some tumour cells grow in the form of cellular aggregates in suspension in liquid medium. These spheroids show a degree of cellular organization, and larger spheroids may have a necrotic centre, thus mimicking *in vivo* tumour structure.

Cancer cells in culture vary depending on the tissue of origin. However, many have features common to transformed cells. The process of cellular transformation will therefore be considered at this point.

Cellular transformation

General consideration

A small number of different stimuli may alter normal cells in culture in such a way that they either become cancer cells or acquire some of the characteristics of cancer cells. Cells altered in this way are said to be transformed. There is, however, no simple definition of *cellular transformation*. Strictly, for cells to be 'fully transformed' they must be capable of producing tumours on inoculation into appropriate hosts. However, it is not always easy to prove tumourigenicity *in vitro*; some transformation events lead to populations of cells which have all the *in vitro* characteristics of transformation but which do not produce tumours in animals. In practice, therefore, if cells have a number of these characteristics, they may be considered transformed. It must be made clear that there is no general agreement on this point; this causes considerable difficulty in interpreting work in this field.

Transforming agents

Oncogenic viruses Transformation *in vitro* was originally described after infection with *oncogenic viruses*. Treatment of a culture with a relatively high dose of virus may lead to transformation of many cells which then outgrow and replace the normal cells. Use of lower virus doses results in the transformation of relatively small numbers of cells which then grow more rapidly to form discrete *foci*. These foci stand out clearly from the background normal cells; counts of foci give a quantitative assay of transformation.

The processes are somewhat different for RNA and DNA viruses. Transforming RNA viruses are all *retroviruses*, i.e. viruses that require a reverse transcription step of the RNA genome to a DNA intermediate. Some retroviruses may, however, infect cells in culture with no obvious cellular alteration. *Fast-transforming retroviruses*, such as Rous sarcoma virus, contain within the *genome* a sequence or sequences that have been acquired by recombination with a cellular host. These sequences, derived by evolution, may be important in the regulation of growth and division of tumour cells. These viral genes are acquired and modified from normal mammalian genes. They are designated *proto-oncogenes*. Proto-oncogenes, which are components of the normal genome, may also be *activated* in a variety of human tumours without viral intervention. This occurs by single base mutation, by translocation, partial deletion or truncation, or in some other way bringing the gene under the inappropriate influence of an active promoter sequence. In a cellular environment, they are termed *c-onc genes*. When they are integrated into a retroviral genome and come under the influence of a viral promotor they are termed *v-onc genes*.

Cellular transformation by fast transforming RNA viruses is a very high-efficiency process which gives foci within a few days of infection. The transformed cells may or may not produce infectious virus. New cells may be recruited to the focus by infection and they seldom form stable cell lines. *Slow transforming retroviruses* do not transform cells in culture. They appear to exert their effect by integration near *c-onc* genes *in vivo*.

Oncogenic DNA viruses, on the other hand, tend to transform with low efficiency (1 in 10^6 cells). The foci take many weeks to appear; they do not normally produce virus and sometimes give rise to established stable cell lines. The viral genome may be integrated, in whole or in part, in the transformed cells but may also exist in an episomal form.

Chemicals There are relatively few reports of *in vitro*

transformation by chemical agents. These are usually polycyclic hydrocarbons. The difficulty here (and this also applies to radiation transformation), is that the criteria used for assessing transformation are extremely variable and correlation of different reports is difficult.

Radiation Similarly, there are relatively few reports of *in vitro* cellular transformation by either ionizing or UV radiation. However, in those cases where this has been achieved, the transformed cells show many of the characteristic features outlined below.

DNA and chromosome-mediated cellular transformation It has been known for many years that the DNA from oncogenic viruses can transform cells but at lower efficiency than for the whole virus. It is now clear that any DNA that contains an *activated oncogene* has the potential for cellular transformation, whether it is derived from the virus, from cells transformed by that virus, or indeed from primary human cancer cells. This process is termed *transfection*. Various means have been devised for facilitating DNA entry into the cell, e.g. by co-precipitation of the DNA with calcium phosphate which is then engulfed by the cell, or by *electroporation* whereby the cells are momentarily exposed to a high current which causes the integrity of the cell membrane to be disrupted and permits entry of exogenous DNA. Not all cells are suitable targets for *DNA transfection* and this appears to be related to the ability of the cells to take up DNA successfully. NIH 3T3 and C127 mouse cell lines are widely used as transfection recipients. These established cell lines, however, appear to be particularly responsive to the 'ras' family of oncogenes. It is likely that other cell lines will detect other 'families' of oncogenes.

Similarly, whole chromosomes, and thereby the oncogenes they contain, may be used for *chromosome transfection* using calcium phosphate precipitation and electroporation. While it is not usual for the donor chromosome to be integrated whole into the host cell, it is clear that large chromosome segments become integrated into the host cell genome. Cellular transformation can then be used as a *selectable marker* for cells that have integrated oncogenes.

The development of plasmid or retroviral vectors, incorporating oncogenes or other genes, has extended greatly the range of cells that may be transfected.

Spontaneous transformation Many reports of *spontaneous transformation* have proved to be the result of contamination with already transformed cell lines. It is therefore vitally important to check the origin of newly transformed cell lines by using immunological, cytogenetic, or DNA marker techniques. There are, however, many well-documented examples of spontaneous transformation of animal cells, while human cells rarely, if ever, spontaneously transform. Indeed, human cells *in vitro* are hard to transform by any agent.

Nomenclature of cell lines

Cultured cells of normal tissue origin usually have a finite length of life in culture; they are sometimes said to have reached the *Hayflick limit*. These are termed *cell strains*. After a period of cell division the growth rate slows down. They become *senescent* and eventually die out. When a cell acquires the potential for indefinite growth in culture it is said to have been *immortalized* and is referred to as an *established cell line*. Immortalization is a common feature of transformation, but may occur in the absence of transformation. Immortalized cell lines do not form tumours on inoculation into animals but they are unusually good targets for transformation by transforming viruses or other agents. They may show some but not all of the characteristics of transformed cells. They may represent a 'half-way house' between a cell strain and a fully transformed cell line.

Human cells of lymphoid origin may be transformed *in vitro* using Epstein–Barr virus (EBV) or by co-cultivation of normal lymphoid cells with cells already transformed by EBV which shed virus. These are termed *lymphoblastoid cell lines* and have similar characteristics to cell lines derived directly from lymphomas, usually termed *lymphoma lines*. Some leukaemias have been cultured to yield established cell lines.

Characteristics of transformed cells

As with tumour cells *in vivo*, cultured transformed cells show considerable variation in both cellular and nuclear morphology. This *pleomorphism* is akin to that observed *in vivo*. It seems quite possible that many of the more bizarre forms are dying cells with little proliferative potential. On the other hand, stable cells with abnormal amounts of DNA often form the major proliferating component of a transformed cell line. Transformed cells often stand out clearly from a background of untransformed cells because they heap up to form a *focus*.

Nucleocytoplasmic ratio

Again, as with many cancer cells *in vivo*, the size of the nucleus relative to the cytoplasm is increased. This may be a reflection of the commitment of these cells to proliferate rather than a consequence of differentiation, although these two functions, and concepts, are difficult to distinguish *in vitro* and *in vivo*.

Chromosome complement

Many transformed cell lines have abnormal individual chromosomes and some have a bizarre number of chromosomes. Cell lines with the normal somatic cell number of chromosomes are *diploid* (i.e. they have twice the *haploid* number found in germ cells). Multiples of the haploid number are *euploid* (i.e. *triploid*, *tetraploid*, etc). Any deviation from euploidy by loss or gain of chromosomes is referred to as *aneuploidy*. Many transformed cells are aneuploid. Commonly, aneuploid cell lines contain slightly more chromosomes than a diploid cell and are referred to as *hyperdiploid* or *hypotetraploid*. *Hypodiploid* cell lines are rare.

In addition to numerical abnormalities, transformed cells often have chromosome rearrangements. Sometimes the number of chromosomes is diploid but the cell is abnormal because of chromosome rearrangements. Such cells are *pseudodiploid*.

Once a cell line has been established for a time, and

sometimes from the moment of establishment, cells with one particular chromosomal abnormality predominate. This is said to be a *stem line*. Variants of this line are *side lines*.

While some transformed cells show great instability of karyotype, others show remarkable consistency with abnormal *marker chromosomes* which characterize that cell line.

Alterations in antigenic structure

Viral transformed cells, in particular, acquire new antigenic determinants on the cell surface and within the cell. These are coded for by the viral genome and are specific for a particular virus, regardless of the cell type. There may be one or many new antigens, depending on the transforming virus.

Chemically transformed and radiation-transformed cells may also bear new antigens, but these are likely to differ with each line of transformed cells. There may also be modification in expression of antigens of the major histocompatibility complex.

Tumour cells *in vivo* and transformed cells frequently also lose antigenic determinants which are expressed on their normal counterparts.

New cell-surface characteristics

In addition to alteration in antigenic structure, modifications in the cell-surface structure may be detected by modifications in the binding properties of other molecules, such as plant lectins. This is almost certainly a reflection of alterations in the structure of cell-surface glycoproteins. Similarly, there may be alterations in cell-surface receptors for growth factors.

Cell membrane transport and permeability may be impaired. Cell surface charge (or ion density), endocytosis, and intercellular communication, may all be altered. Tumour and transformed cells may also have an altered sensitivity to cellular lytic mechanisms, such as killing by *natural killer (NK) cells*.

Loss of contact inhibition of movement

Normal cells interact with the cells around them, whether they are of the same or of different types. Normal fibroblastic cells do not normally move over or under similar cells but reorient to lie parallel to each other, thus forming a highly ordered often 'swirled' pattern. While normal fibroblasts can grow in multiple layers, they do so in an orderly manner. On the other hand, transformed fibroblasts do not respond to adjacent cells in this way and readily move over or under other cells, thus forming a disordered multilayered structure. When stained, these show up as a dense focus against the more uniform normal cells. They are said to have *lost contact inhibition*.

Normal skin epithelial cells (keratinocytes) have a quite different growth pattern. When grown in primary or secondary culture only a proportion of the cells form a colony. Since they do not normally move around, as fibroblasts do, this criterion of loss of contact inhibition does not apply. This poses problems in recognizing transformation in keratinocytes.

Epithelial cells of other origins (e.g. kidney) grow more or less in a uniform monolayer. While they do not migrate as efficiently as fibroblasts, the degree of movement, together with their altered morphology, give a striking focus morphology.

Anchorage independence

Many transformed cells are capable of growing in suspension in soft agar or methylcellulose-containing culture media. This is not a property of normal cells. Immortalized cells acquire this property to a limited extent. Transformed cells that grow in agar are said to show *anchorage independence*. Not all the cells of a transformed cell line grow under these conditions. However, any culture that shows even a low proportion of cells capable of growth in agar is almost certainly transformed. The reverse is not, however, true. Some cells that show many of the other characteristics of transformation do not grow in agar. So, it is not, as claimed by some, an unequivocal method of discriminating normal from transformed cells.

Density-dependent growth

Normal cells grow exponentially in culture until a *saturation density* is reached; even renewal of medium does not permit growth much beyond this density. Transformed cells usually grow to a much higher saturation density under identical conditions. If the amount of serum in the medium is reduced, a point is usually reached where normal cells remain alive but grow little or not at all, while transformed cells grow to relatively high saturation densities.

It is now clear that these different behaviour patterns are largely due to a combination of growth-factor requirements, together with exhaustion of nutrients. However, for some cells at least, a genuine restriction on growth is caused by contact with other cells.

Many cells require specific growth factors. Transformed cells appear to have a lower requirement for these growth factors, for several reasons. For example, the *growth-factor receptor*, to which the growth factor specifically binds on the cell surface, may be modified in such a way that it triggers the internal signalling pathway, which leads to cell growth and division without the necessity for growth-factor binding. Alternatively, the transformed cell may itself secrete the growth factor which stimulates its own growth. This is termed *autocrine stimulation* (see Section 9.6).

Immortalization

Transformed cells have an extended life in culture. Some have acquired the capacity for unlimited growth, viz. *immortalization*. Others, however, while they have an extended life-span, do not grow indefinitely, e.g. human cells transformed by SV40 virus. The latter are transformed by most criteria and then enter a *crisis phase* when growth slows down and many, sometimes all, of the cells die. A small number of cells may come through this crisis and, if they do, they generally form stable, truly immortal cell lines.

Tumourigenicity

Cells that have acquired the above *in vitro* characteristics usually grow into tumours when inoculated into appropriate hosts. Such cells are considered fully transformed. Other cells, which have many of the characteristics of transformed cells, will not produce tumours *in vivo*. In the case of some virus-transformed cells, it can be shown clearly that this is because the new virus-specific antigens acquired by the cells have rendered them immunogenic, even in the syngeneic host. The cells are recognized by the host as foreign and are rejected by an immune mechanism. This process of immune rejection has been termed *immune surveillance* (see Section 9.10). While the existence of this phenomenon has been questioned for other systems, it clearly is very real for virus-transformed cells. Some cells can thus be considered transformed even if not tumourigenic.

What then is cellular transformation?

This is by no means simple. It is accepted that immortalization alone is not enough. At the other extreme, any cells that produce tumours *in vivo* are considered transformed. In practice, many would accept that cells that show anchorage-independent growth and have some of the behavioural and morphological characteristics described above are transformed, even if they fail to produce tumours in animals, e.g. adenovirus type 2 transformed rat embryo cells.

Relationship of cancer cells in culture to transformed phenotype

If cancer cells can be grown in culture they tend to show many of the characteristics of transformed cells, but not all cancer cells show all the features of transformation. Some cancer cells (e.g. ovarian carcinoma) will grow in soft agar, and this has been used as the basis of a drug sensitivity test, but other carcinomas will not grow in agar. Even when a particular kind of cancer has been found to exhibit a specific characteristic, not all tumours of the same kind exhibit that characteristic and, indeed, the usual finding is that a relatively low proportion of cancers of a given type can be adapted to grow in culture.

One must be particularly aware that cancer cells in culture may not be representative of the original tumour. First, not all cell types represented in the original tumour are established in culture; and secondly there may be considerable selection for cell types that are favoured by the particular growth conditions. Nevertheless, some interesting findings have come from the study of tumour cells in culture. For example, a deletion of the short arm of chromosome 3 was found in cultures of small cell carcinoma of the lung. This has now been confirmed as a feature of the primary tumours.

Oncogenes and growth factors

From studies of transforming retroviruses, and DNA transfections, a number of cellular genes have been discovered that are important in cellular growth and/or differentiation, which, when activated so that they function abnormally or inappropriately, play a part in the development of neoplasia. These *proto-oncogenes* are the cellular equivalents, *c-onc genes*, of the *v-onc genes* found in transforming retroviruses. They are all known by three-letter codes, derived most often from the virus in which they were first recognized, e.g. v-*myc* from the virus of myelocytosis has a cellular counterpart, c-*myc*. These proto-

oncogenes belong to a series of families of genes with a close structural and functional relationship. The products of these genes have different functions. Some have homology to growth factors, for example the product of c-*sis* is similar to platelet-derived growth factor (PDGF), and that of c-*erb* B2 is partially homologous to epidermal growth-factor (EGF) receptor. Others appear to be part of, or influence, intracellular signalling pathways which transmit stimuli from the cell surface to the nucleus, while another class (e.g. c-*myc*) are DNA-binding proteins apparently concerned with gene regulation. This is more fully discussed in Section 9.6.

9.2 Morphology of neoplasms

K. C. Gatter

9.2.1 The classification of tumours

Classifying tumours forms a large part of what histopathologists do, and is an obsession for many. Current classification has remained largely unchanged for more than a century and is based on the cell or tissue from which the tumour is believed to have arisen. This is usually referred to as a histogenetic classification and is now so entrenched that it is difficult to believe that it took many years to become established. In 1923 Mallory had to take the time in his textbook of pathology to argue that 'Tumours are classified like normal tissues on a histologic basis . . . The type of cell is the one important element in every tumour. From it the tumour should be named, not from some peculiarity of minor importance, such as method of growth, or arrangement of cells or form of retrograde change.' Even as late as 1948 Willis in his *tour de force*, *Pathology of Tumours*, felt the need to snap at the dwindling band of critics: 'Criticisms of the histogenetic basis of tumour classification such as MacCallum's (1940) are groundless. MacCallum wrote, "Classification is at best unsatisfactory on a histogenetic basis since so often we cannot make a good guess at the tissue which the tumour most resembles, or the point from which it actually sprang." Such a statement from an experienced pathologist is incomprehensible.' MacCallum was a student of the great American pathologist Welch, professor of pathology at Columbia, and then followed Welch as professor at Johns Hopkins.

As we enter a new era of powerful techniques, which threaten to change or modify the basis of our classification of tumours, it is useful to consider the purpose of this classification and why we have stuck to histogenesis for so long. A full discussion of this is beyond the scope of this section but the first few chapters of Willis's book quoted above will provide an excellent foundation and have the advantage that the arguments are not complicated by consideration of current technical advances. Basically, there are as many ways to classify tumours as there are tumours themselves or pathologists to perform the task.

This can be by aetiology, geography, epidemiology, age, sex, or even tumour size. However, in practice none of these has been nearly as useful as a classification based on histogenesis, and a classification will only survive if it is useful to pathologists in their daily duties. Thus one needs to bear in mind the information required of a pathologist about a particular tumour, which can be summarized as follows:

1. What is the origin of the tumour?
2. What is the likely behaviour of the tumour?
3. What is the extent of the tumour?

A histogenetic classification, in spite of its predominant position, only addresses the first of these questions. Therefore it is necessary to obtain additional information, which new techniques and reagents are beginning to provide, as discussed later in this section.

9.2.2   Histogenetic classification of tumours

The histogenetic classification currently in use divides tumours into two large groups, epithelial and non-epithelial (or connective tissue), with further subdivision by behaviour into benign and malignant. The principles of this system are outlined in Table 9.1. Similarly, a table can be constructed giving the main features by which a benign tumour is distinguished from one which is malignant (Table 9.2).

All textbooks of pathology have similar tables, many far more detailed than Tables 9.1 and 9.2. However, it is important to emphasize that all such systems that attempt to be logical are at best approximations to the truth and are often far removed from what is observed in practice. Tumour classification is subject to the rigours of daily life (where it is most easily learned) and consists of a mishmash of eponymous, archaic, or descriptive terms tacked on to the histogenetic structure given above. Many tumour types cannot be divided simply into those that are benign and those that are malignant. Neuroendocrine tumours are an example in which morphologically similar tumours may be either benign or malignant, e.g. carcinoid tumours and paraganglionomas.

The reason that our current classification is so imperfect reflects views, such as those of MacCallum, that our knowledge of a tumour's histogenesis is often a guess. In spite of his stinging attack, Willis gives a classification of tumours 'based solely on histogenesis and behaviour' which includes Hodgkin's disease (cell of origin unknown), myeloma (wrong guess), and chloroma (a purely descriptive term). All of these terms are still in current use.

9.2.3   What is the origin of a tumour?

Much research in pathology over the past 50 years has been aimed at improving histogenetic classification. Until the advent

Table 9.1   Classification of tumours

Tissue type	Behaviour	
	Benign	Malignant
Epithelium		
Stratified squamous	papilloma	squamous cell carcinoma
Glandular	adenoma	adenocarcinoma
Transitional	papilloma	transitional cell carcinoma
Non-epithelium (including connective tissue)		
Fibrous tissue	fibroma	fibrosarcoma
Fat	lipoma	liposarcoma
Smooth muscle	leiomyoma	leiomyosarcoma
Striated muscle	rhabdomyoma	rhabdomyosarcoma
Synovium	synovioma	synovial sarcoma
Cartilage	chondroma	chondrosarcoma
Bone	osteoma	osteosarcoma
Blood vessels	haemangioma	angiosarcoma
Germ cells	benign teratoma	malignant teratoma
Neuroectoderm	naevus	melanoma

Table 9.2   Distinction of benign from malignant tumours

Characteristic	Benign	Malignant
Growth rate	low mitotic rate normal mitoses normal nucleoli	high mitotic rate abnormal mitoses large nucleoli
Differentiation	resembles normal maintains normal functions	often poor lost or altered function
Spread	encapsulated no invasion no metastases	no capsule locally invasive metastases common

of electron microscopy in the 1950s, the origin of a tumour was generally based on where it was and what it looked like microscopically. A keratinizing tumour in the skin is likely to have arisen there from squamous epidermal cells. And indeed, early studies of carcinogenesis, using noxious materials on rabbits' ears, showed a gradual transition from hyperplastic changes through to invasive squamous cell carcinoma. In practice, a proportion of tumours bears so little resemblance to their presumed tissue of origin that morphological analysis alone only provides a diagnosis of malignant tumour.

It could be argued that such undifferentiated neoplasms have an aggressive course so that it is unnecessary to define them further. Advances in therapy have made it important that pathologists improve the accuracy of diagnosis of such tumours. The differential diagnosis of undifferentiated tumours is different in adults and children, as outlined in Fig. 9.1.

It can be seen that carcinoma is the commonest adult malignancy, with lymphoma only 9 per cent of the total. However, when undifferentiated adult tumours are considered, the picture changes and lymphoma becomes the predominant tumour type (67 per cent). Leukaemia and lymphoma are the commonest paediatric neoplasms, both in cases which are straightforward to diagnose and in those requiring immunocytochemical

diagnosis. Thus, in both situations it is essential to recognize these tumours, which are rarely cured by surgery alone, respond to chemotherapy, and have been shown to have a better prognosis than other tumour types (Robinson *et al.* 1988) (see Fig. 9.2).

9.2.4 The diagnosis of tumours of uncertain origin

Electron microscopy held great promise of assisting in the diagnosis of poorly differentiated tumours. It has failed to achieve that goal and is rarely considered an essential investigation today. Its 'downfall' is of interest because it highlights the essential problem of these difficult tumours. Electron microscopy allows a detailed view of the ultrastructure of cells and can reliably distinguish one cell type from another based on the presence of particular features such as melanosomes (melanoma), desmosomes (squamous tumours), or dense core granules (neuro-endocrine tumours). Unfortunately many, if not most, anaplastic tumours do not possess many of these organelles, which means that their poor architectural differentiation is reflected by an underlying lack of cellular differentiation. It therefore becomes a time-consuming task looking for one

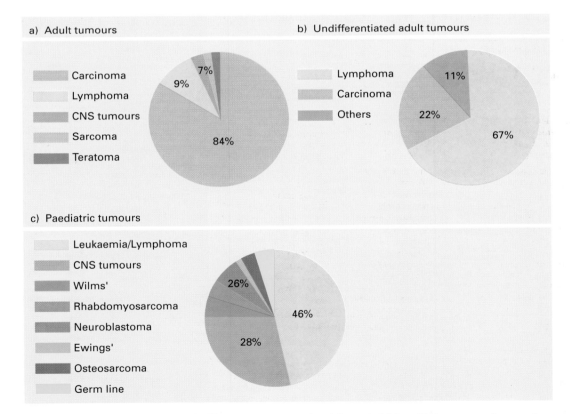

Fig. 9.1 The relative proportions of different tumour types in adults and children. There are two diagrams for adult tumours: (a) represents the overall proportions of different tumours; (b) indicates the distribution of tumour types in a group of neoplasms originally diagnosed as undifferentiated, i.e. they could not be separated into the major tumour types by conventional analysis but required further investigation by immunocytochemical means as detailed below. (Drawn after Gatter *et al.* 1985, with permission.)

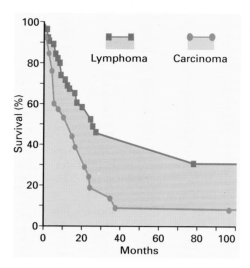

Fig. 9.2 Survival of patients initially diagnosed as having undifferentiated tumours, which were characterized by immunocytochemical labelling. The survival of patients with lymphoma is contrasted with those having carcinoma, illustrating the better prognosis of the former. (Drawn after Robinson *et al.* 1988, with permission.)

granule in a thousand cells. Added to this is the fact that other cell types, both normal and malignant, may possess occasional organelles indistinguishable ultrastructurally (and indeed func-

tionally) from those being sought in a particular tumour. Further problems arise when only small amounts of material are available for analysis, particularly if the morphology is distorted by crushing at biopsy or by poor fixation. Such biopsies are becoming more frequent due to the increasing use of techniques such as endoscopy or fine-needle aspiration.

A great advance in this field has been made in the past 10 years by the application of immunocytochemical techniques and monoclonal antibodies (see Section 30.2). There is now available a small panel of reagents with which the average pathology laboratory can diagnose more than 90 per cent of such problem tumours. This approach has achieved widespread acceptance amongst histopathologists, particularly with the availability of monoclonal antibodies able to recognize their antigens reliably in routinely processed and paraffin-wax-embedded sections. Previously, frozen sections were required, necessitating a separate biopsy (and often the reason for the problem in the first place was that a good biopsy could not be obtained). The simple flow chart in Fig. 9.3 summarizes the way in which the histogenetic origin of a tumour may be shown by immunocytochemical staining when its nature is not apparent on routine histological examination. This scheme refers to immunocytochemical analysis of routinely processed paraffin sections where the number of reagents available is limited (for further details see Mason and Gatter 1987). Table 9.3 gives details of antibodies available commercially as of August 1989.

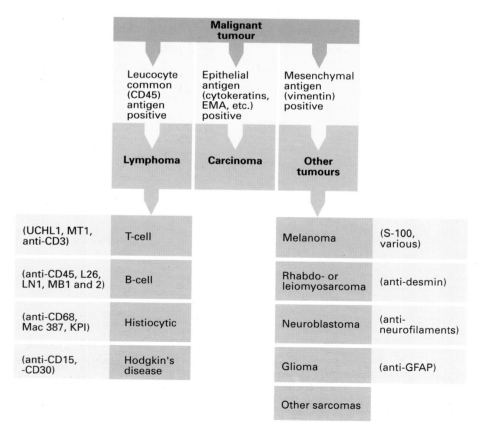

Fig. 9.3 Flow chart illustrating how a malignant tumour of uncertain origin can be investigated immunocytochemically. The antibodies suggested all perform reliably on routinely processed material; further information about them is given in Table 9.3.

Table 9.3 Antibodies reactive with formalin-fixed tissues useful for routine pathological diagnosis

Tumour type	Antibody specificity	Source*	Comment
Carcinoma	Cytokeratin	Various including Becton-Dickinson DAKO, Hybritech, Immunotech	Cytokeratin expression has been reported in a number of sarcomas, including synovial, epithelioid, and leiomyosarcoma
	Epithelial membrane antigen (EMA)	DAKO, Miles, Serotec	EMA has also been identified in a number of high-grade lymphomas, particularly of anaplastic type
Lymphoma	Leucocyte common antigen (LCA) CD45	DAKO	Some high-grade lymphomas (anaplastic and lymphoblastic) may be unstained
Melanoma	HMB45, anti-S100	Enzo, DAKO, Serotec	Specificity for melanoma is questionable; do not distinguish benign from malignant melanocytic lesions
Neural tumours	Neurofilaments	Amersham, DAKO, Boehringer	A proportion of poorly differentiated carcinomas and sarcomas also express neurofilaments
Muscle tumours	Desmin, actin, myoglobin	Amersham, DAKO, Boehringer, Enzo, and others	Desmin is currently regarded as the most useful muscle marker
Glial tumours	Glial fibrillary acidic protein (GFAP)	Amersham, DAKO, Boehringer	For astrocytomas and oligodendrogliomas
Endocrine tumours			
thyroid	Thyroglobulin	DAKO	For most thyroid cancers
prostate	Prostatic acid phosphatase Prostatic specific antigen	DAKO	For prostate cancer
medullary	Calcitonin		For medullary carcinoma of thyroid
neuroendocrine	Serotonin, synaptophysin	DAKO	For neuroblastomas, carcinoid, etc.
Germ-cell tumours	Placental alkaline phosphatase	DAKO	For teratomas and choriocarcinomas
For lymphoma typing			
B-cell	L26 (CD20) CD45RA	DAKO DAKO, Eurodiagnostics, Clonab, Serotec	A small number of T-cell lymphomas have been reported positive with both L26 and CD45RA; L26 also stains many cases of Hodgkin disease
T-cell	CD43 CD45RO (UCHL1)	DAKO, Eurodiagnostics, Clonab DAKO	CD43 antibodies also react with some B-cell lymphomas; both CD43 and CD45RO stain granulocytes and macrophages
Macrophage/monocyte	CD68 (KP1)	DAKO	CD68 labels weakly a number of B-cell malignancies and some cases of melanoma
Granulocytic	Elastase (NP57)	DAKO	Labels most chronic myeloid and approximately half of the cases of acute myeloid leukaemias
Hodgkin disease	CD15	Becton-Dickinson, Clonab, DAKO, Eurodiagnostics	Both CD15 and CD30 antibodies recognize a subset of non-Hodgkin lymphomas
	CD30 (BerH2)	DAKO	
Megakaryocytic	CD61 (Y2/51)	DAKO	Antigen is platelet glycophorin IIIa
Erythroblastic	Anti-glycophorin C (Ret 40f)	DAKO	

* This table of commercial sources is by no means comprehensive, and interested pathologists are advised to contact their local representatives for particular details.

This is an area of great activity so that newer, better reagents can be expected to be produced continuously and interested pathologists should consult the individual companies for further details.

It will be immediately obvious that the greatest detail can be obtained from immunocytochemical study of lymphoma and that the amount of information to be gained from carcinomas and sarcomas is limited. It may seem odd that tumours arising from tissues looking as different as colon and ovary, or fat and bone, cannot be separated immunocytochemically whereas lymphocytes, which all look so similar, can be subdivided so comprehensively. At first there was a tacit assumption that since immunologists were the earliest producers of monoclonal antibodies it was only a matter of time for the solid-tumour specialists to catch up. However, in spite of numerous attempts and many reports of interesting antibodies, no truly tissue-specific antibody, other than those mentioned in Table 9.3, has yet achieved general acceptance and agreement.

For the investigation of unfixed material, the number of antibodies now in existence is large and can be confusing for both novice and expert. A series of international workshops devoted to monoclonal antibodies directed against antigens present on human leucocytes has brought considerable order to the white-cell field by characterizing monoclonal antibodies in groups (CD groups) according to the molecules they recognize. Details of these workshops and the 78 CD groups currently identified are given in Chapter 4 (see McMichael 1987 for information on the first 45 CD groups). Similar classification schemes for other monoclonal antibodies (e.g: against epithelial or mesenchymal antigens) have been more difficult to achieve, due to the difficulties of performing biochemical analyses on solid tissues. However, progress is being made in such fields as cytokeratins, small cell carcinoma antigens and melanoma-associated antigens.

9.2.5 Tumour markers and the subclassification of malignancies

Most tumours are classified as arising in a particular organ or tissue because that is where they are found and they bear some type of resemblance to it. A squamous cell carcinoma in the skin can often be found arising imperceptibly from the epidermis and

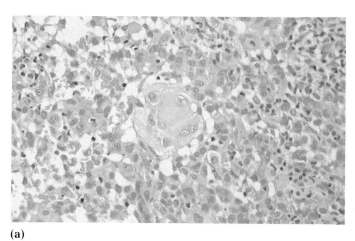

(a)

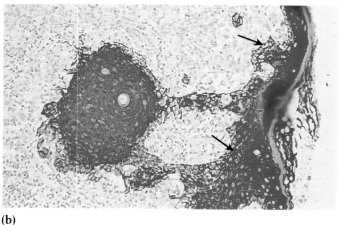

(b)

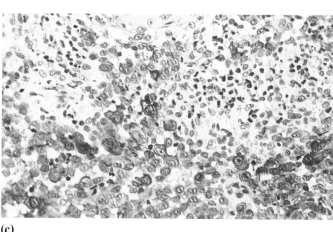

(c)

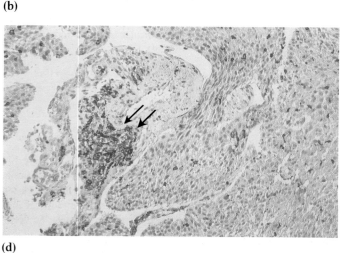

(d)

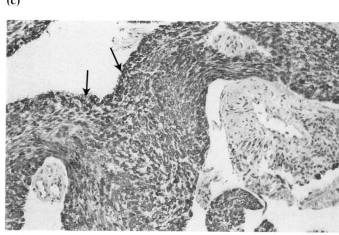

(e)

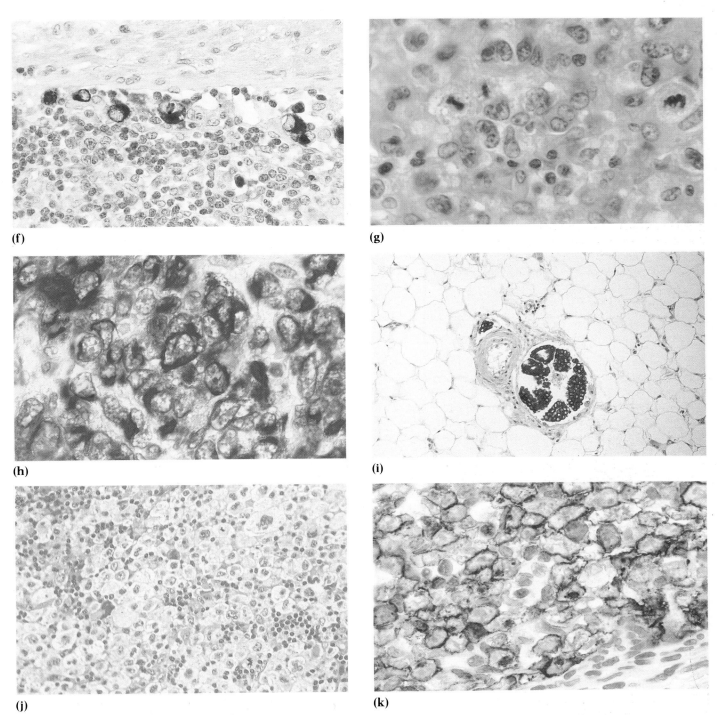

Fig. 9.4 (a) A poorly differentiated tumour initially thought to be a squamous cell carcinoma because of focal areas of keratinous differentiation such as that shown in the centre of the figure. However, immunostaining for high molecular weight cytokeratins (b) shows positivity in the stratified epithelium (arrow) whereas the tumour cells are unstained. The tumour is, in reality, a malignant melanoma, which is confirmed by positive immunostaining for melanoma-associated antigens, such as that shown in (c). (d) and (e) A bronchial biopsy contains a crushed tumour which is clearly malignant but caused uncertainty whether it was a lymphoma or a small cell carcinoma. Immunostaining in (d) shows the tumour to be unstained for leucocyte antigens (only reactive lymphocytes, as arrowed, are positive) whereas the tumour is strongly stained for epithelial cytokeratins (arrowed in (e)). This indicates that the malignancy is a small cell carcinoma. (f) and (i) Immunostaining techniques are able to pick out single or small numbers of malignant cells in lymph nodes (f) or arterioles (i). This may be valuable when looking for micrometastases. A poorly differentiated paediatric tumour (g) is identified as a rhabdomyosarcoma by immunocytochemical staining for desmin intermediate filaments (h). (j) A malignant tumour initially diagnosed as a clear cell carcinoma of the kidney on morphological grounds. However, it was negative when stained for epithelial markers but positive for a range of white-cell markers including the CD30 antigen (k) which is characteristic of a subgroup of large-cell non-Hodgkin lymphomas.

showing stratification and keratinization. It must, therefore, be originating from the epidermis. This holds for many tumours found in epithelial-lined structures, e.g., gut, ovaries, cervix, bladder, etc. Yet there are examples where tumours bear no resemblance to the host organ. For instance, there is no squamous epithelium in the normal lung to account for the commonest carcinoma apparently arising there. It is customary to explain this phenomenon by invoking metaplastic change in the pseudostratified ciliated columnar bronchial epithelium. But there is no proven cell or tissue type that looks like oat (or small) cell carcinoma. Indeed, very few pulmonary adenocarcinomas bear much resemblance to bronchial or alveolar epithelium, and primary tumours are often morphologically indistinguishable from secondary adenocarcinomas.

Tumour classification becomes more difficult when the primary site is unclear. Examples are:

1. secondary carcinoma in lymph nodes or effusions;

2. where the tumour is large and involves several adjacent structures; and

3. when modern biopsy techniques have procured a small sample of tumour with no normal tissue attached.

It is in these instances that pathologists have looked for tumour markers. In the past 20 years many papers and books have been written on this subject but the reader usually searches in vain for a definition of what is being described. Tumour markers represent a theoretical idea that differs, like relativity, depending on the position of the observer. For a pathologist there are two ideal types of tumour marker. Those which distinguish malignant from benign cells (discussed below) and those which distinguish one tumour type from another.

The current history of tumour markers is generally held to date from the mid-1960s with the description of carcinoembryonic antigen, or CEA as it is universally abbreviated. This is a complex glycoprotein whose structure is still not completely elucidated. It was demonstrated biochemically in embryonic tissues and in malignancies of the gastrointestinal tract but not in normal mature tissues. Even more exciting was the fact that it could be demonstrated in the serum of patients with colonic cancer. Subsequent investigation has shown the situation to be considerably more complex. CEA turns out to belong to a family of molecules (frequently confused in many studies) some of which are present in high levels in normal cells and in the serum of patients without malignancies. Furthermore, CEA itself is found in low levels in normal colonic tissue and is absent in a certain proportion of cancers. Borderline lesions have variable levels of CEA and thus cannot, in practice, be distinguished from malignancies. Many other malignancies, including both adeno- and squamous carcinomas, also have high levels of CEA. In summary, CEA is not of practical use as a tumour marker for the distinction of benign from malignant gastrointestinal lesions nor in the separation of tumours of the gut from those of other organs. Research continues to analyse the value of CEA in tumour staging or as a marker of tumour recurrence after sur-

gery. At present the value of CEA as a tumour marker remains unclear.

There is a large number of other tumour markers, many of which are little more than one-paper wonders. The most important with established clinical usage are α-fetoprotein (AFP) and human chorionic gonadotrophin (HCG). Neither has proved reliable for histopathological diagnosis using immunocytochemical techniques and antibodies against them. Like CEA, both can be demonstrated in a wider range of malignancies than originally thought and in some normal tissues. However, AFP is considered valuable in the serological monitoring of testicular tumours and HCG for choriocarcinomas. There is also some evidence that AFP is a practical marker for screening populations at risk of developing hepatocellular cancer, e.g. in China and South-East Asia or amongst Alaskan Eskimos with hepatitis B infection. However, similar screening protocols in Western nations where hepatocellular cancer is rare have not shown AFP to be sufficiently sensitive for routine use.

So, tumour markers in the purist sense do not exist at present for pathological use. However, there has been a great deal of interest in the use of differentiation markers for tumour identification and these are often loosely referred to as tumour markers. The best-known examples are from endocrine tumours. A secondary carcinoma containing thyroglobulin or calcitonin is likely to have arisen in the thyroid, or one expressing prostatic acid phosphatase to have come from the prostate. Even these need interpreting with care, since tumours arising in other sites can produce and secrete hormones not normally associated with their tissue of origin, e.g. carcinoma of the lung is a well-known example of inappropriate or ectopic hormone production.

One group of such differentiation markers which illustrates well the pitfalls and difficulties in this field is that comprising the intermediate filaments. This is a group of intracellular proteins approximately 10 nm in diameter, midway in size between microtubules and structural filaments like actin and myosin. They comprise a number of different proteins, which appear to be specific for the major cell and tissue types, as indicated in Table 9.4.

When monoclonal antibodies were first employed in the investigation of tumours it appeared that neoplasms maintained the intermediate filament pattern of their tissue of origin regardless of the degree of differentiation. Since the cytokeratins had been shown to be a family of at least 19 polypeptides with unique distributions in different epithelial tissues, it seemed that the problem of unclassifiable malignancies was at an end. Un-

Table 9.4 Intermediate filaments as differentiation markers: protein components and cell specificity

Intermediate filament	Cell type recognized
Cytokeratin	epithelial cells
Vimentin	mesenchymal cells
Desmin	muscle cells
Neurofilaments	neural cells
Glial fibrillary acidic protein	glial cells

fortunately, further investigation revealed inconsistencies, e.g. epithelial cells in effusions co-expressed two different intermediate filaments and certain embryonic tissues displayed different intermediate filaments at certain times during development. At first these observations were incorporated into the hypothesis as exceptions or special situations. However, the list of exceptions became so large that intermediate-filament typing alone could not be relied upon to provide histogenetic information, particularly in the very situations where it was most needed, the differential diagnosis of anaplastic tumours. Interestingly, further study of normal and embryonic tissues showed much greater overlap of intermediate filament types than the early studies had indicated.

9.2.6 What is the likely behaviour of a tumour?

'Is it benign or malignant?' is the most important question asked of a pathologist by the clinician. The essence of this is captured by the story of the old-timer pathologist who was immensely popular with his clinical colleagues. He never issued written reports but merely rubber-stamped the request forms BENIGN or MALIGNANT. It may therefore seem surprising that over the past 100 years or so we have made so little technical progress in the pathological distinction of benign from malignant tumours. This still depends almost exclusively on the examination of formalin-fixed paraffin-wax-embedded sections stained with dyes such as haematoxylin and eosin. It is true that we have learned a great deal about the interpretation of such sections, allowing one to give more information about the likely behaviour of a tumour than 50 years ago, but the major technical advances in other disciplines seem at times to have evaded pathology altogether. Perhaps this can be illustrated by imagining the return of the great founding fathers Virchow, Röntgen, and Lister to our modern hospital. Who would be the most amazed? I suspect that the first would be helping us out in our daily work after a short period of acclimatization.

This is not to suggest that pathologists have been complacent in their search for improvement and, in particular, for a cancer test. Since the late nineteenth century virtually every advance in biological science has been examined for its potential as a discriminator of neoplastic and normal tissue. For example, soon after the descriptions of antigen–antibody reactions pathologists were claiming tests based on complement-fixation tests or the haemolytic properties of cancer serum as 100 per cent accurate in distinguishing patients with cancer from those without. One interesting example is the intradermal test for malignancy described by Dr Gruskin from Philadelphia in 1932. He extracted antigen from embryonic liver for a carcinoma test and from Wharton's jelly and red bone marrow of calf embryo for sarcoma. These were then injected intradermally, like a skin allergy test, into the patient. An inflammatory reaction indicated either carcinoma or sarcoma, depending on the antigen used. One receives the impression that Dr Gruskin envisaged a fundamental change in pathological testing, with patients arriving for a battery of skin tests designed to identify carcinoma of the pancreas or osteosarcoma. Of his normal con-

trols, 107 students in good health, nine showed a positive reaction, in which cases Dr Gruskin found a family history of malignancy. As his critics pointed out 'such an unfortunate admission destroys the value of the test. We want to know whether the patient has cancer now, not that he may get it in twenty years hence. As out of any number of normal persons questioned, some would undoubtedly be found to descend from carcinomatous ancestors, the assumption that such descent is sufficient to explain the paradoxical positive reactions in the healthy, seems to be no more than a forced attempt to escape from a difficulty.'

Such comments could apply equally well to the host of serological, histochemical, ultrastructural and, more recently, immunocytochemical tests for cancer. All have burst into the literature on a wave of enthusiasm only to flounder as others try to confirm the work. Why should this be? Why is it so hard to answer such a straightforward question? Obviously there are many factors. Partly, it is a reflection of our continued ignorance about the nature of malignancy. We still have no hard criteria on which to judge our test. A broken bone or an obstructed artery are definite endpoints which can be measured. But what is a malignancy? We recognize it by its effects, such as invasion or metastasis which are advanced events; hence the quip comparing pathologists with other clinicians that 'Pathologists know everything but they're too late!' Thus any test for malignancy comprises two unknowns, the test and the malignancy. If this is applied to any system, it soon becomes evident how difficult it is to improve on the routine stains. The new techniques in molecular biology and the oncogene hypothesis have already run into this problem. It will be fascinating to see whether they can improve on all the previous attempts at a cancer test.

9.2.7 What is the extent of the tumour?

This question is often forgotten in pathological reasearch but is important in clinical practice. For many tumours this information equates with curability. If a carcinoma can be surgically excised before it has extended too far locally or metastasized, then it is generally believed the patient will be cured. Certainly, the evidence from tumours of skin, bowel, and breast would appear to support this thesis. In fact, if a patient with, for example, a completely resected carcinoma of the breast dies some years later with metastatic disease (and no new primary tumour), it is widely held that she must have had occult tumour in lymph glands or bone marrow at presentation.

There have been many studies designed to detect these tumour deposits. Routine removal of impalpable lymph nodes and multiple bone marrow biopsies have been performed in a number of tumour types. None of these has really proved useful. Yet the need to detect occult micrometastases would seem to be more pressing as screening programmes begin to detect earlier, smaller tumours and therapy becomes potentially more efficacious. Conventional radiological and biochemical investigations reveal secondary tumours at a relatively advanced stage. New developments in computerized tomography and magnetic resonance hold promise, but are as yet insufficiently developed even for research into this problem.

Antibodies, particularly monoclonal antibodies, have considerable potential in the detection of small, even single-cell, metastases. Antibodies against epithelial antigens have been shown to detect tiny tumour deposits in both lymph nodes and bone marrow in a variety of carcinomas. Recent studies have indicated that these findings correlate with the patient's clinical course, i.e. tumour recurrence, overt metastatic disease, and survival are all worse in those with micrometastases. It now needs to be established whether this information can be manipulated therapeutically to improve patient survival. Indeed, antibodies themselves are being evaluated as carriers of radioactive or cytotoxic agents to the tumour cells *in vivo*.

9.2.8   Bibliography

Gatter, K. C., Alcock, C., Heryet, A., and Mason, D. Y. (1985) Clinical importance of analysing malignant tumours of uncertain origin with immunohistological techniques. *Lancet* i, 1302–5.

McMichael, A. (ed.) (1987). *Leucocyte typing III*. Oxford University Press, Oxford.

Mason, D. Y., and Gatter, K. C. (1987). The role of immunocytochemistry in diagnostic pathology. *Journal of Clinical Pathology* 40, 1042–54.

Robinson, M., Alcock, C., Gatter, K. C., and Mason, D. Y. (1988). The analysis of malignant tumours of uncertain origin with immunohistological techniques: Clinical follow-up. *Clinical Radiology* 39, 432–4.

Siefert, G. (ed.) (1987). *Morphological tumour markers*. Springer-Verlag, Berlin.

Wick, M. R. and Siegal, G. P. (eds) (1988). *Monoclonal antibodies in diagnostic immunohistochemistry*. Dekker, New York.

Willis, R. A. (1948). *Pathology of tumours*. Butterworths, London.

9.2.9   Nucleolar organizer regions (NORs) in neoplasms

J. Crocker

Nucleolar organizer regions

Nucleolar organizer regions (NORs) are structures of central importance in the transcription of DNA to ribosomal RNA. This latter then forms ribosomes and these ultimately assemble proteins. The NORs consist of strips or loops of ribosomal DNA (rDNA; ribosomal cistrons) and may be regarded in simple terms as 'ribosome factories'. Their molecular nature can be demonstrated by the binding (hybridization) of radiolabelled ribosomal RNA (rRNA), which localizes on the NOR sites. The rDNA transcribes to rRNA under the catalytic influence of RNA polymerase I (RPI). Using specialized ultrastructural techniques, in spreads of chromosomes the nascent RNA molecules can be seen to form from the DNA cores; when this method is

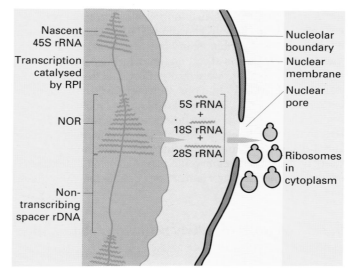

Fig. 9.5   NORs in the assembly of ribosomes (from Crocker 1988).

used the RNA appears in the form of lengthening 'branches' of 'Christmas tree'-like structures, representing the NOR complex (Fig. 9.5). Indeed, the NORs lie in tandem, with non-transcribing spacer regions lying between them. The first RNA moiety to appear at the NORs is the 45S unit, which is then converted to the 18S and 28S subunits, about half of the 45S material being lost or degraded in the process. This temporal sequence of ribosomal assembly has been elucidated by radioactive pulse-labelling. Once the various components of ribosomes are constructed (including some fragments not made in the nucleolus), they are assembled in the cytoplasm, the components having passed through nuclear pores.

Thus, the sequence of ribosomal assembly, from the NORs onwards, is fairly well understood. The role of the NOR-associated proteins (NORAPs) in this sequence is currently being investigated (see below).

NORs and chromosomes

Structures regarded as NORs have been observed on chromosomes for some years. They can be seen in conventionally prepared chromosomes as so-called 'secondary constrictions', observed as unstained 'gaps'. Not surprisingly, these are not true breaks in chromosomal integrity and the areas can be shown to possess an unusual ultrastructural configuration. The secondary constrictions hybridize with radiolabelled rRNA. These regions occur, in humans, on the short arms of the five acrocentric chromosomes, namely 13, 14, 15, 21, and 22. The NORs can be seen close to the centromere as a 'secondary constriction', or by hybridization methods, but are usually (and more conveniently) demonstrated by the binding of their associated proteins to silver (Ag⁺) ions. The silver-binding reaction is relatively simple and can easily be applied to several types of preparation. The latter are exposed to a silver formate colloid stabilized by gelatin, which enables the Ag^+ ions to bind to the NORAPs. This reaction, traditionally run at 60 °C, is now performed at 20 °C and can be applied to chromosome preparations, cells, or paraffin tissue sections. For convenience, this is called the 'AgNOR' reaction and the reaction sites 'AgNORs'.

NOR-associated proteins (NORAPs)

There are numerous proteins associated with the rDNA cistrons. Indeed, some 70 different proteins may lie on the 5' end of nascent rRNA at the NOR sites. Determination of the role and characterization of the proteins has now begun and the properties of some are now known. The major NORAP, C_{23} protein ('nucleolin') is perhaps the best characterized. It can be demonstrated by means of Ag^+ binding or by immunohistochemical techniques using antibodies to nucleolin. The basis for the silver binding (argyrophilia) of NORAPs is fairly well understood and appears to be dependent upon sequential uptake of silver ions by carboxyl, disulphide, and sulphydryl groups. This feature is common to all known or characterized NORAPs, which are rich in these chemical groupings, and has been shown by silver and fluorescent probes. When histone proteins are removed from chromosomes or nuclei, the sites of argyrophilia remain, implying that the silver binding is independent of histones. The same is true of purified DNA and RNA. It seems likely that nucleolin is involved intimately in the regulation of rDNA transcription. Thus, for example, it has been shown to bind to non-transcribing ('spacer') regions of rDNA, next to the area that initiates transcription to pre-rRNA. Indeed, there is evidence that nucleolin may regulate the activity of RP I. If rRNA genes are transfected into foreign cells and amplified, it is possible for them to be transcribed under the influence of RP II (instead of RP I). If this occurs, there is no silver binding at the NOR sites; this strongly sugests that nucleolin controls or even 'selects' RP I activity.

Other NORAPs include B_{23} protein, 100 kDa and 80 kDa proteins, and phosphoproteins pp 105 and pp 135. These have yet to be fully characterized but may be demonstrated cytochemically or immunohistochemically in NOR sites. Nucleolin may, in fact, be pp 105. The role of these proteins is not yet known. Antibodies to pp 105 can be used to label proliferating cells in tissue sections of tumours.

NORs in cytogenetics

The presence of silver-stained NORs on the five acrocentric chromosomes has been used by cytogeneticists for more than a decade for the investigation of chromosomal aberrations. Thus, breakages or translocations involving parts of chromosomes 13, 14, 15, 21, and 22 may result in abnormal positioning of NORs, which can then be used as 'markers' for the areas of the chromosome being studied (Fig. 9.6). This may be seen in meiotic nondysjunctions, such as Down's or Patau's syndromes, where extra inappropriately placed NORs can be seen in metaphase spreads. It is of interest that where the number of NORs is increased, there is a concomitant increase in biochemically assayed DNA in the affected cell. If, as may occur, NORs are lost as a result of chromosomal fusion, the amount of DNA per cell nucleus is diminished.

In human cells, the degree of argyrophilia on individual

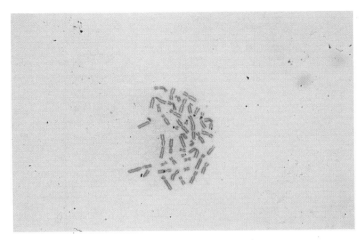

Fig. 9.6 A human trisomy 21 karyotype, stained by the AgNOR technique, showing NOR sites. (From Crocker 1988.)

NORs on chromosomes is constant and inheritable. The size of silver-stained NORs is also related to the degree of transcriptional activity of the rDNA concerned. Thus, larger AgNOR sites on chromosomes are more transcriptionally active than those of small size. This may not be true in interphase nuclei (see below) in malignant cells.

Gene amplification and NORs

When gene amplification occurs, additional copies of that gene are made and these are positioned in tandem. This may result from a variety of stimuli. Thus, AgNOR sizes or numbers might vary with cell activation resulting from external changes. Gene amplification may also be regular at a particular site, and inherited. For example, a human family has been described with inherited gene amplification on chromosome 14; the latter is one of the NOR-bearing acrocentrics and this variant has been named '14p +'. The AgNOR reaction shows enlarged NORs on the chromosome and is associated with 6–8 times more rDNA than usual. Interestingly, much of this area is non-transcribing DNA. It is also highly methylated, containing much methylcytosine (MeC). There is profound gene amplification in transformed or malignant cells, and this may be significant when NOR methodology is applied to analysis of cells in tumours.

NORs and cell proliferation

The behaviour of NORs and nucleoli throughout the cell cycle is fairly clearly defined. Before this can be understood, a description is necessary of the structure of NORs in interphase nuclei. The morphological interphase equivalent of metaphase (chromosomal) NORs is the fibrillar centre. This can be visualized in conventional electron microscope preparations and has three main layers. First, the fibrillar centre itself, which is electron-lucent and sometimes multiple in the nucleolus. This area is argyrophilic and contains nucleolin and other NORAPs (Fig. 9.7). It corresponds to the silver-stained nuclear 'dot' seen by light microscopy. Surprisingly, the numbers of fibrillar

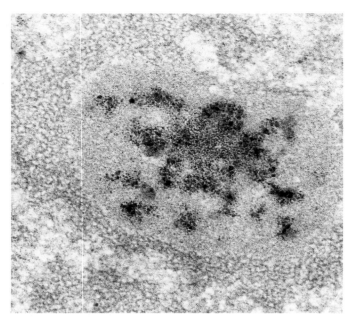

Fig. 9.7 Electron micrograph of a fibrillar centre, strongly stained with the argyrophil method. (From Crocker 1988.)

centres in a nucleus do not necessarily correspond to the number of chromosomes. Secondly, outside the fibrillar centre itself, is the dense fibrillar component and certain RNA-precursors and DNA. Thirdly, a granular component surrounds these two areas. The granules represent pre-ribosomes. Thus, there is apparently a sequence of ribosomal pre-assembly, commencing centrally and progressing outwards in these structures.

NORs and the cell cycle

The structure of fibrillar centres/NORs has been looked at electron microscopically. In prophase there is disappearance of the dense fibrillar and granular components, with concomitant diminution in nucleolar volume. In metaphase and anaphase, the nucleolus does not exist but argyrophilic NORs can be seen on some acrocentric chromosomes. In telophase, the dense fibrillar component/fibrillar centre complex reappears, followed by the granular component, and then the nucleolus can be visualized.

When lymphocytes are stimulated by phytohaemagglutinin, they enlarge, become morphological 'lymphoblasts' and show increased nuclear and protein synthetic activity. Resting lymphocytes have one large fibrillar centre. During blast 'transformation' in the second and third divisional generations, multiple smaller argyrophilic nuclear granules appear. These might be expected to be of value in rapidly dividing cells, to render rDNA transcription more efficient. These findings are reflected in human tumours in histological preparations.

Cell activation, differentiation, and NORs

It might be expected that certain substances would affect NOR activities or numbers. Indeed, this would be an important part of any protein synthetic control system. *In vivo*, certain natural and synthetic hormones, including growth hormone and dexamethasone alter rRNA synthesis. Both increase NOR numbers in human fibroblasts.

In vitro, there have been several studies of cell differentiation and NORs. The cell line HL60, derived from promyelocytic leukaemia, has useful properties in relation to cell differentiation. If HL60 cells are treated with dimethylsulphoxide (DMSO), they take on the morphology, cytochemistry, and functions of granulocytic cells. If, however, they are treated with phorbol esters or vitamin D, they become monocyte-like. This process is called 'induction' and the uninduced HL60 cells are less differentiated. When induction occurs in this cell line, the average number of AgNORs per nucleus drops from 5–6 (uninduced) to 1–2 (DMSO-induced). It appears, therefore, that as cells become more well-differentiated, their NOR numbers decline. Similar effects have been shown in other normal and neoplastic haemopoietic cells. This has obvious implications in human tumour biology and pathology.

NORs and neoplasia

Many neoplastic cells have chromosomal abnormalities. Inevitably, in some instances these abnormalities involve the NOR areas of the five acrocentric chromosomes. Abnormally positioned (ectopic) NORs have been observed on the chromosomes of several types of malignant tumours. For example, rRNA genes have been shown to be both rearranged and amplified in a human chronic myeloid leukaemia cell line (K 562), *in vitro*. Ectopic chromosomal NORs have also been observed in some human testicular tumours, although there was no evidence of amplification in these tumours. Conversely, greatly amplified (10–30 ×) rRNA genes have been noted in some squamous cell carcinomas. It is clear, then, that ectopic and/or amplified NORs are not constant in malignant tumours and are not always present together. This is perhaps not surprising because of the many factors that may modify NOR activity.

NORs in pathology of human tumours

The degree of malignancy of an individual neoplasm cannot be predicted with certainty by simple microscopic analysis alone. This is unfortunate, since this assessment is often essential for accurate prognostication and institution of suitable therapy and management. The subjective means by which degree of malignancy is assessed (e.g. nuclear pleomophism, nucleocytoplasmic ratio, polarity loss, and mitotic frequency) are often unsatisfactory in individual tumours. Accordingly, newer methods have been developed for describing malignancy more objectively.

One of the newer methods is DNA flow cytometry, where the amount of DNA per nucleus, in suspended whole nuclei, is assessed. The number of proliferating cells can also be calculated by means of this method. However, the hardware is expensive and space-consuming, the analytical procedures are time-consuming, and the level of technical expertise required is high. The technique can be applied to fresh and archival (paraffin-embedded) tissue. The results of some studies, in different tumour types, have had some predictive value.

An alternative approach has been the application of certain monoclonal antibodies (e.g. Ki-67; BK19.9; anti-transferrin receptor) which 'label' replicating, but not resting, cells. These have the disadvantage that they can only be applied to frozen material, since they do not react with archival tissue. (Newer antibodies such as those against 'PCNA' or pp105 may, however, react with paraffin sections.)

In an attempt to study tumour cell proliferation, the AgNOR technique has been applied to a wide range of normal and malignant human lymphoid tissues. Conventionally processed paraffin sections were used and it was found that the numbers of AgNOR 'dots' per cell nucleus was far greater in highly malignant lesions than in those of a less aggressive type (Fig. 9.8). This has led to the application of the AgNOR method to a wide range of diagnostic problems, often with useful results. The following are some examples:

1. Benign melanocytic lesions usually contain one AgNOR, while malignant melanomas contain many more. Other skin tumours (basal cell carcinomas) also have characteristic AgNOR counts.

2. Breast carcinomas tend to have much higher AgNOR scores than benign lesions but there is considerable 'overlap' between them. This tends to be generally true of endocrine stimulated tissues and may result from non-neoplastic tissue undergoing hormonal stimulation.

3. Malignant mesotheliomas contain significantly more AgNORs than normal and 'activated' pleural mesothelial cells.

4. Various benign and malignant tumours of childhood can be distinguished on the basis of their AgNOR counts.

5. AgNOR counts distinguish benign and malignant salivary gland neoplasms.

6. Hepatocytes in hepatic cirrhosis, primary liver cancer, and adenoma can be distinguished from one another by AgNOR counts.

Other studies of AgNORs in different situations have given varying results. The technique is most useful in diagnostic pathology if there is a good cut-off between high- and low-grade malignant tumours and especially when it is predictive of outcome in 'borderline' lesions. This is the case in lymphomas, mesothelial lesions, paediatric tumours, salivary gland neoplasms, and liver lesions. Recent evidence suggests that measuring AgNOR size may be a useful adjunct to AgNOR counts. In addition, the method is suited to automated measurement.

AgNORs and other measurements of cell proliferation

A question that has yet to be fully answered is whether the numbers of AgNORs in a cell nucleus are directly related to its ploidy, or to other factors. In non-Hodgkin's lymphomas, there is no demonstrable relationship between AgNOR numbers and DNA ploidy but there is a very high correlation between AgNOR

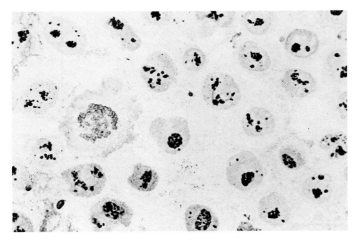

Fig. 9.8 A cytocentrifuge preparation of HL60 cells, with many AgNORs in each nucleus. (From Crocker 1988.)

scores and the number of proliferating cells measured by DNA flow cytometry. A similar correlation has been demonstrated by labelling with antibodies which bind to proliferating cells. Most significantly it has been shown that there is no relationship between interphase and metaphase AgNOR scores. Studies of other tissue types will be necessary to further clarify the relationship between AgNOR counts and other parameters of cell proliferation.

Future prospects

The clinical/biological value of this method in pathology is still being assessed. It has shown promise in many areas. Perhaps the most fruitful clinical studies will come from combined histo logical/cytogenetic investigations. There is little doubt that increased understanding of the roles of NORAPs will be of fundamental biological interest.

9.2.10 Further reading

General reviews

Alberts, B., Bray, D., Lewis, J., Raff, M., Roberts, K., and Watson, J. D. (1983). *Molecular biology of the cell.* Garland, New York.

Crocker, J. (1990). Nucleolar organizer regions. In *Current topics in pathology* (ed. J. C. E. Underwood), Springer-Verlag, Heidelberg.

Goessens, G., Thiry, M., and Lepoint, A. (1987). Relations between nucleoli and nucleolus-organizing regions during the cell cycle. In *Chromosomes today*, Vol. 9 (ed. A. Stahl, J. M. Lucini, and A. M. Vagner-Capodano). Allen and Unwin, London.

Specific references

Crocker, J. and Egan, M. J. (1988). Correlation between NOR sizes and numbers in non-Hodgkin's lymphomas. *Journal of Pathology* **156**, 233.

Crocker, J. and Nar, P. (1987). Nucleolar organizer regions in lymphomas. *Journal of Pathology* **151**, 111.

Crocker, J. and Skilbeck, N. Q. (1987). Nucleolar organizer region-associated proteins in cutaneous melanotic lesions: a quantitative study. *Journal of Clinical Pathology* **40**, 885.

Crocker, J., Macartney, J. C., and Smith, P. J. (1988). Correlation between DNA flow cytometric and nucleolar organizer region data in non-Hodgkin's lymphomas. *Journal of Pathology* **154**, 151.

Derenzini, M., Pession, A., Farabegoli, F., Trere, D., Badiali, M., and Dehan, P. (1989). Relationship between interphasic nucleolar organizer regions and growth rate in two neuroblastoma cell lines. *American Journal of Pathology* **134**, 925.

Hall, P. J., Crocker, J., Watts, A., and Stansfeld, A. G. (1988). A comparison of nucleolar organizer region staining and Ki67 immunostaining in non-Hodgkin's lymphoma. *Histopathology* **12**, 373.

Smith, R. and Crocker, J. (1988). Evaluation of nucleolar organizer region-associated proteins in breast malignancy. *Histopathology* **12**, 113.

9.2.11   Interphase cytogenetics and tumour pathology

C. S. Herrington and James O'D. McGee

History

Cytogenetics is a hybrid science which arose at the beginning of the twentieth century from the union of cytology, which had gained acceptance in the late nineteenth century, and genetics. Although there was interest in the interphase nucleus at this time, cytogenetics has to date been virtually confined to the study of the chromosomal basis of heredity through analysis of metaphase chromosomes. Chromosomes are only identifiable as distinct entities during metaphase, when the nuclear membrane has disappeared and the chromosomes are at their most condensed. However, until banding techniques were introduced in the 1970s, chromosomes were only distinguishable on the basis of relative length and the position of the centromere. This allowed the construction of several morphologically distinct chromosome groups, but the precise identification of, for example, chromosome 21 from 22, was extremely difficult. Banding techniques allow this distinction by exploiting properties of the chromosome other than their size. The intercalation of dyes between the bases of DNA depends on the nucleotide sequence of a particular segment of DNA, as some compounds have a greater affinity for GC pairs than for AT. Thus, GC-rich DNA has the reverse banding pattern of AT-rich sequences. This allows chromosomes to be identified on the basis of their sequence structure. Refinement of banding techniques has provided accurate information regarding the nature of chromosome abnormalities in a variety of situations, particularly tumour-related translocations and deletions (see Section 2.1). In the past 20 years, the application of *in situ* hybridization to metaphase cytogenetics has provided direct visual confirmation of the anatomical localization of specific nucleic acid sequences. Initially, probe preparations were crude and detection methods insensitive, and only highly repetitive sequences were detectable. Advances in both recombinant DNA technology and *in*

situ hybridization allowed the direct visualization of single-copy genes on metaphase chromosomes using first isotopic and then non-isotopic detection methods. Further refinements have increased the sensitivity of these methods such that probes as small as 0.8 kb and 1.4 kb can be detected using fluorescent and non-fluorescent non-isotopic detection procedures, respectively. However, this approach is limited to cells in metaphase. In the context of tumour pathology, metaphase cytogenetics requires either the selection of dividing cells from the tumour, where they constitute only a small and probably unrepresentative portion of the whole, or limited cell culture with the artificial arrest of cells in metaphase using colchicine. Both these approaches only allow the study of a small proportion of tumour cells.

Throughout the 1970s, the interest shown by nineteenth-century investigators, Rabl and Boveri, in the interphase nucleus was rekindled as technological advances allowed its structure to be investigated in more detail. Their suggestions, based on microscopic observations of metazoal cells, were analysed in the light of the knowledge gained through metaphase cytogenetics and using the technique of UV-microbeam irradiation. Data produced in this way were consistent with the original hypothesis that chromosomes occupy discrete nuclear territories throughout the cell cycle. The success of *in situ* hybridization prompted its use in this context, initially using total human genomic DNA to label the residual human chromosomes in mouse–human hybrids and then, with the cloning of chromosome-specific sequences, for the direct visualization of individual chromosomes in both normal and abnormal interphase nuclei. It is the latter approach which has more recently been applied to the analysis of human tumours, in particular solid tumours. This is termed 'interphase cytogenetics', a term coined by Cremer in 1986.

Probes used for interphase cytogenetics

The major criterion for selection of a particular DNA sequence for use as a probe in interphase cytogenetics is chromosome specificity. Ideally, this should be absolute but, as most sequences used are repetitive and therefore derived from the families of repetitive sequences, e.g. the Alu repeats, some cross-hybridization with non-target chromosomes does occur. This can be removed by establishing stringency conditions prior to use in interphase cytogenetics using metaphase chromosome spreads. This approach has been used with probes generated from the alphoid group of repetitive sequences, which are at centromeric sites. These probes therefore provide information regarding numerical chromosomal aberrations (as the centromere is duplicated only late in mitosis) but do not detect structural abnormalities which do not involve the centromere. More recently, an oligonucleotide derived from an alphoid repeat has been used to label the chromosome 17 centromere specifically, without the need for high-stringency conditions. Other repetitive sequences, specific for non-centromeric sites, have been selected using mini-satellites by selection for chromosome-specific variable number tandem repeats (VNTRs). These probes label telomeric sites and have been used individually and in conjunction with alphoid repeats to visualize structural abnormalities. However, the use of several different classes of probe which label discontinuous chromosomal sites provides no information regarding the intervening sequences.

The alternative approach to delineation of individual chromosomes involves the use of chromosome-specific DNA libraries. These libraries have been prepared from flow-sorted individual chromosomes and exhibit relative chromosome specificity. The inevitable cross-hybridizing signal generated from other chromosomes can be selectively removed by the prehybridization of the labelled library sequences with unlabelled human genomic DNA to low C_{ot} value. This procedure has been termed 'in situ suppression hybridization' or 'chromosome painting'. Thus, whole chromosomes, both normal and abnormal, can be specifically labelled in intact nuclei. Application of these techniques to metaphase chromosomes allows more precise characterization of structural abnormalities and the identification of the chromosome(s) of origin of markers.

All of the chromosome-specific sequences discussed above are repetitive and hence present in multiple copies per haploid genome. Thus, these probes can be detected easily using detection systems of limited sensitivity. However, the techniques presently available give information only about gross structural and numerical aberrations. Abnormalities involving shorter stretches of DNA, in particular single-copy genes, require more sensitive methods for their detection. To date, this level of sensitivity has only been achieved for viral sequences in isolated nuclei, using non-isotopic detection systems. However, the analysis of the genome of malignant cells at the single-gene level by in situ hybridization remains the only way in which the genome of malignant cells can be defined precisely, in conjunction with cell and tissue morphology.

Thus, a combined approach to the detection of chromosomes in interphase cells is required. The use of several classes of probe, designed to detect a variety of different abnormalities, both numerical and structural, will allow the description of the malignant cell genome in interphase cells. The application of these systems to tumour pathology will hopefully create some order in the jungle of chromosomal aberrations hitherto described in these lesions.

Application of interphase cytogenetics to tumour pathology

The study of the DNA content of intact tumour cell nuclei has to date been performed by flow cytometry (FCM). By staining cell nuclei using DNA-specific fluorescent dyes, the DNA content of tumour cells can be measured and compared with known diploid standards (see Section 30.6). The resultant ratio is known as the DNA index and provides a measure of the deviation of a population of cells from the normal diploid DNA content. This measure of ploidy has been shown to correlate with patient survival for some tumours but the relationship between these two parameters is less simple for others, for example breast carcinoma. Tumour ploidy measured by FCM provides no information about the nature of the DNA, it simply reflects total DNA

content. Therefore, apparently diploid cells may in reality be markedly abnormal, with deletions and reduplications balancing one another to produce a normal total DNA content. The dissection of the abnormalities in these pseudodiploid cells is one of the strengths of interphase cytogenetics as the number and position of individual chromosomes (both normal and abnormal) can be counted and mapped. In addition, chromosome number, position, and to a lesser extent structure can be correlated with nuclear morphology. As the techniques are refined, correlation with tissue morphology will allow the investigation of the synchronicity of tumour cells and their relationship with each other and the normal stroma, in addition to the description of chromosome content. The use of multiple labelling techniques of in situ hybridization also allow the identification of more than one chromosome within the same nucleus. This has been performed primarily using fluorescent techniques, with the successful identification of up to three separate chromosomes within the same nucleus. The recent development of a non-fluorescent double labelling technique should allow application to cells and tissue sections in a routine clinical setting.

The investigation of human tumours using interphase cytogenetics requires both a tissue sample and the appropriate probe/detection system for the demonstration of the chromosomes of interest. A variety of cell and tissue samples have been used for analysis, but most methods have been applied to either cultured cell lines or disaggregated tumour cells. Although these preparations ensure that intact nuclei are used, their preparation involves either cell culture or isolation. Both these processes are likely to produce a biased cell sample and hence interpretation must be carried out with this in mind. In addition, the morphology of the lesion is destroyed and hence the relationship of tumour cells to one another and to the surrounding stroma cannot be analysed. The use of tissue sections, either frozen or aldehyde-fixed and embedded in paraffin wax, would provide morphological information, but section cutting produces a cell sample containing partial nuclei. Thus, errors occur due to loss of nuclear material, in particular the underestimation of polysomy.

Despite these problems, several tumour types have been investigated using these techniques, including transitional carcinoma of the bladder, carcinoma of the breast, and neuroectodermal tumours. The development of interphase cytogenetics and its application to these particular tumours will now be discussed.

Prior to the application of chromosome-specific probes to the study of tumours, their ability to detect the appropriate chromosome and produce the correct number of signals per nucleus must be evaluated using normal cells and those with known and stable chromosomal aberrations. Hybridization of normal human fibroblasts with a chromosome 18 specific alphoid clone produced a distribution of dot number per nucleus around a modal value of 2. Only 65 per cent of nuclei, however, contained this number of signals. Nuclei containing three or more signals may represent minor hybridization sites: fewer than two dots may be produced by a variety of mechanisms, including poor probe penetration and inefficient hybridization. Data generated by these probes has therefore to be interpreted by statistical analysis rather than by merely counting signal number. This also emphasizes the importance of the optimization of cell pretreatment prior to hybridization in order to maximize probe penetration. Following the analysis of normal cells, trisomy 18 was investigated by the same method. This produced a distribution with a modal signal number per nucleus of 3, again with about 65 per cent of nuclei containing this number of dots. These preliminary investigations paved the way for the application of alphoid clones to tumour-derived cell lines and disaggregated cells.

The method for *in situ* suppression hybridization was evaluated using normal metaphase spreads and interphase nuclei and cell lines with balanced translocations before its application to tumour cells. Chromosomes could be visualized easily and translocations identified in interphase cells.

The interphase cytogenetics of bladder tumours and tumour-derived cell lines has been approached by studying lesions designated diploid by FCM. Using an alphoid clone specific for the heterochromatin of chromosome 1q, many cells were found to be trisomic for chromosome 1. Monosomy 15 and 17 were also identified. The analysis of paraffin sections taken from a diploid transitional cell carcinoma, which had a modal number of signals per nucleus of 3, demonstrated 1–4 spots per nucleus using the probe for 1q. However, in the investigation of aneuploid tumours, where disaggregated cells contained 6–8 signals with this probe, the hybridization of paraffin sections produced a wide variation in signal number with no clear peak. Thus, near-diploid tumours can be analysed more reliably, although aneuploidy can be detected in paraffin sections.

Metaphase cytogenetic analysis of breast carcinoma has demonstrated a variety of abnormalities. Many of these are inconsistent both between lesions investigated by the same workers and between workers. However, several studies of near-diploid tumours have shown consistent polysomy of chromosome 1q. It has been suggested that overrepresentation of chromosome 1q and, to a lesser extent, underrepresentation of chromosome 1p, can be found in the majority of breast tumours. The analysis of the breast-carcinoma-derived cell line MCF-7 has shown trisomy 1 and trisomy 18 using alphoid probes. Diploid tumours also contained a subpopulation of cells with trisomy 1, although the modal signal number per nucleus was 2: aneuploid lesions were associated with polysomy 1.

The analysis of cell lines derived from neuroectodermal tumours using both alphoid probes and *in situ* suppression hybridization (ISSH) has provided more insight into the precise nature of the information provided by interphase cytogenetics. A near-diploid cell line was found to be trisomic for chromosome 1 but ISSH demonstrated four chromosomes and markers derived from chromosome 1. Chromosome analysis showed that there were two normal chromosomes 1, with part of a third having been translocated to another chromosome. Thus, although there were four chromosome 1 derivatives, only three centromeres were present, explaining the modal signal number of 3 with the alphoid probe. With increasing aneuploidy, hybridization with the alphoid chromosome 1 probe produced

signal distributions with peaks shifted to higher modal values (up to 5 for the TC593 cell line). In addition, the number of cells containing this modal number was reduced to a minimum of 35 per cent in this line. ISSH analysis showed that TC593 cells contain six chromosome 1 derivatives. Chromosome analysis shows one of these to be an isochromosome 1p and the resultant five centromeres correspond to the modal number of 5 using the alphoid clone.

Conclusion

Interphase cytogenetics is still in its infancy, but the information that it is capable of providing will lead to a greater understanding not only of the interphase nucleus but also of the genetic content of tumour cells. Application to tissue sections will provide the ability to correlate chromosome complement with tissue morphology and clinical tumour behaviour, perhaps providing prognostic information. Specific data regarding individual tumour types is scanty but this is likely to be generated rapidly as technical advances are made. Indeed, the use of a chromosome 4 specific library has shown abnormalities of this chromosome in neuroectodermal tumours: this points to an area warranting further investigation.

9.2.12 Further reading

Cremer, T., *et al.* (1982). Rabl's model of the interphase chromosome arrangement tested in Chinese hamster cells by premature chromosome condensation and laser-UV-microbeam experiments. *Human Genetics* **60**, 46–56.

Cremer, T., Lichter, P., Borden, J., Ward, D. C., and Manuelidis, L. (1988). Detection of chromosome aberrations in metaphase and interphase tumour cells by *in situ* hybridization using chromosome specific library probes. *Human Genetics* **80**, 235–46.

Herrington, C. S., Evans, M., Graham, A., and McGee, J. O'D. (1991). Interphase cytogenetics III. *Journal of Clinical Pathology* **44**, 33–8.

Herrington, C. S. and McGee, J. O'D. (1990). Interphase cytogenetics. *Neurochemical Research* **15**, 467–74.

Hopman, A. H. N., Ramaekers, F. C. S., and Vooijs, G. P. (1990). Interphase cytogenetics on solid tumours. In In situ *hybridization: principles and practice*, (ed. J. Polak and J. O'D McGee). Oxford University Press, 165–86.

Pinkel, D., *et al.* (1988). Fluorescence *in situ* hybridization with human chromosome specific libraries: detection of trisomy 21 and translocations of chromosome 4. *Proceedings of the National Academy of Sciences, USA* **85**, 9138–42.

9.3 Preneoplasia

R. L. Carter and B. A. Gusterson

9.3.1 Introduction

Preneoplasia is an evolving concept which is difficult to define. It connotes a set of clinical or experimental circumstances associated with an increased risk of developing a tumour, but even a simple statement of this kind requires clarification. 'Clinical or experimental circumstances' may indicate local morphological or other changes present in a target organ, or constitutional changes, often associated with genetic abnormalities and/or a predictable pattern of inheritance. Examples of the first group include atypical hyperplasia of the endometrium, intestinal metaplasia in the stomach, and hypoplasia of seminiferous tubules. The second group is illustrated by conditions such as ataxia telangiectasia, Down's syndrome, the congenital immunodeficiency disorders, and xeroderma pigmentosum. Local morphological changes may be genetically determined, as in familial adenomatous polyposis and the dysplastic naevus syndrome, and the two categories clearly overlap. 'Increased risk' implies a consistent and statistically significant figure but, for reasons that will soon be apparent, recorded orders of risk are frequently variable in a given condition and are difficult or impossible to predict for an individual patient unless the condition is genetically determined and shows a clear pattern of Mendelian inheritance. 'Neoplasm' covers both benign and malignant tumours, but emphasis is concentrated here on the antecedants of malignant lesions, particularly carcinomas.

This section deals with four main topics: preneoplastic implications of hyperplasia, hypoplasia, and metaplasia; the development of dysplasia from mixed antecedents; de novo intra-epithelial carcinomas; and the precancerous (as opposed to preneoplastic) potential of benign tumours. The contentious term dysplastia is briefly considered in the concluding section.

9.3.2 Hyperplasia

Hyperplasia of epithelial and other cells is a common, nonspecific, and potentially reversible response to a variety of inflammatory and other stimuli. In specified circumstances it provides a context in which other changes may develop and evolve into a neoplasm. Laryngeal hyperplasia and hyperkeratosis, for example, is a familiar biopsy finding which is potentially reversible and may be of little consequence. But if these changes occur in a patient who is at risk of developing laryngeal cancer and/or atypical cells are already present in the mucosa, the lesion has to be interpreted as a potential preneoplastic change. A similar situation is illustrated by chronic oesophagitis with mucosal hyperplasia. Identical morphological changes may carry quite difficult connotations in different parts of the world. In patients from high-risk regions for eosophageal carcinoma the appearances should be interpreted as preneoplastic, while in low-risk patients their importance is likely to be much less. Supervening dysplasia, in both these examples, is conventionally classified by the pathologist as mild, moderate, or severe. The more intense dysplasias are more likely to persist and/or progress to carcinoma. Cellular atypia is, however, sometimes minimal, as in the verrucous hyperplasias which precede verrucous carcinomas in the oral cavity and other sites. Similar considerations apply to the transitional epithelium of the bladder where simple, nodular, and papillary hyperplasia are readily identified. The implications of such changes will vary according to the clinical context. Dysplasia is again graded

as slight, moderate, or severe. Mucosal dysplasia often occurs focally throughout the urothelium, suggesting the development of a diffuse 'field' change; transitional cell carcinomas are frequently multiple.

The hyperplasia and related changes seen in more complex glandular epithelia are often difficult to assess, notably in the endometrium where normal appearances vary with age and hormonal stimulation. Atypical hyperplasia, a clear precursor of endometrial adenocarcinoma, is characterized by changes in overall glandular arrangement and architecture, and by progressive cytological atypia. Increasingly dysplastic lesions are more likely to recur and/or persist and to evolve into carcinoma; dysplasia and cancer frequently co-exist. The status of in situ carcinoma in the endometrium is questionable. Adenocarcinomas associated with atypical endometrial hyperplasia tend to develop in perimenopausal women as slowly growing, well-differentiated neoplasms, which seem to be related to chronic unopposed oestrogenic stimulation. Other forms of endometrial cancer, particularly those found in older women, are less clearly related to antecedent hyperplasia or oestrogen excess.

Hyperplasia is rarely seen as a precursor of endocrine neoplasms in man (in contrast to rats and mice) except in the multiple endocrine neoplasia syndromes; MEN types I, IIA, IIB/III (see Chapter 21). These conditions occur in sporadic and familial forms, the later inherited as an autosomal dominant with variable penetrance. The tumours are multicentric and arise mainly in neuroectoderm and foregut endoderm. Hyperplasia is well documented in G-cells in the gastric antrum, pancreatic islet cells, parafollicular C-cells in the thyroid, and in parenchymal cells in the adrenal cortex and medulla—the sites at which tumours develop (in the MEN syndromes). Distinction between hyperplasia and neoplasms is sometimes very difficult. Secretion of several peptide hormones is demonstrated by immunohistochemistry and by elevated plasma levels. Recent investigations have described deletion of a hypervariable region of DNA on the short arm of chromosome 1 in both familial and sporadic cases of MEN type II. A linked genetic marker for familial MEN type IIA has been localized to chromosome 10, and identification and cloning of the predisposing gene are now feasible.

Particular problems are posed by regenerative hyperplasias, exemplified by the cirrhotic liver (Section 17.11). Macronodular or mixed cirrhotic nodules in a varying proportion of patients contain large aberrant hepatocytes with pleomorphic and sometimes multiple nuclei occurring in foci or throughout the nodules. Hepatocellular carcinoma and dysplastic liver cells frequently co-exist. The dysplastic hepatocytes often lack glycogen, and analogies are sometimes drawn between these lesions and the glycogen-depleted nodules that develop in rats exposed to various hepatocarcinogens. Despite their apparent morphological homogeneity, the natural history of the liver nodules in rats is variable; some regress, some persist unchanged, and some progress to form new glycogen-depleted nodules. Only a few cells within a few nodules, perhaps a single clone, eventually give rise to hepatocellular carcinoma.

9.3.3   Atrophy/hypoplasia

Progressive atrophy of the buccal mucosa is a consistent feature of submucous fibrosis, a common preneoplastic condition in the Indian subcontinent and parts of South-East Asia. Frequently associated with exposure to oral tobacco, it is characterized by submucosal inflammation followed by a dense overgrowth of collagen and elastic fibres in the lamina propria. The overlying squamous epithelium becomes atrophic, probably as a result of decreased vascularity. Increasing dysplasia is seen in the mucosa and squamous carcinoma eventually develops. The atrophic epithelium is perhaps more sensitive to the carcinogenic effects of tobacco. It is also likely that normal epithelial/stromal interactions are progressively deranged and that mucosal turnover and maturation are impaired.

Chronic atrophic gastritis is a major precursor of the intestinal form of gastric adenocarcinoma, mainly because it predisposes to the development of intestinal metaplasia (see below). Atrophy is particularly prevalent among high-risk populations, where it develops in younger people compared with low-risk regions. The changes occur mainly in the antrum and consist of loss of glands associated with hyperplasia of residual neck cells; there is variable chronic inflammation. Secretion of hydrochloric acid falls and there is a rise in the concentration of nitrites in gastric juice which, through nitrosation, may generate carcinogenic N-nitroso compounds.

Atrophy or hypoplasia of germinal epithelium in the seminiferous tubules of the testis is well recognized as a preneoplastic change for germ cell tumours. The principal high-risk conditions are cryptorchidism and infertility. The presence of malignant tumour in the opposite testis is recognized as another predisposing factor, and there is evidence that cryptorchid males have an enhanced risk of developing a germ cell tumour in the contralateral descended testicle. *In situ* (intratubular) tumours are increasingly identified in the various high-risk groups. The reasons why neoplasms are more likely to develop in the cryptorchid and/or infertile testis are unclear, but the contributions made by dysgenesis and hormonal imbalance are probably large.

9.3.4   Metaplasia

Like hyperplasia, metaplastic changes are common, nonspecific tissue responses to various pathological stimuli; they frequently arise in mucosa that is already hyperplastic. Two simple examples are provided by squamous metaplasia developing in the respiratory epithelium of the bronchus and in transitional epithelium lining the bladder. It may be present as a result of chronic inflammation or chemical irritation, but squamous metaplasia (with or without dysplasia) commonly co-exists with squamous carcinomas of the bronchus and bladder, the latter associated particularly with bilharzial infestation.

Intestinal metaplasia in the stomach is more complex. It is clearly established as an important antecedent change in the development of the intestinal form of gastric adenocarcinoma. (The mode of origin of diffuse gastric carcinomas is unknown.)

Intestinal metaplasia is usually superimposed on chronic atrophic gastritis (see above) and may be widespread or focal. Residual gastric glands are replaced by highly organized cells of intestinal phenotype, arranged as short, straight crypts lined by absorptive and globlet cells. Histochemical studies have demonstrated a progressive shift in the pattern of mucin production, so that synthesis of small-intestinal-type sialomucins is gradually replaced by mucins associated with the large-bowel sulphomucins and a colon-specific mucin containing O-acylated sialic acid. Regions of intestinal metaplasia producing sialomucins or sulphomucins are in other respects similar, but this functional difference is important because production of sulphomucins may predict malignant progression. The evidence rests mainly on the demonstration of sulphomucins in zones of intestinal metaplasia in stomachs which also contained carcinoma, in contrast to the infrequent finding of sulphomucins in intestinal metaplasia associated with peptic ulcer. Further evidence of the heterogeneity of intestinal metaplasia comes from studies with a series of immunohistochemical markers. Different patterns of staining were found in histologically identical examples of intestinal metaplasia in stomachs with and without carcinoma; co-existing intestinal metaplasia and cancer showed common staining patterns.

The dysplastic changes which lead eventually to carcinoma develop principally in regions of intestinal metaplasia, although they can occur in normal gastric epithelium (and also in adenomatous polyps, see below). The changes consist of abnormal mucosal architecture, abnormal cellular differentiation, and cytological atypia, and are conventionally graded as slight, moderate, and severe. The origin of intestinal metaplasia is unclear. Such changes may be the consequence of gene derepression in neck cells in atrophic mucosa, or of a true mutation induced by local genotoxic carcinogens.

9.3.5   Dysplasia with mixed antecedents

Dysplasia that is apparently associated with mixed antecedent lesions may be illustrated in two rather different contexts—breast and large intestine.

A number of pathological (but non-neoplastic) changes are commonly found in breast ducts and lobules which are included in the unsatisfactory entity of 'benign breast disease' (Chapter 22). Many of them co-exist with *in situ* or invasive ductal or lobular carcinomas; some may be related to tumour development, while others are irrelevant. It is difficult to identify genuine preneoplastic lesions in the breast because of the range of normal tissue appearances at different ages, the pathologist's problems of sampling and nomenclature, the choice of suitable control groups of patients, and the inherent difficulties of studying a disease that develops over a long time-span. The main pathological risk factors that emerge are ductal hyperplasia, atypical lobular hyperplasia, and probably papillary apocrine metaplasia. No increased risks for cancer have been consistently identified with cysts, duct ectasia, sclerosing adenosis, or nonpapillary apocrine metaplasia. In ductal hyperplasia (syn. epitheliosis) the cells are typically polymorphic and lack the cytological features of malignancy. Increasing atypia may supervene (atypical epitheliosis, ductal dysplasia), the cells becoming large and more monomorphic. *In situ* carcinoma is characterized by more intense cytological atypia, necrosis, and frequent and abnormal mitoses, the tumour cells being arranged in various distinctive growth patterns. Broadly comparable changes are seen in atypical lobular hyperplasia, where rather loosely arranged polymorphic cells predominate, varying in size, shape, and staining intensity. Cells in *in situ* lobular carcinomas are larger and often strikingly uniform, filling and distending the lobules. The distinction between *in situ* carcinoma and atypical hyperplasia is, in both circumstances, sometimes very difficult. Dysplastic ductal and lobular breast epithelium has no distinctive features in the electron microscope. A few karyotypic analyses of ductal hyperplasia have indicated the presence of variable numbers of aneuploid cells with (occasionally) structurally deranged chromosomes. Normal and abnormal breast lobules, transplanted into the cleared fat pads of athymic *nude* mice, have failed to grow progressively or undergo malignant change.

Patients with long-standing inflammatory disease in the large intestine, exemplified by ulcerative colitis, have an increased risk of developing progressive mucosal dypsplasia and colorectal adenocarcinoma; the two changes frequently co-exist. The antecedent lesions are diverse and include polyps, nodules, and flat plaques, which may be extensive and difficult to recognize. All these changes have a clear preneoplastic potential. The polyps are typically villous, poorly circumscribed, and lack a stalk. The diagnosis of dysplasia is based on a combination of altered glandular architecture and increasing cellular atypia. The pathologist's assessment is not materially aided by additional techniques such as immunohistochemistry, determination of nuclear ploidy or the use of computer-aided morphometry. Recognition of dysplasia raises three sets of problems: exclusion of changes attributable to concurrent infection, inflammation, and tissue destruction and repair; grading of dysplasia; and recognition of the early stages of carcinoma. Mucosal dysplasia in the large bowel is classified as low grade or high grade, the latter conventionally including intramucosal carcinomas. The disordered mucosa may thus be a marker or precursor of malignant change, or may itself denote an early cancer. This approach has fundamental implications with respect to concepts of dysplasia and preneoplasia, which are discussed later.

9.3.6 De novo, intra-epithelial cancer

Generally, the notion of dysplasia preceding carcinoma has been discarded in the context of the cervix uteri, where previous categories of cervical dysplasia are now replaced by the entity of cervical intra-epithelial neoplasia, graded as I–III (CIN I–III). CIN I, formerly described as mild dysplasia, is associated with nuclear abnormalities throughout the full thickness of the epithelium, but the superficial two-thirds shows maturation. CIN III, corresponding to previous categories of severe dysplasia/*in situ* carcinoma, shows full-thickness loss of the nor-

mal stratified layers of differentiating squamous epithelium, a loss of normal cell polarity, intense pleomorphism, and the presence of mitoses at all levels. The morphological appearances of CIN II are roughly intermediate between those of CIN I and

The risk of progression to invasive carcinoma rises from CIN I, where it is very low, to CIN III. The factors responsible for progression are ill-understood but an association with human papilloma virus (HPV)—a potential aetiological agent for cervical carcinoma—seems increasingly likely. Several different HPV genotypes are now implicated. HPV-6 and HPV-11 are associated with CIN I, where HPV antigens have been localized to the nuclei of koilocytes in the upper layers of the epithelium. Many examples of CIN I are now regarded as flat condylomata, most of which regress. HPV-16 and HPV-18 are associated mainly with CIN III and invasive carcinoma. A distinction should be drawn between the presence of the virus in neoplastic cells and its integation into the tumour cell genome, expression as mRNA, and synthesis of a virus-encoded protein. It appears that the HPV-16 genome is only integrated in tumour cells from invasive carcinomas, an observation which raises questions about the role of HPV proteins in the phase of tumour progression in this system. Other changes which appear to evolve *pari passu* from CIN to invasive cancer include karyotype abnormalities.

9.3.7 Malignant change in benign tumours

True adenomatous polyps in the large intestine provide well-documented examples of the malignant potential of certain benign tumours. Sporadic adenomas occur in the large intestine in *c*.10 per cent of middle-aged and elderly individuals in the West, and are regarded as the site of origin for most colorectal adenocarcinomas. Their morphology is commonly described as tubular, tubulovillous, or villous; mixed forms predominate. The different growth patterns may, in part, be determined by loss of control of crypt cell kinetics. In normal and colonic epithelium, proliferating cells are confined to the lower two-thirds of the crypts where *c*.15–20 per cent are in DNA synthesis. Cells leave the proliferative cycle as they move upward and differentiate. In mucosa near adenomatous polyps, by contrast, there is often a failure of the adjacent epithelial cells to repress DNA synthesis, which continues as cells migrate into the upper segments of the crypts and on to the luminal surface. Various abnormal proteins, such as α-fetoprotein and human placental lactogen, have been demonstrated in adenomatous polyps and this aberrant activity may also reflect local gene derepression. The two most important determinants for impending or actual malignant change are increasing size and increasing cellular atypia. Co-existing adenomatous polyps and carcinomas show a similar nuclear ploidy, and recent investigations have demonstrated common mutations at codon 12 of the c-Ki-*ras* gene. The role of *ras*-encoded proteins (p21^{ras}) in the development and evolution of adenomatous polyps is unclear, and immunohistochemical studies of the cellular distinction of p21^{ras} proteins in normal colorectal mucosa, adenomas, and carcinomas have given conflicting results.

The features of sporadic or non-familial adenomatous polyps are reproduced on a larger scale in familial adenomatous polyposis (syn. polyposis coli), an autosomal dominant condition with almost 100 per cent penetrance and no sex-linkage. The large intestine in these patients contains hundreds or thousands of adenomatous polyps, which appear in the second and third decades; single or multiple adenocarcinomas supervene in the next 10 years. The morphology of the adenocarcinomas is similar in the two conditions, and the same defects are present in crypt cell kinetics. Total colectomy specimens from patients with familial adenomatous polyposis provide ideal material for studying the development of adenomatous polyps down to the level of morphological changes in a single crypt. Macroscopically normal mucosa from such patients shows minor ultra-structural changes, which are consistent with the presence of incompletely differentiated cells in the upper crypts and luminal surface described in previous kinetic studies (see above). Cells with the same distribution within colorectal mucosa also show persistent expression of the c-myc oncogene product (p62$^{c\text{-myc}}$). The adenocarcinomas that arise in association with sporadic and familial adenomatous polyps are similar with respect to their morphology and patterns of spread. Recent studies have strengthened this association by localizing the gene for familial adenomatous polyposis on chromosome 5 and by demonstrating loss of the allele for this chromosome in the development of sporadic forms of colorectal adenocarcinoma. Both sporadic and familial forms of adenocarcinoma in the large bowel may thus result from mutations in the same gene. Loss of all or part of chromosome 5 appears to favour tumour progression, and it is clearly important to isolate the familial adenomatous polyposis gene, clarify its function, and identify the related gene product. In sporadic colonic cancer, loss of heterozygosity (LOH) on chromosome 17 and 18 are more frequently implicated than lesions on chromosome 5. LOH is also associated with (or follows) mutations in Ki-ras and p53 genes.

True adenomatous polyps in the stomach, by contrast, are rare except in patients with pernicious anaemia where they may coexist with chronic atrophic gastritis and intestinal metaplasia (see above). Some authors have demonstrated large amounts of sulphomucins in these tumours and claimed that they are a marker of potential malignant change. Other adverse factors include large size and cytological atypia.

Malignant change in other benign epithelial tumours and in non-epithelial neoplasms, is uncommon. The best-documented examples occur in uterine leiomyomas and in the schwannomas associated with von Recklinghausen's disease.

9.3.8 Conclusions

A few concluding comments remain to be considered. It is worth re-emphasizing the importance of assessing putative preneoplastic changes within their specified clinical context, and the variable natural history (despite clear trends) of such lesions. The changes that occur may form a natural sequence

that is likely to result in a neoplasm, but it is also clear that such sequences are not inevitable and that tumours in the same target organ may develop from other precursor lesions or arise apparently de novo. The variable natural history of preneoplastic lesions becomes less puzzling with the growing recognition that morphologically similar lesions may be functionally heterogeneous—a conclusion that emphasizes the need to supplement standard light and electron microscopy with techniques such as immunohistochemistry, in situ hybridization, and other procedures developed by geneticists and molecular biologists. The association between preneoplasia and in situ/intra-epithelial carcinoma remains a very difficult issue, varying in different types of epithelium and in different organs. In some tissues the distinction can be made by an experienced pathologist, while in others it is difficult or impossible. Much of the confusion stems from the term 'dysplasia': are dysplastic cells abnormal but not neoplastic, are they truly neoplastic, or are they in some kind of intermediate state? Resolution of this question would transform the study of preneoplasia, and it is possible that some clarification may come from current work on human tumours associated with oncogenic viruses. Confusion is likely to remain until carcinogenic mechanisms in man are better understood. It is, however, important to stress that preneoplastic changes (despite self-evident problems and limitations) are of considerable practical value in clinical medicine as a means of identifying individuals in families or in occupations who are at an increased risk of developing a neoplasm, and providing a basis for screening, counselling, and early diagnosis and treatment.

9.3.9 Further reading

Bodmer, W. F., et al. (1987). Localization of the gene for familial adenomatous polyposis on chromosome 5. Nature 328, 614–16.

Bos, L. (1989). Ras oncogenes in human cancer: a review. Cancer Research 49, 4682–9.

Buckley, C. H., Butler, E. B., and Fox, H. (1982). Cervical intra-epithelial neoplasia. Journal of Clinical Pathology 35, 1–13.

Carter, R. L. (1984). Precancerous states. Oxford University Press, Oxford.

Fearon, E. R. and Vogelstein, B. (1990). A genetic model for colorectal tumorigenesis. Cell 61, 659–67.

Henderson, D. E. and Albores-Saavedra, J. (1986). The pathology of incipient neoplasia. W. B. Saunders, Philadelphia.

Koss, L. G., Tiamson, E. M., and Robbins, A. (1974). Mapping cancerous and precancerous bladder changes. Journal of the American Medical Association 227, 281–6.

Kurman, R. J., Kaminski, P. F., and Norris, H. J. (1985). The behaviour of endometrial hyperplasia. A long-term study of 'untreated' hyperplasia in 170 patients. Cancer 56, 403–12.

Lipkin, M. (1975). Biology of large bowel cancer. Present status and research frontiers. Cancer 36, 2319–24.

Mathew, C. G. P., et al. (1987). Deletion of genes of chromosome 1 in endocrine neoplasia. Nature 328, 524–6.

Mathew, C. G. P., et al. (1987). A linked genetic marker for multiple endocrine neoplasia type 2A on chromosome 10. Nature 328, 527–8.

Morson, B. C., Sobin, L. H., Grundmann, E., Johansen, A., Nagayo, T., and Serck-Hanssen, A. (1980). Precancerous conditions and epithelial dysplasia in the stomach. Journal of Clinical Pathology 33, 711–21.

Riddell, R. H., *et al.* (1983). Dysplasia in inflammatory bowel disease: standardized classification with provisional clinical applications. *Human Pathology* **14**, 931–68.

Skakkbaek, N. E. (1987). Carcinoma *in situ* of the testis: frequency and relationship to invasive germ cell tumours in infertile man. *Histopathology* **2**, 157–70.

Solomon, E., *et al.* (1987). Chromosome 5 allele loss in human colorectal carcinomas. *Nature* **328**, 616–19.

Stanbridge, E. J. (1990). Identifying tumor suppressor genes in human colorectal cancer. *Science* **247**, 12–13.

Wallace, R., *et al.* (1990). Type 1 neurofibromatosis gene: identification of a large transcript disrupted in three NF1 patients. *Science* **249**, 181–6.

9.4 Tumour cell differentiation and its control

C. F. Graham

9.4.1 Introduction

Tumours with differentiating cells

Solid tumours often contain a variety of visually recognizable cell types. Many of these are presumed to be normal cells responding to the presence of the tumour: vascular endothelial cells, lymphocytes, and macrophages may congregate in and around tumours, and solid tumours are frequently enclosed in connective tissue capsules (see Section 9.1). The remaining cells usually fall into two categories. There are the cells that look like rapidly dividing stem cells, and there are differentiated cells resembling specialized cell types found both in the adult and in the conceptus (e.g. keratinocytes, chondrocytes, and trophoblast cells); these differentiated cells are believed to develop from the stem-like cells. Much of histopathology depends on recognizing and staging tumours with regard to the type and the proportion of the differentiated cells; in general, the more differentiated the appearance of these cells and the more mature their anatomical organization, the better the prognosis. Experimental studies with mouse tumours provide an explanation of this pragmatic observation: many of the mouse stem-like cells can form transplantable tumours, while most mature differentiated cells cannot (see below).

The demonstration that malignancy is frequently lost as tumour stem cells differentiate, suggests new methods for treating cancer. Currently, most cancers are treated with cytotoxic agents, which are designed to kill tumour cells. The new methods are called 'differentiation therapy', and the proposal is to treat cancer cells with agents that convert the malignant tumour stem cells into non-malignant differentiated cells (see below).

Normal and tumour stem cells

Stem cells are literally the cells from which a set of specialized cells stem: the stem cells divide and some of their progeny form the specialized cells. Initially, the stem cells in the conceptus can form all its tissues: they can each contribute to both the cells of the fetal membranes (extra-embryonic tissues) and to all the cells of the fetus (embryonic tissues). Subsequently, distinct stem-cell populations arise, each population only contributing to a limited range of these tissues (Fig. 9.9). Some stem cells of the early conceptus have a very limited life-span: the fertilized egg divides about five times before its progeny lose the potential to form all parts of the conceptus, and this totipotential stem-cell population disappears from the organism until new gametes are formed. Some of the progeny of these divisions then become stem cells of the extra-embryonic structures, the placenta and the fetal membranes: they are sometimes called progenitor, or precursor, cells to emphasize the developmental limits on their existence. In contrast, other stem cells continue into the adult and form self-renewing populations which persist through the life-span of the adult. These persistent stem-cell populations are defined by the following properties:

1. They produce differentiated progeny. The progeny of unipotent stem cells form only one differentiated cell type (e.g. skin keratinocytes), while the progeny of pluripotent stem cells include several cell types (e.g. the lymphoid–myeloid cells; see Section 1.3).

2. There is no intrinsic limit to the number of times that stem-cell populations can divide, and transplantation studies show that they can remain stem cells for longer than the

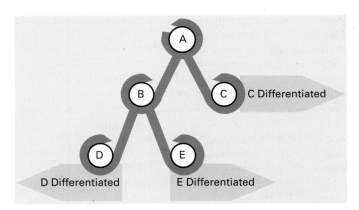

Fig. 9.9 Progression of stem cells. The diagram illustrates a progression of stem-cell populations. All the populations in the diagram are ultimately derived from the pluripotential stem cell A. In a determination step, stem cell A populations produce two progeny stem cells (B and C populations), which have a more limited range of differentiation options. Stem cell C populations are unipotential and they can only differentiate to form type-C differentiated cells. Stem cell B populations are bipotential and, in a determination step, they produce two different unipotential stem-cell populations, D and E. In the diagram, all the stem-cell populations have the capacity to renew their stem-cell population.

life-span of the organism in which they originated. The mature differentiated cells formed from stem cells may continue to divide for a period, but they have a limited life-span.

3. When a stem-cell population multiplies, the progeny cells may either be identical stem cells, or stem cells with more limited differentiation options, or differentiated cells. In many adult systems, the stem-cell populations are self-renewing and the homeostasis of tissues depends on regulated proliferation and differentiation of these cells.

The formation of stem cells involves 'determination', a series of events that limits the type of differentiated cells that may be produced by the stem cell in most biological circumstances. Two tests can be used to discover if a new stem cell has become determined. The first is to isolate the cell in culture, and study the range of differentiated progeny that it forms. The second is to introduce the cell into an organism, and monitor the range of differentiated cell types that it produces after cell interactions in the organism. When an experimenter can no longer extend the subsequent development of the cell in either test situation, then that cell is described as an irreversibly committed, or determined, cell. This is an operational definition, and it is often more informative about the determination of the experimenter than of the cell: clearly, no cell has been tested in all the environments that it might encounter in a solid tumour. Nevertheless, such studies show that development consists of the progressive formation of new stem cells with increasingly more limited differentiation capacity.

Determination causes pluripotential stem cells to give rise to other stem cells whose progeny have a more limited range of differentiation options. When such progressions of stem cells have been studied, it is found that the cellular environment provides combinations of regulatory substances that control the growth and differentiation of each stem-cell population (Section 1.3). Thus, in a progression of stem cells (Fig. 9.9), when one stem-cell population produces progeny that are determined to be a new stem-cell population, the new stem cells are under the control of a novel set of extrinsic molecules.

The phenotypes of tumour stem cells are usually shared with one or other of the various stem-cell populations that are relatively abundant in prenatal life (e.g. onco-fetal antigens and isozymes), and they may also be shared with stem cells in the adult (e.g. leukaemias). There is no evidence that tumour stem cells display unique 'marker' antigens that distinguish them from normal stem cells (Sections 9.2.5 and 9.8.4). The apparent exception to this rule is the immunoglobulin idiotype peculiar to a B-cell leukaemia in any one individual; the particular idiotype is not a marker of leukaemia in general, but its presence in the malignant cells indicates that a particular clone of cells has become expanded during the formation of the leukaemia in that individual.

The common properties of tumour and normal stem cells immediately suggest cancer therapy by the imposition of signals on tumour stem cells to become determined and to differentiate. Such differentiation therapy is only limited by the slow progress in characterizing these signals in normal development.

9.4.2   Determination, differentiation, and growth in early mammalian development

Introduction

A brief sketch of early mammalian development illustrates some general features of the growth, determination, and differentiation that are likely to occur in solid differentiating tumours with many cell types (see Fig. 9.10). These early stages of development have their counterparts in teratomas (see below), and the analysis of normal development helps to interpret all differentiating tumours. Here, 'growth' means cell multiplication and the term 'differentiation' is used broadly to mean the process by which cells become distinct from each other and from their embryonic progenitors: differentiated cells are distinct from their progenitors and from other types of differentiated cells.

The important conclusion from studies of the mammalian conceptus is that local and mutual cell interactions regulate both the growth, determination, and the final differentiation of cells: cell behaviour flows from the inherent characteristics of cells and their immediate environment. The growth of tumours involves emancipation from these regulators of proportional growth and it is important to characterize the normal systems. These normal cell interactions are now reviewed briefly.

Cell interaction and tissue formation

Trophectoderm

The first differentiated cell type to appear during development is trophectoderm, which forms an epithelium, enveloping the other cells of the conceptus (Fig. 9.10). Transplantation studies in the mouse show that this layer contains the stem cells of the trophoblast part of the mature placenta. The trophoblast layer of the mature placenta is the external limit of the tissues of the conceptus, and it is embedded in the uterus. It consists of a rapidly dividing cyto-trophoblast layer which transforms into an external syncytio-trophoblast layer where DNA synthesis no longer occurs. The cells that contribute to the trophectoderm have been identified by short-term cell lineage analysis in the intact conceptus developing in culture. Visible markers are injected into individual cells, and the development of these marked cells is observed at later stages of development. It is clear that trophectoderm progenitor cells are not set aside at a particular moment, but increasingly the descendants of the outside cells of the conceptus contribute only to the trophectoderm as development proceeds from the 8- to 64-cell stage. By the late blastocyst stage, the outside cells only contribute to trophectoderm while the inside cells no longer contribute to this tissue.

The behaviour of cells in the intact conceptus can be compared with their behaviour in unusual environments. In the intact conceptus, the individual cells of the 8-cell stage usually contribute progeny cells to both the outside trophectoderm and the 'inner cell mass' precursors of the fetus (see Fig. 9.10d). However, when the individual cells are isolated from each other at the 8-cell stage and grown apart, then the cells continue to divide two or three times but they only form trophectoderm.

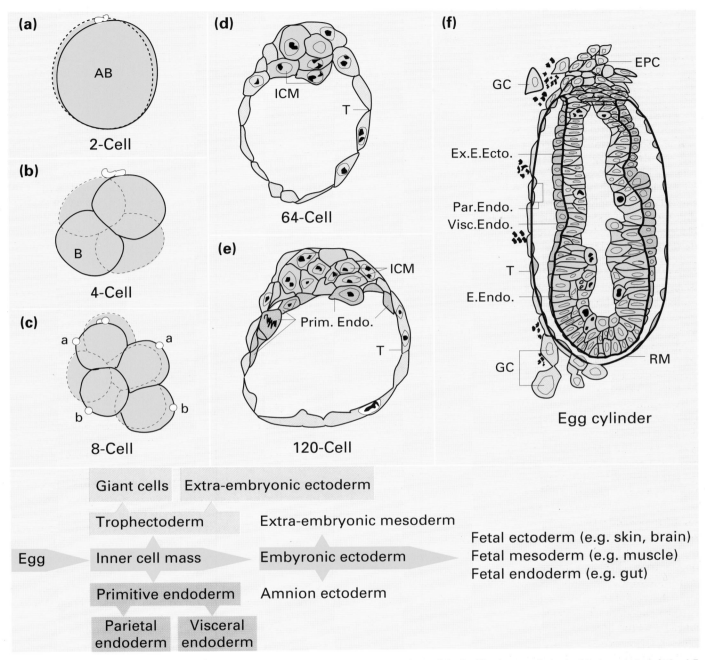

Fig. 9.10 The development of the mouse conceptus. (a)–(d) Illustrate the cell divisions of the fertilized egg to form the blastocyst, during the 4.5 days that the conceptus takes to move down the oviduct and into the uterus. At the blastocyst stage (d), the conceptus is enveloped by the trophectoderm layer (T) and contains a group of inner cell mass (ICM) cells. On the fifth day after fertilization, the trophectoderm layer attaches to the wall of the uterus (implantation), and it is at this time that the primitive endoderm (Prim. Endo.) is formed from the ICM (e). On the seventh day after fertilization, the egg cylinder is formed (f). This contains derivatives of the trophectoderm layer: extra-embryonic ectoderm (Ex.E.Ecto.), the ectoplacental cone (EPC), trophoblast (T), and trophoblast giant cells (GC). The primitive endoderm has formed the parietal endoderm (Par.Endo.) and the visceral endoderm (Visc.Endo.). The ICM has proliferated extensively to form all the fetal precursor cells in the embryonic ectoderm (E.Ecto.). The lineage relationships between these layers is illustrated in the flow diagram.

The same effect can be achieved by reducing the contact between the cells with an antibody directed against the E-cadherin adhesive protein displayed on the cell surface: in this case the conceptus still develops as a ball of cells, but the majority of the cells form trophectoderm. When 8-cell-stage cells are surrounded by other cells, then there is an increased tendency for their progeny to be found in the inner cell mass. The final differentiation of cells clearly depends on cell interactions, and the conclusion is that close cell contacts suppress the tendency of these cells to form trophectoderm.

It is also important to discover when cells acquire the property of only forming one cell type in later development, because cells are likely to experience a wide range of unusual cell interactions in an adult tumour. Studies of determination have been carried out on trophectoderm. The following experiments show that the trophectoderm of the blastocyst is determined to form placental trophoblast. The trophectoderm cells form only this tissue when they are grown:

1. alone in culture or in the uterus;

2. in combination with the inner cell mass cells of another blastocyst, with the chimera returned to the uterus for normal development; and

3. when transplanted beneath the capsule of the adult testis or of the kidney.

The inner cell mass cells of the blastocyst do not have such a fixed future in different environments. When transplanted back into another blastocyst or beneath the capsule of the kidney, then they indeed lack the capacity to form trophoblast: they form the tissues of the fetus, the fetal membranes, and all parts of the placenta except the trophoblast. However, they may retain the capacity to form trophectoderm cells in culture until the very late blastocyst stage, and it is not clear when or whether they completely loose this property.

Primitive endoderm

At the blastocyst stage, a new differentiated cell type appears on the surface of the inner cell mass that faces the cavity (Fig. 9.10e). This cell layer is called the 'primitive endoderm', and transplantation studies show that these cells subsequently form the endoderm of the fetal membranes, the parietal and visceral endoderm. In particular, the yolk sac endoderm cells function as the hepatocytes of early development (see below). When the inner cell mass is grown in isolation from the trophectoderm cells, then the primitive endoderm quickly develops around the whole of the outside surface of the little ball of cells to form a distinct surface layer. It appears that trophectoderm suppresses primitive endoderm formation in normal development, so that it only appears on the free surface of the inner cell mass.

The determination of primitive endoderm cells and their derivatives has been studied by transplantation and cell isolation. The primitive endoderm and its derivatives only form the endoderm of fetal membranes on transplantation back to another blastocyst. When cultured apart from the rest of the conceptus

the parietal and visceral endoderm cells retain their characteristic morphology, but the expression of the differentiated phenotype of the visceral endoderm cells is labile: for instance, all regions of this layer synthesize α-fetoprotein when isolated at the egg cylinder stage (Fig. 9.10f), while tissue interactions limit this synthesis to particular regions of the layer in the intact conceptus.

Conclusions

1. The first two differentiated cell types of the mammalian conceptus arise by progressively escaping suppressive interactions with their neighbours.

2. The trophectoderm and primitive endoderm stem cells become determined in turn, and it is necessary to suppose that their progenitor cells in the conceptus progress through still mysterious states so that they form distinct determined stem cells in response to the similar environment of reduced contact with other cells in the conceptus.

3. These extra-embryonic stem cells form a very small range of specialized cell types in a variety of circumstances. However, it is not certain that the same limitations will apply in the jungle of cell interactions that may be found in a tumour.

Cell interactions and tissue growth

Environmental requirements for cell multiplication

There are two phases of cell multiplication in early mammalian development. The first five or six cell divisions of the conceptus can proceed in a simple salt solution with an energy source (e.g. lactate and pyruvate). This is the period when the conceptus is moving down the oviduct and into the uterus. The second phase starts at about the implanting blastocyst stage, when progressive cell multiplication of individual tissues depends on cell interactions with the other tissues of the conceptus: most tissues will not grow progressively by themselves, and those that do grow require 'rich' culture media. The culture environment must now be enriched with amino acids and serum: serum can be replaced by trace elements, carrier proteins such as transferrin and apolipoproteins, attachment factors, and growth factors (media with serum or with these cocktails of additives are subsequently called 'rich' media: Section 9.6.7).

Trophectoderm and inner cell mass interactions

Inner cell mass action on trophectoderm The trophectoderm and the inner cell mass interact with each other to promote cell multiplication and cell survival. Once the trophectoderm layer is formed around the blastocyst, then it is clear that the most rapid trophectoderm cell multiplication occurs in the part that lies over the inner cell mass. This proliferative zone contributes cells to the expanding roof of the blastocoel and to the ecto-placental cone, a structure that protrudes from the conceptus and penetrates deep into the uterine stroma (see EPC in Fig. 9.10f). When trophectoderm cells are isolated from the inner cell mass cells, then cell multiplication soon stops whether the cells are kept in rich culture media, or transplanted into the uterus or beneath the kidney capsule. The trophectoderm has not been irrevocably damaged by the operation, for it can reform a viable blastocyst when provided with inner cell mass cells from another blastocyst. Indeed, it is possible to induce two proliferative centres by adding an extra inner cell mass at the opposite end of the blastocyst cavity to the resident mass. The conclusion is that the inner cell mass is required to promote the multiplication of trophectoderm cells both in the intact conceptus and in rich culture media: the effect of the inner cell mass is local and not systemic.

Trophectoderm effects on the inner cell mass Trophectoderm has a reciprocal action on the inner cell mass: it provides conditions for the survival of the inner cell mass in the uterus and it probably also promotes inner cell mass growth. Inner cell mass cells do not require the trophectoderm in order to proliferate in rich culture media, but differentiation-inhibiting factors must be added to maintain the stem-cell population, and they do not survive if they are returned to the uterus denuded of their trophectoderm coat.

Primitive endoderm and inner cell mass interactions

The mouse primitive endoderm layer can proliferate and form liquid-filled vesicles in rich culture media, while the immediate derivatives of the inner cell mass quickly die. If these two layers are recombined, then the inner cell mass derivatives grow, and the endoderm enlarges. It is clear that in these conditions, the two layers collaborate to sustain each other's growth.

This co-operative growth is likely to depend on the products of the endoderm, for this tissue produces many of the components required by cells for growth in the absence of serum. As the primitive endoderm originates, so its cells express a wide variety of cell-attachment factors and extra-cellular matrix components: these include type IV collagen, laminin, entactin, and fibronectin. It is probable that these products promote the adhesion of the inner cell mass derivatives. Between the first and second weeks of mouse development, the visceral yolk sac endoderm is, or has the potential to be, the major source of the serum proteins, which are secreted by the liver in the adult. Some of these proteins are known to sustain the growth of early embryonic cells in culture: these include carriers of lipids (apolipoproteins), and the iron transporter, transferrin. The ability to secrete these proteins probably develops early in the human yolk sac as well: transferrin is found concentrated within the yolk sac endoderm of the 21-day-old conceptus, and the endoderm of yolk sacs from later stages of development secrete albumin, transferrin, α-fetoprotein, and apolipoprotein. Lastly, the human yolk sac taken as a whole is known to secrete cell-attachment factors, such as fibronectin, and insulin-like growth factor II (IGF-II). It is a reasonable assumption that some of these yolk-sac products account for the ability of the primitive endoderm and its derivatives to sustain inner cell mass growth and survival in cell culture.

General conclusions

1. The environmental requirements of cell multiplication change from a phase which does not require rich media to one which does.

2. Cell determination is restricted by interaction with other cells.

3. The expression of differentiated characters, such as α-fetoprotein, depends on other cell types in the immediate neighbourhood.

4. The growth of one cell type often depends on close proximity with another cell type. Local cell interactions appear more important than the systemic milieu.

9.4.3 Differentiating tumours

Introduction

Differentiating tumours are tumours that contain a variety of cell types, which are presumed to be, or have been shown to be, derived from a single stem cell. The best test for such tumours is to isolate the putative stem cell, transplant it back to a host, and demonstrate that it can form all the cell types that are characteristic of the mature tumour. This test distinguishes the tumour cells from the host cells, and simultaneously identifies the stem cell of the transplantable tumour. The stem cell of the transplantable tumour need not be identical to the cell from which the tumour originated (see below). Such developmental tumours typically contain rapidly dividing stem cells and more slowly dividing differentiated derivatives. Frequently, the differentiated derivatives of the stem cells cannot by themselves form transplantable tumours. The association between differentiation and the loss of the ability to form tumours is strengthened by the co-segregation of these two properties during chromosome elimination in some hybrid cells. These results suggest new forms of cancer treatment, in which agents are chosen for their ability to promote the differentiation of the tumour stem cells, rather than for their ability to kill the cells.

Unipotential and pluripotential stem-cell tumours

The simplest differentiating tumours are those that only consist of stem cells and one differentiated cell type. The stem cells are called 'unipotential' and they are determined (the operational definition). Squamous cell carcinomas, which only form keratin 'pearls' mimic the limited behaviour of the basal layer of the skin, which only forms keratinocytes. It has been shown clearly that when squamous cell carcinoma differentiates, so the cells' nuclei degenerate and their cytoplasm fills up with keratin; groups of the differentiating cells aggregate in spheres to form the characteristic keratin pearls. As this differentiation proceeds, so the cells lose the capacity to grow progressively. Despite the intense search for the factors that regulate skin growth, such knowledge has yet to be applied in detail to the regulation of squamous carcinoma differentiation.

In contrast, pluripotential stem-cell tumours contain a variety of differentiated cell types, which are ultimately derived from a single pluripotential stem cell. This pluripotential stem cell will often form unipotential stem cells prior to the development of the differentiated cells (Fig. 9.9). The most obvious pluripotential stem-cell tumours are teratomas, which may contain the majority of the cell types that are found in the conceptus: however, tumours of the primitive stem cells of the haemopoietic system also have the possibility of forming a wide range of differentiated cell types in this tissue system (see Fig. 9.11).

Developmental limits on tumour formation

One puzzling feature of some pluripotential stem-cell tumours is that they can be generated at high frequency by transplanting parts of the early mouse conceptus to ectopic sites in adult animals; for instance, over half the transplanted egg cylinders (see Fig. 9.10f) of the mouse develop into teratomas. This contrasts with the situation in the rat, in which the transplanted egg cylinders only form parietal endoderm tumours. Transplanted embryonic cells can only form transplantable teratomas and related tumours during a brief period of development, while similar tumours originate spontaneously from the germ cells in the gonads of adults (see below). The short time-interval during which transplanted embryonic cells can form these tumours suggests that the tumours originate from cells that have a brief life-span in the conceptus.

Developmental limits on tumour differentiation

The capacity to regulate the determination and differentiation of tumour cells appears to be greatest in the conceptus. Thus some stem cells of teratoma, leukaemia, neuroblastoma, and melanoma have been shown to differentiate when transplanted into the conceptus but to show little differentiation when placed in the adult. This phenomenon is not understood.

Teratomas

Characteristics in man and mouse

Teratomas are tumours that occur spontaneously in the gonads of man and mouse. In humans, the tumours characteristically contain cells that resemble those of fetal membranes, for example placental trophoblast and yolk-sac endoderm: these tumours may also contain groups of cells that look like embryonic and adult tissues, such as muscle, nerve, and cartilage. The properties of these tumours have been reviewed in the following collections of articles (human, Anderson *et al.* 1981; Gardner 1983; Jones *et al.* 1986: mouse, Silver *et al.* 1983; Robertson 1987).

Origins and lineage relationships in spontaneous teratoma

Teratoma origins The cell type that first shows abnormal growth in the testis is different from that in the ovary. Using a mouse strain with a high incidence of spontaneous testicular teratomas, it is possible to trace the first histological abnormality to a proliferation of germ cells in the fetal testis. Similarly, when abnormal germ cells are observed in the testis of patients attending infertility clinics, then a very high proportion of such patients subsequently develop teratoma and related

germ cell tumours. In humans, the testicular teratoma cells are characteristically aneuploid, but they often contain both the X- and Y-chromosomes and the same pairs of alleles as are present in the normal cells of the patient's body: these teratomas must therefore originate before the first meiotic division of the germ cells.

In contrast, over half of human ovarian teratomas are homozygous for alleles which are heterozygous in the somatic cells of the host: these tumours must develop from eggs that have completed meiosis. A smaller proportion of the ovarian teratomas originate from developing eggs either before or after the first meiotic division, for partial or complete heterozygosity of alleles may be retained. In all cases, the karyotype of ovarian teratomas is usually normal 46, XX. The origin of ovarian teratomas between the first and second meiotic divisions is also observed in mice: using a strain of mouse with a high incidence of ovarian teratomas it has been possible to associate tumour formation with the appearance of oocytes which start to develop parthenogenetically. Studies of the chromosomes of these embryos and the alleles of these teratomas suggest that they originate from diploid oocytes in metaphase I of meiosis. Thus, the bulk of the ovarian teratomas of mouse and human originate from eggs that have started to proceed through meiosis.

In summary, the spontaneous testicular and ovarian teratomas arise from germ cells at various stages of their progression to mature gametes.

Lineage in spontaneous teratoma Although there is general agreement about the cell types in which abnormal behaviour is first seen in teratoma formation, there is controversy about the lineage relationship between the cell types that are observed in human testicular germ cell tumours. It is difficult to resolve these controversies because one malignant cell type may progress to another in differentiating tumours. Many of the human germ cell tumours are mixed tumours which contain combinations of seminoma, embryonal carcinoma, endoderm sinus tumour, choriocarcinoma, and immature fetal tissues. When each of these kinds of carcinoma are the only cell type in a tumour, they can be characterized by the kind of differentiated cells that they produce, and they may be matched to the stem cells in the gonads and the early conceptus (Table 9.5). Thus a rare subset of seminomas are called spermatocytic seminoma, and some of the cells engage in abnormal spermiogenesis: this suggests that common seminoma is a tumour of pre-meiotic germ cells. Choriocarcinoma consists of cells with similar properties to cyto- and syncytio-trophoblast, and endoderm sinus tumour contains α-fetoprotein-producing cells which are similar to yolk-sac endoderm cells: thus, choriocarcinoma and endoderm sinus tumour appear to contain the transformed counterparts of stem cells of extra-embryonic tissues. Many of these cell types may form transplantable tumours in nude mice, but only human embryonal carcinoma has been rigorously studied: some cloned human embryonal carcinoma cells can form cells producing human chorionic gonadotrophin, neurones, and complex epithelia. Thus these cells are probably the stem cells of the teratoma parts of these germ cell tumours.

Table 9.5 Development levels of dominant tumour type

Development stage	Normal stem cell	Normal differentiated product	Dominant tumour cell type
Germ cell in gonad	Germ cell	Sperm and eggs	Seminoma and dysgerminoma
8-cell embryo	All cells	Whole conceptus	Embryonal carcinoma
Early blastocyst	Trophectoderm	Trophoblast	Choriocarcinoma
	Inner cell mass	All conceptus except trophoblast	Embryonal carcinoma
Late blastocyst	Primitive endoderm	Visceral yolk-sack endoderm; Parietal yolk-sack endoderm	Endoderm sinus tumour Parietal yolk-sack tumour
	Primitive ectoderm	All conceptus except trophoblast and membrane endoderm	Embryonal carcinoma

The dominant tumour cell is recognized by the products of its differentiated cells: choriocarcinoma by the production of human chorionic gonadotrophin, and endoderm sinus tumour by the production of α-fetoprotein: neither the normal nor the tumour stem cells are yet defined by a unique set of antigen products. It is assumed that once a tumour stem cell becomes determined to form a limited class of differentiated cells then it cannot proceed backwards in development and form all the cell types of the conceptus. On the other hand, there is no developmental reason why a seminoma should not give rise to all the other types of tumour in the list.

Embryonal carcinoma is placed at several developmental levels: this is because some embryonal carcinoma cells of the human can differentiate into trophoblast-like cells, while others have not been reported to do so. Again, some embryonal carcinoma cells can produce cells like visceral yolk-sack endoderm, while others have not been reported to do so. It therefore appears that embryonal carcinoma cells can correspond to normal stem cells at the 8-cell, inner cell mass, or primitive ectoderm levels.

Derivation from embryonic cells

Transplantable teratomas are formed in mice by transplanting either embryo precursor cells, or primordial germ cells contained in genital ridges, beneath the capsules of the kidney or testis. The tumours consist of rapidly dividing embryonal carcinoma (EC) stem cells and many of the cell types that are found in the fetal rodent body. The EC cells are selected for tumour formation, but very similar cells are produced when embryo stem (ES) cells are grown out from explanted mouse blastocysts. The ES cells will also form teratomas when injected back into an adult mouse after growth in plastic culture flasks. The major difference between ES cells and EC cells is their behaviour when injected back into a mouse blastocyst: ES cells form a large part of the chimeric body, and they frequently develop into viable germ cells, while EC cells rarely form germ cells and sometimes form teratomas in the chimera. It is helpful to regard EC cells as ES cells that have undergone some change which reduces the probability of determination and differentiation. In both cases, these studies show that cell interactions with the normal conceptus suppress the capacity of these stem cells to form tumours.

When mouse teratocarcinomas are transplanted from one mouse to another for long periods, the range of differentiated cell types in the tumours decrease: in some, differentiation may be restricted to one cell type, such as neural ectoderm (like the neural tube), or striated muscle, or parietal yolk-sac endoderm, while in others only the EC stem cells are apparent. It also seems that different tumours may develop directly from the embryo, for yolk sac carcinoma may be the only differentiated cell type that can be found when a tumour first becomes obvious. These observations demonstrate that it is not always possible to identify the cellular origin of a tumour by studying the characters of the predominant cell type when the tumour is first detected.

Differentiation and transplantation

Single mouse EC cells can form all the cell types of a tumour when transplanted back to a host, an experiment which establishes the stem cell of the mouse tumour. The differentiated cells that develop from the EC cells rarely form transplantable tumours. These results were established by Pierce and his colleagues around 1960: they have been confirmed frequently, and they are the basis for a close study of the factors that regulate the growth and differentiation of EC cells. Note that there is less certainty about the stem cells of human teratoma: cells have been cloned from human teratoma which form a subset of the cells that are found in the tumour. These cells are called embryonal carcinoma, but note that the human gonad tumours may also contain other multipotential stem cells: there is no developmental reason why seminoma might not give rise to the other cell types seen in germ cell tumours (Table 9.5).

Determination, differentiation, and growth control

The cultured stem cells of pluripotential tumours provide an opportunity for studying the factors that control growth, determination, and differentiation in defined culture conditions. Such studies can be rigorously controlled, but the application of these results to tumour behaviour in the body has only just begun. Cell lines from both human and mouse teratomas have been analysed, and it is clear that the growth of the cell populations depends on the relative rates of stem cell multiplication, survival, determination, and differentiation. In general, the stem cells traverse the cell cycle in less than a day, and the cell cycle lengthens progressively as their differentiated progeny are formed; thus differentiation of all the stem cells eventually leads to a nearly non-dividing population of differentiated cells.

Environmental requirements for growth

Established cultured stem cells of mouse and human teratoma have rather undemanding environmental requirements for cell multiplication: both require attachment factors and transferrin, and both will proceed through the cell cycle in the absence of exogenous growth factors. Without added growth factors, cell multiplication is balanced by cell death and the population numbers hardly increase.

The addition of growth factors to serum-free medium promotes cell survival and the cell population enlarges. Mouse EC and human embryonal carcinoma cell populations respond to IGF-II in this way. The human embryonal carcinoma cells also have the potential to respond to a wide variety of growth factors (see Section 9.6), for they display receptors for epidermal growth factor (EGF), basic fibroblast growth factor (bFGF), insulin-like growth factors (IGFs), and platelet-derived growth factor (PDGF). Amongst these growth factors IGF-II is known to be secreted by human embryonal carcinoma cells. Despite the production of this growth factor, the cells are not self-sufficient and in culture they still require an exogenous source of either IGFs or bFGF to reduce cell death and allow the population numbers to increase rapidly (Biddle et al. 1988). In summary, the human embryonal carcinoma cells exploit several growth factors to build up large cell populations.

Determination and differentiation signals

Naturally occurring molecules have been discovered which both prevent and promote the determination and differentiation of teratoma stem cells. These molecules must determine stem cells of the new differentiated cells and the consequence of this event is monitored by scoring the appearance of differentiated cells.

Inhibiting determination and differentiation Two factors inhibit the determination and differentiation of EC cells: one is produced by the EC cells and the other is a product of differentiated cell types. There is a heparin-binding protein secreted by mouse EC cells that has the dual properties of blocking the differentiation of some EC cells and stimulating the cell cycle of their differentiated progeny: thus, it can potentially regulate the growth of the teratoma population as a whole; it is a member of the basic fibroblast growth factor family (Delli-Bovi et al. 1988). The second is a single-chain glycoprotein with differentiation inhibiting activity (DIA) which is secreted by liver cell lines and other cell types (Smith et al. 1988).

Thus, the mouse EC cells secrete molecules that can regulate

their own determination and differentiation and the growth of their differentiated derivatives, while their differentiated derivatives can secrete molecules that regulate the determination and differentiation of their EC cell progenitors. These collaborations may mimic the co-operative growth interactions observed in the early conceptus.

Promoting determination and differentiation: in culture It is often difficult to establish cell cultures from the stem cells of mouse and human teratomas: the stem cells tend to differentiate. After a time, small foci of stem cells grow up and it is likely that these are rare cells with an unusually low rate of determination and differentiation in cell culture.

Differentiation is promoted by reducing the contact between the stem cells, either by separating the cells from each other or by exposing the bulk of the cell surface to the culture medium; a layer of endoderm cells form around isolated clumps of EC cells. It is likely that the dilution of endogenous and exogenous differentiation inhibiting factors partly accounts for differentiation by cell isolation (see above).

A common differentiating agent is the vitamin A analogue, retinoic acid. Retinoids are natural regulators of morphogenesis (morphogens) in some developing systems. The effect of retinoic acid on differentiation depends on its interaction with the cytoplasmic retinoic acid binding protein. In response to retinoic acid, sparse cultures of mouse EC cells form cell populations that resemble parietal yolk-sac endoderm, a cell type which characteristically secretes large quantities of laminin, fibronectin, entactin, and one form of plasminogen activator. In high-density cultures, the EC cells form another cell type, similar to the endoderm layer of the visceral yolk sac. These visceral endoderm-like cells secrete α-fetoprotein, transferrin, and many of the serum proteins characteristic of adult hepatocytes.

Some human embryonal carcinoma cell lines also differentiate in response to retinoic acid, leading to the formation of static cell cultures. In this case, the bulk of the differentiated cells cannot be classified as known cell types but neurones are obvious.

Promoting determination and differentiation: in hosts When retinoic acid is given in pharmacological amounts to mice bearing transplantable teratocarcinomas, then the growth of the tumours is slowed. In some experiments this was the major effect of the treatment, while in other experiments the majority of the tumours differentiated and were no longer transplantable (Speers 1982). When retinoids have been given to patients with advanced teratoma, then the tumours continued to grow. It is possible that the poor response of human teratomas to retinoids is related to the lack of responsiveness of many of the cell lines to these vitamin A analogues in culture; it may not be an appropriate differentiating agent for the human form of this cancer.

Leukaemias

Relationship with normal lymphopoiesis

The progression of stem cells in normal lymphopoiesis is well characterized: the process begins with division of a rare stem

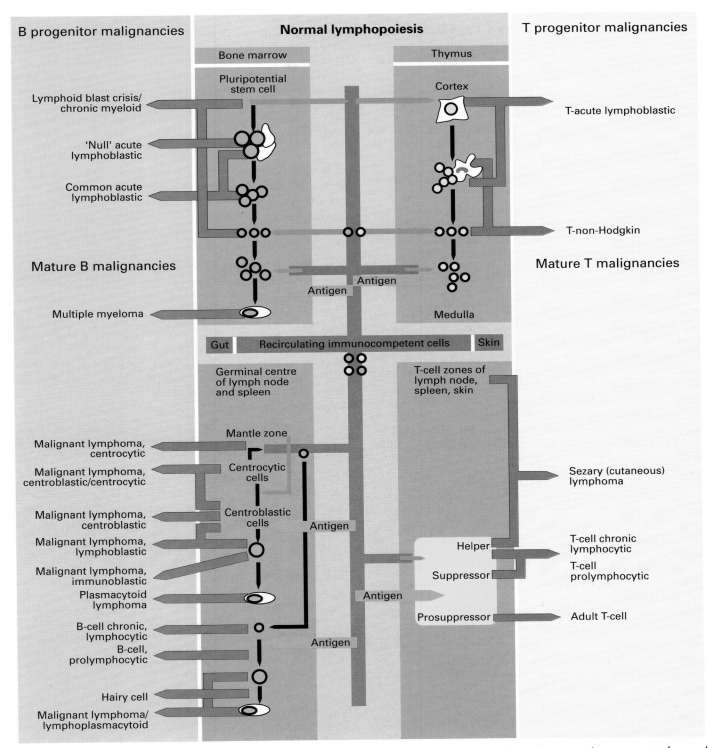

Fig. 9.11 Developmental levels of clonal amplification in lymphoid malignancy. Black pointers indicate the maturation sequence of normal lymphopoiesis, while continuous lines with arrows indicate the movement of cells from one organ to another. Normal lymphocyte and malignant cell subset heterogeneity, anatomical compartmentalization, and precise correspondence of leukaemia/lymphoma cell phenotype to normal has been considerably simplified for presentation of major relationships. In the nomenclature of the malignant cells, the word leukaemia has been omitted from the end of each description to save space. (The figure is adapted from Greaves 1986, with permission.)

cell of the whole haematopoietic system (see also Section 1.3). It is found that cells which are expanded in leukaemias and lymphomas share phenotypes with different subsets of normal haemopoietic cells (Fig. 9.11). This concordance prompts some general conclusions:

1. Many of the malignancies correspond to rare stem cells in the adult.

2. The malignant cells can be regarded as cells in which the probability of progression along the normal lineage of development is reduced.

3. Many of the malignancies may exploit the soluble regulators of the normal lineage in their expansion.

4. The factors that regulate the normal lineage do not act on one stem cell type in the lineage: a single colony-stimulating factor may promote the proliferation of some normal stem cells but stimulate the differentiation of others (see Sections 1.2, 1.3).

Induction of differentiation

In culture In the animal, granulocyte–macrophage colony-stimulating factor (GM-CSF) and granulocyte colony-stimulating factor (G-CSF) regulate several steps in haematopoiesis. In culture, GM-CSF and G-CSF can induce the differentiation of particular acute and myeloid leukaemia cell lines to granulocytes and macrophages. The resulting cells no longer grow progressively. Unfortunately, when acute myeloblastic leukaemia cells are taken fresh from patients and treated with these agents in short-term culture, the cells mainly respond by proliferation, and there is only limited differentiation; there is also great patient-to-patient variation in the response (Miyauchi *et al.* 1987).

In hosts The increasing availability of pure lymphokines has greatly improved cancer therapy because it is possible to use them to expand and activate the normal cells involved in immune responses, when the primary treatment of the tumour is with cytotoxic agents. The hosts can tolerate concentrations of lymphokines that saturate the receptors on the cell surface. However, in differentiation therapy, the pleiotropic effects of the lymphokines makes it difficult to design treatments that induce the differentiation of the malignant cells: in an early study with GM-CSF in patients with pre-leukaemic symptoms (mylodysplastic syndromes), the treatment appeared to accelerate the transformation to leukaemia (Hoelzer *et al.* 1988). It is probable that regimens of lymphokine cocktails will have to be used to pick out the differentiation response.

Differentiation therapy

A variety of agents promote the determination and differentiation of tumour cells in cell culture so that tumourigenicity is lost. Most of these agents induce less differentiation when the tumour is in a host. This is partly because large doses of all these agents are toxic, and at present none are very effective differentiation inducers when applied systematically.

There are four main problems with differentiation therapy.

1. The identification of the natural substances which inhibit and promote stem cell determination and differentiation has only just begun. When many more of the molecules involved in stem-cell regulation are discovered, it will be possible to start a rational differentiation therapy. From studies with leukaemia and teratomas, it is already clear that such regulators will have pleiotropic effects and the problem will be to limit the action of these agents so that they mainly accentuate the determination and differentiation of tumour cells.

2. The therapy will have to be applied locally to tumour stem cells. The lesson of cell interactions in the mammalian conceptus is that close-range and confined interactions regulate the determination, growth, and differentiation of stem cells, and similar interactions are probable in differentiating tumours. Further progress will depend on developing targeted delivery of the determination and differentiating agents.

3. Stem cells of tumours may show variable responses to differentiating agents. For instance, it is possible to select EC stem cells which are resistant to determination and differentiation agents such as retinoic acid.

4. Determination and differentiation may not always suppress the malignant phenotype. For instance, some EC pluripotential tumours may develop into tumours with only single unipotential stem cells: determination must have occurred, and either malignancy has been retained or it has originated again in the new stem cell.

9.4.4   Acknowledgements

The Oxford Cancer Research Campaign Growth Factor Group and the Imperial Cancer Research Fund Developmental Biology Unit contributed both to the work and this analysis. The scope of this section precludes reference to many important contributors to this field.

9.4.5   Bibliography

Alberts, B., Bray, D., Lewis, J., Raff, M., Roberts, K., and Watson, J. D. (1983). *The molecular biology of the cell* (1st edn), pp. 911–50. Garland, New York.

Anderson, C. K., Jones, W. G., and Milford Ward, A. (eds) (1981). *Germ cell tumours*. Taylor and Francis, London.

Biddle, C., *et al.* (1988). Insulin-like growth factors and the multiplication of Tera-2, a human teratoma derived cell line. *Journal of Cell Science* 90, 475–84.

Bloch, A. (1984). Induced cell differentiation in cancer therapy. *Cancer Treatment Reports* 68, 199–205.

Delli-Bovi, P., *et al.* (1988). Processing, secretion, and biological properties of a novel growth factor of the fibroblast growth factor family with oncogenic potential. *Molecular and Cellular Biology* 8, 2933–41.

Fresney, R. I. (1985). Induction of differentiation in neoplastic cells. *Anticancer Research* 5, 111–30.

Gardner, R. L. (ed.) (1983). Embryonic germ cell tumours in man and animals. *In Cancer surveys*, Vol. 2, pp. 1–219. Imperial Cancer Research Fund/Oxford University Press.

Gardner, R. L. (1985). Regeneration of endoderm from primitive ectoderm in the mouse embryo: fact or artifact. *Journal of Embryology
and Experimental Morphology* **88**, 303–26.

Greaves, M. F. (1986). Differentiation-linked leukemogenesis in
lymphocytes. *Science* **234**, 697–704.

Harland, R. (1988). Growth factors in mesoderm induction. *Trends in
Genetics* **4**, 62–3.

Harris, H. (1985). Suppression of malignancy: the mechanism. *Journal
of Cell Science* **79**, 83–94.

Hill, D. J., Strain, A. J., and Milner, R. D. G. (1987). Growth factors in
embryogenesis. In *Oxford reviews of reproductive biology*, (ed.
J. Clarke), Vol. 9, pp. 398–445, Oxford University Press.

Hoelzer, D., Ganser, A., Greher, J., Volkers, B., and Walther, H. (1988).
Phase I–II study with GM-CSF in patients with mylodisblastic syndromes. *Behring Institute, Mitteilungen*, **83**, 134–8.

Hopkins, B., Sharpe, C. R., Baralle, F. E., and Graham, C. F. (1986).
Organ distribution of apolipoprotein gene transcripts in 6–12
week postfertilization human embryos. *Journal of Embryology and
Experimental Morphology* **97**, 177–87.

Jones, W. G., Milford Ward, A., and Anderson, C. K. (eds) (1986). *Germ
cell tumours II*, Advance in the biosciences, No. 55. Pergamon
Press, Oxford.

Kaufman, M. H. and Howlett, S. K. (1986). The ovulation and activation of primary and secondary oocytes in LT/Sv strain mice.
Gamete Research **14**, 255–64.

Kleinsmith, L. J. and Pierce, G. B. (1964). Multipotentiality of single
embryonal carcinoma cells. *Cancer Research* **24**, 1544–51.

Lord, B. I., Potten, C. S., and Cole, R. J. (eds) (1978). *Stem cells and
tissue homeostasis*, 2nd Symposium of the British Society for Cell
Biology. Cambridge University Press.

Metcalf, D. (1982). Regulator-induced suppression of myelomonocytic
leukaemia cells: clonal analysis of early cellular events. *International Journal of Cancer* **30**, 203–10.

Miyauchi, J., *et al.* (1987). The effects of three recombinant growth
factors (IL-3, GM-CSF, and G-CSF) on the blast cells of acute myeloblastic leukaemia maintained in short-term suspension culture.
Blood **70**, 657–63.

Pierce, G. B. and Speers, W. C. (1988). Tumours as caricatures of the
process of tissue renewal: prospects for therapy by directing differentiation. *Cancer Research* **48**, 1996–2004.

Rizzino, A. (1987). In *The mammalian preimplantation embryo: regulation of growth and differentiation in vitro* (ed. B. D. Bavister),
pp. 151–74. Plenum Press, New York.

Robertson, E. J. (ed.) (1987). *Teratocarcinoma and embryonic stem cells: a
practical approach*. IRL Press, Oxford.

Rossant, J. and Pedersen, R. A. (eds) (1986). *Experimental approaches to
mammalian embryonic development*. Cambridge University Press.

Rustin, G. J. S. and Bagshawe, K. D. (1982). Trial of an aromatic
retinoid in patients with solid tumours. *British Journal of Cancer* **45**,
304–8.

Sachs, L. (1982). Normal development programmes in myeloid leukaemia: regulatory proteins in the control of growth and differentiation. *Cancer Surveys* **1**, 321–42.

Sherman, M. I. (ed.) (1977). *Concepts in mammalian enbryogenesis*. MIT
Press, Cambridge, Mass.

Silver, L. M., Martin, G. R., and Strickland, S. (eds) (1983). *Teratocarcinoma Stem Cells*, Cold Spring Harbor Conferences on Cell Proliferation. Cold Spring Harbor Press, New York.

Slack, J. M. W. (1987). We have a morphogen. *Nature* **327**, 553–4.

Smith, A. G., *et al.* (1988). Inhibition of pluripotential embryonic stem
cell differentiation by purified polypeptides. *Nature* **336**, 688–90.

Spangrude, G. J., Heimfeld, S., and Weissman, I. L. (1988). Purification
and characterization of mouse hematopoietic stem cells. *Science*
241, 58–62.

Speers, W. C. (1982). Conversion of malignant murine embryonal
carcinoma to benign teratomas by chemical induction of differentiation *in vivo*. *Cancer Research* **42**, 1843–7.

Strickland, S. and Sawey, M. J. (1980). Studies on the effect of retinoids
on the differentiation of teratocarcinoma stem cells *in vitro* and *in
vivo*. *Development Biology* **78**, 76–85.

Takeichi, M. (1988). The cadherins: cell–cell adhesion molecules controlling animal morphogenesis. *Development* **102**, 639–55.

Watt, F. M. (1988). Keratinocyte cultures: an experimental model for
studying how proliferation and terminal differentiation are co-
ordinated in epidermis. *Journal of Cell Science* **90**, 525–9.

9.5 Tumour metastasis

D. Tarin

Tumours are remarkable forms of life which parasitize the host, with which they share near complete genetic identity, and manifest a complex variety of biochemical, histopathological, and clinical characteristics which distinguish each example as unique. Their detrimental effects can be mediated by diverse mechanisms ranging from simple mechanical compression or erosion of an important viscus to subtle endocrine effects includ-ing paraneoplastic syndromes (such as neuropathies, myo-pathies, and cachexia) mediated systemically (see Sections 9.8, 9.9, and 9.12). Most enigmatic of all is the capability inherent in some tumours of spreading by lymphatic or blood vascular channels to distant sites and organs, to form disseminated secondary tumours within the host, a process known as meta-stasis. Not all tumours are capable of this behaviour and, indeed, even among those that are, the metastatic process itself is not invariably the cause of death. When there is overwhelm-ing growth of secondary tumours in vital organs such as the liver or the brain, death can be directly attributed to metastases or to massive tumour burden competing for limited essential resources. However, in many cancer patients the extent of metastasis by the time of death is insufficient to account for mortality, and they succumb to intercurrent disease such as infection. The *clinical* significance of metastasis, therefore, is that this property confers upon the tumour cell population the ability to survive excision of the primary tumour and thus makes treatment and prognosis uncertain, because of the pos-sibility of disseminated cells lying dormant or growing slowly in numerous sites. The *biological* significance of metastasis is some-what different. It demonstrates unequivocally that the mainten-ance of metazoan body organization and function depends upon tight regulation of cellular growth control and upon localization of different cell lineages in separate territorial domains.

The detection of metastases constitutes decisive evidence for categorizing a proliferating primary lesion, previously of uncertain potential, as neoplastic and 'malignant', and the phenomenon is a topic of unparalleled importance in cancer medicine and biology. Recognition of this and of the feasibility of investigation of this problem by modern techniques, is resulting in increasing momentum in understanding the process.

The information in this section is organized into three main subsections, which should be read sequentially by those new to the topic, but which will serve as independent sources of reference for those more familiar with the field. The first section is a description of the clinical and biological manifestations of the process, the second a review of experimental analysis of the mechanisms involved, and the third a discussion of the prospects for therapy.

9.5.1   Description of the metastatic process

Metastasis and how it came to be recognized

Tumour metastasis is the process by which discrete secondary tumours form in a new site, often remote from the original 'parent' neoplasm. It consists of seeding of the new site with tumour cells, which arrive in the new location by active locomotion or by passive transport in body fluids and subsequently grow progressively. Although the shedding of tumour cells into coelomic or other body cavities and their subsequent implantation on a new surface is included in the overall concept, the term 'metastasis' more frequently refers to the formation of secondary neoplasms after dissemination by lymphatic or blood vascular channels. Its first use, in relation to tumours, is attributed to Recamier (1829), who applied it to a tumour in the brain he had noted in a patient with breast cancer. The term is Greek in origin and means a change of location or a transfer from one place to another, but there was considerable argument amongst nineteenth-century physicians interested in cancer, including Virchow, Waldeyer, Thiersch, and others, as to exactly what was being transferred. Some, led by Virchow, believed that substances or agents released by the primary tumour resulted in the conversion of normal cells elsewhere into tumour cells, which then formed separate neoplasms; while others contended that metastasis was due to the transfer of actual cells from the primary tumour, which then set up secondary tumours where they lodged. With the development of good compound microscopes and reliable histological techniques the process was unequivocally recognized as being due to dissemination and seeding of living tumour cells from the primary tumour, so that by 1889 Paget was confidently advancing his 'seed and soil' hypothesis, to account for the observed clinical patterns of secondary tumour distribution in metastasis (see below).

The early microscopists soon described clearly all the morphological aspects of the process, including invasion, entry into vascular channels, arrest in a distant site (Schmitt 1903), extravasation into the tissues of a new site, and formation of a secondary tumour. They also recognized that the new lesion frequently had close histological resemblance to the original (primary) tumour (see below). Therefore, by the early part of this century, cancer physicians clearly understood the potential of a proportion of tumours to spread and form seedlings, often before the primary had been detected. This led to the design of surgical procedures, such as the radical mastectomy developed by Halstead, to try to remove the disseminated tumour cells. Of course, as we now know, tumour cells can enter the blood and the lymphatics independently and, once in the blood, are disseminated to every organ in the body within 15 min (Fidler 1970; Fidler and Nicholson 1977; Potter *et al.* 1983). Radical surgery even when there are no obvious metastases at the time of presentation is, therefore, often no more effective in terms of length of patient survival or of disease-free interval before recurrence, than more conservative procedures (Baum 1980).

Recognizing this, modern surgical management tends towards less extensive operations, aimed at removing only the primary growth and accessible secondaries, with reliance on adjuvant radiotherapy, chemotherapy, or hormonal therapy to eliminate or suppress possible residual cancer cells in the body.

'Benign' and 'malignant' tumours

The appreciation of the potential virulence of some neoplasms led to the development of the somewhat vague clinical terms 'benign' and 'malignant' to describe tumours. Although they may be useful as a form of shorthand, between members of clinico-pathological units familiar with each other's terminology, they are not helpful to those investigating the underlying nature of the process. For instance, malignant gliomas are very rarely metastatic outside the confines of the meninges, whereas individual tumours of other organs can display a remarkably benign circumscribed appearance and well-differentiated histology but produce multiple metastases. For scientific purposes it is more accurate to speak of expansive or invasive tumours, which are believed to be still localized, and of weakly metastatic or heavily metastatic tumours when they are known to have formed secondary growths elsewhere.

9.5.2   Modern concepts of tumour metastasis

The major pathways of metastasis

Living tumour cells can be transferred from the primary site, to other locations, in a variety of ways, listed in Table 9.6. While the shedding of tumour cells, from the surface of a body cavity and their subsequent implantation to form a separate tumour elsewhere on the same surface, is a true example of metastasis, it is a less complex phenomenon than metastasis occurring via the lymphatics or the blood. In vascular metastasis, the cells forming the secondary tumour have completed a complicated series of manoeuvres, which must be executed in the right

Table 9.6   Pathways of tumour metastasis

Seeding across cavities	
Cerebrospinal spaces	in CSF
Transcoelomic	in effusions, e.g. peritoneal, pleural
Urinary tract	in urine
Bronchial	airborne
Lymphatic/venous permeation	direct growth along the lumen
Vascular	
Lymphatic	
Haematogenous	

sequence, and have demonstrated the ability to survive in unfamiliar environments, indicating that the formation of the metastatic deposit is not a casual or fortuitous event.

The timing of metastasis

Several clinical studies (Sugarbaker *et al.* 1982) have demonstrated that there is a good statistical correlation between the size of the primary tumour and the incidence of metastasis for a number of common tumours, including carcinomas of the breast, colon, lung, and malignant melanoma. However, there are a significant number of patients in all of these tumour groups who either have small or clinically undetectable primaries with widespread large metastases, or who have massive tumours and no secondaries. For the individual tumour or patient, therefore, there is (as yet) no way to ascertain whether metastasis has just occurred, or is imminent but undetectable, and no firm biological evidence for assuming that metastasis occurs at any particular stage of tumour development. The only antecedent conditions that must exist are that the cells involved must have become capable of indefinite replication and of survival in a distant site, because cell migration alone will not result in true metastasis.

Kinetic sequence of events in metastasis

The life history of a metastatic deposit can be reconstructed from detailed studies on large numbers of surgical biopsy and post-mortem specimens. It begins with tumour cells, which have been proliferating *in situ* (Fig. 9.12), breaching the boundaries of the tissue compartment in which they normally reside and eroding or infiltrating, either as mass populations of cells (Fig. 9.13) or as single autonomous units (Fig. 9.14), through the surrounding tissue (Tarin 1967, 1972). This process of invasion and infiltration is associated with considerable destruction of intercellular elements, such as basement membranes (Fig. 9.15), collagen fibres (Fig. 9.16), and the amorphous matrix of the local connective tissue. Any tightly

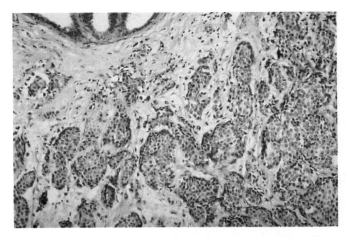

Fig. 9.13 Infiltrating ductal carcinoma of the breast invading adjacent fibrous tissue. These cancer cells migrate in clumps and sheets. A portion of the circumference of a residual duct is seen at the upper edge of the picture.

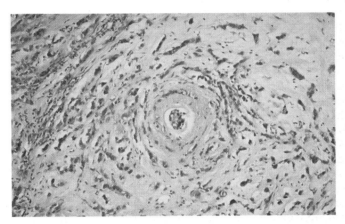

Fig. 9.14 Infiltrating lobular carcinoma of the breast. These cancer cells typically invade as dissociated single cells or in 'Indian file' pattern. The tumour cells are swirling around a residual small degenerating ductule.

compacted normal tissue in the path of the invading tumour, e.g. muscle (Fig. 9.17), bone, liver, kidney (Fig. 9.18), or other parenchymal organ, is either circumvented, with its cells being pushed aside, or destroyed by cytolysis, following direct membrane-to-membrane contact with invading tumour cells (Tarin 1972, 1976).

Sooner or later, the invading tumour cells collide with the basal lamina investing capillary blood vessels, or the exterior surface of endothelium lining lymphatics. These are the first natural obstacles to rapid large-scale dissemination, and only cells that can unleash the appropriate response from their genetic complement will move on to enter the lymph or the jet-stream of the blood and be carried rapidly to distant organs. Tumour cells that manage to enter the blood jostle in a series of high-speed collisions with their neighbours and the wall of the vessel, and are then slammed into a set of narrow exits, which

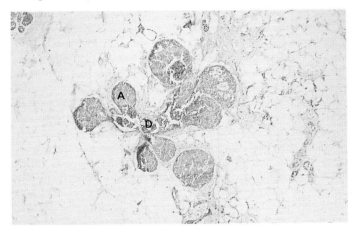

Fig. 9.12 Histological section of a human mammary lobule showing lobular carcinoma *in situ*. The proliferating neoplastic cells are poorly cohesive and distend the ductule (D) and acini (A) but are still within the boundaries of the duct system.

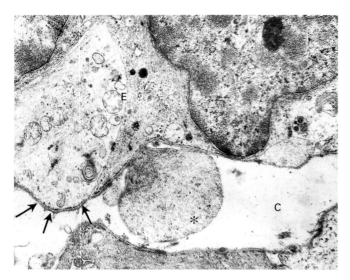

Fig. 9.15 An electron micrograph showing invading mammary carcinoma cells breaching the boundary of the duct. The basement membrane (arrows) which delineates the boundary between epithelium (E) and adjacent connective tissue (C) has been breached, and a finger-like epithelial cell protrusion (asterisk) extends through. Lysis of collagen I is so advanced that the connective tissue is completely devoid of collagen fibres.

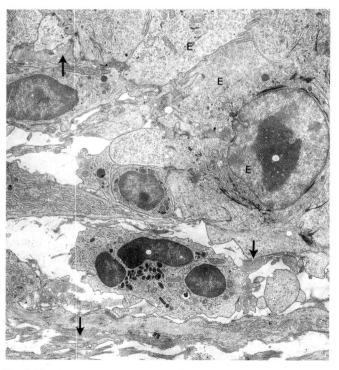

Fig. 9.16 An electron micrograph of the advancing edge of a deeply invasive skin carcinoma. In this portion of the invasion zone there is extensive disorganization of connective tissue, extending several microns in advance of the neoplastic epithelium (E) which is extending clear pseudopodia into the vacant space created by lysis of adjacent tissue. There are few remaining collagen fibres (arrows) and the basement membrane has been demolished.

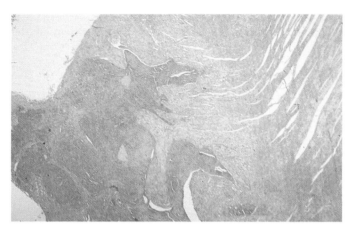

Fig. 9.17 Mouse mammary carcinoma invading skeletal muscle. A sheet of tumour cells is pushing fingers between muscle bundles.

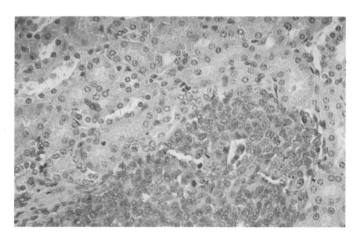

Fig. 9.18 Mouse mammary carcinoma invading the kidney. A sheet of tumour cells is pushing between renal tubules.

of course correspond to the lumina of the capillary network. Those cells that are robust enough to survive this experience now have the opportunity to insinuate their way through the vessel wall into the parenchyma of the lung or liver, or to grow within the vascular lumen (Fig. 9.19) and eventually burst through the wall, or to traffic through into the arterial circulation and be hurled into the capillary network of yet another organ, where the same possibilities arise again. Tumour cells entering the tissues of a fresh host organ now have to be able to multiply in that environment and induce the local non-neoplastic cells to provide them with a fibrovascular framework (Figs 9.20a, b and 9.21), otherwise the size of the colony will be limited to a millimetre or two because of the inefficiency of diffusion as a transport process over larger distances. If all of these conditions are satisfied, metastatic deposits can grow to enormous sizes, sometimes bigger than the primary tumour (Fig. 9.22).

It is important to appreciate that, because of the sequential nature of the process and its complexity, if the disseminating cells cannot mobilize the appropriate activity at the correct time

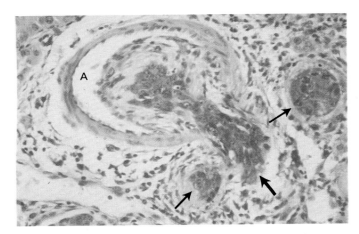

Fig. 9.19 Histological section showing tumour cells (large arrow) extravasating through the wall of a small renal artery (A) into the renal parenchyma. Two adjacent arterioles (small arrows) are blocked with tumour cell emboli.

and place, the whole metastatic process is aborted, even if the cells have the capabilities to perform the rest of the sequence. In fact, experimental studies discussed below show that there is an enormous redundancy in the metastatic process, with numerous cells being eliminated at each step in the sequence, because of inability to proceed to the next.

It is important to recognize that tumour emboli differ significantly from fully formed metastases. Viable clumps of tumour cells are not infrequently seen in the capillaries of the lungs in patients who had metastases in other organs, and the degree of organization of the tumour cell clump often indicates that it is not a recent arrival. In such circumstances it seems that the tumour cells either did not have the capability to escape from the vessels or to survive in the extravascular tissues, or both.

The train of events in metastasis via the lymphatics is much the same, except that lymph flow is more sluggish. Also, the tumour cells it transports often become entrapped in the interstices of the draining nodes (Fig. 9.23) in which they grow, to form secondary deposits which, in turn, shed cells downstream. Eventually, tumour cells enter the bloodstream, if the patient survives long enough, by being released via the thoracic duct into the innominate vein. Retrograde spread from the thoracic duct, along the peribronchial lymphatics, also occurs, resulting in an alternative mode of formation of pulmonary metastases, assuming that the cells of the particular tumour concerned can grow in this environment. It is self-evident that, as in haematogenous metastasis, the tumour cells must be able to complete every step in the sequence to be able to form any metastases.

The process of metastasis does not necessarily cease with the formation of the first shower of deposits. Superimposed metastatic cycles can result from secondary tumours now acting as foci for further shedding into the blood or lymphatics.

Patterns of metastasis

The release of cells into the lymphatic, or blood circulation,

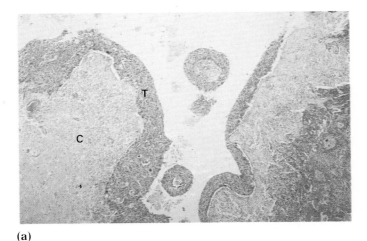

(a)

(b)

Fig. 9.20 (a) Metastatic human bronchial carcinoma (T) growing in the meninges as a thick sheet covering the cerebral grey matter (C). In the underlying white matter on the right there is a further tumour deposit. (b) The same field of view as in (a). This section has been stained with silver techniques for reticulin and shows that the tumour cells have attracted blood vessels (arrows) and stimulated the deposition of collagenous fibrovascular scaffolding for themselves.

systems might be expected to result in more or less uniform distribution of seedlings in all tissues and organs, if the process were entirely random. However, the distribution of metastases is certainly not even and uniform and bears some relationship to the site and type of the primary tumour. It has also been noted that some organs (such as liver, lungs, bone, lymph nodes, and adrenals) are frequently the site of tumour colonization, whereas others (such as the kidney and muscle, either skeletal or cardiac) are rarely involved, despite the fact that they have a rich blood supply (Tarin 1976). Paget (1889) reviewed the autopsy records of 735 patients dying of breast cancer at the Middlesex Hospital and noted that 241 (33 per cent) had metastases in the liver, whereas only 17 (2 per cent) had them in the spleen, although the spleen has a bigger artery. From this and similar information, he drew the analogy that disseminating

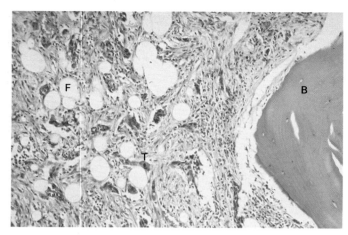

Fig. 9.21 Metastatic bladder carcinoma (T) cells in bone marrow have stimulated proliferation of fibroblasts and capillaries (a desmoplastic response) between bone trabeculae (B) and fat cells (F) of the marrow.

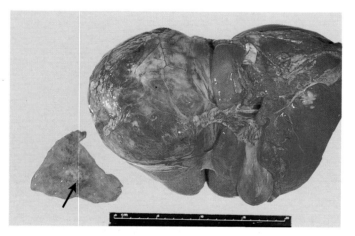

Fig. 9.22 Massive metastases distending the right lobe of the liver. Adjacent is a piece of gastric mucosa, in the centre of which is the tiny carcinoma (arrow) from which they originated (seen as an area of slight roughening of the surface).

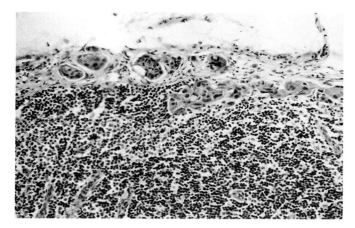

Fig. 9.23 Histological section of a lymph node draining a carcinoma of the breast showing metastasizing tumour cells trapped in the cortical sinus of the node.

cancer cells are like seeds, which, after being scattered on the wind, grow only in sites ('soil') that are congenial, and this therefore came to be known as his 'seed and soil' hypothesis of metastatic spread.

In 1928 Ewing presented the alternative view, that the distribution of metastases could be explained on the basis of circulatory anatomy and that there was no need to postulate special affinities of certain tumours for particular tissues to explain patterns of metastasis. He gave no supporting evidence from autopsy studies or experimental work to justify this conclusion, which was stated in a single sentence. By 1940, in the next edition of his book, he had removed this statement. Some years later the concept was resurrected and embraced more enthusiastically by Coman (1951, 1953), who reported experiments involving intravascular injection of VX2 carcinoma cells in rabbits. He contended that the results were entirely explicable in

terms of circulatory anatomy and extrapolated that they excluded the need to invoke preferential growth in certain sites to explain the distribution of metastases. He did not proceed, however, to offer detailed explanations of the different clinical distribution patterns associated with different human tumour types or of those associated with serially propagated animal cell lines.

Since then, there have been numerous autopsy studies on the distribution of metastases from various types of primary cancer (Lee 1983; de la Monte *et al* 1983; Weiss *et al.* 1984; Noltenius and Noltenius 1985), and the data from these strongly support the interpretation that the distribution of metastases is not random; some organs are much more frequently colonized than others, and common types of primary cancer have typical patterns of secondary tumour distribution, although individual patients do have sporadic deposits in other organs. Collectively, this information also demonstrates that vascular drainage patterns and organ-specific factors both contribute to the observed distribution patterns of secondary tumour deposits. For example, the frequent presence of metastases in the liver, in patients with primary cancer in the catchment area of the hepatic portal vein (about 50 per cent of such patients), and in the lungs, in patients with primary tumours draining into the systemic veins (about 40 per cent), strongly support the interpretation that vascular drainage patterns influence the distribution of secondary tumour deposits.

Conversely, the well-known tendency of bronchial cancers to selectively form bilateral metastases in the adrenals (about 30 per cent) cannot be satisfactorily explained purely in terms of circulatory anatomy. Also unlikely to be explicable on haemodynamic or lymphodynamic principles alone is the recent observation that diffuse seeding of the peritoneal cavity in patients with cancer of the breast is much more often associated with lobular carcinoma than with ductal carcinoma, which tends to form large deposits in the liver (Howell and Harris 1985). Such specific pathological observations constitute strong evidence that subtle, organ-specific factors, perhaps local paracrine hormones or general microenvironmental metabolic conditions in the sites of tumour cell lodgement, powerfully affect the survival and growth of the disseminated cells and therefore the pattern of metastasis seen clinically (see below). Other examples supporting this interpretation are the unusually high incidence of metastases in the brain, in patients with carcinoma of the lung (approximately 30 per cent of patients, compared with an overall incidence of about 5 per cent for carcinomas generally), and of deposits in bone (approximately 70 per cent) in patients with breast cancer (Lee 1983; Paget 1989), compared with a figure of about 20 per cent for malignant tumours overall. These distributions cannot be explained solely on patterns of vascular supply and drainage, and it is therefore difficult, even on solely clinical grounds, to refute the conclusion that metabolic conditions in certain sites favour the growth of particular types of secondary tumour. As will be seen below, there is also direct experimental evidence from studies on metastasis in humans, endorsing this interpretation.

Paradoxically, the findings in individual patients with unusual patterns of metastatic spread, lend further strong support to the conclusion that site-specific factors can encourage or discourage the growth of disseminated tumour cells. To illustrate this, the data from two recent autopsies on patients with malignant melanoma will be compared and contrasted. In the first patient, who died 18 months after excision of a primary melanoma on the lower leg (Fig. 9.24), metastases were found in the iliac and para-aortic lymph nodes and in the skin of the leg and foot (Fig. 9.25), all resulting from spread via lymphatics. However, the only other site in the body in which metastases could be found, was the brain (Fig. 9.26). Therefore, although the brain deposits provided incontrovertible evidence of haematogenous dissemination of the melanoma cells and of their entry into the systemic arterial blood, there were no detectable colonies (even histologically) in the lungs, through which the tumour cells must have transitted.

In the other patient there were multiple seedlings in the liver, spleen, lungs, bone, muscle, breast, heart, bladder, and many other tissues (Figs 9.27, 9.28, and 9.29), but the brain (Fig. 9.30) was completely free of macroscopic or microscopic

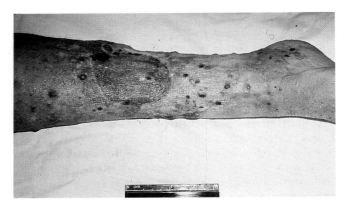

Fig. 9.24 Pigmented metastases in the leg of a patient (MM1) with malignant melanoma. The site of resection of the primary tumour can be seen and deposits are even present in the skin graft covering the deficit.

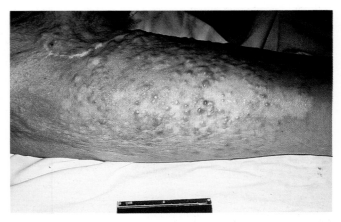

Fig. 9.25 Thigh of the same patient (MM1) as in Fig. 9.24, showing numerous cutaneous metastases, some of which are pigmented. A pale scar can be seen in the groin at the site of previous resection of deposits in the inguinal nodes.

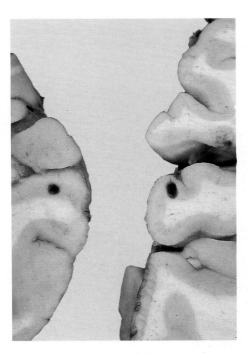

Fig. 9.26 Portions of two slices of the brain of patient (MM1). Pigmented metastases can be seen in the grey matter of the cerebral cortex.

involvement, although tumour cells had clearly been disseminated to this organ by the systemic arterial circulation.

Even in individual cases, therefore, there is evidence that site-specific factors interact with inherent properties of individual tumour cells, to influence whether the scattered cells grow to form secondary tumours or not.

In summary, these studies on the distribution of metastatic deposits in patients with cancer have indicated beyond reasonable doubt that:

1. There are recognizable patterns of metastatic spread, which

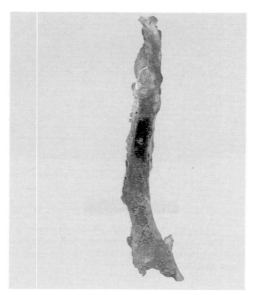

Fig. 9.27 A slice through the sternum of another patient (MM2) with proven malignant melanoma, showing heavily pigmented metastasis.

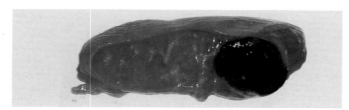

Fig. 9.28 A pigmented metastasis in the spleen of patient MM2.

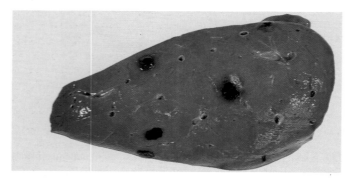

Fig. 9.29 Pigmented metastases in liver of patient MM2.

are related to the site and even the histological type of the primary tumour.

2. Regional venous and lymphatic drainage pathways play an important role in contributing to these patterns.

3. Tumour cells will not necessarily grow in every tissue in which they become entrapped and clinical observations indicate that the growth of secondary tumours is dependent upon complementation between intrinsic properties of the tumour cell and those of the tissue in which it lodges.

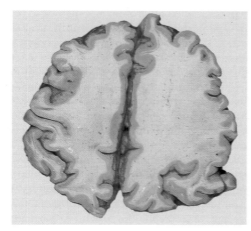

Fig. 9.30 A slice across the cerebral hemispheres of patient MM2 showing absence of deposits.

4. Sporadic variations from the general metastatic pattern for a given tumour are seen in individuals, as would be expected in a genetically heterogeneous population.

5. Some types of tumours (for instance melanomas) have much more latitude than others in the variety of tissues that they can colonize.

The knowledge that tumours of various organs and histological types exhibit more or less characteristic patterns of metastatic spread is important, both in clinical management, where such information guides patient evaluation and choice of therapy, and in basic understanding of the metastatic process, because it reveals that disseminating cancer cells are not invincible units, capable of replicating autonomously, wherever they alight.

The histological structure of metastases reflects their tissue of origin

The microscopic structure of metastases conforms closely to that of the parent tumour (Figs. 9.31 and 9.32) and this correspondence in histological pattern is used diagnostically in trying to identify the site of an unknown primary, when the metastases are responsible for the clinical presenting features. Sometimes the structure of the metastasis seems to differ from that of the primary, in degree or type of differentiation, but it is almost always possible to find comparable areas within the primary tumour, if enough tissue is examined. Likewise, separate metastases from the same primary tumour sometimes differ from one another in histological pattern, but examples of both histopathological appearances will be found in the primary tumour, if sufficient samples are taken. Therefore, although the tumour cells have translocated to a different organ, they retain the appearances of the tissue and the tumour from which they arose, and are not induced by local tissue factors to change their intrinsic characteristics (see further discussion in Tarin 1972, 1976).

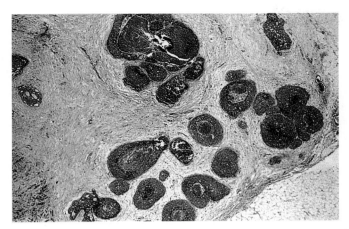

Fig. 9.31 Histological section of an infiltrating ductal carcinoma of breast showing 'comedo pattern' of growth, with central necrosis in many islands of tumour cells.

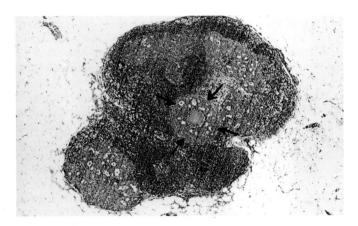

Fig. 9.32 Histological section of a lymph node draining the breast carcinoma illustrated in Fig. 9.31. The node contains a metastatic carcinoma deposit which retains a similar comedo pattern to the primary tumour.

The clinical effects of metastasis

In general, the deleterious effects of secondary tumours parallel those of primary tumours in corresponding sites but, because of the frequent multiplicity of metastases, their clinical effects can combine to accelerate the debilitation of the patient. Individually, metastases can, depending on their location, cause pain, fractures, neurological and psychiatric effects, and compression or rupture of other vital organs with consequent mechanical obstruction or haemorhage. Multiple metastases in the coelomic cavity can cause massive effusions with associated loss of protein and trace elements sequestered in the fluid, and consequent gross metabolic imbalance. The mechanism of production of malignant ascites is still unknown. Similarly, multiple metastases can also create severe systemic effects by permeation and blockage of lymphatics (lymphangitis carcinomatosa) (Fig. 9.33) and, by massive expansion of total tumour burden, result in wasting. If the tumour is metabolically or endocrino-

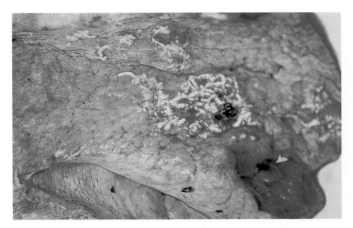

Fig. 9.33 Lymphangitis carcinomatosa. Surface lymphatics of the lungs are focally distended with propagating tumour cells giving the appearance of a 'bag of worms'.

logically active, severe paraneoplastic syndromes (see Sections 9.8 and 9.9) may occur and cause death by marked disturbances in electrolyte balance, by muscle weakness and consequent respiratory failure, or by cardiac arrhythmias.

9.5.3 Mechanisms of metastasis

General principles of investigation

The above information is derived from observations on the natural history of tumour metastasis, without experimental intervention. This section considers what has been learned about the phenomenon from experimental analysis of the process in humans and laboratory animals. In spite of its clinical and biological importance and the allure of trying to understand a unique and enigmatic phenomenon, whose mechanisms are shrouded in mystery, the field attracts only a trickle of new workers and of the financial resources lavished on the cancer problem. Perhaps it is because of the technical difficulty involved: metastasis is a kinetic process occuring in a living organism and it therefore has anatomical and temporal coordinates that cannot be reproduced *in vitro*. Furthermore, assays are relatively slow, because the only reliable endpoint is the detection of secondary tumours at autopsy, some weeks later, and the incidence of metastasis in many cell lines is not 100 per cent. Hence, investigation of the problem is expensive in time, effort, and resources, but its appeal lies in the synthesis of molecular, cellular, and clinical observations to try to explain the pathogenesis of this unusual behaviour pattern displayed apparently only by neoplastic cells. As an interesting aside, it should be noted that metastasis of other organisms, such as tubercle bacilli, toxoplasma, and parasitic worms, e.g. *Trichinella spiralis*, is occasionally seen in non-neoplastic diseases.

A working scheme for consideration of tumour metastasis

Research data enable the construction of a coherent blueprint for the metastatic process. This will need modification as further information accrues, but will serve as a framework for the ensuing discussion of experiments and for the formulation of conclusions on the mechanisms of the metastatic process.

This scheme proposes that metastasis results from the development of regulatory genomic disturbances in a small proportion of the tumour cell population. These cells consequently develop migratory and other properties that are the driving force of the metastatic process. However, metastasizing tumour cells are not invincible and their eventual success or failure to set up secondary colonies elsewhere, depends on whether they survive mechanical destruction during dissemination and can grow in the organs in which they come to rest. Superimposed on this interaction between the properties of the tumour cell and the new organ environment, are systemic effects exerted by the immune and endocrine systems, the magnitude of which depends on the quantity and type of exposed antigens and receptors on the neoplastic cell surface, and on the vigour of the host response (see Section 9.8).

Some methodological considerations

Before proceeding to consider the evidence on which our current understanding of the metastatic process is based, it is important to outline experimental approaches that have been used to study the problem.

The simplest method for studying some aspects of metastasis via the bloodstream, is to inject suspensions of cells from freshly disaggregated tumours, or serially propagated cell lines, directly into the veins, and to study the result at autopsy some weeks or months later. This method is known as experimental metastasis, or the lung colony assay (because, following this procedure, most, but not all, tumours appear to make colonies predominantly in the lungs). Clearly, it is not an exact simulation of natural metastasis, but has the advantage that the dose of tumour cells and the timing of their release into the bloodstream are controlled by the investigator. In such experiments the method of cell dissemination is deliberately artificial, because the critical endpoint of enquiry is colony formation. Circulating tumour cells are not a significant clinical problem if they cannot colonize. The main objective of this approach is to focus attention solely on events after blood-borne dissemination and to cut away all interfering phenomena.

An alternative method is to inject suspensions of tumour cells subcutaneously (or in some other site) and to await the development of a primary tumour, after which the animal is autopsied at a specified interval or when it first shows signs of morbidity. This technique has been referred to as 'spontaneous' metastasis, but it, too, does not exactly simulate natural metastatic spread from an undisturbed tumour, because the process of inoculation could release cells into small vessels at the injection site and the tumour is often induced, for the sake of convenience, in an inappropriate site to its histogenetic origin. (Naito et al. 1986 and Bresalier et al. 1987 have provided interesting information indicating that primary growth in an appropriate site, i.e. the organ from which the tumour cell line is derived, may be necessary for recapitulation of expected patterns of metastasis). Nevertheless, with appropriate controls, this approach is the nearest one can get to studying the natural phenomenon, especially if the cells are obtained from a fresh, naturally occurring tumour.

One of the major points to clarify at the outset, is that it can be misleading to seek to 'model' or simulate human metastatic spread in animal counterparts. Unless such models are first demonstrated by experiment and observation to be homologous with the subject of study, they usually reflect the bias of the observer, leading to circuitous investigation of one's own preconceptions. Animal experiments, therefore, need to be regarded as of interest in their own right; but factors found to be important in metastatic colony formation need to be validated separately in a human context.

A further important point is that it is advisable to confirm metastasis by histology. When there is heavy colonization of the lungs, it is possible to be reasonably certain that the large numbers of nodules are composed of tumour tissue, but it is essential to monitor all weak colonization and non-colonization results, histologically. Representative sections from the organs of such animals should always be examined, to verify that any nodules seen are indeed tumour deposits from the grafted cells and not pulmonary adenomas, foci of lymphoid infiltration, or inflammatory lesions. This is indispensable, because animals thought to have deposits in the lungs, liver, and spleen have sometimes been found, on microscopy, to have quite unrelated conditions, such as fibrous scars and focal granulomata due to *Yersinia* infection, sometimes associated with amyloidosis (see Price *et al.* 1982).

Lastly, as tumour cells preserved in liquid nitrogen retain their original metastatic capability indefinitely, it is possible to conduct reproducible experiments on banked pre-selected cells of known metastatic potential from naturally occurring tumours, or from clones of serially propagated lines.

The metastatic drive of tumour cells—cell biological aspects

When cells from freshly disaggregated spontaneous mammary tumours are inoculated into batches of syngeneic mice, it is found reproducibly that some tumours colonize the lungs of all inoculated animals heavily, whereas other tumours do so weakly, or not at all (Tarin and Price 1979). A few tumours are intermediate in their behaviour, but there is sufficient disparity between the two major types of behaviour to warrant separation of primary mammary tumours in these donor animals, into two major groups: those with high colonization potential (HCP) and those with low colonization potential (LCP). Spontaneous metastasis from undisturbed mammary tumours occurs in about 30 per cent of tumour bearers in the strain of mouse (C_3H/Avy) used for these studies (Price *et al.* 1982).

Only neoplastic cells have these colonizing properties, as demonstrated by the observation that even rapidly proliferating mammary epithelial cells, from glands of pregnant or lactating animals, could not do so (Price *et al.* 1982). From this it can be inferred that the ability to colonize distant sites, after blood-borne dissemination, is a property possessed only by neoplastic cells, but not all tumour cells have this property. In short, neoplasia is a necessary precondition, but not by itself sufficient to confer the metastatic phenotype.

In 1978, Fidler published an account of his important work with Kripke, demonstrating that individual cells within a tumour are heterogeneous for their capability to form blood-borne metastatic deposits (Fidler 1978; Fidler and Kripke 1977). They showed that clones of B16 melanoma tumour cells, grown from single cells, differed substantially from one another and from the parental population in their metastatic capability and advanced the notion, heretical for the time, that neoplasms are composed of heterogeneous cell populations. Their work was subsequently amply corroborated by others working with serially propagated cell lines (Chambers *et al.* 1981; Poste *et al.* 1982b) of various types, and with freshly disaggregated spontaneous neoplasms (Price *et al.* 1984). The corollary of confirming that tumours and their constituent cells are heterogeneous with regard to metastatic capabilities, is that metastasis is initiated by driving forces within some of the tumour cells and is not *primarily* the consequence of some failure in the host organism.

Further work by Poste and colleagues (1981, 1982a) with the B16 melanoma has indicated that the metastatic capabilities of individual clones within a tumour not only differ from one another, but can change with time, if circumstances are appropriate. Thus, it was found that isolation and separate culture of clones derived from a single tumour led to greater instability in their behaviour and other characteristics, such as drug sensitivities, over time, so that some became more metastatic and others less so. Pooling of clones resulted in stabilization of the behaviour of the group population. Similar observations have been recorded by Hill *et al.* (1984) and by Neri and Nicolson (1981) for different cell lines. Also, Price *et al.* (1984) found that when spontaneous pulmonary metastases were transplanted back into the mammary fat pads of fresh recipients, the constituent cells were nearly always tumourigenic (95 per cent), but not necessarily able to recapitulate the metastatic process (35 per cent). This suggests that the progeny of cells that have already shown their fitness for the metastatic process, do not necessarily all inherit or retain this capability, although repeated selection of metastases and reinoculation of their cells (Fidler 1973a) can eventually lead to the development of cell lines that have high metastatic potency. As with the evolution of multicellular organisms, therefore, it appears to be necessary to exert a selection pressure to stabilize new properties. The significance of the observations of Hill *et al.* (1984) and of Price *et al.* (1984) is that metastasis is not necessarily the endpoint in the line of tumour 'progression' and generation of heterogeneity. In effect, therefore, the clone can be 'progressing' away from metastatic behaviour as well as towards it, over the course of time.

Confirmation that metastatic behaviour of tumour cells is initiated and sustained by intrinsic properties of the tumour cells concerned, led to an avalanche of work, comparing metastatic cells with non-metastatic counterparts. In this field the best studies compared metastatic and non-metastatic variant cell lines derived from a common origin, but the quest for a universal property or biochemical marker, which would invariably distinguish cells with metastatic capability in all tumours, and thus target research towards underlying causal mechanisms, has so far been in vain. However, several cellular properties are associated strongly with metastatic behaviour and it is useful to review some of these briefly.

Clonogenicity

Metastasis can be regarded, at least in part, as a highly selective form of clonogenicity (see Section 9.1). Once disseminating cells have arrested in the target organ, they require the proliferative potential to establish a new colony and grow into a secondary tumour. There is also experimental evidence that individual metastases of transplantable mouse tumour lines (Poste *et al.* 1982a; Talmadge *et al.* 1982) can be clonal in origin, i.e. derived from single cells, or oligoclonal (Poste *et al.* 1982b). Clonogenicity and stem-cell content of a tumour cell population capable of metastasis are therefore pertinent intrinsic properties to study in attempts to identify important elements of the metastatic process. Direct examination of the clonogenicity of cells from undisturbed mammary neoplasms (Price 1986) showed that colony-forming efficiency in agar varied between individual primary mammary tumours and correlated well with experimental metastatic potential, supporting the view that the stem-cell content of primary tumours is one of the important determinants of metastatic capability. However, there was no direct relationship between colony-forming efficiency *in vitro* and *spontaneous* metastatic behaviour. Thus, while clonogenicity is an essential element in forming distant tumour colonies, it is only one of the properties required for tumour cells to successfully complete the multiple rate-limiting steps of the metastatic process (for further discussion see Price 1986; Price *et al.* 1986).

Cell-surface properties

Many studies have been conducted on the cell membranes of metastatic cells and there have been several reports that the surface glycoprotein composition of metastatic variants derived from cultured lines differs significantly from their non- or weakly metastatic counterparts (reviewed by Nicolson 1982; 1988). Metastases in different organs have also been reported to have different surface glycoprotein compositions (Chan *et al.* 1985). However, other investigations (e.g. Sargent *et al.* 1987) have not found any consistent differences in membrane glycoprotein composition between cells from naturally occurring tumours that could heavily colonize the lungs and cells from ones that could not. Even among reports of differences in cell-surface composition between metastatic and non-metastatic subtypes of defined cell lines, there is no concensus regarding the size or chemical composition of the molecules involved and many of the dissimilarities observed could be coincidental to differences in metastatic capability. Such discrepancies can only be resolved by experiment, but very few studies have involved direct modification of the glycosylation patterns of surface molecules to investigate whether they are causally involved in success or failure of the metastatic process. The most cogent evidence that the surface glycoprotein composition of tumour cells may affect their metastatic capability has been provided by the work of Irimura *et al.* (1981), Kerbel *et al.* (1983), Larizza and Schirrmacher (1984), Olsson and Forschhammer (1984), and Humphries *et al.* (1986). All these groups observed alterations in capability to make metastatic tumour colonies in distant organs following procedures that concomitantly altered surface glycoprotein composition.

Irimura *et al.* (1981) used tunicamycin, an antibiotic that blocks glycosylation of proteins and lipids, and Humphries *et al.* (1986) used swainsonine, which also affects glycosylation but at a different stage. Olsson and Forschhammer (1984) used 5-azacytidine, which alters DNA methylation and hence gene expression, and showed the appearance of a novel cell-surface protein; whereas Kerbel *et al.* (1983) obtained cells with altered metastatic capability by use of *in vitro* selection for resistance to lectin toxicity. Larizza and Schirrmacher (1984) fused non-metastatic lymphoma cells with macrophages and the hybrids were metastatic and expressed macrophage surface markers. However, the issue remains that none of these experimental procedures can be confidently assumed to have specific effects on the metastatic process *solely* via effects on the surface glycoprotein composition. Further, recent experiments (Sargent *et al.* 1987) involving the treatment of tumour cells with a variety of agents (tunicamycin, swainsonine, trypsin, neuraminidase, or succinylated lectins) known to cause specific disturbances in the composition and glycosylation of tumour cell membranes did not cause any significant change in the lung colonization performance of cells from murine mammary tumours. These results indicated that either these cells are extremely robust and reconstitute their surfaces rapidly, or that the surface glycoprotein components deranged by these treatments are not decisively involved in metastatic colonization and growth. However, as the cell surface is the interface between the environment and the metastasizing cell, and is thus the organelle by which it receives information about its surroundings, it is hard to imagine that it does not have an important role in the metastatic process.

Recently, an endogenous lectin has been isolated from the surfaces of highly metastatic variants of the B16 melanoma, and other rodent and human tumours. It is a fucose-binding protein and causes marked cellular aggregation when the cells are placed in serum-containing media (Meromsky *et al.* 1986; Raz *et al.* 1986). The lectin is not present in sufficient quantity on non-metastatic cells to have the same effect. Earlier it had been noted by Fidler (1973b) that intravenous inoculation of aggregated or clumped suspensions of B16 melanoma cells caused much more pulmonary colonization than inoculation of similar suspensions which were monodispersed. Hence, this work suggests that expression or up-regulation of this endogenous lectin in the tumour cell membrane could contribute to the cell acquiring enhanced metastatic capability. The gene for this cell surface component has recently been cloned and this could provide a probe to test whether there is increased expression of the gene in other types of metastatic cells.

Collagenase secretion

Collagen fibres and other proteins form the scaffolding of the connective tissue, which supports the epithelial and vascular elements of organs with complex histology. Invading primary and metastatic tumour cells readily demolish these structural elements as they cross and colonize new territory. Many different types of collagen are now recognized, but collagen type I is the main structural protein in most tissues and exists in the form of cross-striated fibres with a periodicity of 64 nanometres (see Section 1.4). Under normal conditions of body pH and temperature, collagens are only cleaved by a single enzyme family, the collagenases. These enzymes are metalloproteases, needing calcium ions in order to function, and show strong substrate specificity for individual types of collagen. As one might expect, many invasive and metastatic tumours in humans and animals produce elevated amounts of these proteases. However, although we found a very strong statistical correlation ($P < 0.001$) between lung colonization capability and metalloprotease activity against type I collagen (collagenase type I), in a group of *murine* mammary tumours, the concordance was not complete for every tumour studied. Also, we did not find any direct relationship between invasive and metastatic behaviour and collagenase I activity in a series of *human* breast tumours (Ogilvie *et al.* 1985). Breast carcinomas exhibited a wide quantitative spectrum of collagenase secretion, showing no correlation with histological type but, strangely, fibroadenomas, which are non-invasive 'benign' proliferations of mammary lobular connective tissue (Chapter 22), had uniformly high levels of enzyme output. The interim data, from clinical follow-up studies on patients with invasive and metastatic breast cancer in this study, show no detectable correlation between enzyme output by the sample of tumour obtained at mastectomy and subsequent local recurrence or metastasis.

Such studies are fraught with technical difficulties, including sampling complications caused by zonal and temporal variations within the tumours. Absence of an obvious correlation between clinical observations and laboratory data, therefore, does not exclude a role for the enzyme in invasion and metastasis. The findings merely indicate that measurements of activity of this enzyme, on tumours at the time of resection, are not a useful indicator of the prognosis of individual patients.

On the other hand, studies on the Lucke renal adenocarcinoma of the Leopard frog provided intriguing new data supporting a causal involvement of collagenase in metastasis (McKinnell and Tarin 1984). The frog is a poikilothermic vertebrate whose internal body temperature closely follows that of the environment, and Lucke and Schlumberger (1949) observed that tumour-bearing frogs living in a warm (28 °C) environment have a much higher incidence of metastasis (>75 per cent) than those in cold (4 °C) conditions (<6 per cent). This means that one can use alternation in the ambient temperature at which the cells or animals are maintained as a technique to search for cellular properties that correlate exclusively with, and may be important in, metastatic behaviour. For example, it was found that explants of Lucke tumours cultured at 28 °C

(Ogilvie *et al.* 1984) had high levels of secretion of collagenase type I. This activity was found to be reproducibly and specifically associated with metastasis-permissive conditions because, when the ambient temperature was switched backwards and forwards between permissive and inhibitory values, the output of collagenase into the surrounding medium rose and fell accordingly. In contrast, normal frog renal tissue had low levels of output of this enzyme, unaffected by temperature.

Liotta *et al.* (1979) described increased release, by metastatic tumour cell lines, of a protease that specifically digests collagen type IV, one of the main structural components of basement membranes. Such membranes play an important part in maintaining histological organization, by providing suitable substrata for epithelia or by separating different tissue domains. They also invest blood vessels and nerves. Metastasizing cells have to breach many such membranes to migrate from their original location (see Figs 9.15 and 9.16), transit vessel walls, and grow elsewhere. Hence, ability to degrade basement membranes may be a rate-limiting requirement for the metastatic process, but the amount of collagen I that is seen to be destroyed by advancing tumour cells in histological sections (Fig. 9.16) is orders of magnitude greater and, perhaps correspondingly more important, biologically. Even with collagenase IV, the correspondence with invasive and metastatic capability is not absolute, probably because control of synthesis of the enzyme fluctuates in a disorderly manner in tumour cells.

Other biochemical properties and metastatic capability

Thrombogenic and thrombolytic activity of metastatic cells Despite considerable research, the question of whether interactions between metastasizing tumour cells and the blood coagulation and fibronolytic systems affect secondary tumour formation, remains controversial. Some argue that metastatic variants of tumour cells are more prone to cause activation of the coagulation cascade than non-metastatic ones, whereas others contend that cells with greater fibrinolytic activity are more metastatic (see also Chew *et al.* 1976; Donatti and Poggi 1980; and Gaspar 1982 for reviews). Those subscribing to the former view suggest that induction of platelet aggregation and thrombosis by tumour cells is conducive to their arrest in small capillaries, and hence to metastasis. Conversely, those contending that metastasis correlates with increased fibrinolysis and output of plasminogen activator suggest that such properties would aid tumour cells to remain free of enmeshment in fibrin thrombi or to extricate themselves from such entanglement and burrow through the wall of the vessel. The evidence therefore is contradictory but the findings are not necessarily mutually exclusive, because it is possible that inappropriate release of both thrombogenic factors and fibrinolytic enzymes could occur simultaneously, as a result of discoordinated gene activity in tumour cells. Attempts to examine experimentally whether coagulation-related processes are causally involved in metastasis have included the use of drugs (such as aspirin and heparin) known to interfere with the coagulation cascade. The results have proved difficult to interpret because of the problems of attributing any effect on metastasis solely to the action of the drug on the coagulability of the blood.

Cytoskeletal elements of metastatic cells Sporadic studies on other properties of tumour cells which might be implicated in metastasis, such as intermediate filaments, microtubules, prostacyclin/prostaglandin production, and tumour cell motility factor have been performed on too few cell types or by only single laboratories. This makes it difficult to judge the general applicability of the findings. However, the results on the cytoskeleton are of potential importance and will be reviewed briefly. Hart *et al.* (1980) observed that treatment of B16 melanoma cells with cytochalasin B and colchicine, which disrupt or disperse microfilaments and microtubules respectively, caused reduction in their capability to colonize the lungs after i.v. injection. Concomitant studies with labelled cells showed that treatment reduced the numbers retained in the lungs and their adhesion to each other. A further study (Ben Ze'ev and Raz 1985) involving cyclohexamide treatment of B16 cells showed that, when the dosage was sufficient to disorganize cytoplasmic intermediate filaments, the numbers of pulmonary metastases were reduced. Similarly, treatment of B16 melanoma cells with local anaesthetics resulted in reduction in the number of stainable actin microfilaments in the cytoplasm and in fewer pulmonary colonies after i.v. inoculation (Nicolson *et al.* 1986). Isotopic labelling studies showed that fewer cells were retained in the lungs of these animals 1 h after inoculation, and the corresponding increase in numbers trafficking through to recirculate to other organs was associated with some increase in extrapulmonary metastases. Other data pertinent to this suggestion (McKinnell *et al.* 1984) were derived from studies on frog renal adenocarcinoma cells (see above). At metastasis-permissive temperatures, the Lucke carcinoma cells had a complex microtubular system, whereas in cells kept at low temperatures microtubular assembly was inhibited. Although tubulin could be seen dispersed throughout the cytoplasm, there was no residual microtubular array. In contrast, the cytoplasmic microtubule complex remained intact in chilled normal kidney cells.

Genetic basis of the intrinsic metastatic drive

Since the 1890s it has been recognized that the genes regulating cellular and supracellular hereditary characteristics reside within the cell nucleus, and that all normal somatic cells within the body contain an equal complement of genetic material. Modern research has substantiated that cellular phenotype is the result of the prevailing pattern of gene expression. From the information provided earlier in this section, on the sequential and complex nature of the metastatic process, it follows that manifestation of metastatic behaviour depends upon coordinate, or at least concomitant, expression of genes regulating several different aspects of cell behaviour, for example motility (invasiveness), protease secretion, insinuation into vessels, diapodesis out of vessels, mobilization of appropriate metabolic functions to survive in a foreign organ/environment, and induction of local tissue to make a fibrovascular framework. It also seems, from information given earlier in this section about the instability of the metastatic phenotype, that co-ordinate expression of these properties may be transient. From a global or detached vantage point, individual cellular characteristics of metastasis-competent cells may therefore represent mere epiphenomena, resulting from more profound disturbances in *control* of cellular activities, which would be better understood by examination at a genetic level. (For clarification one may cite Smither's (1962) analogy that a lifetime's study of the workings of the individual parts of the internal combustion engine would not enable one to understand the causes of a traffic jam, because the disorder lies in organization and control of vehicles by humans, although it may have been precipitated by failure of a mechanical component.) The experimental information presented in the following sections suggests that the above analysis is correct and this approach, therefore, forms the framework for our current thinking and research on the nature of metastatic behaviour.

Gene modulation can affect metastatic behaviour

The exposure of dividing cells to the pyrimidine analogue 5-azacytidine (5-aza-C), results in its incorporation in newly synthesized DNA in random substitution for normal cytidine residues; as 5-aza-C cannot be methylated, the treatment results in depression of general levels of DNA methylation. In such cells, genes that were inactive have been observed to become expressed and this led to the realization that methylation is one means of controlling gene expression. Such alterations of expression have been found to be stable and sustained over several cell generations, as a consequence of methylation patterns being carefully copied by maintenance methylases during mitosis. Exposure of weakly metastatic cells to 5-aza-C in some experiments (Trainer *et al.* 1985) increases their capability to colonize the lungs after intravenous inoculation; other work indicates that spontaneous metastatic capability can also be increased by this treatment (Olsson and Forschammer 1984; Kerbel *et al.* 1984; Tarin 1988). In the latter, 5-aza-C-treated cells were injected subcutaneously and must have undergone several divisions to make a local tumour before metastasis occurred, indicating that the change of behaviour was heritable and probably caused by alterations in gene expression. This stable alteration of phenotype by an external agent, without alteration of the genetic code, offers powerful opportunities for further investigation of the genetic basis of metastasis.

Cell fusion between appropriate partners can activate metastatic behaviour

Recent studies have provided strong evidence that fusion between non-metastatic tumour cells and non-neoplastic cells of the host *in vivo* can result in metastatic behaviour by the hybrid (Kerbel *et al.* 1983; Larizza and Schissmacher 1984; Hart 1984; de Baetselier *et al.* 1984), although contrary observations (Sidebottom and Clarke 1983) of inhibition of metastatic capability after fusion with normal cells, counsels some caution in interpretation. Further investigations involving fusion of tumour cells *in vitro* with various types of cells, followed by inoculation of the hybrids, confirmed that fusion with appropriate partners can activate metastasis, and indicated that the host cells involved in conferring metastatic properties after fusion *in vivo* are probably macrophages, lymphocytes, or others derived from the bone marrow.

The cells used in these experiments had drug-resistance markers so that it was possible to eliminate all unfused cells by exposure to appropriate drugs. This work suggested that the genes that are active in migratory haematological cells may, when transferred into tumour cells, enable them to metastasize. However, this need not be the only mechanism by which metastatic cells naturally acquire their migratory capability, and this leads to the following, even more important, concept: all the somatic cells of an organism contain a virtually identical set of genes. Also, all properties manifested by all types of tumour cells have counterparts in normal cells somewhere in the body; consider, for example, ectopic production of the pituitary hormone ACTH by lung tumours (Section 9.8). It could hence be argued that activation of *intrinsic* migratory genes within a tumour cell, and subsequent metastatic behaviour, could occur *without* fusion, the latter being merely a way of introducing a gene which is already derepressed. Cell fusion studies have therefore added impetus to the conception that further investigation of the genetic constitution of the metastatic tumour cells could be illuminating.

Gene transfection from appropriate donors can confer metastatic tendencies

We recently found that transfer of high molecular weight DNA, from highly metastatic cells, into non-metastatic tumour cells by transfection, resulted in the recipients becoming able to colonize many organs (McMenamin *et al.* 1988; Tarin 1988). This approach may allow easier isolation and identification of genes involved in metastasis because, in contrast to methods such as cell fusion and chromosome transfer, each transfected cell takes up only a limited portion of the genome and selection of resulting metastatic clones can be exercised by inoculation into mice. Thus the search can be narrowed to just the incorporated sequences in cells proven to be metastatic.

In one of our experiments, total genomic DNA from a highly metastatic human melanoma cell line (A375M) was co-transfected, with the bacterial gene for neomycin resistance, into non-metastatic mouse fibrosarcoma cells (TR4 Nu). The antibiotic neomycin is severely toxic to most eukaryotic cells, including the cell line we used. Co-transfection with the neomycin-resistance gene, a dominant selectable marker, is therefore a useful procedure for identification of cells that are recpients of successful DNA transfer. After selection in neomycin, which eliminates cells that have not taken up the exogenous DNA, the remaining clones were pooled and injected into nude mice to assay for metastasis. These animals are immunologically incompetent and would be unable to reject transfected cells which conceivably could be expressing human surface antigens.

The results shown in Table 9.7 demonstrated that the transfected cells (designated the AH8 cell line) had acquired

Table 9.7 Total genomic transfer

DNA donor	DNA recipient	Inoculation route	Survival time	Incidence of metastasis*	Distribution of metastases
A375M	TR4 Nu	i.v.	6–8 weeks	18/21 (6/18 extrapulmonary)	Lungs, diaphragm, liver, muscles, skin
—	TR4 Nu	i.v.	8 weeks	6/59	Lungs only (single)
TR4	TR4 Nu	i.v.	8 weeks	26/112	Lungs only (single)
M5076	P574	s.c.	26 weeks	29/63 (46%)	Lungs only (multiple: 5+)
—	P574	s.c.	26 weeks	6/39 (15%)	Lungs only (single)
P574	P574	s.c.	26 weeks	0/32	—

$$* \text{ Incidence} = \frac{\text{Number of mice with lesion}}{\text{Number of mice injected}}.$$

Origin of cell lines: A375M, human malignant melanoma metastatic in the patient and in nude mice; M5076, mouse sarcoma, probably of macrophage origin, heavily metastatic to liver from subcutaneous site; TR4Nu, mouse fibrosarcoma non-metastatic from subcutaneous site (derived from 3T3 fibroblasts); P574, mouse mammary carcinoma, weakly metastatic from mammary fat pad.

overwhelming metastatic capability, compared to control, untransfected TR4 Nu cells or to TR4 Nu cells transfected with their own DNA. Figs 9.34–9.38 show unequivocal pathological evidence of widespread metastasis in the animals inoculated with AH8 cells i.v., and Fig. 9.39 shows an autoradiograph of a Southern blot, demonstrating the presence of human DNA in the transfected cell line, absent in the untransfected control. Further analysis, using specific probes for repetitive sequences (Alu and Kpn) characteristic of human DNA, showed discrete bands confirming uptake and incorporation of human sequences.

This particular transfected cell line (AH8) only showed augmented *experimental* metastatic ability (i.e. ability to colonize the lungs after intravenous inoculation), and subcutaneous inoculations resulted only in localized tumours with no metastases. Interestingly, the melanoma cell line (A375M), which was the donor of the DNA used in the first experiment, was itself only capable of experimental metastasis, whereas the donor in the next experiments to be discussed was spontaneously metastatic.

In the following transfection experiments we produced lines showing a marked increase in *spontaneous* metastasis from a subcutaneous site (see Table 9.7) and analysis of these results is

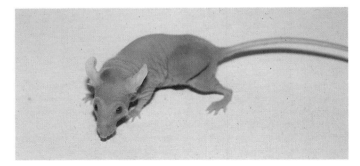

Fig. 9.34 A mouse with subcutaneous tumour deposits on its flank and its head. It had been injected i.v. some weeks before with tumour cells transfected with DNA from metastatic cells.

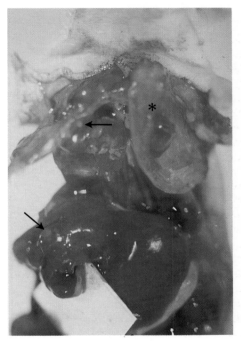

Fig. 9.35 Survey view of the autopsy of the mouse shown in Fig. 9.34. Metastatic tumour deposits are visible in the liver (large arrow), thoracic cage (asterisk), and lungs (small arrow).

still in progress. The DNA transfected was obtained from the highly metastatic M5076 *mouse* histiocytic sarcoma cell line and was cloned into a cosmid library before being introduced into *mouse* cells by transfection. In cell line AH8, the DNA transferred into mouse cells was of *human* origin and therefore could be distinguished from the background mouse DNA because of its highly characteristic repetitive sequences. For transfection experiments involving transfer of DNA between cells of the same species, other techniques are required for identification of incorporated sequences, and this was the reason for creating the cosmid library of M5076 DNA. The cosmid vector used also

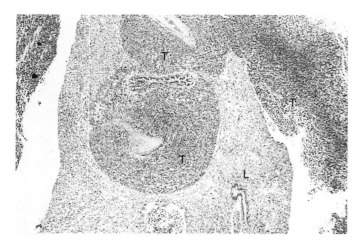

Fig. 9.36 Histological section of the lungs of the mouse in Fig. 9.34 confirming extensive colonization of the lungs (L) and mediastinum by metastatic tumour (fibrosarcoma) cells (T).

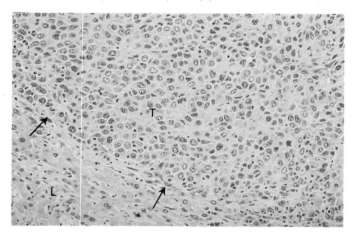

Fig. 9.37 Histological section of the liver of the mouse shown in Fig. 9.34, confirming the presence of metastatic tumour. The picture shows the boundary (arrows) between the tumour deposit (T) and liver tissue (L).

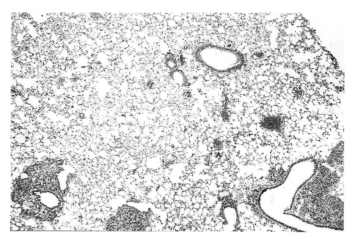

Fig. 9.38 Histological section of the lungs of a mouse inoculated with control (untransfected cells). This field shows, at the same magnification as Fig. 9.36, the heaviest area of colonization in the animal with the most (i.e. two) macroscopically visible deposits.

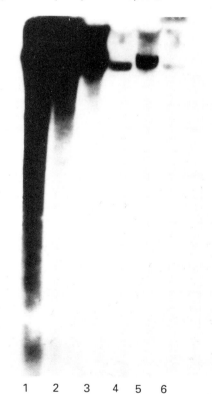

Fig. 9.39 Autoradiograph of a Southern blot of DNAs from various sources probed with ^{32}P-labelled human total genomic DNA. Tracks were loaded with equal quantities of DNA as follows: 1, human total genomic DNA (positive control); 2, total genomic DNA from metastatic donor cell line (A375M); 3, a human–mouse hybrid cell line containing four human chromosomes; 4, a mouse cell line (TR4 Nu) transfected with normal human DNA; 5, AH8 cells, a mouse cell line (TR4 Nu) transfected with total genomic DNA from the human metastatic cell line A375M; 6, the untransfected recipient mouse cell line (TR4 Nu). Note the strong signal showing the presence of human DNA in AH8 cells, absent in untransfected TR4 Nu cells.

contained the bacterial *neo* gene, as an integral part of the construct, to allow selection of transfected cells and to aid identification and recovery of the mouse genes, which have been transferred into the non-metastatic mouse tumour cells. Recent preliminary results confirmed the presence of cosmid DNA in the recipients, demonstrating that some DNA from the donor metastatic cells had also been successfully transferred.

These findings suggest that components of the metastatic phenotype are heritable, highly conserved in evolution and can be conferred on previously non-metastatic tumour cells by transfer of genomic DNA. Interestingly, it would appear that whatever genetic activity is responsible for this new behaviour is not repressed (at least not immediately) by the homologous genes in the non-metastatic partner. The metastatic process is so complex, that, at this early stage, there is need for caution in the interpretation of these results. However, the results of all experiments discussed in this section have demonstrated that direct experimental analysis of the genetic disturbances in the metastatic phenotype is now feasible and a new era of active investigation of the problem has opened.

Host factors affecting survival of metastatic cells and the distribution of deposits

Information from vascular dissemination of labelled tumour cells

From the early studies of Fidler (1970) using isotope-labelled B16 melanoma cells, we know that many of the cells entering the circulation from tumours die within 24 h and that there is a massive redundancy, or inefficiency, in the process of dissemination. Fidler estimated that only about 1 per cent of the tumour cell population remained alive 24 h after i.v. inoculation. His data also indicated that numerous cells arrived in all organs sampled, soon after injection. Although the lungs, being the site of the first capillary bed encountered after injection of tumour cells into the tail vein, naturally exercised a significant sieving effect on cells in the circulation, enough cells reached other organs to represent adequate seeding. For example, two weeks after i.v. inoculation of 200 000 tumour cells, approximately 400 survived in the lungs and eventually formed about 80 deposits. Other organs had received several thousand cells a few hours after inoculation, but they had either not been retained or had not survived, and no extrapulmonary deposits were formed.

These findings with radioactive cells have been confirmed and extended. For example, we (Potter *et al.* 1983) observed substantial numbers of whole living cells labelled with fluorescein isothiocyanate in all organs examined within 15 min of intravenous inoculation of murine mammary tumour cells (Fig. 9.40). The viability of cells labelled in this way was confirmed by their ability to form metastatic deposits in the usual sites in simultaneously injected animals of the same batch.

Thus, direct visual observation and indirect, but quantitative, radioactive measurement mutually confirmed that numerous living tumour cells, not just disembodied isotope or cell fragments, speedily arrived in all organs of animals injected intravascularly. Hence, the number of living cells distributed to each organ is not the only, nor the most decisive, factor affecting sites of secondary tumour formation. Even when larger numbers of viable tumourigenic cells are delivered directly to certain organs by arterial inoculation, growth is still not guaranteed (see Tarin and Price 1981).

Organ-specific patterns of metastasis

The B16 melanoma and the naturally occurring murine mammary tumours used in the above experiments, both have specific, non-random patterns of organ colonization after intravenous inoculation. The B16 melanoma preferentially colonizes the lungs and ovaries and does not colonize the brain, even when cells are inoculated directly into the carotid artery, although in such circumstances it will colonize the meninges (Schackert and Fidler 1988). Spontaneous metastasis from B16 tumours in the footpad or the subcutaneous tissue are seen mainly in regional lymph nodes and in the lungs. The naturally occurring mouse mammary carcinomas spontaneously metastasize exclusively to the lungs and favour this organ for growth, if inoculated intravenously. If inoculated intra-arterially, cells from some mammary tumours will colonize the lungs, kidneys, and ovaries, but not other organs, especially not the brain, even after intra-carotid injections (Price *et al.* 1984; Juaçaba *et al.* 1983), nor the marrow or bone of the femur after injection into the lower abdominal aorta. The conclusion that organ-specific effects influence tumour colony formation seems inescapable.

It has been reported (Nicolson 1988) that sublines with organ-specific patterns of colonization have been isolated from mixed, unselected 'parent' stocks of commonly used cell lines which are known to be metastatic. These sublines were derived from repeated cycles of intravenous or arterial inoculation of tumour cells obtained from experimental metastases in the appropriate organ and harvesting of subsequent metastases to grow more cells for re-inoculation. After 10–15 cycles the cell lines obtained had increased potential for colonizing the appropriate organ. These observations suggest the pre-existence within the original tumour of subpopulations with the corresponding organ affinities and that these are selectively enriched by the protocol. The alternative possibility, that the cell line gradually adapted to growth in the chosen organ, has been rendered unlikely by Nicolson and Custead's (1982) attractive experiment of binding the cells to Biobeads before inoculation. After several cycles of recovering and re-inoculating the beads, the attached cells were found to have no more capability for colonizing the organ than the original populations. These observations, by definition, support the interpretation that tumours have organ-specific patterns of metastasis.

Even more powerful evidence of organ selectivity in metastasis of animal tumour cell lines is the remarkably consistent and characteristic propensity of the M5076 murine cell line to form many hepatic metastases spontaneously after subcutaneous tumour growth. Deposits are rarely seen in the lungs,

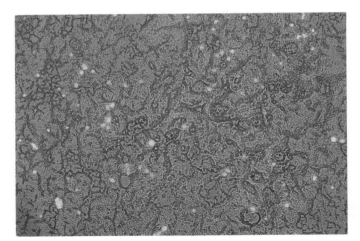

Fig. 9.40 Murine mammary carcinoma cells, labelled with fluorescein isothiocyanate fluorescing in a frozen section of liver viewed in a UV microscope.

although on histological sections we have found that the pulmonary capillaries are invariably congested with tumour cells.

Thus, the results of experiments on *animals* are in accordance with Paget's 'seed and soil' hypothesis based on analysis of *human* autopsy records. Restated in modern terms, the hypothesis proposes that environmental conditions in certain organs might favour or permit the growth of particular types of tumour cells, and that this is the primary selective pressure which determines the differential pattern of organ colonization. The data, incidentally, also confirm that mechanical sieving effects can influence patterns of vascular dissemination of tumour cells and therefore have some influence on the distribution of metastasis.

Patients with circulating tumour cells

Although animal experiments were informative, there was no way to judge, until recently, whether they were significant for understanding mechanisms of metastasis in man. However, owing to a remarkable set of circumstances, arising from introduction of a new form of therapy for intractable ascites in patients with inoperable abdominal cancer, direct evidence became available that the fundamental principles of cancer metastasis in humans are broadly the same as those revealed by animal experiments. The mode of treatment which allowed these insights was peritoneo-venous shunting, a more satisfact-

ory method of removing the rapidly accumulating abdominal fluid, which otherwise causes pain and discomfort in patients with neoplastic ascites. The main advantage of this over previous methods is that it causes symptomatic relief, without causing metabolic imbalance due to loss of proteins, salts, and other essential substances. This was an effective palliative procedure for patients who were unresponsive to antineoplastic treatment and brought relief and improvement in quality of life to otherwise moribund people. It also, incidentally, provided a unique opportunity for observing the results of direct infusion of viable tumour cells into the circulation, and thus for studying some aspects of haematogenous metastasis in humans. Much to everyone's surprise, the patients were not speedily overcome by indiscriminate synchronous growth of diffuse metastases. In fact, it was found that in half the patients (see Table 9.8) there was no evidence of any extra-abdominal metastatic tumours whatsoever, even in those who survived as long as 27 months after insertion of the shunt (Tarin *et al.* 1984,b,c). In some of these patients inert tumour cells identifiable by natural biological markers (Figs. 9.41 and 9.42), were recognized in the tissues, although growing metastases were absent, confirming that effective dissemination and sequestration of cells in distant organs does not necessarily result in metastasis. In the group of patients in whom extra-abdominal metastases were found

Table 9.8 Summary of clinical and pathological findings

Patient		Sex	Age	Site of primary tumour	Survival time after shunting (months)	Distribution of haematogenous metastases
Group 1: No haematogenous metastases						
1	DG	F	53	Ovary	27*	None
2	EH	F	66	Ovary	2	None
3	RH	F	68	Stomach	1	None
4	DJ	M	60	Unknown	2.5	None
5	AR	F	57	Ovary and breast	7	None
6	HM	F	48	Ovary	2	None
7	JB	F	76	Ovary	4	None
8	BB	F	46	Ovary	1	None
9	GP(1)	F	73	Ovary	2	None
10	GP(2)	F	72	Ovary	7	None
11	FC	F	62	Ovary	3	None
Group 2: Haematogenous metastases present						
12	MM	F	49	Vagina	2.5	Lungs, liver
13	WA	F	82	Ovary	4	Several organs†
14	ER	F	55	Ovary	3.5	Lungs
15	FG	M	67	Pancreas	9	Lungs, liver
16	DJ	F	59	Unknown	5	Liver, vertebrae‡
17	WH	M	51	Bronchus§	1	Other lung
18	EJS	F	61	Colon	4	Lungs
19	EES	F	76	Ovary	5	Several organs‖
20	FM	F	79	Colon	10	Liver, ovary¶
21	LD	F	63	Ovary	8	Lungs, liver, spleen
22	BR	F	41	Ovary	2	Myocardium pericardium
23	ES	F	76	Ovary	5	Liver, adrenals

* First shunt functioned freely for 5 months and second for 6 months, with an interim period of 16 months with intermittently functioning shunt.

† Lungs, liver, spleen, brain, chroid, plexus, intestinal wall, adrenals; all tiny deposits.

‡ Large hepatic and vertebral deposits before shunt inserted. More deposits were present in these organs at autopsy, but the lungs and other organs were completely negative.

§ Pleurovenous shunt.

‖ Adrenals, lungs, and liver.

¶ No pulmonary metastases despite colonization of liver and ovary.

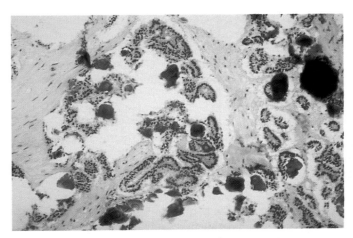

Fig. 9.41 Histological section of the primary papillary cystadenocarcinoma of the ovary in patient DG. Note the small, dark calcified psammoma bodies produced by this tumour.

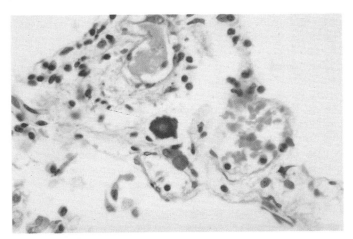

Fig. 9.42 Histological section of the lungs of patient DG who was treated with a peritoneo-venous shunt for malignant ascites and survived 27 months. The presence of psammoma bodies in the extravascular tissues confirms that tumour cells have not only disseminated but have also migrated through capillary walls.

(sometimes within as short a period as a month), the lesions were small and clinically asymptomatic.

This diversity of behaviour among tumours in different patients was not due to differences in treatment, because this palliative procedure was only undertaken as a terminal measure in patients in whom all other means of treatment had failed and had been discontinued. Also, failure to form detectable metastases was not solely a function of time, since their presence in some patients, who survived very short intervals, indicates that cells with the necessary potential can metastasize quickly. As entry of substantial numbers of viable cells into the circulation is guaranteed in all patients successfully treated with this technique, the findings indicate that the metastatic competence of these human tumours was determined by intrinsic properties of their constituent cells. These conclusions on human tumour behaviour, therefore, are extremely similar to

earlier ones based on studies on naturally occurring mammary tumours in mice (Tarin and Price 1979; Price *et al.* 1982, 1984), and imply that metastasis is not a random process, but is the reproducible outcome of systematic disturbances in control of cellular activities.

Among the patients in whom metastases were observed, the distribution of secondary deposits was sometimes unexpected, in that metastases did not necessarily form in the organ containing the first capillary bed encountered, although haematogenous metastases had formed in other organs. Thus, tumours could not colonize all sites to which substantial numbers of viable tumour cells were known to have been transported, and this experimentally confirms, in living human subjects. Paget's (1889) deductions based on autopsy data as well as validating the results from animal experiments involving i.v. inoculation of tumour cells. In this connection, the findings in two patients with colorectal cancer in this series treated with p-v shunts are of particular interest. Patient 1 (EJS) and patient 2 (FM) both had well-differentiated mucin-secreting adenocarcinomas of the colon. The former (EJS) had formed microscopic metastases in the interstitial tissues of the lungs (Fig. 9.43) within 2 months of shunt insertion. Although it cannot be categorically stated that these tiny secondary lesions resulted from the vascular infusion of tumour cells via the shunt, rather than by spontaneous haematogenous metastasis, their uniformly small size makes it as certain as anything can be in clinical medicine that this was the case. In this patient, the liver had no microscopic or macroscopic tumour deposits, but tumour growth was extensive in the abdominal lymph nodes and in the lymphatics permeating the diaphragm. In contrast, patient FM had obvious macroscopic haematogenous metastases in the liver (Figs 9.44 and 9.45), but the lungs and other organs were free of haematogenous metastases, even though she had survived 10 months with a functioning shunt and small clumps of mucin-secreting tumour cells could be identified in the pulmonary vessels (Fig. 9.46). In this patient, therefore, cells proven to be capable of forming haematogenous metastasis in the liver failed

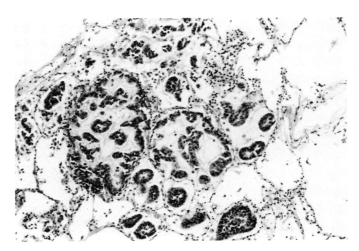

Fig. 9.43 Histological section of a metastatic deposit of mucin-secreting adenocarcinoma in the lung of patient EJS.

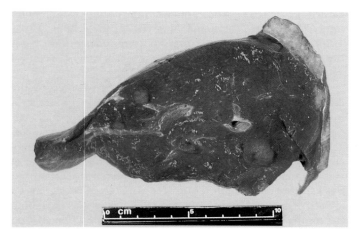

Fig. 9.44 A slice of the liver of patient (FM) showing liver metastases.

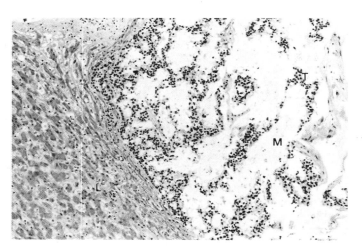

Fig. 9.45 Histological section of the liver of patient FM showing mucin-secreting colonic adenocarcinoma deposits. M, mucin; T, tumour cells; L, liver.

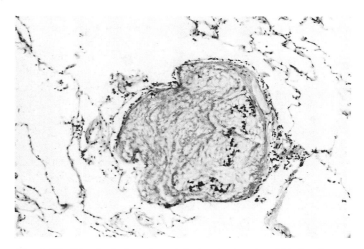

Fig. 9.46 Histological section of the lungs of patient FM showing an intravascular embolus of tumour cells and mucin but no parenchymal tumour growth.

to establish detectable metastases in the lungs, although large numbers of them were being infused directly into the capillaries of this organ, for several months. The cells being infused into the systemic veins in this patient were undeniably viable and tumourigenic, because small tumour deposits were observed in the track of the shunt (Fig. 9.47). These resulted from implantation of cells in this site by leakage of malignant ascites along the subcutaneous tunnel housing the shunt, owing to slackening of the purse-string suture around the tubing of the shunt where it emerged from the peritoneal cavity.

Again, therefore, the findings in humans are in close agreement with our results on naturally occurring murine mammary tumours (Tarin and Price 1981). Using homologous techniques of intravascular infusion of tumour cells, we had demonstrated that cells from animal tumours, known to be capable of forming metastases in the lungs, would not necessarily form haematogenous deposits in other organs, such as the liver, even if injected directly into the supplying vessels. Furthermore, mouse and rat tumour cell lines known to grow preferentially in the lungs and ovaries after vascular dissemination, still do so, even when the organs are transplanted to an anatomically unusual location *before* intravenous inoculation of the tumour cells.

The findings in all three species are therefore mutually complementary and reinforce the interpretation that microenvironmental influences in the sites where tumour cells lodge can modulate whether cells with proven metastatic capability can express this potential. It may, therefore, be safely concluded that tumour cells, even ones that are capable of high growth potential in some sites, are not invincible everywhere, and the clinical significance of this knowledge is that metastasis is not an inevitable consequence of tumour cell dissemination.

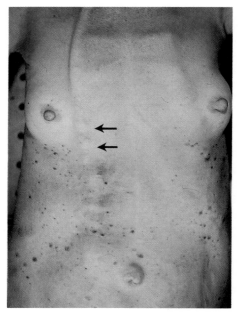

Fig. 9.47 The abdomen and chest of patient FM showing the subcutaneous path of the shunt, containing nodules (arrows) histologically confirmed as tumour.

Interactions affecting survival of disseminated cells

Such vindication of the 'seed and soil' hypothesis of Paget has implications both for clinical issues, like knowing where to look for residual systemic disease after therapy, and also for understanding mechanisms underlying metastatic spread. Once it is accepted that tumours are composed of heterogeneous populations of tumour cells (see above) with differing metastatic potentials, scattered in more or less representative proportions throughout the body after mixing in the vortex of the blood, and that they reproducibly grow in some sites and not others, it follows that individual organs permit, or inhibit, secondary tumour formation by metastasis-competent cells. Hence, cells of normal organs can, on occasion, suppress or at least fail to support malignant growth. Verification of this interpretation requires demonstration of the mechanisms of the microenvironmental effects, deduced to be operative *in vivo*. Recent work (Horak *et al.* 1986; Nicolson and Dulski 1986; Naito *et al.* 1987) suggests that these effects may be exerted, at least in part, by soluble factors released by the constituent cells of each organ. We found that co-culturing mouse mammary tumour cells, which normally only form pulmonary metastases, with fragments of liver or thyroid (Fig. 9.48) resulted in the death of tumour cells, whereas co-culture with pieces of lung resulted in increased survival and adherence of the tumour cells to the

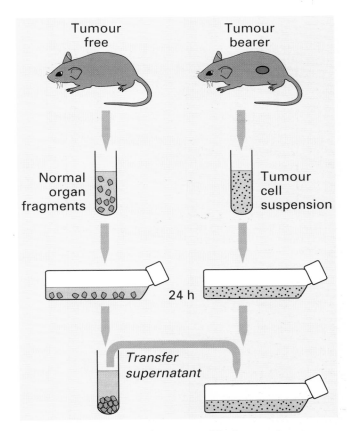

Fig. 9.49 Outline of organ-conditioning experiments.

substratum (Horak *et al.* 1986). These effects could be transferred from one culture to another, with cell-free media 'conditioned' by the organs (Figs. 9.49 and 9.50). The findings *in vitro* were thus in good agreement with *in vivo* observations on the common distribution patterns of deposits of this tumour.

Lactating mammary epithelial cells, the normal counterparts of the tumour cells, were profoundly inhibited by conditioned media from all organs tested (Fig. 9.51). Initially we thought that this was a non-specific effect of the conditioned media on tumour cells. Then we realized that normal cells accidentally or incidentally disseminated by the vascular system do not thrive in ectopic sites, e.g. bone marrow embolized into the lungs after road traffic accidents, and chorionic villi embolizing to the lungs in labour do not grow. Monodispersed lactating murine epithelial cells, likewise, do not grow and colonize other organs in syngeneic animals, even when inoculated intravenously (Price *et al.* 1982), although organ implants can sometimes grow in ectopic sites in appropriate circumstances. It can readily be appreciated that in higher multicellular organisms it is not advantageous to allow cells, shed accidentally, to survive and grow wherever they land. Our observations with normal cells therefore suggest the existence of a homeostatic mechanism that maintains territorial and functional integrity in the organs of higher vertebrates. The evidence further suggests that cells that successfully establish metastases in some organs have acquired or evolved the ability to survive the destructive effects

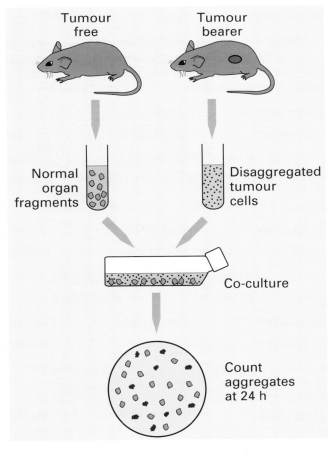

Fig. 9.48 Outline of co-culture experiments.

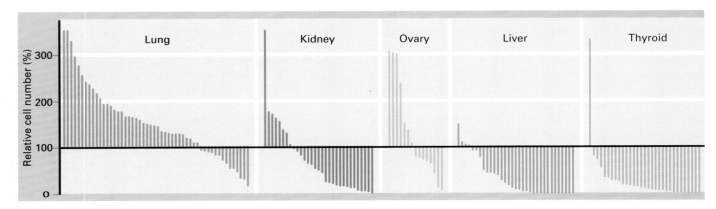

Fig. 9.50 Graphs showing relative increase or decrease of numbers of cells attached to the substratum at 24 h in monolayer cultures of several murine mammary tumours supplemented with conditioned medium from various organs. The baseline (100 per cent) is the number of cells in control cell cultures from the same tumours, not exposed to conditioned medium, and the height of each line expresses the percentage deviation from this value for each separate tumour.

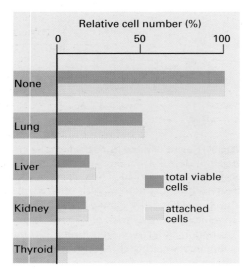

Fig. 9.51 Histogram showing the numbers of non-neoplastic mammary epithelial cells surviving at 24 h in cultures supplemented with organ-conditioned media as indicated. Control cultures (unsupplemented) were assigned a value of 100%.

of normal organs on accidentally displaced non-neoplastic adult somatic cells.

Host immune response and metastasis

From the earliest recognition of the involvement of the immune system in graft rejection, there has been a school of thought that considered that metastasis of malignant tumours might be controlled by immune surveillance, and that the process of metastasis only succeeded when immune defences were partially or completely abrogated. There is substantial evidence that the spontaneous and experimental metastasis of certain tumour cell lines is greatly augmented in animals immunosuppressed by depletion of T-lymphocytes or by bone-marrow ablation (Alexander 1976; Frost and Kerbel 1983; Schirr-

macher 1985). The intriguing findings of Wallich *et al.* (1985) that induction of major histocompatibility complex (MHC) antigen expression in previously metastasis-competent cells by transfection with the appropriate gene could abrogate metastatic properties, provides further evidence of immune regulation of the metastatic potential of cancer cells in some circumstances. Undoubtedly convincing as these studies are, it is also important to be aware that many spontaneous tumours in animals are non-immunogenic or only weakly immunogenic, and remain so if propagated in their original host strain.

Hewitt (1976) pointed out that much of the work demonstrating immunological reactivity to tumours had been done either on tumours of unknown genetic origin, or on tumours transplanted outside the inbred *substrain* of animals in which they arose, or on tumours induced by powerful carcinogenic chemicals. He contended that the forms of host resistance to tumours demonstrated by such experiments were attributable to laboratory artefacts, associated with the methods of tumour induction or conditions of transplantation and, therefore, were not representative of circumstances in hosts developing fresh spontaneous tumours. In support of these conclusions he reported that, after years of effort to detect tumour-specific antigens in 27 spontaneously arising murine tumours of various histogenetic types, his group could not find a single clear-cut case of an immune response excited by any one of the tumours examined. It is surprising to note that despite the compelling logical power of these arguments and the absence of convincing evidence refuting the observations cited, research on immunological aspects of metastasis and tumour biology continues, unabated, to use such unsuitable tumour types as models for the natural situation.

Host immunization to the tumour can sometimes actually enhance its metastatic capability (Fidler 1974; Fidler *et al.* 1979). Thus, the role of active specific immunity in relation to success or failure of metastasis is complex and, in the absence of any conspicuous success in experimental or clinical management of metastatic tumours *in general* by methods involving activation of specific immunity, the cautious reader must reserve judgement. In fact, as the tumour is so genetically similar to the host that it parasitizes, it is not surprising that many spontaneous neoplasms are invisible to the host's immune system. Only when the constituent cells display new antigens coded for by viruses or by genetic recombinations induced by other carcinogenic agents (e.g. chemicals) are they likely to be recognized as foreign by specialized immune cells. Even then, rapid evolution of phenotypic and antigenic diversity can lead to the development of a complex tumour ecosystem of different immunological subtypes, the metastatic behaviour of which could be unpredictably enhanced, or diminished, by the immunological status of the host (see above). Nevertheless, the concept of mobilizing the immune system to kill disseminated neoplastic cells remains very attractive and, because of its proven power in eradicating foreign organisms, is worthy of more exploration.

Because of these considerations, and the known marked heterogeneity amongst cells of a given tumour for practically all properties, including immunogenicity, Fidler and his colleagues have, in recent years, adopted the original and interesting approach of concentrating on large-scale mobilization of host defences which are *non-specific* in nature, such as macrophage tumouricidal activity, for eradication of metastatic tumour burden. Macrophages are capable of recognizing and killing tumour cells, without prior acquaintance with the tumour. Activation of the cytotoxic properties of macrophages by intravenous injection of liposomes containing immunomodulators (such as muramyl dipeptide) is remarkably effective in eradication of established pulmonary and lymph node metastases (Fidler *et al.* 1981; Fidler 1985). These observations prompt cautious enthusiasm about the possible deployment of such approaches for treatment of metastatic disease in humans. The results to date are therefore encouraging but suggest that this mode of therapy, like others, will need supplementation, because there was still significant tumour-related mortality (of the order of 40–50 per cent) when these agents were administered after the metastases were presumed to have formed. This is probably because recruitment of activated macrophages follows arithmetic kinetics, while the tumour cell proliferation is geometric and therefore outstrips the defence capabilities of the host. Therefore, even if immunotherapy of some sort is found to be effective against neoplasms in general, multiple-modality therapy will continue to be the most promising approach for management of established metastatic tumour burden (see Section 9.10).

9.5.4 Prospects for the treatment of metastatic neoplastic disease

Currently, the therapeutic management of cancer depends on surgical resection of the primary lesion wherever technically possible, combined with subsequent radiotherapy for control of loco-regional recurrence, if the neoplasm is known to be radio-sensitive and in an accessible site. In all health care systems efforts are being directed towards earlier detection of primary neoplasms, in the hope that a greater proportion can be detected and treated at an earlier stage, that is before there has been widespread dissemination. However, treatment of those in whom there is already evidence of disseminated cancer at the time of first presentation is difficult and depends largely on cytotoxic chemotherapy, supplementing the other modalities of therapy already mentioned, the idea being that disseminated seedlings can only be reached by agents carried to them in the blood. Such chemotherapeutic drugs are chosen on the basis that they interfere with metabolic pathways involved in cell division and, hence, are more toxic to actively dividing cell populations than to quiescent ones. The natural consequence of this is that, although the drugs are indeed more-or-less toxic to tumour cells, they are also toxic to rapidly dividing normal cell populations, needed for replenishment of cell loss due to natural wastage, such as in the intestinal epithelium, bone marrow, and hair follicles. In fact, normal high-turnover cell populations are often dividing faster than tumour populations, and there is real difficulty in delivering the therapeutic regimen because of the side-effects. There have been some remarkable successes in cancer chemotherapy, notably the virtual cure of choriocarcinoma, testicular cancer, and acute lymphoblastic leukaemia of childhood, but in many other neoplastic disorders the cytotoxic drugs and radiotherapy are poorly tolerated and create considerable morbidity for only a modest prolongation of survival (measured in months). This is particularly so for many common solid tumours, such as gastrointestinal cancer and cancer of the breast, when they have already disseminated. In a proportion of patients with breast cancer, further brief postponement may be gained by endocrine ablation or by administration of Tamoxifen, which competes for and blocks oestrogen receptors (and probably also acts by other pathways because it is also effective in a certain proportion of patients whose tumours have few such receptors).

So far the great hopes placed on raising intrinsic active *specific* immunity to the patient's own tumour and on destruction of tumour cells by administration of tumour-specific monoclonal antibodies, coupled with cytotoxic agents, have not been fulfilled in clinical practice, but the results of current trials involving stimulation of host T-cell activity with biological agents such as interleukin-2 (IL-2) (Rosenburg *et al.* 1985) and by co-injection of BCG with lethally irradiated *live* autochthonous tumour cells (Hanna and Hoover 1987) are awaited with interest.

The potential value of stimulating the tumouricidal activity of the *non-specific* defences provided by host macrophages is perhaps even greater, as suggested by the improved survival of tumour-bearing animals treated with liposomes containing macrophage activator (see above). The results of further studies and of clinical trials with this treatment modality will therefore also be of considerable interest.

While the search for new drugs and more effective combinations of existing treatment modalities continues, it is necessary to periodically review and update the philosophy on which long-term research on antimetastatic therapy is based. The disseminated cancer cell population presents to the host defence systems very much the same sort of problem that a guerilla army presents to orthodox military forces. The disorderly tumour cells are difficult for host defences to distinguish from normal cells and are dispersed in small units in unknown numbers in a large terrain, which is difficult to police effectively. Against such a hazard it is ineffective to use massed concentrations of defences, because as soon as one small unit has been liquidated another can manifest itself elsewhere. The classical strategy against such tactics is to use a dual approach: on the one hand to induce the local population to deny the infiltrating units the support from the local population and environment on which they depend and, on the other, to infiltrate the organization from within and thus to subvert or sap its purpose and drive. In relation to metastasis, eventual success in treatment may depend on deployment of similar ideas. We now have evidence, referred to above, that in certain organs disseminating tumour cells cannot form metastases and that this effect of normal cells upon scattered tumour cells may be chemically mediated. It requires considerable time and imagination to conceive how this knowledge might be used to therapeutic advantage and it is too early to speculate on such details, but the mere realization that metastasis is not an inevitable consequence of tumour cell dissemination is both psychologically and practically valuable, even at present.

The new possibilities opened up by study of abnormalities of genetic regulation and constitution also offer a distant promise of possible application to the management of neoplastic disease. Since the pioneering studies of Harris (1971) there has been tangible evidence that introduction of normal genetic material into a tumour cell (by fusion with a normal cell) can control neoplastic behaviour (see also Stanbridge *et al.* 1982). Harris's conclusion that neoplasia may result from deletion or inactivation of normal regulatory genes and that it can be controlled by the product of the normal homologous locus, is supported by much subsequent information. Modern clinical work has provided further evidence that deletion of genes may be important in the genesis of some neoplasms, retinoblastoma and Wilms' tumour being the best documented so far. On the basis of this information, Knudson (1985) has developed an elegant hypothesis, proposing that cancer results from deletion of both alleles of genes concerned in regulation of cell growth. Still more evidence is accruing that deletions, which may have a causal role in tumour induction, can be detected in a variety of other neoplasms for example, polyposis coli (Bodmer *et al.* 1987), carcinoma of the lung (Kok *et al.* 1987), and renal carcinoma (Zbar *et al.* 1987). Strong evidence that the deletion on chromosome 11 in patients with Wilms' tumour may be causal in inducing neoplasia, is provided by Stanbridge's recent work (Saxon *et al.* 1986) showing that transfer of an undeleted extra copy of chromosome 11 into cells of a tumourigenic renal cell line from a patient with Wilms' tumour rendered them non-tumourigenic in nude mice.

This accumulating body of information is prompting a new appraisal of genetic aspects of cancer and metastasis, and work is now beginning in an increasing number of laboratories (see Sager 1986) to ascertain whether reliable suppression of tumourigenicity by genetic reconstitution is a feasible proposition. A number of different experimental approaches are being adopted, but in our laboratory we have decided to use gene transfection followed by animal inoculation as our experimental protocol (see above). From this work we have recently obtained results suggesting that transfection of DNA from normal human blood leucocytes into tumourigenic mouse cells (TR4 Nu) can inhibit or suppress their ability to form tumours, on re-inoculation into nude mice, for prolonged periods of time (Tarin *et al.* 1988).

It will not escape the reader's attention for long that if this work in many laboratories collectively establishes that tumourigenicity can be abrogated or controlled by introduction of a gene or group of genes, gene therapy of neoplasia may become a reality within the lifetime of students currently reading this book. Bringing the unrestrained proliferation of tumour cells under control by such means would also have obvious implications for the management of metastatic disease: metastatic tumour cells that could not proliferate autonomously would cease to be a therapeutic problem. If these genes can be isolated and cloned, suitable vectors for delivering the genes specifically to the malignant cells and integrating them in a functional position inside their genomes, would need to be explored. We already know that there are viruses with tissue-specific affinities, and targetted correction of specific gene defects in cells *in vitro* has been achieved (Doetschman *et al.* 1987). The idea of infection of the individual with a specially tailored virus, which would bind to tissue-specific receptors on the tumour cell, enter the nucleus and control neoplastic behaviour, therefore does not seem too far-fetched.

A different but not necessarily incompatible concept, involving the possible use of specially constructed viruses in the treatment of metastatic cancer, is suggested by Kobayashi's studies (1982), showing regression of metastases if the tumour cells had been deliberately infected by viruses before i.v. inoculation. This regression occurs as a result of immune recognition and destruction of tumour cells, which are induced by the virus to display new antigens, but would otherwise have been invisible to host defences. The process has been termed viral xenogenization and may have potential for therapeutic exploitation if effective means could be designed for delivering suitable viruses specifically to tumour cells disseminated in the body.

The idea of using such approaches for the therapy of metastasis seems particularly attractive because if the disseminating tumour cells could not proliferate relentlessly in the new site in which they had landed, much of the sinister potential of metastasis would have been neutralized by the strategy, mentioned above, of infiltrating the organization of the cancer cell from within. These goals are not yet within our grasp, but in the interests of reducing the morbidity attendant upon current methods of cancer treatment, it is desirable to retain a mind open to new ideas about cancer metastasis and its control. The complexity of this disease process makes a single solution unlikely and effective management will almost certainly require multi-modality therapy, incorporating several new approaches.

9.5.5 References

Alexander, P. (1976). Dormant metastases which manifest on immunosuppression and the role of macrophages in tumours. In *Fundament aspects of metastasis* (ed. L. Weiss), pp. 227–39. North-Holland, Amsterdam.

Baum, M. (1980). Carcinoma of the breast. In *Recent advances in surgery* 10, 241–58. Churchill Livingstone, London.

Ben Ze'ev, A. and Raz, A. (1985). Relationship between the organization and synthesis of vimentin and the metastatic capability of B16 melanoma cells. *Cancer Research* 45, 2632–41.

Bodmer, W. F., *et al.* (1987). Localization of the gene for familial adenomatous polyposis on chromosome 5. *Nature* 328, 614–16.

Bresalier, R. S., Raper, S. E., Hujanen, E. S., and Kim, Y. S. (1987). A new animal model for human colon cancer metastasis. *International Journal of Cancer* 39, 625–30.

Chambers, A. F., Hill, R. P., and Ling, V. (1981). Tumour heterogeneity and stability of the metastatic phenotype of mouse KHT sarcoma cells. *Cancer Research* 41, 1368–72.

Chan, W.-S., Jackson, A., and Turner, G. A. (1985). The binding of conA and other lectins to surface glycoproteins: a comparison of a subcutaneous tumour and its liver metastases. *Invasion Metastasis* 5, 233–44.

Chew, E. C., Josephson, R. L., and Wallace, A. C. (1976). Morphological aspects of the arrest of circulating cancer cells. In *Fundamental aspects of metastasis*, (ed. L. Weiss), pp. 121–50. North-Holland, Amsterdam.

Coman, D. R. (1953). Mechanisms responsible for the origin and distribution of blood-borne tumor metastases: A review. *Cancer Research* 13, 397–404.

Coman, D. R., DeLond, R. P., and McCutcheon, M. (1951). Studies on the mechanisms of metastasis. The distribution of tumors in various organs in relation to the distribution of arterial emboli *Cancer Research* 11, 648–51.

Conley, F. K. (1982). Murine models of metastatic neoplasia to the central nervous system. *Cancer Metastasis Reviews* 1, 203–13.

De Baetselier, P., *et al.* (1984). Nonmetastatic tumour cells acquire metastatic properties following somatic hybridization with normal cells. *Cancer Metastasis Reviews* 3, 5–24.

de la Monte, S. M., Moore, G. W., and Hutchins, G. M. (1983). Patterned distribution of metastases from malignant melanoma in humans. *Cancer Research* 43, 3427–33.

Doetschman, T., *et al.* (1987). Targetted correction of a mutant HPRT gene in mouse embryonic stem cells. *Nature* 330, 576–8.

Donati, M. B. and Poggi, A. (1980). Malignancy and haemostasis. *British Journal of Haematology* 44, 173–82.

Ewing, J. (1928). *Neoplastic diseases* (3rd edn), p. 86. W. B. Saunders, Philadelphia.

Fidler, I. J. (1970). Metastasis: quantitative analysis of distribution and fate of tumor emboli labeled with ^{125}I-5-Iodo-2′-deoxyuridine. *Journal of the National Cancer Institute* 45, 773–82.

Fidler, I. J. (1973a). Selection of successive tumor lines for metastasis. *Nature New Biology* 242, 148–9.

Fidler, I. J. (1973b). The relationship of embolic homogeneity, number, size and viability to the incidence of experimental metastasis. *European Journal of Cancer* 9, 223–7.

Fidler, I. J. (1974). Immune stimulation—inhibition of experimental cancer metastasis. *Cancer Research* 34, 491–8.

Fidler, I. J. (1978). Tumour heterogeneity and the biology of cancer invasion and metastasis. *Cancer Research* 38, 2651–60.

Fidler, I. J. (1985). Macrophages and metastasis—A biological approach to cancer therapy. *Cancer Research* 45, 4714–26.

Fidler, I. J. and Kripke, M. L. (1977). Metastasis results from pre-existing variant cells within a malignant tumour. *Science* 197, 893–5.

Fidler, I. J. and Nicolson, G. L. (1977). Fate of recirculating B16 melanoma metastatic variant cells in parabiotic syngeneic recipients. *Journal of the National Cancer Institute* 58. 1867–72.

Fidler, I. J., Gersten, D. M., and Kripke, M. L. (1979). The influence of immunity on the metastasis of three murine fibrosarcomas of differing immunogenicity. *Cancer Research* 39, 3816–21.

Fidler, I. J., Sone, S., Fogler, W. E., and Barnes, Z. L. (1981). Eradication of spontaneous metastases and activation of alveolar macrophages by intravenous injection of liposomes containing muramyl dipeptide. *Proceedings of the National Academy of Sciences, USA* 78, 1680–4.

Frost, P. and Kerbel, R. S. (1983). Immunology of metastasis: can the immune response cope with disseminated tumor? *Cancer Metastasis Reviews* 2, 239–56.

Gastpar, H. (1982). Platelet aggregation inhibitors and cancer metastasis. *Annales Chirurgiae et Gynaecologiae* 71, 142–50.

Hanna, M. G. and Hoover, H. C. (1987). Basic and applied principles of active specific immunotherapy in the treatment of metastatic solid tumors. In *Immune responses to metastases* (ed. R. B. Herbeman, R. Wiltrout, and E. Gorelik), Vol. 2, pp. 95–115. CRC Press, Boca Raton, Florida.

Harris, H. (1971). The Croonian Lecture, 1971: Cell fusion and the analysis of malignancy. *Proceedings of the Royal Society of London B* 179, 1–20.

Hart, I. R. (1984). Tumor cell hybridization and neoplastic progression. In *Cancer invasion and metastasis: biologic and therapeutic aspects* (ed. G. L. Nicolson and L. Milas), pp. 133–43. Raven Press, New York.

Hart, I. R., Raz, A., and Fidler, I. J. (1980). Effect of cytoskeletal-disrupting agents on the metastatic behaviour of melanoma cells. *Journal of the National Cancer Institute* 64, 891–900.

Hayle, A. J., Whittaker, P. A., Darling, D., Tutty, B., Gazzard, A., and Tarin, D. (1987). Transfection of metastatic capability with total genomic DNA from metastatic cell lines. *Proceedings of the American Association for Cancer Research* 28, 70.

Heppner, G. H. and Miller, B. E. (1983). Tumor heterogeneity: biological implications and therapeutic consequences. *Cancer Metastasis Reviews* 2, 5–23.

Hewitt, H. B. (1976). Projecting from animal experiments to clinical cancer. In *Fundamental aspects of metastasis* (ed. L. Weiss), pp. 343–57. North-Holland, Amsterdam.

Hill, R. P., Chambers, A. F., Ling, V., and Harris, J. F. (1984). Dynamic heterogeneity: rapid generation of metastatic variants in mouse B16 melanoma cells. *Science* 224, 998–1001.

Horak, E., Darling, D. L., and Tarin D. (1986). Analysis of organ-specific effects on metastatic tumor formation by studies *in vitro*. *Journal of the National Cancer Institute* 76, 913–22.

Howell, A. and Harris, M. (1985). Infiltrating lobular carcinoma of the breast. *British Medical Journal* 291, 1371–2.

Humphries, M. J., Matsumoto, K., White, S. L., and Olden, K. (1986). Oligosaccharide modification by swainsonine treatment inhibits pulmonary colonisation by B16–F10 murine melanoma cells. *Proceedings of the National Academy of Sciences, USA* 83, 1752–6.

Irimuira, T., Gonzalez, R., and Nicolson, G. L. (1981). Effects of tunicamycin on B16 metastatic melanoma cell surface glycoproteins and blood-borne arrest and survival properties. *Cancer Research* 41, 3411–18.

Juacaba, S. F., Jones, L. D., and Tarin, D. (1983). Organ preferences in metastatic colony formation by spontaneous mammary carcinomas after intra-arterial inoculation. *Invasion Metastasis* 3, 208–20.

Kerbel, R. S., Lagarde, A. E., Dennis, J. W., and Donaghie, T. A. (1983). Spontaneous fusion *in vivo* between normal host and tumor cells; possible contribution to tumor progression and metastasis studied with a lectin resistant mutant tumor. *Molecular and Cellular Biology* 3, 523–38.

Kerbel, R. S., Frost, P., Liteplo, R., Carlow, D. A., and Elliott, B. E. (1984). Possible epigenetic mechanisms of tumor progression: induction of high-frequency heritable but phenotypically unstable changes in the tumorigenic and metastatic properties of tumor cell populations by 5-azacytidine treatment. *Journal of Cell Physiology Suppl.* 3, 87–97.

Knudson, A. G. (1985). Hereditary cancer, oncogenes and anti-oncogenes. *Cancer Research* 45, 1437–43.

Kobayashi, H. (1982). Modification of tumor antigenicity in thera-peutics: increase in immunologic foreignness of tumor cells in experimental model systems. In *Immunological approaches to cancer therapeutics* (ed. E. Mihich), pp. 405–40. John Wiley & Sons, London.

Kok, K., *et al.* (1987). Deletion of a DNA sequence at the chromosomal region 3p21 in all major types of lung cancer. *Nature* 330, 578–81.

Larizza, L. and Schirrmacher, V. (1984). Somatic cell fusion as a source of genetic rearrangement leading to metastatic variants. *Cancer Metastasis Reviews* 3, 193–222.

Lee, Y-T. N. (1983). Breast carcinoma: Pattern of metastasis at autopsy. *Journal of Surgical Oncology* 23, 175–80.

Liotta, L. A., Abe, S., Robey, P. G., and Martin, G. R. (1979). Preferen-tial digestion of basement membrane collagen by an enzyme de-rived from a metastatic murine tumor. *Proceedings of the National Academy of Sciences, USA* 76, 2268–72.

Lucke, B. and Schlumberger, H. (1949). Induction of metastasis of frog carcinoma by increase of environmental temperature. *Journal of Experimental Medicine* 89, 269–78.

McKinnell, R. G. and Tarin, D. (1984). Temperature-dependent meta-stasis of the Lucke renal carcinoma and its significance for studies on mechanisms of metastasis. *Cancer Metastasis Reviews* 3, 373–86.

McKinnell, R. G., De Bruyne, G. K., Mareel, M. M., Tarin, D., and Tweedell, K. S. (1984). Cytoplasmic microtubules of normal and tumor cells of the leopard frog. Temperature effects. *Differentiation* 26, 231–4.

McMenamin, M. M., *et al.* (1988). Genetic basis of metastases. *Advances in Experimental Medicine Biology* 233, 269–79.

Meromsky, L., Lotan, R., and Raz, A. (1986). Implications of endo-genous tumor cell surface lectins as mediators of cellular interac-tions and lung colonisation. *Cancer Research* 46, 5270–5.

Naito, S., von Eschenback, A. C., Giavazi, R., and Fidler, I. J. (1986). Growth and metastasis of tumour cells isolated from a human renal carcinoma implanted into different organs of nude mice. *Cancer Research* 46, 4109–15.

Naito, S., Giavazzi, R., and Fidler, I. J. (1987). Correlation between the *in vitro* interactions of tumour cells with an organ micro-environment and metastasis *in vivo*. *Invasion Metastasis* 7, 126–9.

Neri, A. and Nicolson, G. L. (1981). Phenotypic drift of metastatic and cell-surface properties of mammary adenocarcinoma cell clones during growth *in vitro*. *International Journal of Cancer* 28, 731–8.

Nicolson, G. L. (1982). Cancer metastasis: organ colonization and the cell-surface properties of malignant cells. *Biochemica Biophysica Acta* 695, 113–76.

Nicolson, G. L. (1988). Organ specificity of tumor metastasis: role of preferential adhesion, invasion and growth of malignant cells at specific secondary sites. *Cancer Metastasis Reviews* 7, 143–88.

Nicolson, G. L. and Custead, S. E. (1982). Tumor metastasis is not due to adaptation of cells to a new organ environment. *Science* 215, 176–8.

Nicolson, G. L. and Dulski, K. M. (1986). Organ specificity of metastatic tumor colonization is related to organ-selective growth properties of malignant cells. *International Journal of Cancer* 38, 289–94.

Nicolson, G. L. and Poste, G. (1983). Tumor cell diversity and host responses in cancer metastasis—Part II. Host immune responses and therapy of metastases. *Current Problems in Cancer* VII (7), 3–42.

Nicolson, G. L., Fidler, I. J., and Poste, G. (1986). Effects of tertiary amine local anesthetics on the blood-borne implantation and cell surface properties of metastatic mouse melanoma cells. *Journal of the National Cancer Institute* 76, 511–19.

Noltenius, C. and Noltenius, H. (1985). Dormant tumor cells in liver and brain: an autopsy on metastasizing tumors. *Pathology Research Practices* 179, 504–11.

Ogilvie, D. J., McKinnell, R. G., and Tarin, D. (1984). Temperature-dependent elaboration of collagenase by the renal adenocar-

cinoma of the leopard frog, *Rana pipiens. Cancer Research,* 44, 3438–41.

Ogilvie, D. J., Hailey, J. A., Juacaba, S. F., Lee, E. C. G., and Tarin, D. (1985). Collagenase secretion by human breast neoplasms: a clinicopathologic investigation. *Journal of the National Cancer Insti-tute* 74, 19–27.

Olsson, L. and Forschhammer, J. (1984). Induction of the metastatic phenotype in a mouse tumour model by 5-azacytidine and charac-terisation of an antigen associated with metastatic activity. *Pro-ceedings of the National Academy of Sciences, USA* 81, 3389–93.

Paget, S. (1889). The distribution of secondary growths in cancer of the breast. *Lancet* i, 571–3.

Poste, G., Doll, J., and Fidler, I. J. (1981). Interactions among clonal subpopulations affect stability of the metastatic phenotype in poly-clonal populations of B16 melanoma cells. *Proceedings of the National Academy of Sciences, USA* 78, 6226–30.

Poste, G., Tzeng, J., Doll, J., Greig, R., Rieman, D., and Zeidman, I. (1982a). Evolution of tumor cell heterogeneity during progressive growth of individual lung metastases. *Proceedings of the National Academy of Sciences, USA* 79, 6574–8.

Poste, G., Doll, J., Brown, A. E., Tzeng, J., and Zeidman, I. (1982b). Comparison of the metastatic properties of B16 melanoma clones isolated from cultured ell lines subcutaneous tumours and indi-vidual lung metastases. *Cancer Research* 42, 2770–8.

Potter, K. M., Juacaba, S. F., Price, J. E., and Tarin, D. (1983). Observa-tions on organ distribution of fluorescein labelled tumour cells released intravascularly. *Invasion Metastasis* 3, 221–33.

Price, J. E. (1986). Clonogenicity and experimental metastatic potential of spontaneous mouse mammary neoplasms. *Journal of the National Cancer Institute* 77, 529–35.

Price, J. E., Carr, D., Jones, L. D., Messer, P., and Tarin, D. (1982). Experimental analysis of factors affecting metastatic spread using naturally occurring tumours. *Invasion Metastasis* 2, 77–112.

Price, J. E., Carr, D., and Tarin, D. (1984). Spontaneous and induced metastasis of naturally-occurring tumors in mice: analysis of cell shedding into the blood. *Journal of the National Cancer Institute* 73, 1319–26.

Price, J. E., Syms, A. J., Wallace, J. S., Fleming, K. A., and Tarin, D. (1986). Cellular immortality, clonogenicity, tumourigenicity and metastatic phenotype. *European Journal of Cancer and Clinical Onco-logy* 22, 349–55.

Raz, A., Meromsky, L., and Lotan, R. (1986). Differential expression of endogenous lectins on the surface of nontumorigenic, tumorigenic and metastatic cells. *Cancer Research* 46, 3667–72.

Recamier, J. C. A. (1829). *Recherches sur le Traitment du Cancer par la Compression Methodique Simple ou Combinée et sur l'Histoire Générale de la Même Maladie,* Vol. 2, p. 110. Chez Gabor, Paris: cited by Wilder, R. J. (1956). *Journal of Mt. Sinai Hospital* 23, 728–34.

Rosenberg, S. A., *et al.* (1985). Observations on the systemic adminis-tration of autologous lymphokine-activated killer cells and re-combinant interleukin-2 to patients with metastatic cancer. *New England Journal of Medicine* 313, 1485–92.

Sager, R. (1986). Genetic suppression of tumor formation: a new fron-tier in cancer research. *Cancer Research* 46, 1573–80.

Sargent, N. S. E., Price, J. E., Darling, D. L., Flynn, M. P., and Tarin, D. (1987). Effects of altering surface glycoprotein composi-tion on metastatic colonisation potential of murine mammary tumour cells. *British Journal of Cancer* 55, 21–8.

Saxon, P. J., Srivatsan, E. S., and Stanbridge, E. J. (1986). Introduc-tion of human chromosome 11 via microcell transfer controls tumorigenic expression of HeLa cells. *EMBO Journal* 5, 3461–6.

Schackert, G. and Fidler, I. J. (1988). Site-specific metastasis of mouse melanomas and a fibrosarcoma in the brain or the meninges of syngeneic animals. *Cancer Research* 48, 3478–84.

Schirrmacher, V. (1985). Cancer metastasis: experimental ap-proaches, theoretical concepts, and impacts for treatment strategies. In *Advances in cancer research* (ed. G. Klein and S. Weinhouse), Vol. 43, pp. 1–73. Academic Press, London.

Schmidt, M. D. (1903). *Die Verbrietungswege der Karcinome und die Beziehung generalisierter Sarkome zu den leukamischen Neubildungen.*

Jena, Gustav Fischer, Jean: cited by Willis, R. A. (1973).

Sidebottom, E. and Clark, S. R. (1983). Cell fusion segregates progressive growth from metastasis. *British Journal of Cancer* **47**, 399–406.

Smithers, D. W. (1962). Cancer: an attack on cytologism. *Lancet* **i**, 493–9.

Stanbridge, E. J. *et al.* (1982). Human cell hybrids: analysis of transformation and tumorigenicity. *Science* **215**, 252–9.

Sugarbaker, E. V., Weingrad, D. N., and Roseman, J. M. (1982). Observations on cancer metastasis in man. In *Tumor invasion and metastasis* (ed. L. A. Liotta and I. R. Hart), pp. 427–65. Martinus Nijhoff Pubishers, The Netherlands.

Talmadge, J. E., Wolman, S. R., and Fidler, I. J. (1982). Evidence for the clonal origin of spontaneous metastases. *Science* **217**, 361–3.

Tarin, D. (1967). Sequential electron microscopical study of experimental mouse skin carcinogenesis. *International Journal of Cancer* **2**, 195–211.

Tarin, D. (1972). Morphological studies on the mechanism of carcinogenesis. In *Tissue interactions in carcinogenesis* (ed. D. Tarin), pp. 227–89. Academic Press, London.

Tarin, D. (1976). Cellular interactions in neoplasia. In *Fundamental aspects of metastasis* (ed. L. Weiss), pp. 151–87. North-Holland, Amsterdam.

Tarin, D. (1982). Investigations of the mechanisms of metastatic spread of naturally occurring neoplasms. *Cancer Metastasis Reviews* **1**, 215–25.

Tarin, D. (1988). Molecular genetics of metastasis. In *Ciba Foundation Symposium* (ed. G. Bock and J. Whelan) **141**, 149–69. John Wiley & Sons, Chichester.

Tarin, D. and Price, J. E. (1979). Metastatic colonization potential of primary tumour cells in mice. *British Journal of Cancer* **39**, 740–54.

Tarin, D. and Price, J. E. (1981). Influence of microenvironment and vascular anatomy on 'metastatic' colonization potential of mammary tumors. *Cancer Research* **41**, 3604–9.

Tarin, D., Hoyt, B. J., and Evans, D. J. (1982). Correlation of collagenase secretion with metastatic colonization potential in naturally occurring murine mammary tumours. *British Journal of Cancer* **46**, 266–78.

Tarin, D., Vass, A. C. R., Kettlewell, M. G. W., and Price, J. E. (1984a). Absence of metastatic sequelae during long-term treatment of malignant ascites by peritoneo-venous shunting: a clinicopathological report. *Invasion Metastasis* **4**, 1–12.

Tarin, D., Price, J. E., Kettlewell, M. G. W., Souter, R. G., Vass, A. C. R., and Crossley, B. (1984b). Mechanisms of human tumor metastasis studied in patients with peritoneovenous shunts. *Cancer Research* **44**, 3584–92.

Tarin, D., Price, J. E., Kettlewell, M. G. W., Souter, R, G., Vass, A. C. R., and Crossley, B. (1984c). Clinicopathological observations on metastasis in man studied in patients treated with peritoneovenous shunts. *British Medical Journal* **288**, 749–51.

Tarin, D., Hayle, A. J., Taggart, J., and Whitaker, P. A. (1988). Suppression of tumourigenicity in cells transfected with DNA from non-neoplastic cells. *Proceedings of the American Association for Cancer Research* **29**, 456.

Trainer, D. L., Kline, T., Mallon, F., Greig, R., and Poste, G. (1985). Effect of 5-Azacytidine on DNA methylation and the malignant properties of B16 melanoma cells. *Cancer Research* **45**, 6124–30.

Wallich, R., Bulbuc, N., Hammerling, G. J., Katzav, S., Segal, S., and Feldman, M. (1985). Abrogation of metastatic properties of tumour cells by *de novo* expression of H-2K antigens following H-2 gene transfection. *Nature* **315**, 301–5.

Weiss, L., Voit, A., and Lane, W. W. (1984). Metastatic patterns in patients with carcinomas of the lower esophagus and upper rectum. *Invasion Metastasis* **4**, 47–60.

Willis, R. A. (1973). *The spread of tumours in the human body* (3rd edn). Butterworth, London.

Zbar, B., Brauch, H., Talmadge, C., and Lineham, M. (1987). Loss of alleles of loci on the short arm of chromosome 3 in renal cell carcinoma. *Nature* **327**, 721–4.

9.6 Carcinogenesis

9.6.1 General introduction

D. G. Harnden

Methods of approach

Evidence on the causes of cancer comes from a number of sources. Studies on experimental animals have yielded a vast amount of information but often the reason for carrying out an animal study has been information derived from observations on humans. Clues about cancer aetiology arise largely from studies on human populations, though once again the population study may be based on an observation on an individual or a small group of people. The acute observation of the clinician at the bedside or in the clinic has played, and can still play, a vital role in providing the stimulus for larger, statistically valid studies and for animal experimentation.

Human studies are of several kinds. Classical epidemiology (see Section 9.7) has yielded valuable information from observations on the 'natural' incidence of cancer in different geographical areas on a global scale; this may draw attention to the effect of 'lifestyle' of different communities on cancer incidence. On a national or local scale such studies may focus on particular local circumstances that determine the pattern of cancer incidence. A second approach is to focus on a specific population defined in a particular way (e.g. by occupation, by age, by ethnic group, by drug exposure, by exposure to medical radiation) and to compare incidence with that of appropriate control groups. A special case of such studies would be the observation of subjects accidentally exposed to some natural or man-made hazard thought to be carcinogenic (e.g. A-bomb survivors, large-scale chemical accidents such as that at Seveso, or accidental inoculation of live oncogenic virus SV40; see below). A third type of human study is the intervention study, where having identified a putative 'carcinogenic agent' populations are treated in such a way that the hazard is removed or modified (cigarette smokers compared to ex-smokers; dietary modification).

Animal carcinogenicity studies are usually carried out on 'inbred strains' of animals. These were often developed to minimize variation between animals in experiments, but they were also developed to provide strains of animals especially sensitive to a particular carcinogen or with a high spontaneous incidence of cancer or leukaemia. Many chemical carcinogenesis studies on animals, however, have arisen initially because of human observations. Work on polycyclic hydrocarbon skin carcinogenesis in mice followed the recognition that certain workers exposed to tars, soots, and oils developed skin cancer. Similarly, the early observation of skin cancer on the hands of radiologists predated the first observations of radiation-induced cancer in experimental animals. On the other hand, the early work on tumour viruses was carried out almost exclusively on domestic and experimental animals, and it is only relatively recently that it has become clear that viruses are involved directly or indirectly in the aetiology of human neoplasms.

Causal agents

We already know a great deal about the causation of cancer and about the factors involved in the process of carcinogenesis, but for an individual case of cancer it is, more often than not, impossible to say what the cause of that particular cancer was. Indeed, those cases that can be attributed to a precise cause (with the outstanding exception of lung cancer caused by tobacco smoking) are rare and largely confined to cancers that arise as a result of heavy occupational exposure to a known carcinogen.

Causes of cancer can be broadly divided into:

1. factors extrinsic to the patient (environmental factors); and
2. factors intrinsic to the patient, which may be genetic, age-related, or physiological (such as immune status or endocrine balance).

It is important to accept at the outset that these factors do not operate independently.

It is quite clear that not only do environmental factors interact with intrinsic factors, but different environmental factors interact with each other and different intrinsic factors interact with each other. There are several instances where the effect of a specific environmental agent is modified by the genetic make-up of the individual exposed, e.g. the well-known differences in susceptibility to skin carcinomas following exposure to sunlight, of individuals with different degrees of skin pigmentation. An example of interaction between two environmental agents is the synergism between cigarette smoking and exposure to asbestos in the causation of carcinoma of the lung.

It is also important to realize that any one cancer may be caused not only by interacting factors but also by quite different factors. For example, we know that skin carcinomas may be caused by ionizing radiation, ultraviolet light, mineral oils, arsenic exposure, and papilloma viruses. Similarly, particular agents may cause more than one kind of cancer. Cigarette smoking is associated particularly with carcinoma of the lung but smokers also have an increased incidence of cancer of the larynx, oesophagus, bladder, and cervix. Similarly, radiation may cause leukaemias, skin cancers, thyroid cancers, and many others.

So the situation is complex. There are many different cancers, each one possibly caused by a number of different factors (extrinsic and intrinsic), which may be interacting. There are also a variety of causal agents which, though having some specificity, may be involved in the aetiology of several different cancers. In order to understand clearly the aetiology of cancer one must, therefore, ask precise questions about particular cancers or subgroups and about particular causal agents; not about cancer in general.

9.6.2   Causal mechanisms in carcinogenesis

D. G. Harnden

Latent period

There are a few general points that can be made. First, it is quite clear from both human and animal studies that a relatively long period of time elapses between the application of a known stimulus and the emergence of a clinically recognizable cancer. This is known as the latent period (Fig. 9.52). In the case of human leukaemia caused by radiation the minimum latent period is about 18 months; the mean is around 5 years but it can be as long as 15 or 20 years, perhaps more. Even longer latent periods have been reported for solid tumours caused by radiation. In the case of chemically induced human cancers it is harder to determine latent period, since the exposure may be over a substantial period of time, but it is known that cancers may occur many decades after exposure has ceased. For virus-induced cancers, the latent period is almost impossible to measure since the timing of the primary infection may not be known; however, there is no evidence to suggest that a cancer may arise immediately after the initial infection with a virus so, once again, there is a clear latent period.

In experimental animals the latent period may be many weeks or months, or even years, depending to some extent on the species. It is of considerable interest that the length of the latent period appears to be a function of life-span. Short-lived animals have shorter latent periods. This has led to speculation that the mechanisms that have evolved to prevent the development of cancer must be more rigorous in long-lived species, but little hard evidence exists on this point.

Multistage carcinogenesis

The question arises, what is going on during the latent period? There are several possibilities.

1. The causal agent may create one or more cancer cells which

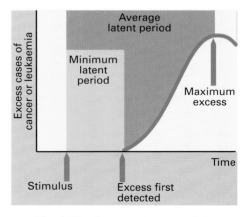

Fig. 9.52   Concept of latent period.

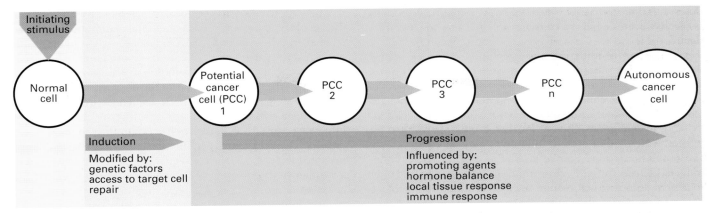

Fig. 9.53 Multistage carcinogenesis.

lie dormant for many months or years but which eventually begin to divide and cause a cancer.

2. The cancer cell or cells do begin to grow immediately, but either this growth is very slow or the increase in cell number is balanced by loss of cells caused by intrinsic instability or by killing of cells by host defence mechanisms.

3. The carcinogenic agent does not cause cells to become cancer cells at one step but alters a normal cell (or cells) in some way that makes them more susceptible to further changes. This latter is therefore, a multistage model of carcinogenesis.

There is some evidence in favour of each of these three models. Undoubtedly cancer cells or potential cells can lie apparently dormant for many years (e.g. metastatic breast cancer). Unless one supposes that they become activated without further stimulus, this really is a special case of the multistage model. Similarly, the concept that the cancer cells are growing against attrition due to cell death is again a special case of the multistage model since, as a result of this process, a more aggressive, more viable cell type is being selected out. So most arguments point towards a multistage model for carcinogenesis and, indeed, the experimental evidence is quite compelling. Similarly, if one examines the increase in incidence of particular cancers with age, either in experimental animals or man, the rate of increase is not compatible with carcinogenesis being attributable to a single event. The human age incidence curves best fit a model which suggests 4–6 stages being involved in development of full malignancy. It must be remembered, however, that not all cancers follow such an age-related pattern. For example, testicular cancer in men appears related strongly to hormonal influences following puberty.

Initiation and promotion

The concept, therefore, has arisen of an initial stimulus producing an altered cell which is not an autonomous cancer cell, followed by a period of progression (promotion), during which further changes take place (Fig. 9.53).

The classic work of Berenblum on skin carcinogenesis in the

mouse, carried out almost half a century ago, provided a model which is still the basis of current concepts of carcinogenesis. He recognized that there were two types of chemical involved in causing cancer, initiating agents and promoting agents. Initiating agents, such as the polycyclic hydrocarbons, will, in high doses, cause both papillomas and carcinomas after application to mouse skin, either as a single dose or as repeated doses. At lower doses they fail to induce a cancer, even after a prolonged period. However, if skin treated with a subthreshold dose of the initiating agent is further treated (repeatedly) with a promoting agent, then a papilloma or cancer will arise (Fig. 9.54). The promoting agent on its own will not induce cancer, even in high

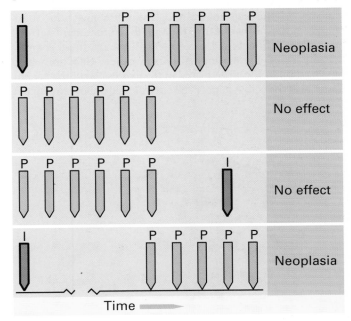

Fig. 9.54 Initiation and promotion. A subthreshold dose of a carcinogen with initiating potential (I) followed by repeated application of a promoting agent (P) will lead to neoplasia. The promoter on its own, or given prior to the initiator, has no effect. However, tumours will still occur even if there is a long lapse of time between the application of the initiator and subsequent application of the promoter.

doses. It is not effective if applied before the initiating agent, but is effective even if applied a considerable time after the initiating agent.

The concept of initiation and promotion has been widely applied in other situations, even to situations which do not involve chemical carcinogens. For example, in the case of radiation-induced cancers one can regard the primary changes caused by radiation as initiating events which do not lead inevitably to malignant disease. Further events precipitated by agents, which are at present unknown, may be thought of as the promotion stage. Similarly, in the case of some virus-induced cancers the early virus-induced changes may lead only to benign lesions which require the intervention of some other agency before full malignancy develops. This is seen in the classic case of benign oesophageal papillomas induced in cattle by bovine papilloma virus; the papillomas are converted to carcinomas of the oesophagus under the influence of a toxin from the bracken fern. Useful though it is, this model should not be thought of as a universal or obligatory mechanism of carcinogenesis.

The nature of the changes in cancer cells

Cancer cells when observed *in vivo* or *in vitro* show many changes that distinguish them from normal cells. The morphological changes affect the cell membrane, cytoplasmic structures and organelles, and the nucleus of the cell. Cell behaviour is dramatically altered. Over many years there has been much speculation as to which cell structures are involved in the fundamental changes that lead a cell to become cancerous. The changes in the cell membrane, the ribosomes, the mitochondria, were all at one time thought to be fundamental. However, there is now broad agreement that while these changes are important, the basic alteration in cancer cells must be a modification in the structure or in the expression of the genetic material of the cell. A cancer cell once altered divides to produce

two new cancer cells and eventually a great many similar cells. This could be the result of either a heritable mutational change or of altered expression of the genome more akin to differentiation. There is now good evidence that both kinds of modification do occur in cancer cells. Mutational changes can be shown experimentally to be responsible for the neoplastic phenotype by introducing specific mutant DNA sequences from cancer or transformed cells into normal cells and thereby changing them into cancer cells. It is harder to be certain that changes in expression of existing genes are fundamental, since such change in expression could be the consequence of a mutational event in a regulatory gene. For example, it is well documented that the insertion of a regulatory sequence from an oncogenic virus in the proximity of a normal cellular gene may cause the abnormal expression of that gene and so lead to neoplastic change.

A number of *tumour suppressor genes* have now been identified which, when reintroduced into appropriate cancer cells, can cause reversion to a normal phenotype. This suggests that in some circumstances absence of a gene product rather than the presence of an abnormal product may be the factor which precipitates malignancy.

Chromosomal abnormalities in cancer cells

Evidence that changes in the genetic material of the cell are fundamental comes from a variety of different sources. It has been known for many years that visible chromosomal damage is observed in many cancer cells. This is often complex and apparently random, and there has been much debate about its significance. Recently, however, specific chromosomal changes have been associated with specific malignancies, so that there can be little doubt that some of these chromosomal abnormalities are close to the basic changes in the neoplastic cell and perhaps are the initiating events. For example in chronic myeloid leukaemia the translocation between chromosomes 9 and 22 (Fig. 9.55) has now been defined in molecular terms as an

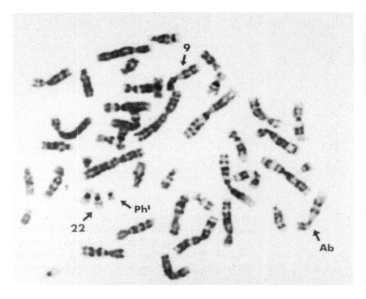

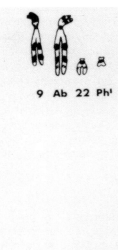

Fig. 9.55 G-banded cell from a patient with chronic myeloid leukaemia showing the Ph¹ chromosome which is derived from a translocation between the long arm of chromosome 22 and the long arm of chromosome 9. (From Mulvihill, J. J. (ed.) (1977). *Genetics of human cancer*. Raven Press, New York, with permission.)

exchange between two specific genes, one known (the *c-abl* oncogene) and one so far unknown (*bcr*, for breakpoint cluster region), which leads to the production of an abnormal *c-abl* gene product of 210 kDa (as compared to 145 kDa for the normal gene product) with enhanced tyrosine kinase activity. Similarly, the chromosome translocations observed in B-cell lymphomas represent exchanges between the *c-myc* gene on chromosome 8 and either the immunoglobulin heavy chain gene (chromosome 14) or the Igκ light chain gene (chromosome 2) or the Igλ light chain gene (chromosome 22) (Fig. 9.56). It appears in this case that the *c-myc* gene comes

under the control of the regulatory sequences of the Ig genes which are activated in antibody-forming B-cells.

Specific chromosomal changes were first identified in leukaemias and lymphomas but now similar specific changes are being recognized in solid tumours. A deletion of the short arm of chromosome 3 is found repeatedly in small cell carcinoma of the lung. It is certain that further specific aberrations remain to be discovered. However, in addition to these highly specific chromosomal changes, cancer cells may contain much apparently random chromosomal damage. It is possible that some of these changes, though not highly specific, may be non-random

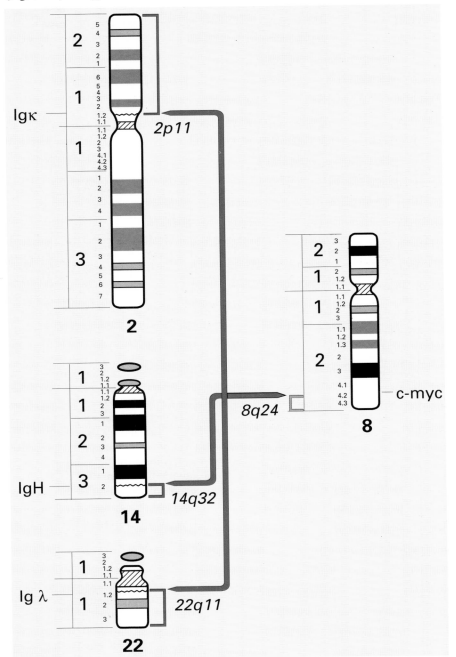

Fig. 9.56 Diagrammatic representation of the human chromosomes involved in specific translocations in B-cell lymphomas. The arrows point to breakpoints at which chromosomes 2, 14, and 22 reciprocally exchange chromosomal segments with chromosome 8.

and play a role in the progression of the cancer. For example, segments of the long arm of chromosome 1 are often present in triplicate in many different kinds of neoplasm, while interstitial deletion of the long arm of chromosome 5 is associated not only with carcinoma of the colon but also with a wide range of leuk-aemias, lymphomas, and other haematological disorders. Nevertheless, it is hard not to conclude that much of the chromosomal damage seen in cancer cells is generated by an increasing instability of the genome. There is a general tendency for more advanced, aggressive neoplasms to have more complex, bizarre chromosome complements; the chromosomes of ascites cells are frequently grossly abnormal in an apparently random manner.

Constitutional chromosomal abnormalities

The chromosomal changes so far discussed are those occurring in cancer cells *per se* but evidence that genetic change is import-ant in cancer also comes from those rare instances where a constitutional chromosomal abnormality (i.e. one inherited from a parent) is associated with a susceptibility to cancer. The classic example is retinoblastoma, a cancer of the neural retina of the eye occurring in children. Cases of retinoblastoma may be familial (about 40 per cent of cases) or sporadic. A small propor-tion (5 per cent) of cases of retinoblastoma have a constitu-tional, microscopically visible deletion of chromosome 13. This has led investigators to focus on this chromosome region, not only in these cases but also in those where there is no visible chromosome lesion. It has been found that mutational change at the region of interest (13q14) is frequent and has led to the notion of 'loss of heterozygosity' as the genetic mechanism in these cases (Fig. 9.57). This idea follows closely the 'two mutation hypothesis' put forward by Knudson in 1971 on the basis of a consideration of the distribution of the occurrence of cases of retinoblastoma. Knudson suggested that sporadic cases required two sequential somatic mutational events but that familial cases inherited one lesion and acquired the second by somatic mutation. It has been shown that loss of chromo-some 13, deletion of 13q14, and translocation or somatic recombination involving 13q14 are all common in retino-blastoma tumours. Where no change can be seen, point mutations may be occurring at this same locus. The concept, therefore, is as follows; hereditary cases have either a deletion or a mutation at 13q14, rendering a specific gene non-functional. While the corresponding normal gene on the homologous chromosome is present and functional the cell behaves normally. If however, the normal gene is lost or inactivated, a vital function is then missing from the cell. Neo-plastic behaviour follows, possibly as a consequence of the mal-function of other genes which are normally regulated by the missing gene function. It is this concept that has led to the suggestion that genes such as the retinoblastoma gene may be 'anti-oncogenes', i.e. genes that, when functioning normally, suppress the neoplastic potential of other genes, the 'onco-genes'. The retinoblastoma gene (Rb1) has been cloned and, while its function is not yet known, it is expressed in many

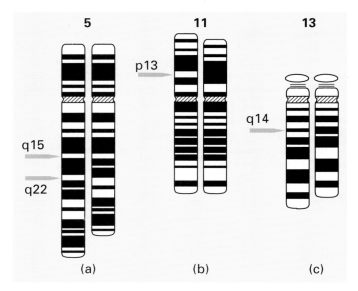

Fig. 9.57 Chromosome deletion in cancer susceptible subjects. (a) Deletion of chromosome 5 in the region q15–q22 is associated with familial polyposis of the colon and with some cases of carcinoma of the colon; (b) deletion of band p13 of chromosome 11 is found in some cases of Wilms' tumour (nephroblastoma, kidney cancer of children); (c) deletion of band q14 of chromosome 13 is found in some cases of the eye tumour, retinoblastoma, in children.

normal tissues but not in retinoblastoma cells. Rb1 has been found to be deleted in a proportion of cases of other malig-nancies and is considered as the prototype of tumour suppressor genes.

If this occurred only in this rare eye tumour it would be of interest but merely a curiosity. There is, however, mounting evidence that this mechanism may play an important role not only in other rare neoplasms such as Wilms tumour (nephro-blastoma) in children, where chromosome 11 is deleted in some cases, but also in some of the commoner adult neoplasms. Using anonymous DNA probes and linked marker enzymes, it has been possible to show that loss of one of two specific alleles (loss of heterozygosity) occurs in a proportion of cases of a variety of cancers. A good example follows the finding that the gene for the rare inherited condition, familial adenomatous polyposis (FAP), which predisposes to carcinoma of the colon, is located on the long arm of chromosome 5. In non-familial cases of car-cinoma of the colon a proportion of the tumours show loss of heterozygosity for this region, implying that a mutational event in this region is important in the genesis of this common 'sporadic' cancer.

Gene mutation

While visible chromosomal change is relatively easy to docu-ment, gene mutation is not easy to demonstrate directly in cancer cells. There is, however, much circumstantial evidence that gene mutation is important in the initiation and progres-sion of neoplasia. First, many, though not all, agents that cause mutations are also carcinogens (see below). Secondly, in a number of instances where patients are unusually liable to mutation induction they are also unusually susceptible to cancer. Patients with the inherited skin disease, xeroderma pigmentosum, are exceptionally sensitive to the effects of UV light because of defective repair of specific promutational lesions (thymine dimers) induced in DNA by UV light. Such patients also have a grossly elevated risk of skin cancers. The precise link between mutation, induction, and the occurrence of cancer in these patients is, however, not known.

Direct evidence that gene mutation is an important part of the neoplastic process comes from two sources: study of repair of induced DNA damage; and study of mutational changes in cellular oncogenes. Carcinogens cause damage of a variety of different types to DNA. Therefore, there exist a variety of different mechanisms for the repair of DNA damage, depending upon the nature of the lesion to be repaired. These systems have been well studied in bacterial cells for many years and are now becoming well known in mammalian, and even human, systems. Some repair systems are 'error free' but others are 'error prone' leading to mutation. Further, if repair is not carried out before replication synthesis occurs, errors in DNA synthesis leading to mutation will arise.

The most direct evidence for mutation in cancer cells comes from the study of the activated 'oncogenes'. These genes are normal cellular genes controlling vital cellular functions. Cells containing mutated oncogenes behave in a neoplastic manner (Fig. 9.58). Moreover, if the DNA of that mutated oncogene is transfected into 'normal' non-malignant cells these are transformed into cells with malignant potential.

Specific mutational changes in cancer cells can be recognized using the polymerase chain reaction (PCR) which amplifies a short sequence of DNA by repeated cycles of denaturing and reannealing. The amplified sequence can then be chatacterized. Since this procedure can be used on fixed material, large series of well characterized cancers can now be studied.

Alteration in gene expression

There are many examples of cancer cells expressing genes inap-

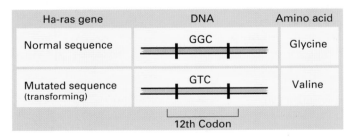

Ha-ras gene	DNA	Amino acid
Normal sequence	GGC	Glycine
Mutated sequence (transforming)	GTC	Valine
	12th Codon	

Fig. 9.58 Gene mutation and oncogene activation. The H-*ras* gene is a cellular proto-oncogene, the product of which is located on the inner side of the cell membrane. It has tyrosine kinase activity but its precise function in the normal cell is unknown. The twelfth codon is normally the triplet GGC, which codes for the amino acid glycine. In some tumour cells a mutation is found in codon 12 giving the triplet GTC which codes for valine. This mutated gene sequence has transforming activity when transfected into suitable cells. The oncogene has therefore been activated by a mutation.

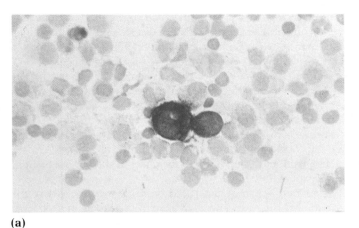

(a)

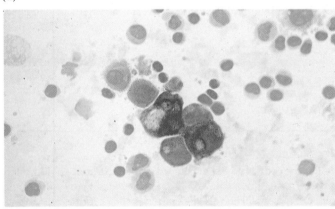

(b)

Fig. 9.59 (a, b) Colon carcinoma cells from an ascitic fluid stained for carcino-embryonic antigen (CEA) using the immunoalkaline phosphatase method. (Courtesy of A. Gosh.)

propriately. Possibly the best-known example is the production of carcino-embryonic antigen (CEA) by carcinomas of the colon and some other neoplasms. CEA is a glycoprotein normally produced during fetal development which is re-expressed inappropriately by these cancer cells (Fig. 9.59). This does not necessarily mean that the abnormal expression plays a part in determining the neoplastic phenotype of the malignant cells. It can, however, be a useful marker for the cancer in some cases. There are many other examples of inappropriate gene expression in cancer, e.g. the production of adrenocorticotrophic hormones by some lung tumours leads to serious and confusing clinical complications but does not necessarily play a causal role in neoplasia (see Section 9.8).

Some alterations in gene expression do clearly have a direct bearing on the behaviour of transformed and cancer cells. (In some of these instances, however, the altered expression may be attributable to mutational events in regulatory genes.) The best examples come from the study of growth-factor-dependent cells. A range of haemopoietic growth factors have been identified and, in many instances, isolated and cloned (see Chapters 1 and 4). These growth factors control either the proliferation of primitive stem cells or, following such stimulation, the differentiation and proliferation of cells of a specific morphological type. One such growth factor, interleukin-3 (IL-3) is a stimulator of primitive cells and of cells from several different lineages.

Normal haemopoietic cell lines, which require exogenous IL-3 for their continued growth, have been developed in the laboratory. Some lines, however, have become 'factor independent' and can grow without external stimulation. It is clear that some of these are producing the factor themselves and are thus being 'auto-stimulated'. It has been suggested that this mechanism may play an important part in the development of some cancers.

It will be apparent from this brief consideration that the alteration in the expression of growth factors or of their cell-surface receptors, will have a dramatic effect on cell behaviour and that this may be central to the development of neoplasia (see below).

9.6.3   Cell lineages in tumours

D. G. Harnden

The clonality of tumours

When the cells of a fully developed cancer are studied, it is often possible to demonstrate that they are the progeny of a single cell, i.e. a clone. The presence of a specific chromosome abnor-mality in all of the cells of a cancer or leukaemia strongly suggests that the cell population is a clone, simply because of the inherent improbability of the same chromosome aberration occurring more than once within a single neoplasm. One can, however, go further than that in determining clonality. Many chromosomes show polymorphic variation, i.e. the two homologues are not identical when examined with particular staining techniques (e.g. fluorescent dyes). It can be shown that in cells with a translocation involving chromosome 14 that it is always the same chromosome 14 that is involved in the translocation—even stronger evidence that the neoplasm is clonal.

The use of genetic polymorphism to determine the clonality of tumours depends upon X-chromosome inactivation in women (Fig. 9.60). Women have two X-chromosomes (compared with one X in men) and one of these Xs is 'switched off' during the course of development as a dosage compensation mechanism. Because this is a random inactivation, all women are mosaics in all tissues, some cells having the maternal X active and other cells having the paternal X active. If a woman is heterozygous for a specific gene on the X-chromosome, some cells will exhibit one allele and some cells will show the other allele. This can be demonstrated readily with the A and B isozymes of gluocose-6-phosphate dehydrogenase (G6PD). If one examines the cells of a neoplasm in a female heterozygous for G6PD, the cells will be all A or all B if the tumour is clonal, but a mixture of A and B, like a normal tissue, if it is polyclonal. The clonality of cancers can also be readily determined using a similar strategy but employing *restriction fragment length polymorphisms* (RFLPs). When normal DNA is cut with a specific endonuclease

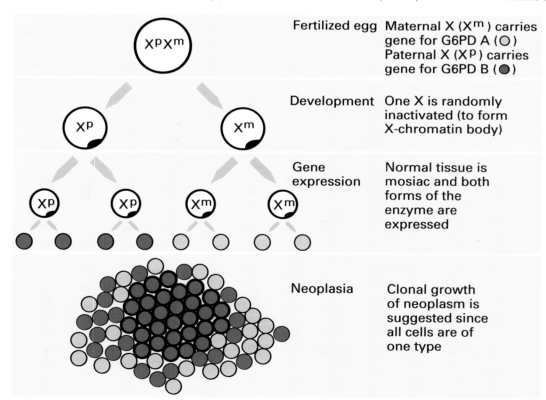

Fertilized egg   Maternal X (X^m) carries gene for G6PD A (○) Paternal X (X^p) carries gene for G6PD B (●)

Development   One X is randomly inactivated (to form X-chromatin body)

Gene expression   Normal tissue is mosiac and both forms of the enzyme are expressed

Neoplasia   Clonal growth of neoplasm is suggested since all cells are of one type

Fig. 9.60 Clonality of neoplasms may be demonstrated in women heterozygous for an X-linked marker gene such as glucose-6-phosphate dehydrogenase (G6PD) by making use of the phenomenon of random inactivation of the X-chromosome during development.

it will yield fragments of a particular size. If a mutation is present it may modify the size of DNA fragments obtained. Human populations are often *polymorphic* for such base changes (without phenotypic effect) so that some individuals are heterozygous for these specific changes having one variant on one chromosome and another at the same locus on the homologous chromosome. In informative (i.e. heterozygous) individuals loss of one specific allele recognized by the RFLP pattern can demonstrate the clonality of the tumour. For many fully developed cancers it is found that they are clearly monoclonal or monotypic. This is not universally true, and some cancers and many benign neoplasms, such as neurofibromas, have been found to be polyclonal.

The idea that a cancer is clonal fits well with the idea that the initiating event was a mutation in a single cell. The variation between cancer cells often observed in tumours then has to be explained by subsequent cellular evolution and selection, possibly on the basis of further mutational events, within a clonal population. Such selection and clonal evolution has been demonstrated dramatically in the course of serial observations in cases of leukaemia, in which further chromosome changes are superimposed upon the initial changes and a new cell type comes to predominate.

It is necessary, however, to sound a warning note. The observation that a cancer is clonal when it is observed as a fully malignant tumour is not necessarily proof that it started from a single cell. It is also compatible with the concept of the selection of one particularly aggressive clone from within a multiclonal population. The observation of multiple clones in benign neoplasms gives some support to this idea, as does the classic observation of pathologists over many decades that a cancer may arise within a tissue which is clearly already abnormal over a wide field. This 'field change' is particularly obvious when skin cancers arise within an extensive field of solar keratosis. Clonal origin is also compatible with multistage carcinogenesis and with the concept of initiation and promotion. One could regard a specific mutational event as the origin of the clone which need not be, at that stage, fully transformed. Further events could then lead to selection of variants within the clone. These could constitute at least some of the additional 'stages'. While it seems probable that in some cases the mutational event is also the initiation event (e.g. following acute radiation exposure), it is possible that steps preceding the origin of the clone which forms the tumour may create a population of cells in which an initiation event is more likely to occur.

The stem cell concept

In rapidly dividing normal tissues, such as bone marrow or skin, the production of new differentiated cells in based upon a hierarchical system in which specific cells, termed stem cells, are capable of generating sufficient progeny to maintain the tissue (see Chapter 1 and Section 9.4). When a stem cell divides, it produces one new stem cell and one committed daughter cell which has the capacity to divide many times to create a population of cells from which terminally differentiated cells are de-

rived (Fig. 9.61). The distinction between stem cells, committed cells, and differentiated cells will not necessarily be absolute, and some committed cells may have a limited potential for regeneration of the tissue. The basic pattern is, however, clear. These tissues are made up of a small number of cells (the stem cells) with an unlimited potential for cell division, and a large number of cells with no potential or only limited potential for cell division. Various assays have been developed for measuring the cells with clonogenic potential (see Section 9.1).

There is evidence to suggest that many tumours have a similar composition. If a tumour is disaggregated, most of the cells will not form colonies either on a solid substratum or in agar suspension culture, but a small proportion will do so. These clonogenic cells are thought to be the counterpart of those cells which *in vivo* maintain the growth of a tumour and which, when a tumour is damaged by chemical or radiation treatment, are capable of causing tumour regrowth. These cells are sometimes referred to as 'stem cells' but 'clonogenic' cells is more appropriate. Thus, a tumour may be composed of many cells with only limited division potential and a relatively small number of clonogenic cells.

9.6.4 Intrinsic factors in carcinogenesis

D. G. Harnden

The growth of a cancer is dependent in part upon the multiplication potential of the cancer cells but also on the response of the host. The use of the word 'host' in this context deserves some comment.

When a parasite invades another animal, the animal harbouring the parasite is referred to as the 'host'. The host is attacked by the parasite and responds to that attack in a variety of ways, e.g. by local tissue response or by immunological response. By referring to the patient or animal in which a cancer is growing as the 'host' we are, often unconciously, equating the cancer with a parasite. While this is helpful in some respects it could be misleading in others. Notably, the parasite is immunologically totally distinct from the host whereas a cancer will be largely immunologically compatible with the host, except for those antigenic changes which, as we have already noted, may occur in cancer cells.

Local response

When a cancer begins to grow there is a complex relationship with the surrounding tissue, and this will vary both in nature and degree between cancers and often between different subtypes of a single cancer. It is important to realize that without the support of the surrounding tissue a cancer could grow to only a very limited extent. Importantly, a growing cancer is supplied by blood vessels. The cancer is said to stimulate angiogenesis and a number of specific and non-specific angiogenic factors have been identified. Some of these are specific cloned

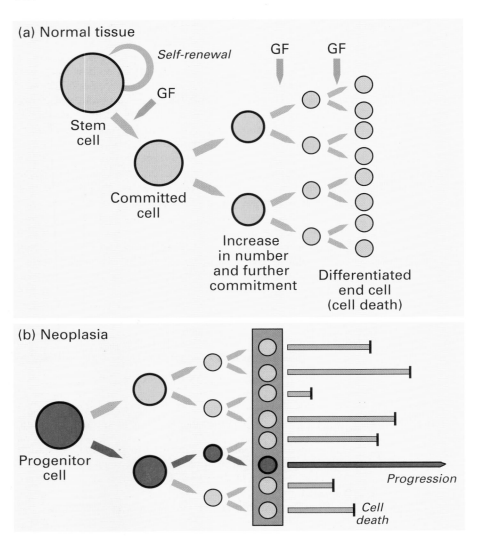

Fig. 9.61 (a) In normal tissues a small number of cells with self-renewal capacity also give rise to committed cell populations which still have considerable potential for cell division. These committed cells expand the population of differentiating cells in response to a series of growth factors (GF). (b) In a neoplasm, 'stem cell' has come to have a different meaning. When cells of a cancer are examined at one moment in time (blue box) they will be comprised of a mixture of cells, some with unlimited division potential and others that are destined to die. If sequential observation is possible, it is found that the unlimited cells are evolving new types (as measured by chromosome changes). This line of cells (red) is termed a stem line. It is composed of clonogenic cells capable of forming clones in culture and permitting regrowth of a cancer *in vivo* following depletion of the population by radiotherapy or chemotherapy.

molecules, such as tumour angiogenesis factor (TAF) and transforming growth factor (TGF-α). Others, however, are simple, apparently non-specific molecules, such as oligosaccharides. Sometimes in large tumours the growth of the tumour outpaces the growth of blood vessels so that areas of the tumour are starved of oxygen and become necrotic. In such cancers the live, active cells are on the periphery of the tumour or surrounding blood vessels to form tumour chords (Fig. 9.62).

Tumours also stimulate the growth of surrounding connective tissue. But this process may be reciprocal, with the stromal cells providing specific growth factors for the support of the tumour cells. It seems probable that this complex interaction between the stroma and the tumour cell may be the basis, in some cases at least, of the selectivity shown in the localization of secondary cancers.

Tumour cells often contain many dead and dying cells, and it is not surprising that many tumours contain large numbers of macrophages and other phagocytic cells. More specific, however, and more varied is the infiltration of lymphocytes. This

may well reflect an immune response to the tumour. As early as the end of the nineteenth century, pathologists talked of tumours being washed away by a flood of lymphocytes. It is certainly true that there is a broad correlation between the degree of lymphocytic infiltration and the prognosis. Lymphocyte-depleted Hodgkin's disease has a poor prognosis. Carcinomas of the breast wih a rich lymphocytic infiltrate tend to do well.

Immune response to tumours

The observation of immunocompetent cells in tumours and the knowledge that both bacterial infections and parasitic infestation provide an immune response led, very early, to the idea of an immune response to cancer and also to the notion that an enhancement of this response could be utilized to treat patients with cancer. This topic is dealt with in detail later (Section 9.10) but one cannot consider the process of carcinogenesis without relating it to the immune response of the host.

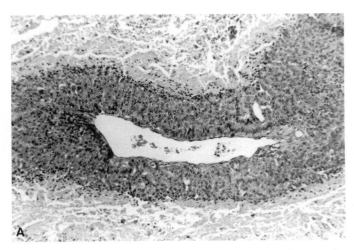

Fig. 9.62 Section of rat hepatoma showing healthy cells around a small blood vessel, a 'tumour chord'. Cells at a distance from the blood vessel have become necrotic. (Courtesy of J. Moore.)

As we have already noted, many cancer cells have new antigenic determinants. This is especially true of tumours induced by viruses. These antigens are usually referred to as tumour-associated transplantation antigens (TATA) or, more fully, tumour-specific antigens with rejection-inducing potential in the autochthonous host (Fig. 9.63). However, 'spontaneous' cancers where a specific stimulus has not been recognized (and that includes the majority of human cancers) tend to be only weakly antigenic in the autochthonous host. It was suggested by Burnett and others that the immune response to those new antigens was one of the major, natural means of controlling tumour growth. This concept of 'immune surveillance' suggested that tumours were initiated in the body with considerable frequency; being antigenically different from the host, they were recognized as foreign, provoked an immune response largely mediated by T-cells and were, most often, eliminated.

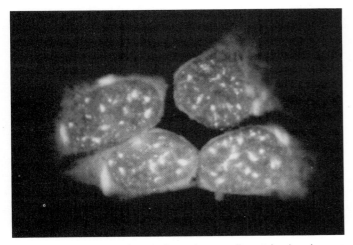

Fig. 9.63 Adenovirus-2 transformed rat cells, stained using an immunofluorescent technique for the virus T-antigen, which shows as a characteristic flecked nuclear staining. (Courtesy of P. Gallimore.)

Only where this immune surveillance failed did the tumour become recognizable as a clinical cancer.

There is little doubt that this concept does not hold good universally, but it may be useful for some cancers, e.g. virus-induced cancers. It is found that some virus-induced neoplasms, such as mouse lymphoid leukaemias, cannot be transferred to immunologically mature animals. Indeed, it was the classic work of Ludwig Gross, in which he transmitted mouse leukaemia by inoculation of cell-free extracts into immunologically immature animals, which marked the beginning of a clear understanding of viruses in the aetiology of neoplasia and also of the role of the immune system in cancer. Where viruses, or virally transformed cells, are inoculated into adult animals, it can be demonstrated that they provoke an immune response even where no growth of the neoplasm occurs, and it is reasonable to infer that these transformed cells are being held in check by immune mechanisms.

Hormonal influences on carcinogenesis

Once a tumour has been initiated and the abnormal cells start to grow there are, as we have seen, local influences that affect the way a tumour may grow. Likewise, there are systemic influences, of which immune response is only one. It is clear that the hormonal balance in the host animal or in the patient has a profound influence on whether or not a cancer will develop. There is some indication that an abnormal hormonal balance may promote the growth of a tumour, but it is not easy to be sure that the hormones actually initiate the cancer. In one classic experiment three groups of animals were set up, each with an ovary transplanted to the spleen. In that site hormones produced by the ovary enter the bloodstream via the portal circulation so that metabolism of the hormones may occur before they reach the pituitary. In the first group no further action was taken; in the second group the other ovary was removed; in the third group the other ovary was removed and an oestrogen supplement was given to the animals. Only in group 2 did the transplanted ovary become neoplastic (Fig. 9.64). The postulated explanation is that in the low-oestrogen environment, caused by the break in the feedback loop to the pituitary, produces excess gonadotrophic hormone, leading to overstimulation of the transplanted ovary and eventually to neoplasia. This suggests that initiation of neoplasia may arise as the result of hormonal imbalance.

There are a few possible examples of similar hormonal effects in man, although it is impossible to distinguish between hormonal initiation and an effect on the progression of an already initiated cell. For example, in phenotypic female patients with gonadal dysgenesis and a 46, XY-chromosome complement, there is a high risk (50 per cent) of dysgerminoma or gonadoblastoma occurring in the dysgenetic gonads. Again, overstimulation of the abnormal gonad by pituitary hormones may be the precipitating factor.

There are also examples in experimental animals of interaction between hormonal balance and environmental factors. Treatment of young female mice with dimethylbenzanthracene (DMBA) leads to the induction of mammary carcinoma in a

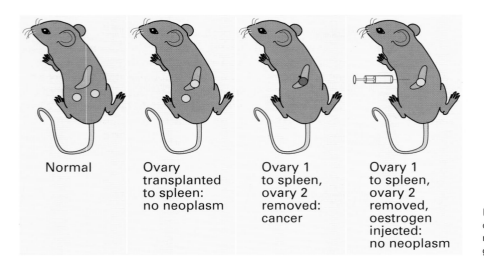

Normal

Ovary
transplanted
to spleen:
no neoplasm

Ovary 1
to spleen,
ovary 2
removed:
cancer

Ovary 1
to spleen,
ovary 2
removed,
oestrogen
injected:
no neoplasm

Fig. 9.64 Hormone induction of cancer. An ovary transplanted to the spleen will become neoplastic in the absence of circulating oestrogen.

proportion of the treated animals. Males are not affected. If, however, the males are castrated and oestrogen-treated, they too get mammary carcinoma. There are many other examples of the incidence of chemically induced cancer being dependent upon the sex of animals treated.

Human examples of hormonally influenced cancers are also numerous, the best documented being carcinoma of the breast. It has been known for many years that the progression of some breast cancers can be delayed or halted by hormone therapy, or removal of the ovaries. Such 'hormone-responsive' breast cancers can now be treated with the drug 'Tamoxifen' which is an oestrogen antagonist, exerting its effect by blocking oestrogen receptors and so making them unavailable to endogenous oestrogens that stimulate tumour growth. Hormone dependency in breast is considered in Chapter 22.

Genetic susceptibility to cancer

Inbred strains of experimental animals

In considering the mode of action of carcinogenic agents it is important to bear in mind the variability of the population exposed to these agents. This fact was recognized by the early experimentalists. They rapidly discovered that in order to carry out meaningful experiments with specific chemicals or viruses the experiments had to be carried out on genetically homogeneous groups of animals. This led to the development of 'inbred' strains of animals, usually mice (Fig. 9.65). Inbred animals are as alike to each other as are identical twins. Experimental variation in carcinogenesis experiments using such strains cannot therefore be due to genetic differences between animals. These inbred strains were also developed because some of them showed a susceptibility to a particular carcinogenic agent, either viral or chemical, and they have played an important role in elucidating the mode of action of these agents. A further advantage of these inbred animals is that they will accept reciprocal skin grafts (i.e. they are syngeneic) and can therefore be used to test whether a tumour induced in one animal provokes an immune response in another syngeneic an-

imal. Some strains will accept transplanted tumours of many kinds because they are genetically immune deficient (nude or *nu/nu* mice).

From these early studies it was concluded that the genetic component in cancer is an important one. In human cancer, however, it is not immediately apparent that this is so, and to understand this we must therefore consider how genetic factors interact with other factors in carcinogenesis.

Interaction of genetic and environmental factors

Many studies have shown that for human cancer, environmental agents, chemicals, radiation, and viruses are very important in the development of cancer; each will now be considered in detail. Evidence for this comes largely from geographical studies and from studies of populations exposed to specific carcinogenic agents (see Section 9.6.1). This epidemiological evidence is backed up by strong experimental evidence which has identified many carcinogenic agents and helped to elucidate their mode of action. It is often estimated that as much as 80 per cent of human cancer is 'due to environmental factors'. However, when we begin to analyse these environmentally induced cancers we not infrequently find that they are only partly attributable to the environment. The most striking example is the induction of skin cancer by UV light. Skin cancers (squamous cell and basal cell carcinoma) have an incidence in the UK of about 30 cases/100 000 of the population per annum. In countries such as South Africa, where exposure to sunlight is much greater, the incidence of skin cancer in the white population is roughly three times that figure, clearly demonstrating the environmental influence. However, the incidence of skin cancers in the black population of South Africa is vanishingly low, so that exposure to sunlight will only cause skin cancer in populations whose cells are not protected from UV by the melanin granules in the skin cells—which is a genetically determined characteristic. It can be shown readily that the degree of skin pigmentation is related to skin cancer incidence and, moreover, that those with red hair (phaeomelanin) are especially susceptible. For some cancers the role of environment

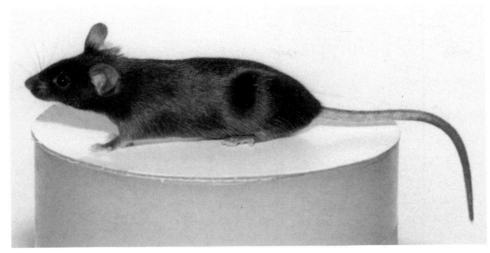

(a)

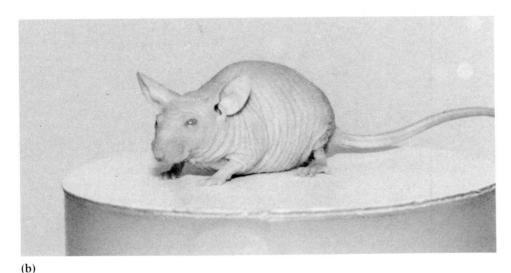

(b)

Fig. 9.65 Inbred mouse strains (a) C57 black/DBA F_1 cross; (b) athymic or nude mouse homozygous for the *nu* gene (*nu/nu*).

is much stronger. In one situation, where workers were exposed to the aromatic amine, 2-naphthylamine, all those exposed in a particular workshop developed bladder cancer. In such a case, where the environmental exposure is overwhelming, genetic factors (or other individual variability) is of little importance. At the other extreme there are some cancers which appear to be inherited as Mendelian dominant traits. This appears to leave little room for the action of environmental factors but it is probable that induced somatic mutation may be important, even in the development of retinoblastoma (see above).

What emerges, therefore, is the concept that there are not environmental cancers on the one hand and genetic cancers on the other, but a situation where environmental factors and genetic factors interact to lead to the development of cancer—just as they do in determining any other biological variable (Fig. 9.66). For many cancers, indeed the majority, it is likely that the environmental component may be the more important. For others, a minority, the genetic factors will be overriding, but

nevertheless interacting with the environment. In between, there will be many types of cancer where the precise aetiology is not clear but where we can be reasonably sure that the process of carcinogenesis will involve complex interactions between different factors, some environmental, some genetic.

Mechanisms of genetic susceptibility to cancer

There are two basic mechanisms of cancer susceptibility. First, the initiation event may be more probable in some individuals than in others; and secondly, progression may be more likely because of some genetically determined variation in the host response to the cancer.

There are a variety of ways in which the probability of initiation may be enhanced. First, the subjects may vary in the likelihood of the carcinogenic agent reaching the target cell. The example of skin pigmentation has already been mentioned. Less obvious, but very real, is genetic variation in the way in

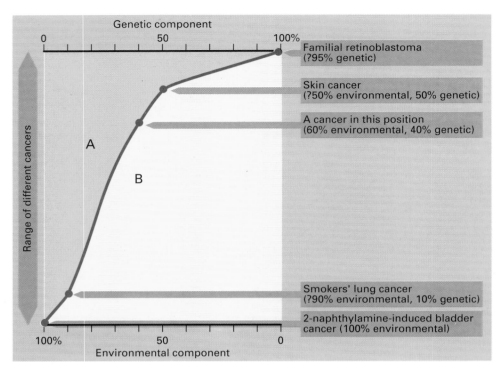

Fig. 9.66 Genetic/environmental interaction in cancer. A diagrammatic representation of the relative importance of extrinsic and intrinsic factors in cancer. The red line (which is somewhat speculative) is made up of a series of points representing a range of cancers, from those that are largely environmental to those that are largely genetic. The area (B) would represent the environmental component in cancer and the area (A) the genetic component. The purpose of the diagram is to encourage the reader to abandon the idea that some cancers are environmental and some are not.

which carcinogens are metabolized. Many carcinogenic chemicals require metabolic activation within the body. In experimental animals metabolic activation of polycyclic aromatic hydrocarbons is clearly under genetic control. There have been a number of suggestions that this is also true in man, but the area has been confused until recently when it was shown that metabolism of debrisoquin by the P_{450} enzyme complex is genetically controlled and, moreover, shows genetic polymorphism in human populations. The principle that people may vary in this way in their response to carcinogens is of great interest and may offer opportunities for cancer prevention.

The second possibility leading to enhanced initiation is that the patient may inherit one of the steps required for the process of carcinogenesis. The example of retinoblastoma has already been considered and may well prove to be a model for other kinds of cancer. If even one of the steps in a multistage process is inherited, the probability of reaching the final stage is enhanced.

Thirdly, conditions are known where an inherited gene leads to a degree of instability in the genome so that further changes are more likely to occur. Such patients are also cancer prone. Most of these rare syndromes are associated with an unusual susceptibility to a specific environmental agent or group of agents. Patients with xeroderma pigmentosum are unusually sensitive to UV light and to a group of chemicals which cause bulky lesions in DNA, while patients with ataxia telangiectasia are unusually sensitive to the effects of ionizing radiation and to a very small group of radiomimetic chemicals.

Some individuals are unusually sensitive to the affects of oncogenic viruses. The ubiquitous Epstein–Barr virus (EBV) is associated with nasopharyngeal carcinoma only in South-East Asia and in people who originate from that region, suggesting that this virus (which for the most part causes only minor infections in people of other regions) has a different, more damaging effect in one genetically distinct group.

Genetic susceptibility due to enhanced progression is harder to document, but the unusually high incidence of lymphoid neoplasms in patients with genetically determined immune deficiency is one possible example.

Examples of genetic susceptibility to cancer in man

There are three areas to consider: (1) association of cancer with normal inherited traits, (2) familial aggregation, and (3) Mendelian syndromes.

Association with normal traits We have already noted that fair-skinned people are more susceptible to skin cancer than are dark-skinned people, but there are other examples of association of cancer with normal traits. Carcinoma of the stomach is commoner in subjects with blood group A than in those with other blood groups. In certain types of leukaemia and lymphoma, specific HLA subtypes are more common. In the future the use of DNA polymorphisms should help to identify populations with an unusual proneness to cancer.

Cancer families There are many well-documented families where there is an unusually high incidence of a particular cancer or of a number of different cancers. While some of these could well be due to chance, especially where the age of the patient is high, it now seems clear that there is a real cancer susceptibility problem in some families. In particular, there are reports of families in which many of the females have developed breast cancer at a very young age (Fig. 9.67). Similarly, families with multiple cases of colonic cancer, occurring in both men and women at young ages, are reported. The latter are described as hereditary non-polyposis colonic cancer (HNPCC) of two types: one where only colon cancer occurs in the family members; and in the second type colonic cancer occurs in some members and other neoplasms, especially carcinoma of the breast, occur in other members. This terminology replaces the unsatisfactory term 'cancer family syndrome'.

Mendelian inheritance of cancer susceptibility It should be noted that what is inherited is 'susceptibility'. Cancer is not obviously inherited in the way that, say, achrondroplasia is inherited. Almost by definition, any organism made up of cells containing a gene which (when expressed), converted them into cancer cells could not survive in any meaningful way as an organism. Therefore, in all the inherited cancer syndromes the tissues are not overtly abnormal during development and early life but only acquire focal neoplastic lesions at a later stage.

There are several classic Mendelian autosomal dominant syndromes. In familial adenomatous polyposis (FAP, also known as polyposis coli) multiple colonic polyps develop during the teenage years and early twenties (see Chapter 16). A high proportion develop carcinoma of the colon by 30 years of age and the lifetime risk of carcinoma of the colon is virtually 100 per cent. Retinoblastoma is also dominantly inherited in about 50 per cent of cases. Patients carrying the gene seldom if ever develop the disease after 10 years of age. Other dominant cancer susceptibility diseases are neurofibromatosis (Fig. 9.68),

multiple endocrine neoplasia types I and II, basal cell naevus syndrome, and dysplastic naevus syndrome. Recessive cancer susceptibility syndromes include xeroderma pigmentosum, ataxia telangiectasia, epidermodysplasia verruciformis (susceptibility to human papilloma virus, HPV), and the various immune-deficiency diseases.

The only X-linked cancer susceptibility diseases are X-linked agammaglobulinaemia (susceptibility to lymphoid neoplasms) and Duncan's disease (susceptibility to Epstein–Barr virus).

Age and carcinogenesis
Experimental animals

In experimental animals it is usual to begin carcinogenesis experiments at a relatively young age. The principal reason is the latent period. Only if sufficient time is allowed to elapse before animals reach the end of their natural life-span will the true carcinogenic potential of an agent be recognized. However, where the effect of age *per se* on chemical carcinogenesis has been examined, it seems clear that it is the potency and dose of the agent that is used that determines the occurrence of cancer, rather than the age at which it is applied. In the case of viruses, however, the result is quite different. Most viruses will only induce leukaemia or other neoplasms if inoculated into young, immunologically immature animals, where the growing clones of cells can reach an advanced stage before the immune system recognizes them as foreign.

In the case of 'spontaneous' animal tumours there is a clear relationship with age. Only if kept in captivity will mice develop cancer because in the wild they do not live long enough for the

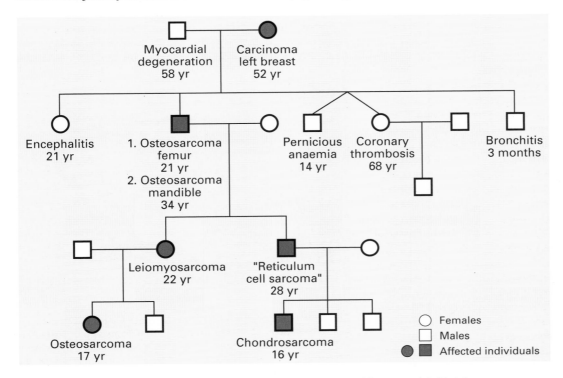

Fig. 9.67 Cancer family pedigree, with no clear pattern of inheritance. (Courtesy of J. Birch.)

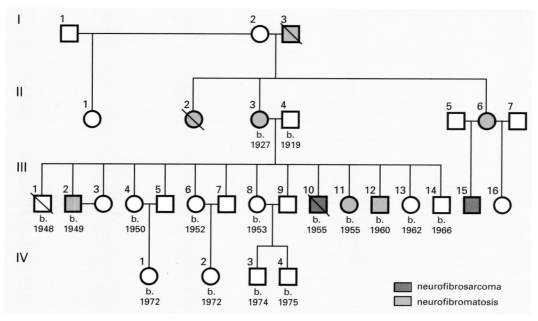

Fig. 9.68 Pedigree of family with neurofibromatosis showing classical Mendelian dominant inheritance of susceptibility, with two members developing cancer (neurofibrosarcoma).

disease, even if initiated, to be recognized as a tumour. The relationship with age is in accord with the concept of multi-stage carcinogenesis. It is improbable that in a young animal all the necessary steps will have occurred; as the animals ages the probability of the sequence of events being completed increases. From the shape of the age incidence curve of spontaneous tumours one can deduce the probable number of events necessary for a neoplasm to be recognized.

Age effects in humans

In humans, age clearly influences cancer incidence; or rather events which occur at particular ages influence cancer incidence. While, as we have already seen, cancer as a whole tends to increase with age, specific neoplasms have quite characteristic age incidence patterns (Fig. 9.69). There is a peak of cancers in early childhood, which means that, though still rare compared with incidence in adults, these cancers are, after accidental death, the commonest cause of death in childhood. Obviously, this has only been true since the major lethal childhood illnesses such as diphtheria, scarlet fever, and others were eliminated. The cancers of children are quite different from those of adults. They often affect cells still undergoing development, e.g. nephroblastoma, retinoblastoma, specific types of lymphoblastic leukaemia, and brain tumours. The reasons for a childhood peak are not clear, but it may be that certain sorts of developing cells are especially susceptible to neoplastic development. There are, indeed, specific instances of the fetus being especially susceptible to the effects of carcinogenic agents. The treatment of women in early pregnancy with diethylstilboestrol may lead to the development of adenomatosis of the vagina and sometimes to carcinoma of the vagina in their daughters during

their early teens, an age at which such neoplasms do not normally occur. This phenomenon of transplacental carcinogenesis is also well documented in experimental animals. For example, treatment of pregnant rats with ethylnitrosurea will lead to the development of brain tumours in a proportion of their offspring.

Cancers during early adulthood are rare. Those that do occur tend to be of particular types, e.g. osteosarcoma, Hodgkin disease, and testicular cancers in young men. It seems possible

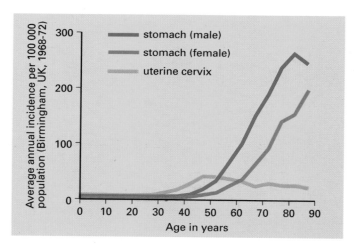

Fig. 9.69 Cancer–age incidence curves. Each cancer has its own age incidence pattern. Some, like stomach cancer, increase progressively in incidence with age, although males have a substantially higher incidence than females at a given age. Cancer of the uterine cervix, on the other hand, increases rapidly from age 25 to 45 years but then levels off and even declines in later years.

that the occurrence of these cancers may be attributable to physiological events occurring at that time, and in particular to the intense hormone stimulation that may be occurring in bone, testis, or other developing tissues.

Age-related social behaviour may also influence cancer incidence. Breast cancer is less common in women who have had their first pregnancy at a young age than in those who had their first pregnancy at a later age or in those who have not had a child (see Chapter 22). Similarly, the incidence of carcinoma of the cervix is clearly related, amongst other influences, to age at first intercourse, being more common in women who have had intercourse at a young age (see Chapter 21). The age pattern of carcinoma of the cervix is also changing, being more common now in younger women than 20 years ago. Carcinoma of the cervix is, however, still much commoner in older women than in younger women.

The increase of most cancers with age is usually attributed to the accumulation of the events required for the several steps in the development of malignancy. These are often thought of as mutational events which become commoner with age, either because of the increased time of exposure to environmental mutagens or because repair systems that normally protect cells from the damaging effects of these environmental agents become less efficient with age. There is, however, little evidence for such a decline in repair efficiency with age.

It is also possible that the steps towards malignancy may be other life events. Damage to certain organs appears to be closely associated with the development of neoplasia. Hepatocellular carcinoma is more likely to occur in a cirrhotic liver, especially following hepatitis B virus infection. Melanoma is more likely to occur following episodes of acute sunburn. Precisely how these events help progression towards neoplasia is uncertain, but the stimulation of cell division in a damaged tissue may permit the expansion of a previously dormant clone. The probability of events such as these increases with age.

Lastly, there is good evidence that immune competence declines with age in both experimental animals and man. It is also possible, therefore, that some cancers held in check by immune mechanisms may become commoner in older people because of a weakening of these constraints. This interesting hypothesis has little firm evidence to support it.

9.6.5 Extrinsic factors in carcinogenesis

D. G. Harnden

There are three principal groups of external causal agents: viruses, chemicals, and radiation.

Oncogenic viruses

For many years it was thought that viruses, while clearly the cause of cancer in animals, were of very little relevance to human cancer. However, viruses are now implicated in many different human cancers and while it is difficult to say that they are the primary cause, the evidence that they play a role in human carcinogenesis is overwhelming.

Cancer-causing viruses are usually referred to as 'oncogenic' viruses, whereas chemicals that cause cancer are termed 'carcinogenic'. The reason for the difference is obscure and unimportant—the words are synonymous.

In the latter half of the nineteenth century it became apparent that a number of diseases of both plants and animals could be transmitted by cell-free filtrates, indicating that bacteria could not be the causal agent. Tobacco mosaic disease and foot-and-mouth disease in cattle were amongst the first to be transferred in this way. It was natural to search for these transmissible agents in neoplasms.

The first demonstration of the transmission of a neoplasm by a cell-free filtrate was when Ellerman and Bang transferred chicken leukosis in 1908. It was two years later, in 1910, that Peyton Rous showed that chicken sarcoma could be transferred by a cell-free filtrate. This discovery of the Rous sarcoma, or chicken sarcoma, virus was rewarded with a Nobel prize 55 years later! The study of oncogenic viruses progressed slowly over the ensuing half century. In the 1930s Bittner discovered the mouse mammary tumour virus, while Shope conducted his classic experiments with rabbit fibroma and rabbit papilloma viruses. The rabbit and chicken viruses were thought of as curiosities and it was not until Ludwig Gross in 1951 discovered murine leukaemia virus that the study of cancer viruses really began in earnest. Since then the progress has been rapid, and new cancer viruses or new associations of viruses with cancer are being discovered regularly. The most recent is the association of the virus of AIDS, human immunodeficiency virus (HIV), not only with Kaposi's sarcoma, but also with leukaemia and lymphomas.

Viruses are intracellular parasites, which have either a DNA or an RNA genome. Many of the groups of DNA viruses, which are well known because they are associated with pathologies other than neoplasia, have oncogenic members. On the other hand, most of the well-known RNA viruses, which cause common diseases such as measles and influenza, are not associated with neoplasia. Indeed, the only RNA viruses known to cause cancer are the retroviruses. This group of viruses, which includes the lentivirus (slow virus) group to which HIV belongs, has a DNA stage in the life cycle. Genomic RNA is used as a template to make a DNA copy under the control of an RNA-primed DNA polymerase (reverse transcriptase) coded by the virus itself.

DNA oncogenic viruses

DNA viruses contain two groups of genes: those involved in early events within the cell, in particular the replication of the virus genome, and those involved with late events. Late events include the synthesis of viral proteins and viral assembly. If the viral life cycle within the cell is completed, large numbers of virus particles are produced, the cell is lysed (except pox viruses), and the virus released. Sometimes, however, a stable relationship is established between the virus and the cell such that only some of the early events take place and the life cycle is not completed. It is under these circumstances that cellular transformation by an oncogenic DNA virus may take place (Fig. 9.70). The nature of the interaction depends crucially on the particular cell type that is invaded by the virus. In transformation, the viral genome persists within the cell. In some cases the whole genome becomes integrated (sometimes in multiple copies) within the host cell genome. In some cases only part of the genome becomes integrated, while in yet other instances the genome persists in an episomal form without integration. In each case, one or more of the viral early genes plays an active role in the cellular transformation process, though the nature of the precise function that brings about transformation is often not known. There are, however, some instances where a DNA virus appears to be capable of effective cellular transformation, and yet viral DNA is not readily demonstrated in the transformed cells. It is suggested, though not proven, that in these instances the virus brings about some

change in the genome, which then persists in the absence of the virus—the so called 'hit and run' mechanism.

Thus for the DNA viruses there appear to be alternative cellular pathways. Either the virus completes its life cycle, leading to cell death and virus release, or a stable, potentially transformed relationship is established. Most often, tumours induced by DNA viruses do not contain infectious virus. In some instances, however, the stable relationship between the virus and the cell may break down in individual cells that go into productive infection, and such a neoplasm contains some infectious virus. In the case of benign lesions, such as warts, the nature of the tumour itself creates conditions where the virus enters the replicative cycle and the wart may contain large amounts of infectious virus.

It can be shown in experimental systems that transformation by DNA viruses is a relatively rare event, perhaps not more frequent than one chance in a million, even when the cell–virus combination and the conditions of infection are appropriate for transformation.

The groups of DNA viruses that contain oncogenic members

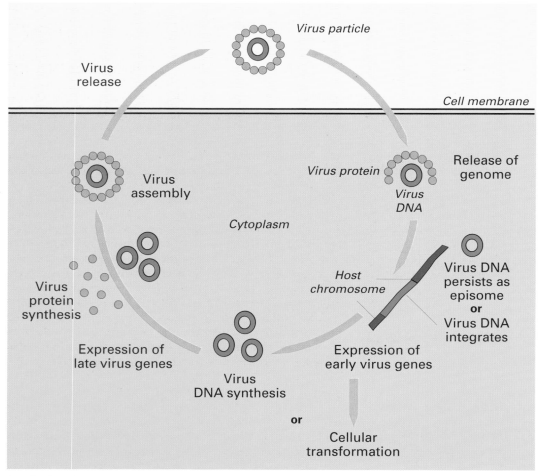

Fig. 9.70 Life cycle of an oncogenic DNA virus. After entry into the cell the DNA may integrate into the host cell genome or persist as an episome. Two alternative pathways then exist: (a) expression of some of the early genes, followed by cellular transformation; or (b) synthesis of viral DNA and protein, followed by virus assembly and release.

are the adenoviruses, the herpes viruses, the papoviruses, the pox viruses, and the hepadna viruses.

Adenoviruses Oncogenic adenoviruses of animals are known, e.g. CELO virus of chickens or simian adenovirus type 5. However, most studies have been carried out with the human adenoviruses, of which there are now over 40 different serotypes, only some of which have oncogenic potential. Some of these viruses are common in human populations causing, for the most part, mild infections of the respiratory tract and upper gastrointestinal (GI) tract. Such infections will pass off as 'colds' or 'gastric flu'. They may be associated with rather more severe infections of the eye (conjunctivitis). There is, to date, no evidence that these viruses can cause cancer in humans, although it is clear that they are capable of transforming human cells in culture. They, therefore, do have oncogenic potential in man and may yet be found to play a role in human cancer.

The different serotypes of adenovirus vary in their oncogenic potency, as measured in experimental systems (usually rat or hamster cells in culture). Adenovirus type 12 (Ad12), for example, is strongly oncogenic, whereas type 2 (Ad2) is only weakly oncogenic. Others have apparently no oncogenic potential. Cells transformed by adenoviruses (Fig. 9.71) do not shed virus; indeed, no infectious virus can be recovered from the cells because transformation is brought about by integration of only part of the adenovirus genome. While the extent of the integrated virus genome varies from one transformation event to another, it always includes the early genes (*E1A* and *E1B*) which are therefore thought to be responsible for transformation. The presence of the virus in the cell can also be demonstrated by immunofluorescence techniques, since adenovirus-transformed cells display strong, new, virus-specific antigens (these are often termed T-antigens or transformation antigens) which are largely (but not exclusively) nuclear in location.

Adenovirus 12 causes tumours of several types on inoculation into rats, the tumour type depending on the site of inoculation. Similarly, rat cells transformed *in vitro* by Ad12 will always grow into tumours in syngeneic animals. However, although Ad2 will transform rat cells in culture, these cells, with rare exceptions, do not grow into tumours when inoculated into syngeneic rats. It can be shown, however, that if Ad2 transformed rat cells are inoculated into immune suppressed animals or into athymic (nude) mice, tumours will be formed, showing that in the case of virus-transformed cells at least, the immune system plays a vital role in controlling tumour formation.

Herpes virus There are several animal herpes viruses with oncogenic potential. Lucke virus causes kidney tumours in frogs while Marek's disease virus causes an economically important disease in the domestic chicken. The main features of Marek's disease are peripheral neuropathy and lymphomatous tumours. A live virus vaccine (originally attenuated by growth in turkeys, but more recently an antigenically related turkey herpes virus) has been in use very extensively for many years. The savings to the poultry industry are substantial. This is of

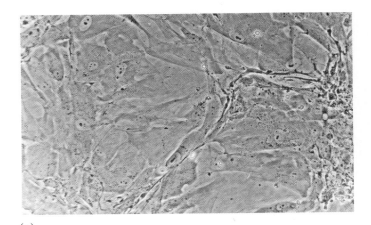

(a)

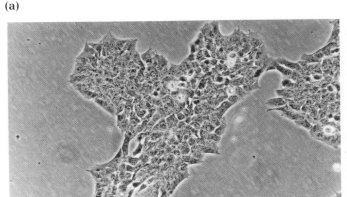

(b)

Fig. 9.71 Cellular transformation by virus. (a) Normal primary human retinoblast cells; (b) the same cells after transformation with the *E1* gene of human adenovirus type 5. (Courtesy of P. Gallimore.)

particular interest in view of the increasing evidence that some human cancers are virus-associated.

There are six human herpes viruses; herpes virus type 1 (labialis or HSV1) herpes virus type 2 (genitalis or HSV2); cytomegalovirus (CMV); varicella zoster virus (VSV or chickenpox); Epstein–Barr virus (EBV); and the recently discovered human herpes virus type 6 (HHV6). There is no evidence that VSV is directly associated with neoplasia. It has been suggested that CMV is associated with some cancers, such as Kaposi's sarcoma in AIDS patients, but there really is no evidence that this is anything other than an opportunistic infection. HHV6 has only recently been recognized, but already there are suggestions that it may play a role in some lymphomas.

The main associations of human herpes viruses with cancer are of HSV1 with oral cancer; HSV2 with carcinoma of the cervix; and EBV with both Burkitt's lymphoma and nasopharyngeal carcinoma. The evidence for association of HSV1 with oral cancer is weak. Reports of the presence of HSV1 genome in oral cancers are hard to distinguish from the presence of infectious virus in these tissues. The suggestion that HSV2 is involved in cervical cancer was based on evidence that is now in some doubt. The current view is that while there is some association, it is more likely that the virus, at most, plays only a supporting role in a cancer caused primarily by other agencies. The epidemiology of carcinoma of the cervix strongly suggests that a sexually transmitted agent is involved in its aetiology. This disease is commoner in women with an early age at first intercourse and in women with multiple sexual partners or whose husbands or consorts have had multiple sexual partners. This evidence, however, does not specifically implicate HSV2. HSV DNA was also sometimes demonstrated in cervical lesions but, once again, it is hard to distinguish this from low-grade productive herpes infection. HSV 1 and HSV 2 do have the potential to transform animal cells in culture, but there are only rare reports of transformation of human cells. Moreover, in HSV-transformed cells persistent DNA cannot normally be demonstrated, suggesting that if the virus is involved in the transformation event it must be by a 'hit and run' mechanism.

Epstein–Barr virus (EBV) is a very common virus with which a high percentage of the population is infected at an early age. In small children it causes inapparent or mild infections, leading to persistent latent infection which ensures long-lasting immunity to further infection.

In previously uninfected young adults EBV causes glandular fever (infectious mononucleosis). For most countries of the world, therefore, this is a relatively innocuous virus, but in two instances EBV is associated with neoplasia. In tropical Africa and some other tropical regions a particular type of malignant lymphoma—African or Burkitt's lymphoma—affects young children living in areas that can be defined fairly precisely by climatic criteria (mean temperature over 60 °C and mean rainfall over 20 inches per annum). These criteria also describe the distribution of the malaria-carrying mosquito. Mr Dennis Burkitt, an English surgeon, documented this distribution and suggested an aetiology involving an arthropod-borne virus. While this proved to be incorrect, the research generated by his observation led to the discovery of EBV, which is closely associated with the disease. Moreover it transforms human B-cells in culture and causes lymphoma in some classes of primates (notably cotton-top tamarins). The viral genome persists within transformed cells, usually in episomal form, though some examples of integration are reported. Usually the entire genome is retained and some transformed lines regularly produce infectious virus. However, in most cells of a transformed population only limited regions of the genome are expressed, and much research is now focused on those genes that are expressed in cancer cells and transformed cells.

The geographic distribution of the disease is thought to be due to an interaction of EBV with cells in individuals where the lymphoid system has been disturbed by the presence of malaria. The precise aetiological mechanisms are not known. Burkitt's lymphoma can, however, occur (though rarely) in subjects who are EBV negative. These B-cell lymphomas have characteristic translocations involving the c-myc oncogene on chromosome 8 and one of the immunoglobulin genes on chromosome 14 (IgH), 2 (Igκ), or 22 (Igλ). This is true of both EBV positive and EBV negative cases. It seems probable that the virus is in some way linked to the translocation process and that it is this translocation that leads on to neoplastic development.

Burkitt's tumour is a disease of children in Africa and not of children of African origin—its aetiology is firmly linked to local environmental conditions. The other EBV-associated cancer, nasopharyngeal carcinoma, occurs in South-East Asia (particularly in SE China) or in people who come from that region and live in other places, e.g. Chinese in Singapore. Again the association with the virus is strong. The virus persists in the cells of nasopharyngeal carcinoma and a specific group of viral genes is expressed in these cells (Fig. 9.72). Recent evidence, however, has shown that in China, and also in the UK, normal individuals may carry EBV in cells of the nasopharynx. It seems likely, therefore, that the aetiology of this disease involves a genetic susceptibility to EBV infection of perhaps twofold in some members of the population. Co-factors enhance the probability of transformation, e.g. plant toxins, smoking, hard drugs, and certain preserved foodstuffs. Workers handling croton oil have a 27-fold increase in incidence of nasopharyngeal carcinoma.

Papova viruses This group of small DNA viruses is named after

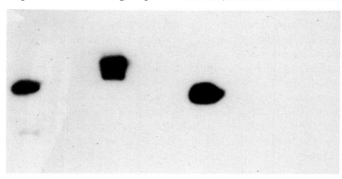

(a)

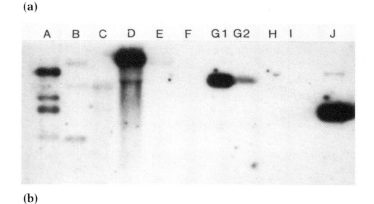

(b)

Fig. 9.72 Expression of EBV genes in nasopharyngeal carcinoma (NPC). Cloned EBV DNA fragments cleaved with restriction enzymes *Eco*RI + *Bam*HI (A–C) or *Eco*RI alone (D–J) and separated by size on an agarose gel by electrophoresis. The DNA hybridized with radioactive RNA from (a) normal lymphocytes from an EBV-negative subject, and (b) nasopharyngeal carcinoma cells. (a) Shows regions of cross-homology with normal cells; (b) all the other bands represent specific expression of EBV genes in NPC. (Courtesy of J. Arrand.)

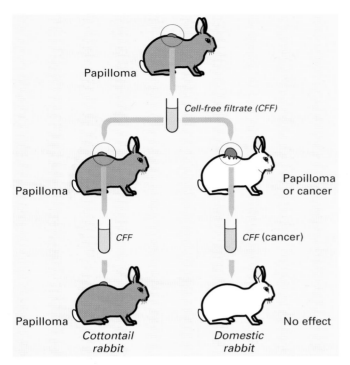

Fig. 9.73 Shope rabbit papilloma virus. The virus from papillomas may be transmitted to other rabbits but the resulting lesion is dependent on the strain of rabbit. Infectious virus is not normally recovered from malignant lesions.

loma virus of the wild cottontail rabbit could also be transmitted in this way (Fig. 9.73). The cell-free extracts also caused papillomas (and not infrequently carcinomas) in the domestic rabbit. Carcinoma formation was uncommon in the natural host and while the papillomas contained the transmissible agent, the carcinomas did not. This difference between strains of rabbit is an excellent example of genetic–environmental interaction.

Little futher work was done with the papilloma viruses until very recently, when two observations stimulated interest. First, Jarrett showed that the bovine papilloma virus (BPV), which was known to be associated with oesophageal papilloma in cattle, was also associated with carcinoma in animals that had grazed on marginal hill-land. Bracken fern, which grows on this land, was known to contain a potent toxin and it seems likely that the development of carcinomas is due to the promoting effect of bracken fern toxin on the pre-existing, benign, virus-induced lesions.

It also proved possible to grow BPV in tissue culture and show that it had transforming potential. This was important since one of the main stumbling blocks to the study of the human papilloma viruses (HPV) was the failure to grow the virus in culture. The second observation was the demonstration, using recombinant DNA techniques, that HPV was commonly associated with human carcinoma of the cervix. It also became possible to subdivide the HPV isolates into classes depending on the degree of DNA homology, and it was found that there were many different HPV strains, each being associated with a particular type of pathology. For example, types 6 and 11 are generally associated with benign lesions of the uterine cervix ('warty atypia') whereas HPV-16 and HPV-18 are associated with cervical intra-epithelial neoplasia (CIN) and frank neoplasia (Fig. 9.74). A causal relationship between HPV-16, HPV-18, and cervical carcinoma is not yet proven, but if it can be shown that those normal women who carry HPV-16 are

three members, *pa*pilloma, *po*lyoma, and *va*cuolating virus (better known as simian virus 40, SV40). The papilloma viruses were first recognized in the early part of this century when human warts (papillomas) were found to be transmissible with cell-free extracts. In the 1930s Shope discovered that the papil-

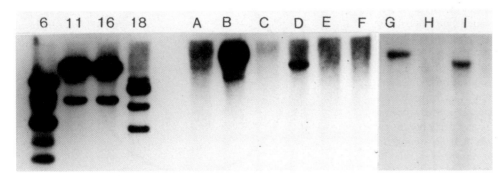

Fig. 9.74 Human papilloma virus (HPV) in lesions of the uterine cervix. DNA from cervical biopsies (A–I) is digested with the restriction enzyme *Bam*HI and the fragments of differing size separated by electrophoresis on an agarose gel. Lanes marked 6, 11, 16, and 18 contain controls of DNA from HPV-6, -11, -16, and -18 and are hybridized with a ^{32}P-labelled mixed human papilloma virus DNA probe. The other lanes are normal cervix (A), squamous cervical cancers (B, G), non-specific inflammatory cervices (E, F, H), cervical intra-epithelial neoplasia stage III (C), CIN II (D), koilocytosis (I). A specific ^{32}P-labelled probe shows that lanes D and I contained HPV-16. Lanes B and G (the carcinoma) also hybridize specifically with HPV-16 but the higher molecular weight suggests that the virus is integrated into the host cell genome. (Courtesy of J. Arrand.)

more at risk of carcinoma of the cervix than those who carry HPV-6, -11, or no virus at all, then there will be a basis for considering HPV to be the cause of cervical cancer. It is very probable, however, that the virus may interact with other known aetiological factors (e.g. cigarette smoking).

The genome of the papilloma viruses normally persists in cells in a non-integrated episomal form. Infectious virus is produced only in cells that are undergoing terminal differentiation, so that keratinocyte cell-culture systems, which do not fully differentiate, will not support growth of the virus. (This problem has recently been overcome by growing epithelial cells on floating rafts of collagen gel containing suitable connective tissue cells.) In some instances, particularly in malignant lesions, the virus becomes integrated into the host cell genome and some lines of cells derived from carcinoma of the cervix (e.g. HeLa cells), which have been cultured for very many years, have been shown to contain integrated HPV genome. Such cells do not produce infectious particles and it seems probable that this explains Shope's observation on rabbit papilloma virus.

Polyoma virus is a mouse virus, which was first recognized as a contaminating virus in preparations of mouse leukaemia virus. First known as parotid tumour virus, its current name—polyoma—indicates that it causes tumours in a variety of tissues of the mouse. It readily transforms cells in culture and the cellular transformation assay using polyoma virus in BHK (baby hamster kidney) cells provided the first truly quantitative system for measuring the oncogenic potential of a virus. While largely an experimental tool, its study has advanced understanding of how tumour viruses exert their effect on cells and how the host animal responds to virus-induced tumours. Its molecular structure is completely known and the transforming genes identified (Fig. 9.75). Attention is now focused on the function of these gene products.

The third member of the papova group is the well known and much studied SV40 virus. Isolated originally as a contaminant of monkey kidney cultures in which poliovirus vaccine was being prepared, it is one of very few viruses which can transform human cells in culture. Such transformed cells are usually highly unstable and after a period of rapid growth enter a 'crisis' phase, when growth slows down and often ceases altogether. However, in some cases clones of SV40-transformed cells emerge from crisis to form stable cell lines of unlimited growth potential. SV40 has not been associated with any human neoplasm, even though large numbers of people are known to have been infected with the virus. In particular, some early batches of 'killed' polio vaccine were contaminated with live SV40 and the inoculated population has been closely monitored but no unusual cancer incidence has been noted. As an experimental tool, SV40 is invaluable. Its molecular structure is fully known and its transforming genes cloned (Fig. 9.76). SV40 has now been used in various truncated forms as a cloning vector and, in particular, the origin of replication and promoter sequences have been incorporated into many vectors now widely used.

Normally SV40 virus and polyoma virus persist in cells by integration into the host cell genome. Unlike the adenoviruses, the whole genome usually integrates so that by using specific

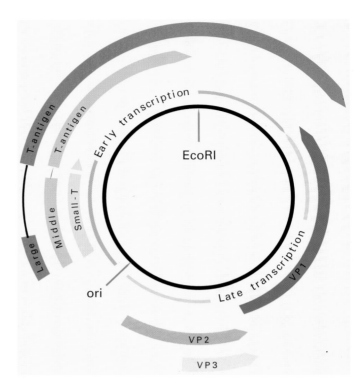

Fig. 9.75 Genome of polyoma virus. *Eco*RI, site of DNA cutting by restriction endonuclease *Eco*RI; ori, origin of replication; VP1, 2, 3, capsid (i.e. outer) proteins.

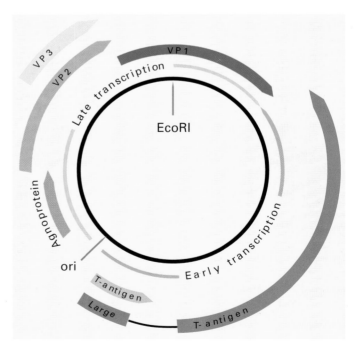

Fig. 9.76 Genome of SV40 virus. *Eco*RI, site of DNA cutting by restriction endonuclease *Eco*RI; ori, origin of replication; VP1, 2, 3, capsid (i.e. outer) proteins.

stimuli, such as iododeoxyuridine, the virus can be 'rescued' from transformed cells. Two human viruses which resemble polyoma and SV40 have been discovered. BK virus was named after the immunosuppressed kidney transplant patient from whom it was first isolated. It has transforming potential in cell culture and, while there is no known human pathology, a proportion of the population have antibodies against the virus, which is isolated only from the urine of immune-deficient patients. Similarly, JC virus, isolated from the brain of a patient with the degenerative brain disease, progressive multifocal leukoencephalopathy (see Chapter 27), transforms rodent cells in culture but has not, so far, been associated with any human neoplasm.

Pox viruses Many members of this group have the potential to stimulate cell growth. Vaccinia virus was first assayed on the chicken chorioallantoic membrane because of 'pocks' caused by focal cellular proliferation. Vaccinia virus, however, is not known to have oncogenic potential. Two viruses of this group are known to cause neoplasms in animals; the Shope fibroma virus of rabbits and the Yaba and Tana viruses of monkeys. The only 'oncogenic' human member of the group is the agent of molluscum contageosum, a benign spreading skin lesion with a raised edge and a flat centre. Sometimes transmitted by sexual contact, it may also be transmitted by other means and affect any part of the body.

Hepadna viruses Hepatitis B virus is a major human pathogen, causing debilitating and often fatal disease in huge numbers of people, particularly in the Third World countries (see Chapter 17). It has been shown in these countries, particularly in South-East Asia, that primary liver cancer is much more common in those who have had hepatitis and who have become chronic carriers than in those who have not. In one study the risk factor was 200-fold—a huge risk that dwarfs even the tenfold elevated risk of lung cancer in cigarette smokers. While this epidemiological relationship is clear, the precise role of the virus in inducing liver cancer is not. The virus DNA has been recognized in primary liver cancer cells in hepatitis-infected patients; however, it has also been found in the non-malignant cirrhotic livers of post-hepatitis patients. While elucidation of the mechanism of oncogenesis would be of considerable interest, it is clear that this information is not necessary to prevent the disease. If hepatitis can be prevented, hepatocellular carcinoma will also be prevented. Vaccines have now been developed against hepatitis. These are of three kinds: subunit vaccines prepared from the blood plasma of infected patients; genetically engineered subunit vaccines; and live vaccines prepared by inserting hepatitis B virus genes into vaccine strains of vaccinia virus (Fig. 9.77). Trials of these vaccines are now in progress, but each of them has problems. The former two vaccines are expensive, relatively unstable (requiring refrigeration), and to be effective multiple inoculations must be given. These features make their delivery in the Third World difficult. The vaccinia-based vaccines overcome these problems, but there is growing anxiety about the use of live vaccines in

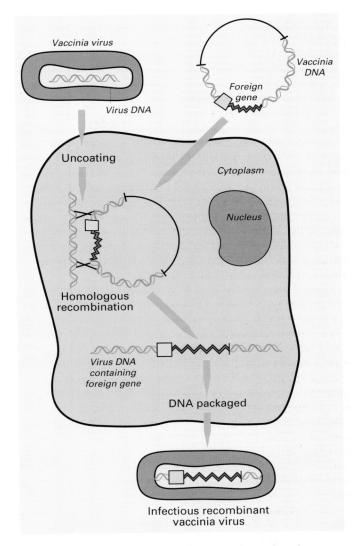

Fig. 9.77 Recombinant vaccinia viruses can be made to incorporate genes of other viruses. A susceptible cell is infected with a vaccine strain of vaccinia virus and a plasmid vector containing the gene to be incorporated and sequences from vaccinia. Homologous recombination within the cell gives a recombinant virus, which is packaged and released as infectious virus.

populations where AIDS is common or may become common in the near future.

These problems must be overcome since, world-wide, viruses are now recognized as one of the most important associations of cancer. As we have seen with Marek's disease in chickens, virus-induced cancers can be prevented.

RNA oncogenic viruses (retroviruses)

The RNA retroviruses are a heterogeneous group of small viruses of man and animals, that are not usually associated with a pathology other than the neoplastic pathology which characterizes the virus. Exceptions to this generalization are the immunodeficiency viruses of the lentivirus group, which appear to be associated with neoplasia only secondarily; and possibly, the feline leukaemia viruses, which also cause immuno-suppression. Many of the retroviruses, however, exist within the host animal apparently causing no pathological lesions at all. These endogenous viruses may play a secondary role in determining patterns of neoplasia.

The genetic material of retroviruses is in the form of single-stranded RNA (Fig. 9.78). In the long-latency leukaemia viruses there are three genes: *gag*, which encodes the internal proteins; *pol*, which encodes the reverse transcriptase; and *env*, which encodes the envelope proteins. These genes are flanked by a short repeat sequence, a 5′ unique sequence (U_5), and a 3′ unique sequence (U_3) which contains the regulatory elements for viral transcription. On integration the U_5 sequence is duplicated at the 3′ end of the genome and the U_3 sequence at the 5′ end. These, now symmetrical, structures flanking the genome are known as the long terminal repeats (LTRs), which contain the virus promoting and enhancing sequences.

Broadly, the transforming retroviruses can be divided into two groups: fast transforming and slow transforming. The latter group (which includes mouse mammary tumour virus, avian leukosis virus, and some mouse leukaemia viruses) do not transform cells readily in culture. *In vivo*, however, it can be shown that they integrate a DNA copy of the virus genome into the host cell genome close to a significant host cell gene to cause neoplasia. It can further be shown that it is not necessary for the entire virus genome to integrate. The critical region is the long terminal repeat (LTR). Thus abnormal expression of a cellular gene under the control of a virus promotor may lead to neoplasia.

The fast-transforming retroviruses are highly efficient at cellular transformation (approaching 100 per cent). They include all the sarcoma viruses of both rodents and birds, and several cell-type-specific leukaemia viruses. It appears that these viruses have been derived in an evolutionary sense from the slow-transforming leukosis viruses. A partial deletion permits the inclusion within the virus genome of a new DNA sequence or sequences, the viral oncogenes (v-*onc*), which show DNA homology to normal cellular counterparts (the cellular proto-oncogenes—c-*onc* genes). These latter have specific functions concerned with the control of cell division. It is generally agreed that these viruses are chimeric, i.e. that the *onc* gene sequence is derived from the cellular homologue at some point in the evolution of the virus. Following transformation by these retroviruses, the v-*onc* gene is integrated into the cellular genome under the direct control of the LTR regions. Cell culture systems using such viruses can be used for the quantitive assay of transformation. Because of the deletion in the genome, these viruses are usually defective in replication functions. In practice, they frequently infect cells in conjunction with a *helper* virus, usually a leukaemia or leukosis virus, which may be endogenous to the cell or animal infected, or may be transmitted along with the fast-transforming virus. The defective virus genome is replicated and becomes enclosed within a virus particle made up of proteins coded for by the helper virus. Thus the specificity of the virus, which depends upon the recognition of specific antigenic determinants on the cell surface, is dependent upon the helper virus and not the fast-transforming virus. This can be used experimentally to alter or extend the host range of the virus.

Retroviruses are released from the cell surface by a process of budding. Thus, unlike the DNA viruses, the RNA retroviruses do not kill the cells they infect, and transformed cells normally continue to shed virus. Non-producer cells also occur.

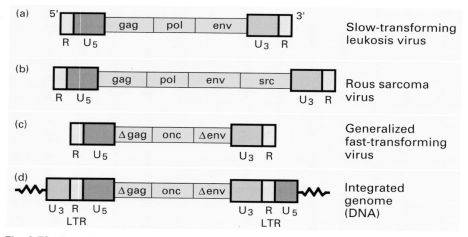

Fig. 9.78 Retrovirus genomes. (a) The basic structure of a slow-transforming retrovirus; R, repeat sequence; U_3 and U_5, unique 3′ and 5′ sequences; *gag*, *pol*, and *env* are virus genes for internal proteins, reverse transcriptase, and envelope proteins, respectively. (b) Rous chicken sarcoma virus (RSV) shows incorporation of *src* gene derived from the c-*src* cellular proto-oncogene. Note that, unusually, some strains of RSV are not deleted. (c) More usually, the virus genes are deleted to accommodate the *onc* gene. (d) When the RNA genome is incorporated into the host-cell genome the U_3 region is duplicated at the 5′ end and the U_5 region is duplicated at the 3′ end to form the now symmetrical long terminal repeats (LTR) which contain promoting and enhancing sequences.

Mouse mammary tumour virus (MMTV) was first recognized as a factor in milk which could transmit mammary tumours from one generation to the next. Some inbred strains of mice have a high spontaneous incidence of mammary tumours while some have a low incidence. It was shown by Bittner, in the 1930s, that if animals from a low-incidence strain were suckled on a high-incidence mother they developed mammary carcinomas. Conversely, offspring of a high-incidence mother failed to develop carcinoma if they were suckled exclusively on a low-incidence mother (Fig. 9.79). The virus proved hard to study because it is difficult to grow in cell culture, but it was demonstrated that the virus could be transmitted not only via the milk but also via germ cells, suggesting an intimate relationship between the virus genome and the genetic material of the host animal. The morphology of the virus is well characterized. The virus particles mature in the cytoplasm of tumour cells (type A particles) and bud through the cell membrane to give mature type B particles (Fig. 9.80). Large numbers of particles may be seen in intercellular spaces. Recent studies on the integration of the virus into the host cell genome of tumour cells show that it occurs in a non-random fashion. Integration sites are found to flank specific host cell sequences, which have been termed *int* genes (which are members of a family of *onc* genes which includes the fibroblast growth factor genes). It appears that the virus genome causes inappropriate expression of these sequences and that this is associated with malignant behaviour of the cells. It is of particular interest that the human *int 2* gene is located in the same chromosome region as the progesterone receptor gene.

Leukaemia/sarcoma complex This large group of RNA retro-viruses is found in many different species, including chicken, turkey, mouse, rat, cat, cattle, monkeys, and man. The basic genomic structure shows variation from one strain to another. In many cases the viruses appear to be carried by the host without any pathological effect. Such endogenous viruses can, however, play an important role by interacting with other retroviruses with which the host becomes infected. Viruses of one species may infect other species. Such xenotropic viruses may show an altered and often more aggressive pathology in the new host species.

Chicken leukosis virus is widespread in chicken stocks and can cause serious loss of stock. The virus replicates by assembling new virus directly beneath the cell membrane to form budding particles which mature to form type C particles (Fig. 9.80). It is a non-defective retrovirus and appears to be the prototype from which both the sarcoma viruses and the fast-transforming leukaemia viruses were derived. These latter viruses have been found to harbour v-*onc* genes and these have become the subject of intensive study, e.g. avian myelocytosis virus (v-*myc*), avian myeloblastosis virus (v-*myb*), avian erythroblastosis virus (v-*erb A* and v-*erb B*). V-*myc* and v-*myb* products are located in the nucleus, v-*erb A* is cytoplasmic while v-*erb B* is in the plasma membrane. The precise functions of *myc*, *myb*, and *erb A* are unknown, but *erb B* is a truncated form of the epidermal growth factor (EGF) gene.

The most widely studied virus is the chicken sarcoma virus, or Rous sarcoma virus (RSV). It is transmissible from one bird to another by inoculation and produces tumours at the site of inoculation. In young birds it may cause large haemorrhagic lesions. It causes a systemic infection, since tumours can be produced at sites distant from the site of inoculation by minor

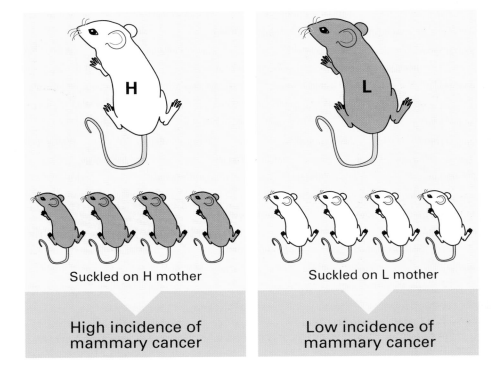

Suckled on H mother

Suckled on L mother

High incidence of mammary cancer

Low incidence of mammary cancer

Fig. 9.79 Mouse mammary tumour virus (MMTV). Bittner's experiment demonstrating transmission of MMTV in the milk (milk factor). H, high-incidence strain; L, low-incidence strain.

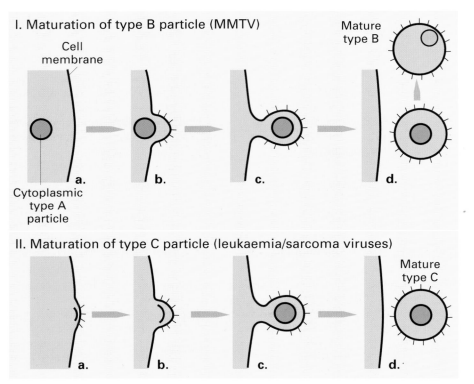

I. Maturation of type B particle (MMTV)

Cell membrane

Mature type B

Cytoplasmic type A particle

a.   b.   c.   d.

II. Maturation of type C particle (leukaemia/sarcoma viruses)

Mature type C

a.   b.   c.   d.

Fig. 9.80 Retrovirus morphology. I (a) The central nucleoid of mouse mammary tumour virus (MMTV) forms in the cytoplasm (type A particle); (b) as it approaches the membrane, modification of the membrane becomes apparent; (c) a 'bud' is formed; and (d) the particle separates from the cell. In the mature form the nucleoid often appears darker and eccentric (type B morphology). II (a) In the case of the type C particle there is no cytoplasmic particle; the nucleoid begins to assemble directly under the plasma membrane, which then becomes modified; (b) a bud begins to form; (c) the now complete nucleoid is within the bud. (d) The mature type C particle usually has a concentric nucleoid.

trauma. Discovered by Rous in 1910, it became amenable to detailed experimentation when Temin and Rubin described a quantitative tissue culture assay in 1958. It was Temin who showed that RSV passed through a DNA phase of its life cycle, thus opening the way to the discovery of 'reverse transcriptase'; the RNA-primed DNA polymerase that characterizes this whole group of viruses (Fig. 9.81). RSV contains within its genome a sequence termed v-src, which is homologous to a cellular sequence c-src that codes for a membrane-associated protein (pp60[src]) with tyrosine kinase activity. The v-src gene has strong transforming activity and confers on RSV the characteristic of a rapidly transforming virus. There are many different strains of RSV, each with slightly different characteristics. Most are defective and require a helper virus (usually one of the chicken leukosis viruses) for successful replication.

The same general pattern emerges from a study of the rodent RNA retroviruses. Mouse leukaemia viruses are non-defective viruses of type C morphology. They are of several different kinds, causing both lymphoid leukaemia (Gross and Moloney viruses) or myeloid leukaemia (Graafi virus and Friend virus). They do not transform mouse fibroblasts in culture. The mouse and rat sarcoma viruses are, on the other hand, defective transforming viruses with incorporated oncogenes. The two best-known strains are those discovered by Harvey and by Kirsten which contain the v-Ha-ras and v-Ki-ras genes, respectively. The cellular homologues of these genes have now been extensively studied in their own right and activation by mutation of the c-Ha-ras gene may be an important step in cellular trans-

formation. The mutant form of the gene is present in some cultured tumour cells and in some specific tumours.

Feline leukaemia virus has been shown by Jarrett to be a horizontally transmissible virus that causes a lymphoid leukaemia, especially in domestic cats in multi-cat households. Experimental infection of kittens by housing them with an infected cat is associated with a viraemic phase, followed, in a proportion of cases, by leukaemia after a latent period of some months. Casual contact of adult cats in a normal outdoors environment may lead to infection, but this is more often followed by immunity, sometimes associated with a virus carrier state, than by leukaemia. Infection with this virus may also be associated with a degree of immunosuppression. A successful vaccine has been developed and is used widely for valuable pedigree cats. Feline sarcoma virus is a strongly transforming defective virus which contains the v-fes oncogene.

Bovine lymphomatosis is an economically important disease caused by bovine lymphomatosis virus (BLV). This non-defective RNA retrovirus is transmissible from animal to animal, but only a proportion of the infected animals develop the disease. It is also of interest that it appears to be related, both in terms of its biological behaviour and its structure, to the human retroviruses HTLV-I and HTLV-II (see below).

There have been many claims that human leukaemia is associated with a virus. Most of the early reports were based on the recognition of 'virus-like particles' using the electron microscope, but these reports can be dismissed as artefacts. Now clear evidence has emerged that at least one kind of human leuk-

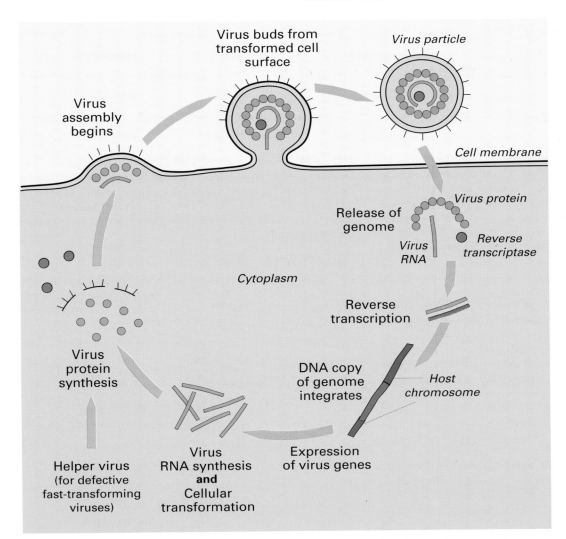

Fig. 9.81 Life cycle of oncogenic RNA virus. The virus enters the cell and then, by means of a reverse transcriptase enzyme contained within the particle, a DNA copy is made which integrates into the host cell genome. A susceptible cell is transformed but may also release infectious virus particles by budding from the cell surface. In the case of defective viruses, the production of new virus is dependent upon co-infection with a non-defective helper virus.

aemia, adult acute T-cell leukaemia, is virus-associated. The virus was first described in patients with mycosis fungoides, a condition that manifests skin infiltration with leukaemic lymphoid cells (see Chapter 28). However, it was soon shown that there was a specific association of this type-C RNA retrovirus with adult acute T-cell leukaemia and the virus was named human T-cell lymphotrophic virus (HTLV-I). This virus is capable of transforming human T-lymphocytes stimulated with T-cell growth factor, interleukin-2 (IL-2). It is endemic in specific geographical regions, notably southern Japan and parts of the Carribean. In these areas a substantial proportion of the population carry the virus, although only a relatively small number of carriers develop the disease. A second related virus, HTLV-II has been isolated from a small number of cases.

Lentiviruses These 'slow viruses' were first discovered in domestic animals, e.g. Visna virus of sheep. They have a long incubation period and are associated with slowly progressing degenerative disease. When the virus associated with human acquired immunodeficiency syndrome (AIDS) was first isolated by Montagnier and by Gallo, it was at first thought to be related to HTLV-I and HTLV-II and was called HTLV-III by Gallo, but lymphocyte-associated virus (LAV) by Montagnier. The virus of AIDS, now termed human immunodeficiency virus (HIV), is now considered to be a member of the lentivirus group. Its association with neoplasia appears to be indirect. Patients with AIDS develop Kaposi's sarcoma, a spreading skin lesion, at multiple sites. It has been suggested that this may be caused by another agent, but enabled to spread because of the patient's immunological incompetence. Evidence is now also emerging that patients with AIDS may have an increased risk of leukaemia and lymphoma; this would be similar to the observed increase of these diseases in the inherited immune deficiency diseases.

Chemical carcinogenesis

Introduction

Much of the evidence that human cancer may be caused by chemical substances comes from classical epidemiological studies beginning in the eighteenth century with the observations by Hill on nasal cancers in snuff takers; and by Percival Pott on scrotal cancers induced by soots and tars in chimney sweeps; more recently there is the demonstration by Doll and Bradford Hill that carcinoma of the bronchus is caused by smoking cigarettes (see Section 9.7).

While epidemiology can point to situations where a chemical is likely to be involved in the aetiology of a cancer, it is only in exceptional cases that the specific carcinogen can be identified. Often in industrial situations complex mixtures are being used and laboratory studies have been necessary to identify the specific carcinogenic compounds. Similarly, in the case of cigarette smoking it has been shown that a large number of different carcinogenic materials are present among the hundreds of chemicals of which cigarette smoke is composed; but it is hard to say which are the important substances for lung cancer induction.

Sometimes materials that are clearly associated with human cancer are not readily demonstrated to be carcinogenic in experimental animals, e.g. 2-naphthylamine, which was clearly shown to be a human bladder carcinogen, is not carcinogenic in rodents and is carcinogenic in dogs only at high dose levels. Similarly arsenic, which has been shown by epidemiological studies to cause skin carcinomas in man, has only recently been shown to be weakly carcinogenic in animals. This highlights one of the principal difficulties of studying human carcinogens in experimental animals—different species handle chemical substances in different ways, and carcinogenic potential in one or more animal species does not necessarily mean that the compound is a human carcinogen. The convention has been adopted, however, that the demonstration of carcinogenicity in one species is an indication that chemicals should be considered as a potential hazard in man. This seems sensible but there are problems even with such a pragmatic solution. Some substances may cause cancer in animals only after the administration of huge doses, so great in fact that human exposure at such dose levels is highly improbable. One such example is saccharin, where there is some evidence of weak carcinogenicity in rodents and where the Food and Drug Administration (FDA) of the USA require a health warning to be placed on packets of saccharin tablets; but the actual risk to human health is almost certainly very small. Similarly, comparable weak evidence of carcinogenicity of the artificial sweeteners, cyclamates, led to their total ban in the UK.

The definition of a chemical carcinogen is not a simple matter. First, some chemicals (promoting agents) enhance the effects of other carcinogens but are not themselves complete carcinogens. Secondly, the range of potency, measured in a standard unit such as weight of compound per kilogram of body weight given at specified intervals, ranges over about seven orders of magnitude from saccharin to aflatoxin B_1, which is a liver carcinogen at exquisitely low doses (Fig. 9.82). Clearly, if a specific chemical has been shown to be associated with human cancer, it is a human carcinogen. However, much of cancer prevention is aimed at identifying potentially carcinogenic compounds to which the human population is exposed or may in the future be exposed, and for which no evidence of human carcinogenicity is available. In practice, several different pieces of information (see below) are considered together to determine carcinogenic risk.

Tests for carcinogenicity

Animal carcinogenicity tests In spite of the difficulties already noted, an important step in attempts to recognize human carcinogens, is to test their carcinogenicity in an experimental

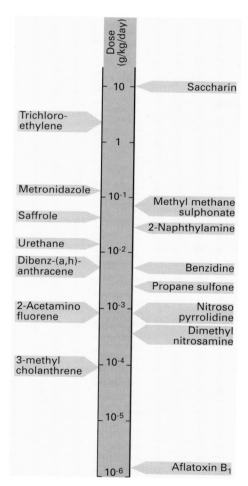

Fig. 9.82 Range of potency of carcinogens expressed as the dose (in g/kg/day) to give 50 per cent of the animals with tumours during lifetime exposure.

animal system. The route of administration may be oral, in food or drinking water; by inoculation into a specific site, e.g. intraperitoneally, subcutaneously, or intradermally; by inhalation; or by painting on to the skin or some other easily accessible organ or tissue. Usually, repeated doses are administered. Normally a group of animals is treated and a similar number kept untreated as controls. The carcinogenicity is then measured in terms of the dose necessary to produce an effect, the number of animals developing tumours, the latent period, and sometimes the rate of growth of tumours. The controls are critical since laboratory animals may have a relatively high spontaneous incidence of cancer. More than one species may be used in these tests. The doses used are often much higher than those to which human populations might be exposed, since cancer induction at low doses may be quite rare even for potent carcinogens, and there are physical and economic limits on the number of animals that can be used.

Nevertheless, a positive result in such a test is taken as evidence of human carcinogenic potential. A full carcinogenicity test on a single species takes at least two years to complete, at enormous cost.

Short-term tests For these reasons much effort has gone into the search for inexpensive, rapid tests, which can predict with reasonable accuracy whether or not a compound is likely to be a carcinogen. A compound may come under suspicion because it is structurally related to a known carcinogen, but that is not enough since it is known that tiny changes in chemical structure may affect carcinogenic potency. There are instances, for example, where one of a pair of stereo-isomers is carcinogenic and the other is not.

Many of the proposed tests have been based on the relationship between mutagenicity and carcinogenicity. If a compound is a mutagen, it is likely to be a carcinogen, since DNA alterations are a critical step in carcinogenesis. Mutagenicity tests in rodents are possible but are again very expensive and slow. At the other extreme, bacterial mutagenicity tests are cheap and rapid, but were at first ruled out because bacteria do not have the capacity to activate carcinogens in the same way as mammals, in which metabolism is a crucial step in the activation of some carcinogens. However, Ames introduced a novel bacterial mutagenicity test which incorporates into the culture medium a liver extract containing microsomal enzymes. This reveals many of the indirect carcinogens that do not show up in conventional bacterial mutagenicity tests (Fig. 9.83). Though not perfect, the Ames test has become one of the useful tests for predicting carcinogenicity and, being quick and cheap, can be used for preliminary screening. It is unlikely that a new material intended for human exposure would go into production if it had a strongly positive Ames test, even without extensive animal testing. However, there are some false negatives and a variety of other tests have been used in conjunction with the Ames test to try to increase accuracy. These include mutation tests in *Drosophila* or yeast, cellular transformation studies, micronucleus tests, and chromosome damage assays. It is now widely accepted that some sort of chromosome damage test,

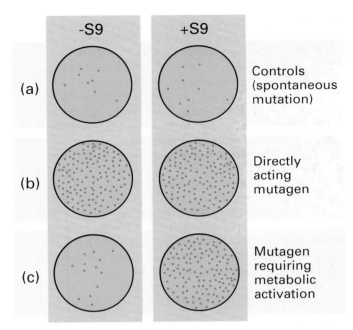

Fig. 9.83 Ames bacterial mutagenicity test. Histidine-requiring mutants of *Salmonella typhimurium* are grown on histidine-deficient medium in the presence of the test chemical with or without the liver microsome metabolizing system (±S9). (a) Spontaneous mutants (colonies on culture medium in Petri dish) which have reverted to histidine auxotrophy; (b) large numbers of mutant colonies with and without the metabolizing system from a directly acting carcinogen; (c) spontaneous mutants only without the metabolizing system, and many mutants with the metabolizing system from a non-direct carcinogen.

preferably in human cells, can complement the Ames test to give an accurate (over 90 per cent) prediction of carcinogenicity that is reasonably quick and inexpensive.

There have been a number of other non-mutation-based tests, e.g. degranulation of the endoplasmic reticulum, but these are of limited usefulness since they usually recognize only specific classes of carcinogen. They may nevertheless be important since the widely used tests based on genotoxicity would miss carcinogens that are non-mutagens, e.g. some promoting agents and agents that cause peroxisome proliferation.

Mode of action of chemical carcinogens

The precise mode of action varies with the particular class of carcinogen. In some cases the mode of action is unknown. For those carcinogens for which we do have some understanding, the carcinogen is known to interact with DNA in one of a number of different ways; for example, by binding to the DNA and causing bulky lesions; by causing specific base alkylation or other specific base damage; by intercalation; by causing double- or single-strand breaks in the DNA; or by cross-linking within or between DNA strands. The cell recognizes DNA damage and uses either constitutive enzymes or enzymes induced as a result of the chemical insult to attempt to repair the damage. Successful (error-free) repair leads to reconstitution of the normal DNA sequence. Some repair systems are 'error prone' and lead to imperfectly repaired DNA, with the insertion of wrong bases or deletions, or even strand switches. This is particularly true when called upon to deal with high levels of damage. Some of these errors will lead to the death of the cell but a proportion of the viable mutations are considered to be the pro-carcinogenic lesions. In some cases repair fails totally, leaving gross chromosome errors and almost certainly cell death. The extent of the ultimate DNA damage following chemical exposure is to some extent dependent upon the replicative state of the cell. If the cell enters a replicative cycle before repair has occurred, the resulting damage as the cell attempts to replicate damaged DNA is likely to be greater. One can demonstrate this experimentally by holding cells in a non-dividing stage for some time after exposure to the carcinogen and demonstrating that fewer cells are killed than if replication is permitted. This measure of repair of potential lethal damage (PLD) is a good general test for cellular repair proficiency (Fig. 9.84). Further details of specific repair pathways are considered below.

Classes of chemical carcinogens

Chemical carcinogens fall into many different structural groups. These include the polynuclear aromatic hydrocarbons, aromatic amines, azodyes, alkylating agents of several different classes, and inorganic carcinogens. Equally, carcinogens may be classified not by their chemical structure but by the way in which they are derived or encountered by the human population, e.g. plant fungal carcinogens; carcinogens in the working environment; carcinogens in food; medicines as carcinogens; and carcinogens in the natural and man-made environment.

Polynuclear (polycyclic) aromatic carcinogens Following the

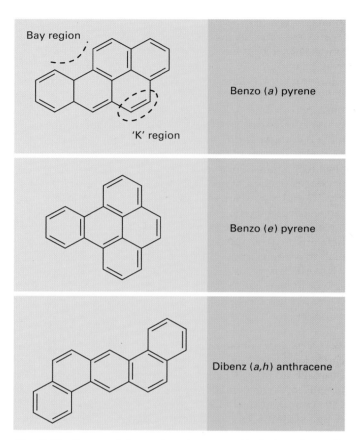

Fig. 9.85 Representative polynuclear aromatic hydrocarbons. For benzo(a)pyrene the 'K region' was thought at one time to be the active site but it is now generally accepted that modification of the bay region is critical for carcinogenic activity.

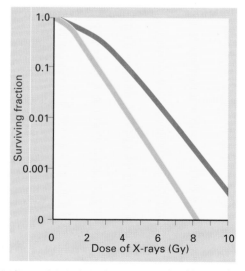

Fig. 9.84 Potential lethal damage repair. Mammalian cells are exposed to X-rays and plated out in growth medium (green line). The surviving fraction is the number of colonies produced at a given dose, expressed as a fraction of the colonies obtained from the same number of unirradiated cells. If plating is delayed for 6 h (red line) some repair occurs before the cells are forced into the cell cycle and hence more cells surive for a given dose of X-rays.

recognition by Yamagiwa and Ichikawa in 1915 that coal tars painted repeatedly on to the ears of rabbits produced cancers, a long search led to the identification of the active constituent as benzo(a)pyrene in 1933. Three years earlier Kennaway had demonstrated the carcinogenicity of dibenz(a,h)anthracene, which was the first chemically pure substance to be shown to be carcinogenic. The polynuclear hydrocarbons vary greatly in their carcinogenic potential (Fig. 9.85). Benzo(a)pyrene is a highly active carcinogen but the closely related benzo(e)pyrene is inactive. Dibenz(a,h)anthracene is a carcinogen of moderate activity.

The polynuclear compounds fall into many different classes and the carcinogenic members of the group are to be found in most of these classes. There is no obvious general structure–activity relationship that extends to all classes of compounds; but within a related group of compounds the structure may give valuable clues to carcinogenic activity. Various properties of the polynuclear carcinogens have been studied in an attempt to identify the critical characteristics of those compounds that exhibited carcinogenic activity. For example, many carcinogenic members have low ionization potentials and many are good electron donors. However, many non-carcinogens also exhibit these properties. One relationship that is, however, of great current interest is the correlation between the reactivities of the dihydrodiol epoxides and carcinogenic activity (see below).

The polycyclic hydrocarbons are not directly acting carcinogens, i.e. they require metabolic activation. They are metabolized in the body principally by the mixed function oxidase system to yield epoxy or hydroxy derivatives. This enzyme system is complex, but the substrate specificity appears to be controlled by the terminal oxidase, cytochrome P_{450} (or more properly, by a family of such cytochromes). The P_{450} enzyme systems are membrane-bound, requiring NADH or NADPH and oxygen; high activity resides in the microsomal fraction of the cell.

The metabolites generated by this system may be further modified by other enzymes, and it is these metabolites that are of particular interest. In the case of carcinogenic members of the group, they are usually termed proximate carcinogens or, if the identity of the metabolite reacting with DNA is known precisely, it is termed the ultimate carcinogen.

Initially, particular interest focused on the metabolites of the 'K region' (Fig. 9.85). It is now widely held that metabolites affecting the 'bay region' are more likely to correlate with carcinogenic activity. In particular, bay region dihydrodiol-epoxides are of interest, though the precise activity varies not only with chemical structure but also with the stereochemistry of different isomers. Thus the (+)-anti-7,8-dihydrodiol-9,10-epoxide of benzo(a)pyrene is the most carcinogenic of the four possible stereoisomers of this metabolite (Fig. 9.86).

It has been known for many years that the polynuclear carcinogens interacted with cellular macromolecules and that covalent binding of benzo(a)pyrene to cellular proteins occurred after metabolism had taken place. Brookes and Lawley in 1964 showed, not only that these hydrocarbons bind to DNA, but that the extent of binding is correlated with carcinogenic potential. This work gives strong support to the somatic mutation hypothesis of cancer induction.

Most of the experimental carcinogenesis studies using polynuclear hydrocarbons were carried out using repeated applications to mouse skin, either alone or in combination with a promoting agent such as the phorbol ester 12-O-tetradecanoyl-phorbol-13-acetate—TPA—(Fig. 9.95), but some work has

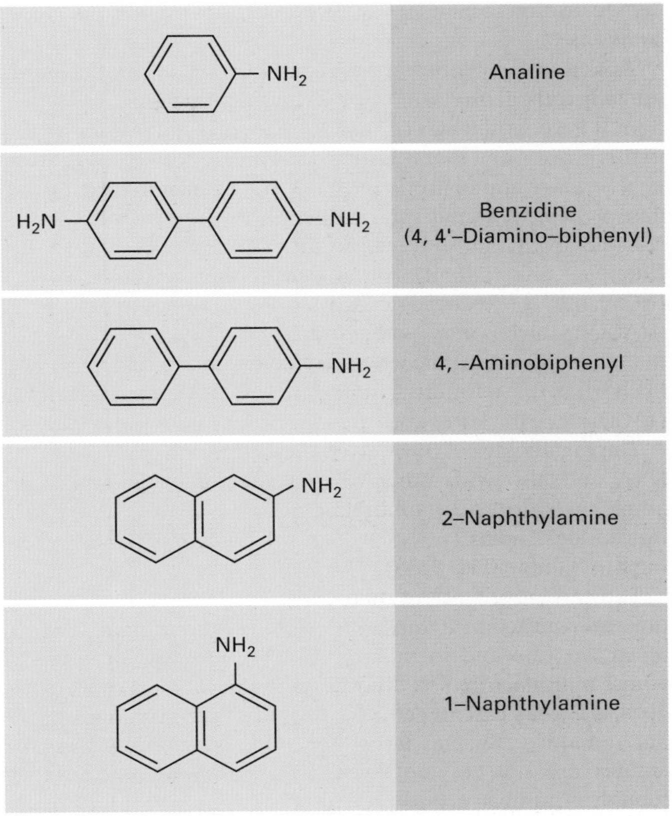

Fig. 9.87 Representative carcinogenic aromatic amines.

also been done using intraperitoneal injections or injection into other tissues. The relative efficacy of many different derivatives of benzo(a)pyrene have been carefully studied. To a lesser extent, the carcinogenic potential of metabolites of other polynuclear hydrocarbons such as benz(a)anthracene, dibenz(a,h)-anthracene and 3-methylcholanthrene have also been studied in these systems. The concept originally derived from the study of benzo(a)pyrene itself, that the bay region dihydrodiol epoxides are of special importance in determining carcinogenic potency, also holds good for these other carcinogens.

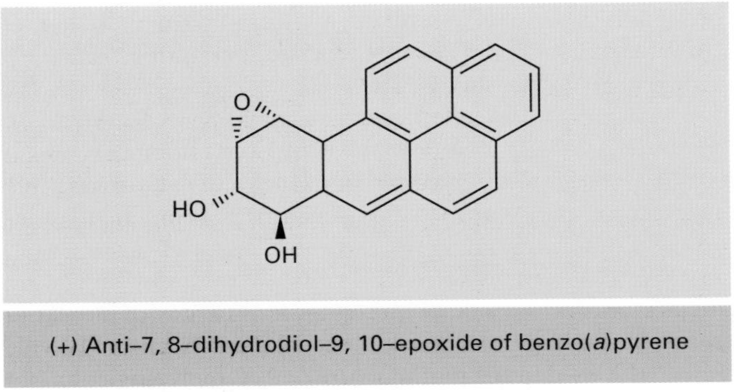

Aromatic amines The early evidence that aromatic amines were human carcinogens came from a study of bladder cancer in workers in the chemical industry in the UK, particularly in the manufacture of analine dyes. Often workers were exposed to several of the suspect chemicals, but in the early 1950s Case and his colleagues showed that 2-naphthylamine (Fig. 9.87) was the most potent bladder carcinogen, while benzidine and 1-naphthylamine were also carcinogenic (though subsequent studies showed that the 1-naphthylamine was probably contaminated with the very potent 2-naphthylamine). Other aromatic amines have subsequently been shown to be human bladder carcinogens (e.g. 4-aminobiphenyl). In addition, experimental studies have shown that some are also carcinogenic in experimental animals systems, although the

(+) Anti–7, 8–dihydrodiol–9, 10–epoxide of benzo(a)pyrene

Fig. 9.86 The most active isomer of benzo(a)pyrene.

demonstration of bladder carcinogenicity has proved difficult in some cases.

As with the polynuclear hydrocarbons, the aromatic amines are indirectly acting carcinogens that require metabolic activation. It is generally agreed that N-hydroxylation is the first step in this process and that this may occur by oxidation of a primary or secondary amino group mediated by the mixed-function oxidase system. Alternatively, reduction of a nitro-, nitroso-, or N-oxide group can also lead to the N-hydroxy derivative. For example, the potent carcinogen 4-nitroquinoline-1-oxide (NQO) may be reduced to 4-hydroxyaminoquinoline-1-oxide (HAQO), which is more potent than the parent compound in the induction of subcutaneous sarcomas in mice. However, it is likely that the ultimate carcinogen is a further metabolite of HAQO, since the latter does not react with nucleophiles *in vitro*.

The metabolites of these aromatic amines react directly with DNA and also with other cellular macromolecules. For example, N-hydroxy-2-naphthylamine reacts with DNA for form nucleoside adducts such as 1-(N-deoxyguanosinyl)-2-naphthylamine (Fig. 9.88).

The carcinogenicity of many different aromatic amines has now been tested in a variety of experimental animal systems, mostly in rats and in mice. Curiously, aniline, the material whose manufacture first drew attention to this class of carcinogens, is a weak carcinogen, causing only spleen tumours in rats but not mice. By and large, the other single-ring aromatic amines are not carcinogenic or only weakly carcinogenic, though a number are potent mutagens. There is no evidence that any are human carcinogens.

The biphenylamines, on the other hand, do contain some human carcinogens, e.g. 4-biphenylamine. However, carcinogenicity of the biphenylamines varies widely in different species and in organ specificity within a single species. 4-BPA is a powerful bladder carcinogen in dogs and rabbits, while in rats it produces mammary and intestinal tumours after a long latent period. There is no evidence of carcinogenicity in the hamster. Benzidine, another human bladder carcinogen, is a weak bladder carcinogen in dogs but causes tumours at other sites in rats and mice; while 2-naphthylamine, possibly the most potent human bladder carcinogen, does not produce bladder cancers

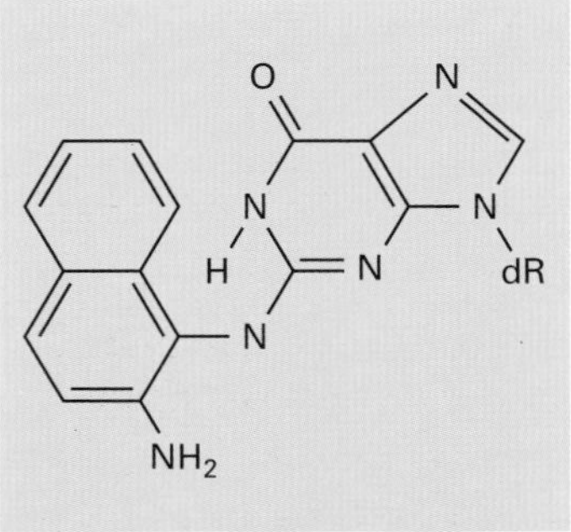

1-(N–deoxyguanosinyl)–2–NA

Fig. 9.88 The DNA adduct formed by 2-naphthylamine(-2-NA).

in mice or rabbits but induces bladder cancers in dogs and monkeys at relatively high doses. These differences almost certainly reflect variation in the metabolism of these compounds in different organs of different species.

Azo dyes The azo dyes are an important group of carcinogens since many have been used in foods, drinks, medicines, and in industrial processes. The best known is probably N,N-dimethyl-4-phenylazoaniline, also called 4-dimethylamino-azobenzene (DAB), or butter yellow, which was commonly used as a colouring material. DAB is a potent liver carcinogen in rats when given orally (i.e. fed continuously in the diet). It also produces bladder tumours in dogs and liver tumours in mice. Tests in other species have been negative, though perhaps the testing was not rigorous. Extensive testing of the derivatives of DAB in liver carcinogenicity tests in rats has shown many to be carcinogenic but others to be non-carcinogens. It appears that the azo group is essential for carcinogenesis.

Many other dyes in common use, such as trypan blue and Evans blue are proven carcinogens, but the closely related vital red appears to be inactive. Amaranth and tartrazine are azo compounds used as food dyes and have been tested for carcinogeneity and found to be negative.

Alkylating agents The alkylating agents, unlike the polynuclear carcinogens and the aromatic amines are direct-acting carcinogens which do not require metabolism for activity. Indeed, many other carcinogens are activated by metabolism to alkylating agents, e.g. nitrosamines and vinyl chloride. The archetypal alkylating agent is mustard gas $ClCH_2CH_2SCH_2CH_2Cl$.

Long known as a mutagen in *Drosophila* and other species, it is now well established as a carcinogen in man and in experimental animal systems. It was also the first carcinogen for which a precise interaction with DNA was chemically defined. Brooks and Lawley in 1960 showed that mustard gas alkylated the N-7 position of guanine both *in vitro* and *in vivo*. The significance of this direct interaction was later strengthened when it was shown that there was a strong positive correlation between alkylation of guanine at the O-6 position by a range of alkylating agents and their carcinogenic potency. O-6 alkylation of guanine appears to be mutagenic by virtue of mispairing with thymine during DNA synthesis, rather than the normal base pairing between guanine and cytosine. *In vitro* there is also a correlation between electrophylic activity and the induction of promutagenic lesions. The more reactive compounds react with the less nucleophilic sites in DNA.

A wide range of alkylating agents have been shown to be carcinogenic. These include many drugs and antibiotics, which have been used or are in common usage; e.g. cytotoxic agents in cancer chemotherapy such as cisplatin, chlorambucil, cyclophosphamide, melphalan, mitomycin-C, as well as nitrogen mustard itself. An even more extensive range of alkylating agents is used in very large quantities in a variety of industrial processes. Perhaps the best known of these is vinyl chloride (CH_2:CHCl) used in the manufacture of PVC (polyvinylchloride) and other plastics; and this causes haemangiosarcoma of the liver in humans (Chapter 17) as well as in experimental animal systems. In practice, any alkylating agent should be regarded as a potential carcinogenic hazard where there is a possibility of human contact, inhalation, or ingestion. This would include alkyl halides and sulphates, diazomethane and its precursors, ethyleneimines, and lactones such as β-propiolactone. Materials which are used as insecticides or which are applied using aerosols are of particular concern. The insecticide, dichlorvos has caused particular concern because of proven mutagenicity in bacteria, but so far the epidemiological evidence that it is a human carcinogen is inconclusive. Other materials that have fallen under suspicion as human carcinogens, either because of mutagenicity or reactivity with DNA, are the chemosterilant, ethylene oxide, and the flame retardant, tris(2,3-dibromo-propyl)phosphate. An interesting situation has now arisen in that use of the latter has been restricted on the basis of short-term tests and animal carcinogenicity tests, so that final proof of human carcinogenicity may never be obtained. This is the objective of testing such materials but it leaves the investigation short of rigorous proof of hazard.

Some lactones must also be included amongst the carcinogenic alkylating agents. Aflatoxin B₁ is a product of *Aspergillus niger*, a fungal contaminant of stored food products especially in tropical regions (Fig. 9.89). The 8,9-epoxide of aflatoxin B₁ reacts with DNA, particularly with the N-7 of guanine. It has a very high DNA-binding index and is one of the most potent carcinogens known in experimental systems. Epidemiological evidence suggests that it may be associated with primary liver cancer in some parts of the world (particularly Africa) but also that it may interact with cofactors such as hepatitis B virus.

Monofunctional alkylating agents appear to exert their effect by the alkylation of specific bases in DNA. The repair of such lesions has been carefully studied in bacteria and in higher organisms and it is clear that a number of different enzymes are involved in repair of DNA alkylation. A well-studied enzyme is one of the products of the adaptive response in *E. coli*, namely the *ada* gene. This is an alkylguanine DNA-alkyl transferase which, in removing the alkyl group from the DNA, binds irreversibly to the alkyl group and is thereby itself inactivated (Fig. 9.90). This irreversibility has been used as the basis of a

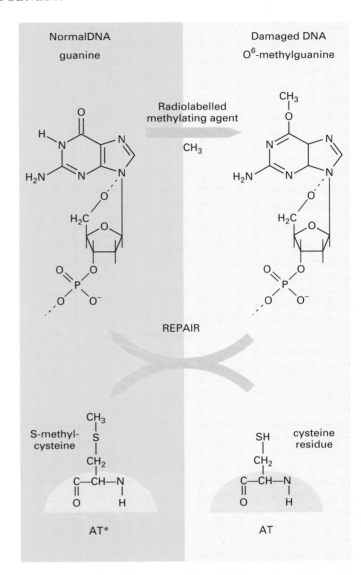

Fig. 9.90 Repair of DNA damaged by an alkylating agent. The methyl group in the O-6 position of guanine binds irreversibly with the cysteine residue of the alkyl transferase (AT) enzyme, thus removing it from the DNA. The process is monitored by using a radiolabelled alkylating agent. The inactivated repair protein is now radiolabelled (AT*). (Courtesy of G. Margison.)

very sensitive test of both enzyme function and extent of DNA alkylation.

Bifunctional alkylating agents, e.g. the nitrogen mustards, diepoxybutane, and mitomycin-C, cross-link DNA. Such lesions can be repaired but the process is more complex and more likely to be error prone.

Inorganic carcinogens The inorganic carcinogens, leaving aside radioactive materials, are the metals and the mineral fibres. Several metals have been firmly established as human carcinogens, e.g. arsenic, beryllium, chromium, and nickel, while others are suspected of being human carcinogens or have

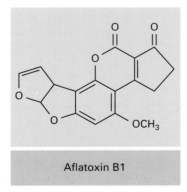

Aflatoxin B1

Fig. 9.89 Aflatoxin B₁, the potent carcinogen derived from *Aspergillus flavus*.

been shown to have carcinogenic potential in short-term tests or in animal assays, e.g. cadmium and cobalt.

Of the established carcinogens, arsenic is probably the best known and longest studied. Agricultural workers, in particular, who have been exposed to arsenical insecticides and fungicides have an excess of cancers of the skin by direct contact, and of lung by inhalation. Similarly, contamination of drinking water has led to population exposure, giving arsenical dermatoses and skin cancer. Medicinal use of arsenic has led to lung, skin, and liver cancers.

Curiously, repeated attempts to demonstrate the carcinogenicity of arsenic in experimental animals have failed. A few studies have given equivocal positive results. In short-term tests, arsenic can be demonstrated to be mutagenic in bacteria and clastogenic in the cultured cells of a variety of different species, including man. By present criteria, therefore, arsenic would be picked out as a potential carcinogen on screening tests in spite of the negative results in animal carcinogenicity tests. Though there is no direct evidence on the mode of action of arsenic as a carcinogen, these results also suggest that its genotoxic activity is important.

Beryllium, chromium (particularly hexavalent chromium), and nickel are all associated with lung cancer in occupationally exposed groups. Chromium has also been associated with gastrointestinal cancers, and nickel additionally with cancers of the nasal sinuses, larynx, and kidney. The nasal cancer risk for nickel workers is particularly high (80-fold). All three have been shown to be genotoxic, e.g. nickel and chromium induce infidelity of DNA synthesis.

For mineral fibre carcinogenesis the principal focus of attention has been on hazards arising from the use of different forms of asbestos for a whole range of purposes in the manufacturing and construction industries and in the home. However, naturally occurring mineral fibres such as the zeolites (especially erionite) are currently of interest as possible environmental carcinogens.

There are several types of asbestos, with different physical characteristics (Fig. 9.91). The most commonly used is chrysotile (white asbestos) which is composed of magnesium and silica. It tends to form rather large hollow fibres. Crocidolite (blue asbestos), on the other hand, is a chain silicate rich in iron. Its fibres are finer and shorter. Crocidolite has been used particularly in ship construction and for the insulation of steam boilers, but significant quantities were used in the construction industry.

Ultrastructural studies have shown that the fibre diameter is critical in determining the carcinogenic hazard. The fibres responsible for mesothelioma (see Chapter 10) are less than 0.25 μm in diameter and more than 0.5 μm in length and these are most commonly found in crocidolite. The fibres responsible for pulmonary fibrosis, on the other hand, may be up to 3.0 μm in diameter and the most effective length is over 10.0 μm.

Asbestos exposure is associated with diffuse pleural fibrosis, interstitial pulmonary fibrosis (asbestosis), carcinoma of the lung, mesothelioma of the pleura and peritoneum, and possibly increased incidence of gastrointestinal and laryngeal cancers.

There is a very strong synergism between cigarette smoking and asbestos exposure in the induction of carcinoma of the lung.

Non-genotoxic carcinogens It has been implied for much of the preceding discussion of chemical carcinogens that they are carcinogenic by virtue of their genotoxicity. In many cases this is almost certainly correct, but in other cases the role of genotoxicity in carcinogenesis is not proven. There are, however, a number of cases where a compound plays a part in the development of a neoplasm, and could therefore reasonably be termed a 'chemical carcinogen', but where the effect appears to be mediated by some mechanism other than genotoxicity. These fall into a number of different groups.

The organochlorine pesticides, such as lindane (1,2,3,4,5,6-hexachlorocyclohexane,HCH), dioxin (2,3,7,8,-tetrachlorodibenzo-para-dioxin), heptachlor (Fig. 9.92), and heptachlorepoxide, are carcinogenic in experimental systems, producing a variety of different types of liver cancer in mice and rats. However, extensive testing has failed to show mutagenicity and it is concluded that these and similar polychlorinated hydrocarbons exert their effect by a mechanism that does not require direct interaction with DNA. One suggestion is that their toxicity alone stimulates cell proliferation which would promote the growth of cells initiated by some other agent. Dioxin received wide publicity because of its presence in defoliants used in Vietnam and in the emissions following the accident at Serveso in Italy.

Brief mention has already been made of carcinogenicity of polymer or metal foils and mineral fibres that appear to exert their effect by virtue of their physical characteristics rather than by their chemical composition.

Promoting agents are chemical substances which, though not capable of inducing cancers directly, will interact with other classes of carcinogen to augment their effects. The best known are the phorbol esters, such as phorbol myristate acetate (PMA) also known as 12-O-tetradecanoyl phorbol-13-acetate (TPA) (Fig. 9.93). The phorbol esters were classically used in mouse skin carcinogenesis experiments where a polycyclic hydrocarbon was used as the initiator and the phorbol ester as the promoting agent. It was originally postulated that the promotor stimulated cell division and thus enhanced the effect of the initiator. More recent experiments show that phorbol esters induce normal cells to undergo changes that closely resemble terminal differentiation. They do not, however, have this effect on already transformed or tumorgenic cells. Their promoting effect may therefore be due to the switching off of normal cells, thus permitting initiated cells on which they would have no effect to proliferate freely. Other examples of promoting agents are: phenol, anthralin, bile acids, and saccharin.

Many hormones act as carcinogens and this has been discussed in detail (see above). It should be noted in the present context that they appear to exert their effect without genotoxicity. Most likely, their effect is exerted simply by the stimulation of cell division.

Similarly, immunosuppressive agents such as azothrioprine

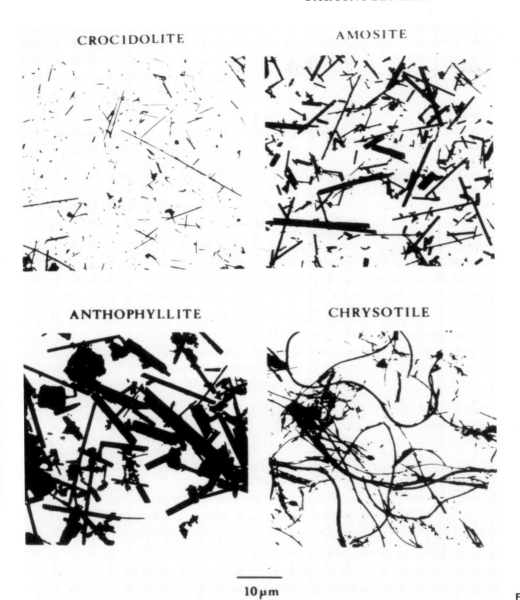

CROCIDOLITE

AMOSITE

ANTHOPHYLLITE

CHRYSOTILE

10 µm

Fig. 9.91 Asbestos fibres.

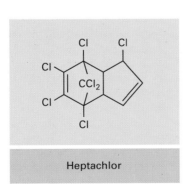

Heptachlor

Fig. 9.92 An organochlorine pesticide.

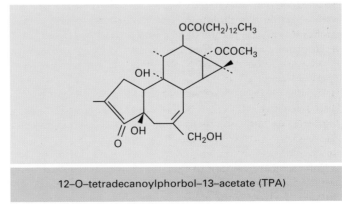

12–O–tetradecanoylphorbol–13–acetate (TPA)

Fig. 9.93 TPA, a phorbol ester promoting agent.

and 6-mercaptopurine are associated with increased incidence of lymphomas in patients, and virally induced and other neoplasms in experimental animals. The mechanism is unknown. But it is not the direct consequence of their effect on the genome of the tumour cells.

Radiation-induced cancer

Cancers in man may be induced by both ionizing and non-ionizing radiation. Most of the evidence comes from epidemiological studies which are considered in Section 9.7. A brief outline of these studies will help to put the experimental studies into context.

Ionizing radiation

Epidemiological evidence In the early years of the use of medical X-rays it was recognized that cancers of the hands occurred with unusual frequency amongst radiologists. Safety regulations introduced in 1920 largely solved that problem. Since then medical X-rays have been associated with cancer induction in patients treated for both malignant and non-malignant conditions. The medical practitioner, therefore, must still exercise great care in prescribing and administering radiation treatment to patients to ensure that harm that will inevitably be caused by radiation is kept to a minimum. The classic study by Court Brown and Doll of patients given X-ray treatment to the pelvis and spinal axis for the treatment of ankylosing spondylitis showed an increased risk of leukaemias, peaking at between 5 and 7 years after irradiation and showing a clear dose-dependence. Follow-up of these patients showed that the incidence of a number of solid tumours also increased but that the latent period was much longer, and in some cases exceeded 30 years. Therapeutic radiation treatment has been associated with cancers in a number of other situations, e.g. cancers of the thymus following radiation for enlargement of the thymus or for acute acne; skin cancers following irradiation of the scalp for tinea capitis (ringworm). Though radiation is not used in these conditions now, it is still possible that leukaemias and cancers may still arise from these causes because of the long latent period. Diagnostic X-rays have also been associated with leukaemia and cancer induction. Stewart first reported a roughly 1.4-fold increase in leukaemia in children whose mothers had been exposed to diagnostic X-rays (pelvimetry) during pregnancy. While this finding has been disputed by some other studies it is now generally agreed that the risk to the fetus may be unusually high and that special care must be taken when deciding whether or not X-ray diagnosis is appropriate in pregnant women.

The use of the radioactive contrast medium, thorotrast, has been associated with cancers of the liver. The practice of using thorotrast for angiography has long since stopped and very precise regulations now exist for the control of the use of radioisotopes for both treatment and for diagnostic purposes.

Non-medical exposure to radiation has also revealed much about radiation carcinogenesis. Careful follow-up of the exposed survivors of the atomic bombs at Hiroshima and Nagasaki shows a pattern of increased leukaemia and cancer incidence remarkably similar to those found in medically exposed groups. In addition, fallout of radioactive material from nuclear test explosions is also associated with increased cancer risk. The classic case being the high incidence of thyroid cancers among the population of the Marshall Islands as a result of the large deposition of radioiodine following bomb tests in the South Pacific Ocean.

Industrial exposure to ionizing radiation has also been observed. An excess of lung cancers in uranium miners due to exposure to radon in the atmosphere was one of the very early industrial cancer risks to be recognized. Similarly, workers who painted the luminous dials on clocks and watches were found to develop bone sarcomas as the result of ingestion of radium (a bone-seeking isotope) through the habit of placing the brush in the mouth to obtain a fine point. There has recently been controversy about the possible increase of leukaemia in the vicinity of nuclear waste reprocessing plants. Though the number of cases is small, there is now little doubt that these clusters are real; however, the doses of radiation to which the population have been exposed are much too low to account for these leukaemias if the conventional models of exposure and risk are correct. Either there is an as yet undiscovered cause or else there may be much more to learn about the mechanisms of radiation carcinogenesis and leukaemogenesis.

Increased risk may be considered either as:

1. the additive risk, i.e. the additional number of cases occurring per unit time per unit dose for a specified number of individuals at risk; or
2. the multiplicative risk, which is the ratio of the risk in the exposed population compared to the risk in a comparable control population.

The United Nations Scientific Committee on the Effects of Atomic Radiation (UNSCEAR) use the additive model.

Doses of radiation are measured in terms of the absorbed energy per unit mass. The current basic unit is the gray (Gy) which is 1 joule/kg. The more familiar but now outdated unit, the rad, is equivalent to 0.01 Gy. Different types of radiation differ in their relative biological efficiency (RBE) so that, for example, neutrons (high LET) are five times more effective than γ-rays (low LET) for a given dose (Fig. 9.94). However, there is now much evidence that, over a lower dose range, high LET radiation may be relatively even more effective. The doses of radiation found to be carcinogenic vary greatly, depending on the quality of radiation, the dose rate, and the site of irradiation. The spondylitis patients referred to above received an estimated average dose of 3.4 Gy to the bone marrow, though the dose distribution was very uneven. The Marshall Islanders received thyroid doses between 0.15 and 15 Gy.

Animal models Very early studies showed that ionizing radiation caused both leukaemia and solid tumours in experimental animals, particularly in mice. Leukaemia has been particularly well studied and it has been shown that leukaemia induction is critically dependent on both the dose and the dose rate.

Most of the leukaemias induced in mice are lymphoid and this

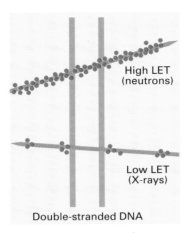

Fig. 9.94 Linear energy transfer (LET). Radiation of different types may cause dense ionization or sparse ionization along its track. This will affect the type of damage caused to DNA.

High LET (neutrons)

Low LET (X-rays)

Double-stranded DNA

has led to some difficulties in interpreting results since many strains of inbred mice have a high spontaneous incidence of lymphoid neoplasms, and furthermore many of these are virus associated. It is now clear that virus and radiation can interact synergistically to give an exceptionally high leukaemia incidence in some mouse strains. Moreover, in some cases, viruses appear to be activated by radiation exposure so that radiation-induced leukaemia may be subsequently transmitted by virus-containing extracts of leukaemia cells. More recently, Mole has developed a radiation-induced myeloid leukaemia model in the mouse which does not appear to be virus associated.

Radiation has also been shown to cause many different types of solid tumours in experimental animals. Lung tumours can be induced with X-rays, γ-rays, and neutrons. The incidence of tumours is low, and perhaps of more interest are respiratory-tract cancers induced in mice, rats, and dogs by α-particle emitting radionuclides, such as radon and its decay products. An increase in lung cancer incidence has been observed in rats with cumulative lung doses as low as 0.1 Gy, though doses of around 20 Gy give maximum incidence. Estimates of incidence related to dose vary from 25–50 cases per 10^4 animals per Gy.

Similarly, mammary tumours have been induced in dogs, mice, and rats by both external beam irradiation and by ingested or injected radionuclides. In the case of the mouse there is apparently an interaction with mouse mammary tumour virus (MMTV) and it has even been suggested that the induction of radiation mammary tumours in mice depends upon the activation of MMTV. In the rat, ionizing radiation of several different types led to mammary neoplasia. A strong synergism between radiation and steroid hormone stimulation in the induction of neoplasia has been reported. Similarly, in thyroid cancer induced in experimental animals there is an interaction with exposure to thyroid-stimulating hormone. It is of particular interest that lower doses, where the lethal effects of the radiation were less, were more likely to give rise to tumours. This has particular implications for radiation therapy in man where the thyroid is at the edge of the irradiation field.

Radiation-induced cancers in experimental animals have also been reported in skin, bone, and the digestive and genito-urinary tracts.

Radiation transformation of cells in culture While fewer studies have been carried out with radiation transformation than virus transformation of cells in culture, they have yielded useful information. The two main systems are Syrian hamster embryo cells and the mouse C3H 10T$\frac{1}{2}$ cell lines, which both show a direct dependence of transformation upon dose. However, at higher doses where lethality is high, the number of transformation events declines with increasing dose. Transformation is also dependent upon the quality of radiation. Low LET radiations have a lower transforming efficiency than high LET radiation (and also lower cell killing, chromosome damage, and mutation-inducing potential). Dose rate is also important. Low dose radiation gives fewer transformation events per unit dose, which implies repair of radiation-induced damage.

Mechanism of radiation carcinogenesis Ionizing radiation is known to cause a wide range of different types of damage to DNA, in particular single- and double-strand breaks but also base damage. Some of this damage leads to cell death and one can demonstrate a dose–response relationship between cell killing and radiation exposure which depends both on the quality of the radiation and on the dose rate. There is agreement that this cell killing is due to the production of double-strand breaks in DNA. Ionizing radiation is also known from studies on lower organisms, such as bacteria, fungi, and *Drosophila*, to be a potent mutagen. Cell culture studies show that ionizing radiation also induces mutations in mammalian cells, and many of these mutations are deletions. As with chemical damage to DNA, the phenomenon of potential lethal damage repair can be demonstrated following exposure to ionizing radiation. Therefore, there exists within cells repair pathways capable of repairing these different types of radiation-induced DNA damage and, as with repair of other types of damage, some of them are error free but some are error prone. Where the DNA lesion affects a single DNA strand the opposite undamaged strand can be used as a template for the synthesis of a new second strand after the excision of the damaged region. Such repair involves several different enzymes: an exonuclease, a DNA polymerase, and a DNA ligase. This has the potential of error-free repair. However, where a double-strand break occurs there is no template for repair synthesis and therefore errors are more likely to occur.

Some of the DNA damage caused by ionizing radiation can be visualized as chromosome damage. Where irradiation is given in the G$_1$ phase of the cell cycle, it classically causes 'chromosome' lesions (i.e. involving both chromatids of the metaphase chromosome). This leads to the formation of chromosome breaks, chromosome deletions, dicentric chromosomes, and ring chromosomes (Fig. 9.95). Irradiation at later stages of the cell cycle may lead to 'chromatid' aberrations (involving only one chromatid of the metaphase chromosome), giving chromatid gaps and breaks, chromatid deletions, and chromatid interchanges, leading to triradial and quadriradial configurations.

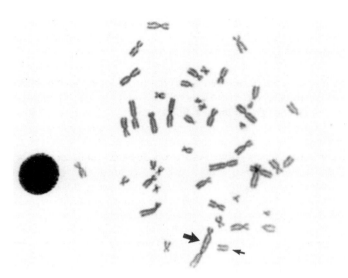

Fig. 9.95 Chromosomes from a human cell showing typical radiation damage. Large arrow, dicentric chromosome; small arrow, acentric fragment. (Courtesy of D. Scott.)

Such damage is quite characteristic of ionizing radiation (and a small number of radiomimetic chemicals).

It is not possible to state firmly that mutations arising from incorrect repair of DNA damage caused by ionizing radiation is the direct cause (initiation) of the neoplastic process, but the circumstantial evidence is strong. Patients exposed to medical X-rays, or accidentally exposed to ionizing radiation where we know there is an unusual cancer and leukaemia risk, show a dose-related elevation of chromosome damage. In the recessively inherited condition ataxia-telangiectasia, where there is an inherited increase in sensitivity to X-rays (and other ionizing radiation), there is also an increase in the incidence of cancers, particularly of the lymphoid system. It has been shown clearly that there is a defect of DNA repair which is attributable at least in part to infidelity of the repair of double-strand DNA breaks. In another inherited condition, basal cell naevus syndrome, there is an unusual sensitivity to radiation-induced skin cancers. There is a tendency for the cancers to arise at the edge of the radiation field, suggesting that it is in the regions receiving relatively low doses of radiation, where survival following DNA repair is presumably highest, that the cancers are most likely to occur.

Most studies on radiation damage to DNA and on the induction of neoplasms in animals and man have been done using radiations of low LET, such as X-rays or γ-rays. Most mathematical models of radiation-induced cancers and leukaemias are based on low LET radiation. Studies are now being carried out on leukaemia induction by high LET radiation (such as α-particles). Furthermore, high LET radiation may come from particulate material, and the chemical nature of the isotope will affect the distribution of the isotope in the body: e.g. radium and strontium are both bone-seeking isotopes but their behaviour and distribution in bone is quite different. We also know that stem cells (the presumed target cells for leukaemogenesis) are not uniformly distributed in bone marrow so that the dose to the target cell will depend on the chemical nature of the isotope as well as its radioactivity. Recent studies suggest that high LET radiation may be unexpectedly efficient in inducing leukaemia at relatively low doses. Furthermore, most work has been carried out on adult animals or at least animals in postnatal life. The effects on the fetus are little known and urgently require consideration.

Ultraviolet radiation

Effect of sunlight on human populations Much of the evidence for the carcinogenic potential of non-ionizing radiation comes from epidemiological studies (see Section 9.7). Briefly, skin cancers (basal cell and squamous carcinomas) are more common in those areas of the world where the population is exposed to more intense and longer hours of sunlight. The increase is, however, confined to the white population—the indigenous black populations have low levels of skin cancer, even in the sunniest climes. It is likely that this is one of the factors determining the evolution of racial differences and their global distribution. Mention has already been made of the correlation of skin cancer incidence with degree of skin pigmentation even among the 'white' skinned races, with the red-haired, fair-skinned types being most susceptible. The evidence for sunlight being the major factor in determining the pattern of skin cancer also comes from studying its occurrence within a population and its anatomical distribution. Squamous and basal cell carcinomas are commoner in those with outdoor occupations, such as farmers, fishermen, and labourers. These cancers occur most commonly on the face, neck and, where exposed, the forearms. The third major skin cancer malignant melanomas, is perhaps less obviously sun related. There is a gradient of incidence, however, from rare in North USA to common in the South. There is now compelling evidence linking exposure to sunlight (intense enough to cause sunburn) with the occurrence of malignant melanoma. Those most at risk appear to be those who normally do not get much sunlight exposure but who, perhaps on holiday, get short periods of intense exposure. As with the other skin cancers, there is also some evidence of an influence of sunlight on anatomical distribution, with melanoma being commoner on the legs in women than in men.

Interaction of sunlight with the genome The interaction between the genetic make-up of the individual and sunlight exposure has already been stressed. Two extreme cases are of particular interest. In the rare recessive condition, epidermodysplasia verruciformis, there is genetic predisposition to HPV infection. In these patients skin warts, which are normally entirely benign, tend to develop into carcinomas. However, they do so particularly on sun-exposed parts of the body, suggesting a triple interaction between causal factors in the development of malignancy.

Better known, though still rare, xeroderma pigmentosum (XP) is an autosomal recessive condition in which the patient is unusually susceptible to all the damaging effects of sunlight. XP patients are apparently normal at birth but as sunlight exposure increases with age they develop severe actinic keratosis. They usually show severe photophobia. By the age of 20 years the skin is already severely damaged and, in addition, shows both pigmented and depigmented areas. The severity of the lesions varies from family to family and it is now known that the disease is genetically heterogeneous (Table 9.9); the most severely affected are those with the de Sanctis Cacchione syndrome who also have severe mental retardation. Most patients develop multiple skin carcinomas. The age of onset is dependent both upon the degree of skin pigmentation and the exposure to sunlight. Cases diagnosed early and protected totally from sunlight can be kept symptom free.

Mode of action of ultraviolet light Exposure of DNA to UV light causes a number of different lesions but does not cause strand breakage. The most common lesion is the thymine dimer where two adjacent thymine molecules become linked together to form a bulky lesion in the DNA helix. Such lesions are repaired (Fig. 9.96) by the excision-repair process, which involves an incision being made by endonucleases in the DNA adjacent to the lesion. An exonuclease then removes the segment DNA containing the damage. A new strand is synthesized by a DNA polymerase, using the second strand as a template, and finally the new DNA is linked in by a DNA ligase, giving potentially an error-free repair. In XP patients the incision step is defective but all the other steps can be carried out competently. It can be demonstrated experimentally that cells from different XP patients vary considerably in their excision-repair capacity and, moreover, the patients belong to several different 'complementation' groups, i.e. caused by different genes (Table 9.9). When cells from a patient in one complementation group are fused to those from a patient in another group it is found that the hybrid cells are now repair proficient. In this way it can be deduced that the incision step in the repair process is under the control of several different genes.

Cells from XP patients show an increased susceptibility to killing by UV light but also an increased susceptibility to mutation induction by UV, which is dose dependent. The link between this increased mutability and the increased susceptibility to cancer induction is not clear, but it seems reasonable to assume that errors made in repair of UV-induced DNA lesions are the initiation events in carcinogenesis.

9.6.6 Oncogenes, growth factors, and cell regulation

D. G. Harnden

One of the exciting features of recent research into carcinogenesis has been the realization that, though we have identified many different causal agents, a common theme is beginning to emerge. All of these agencies act directly or indirectly on DNA. The DNA changes affect a pathway that leads from a stimulus to a cell to divide, through receptors and activation of membrane molecules, through second messages to DNA-binding proteins, the regulation of specific gene sequences, and the replication of the DNA, the chromosomes, and the cell. Two key discoveries have been the recognition of 'oncogenes' and the recognition of the key role of specific growth regulatory molecules or 'growth factors' (see Section 9.6.7). Oncogenes have been referred to on several occasions already in this chapter but it may be useful to summarize briefly the state of our present knowledge.

Oncogenes were recognized in two different situations. First,

Table 9.9 Genetic heterogeneity in xeroderma pigmentosum (XP)

Complementation group	Percentage of normal excision-repair proficiency after UV	Cell killing by UV	Clinical symptoms
XP-A	<10	+ + + +	severe, neurological
XP-B	5	+ +	severe but patient also has Cockayne syndrome
XP-C	10–30	+ +	severe, skin only
XP-D	10–50	+ + + +	severe, neurological
XP-E	40–60	+	moderate
XP-F	10–20	+ +	moderate
XP-G	<10	+ + +	severe
XP-variant	100*	+	variable, skin only

* Daughter-strand repair is severely deficient.

The single clinical entity, DNA repair-deficient XP is found to be due to several different mutations. These are recognized by fusing repair-deficient cells from different patients in culture. If the hybrid cells so formed are repair proficient, the patients must carry different mutations which complement each other. Cells from patients which do not complement are said to be in the same complementation group, i.e. are due to the same mutation. Groups A–G differ in excision-repair capacity, sensitivity to UV, and in severity of clinical symptoms. The XP-variant group is proficient at excision repair but deficient at post-replication (daughter-strand) repair.

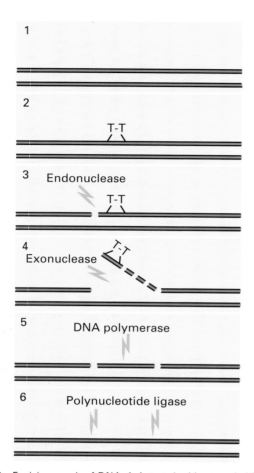

Fig. 9.96 Excision repair of DNA. 1, Intact double-stranded DNA. 2, Induction of a thymine dimer by UV. 3, An incision made close to the dimer by an endonuclease enzyme. 4, Removal of the sequence of DNA containing the damage. 5, Synthesis of a new strand using the other strand as a template. 6, The new strand is completed by a polynucleotide ligase enzyme.

the study of the oncogenic retroviruses revealed the presence of sequences which were capable of cellular transformation on DNA transfection into appropriate cells. These sequences known as v-*onc* genes proved to have cellular homologies, the c-*onc* genes, which are also in their non-initiated form referred to as proto-oncogenes (Table 9.10). The v-*onc* genes are present only in the fast-transforming, short-latency retroviruses which (with the exception of some strains of chicken sarcoma virus) are defective in replication function. The v-*onc* sequences are thought to have been derived in an evolutionary sense from the c-*onc* sequences, a situation made possible by the fact that the RNA retroviruses must integrate into the host cell genome and be transcribed from these integrated sequences to make new viruses. It should be noted that the v-*onc* genes do not contain introns as do the genomic c-*onc* sequences, i.e. they resemble eukaryotic m-RNA.

The second type of experiment which led to the recognition of the oncogenes also involved DNA transfection. In this case, however, the transfection of DNA from transformed or cancer cells into suitable recipients, such as mouse NIH 3T3 cells or mouse C127 cells, led to the formation of transformed foci which proved to be tumourigenic on injection into mice (Fig. 9.97). It was shown that specific DNA sequences were responsible for this transforming activity, and initially there was some surprise that these sequences proved to be the same sequences whose transforming activity had been recognized in RNA retroviruses. While these transformation assays have limitations, in that not all cells are suitable targets and only particular classes (e.g. the *ras* family) of oncogenes can be detected by this method, they have served to extend very considerably our knowledge of oncogenes. New oncogenes, unrecognized as v-*onc* genes, have been detected and a molecular analysis of the transforming sequences has led to a precise knowledge of the mutational events that confer transforming activity. More recently, assays have been used that bypass the cell-culture stage by direct inoculation of the transfected cells in immune

Table 9.10 Examples of oncogenes

Symbol	Species of origin of retrovirus	Product function	Cellular location	Human chromosome location
src	chicken	PK	plasma membrane	20q12–q13
fes	cat	PK	plasma membrane	
abl	mouse	PK	plasma membrane	9q34–qtr
erb A	chicken	?	cytoplasm	7p13–q11.2
erb B	chicken	truncated EGF receptor	plasma membrane	7p11–q21
fos	mouse	?	nucleus	14q21–q3
sis	monkey	truncated PDGF (B-chain)	membranes	22q11–qter
myc	chicken	DNA binding	nucleus	8q24
myb	chicken	?	nucleus	6q22–q24
Ha-ras	rat	GTP binding, GTPase	plasma membrane	11p15
Ki-ras	rat	GTP binding, GTPase	plasma membrane	12p12–pter
cts	chicken	?	nucleus	11q23–q24

PK, protein kinase; EGF, epidermal growth factor; PDGF, platelet-derived growth factor.

impaired (nude) mice. The transfected genes can be recovered directly from the tumour cells.

A very large number of oncogenes have now been recognized. These tend to fall into families of related genes which shown some DNA homology and have a similar function. While the precise function of the oncogene product is often not known, its cellular location can usually be determined, and also its general nature is known in many cases (e.g. a protein kinase or a DNA-binding protein). In a small number of instances the function is known, e.g. c-*erb B* is a truncated form of the epidermal growth factor receptor and c-*sis* shows strong sequence homology to platelet-derived growth factor. The proto-oncogenes, therefore, are cellular genes that have a function vital to the normal process of cell stimulation, and nuclear and cellular division.

These are associated with neoplasia, however, only when they are 'activated' and this may come about in several different ways. First, mutation of the proto-oncogene at specific positions in the DNA may confer on the gene cell-transforming activity, e.g. H-*ras* may be activated by mutation at codon 12, 13, or 61, depending on the particular situation. Second deletion of specific sequences at the 5′ end of the genome may lead to inappropriate expression of the gene. Translocation of the *onc* gene sequence to a new location may lead to the production of a new gene product with altered properties [e.g. c-*abl* in the t(9;22) translocation in chronic myeloid leukaemia] or place the *onc* gene under the influence of new regulatory sequences. This alteration in expression of a proto-oncogene may also be effected by its coming under the control of viral promoting sequences, as in the insertion of LTR regions near c-*myc* in avian B-cell lymphomas. In this case the structure of the proto-oncogene is not altered. The oncogenic effect comes from the inappropriate expression of the gene under the influence of the viral promoter.

Growth factors are molecules that bind to specific receptors on the surface of target cells, leading to specific changes in the development of those cells and their descendants. Some have been known for many years, e.g. epidermal growth factor, which stimulates the growth and division of epidermal cells. A whole range of growth factors have been identified which control the proliferation and development of haemopoietic cells: from interleukin-3 (IL-3), which stimulates primitive stem cells, through lineage-specific growth factors, such as granulocyte/macrophage colony-stimulating factor (GMCSF), to those that control the production of terminally differentiated cells, such as erythropoietin (EPO). Some, such as EPO, are produced at a site distant from the cell to be controlled, but others operate over very short distances and, indeed, may only be effective when presented on the surface of a cell actually in contact with the target cell. Many other growth factors have been, and are being, discovered: T-cell growth factor (IL-2), fibroblast growth factor, transforming growth factor α and β, insulin-like growth factor. Currently the origin of these factors and their mode of action is under intensive investigation. Their relationship to well-known hormones, such as insulin, is also a matter of great interest (see Section 9.6.7).

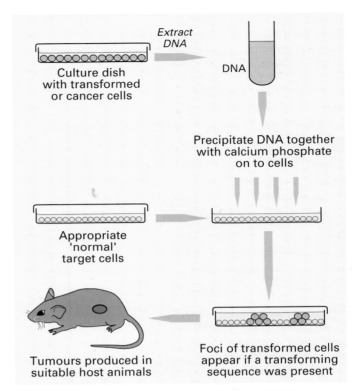

Fig. 9.97 DNA transfection. High molecular weight DNA is extracted from transformed or cancer cells. It is then transfected into suitable recipient cells (such as NIH 3T3 mouse fibroblasts) by co-precipitation with calcium phosphate on to the surface of the cells. After some weeks, foci of transformed cells appear and may be shown to be tumourigenic by inoculation into suitable animals.

Inhibitory molecules as well as stimulatory molecules have been discovered. Indeed, some 'growth factors' may stimulate one cell type but regulate and slow down another cell type. These molecules are therefore vital in the maintenance and function of tissues throughout the body. They are the signals that activate the pathways where the proto-oncogenes have been found to play an important role. An understanding of their role and how they may be inappropriately expressed will be vital in developing our knowledge of carcinogenesis.

9.6.7 Growth factors

J. Lorenzen, L. Pusztai, and James O'D. McGee

Introduction

In a multicellular organism, strict controls of basic cellular functions such as differentiation, mitosis, and locomotion are necessary for survival. During morphogenesis, signal substances are required to inform every single cell about its position in relation to the entire organism, when to enter the mitotic cycle and when to switch from the proliferation to the differentiation programme. To maintain the integrity of the organism, many of these mechanisms have to remain operational during later life. They regulate cell renewal in response to normal cell loss as well as in wound healing and have to prevent 'mitotic anarchy'.

Early this century, it was noted that in order to propagate eukaryotic cells outside their normal environment, the addition of serum was required apart from basic nutrients and vitamins. Various serum subfractions were found to support cell growth better than others, which lead to the isolation of 'agents' and—where isolation to apparent homogeneity could be achieved—of 'growth factors'; These factors and agents were named according to their source or to the system used to monitor their isolation such as 'retina-derived growth factor', 'colony-stimulating factor', or 'multiplication stimulating agent'. With the more recent developments in protein chemistry, DNA sequencing, and immunological assays, our knowledge has increased dramatically. These developments have also led to a kind of converging evolution in the terminology of growth factors, and has provided revealing insights linking areas of embryology, cancer research, immunology, and endocrinology. This process is still under way and our understanding of important issues of cell-cycle control is far from complete.

Definition

Growth factors are polypeptides that interact with specific cellular membrane receptors, thus stimulating target cell proliferation and often promoting differentiation. We exclude basic nutrients such as glucose, amino acids, and vitamins, as well as essential minerals necessary for cell metabolism. Growth factors differ from hormones in that they act on a microenvironmental level through paracrine and autocrine mechanisms. Paracrine secretion is the active release of substances into the extracellular space, where they diffuse to their target cells. This mechanism only functions in the close proximity, the 'microenvironment', of the secreting cell. Autocrine secretion is present if the secreting cell itself can act as target, expressing receptors for the secreted substance.

Growth factors and neoplasia

Autocrine stimulation of neoplastic cells

Neoplastic growth can be defined as proliferation of cells that have escaped the normally tight regulatory system of the host. Neoplastic cells differ from their normal counterparts in their capability to enter the mitotic cycle without the requirement of certain growth signals. This is exemplified in the less refined serum requirements of malignant cells in culture. In this context, it was of chief importance to notice that the transformation of cells by oncogenic retroviruses leads to the secretion of a growth factor, for which receptors are already expressed on the cell membrane. The concept that neoplastic cells evade the host control by *autocrine stumulation* applies to a whole range of tumours.

Two growth factors, that are often involved, are platelet-derived growth factor (PDGF) and transforming growth factor (TGF-α). PDGF is present in the α-granules of platelets, from where it is released during aggregation and clotting. It accounts for the fact that platelet-deficient plasma supports the growth of cell cultures less well than serum. PDGF is secreted by various transformed cells and acts on mesenchymal cells via a well-described receptor (PDGFr). On its own, PDGF is not sufficient to induce a mitogenic response, but requires the co-operation of other growth factors, among which are epidermal growth factor (EGF) and insulin-like growth factor 1 (IGF-I = somatomedin C). PDGF induces the *competence* to enter the S-phase of the cell cycle. Other plasma constituents, the most potent factors being the IGFs, are then needed to stimulate the actual *progression* through the G_1- to the S-phase.

TGF-α, which is assayed by its ability to promote anchorage-independent growth of normal rat kidney (NRK) cells, has generally the same biological properties as EGF and binds to the same receptor. However, it sequence homology is not sufficient to cause immunological cross-reactions with EGF. TGF-α plays a role in the normal neonatal development and its expression by tumour cells might serve as another example of derepression of silent fetal genes during oncogenesis.

Together with TGF-α, another transforming growth factor, TGF-β, was isolated. TGF-β has essentially no sequence homology to TGF-α or EGF, does not bind to the same receptor, and is quite distinct in its biological properties. Depending on the target cell and the presence of other growth factors, TGF-β promotes or inhibits proliferation. High-affinity receptors are present on virtually every cell. TGF-β is an important differentiation signal for bronchial epithelial cells and is noteworthy for its effects on the production of collagen and fibronectin by fibroblasts. It is suspected of playing a key role in bone metabolism and has been linked to the regulation of the immune response.

Interaction with the immune system

Malignant neoplasms escape the host's immune surveillance by various means. During recent years it has emerged that growth factors secreted by cancer cells interfere with the cellular immune system.

TGF-β deserves particular interest. TGF-β can be produced in a tumour by different mechanisms. Metastatic tumours release coagulant factors that induce the aggregation and the release of TGF-β by platelets. TGF-β is also secreted by tumour cells themselves in relatively large amounts. TGF-β acts as a strong chemotactic factor for monocytes and macrophages stimulating them to secrete interleukin-1 and, among other growth factors, again TGF-β. Monocytes can make up for more than 50 per cent of cells present in solid tumours. The IL-1-dependent proliferation of lymphocytes is inhibited by TGF-β at picomolar concentrations. By this mechanism, the effects of IL-1 are channelled towards fibroblasts. Thus, TGF-β 'paralyses' B- and T-lymphocytes and encourages fibrosis in malignant neoplastic growth. The same mechanism is involved in the formation of fibrous tissue in the late stages of wound repair. PDGF has been shown to impair natural killer cell activity and is another example of the interactions between growth factors and the immune system.

Interaction with tumour stroma

The morphology of many different malignant neoplasms is characterized not only by the appearance of the neoplastic cells, but also by the presence and pecularities of the non-neoplastic tumour stroma. Characteristic features of tumours are established by the secretion of appropriate growth factors.

Neoplasms are able to create a suitable microenvironment (tumour stroma) to support their growth by the secretion of growth factors. For example, solid tumours cease to grow once they have reached a size of $1–2$ mm^2, if the formation of new capillary vessels is prevented. The induction of *neovascularization* is therefore a necessary feature of malignant neoplastic growth. It is interesting to note that, apart from processes during ovulation, physiological angiogenesis is infrequent. Great efforts have been undertaken to isolate the responsible angiogenic substances from tumour extracts. The fact, that many of these angiogenic factors share an affinity for heparin greatly facilitated their purification. A whole family of growth factors was found to be capable of interacting with two basic steps of angiogenesis: endothelial cell locomotion and proliferation. This family includes the acidic and basic fibroblast growth factors (aFGF, bFGF), the endothelial growth factors (ECGFa, ECGFb), an eye-derived growth factor (EDGF-II), the retina-derived growth factor (RDGF), and the corpus luteum angiogenic factor. The angiogenic activity of the transforming growth factors appears to be mediated by their chemotactic properties, attracting macrophages and causing them to release different growth factors.

More recently, it was shown that the transforming agent of Kaposi sarcoma, a tumour generally considered an angiosarcoma of endothelial–mesenchymal origin, shares sequence homology to this group of endothelial cell mitogens.

The picture of various malignant neoplasms is dominated by the prevalence of fibrous tissue (for example scirrhous carcinomas). This appears to be the response of normal stroma to cancer cells secreting certain growth factors, such as TGF-β or PDGF.

Relation to oncogenes

Only weeks after the amino-acid sequence of PDGF had been described, its strong similarity to the transforming agent of the simian sarcoma virus, the *sis* oncogene, was noticed. The amino-acid sequence of this oncogene is virtually identical to the 109 *N*-terminal amino acids of the PDGF B-chain. The implication of this discovery led to a boost in our understanding of tumour biology. The picture emerging is that oncogenes can be grouped according to the level of interference with the regulation of cell proliferation by growth factors.

1. Oncogenes encoding growth factors: *sis* is homologous to PDGF; *hst* (similar to Kaposi sarcoma oncogene) is homologous to FGF.

2. Oncogenes encoding growth factor receptors: *fms* is related to the mCSF or CSF-1 receptor; *erb B* shows the structure of an EGFr, whose extracellular domain has been lost; *erb A* is a receptor for thyroid hormone.

3. Oncogenes interfering with signal transduction: *ras*, *myc*, *ros*, etc.

Growth factor genes in chromosomal deletions

Certain tumours are associated with specific chromosomal deletions. The following two examples illustrate possible links between growth factor expression and chromosomal deletions, although at present the molecular mechanisms are not well understood.

Insulin-like growth factor II (IGF-II) is predominantly found during fetal development, but is also expressed in adult mesenchymal tissues, although in much lower levels. It has been shown to be secreted by certain human tumours of embryonal type, such as Wilms tumour, rhabdomyosarcoma, and hepatoblastoma. These tumours have been associated with a karyotypic anomaly involving chromosome 11. As similar deletions have been described for breast cancers, it was interesting to detect IGF-II secretion and IGF-receptors in human breast cancer tissues as well.

Another association between chromosomal deletion and growth factors has been described for the 5q-syndrome, which is associated with a high prevalence of myelodysplasia and acute myeloid leukaemias. The genes encoding EGFR, PDGFr, CSF-1, GM-CSF, c-*fes*, and interleukin-5 are all located on chromosome 5q and are reduced to homozygosity in this syndrome.

Regulation of the growth factor system

In order to fulfil their activities in a useful manner and to avoid possible deleterious effects for the entire organism, the growth factor system is controlled tightly. Here various systems interact with each other, forming a co-operative network regulating cellular events.

As with other ligand/receptor interactions, several events can be distinguished in the action of growth factors and their receptors. The first event is the actual binding of the factor to its specific receptor, leading to conformational changes in the receptor and so to the activation of an enzymatic activity (*signal transformation*). Secondary membrane events take place and induce a change in the local density and distribution of the membrane-bound receptors (*receptor clustering*). A cascade of enzymes is activated and changes the cytoplasmic concentration of messenger substances (*secondary messengers*) leading to the expression of certain genes (*signal transduction*). Feedback loops are activated to decrease the stimulatory input, either by diminishing the affinity of the receptor for its ligand or by reducing the number of membrane-borne receptors (*downregulation*). As an example, these steps can be recognized in more detail in the regulation of EGFR (Fig. 9.98).

1. Binding of EGF or TGF-α to the receptor induces the tyrosine-specific kinase activity by intramolecular events leading to

Table 9.11　Some growth factors and their receptors*

Factor	MW	Source	Target cell	Receptor/ oncogene	MW
Insulin	6000	β-cell of pancreas	general	insulin receptor	430 000
Insulin-like growth factor I (IGF-I) = somatomedin C	7650	plasma	general	IGF-I receptor	350 000 320 000 290 000
Insulin-like growth factor II (IGF-II) equivalent to multiplication stimulating agent (MSA) of rat	7500	plasma	general	IGF-II receptor	268 000
Nerve GF(NGF)	26 500	cobra venom, sub-maxillary gland	sympathetic ganglia cells, sensory neurones, melanoma cells	NGF receptor	75 000
Acidic fibroblast GF (aFGF)	17 000	bovine pituitary	fibroblasts, smooth muscle, chondrocyte, vascular endothelium, glial cells	FGF receptor	125 000 145 000
Basic fibroblast GF (bFGF)	14 000	brain, pituitary, retina, kidney, adrenal gland	mesodermal cells, vascular endothelium	FGF receptor	125 000 145 000
Kaposi sarcoma GF (ks) equivalent to *hst* oncogene	24 000	Kaposi's sarcoma	3T3-cells	?	?
Angiogenin	14 000	human colon cancer line	capillary endothelium	?	?
Endothelial cell GF (ECGF)	20 000	endothelial cells	vascular endothelium	ECGFR	150 000
Eye-derived GF II (EDGF-II)	17 000	bovine retina	vascular endothelium	?	?
Platelet-derived GF (PDGF)	24 000–31 000	α-granule of platelets	fibroblasts, glia, smooth muscle	PDGF receptor	180 000
Epidermal GF (EGF) equivalent to urogastrone	6000	submaxillary gland of male mouse, human urine	epidermal cells, chondrocytes, fibroblasts, endothelial cells	EGF receptor *erb B*	170 000
Transforming GF-α (TGF-α)	6000	virally transformed cells	similar to EGF	8EGF receptor	170 000
Transforming GF-β (TGF-β)	25 000	platelets, bone, placenta, kidney, monocytes	general	TGF-β receptor	500 000–600 000
Colony-stimulating factors: Human: CSF-α Mouse: GM-CSF	22 000 23 000	placenta	granulocyte/ macrophage progenitor cells	CSF-α receptor	51 000
Human: CSF-β Mouse: G-CSF	30 000 25 000	placenta	granulocyte progenitor cells	CSF-β receptor	150 000
Human: urinary CSF Mouse: CSF-I	45 000 70 000	urine	macrophage progenitor cells	M-CSF receptor *fms*	165 000
The interleukin group: Interleukin-1 (IL-1)	15 000	macrophages, keratinocytes, astrocytes	lymphocytes, fibroblasts, chondrocytes, hypothalamic fever centre, osteoclasts	IL-1 receptor	79 500
T-cell GF (TCGF) = IL-2	15 400	T-lymphocytes	CD4-positive T-cells	IL-2 receptor = CD25 = Taq Ag	55 000
Multi-CSF (= IL-3)	28 000	T-lymphocytes	T-cells, eosinophils, mast cells, granulocyte and macrophage progenitor cells	IL-3 receptor	55 000–75 000
B-cell stimulation-factor-I = IL-4	18 000	activated T-cells	early B-cells CD4+ T-cells	IL-4 receptor	?

Table 9.11 *Continued*

Factor	MW	Source	Target cell	Receptor/ oncogene	MW
Eosinophil differentiation factor = T-cell replacing factor = B-cell growth factor II = IL-5	45 000–55 000	stimulated T-cells, HTLV-transformed T-cells	activated B-cells, eosinophil precursor cells	IL-5 receptor = BCGFR	90 000
B-cell stimulation-factor II = IL-6 = interferon-β_2 = hepatocyte stimulating factor	26 000	fibroblasts T-cells, tumour cell lines	activated B-cells, lymphoblastoid cells, plasmocytoma, hepatocytes	IL-6 receptor	128 000 103 000

* This is a list of examples and is not comprehensive; see Bishop 1991 for review.

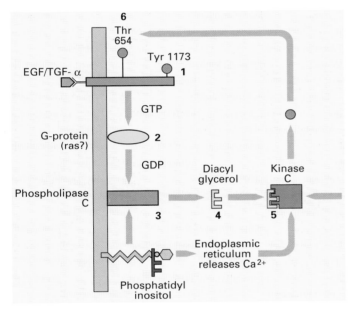

Fig. 9.98 Regulation of the epidermal growth factor receptor (for explanation, see text).

the *autophosphorylation* of the Tyr residue 1173 in the vicinity of the carboxyl terminus. Activated EGFR phosphorylates a number of substrates at Tyr, many of which are believed to be intracellular messenger substances and are targets of other mitogens (like PDGF, FGF) and oncogenes of the tyrosine kinase group (*src, ros, erb B, neu, trk*).

2. One of the substrates phosphorylated by EGFR is the oncogene Ha-*ras*, which belongs to the family of GTPases known as G-proteins. These proteins play a significant role in membrane signalling (Neer and Clapham 1988). Among other reactions, G-proteins stimulate phospholipase C. PDGF and FGF are also known to activate phospholipase C.

3. Phospholipase C controls the production of two cellular messenger substances: diacyl glycerol (DAG) and inosityl

triphosphate. Inosityl triphosphate causes an increase of cytoplasmic Ca^{2+} ions, which are released from the endoplasmic reticulum.

4. DAG, together with Ca^{2+}, activates protein kinase C (Nishizuka 1984). DAG shows close structural relations to phorbol esters, which are known for their tumour-promoting effects *in vitro* and *in vivo*. The main substrate for protein kinase C is EGFR, which is phosphorylated at the threonine residue 654.

5. The phosphorylation of EGFR at Thr 654 in turn diminishes its affinity for EGF and TGF-α. This negative regulatory event can also be induced by the activated PDGFr or FGFR via the activation of kinase C.

6. Together with other yet unknown mechanisms, the phosphorylation of Thr 654 induces the clustering of the EGFR on the cell membrane and its *internalization*. This event, which is also seen with other receptors, is known as *down-regulation*.

Apart from the direct regulation of the EGF/EGFR system, other functional negative-feedback loops exist and are mediated via the expression of gene products like TGF-β and IFN-β, which promote cellular differentiation and remove cells from the proliferation pool. There is evidence that the production of the EGFR is orchestrated with the expression of other genes at the DNA level. The transcription of the EGFR gene is in part regulated by the transcription factor Sp1. This transcription factor recognizes a concensus sequence known as the GC box in the promoting regions of several other genes, among which the H-*ras* oncogene, the SV40 early antigen, and the HMG-reductase are the best known.

Negative regulators

The regulation of organized growth in tissues has intrigued scientists for a long time. Earlier this century the regeneration of kidney and liver were studied in adult rats. It was theorized that every tissue contained mitotic inhibitors. In the case of tissue

Table 9.12 Negative regulators of cell growth*

Factor	Source	Target cells	Molecular weight
p105-RB	Retinoblasts (and others)	many cell type	105 000
p53	many cell types	lung, colon, etc., cells	53 000
BSC-1 growth inhibitor (= TGF-β?)	BSC-1 conditioned medium	BSC-1 cells, CCL64 mink lung cells	25 000
Interferon-β	fibroblasts	HeLa cells	28 000–35 000
Fibroblast growth regulator (FGRs(13 k))	3T3 conditioned medium	fibroblasts	10 000–15 000
Hepatic proliferation inhibitor (HPI)	rat liver	rat hepatocytes	26 000
N.N.	bovine mammary gland	Ehrlich ascites mammary cells	13 000
Bovine glycopeptide inhibitor (BCSG)	bovine cerebral cortex	mouse fibroblasts	16 000–18 000

* This list is representative and not comprehensive; see Bishop 1991.

loss, the concentration of these substances would be reduced, thus allowing proliferation and wound repair. For these inhibitors the name chalone was coined ($\chi\alpha\lambda\sigma\nu = I$ prevent). Chalones are defined by their cell specificity, their autocrine secretion, and their capability to induce cell differentiation. The chalones are the conceptual opposite of growth factors. The rapid advance in isolating and characterizing growth factors was unparalleled in the field of chalones during the past decade, but still some progress has been made on this subject (see Table 9.12).

Although TGF-β was originally described together with TGF-α as promoting anchorage-independent growth of fibroblasts, subsequent investigations have discovered its role in differentiation and growth inhibition for various other cells. The growth factors IL-2 and IL-4 are secreted in an autocrine manner by CD4$^+$ T-cells and are important differentiation signals. IFN-β expression is stimulated by the activated PDGFr and exerts negative growth modulatory effects to a whole range of cells. So it can be concluded that the autocrine secretion of growth factors is not a neoplastic feature *per se* and that there is an intriguing dichotomy in the actions of growth factors and their differentiation promoting effects. In fact, some growth factors act on specific cells in such a manner that they could be categorized as classical chalones.

The best studied tumour suppressor genes (antioncogenes) are the retinoblastoma (RBI) and p53 genes. There is evidence that both act in a dominantly negative way on cell growth in the appropriate cell lines. The possible mechanism of actions are reviewed elsewhere (Bishop 1991; Marshall 1991) but at this time there is no clear understanding of how their protein products work mechanistically. In fact a myriad of growth factors and tumour suppressor products have been isolated in the same and different experimental systems. This is not surprising. 'Homeostasis' of normal and malignant cell growth is predictably going to be more complex than blood coagulation homeostasis.

9.6.8 Bibliography

Bishop, J. M. (1991). Molecular themes in oncogenesis. *Cell* 64, 235–48.

Broder, S (ed.) (1991). *Molecular foundations of oncology*. Williams and Wilkins, London.

Centrella, M., McCarthy, T. L., and Canalis, E. (1988). Skeletal tissue and transforming growth factor β. *FASEB Journal* 2, 3066–73.

Cooper, C. S. and Grover, P. L. (eds) (1990). *Chemical carcinogenesis and mutagenesis*, Vols I and II. Springer-Verlag, Berlin, Heidelberg.

Crepin, M. (ed.) (1988). *Research in retroviruses and oncogenes*. John Libbey, London.

Deuel, T. F. (1987). Polypeptide growth factors: Roles in normal and abnormal cell growth. *Annual Review of Cell Biology* 3, 443–92.

Fields, B. N. and Knipe, D. M. (eds) (1990). *Field's virology* (2nd edn). Vol. 1 (Chap. 14) and Vol. 2 (Chaps 52, 57–61, 68). Raven Press, New York.

Folkmann, J. and Klagsbrunn, M. (1987). Angiogenic factors. *Science* 235, 442–7.

Franks, L. M. and Teich, N. (eds) (1986). *Introduction to the cellular and molecular biology of cancer*. Oxford University Press.

Marshall, C. (1991). Tumour suppressor genes. *Cell* 64, 312–26.

Moossa, A. R., Schimp, F. F., and Robson, M. C. (eds) (1991). *Comprehensive textbook of oncology* (2nd edn). Williams and Wilkins, London.

Neer, E. J. and Clapham, D. E. (1988). Roles of G protein subunits in transmembrane signalling. *Nature* 333, 129–34.

Nishizuka, Y. (1984). The role of protein kinase C in cell surface signal transduction and tumour promotion. *Nature* 308, 693–8.

Ruddon, R. W. (1987). *Cancer biology* (2nd edn). Oxford University Press, New York.

Sporn, M. B. and Roberts, A. B. (1985). Autocrine growth factors and cancer. *Nature* 313, 745–7.

Sporn, M. B., Roberts, A. B., Wakefield, L. M., and Assoian, R. K. (1986). Transforming growth factor-b: Biological function and chemical structure. *Science* 233, 532–4.

Todaro, G. J. and De Larco, J. E. (1976). Transformation by murine and feline sarcomaviruses specifically blocks binding of epidermal growth factor to cells. *Nature* 264, 26–30.

Wang, J. L. and Hsu, Y. M. (1986). Negative regulators of cell growth. *Trends in Biochemical Sciences* 11, 24–6.

9.7 Epidemiology of human neoplasia

Richard Doll

9.7.1 Introduction

Epidemiology, that is the study of the incidence of disease in groups of people with defined characteristics, has been one of the principal means of obtaining knowledge about the causes of cancer. It has shown, first, that every type of cancer that is at all common anywhere varies in incidence at least fivefold, often fiftyfold, and occasionally a thousandfold, and that very little of this variation can be explained by differences in genetic constitution. Secondly, it has obtained clues to causation by showing that the incidence of a particular cancer correlates with the prevalence of some potential agent. Thirdly, it has identified causes by comparing the personal characteristics and past experience of people with and without a particular type of cancer, or by following up groups of people whose characteristics have been recorded and observing the incidence of cancer in subgroups whose characteristics differed; and it has checked the validity of the conclusions that have been reached by monitoring the effect of changes in exposure or behaviour that the tentative conclusions have caused. Fourthly, it has provided information about the biological relations between cause and effect that has helped to test hypotheses about the mechanism by which cancer is produced.

To make these contributions, epidemiologists have frequently required information about large numbers of cases and they have often had to use the numbers of deaths certified as being due to particular causes, or the numbers of cases recorded in cancer registries or in hospital series. With such data, the possibility of diagnostic error and the probability that the amount of error varies from place to place and from time to time has always had to be taken into acount. With such data, too, epidemiology has often been limited to the study of cancer of a whole organ, without distinction between the different histological types or between the parts of the organ in which the cancer arises. This, however, is less limiting than might be supposed, as most cancers in a particular organ tend to have the same group of causes, when cancer in that organ is at all common, and it has not prevented many causes from being discovered.

When, however, precise pathological information has been available, the productivity of epidemiological research has been greatly enhanced. In these circumstances it has often shown that the incidence of a pathologically defined type of cancer varies a great deal more than the incidence of all cancers of the organ grouped together, and this has led to the discovery that precisely characterized types of cancer may each have their own specific causes. For the epidemiologist, however, the limitation of a study to pathologically confirmed cases is not always an advantage; for account then has to be taken of variation in the availability of pathological services, in the readiness of clinicians to make use of them, and in the criteria for pathological diagnosis; and these sources of variation may introduce greater confusion than the pathological confirmation avoids.

In this section, we examine first the biological relationship between the incidence of cancer and the individual's sex and age, and the temporal relationship between exposure to a carcinogen and the development of the disease. We then review the evidence relating to the causes of each type of cancer. Many were discovered by clinical acumen or by laboratory investigation rather than by epidemiological enquiry; but only those causes of cancer are included that have been confirmed by epidemiological evidence.

9.7.2 Biological relationships

Age

Cancer occurs at all ages, but the different types, defined by the type of cell from which they arise and the organ in which they occur, have different relationships with age, and each of these relationships provides a clue to the causes of the disease. For some types of cancer the general pattern is invariant; for others it varies in different places and at different times.

By far the most common pattern is a progressive increase in incidence from near zero in late adolescence to a high figure in old age. The rate of increase is rapid, being typically proportional to the fourth, fifth, or sixth power of age, so that cancers that affect only 1 or 2 individuals per 1 000 000 persons each year at around 20 years of age may affect 1 or 2 per 1000 at age 80. This pattern is shown by most carcinomas of the buccal cavity, pharynx, digestive tract, urinary tract, and skin, and by myelomatosis and chronic lymphatic leukaemia. With most of these cancers the recorded rate of increase diminishes after about 75 years of age; but this seems likely to be an artefact, due to incomplete investigation of the terminal illnesses of old people. With continued improvement in diagnosis and the more intensive investigation of old people, cancer incidence rates in old age must be expected to increase further, even in the absence of any secular change in the risk of developing the disease.

The pattern of a progressive increase in incidence with age has sometimes been thought to be due to the 'ageing' of the immune system, with a consequent progressive ease of escape of malignant clones from immunological control. This concept is given some support by the fact that in adult life the risk of cancer induced by many chemical carcinogens or by ionizing radiation increases with age, but it is not supported by the effect of congenital or induced immunodeficiency on the incidence of cancer, which is marked for only a few specific types of the disease. An alternative explanation is that the pattern reflects prolonged exposure to small doses of carcinogens. This pattern is observed for skin carcinomas produced by ultraviolet light, for bronchial carcinomas in both non-smokers and in men who regularly smoke a constant number of cigarettes a day, and in skin-painting experiments on mice. In all these circumstances the incidence of the induced cancer increases approximately with the fourth power of the duration of exposure. If exposure begins at birth, the incidence also increases with the fourth power of age, but if it begins later in life, the same relationship with duration of exposure has the effect of making the incidence appear to increase with a higher power of age, the power becoming progressively higher as the age of first exposure is postponed.

Another, but much less common, pattern is shown by retinoblastomas, nephroblastomas, and medulloblastomas: namely, a peak incidence in childhood followed by a decline virtually to zero. This pattern is presumably due to the action of carcinogenic agents *in utero*, or in the first few years of life, on tissues that soon become too differentiated to be capable of initiating a malignant clone. When there is a family history, retinoblastomas nearly always affect both eyes, and they tend to occur a year or so earlier than the sporadic cases, which are usually unilateral. This, Knudson (1985) has pointed out, accords with the idea that the development of the disease requires two mutations, one of which is present prezygotically in hereditary cases, while both mutations have to occur postzygotically in sporadic cases.

The remaining cancers show a bewildering variety of patterns. Carcinoma of the breast behaves initially like the common cancers of the digestive tract; but the incidence stabilizes for a few years around the menopause before increasing again at a slower rate. In many parts of Africa and Asia, however, the incidence falls after the menopause. Carcinoma of the cervix behaves in an intermediate way, increasing in incidence until shortly after the menopause and then stabilizing. Hodgkin's disease begins to occur in childhood (particularly in undeveloped countries) and then continues to occur throughout life, with minor peaks in young adult life and old age. Osteosarcomas show a sharp rise in incidence to a peak in late adolescence and then decrease in incidence, only to rise again in old age in association with Paget disease.

Many cancers are recorded as decreasing in incidence in old age in developing countries, but this is often an artefact due to the lack of services for old people. Alternatively the pattern may, sometimes, reflect a cohort effect, like the effect that used to be seen with bronchial carcinomas in Europe and North America after the spread of cigarette smoking. The disease, which had been rare, became progressively more common, first in early adult life, then in middle age, and many years later in old age when there began to be old people in the population who had smoked cigarettes all their adult lives. As a result, the pattern changed from one with a peak mortality at about 60 years of age to one showing a progressive increase with age to 80 years and over, as shown in Fig. 9.99. The figure, it will be noted, also shows the beginning of the reverse process, with a decline occurring first at relatively young ages, at which the effects of reducing the amount smoked and the reduction in the amount of tar delivered per cigarette are already having an effect.

Sex

Cancer used to be more common in women than in men in nearly all countries, due to the great frequency of carcinoma of

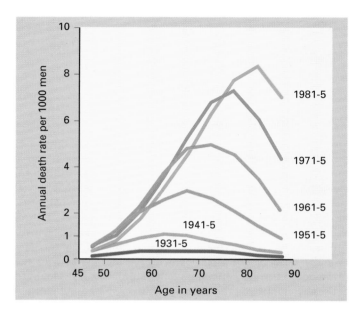

Fig. 9.99   Mortality from lung cancer by age in different periods.

the cervix and the rarity of carcinoma of the bronchus, and it still is in populations in which these conditions continue to hold, as in parts of Latin America. Elsewhere, cancer is now more common in men. The overall male preponderance hides, however, a wide range of sex ratios. This is shown in Table 9.13, which gives the male incidence rate divided by the female rate (both standardized for age) for 34 types of cancer in England and Wales. If the sites that are peculiar (or almost peculiar) to one sex are omitted, the ratio is seen to vary from 7.0:1(M:F) for carcinoma of the lip to 0.4:1 for carcinoma of the thyroid.

For some types of cancer, the sex ratio is always much the same everywhere. For others, however, the sex ratio may be extremely variable—not only between countries, at different times, and at different ages, but also with different cell types and in different parts of the organ. Cancer of the oesophagus, for example, may be very common and affect both sexes equally (as in parts of China) or be 20 times more common in men than in women (as in parts of France). As with the various patterns of incidence with age, these different sex ratios and the variation between countries, times, and ages can provide clues to the causation of the different types of the disease.

Latent period

One reason why it has been difficult to recognize the causes of human cancer is the existence of a long interval between first exposure to the cause and the clinical appearance of the disease. This is commonly 20–40 years, but it may be as long as 60 years or as short as 1 year. To call this interval a 'latent period' is misleading, because there is no reason to suppose that the cancer is present in a latent form from the start of exposure. It is better thought of as comprising three elements: a pre-induction

Table 9.13 Ratio of male to female incidence rates (standardized for age) in England and Wales

Type of cancer (organ of origin)	Male rate divided by female rate	Type of cancer (organ of origin)	Male rate divided by female rate
Lip	7.0	Hodgkin disease	1.6
Larynx	5.7	Non-Hodgkin lymphoma	1.5
Pleura	4.0	Brain	1.5
Bronchus	3.8	Chronic lymphatic leukaemia	1.5
Bladder	3.8	Myelomatosis	1.4
Mouth	2.4	Salivary glands	1.3
Stomach	2.4	Small intestine	1.3
Tongue	2.0	Extrahepatic bile ducts	1.3
Nasopharynx	2.0	Bone	1.3
Pharynx	2.0	Connective tissue	1.3
Liver	2.0	Acute leukaemia	1.2
Nose and nasal sinuses	2.0	Chronic myeloid leukaemia	1.2
Kidney	2.0	Colon	1.1
Oesophagus	1.9	Eye	1.0
Rectum	1.7	Gall-bladder	0.6
Pancreas	1.6	Skin (melanoma)	0.6
Skin (squamous and basal cell)	1.6	Thyroid	0.4

period before any change is produced, a 'promoting' period in which 'initiated' cells are multiplied or in which a succession of further changes in initiated cells is produced, and a development period in which a genuine malignant clone grows large enough to be recognized as a cancer clinically or pathologically.

The total 'latent period' varies greatly from one subject to another and, to some extent, also from one type of cancer to another. For acute myeloid and acute lymphatic leukaemias it may be as short as 18 months, but the modal period is 5–10 years and it may be as long as 25 or 30 years. In contrast, the 'latent period' for mesotheliomas and for nasal sinus cancers is seldom less than 15 years (except for those few that occur in childhood and may be due to prenatal factors) and it is commonly more than 30 years. Most other tumours begn to appear within 10 years of exposure and reach a peak about 10 years later. Estimation of the length of time it takes to produce a cancer is complicated, however, by the fact that few human tumours are known to have been induced after only brief periods of exposure, apart from those induced by ionizing radiations, and there is no way of knowing when, during a long period of exposure, the induction of the tumour actually begins. With some occupational carcinogens, the picture is further obscured by the retention of the carcinogenic agents within the body, so that cellular exposure and environmental exposures are not necessarily coterminous.

With long 'latent periods' it is only to be expected that the incidence of cancer may continue to increase for many years after exposure to the carcinogenic agent has ceased. This, however, is not always the case. It does not happen with cigarette smoking, the cessation of which leads to the stabilization of the incidence of bronchial carcinoma, if not to an actual decline, within 2–3 years. This presumably implies that cigarette smoke acts to promote the process of carcinogenesis as well as to initiate it.

9.7.3 General causes of cancer

Some few agents cause or prevent (or help to cause or prevent) a wide variety of cancers in many different organs and it is convenient to consider some of these separately, before considering the specific causes of particular types of the disease.

Ionizing radiations

Ionizing radiations of all sorts penetrate animal tissues and damage DNA and it is not surprising that they have been shown to cause cancer in many organs. The survivors of the Hiroshima and Nagasaki atomic bomb explosions and patients treated by radiotherapy have been found to have an increased incidence of all cancers that are common enough to be observed at all frequently in several thousand subjects followed for 30–40 years, and it seems only reasonable to assume that an increased incidence of other rarer types of cancer would also be observed if a large enough group of people were exposed. Chronic lymphatic leukaemia may, however, provide an exception, due perhaps to the extreme sensitivity of the relevant stem cells to the effects of ionizing radiations, so that the cells are killed by doses that would be large enough to produce a detectable increase in the incidence of the disease.

Theoretical considerations and the observed effects of exposure to moderate and large doses both indicate that there is unlikely to be any threshold below which no effect is produced, and this conclusion is reinforced by the observation that children who received doses of only 10–20 mSv (1–2 rem) *in utero* (because their mothers were irradiated for diagnostic purposes while pregnant) were subject to an added risk of developing cancer in childhood of about 1 in 2000. At very low doses it seems probable that the carcinogenic effect is likely to be proportional to the dose, but it is still uncertain whether it is proportional to the dose or to the square of the dose at the higher levels at which most of the observations have been made. Quantitative estimates of the effect, derived primarily from observations on the survivors of the Hiroshima and Nagasaki atomic bomb explosions, vary with sex and age, the figures being slightly higher for men than for women and higher for the young than for the middle-aged and elderly. For persons with the sex and age distribution of the population of the UK, the National Radiological Protection Board estimated in 1988 that the lifetime risk of fatal cancer was about 130 per 1000 per Sv and for persons of working age (20–64 years) about 100 per 1000 per Sv. For low doses spread out over a long period, as are received from occupational or natural exposure, the risks may be somewhat lower and were estimated by the National Radiological Protection Board to be respectively about 45 and 40 per 1000 per Sv.

These estimates are liable to be revised as more information is obtained about the effects four or five decades after exposure and about the relative effects of acute and chronic exposure. On the current basis it would appear that an average dose of about 2500 μSv a year (averaging about 2200 μSv a year from radionuclides in soil, air, and body tissues; 300 a year from medicines and medical procedures; 10 μSv from fall-out from past bomb tests and nuclear accidents; 10 μSv from air travel; 5 μSv from occupational exposure; and 1 μSv from all other sources) would produce about 6200 fatal cancers a year in a population of 55 million (or a few hundred less if allowance is made for the short expectation of life of some medically irradiated patients): that is, about 5 per cent of all fatal cancers.

Overnutrition

Experiments leave no doubt that overnutrition increases the incidence of spontaneous tumours of the lung and breast in laboratory animals, and that the restriction of the intake of food can halve the number of tumours produced by a wide range of carcinogens. The relevance of these results to human cancers is, however, uncertain. In the American Cancer Society's massive follow-up study of a million Americans, the mortality from several types of cancer (that is, from cancers of the cervix, breast, and kidney in women and from cancer of the colon in men) was increased in people who were 40 per cent or more above the standard weight and approximately double that in people who were more than 20 per cent below the standard weight; but it is not clear whether this was because obesity increased incidence, delayed diagnosis, and hence led to an increased fatality, or was associated with socio-economic factors that affected the incidence of cancer for other reasons. A marked and progressive increase in mortality with increasing obesity was observed only for cancers of the endometrium and gall-bladder, and it is only these two types of cancer that are consistently associated with obesity in clinical series. Overnutrition (or what in developed countries has come to be regarded as a high standard of nutrition) may, however, play a major part in the production of breast cancer by causing greater growth in childhood, a greater mass of breast tissue, and an early menarche.

Nutritional deficiency

Vitamins

Several other aspects of diet may have non-specific effects on the incidence of a wide variety of cancers, the most important of which may be the dietary content of vitamin A (retinol) and β-carotene. Experiments on animals and on cell cultures have shown that retinol and its esters and analogues may, in appropriate circumstances, reduce the risk of cancer by reducing the probability that partially transformed cells become fully transformed and proliferate into a clinically detectable tumour while, in other circumstances, they appear to have opposite effects. Epidemiological studies seemed at first to support the idea that vitamin A-rich diets might protect against many different cancers, including most notably cancer of the lung; but this was difficult to understand as, in the absence of gross deficiency, homeostatic mechanisms mantained the amount of retinol in the blood at a steady level. What had been classed as vitamin A in most diets was, however, β-carotene, some of which is converted into vitamin A *in vivo*, while the rest circulates in the blood and is deposited in tissues or excreted. Follow-up studies have now shown that the amount of retinol in the blood bears no relationship to the subsequent incidence of cancer, while the amount of β-carotene sometimes does. Evidence of a prophylactic effect in laboratory animals is less impressive for β-carotene than for retinol, and the epidemiological evidence of the effect of β-carotene is not wholly consistent. On current knowledge, however, β-carotene seems to be the most likely candidate for a dietary agent of prophylactic value against a wide spectrum of cancers.

Two other vitamins have also been thought to have a protective effect: namely vitamin C (ascorbic acid) and vitamin E (α-tocopherol). A high intake of vitamin C, indicated by a dietary history of frequent consumption of fresh vegetables and fruit, seems likely to protect against the development of both oesophageal and gastric cancer, as these items are characteristically deficient in the diet of affected patients. That this might be so is, moreover, suggested by the fact that vitamin C inhibits the formation of nitrosamines both *in vivo* and experimentally *in vitro*. Unfortunately, however, there is no clear evidence that nitrosamines formed *in vivo* are responsible for either disease in man.

Vitamin E has been thought to be protective because of its role in catalysing the removal of peroxides in conjunction with glutathione peroxidase. A few studies have reported an increased risk of cancer in people with low levels of serum vitamin E, but others have not and the present evidence is inconclusive.

Trace elements

Several trace elements have been thought to have a role in the production or prevention of cancer, including iodine, zinc, copper, molybdenum, and selenium, but material human evidence has been produced only in relation to the last. Selenium occurs at the active site of the enzyme glutathione peroxidase, referred to in relation to vitamin E, and deficiency of selenium leads to a deficiency of the enzyme. Selenium levels have sometimes been found to be lower in cancer patients than in controls and inverse correlations have been reported between selenium intake and cancer risk in North America. It is notable, however, that there is no general excess of cancer in the Keshan province of China in which selenium deficiency is so gross that it results in the development of a specific form of heart disease. Cohort studies, in which blood has been stored and the selenium content subsequently examined in individuals who have or have not developed cancer, should eventually show whether the variation that occurs between individuals in developed countries is of any clinical significance. Present results are inconsistent.

9.7.4 Causes of specific cancers

Lip, buccal cavity, and pharynx

Carcinoma of the lip accounts for about 0.2 per cent of all cancers in Britain. It was one of the first types of cancer to be related to an extrinsic cause when, more than 200 years ago, it was noted to occur characteristically in pipe-smokers. Many years later it was realized that the disease could also be produced (though less easily) by smoking in other ways. It must, therefore, be produced by the chemicals in smoke rather than by local heat. It is more common in outdoor than in indoor workers, and is evidently induced by ultraviolet light in the same way as carcinoma of the exposed skin. Ultraviolet light and tobacco account between them for the great majority of all cases in Britain; but it is uncertain whether they act independently or synergistically. The disease is now much less common than it used to be, due presumably to the decrease in both pipe smoking and outdoor work.

Carcinomas of the tongue, mouth, and pharynx (other than nasopharynx) account for about 0.8 per cent of all cancers in Britain. All are related to smoking (of pipes, cigars, and cigarettes) and to the consumption of alcohol. The two factors act synergistically and very few cases occur in Europe and North America unless both factors are present. All these cancers are much more common in parts of South-East and Central Asia where quids composed of various mixtures of tobacco, lime, and betel nut or betel leaf are chewed. In some areas they are so common that they account for 20 per cent of all cancers. Most originate in the part of the mouth in which the quid is usually held, something which varies between communities and between individuals. The materials chewed also differ and, although the disease is often described as 'betel chewers' cancer', betel is not an invariable component.

Carcinoma of the tongue is much less common in Britain than it used to be. It tended to be associated with syphilitic leukoplakia, and the reduction in incidence has been due in part to the reduced prevalence of syphilis. It has become more common in the United States in recent years in young men, following the increased use of oral snuff.

In parts of India, Sardinia, and South America where women tend to smoke small cigars and cigarettes with the burning ends inside their mouth to prevent them going out, the habit is associated with the development of carcinoma of the palate, a disease that is extremely rare everywhere else.

Carcinomas of the nasopharynx (which account for 0.1 per cent of all cancers in Britain) and cancers of the salivary gland (which account for 0.3 per cent) alone in this group are unrelated to either smoking or alcohol, and have not (in Britain) been related to any specific cause. In some other countries, however, the position is different.

Nasopharyngeal cancer is very common in Chinese who live in, or emigrated from, the region near Guangdong, and moderately high rates have been observed in Alaskan Eskimos, American Indians, and in Malaysia, Kenya, and North Africa. In most of these areas DNA characteristic of the Epstein–Barr (EB) virus has been detected in the nuclei of nasopharyngeal cancer cells, and patients with the disease have high levels of antibodies against EB virus-related antigens in their serum. It is clear, however, that the EB virus alone is not sufficient to cause the disease and that some other agent is required to interact with it. In the high-risk Chinese this is a chemical in the salted fish which is a favourite food and is commonly given to children when they are weaned. Nitrosamines extracted from the fish have caused nasopharyngeal cancers in rats, but this finding has yet to be confirmed.

Cancers of the salivary glands are not common anywhere but they are relatively more common in the Asiatic populations of Hawaii and in Canadian Indians than in other people. No special cause is known, apart from a genetic factor that increases susceptibility to cancer in both the salivary glands and breast.

A rare cause of all these cancers (apart from cancers of the lip and salivary gland) is exposure to mustard gas. Excess cases were not observed in combatants exposed acutely in the First World War, but they have been observed in manufacturers of mustard gas in Britain and Japan.

Digestive tract

Cancers of the digestive tract have one feature in common, the suspicion that they are caused by components of the diet. On present evidence, however, the causes of cancer in each organ appear to be largely different.

Oesophagus

Carcinoma of the oesophagus accounts for about 1.9 per cent of all cancers in Britain. Like cancer of the buccal cavity and pharynx, it is closely related to both smoking (of all types) and the consumption of alcohol. In the absence of either, the incidence of the disease in Britain is reduced by about three-quarters. A few cases originate from the scars resulting from poisoning with corrosive chemicals, and a very few in conjunction with a particular hereditary form of tylosis, which presents with keratoses of the palms and soles.

In Africa and Asia the epidemiological findings are striking, but they have yet to be explained. In parts of China (particularly in Shanxi and Henan provinces) and on the east coast of the Caspian Sea the oesophagus is the most common site for cancer and the incidence rates in both sexes are equal to the incidence of lung cancer in European cities in men. Very high rates are also found in parts of Africa, particularly in the Transkei regions of South Africa and on the east coast of Lake Victoria in Kenya, sometimes equally in both sexes and sometimes only in men. In these areas the high incidence zones are strictly localized and the incidence falls off rapidly over distances of 200–300 miles. When tobacco and alcohol are used they increase the hazard, but they are not the principal agents. Many causes have been proposed, but none has been established and the only factor common to all the high-incidence areas is a restricted diet, particularly poor in animal protein and green vegetables. In some parts of China mycotoxins produced by fungi of the *Fusaria* species are a possible cause, and in Japan a few cases may be attributable to the consumption of bracken fern. Despite much intensive research it has not been possible to connect any of the high risks of the disease to the nitrosamines that have been such a prolific cause of oesophageal cancer in animal experiments.

Stomach

Until the mid-1970s, cancer of the stomach was responsible for more deaths in the world each year than any other type of cancer. Over the past 50 years, however, the incidence of the disease has progressively declined, particularly in Western Europe, North America, and Australasia, and the decline is still continuing. High rates are confined to China, Japan, the USSR, and Central and South America, while very low rates are found perhaps surprisingly in some of the least developed parts of Africa, with only slightly higher rates in North America, Australia, and New Zealand. In Britain, the incidence is intermediate and the disease still causes approximately 7 per cent of all cancers.

Within Britain, cancer of the stomach is most common in North Wales and becomes progressively less common from north to south and from west to east. It has consistently been more common in manual labourers than in members of the major professions and the gradient with social class has been one of the most marked for any disease. Occupational hazards have been suspected in coal mining, some sections of the rubber industry, and from exposure to asbestos; but none has been proved. In the asbestos industry it seems probable that the excess rates have been an artefact due to the misdiagnosis of peritoneal mesotheliomas and lung cancers with secondary abdominal spread.

The principal causes seem likely to be dietary, but it is still uncertain what they are. Smoking food and cooking it in ways that produce polycyclic hydrocarbons or mutagenic substances are, at the most, of minor importance, and modern methods of food preservation, particularly by refrigeration, are more likely to have reduced the hazard than the reverse. Despite intensive research it has not been possible to link the disease with the consumption of nitrites or nitrates or with the formation of nitrosamines *in vivo*. There is, however, good evidence that the disease is relatively uncommon when the diet is rich in fruit and green vegetables.

The incidence is consistently 20 per cent higher in people belonging to blood group A than in people belonging to other blood groups, irrespective of whether they live in high- or low-incidence areas. Pathologically, the disease tends to be preceded by intestinal metaplasia of the gastric mucosa or atrophic gastritis. Gastroenterostomy increases the risk of the disease, but, given an accurate initial diagnosis, it does not occur as a complication of chronic gastric ulcer more often than would be expected from the association of both diseases with low socioeconomic status.

Large bowel

Cancers of the colon and rectum are commonly classed together, partly because cancers often occur at the rectosigmoid junction and the correct allocation may be arbitrary, and partly because they have many aetiological features in common. There are, however, also important differences. Cancer of the colon tends to occur more often in women than in men, particularly when it occurs on the right side, while cancer of the rectum is more common in men. The geographical distribution also differs slightly, colon cancer varying in incidence more than rectal cancer. Both diseases are much more common in developed countries than in Africa and Asia, and they are more common in Western than in Eastern Europe. In developed countries incidence rates have changed very little over the past 50 years, apart from a slight decrease in some countries in the immediate post-war period and in early middle-age in Britain in the last two decades. The incidence used to be low in Japan, but the rate in Japanese who migrated to Hawaii rapidly came to equal the rate in Caucasians and it is now increasing steadily in Japan itself.

In Britain, rates are moderately high and the two large bowel cancers together account for 12.4 per cent of all cancers. Within Britain there is no clear relationship to socio-economic class and no occupational hazards have been established. An increased incidence has been reported in some groups of asbestos workers; but, as with gastric cancer, this may have resulted from the misdiagnosis of peritoneal mesotheliomas and lung cancers with secondary abdominal spread. International comparisons have suggested that the incidence of both diseases is positively correlated with the amount of fat in the diet. The evidence is, however, inconclusive, possibly because there is relatively little variation in dietary habits within a single cultural group and partly because it is so difficult to obtain accurate histories of the dietary habits of individuals. One way in which fat might cause the disease would be by stimulating the secretion of bile acids, metabolites of which can act as promoting agents in animal experiments. Other factors that appear to affect the risk of the disease are cruciferous vegetables (typically cabbage and Brussels sprouts) and fibre and resistant starch which may reduce it substantially, and beer, and to a less extent other alcoholic drinks, which may increase it. Various mechanisms have been proposed by which these effects might be produced, but none has been substantiated.

Two chronic diseases that increase the risk of large bowel cancer are ulcerative colitis and rectal infection with *Schistosoma japonicum*. The latter is still very common in the Yangtze valley of central China and is a major cause of what is, otherwise in China, a rare disease. In developed countries, carcinomas of the large bowel usually arise from adenomatous polyps, whether present singly, in small numbers, or in the large numbers that are characteristic of polyposis coli and Gardner's syndrome. In the former, polyps and carcinomatous degeneration occur so early in life and are so common that few affected people survive to middle-age without colectomy.

In a few cases, anal intercourse, leading to infection with some types of the human papilloma virus, may possibly be a cause of anal carcinoma, in the same way as a similar infection will cause carcinoma of the cervix.

Liver

The incidence of primary carcinoma of the liver tends to be overestimated in developed countries, particularly at ages over 65 years, when hepatic metastases from primary cancers in the respiratory and gastrointestinal tracts are common and may be mistaken for it. In Britain and the United States, where current rates are among the lowest in the world, the disease accounts for about 0.4 per cent of all cancers and the incidence is static, except perhaps in women, in whom some small increase has been recorded recently. In tropical Africa and parts of China and South-East Asia the position is very different, and carcinoma of the liver is so common that it may be the principal type of cancer in men.

Most liver cancers are hepatocellular carcinomas and are due to the combined effects of infection with the hepatitis B virus and exposure to aflatoxin, a metabolite of the fungus *Aspergillus flavus*, which commonly contaminates peanuts, maize, and other oil-bearing foods, when they are stored under hot and humid conditions. Just how these two agents interact is unclear. The risk of the disease is particularly great in carriers of the virus who are infected in infancy, and efforts to prevent the disease will require immunization within a few days of birth, as is now being attempted in Japan, Singapore, and the Gambia. The incidence is never high, however, unless the diet contains large amounts of aflatoxin.

In Britain and other developed countries where very little aflatoxin is consumed and the hepatitis B carrier state is uncommon, a more important cause is cirrhosis of the liver, irrespective of whether it is due to hepatitis, alcoholism, or haemochromatosis. Occasional cases are also produced by drugs, particularly by the use of steroid contraceptives or anabolic steroids taken to increase muscular strength.

Cholangiocarcinomas are less common and tend to occur at later ages than hepatocellular carcinomas. In China they occur as a complication of chronic infection with liver flukes (clonorchiasis).

A third histological variety, variously described as reticuloendothelioma or angiosarcoma, is extremely uncommon, affecting about 1 in 20 000 000 people a year. Its rarity, however, made it particularly easy to recognize its causes. Two have now been eliminated: namely inorganic arsenic, which was commonly prescribed for a variety of chronic diseases of unknown aetiology, and thorotrast, a contrast medium that was used in neuroradiology and which led to the retention of insoluble radionuclides in the marrow, liver, and spleen. The third, exposure to vinyl chloride, is now largely controlled. An occupational hazard was discovered in 1973, shortly after the discovery of the carcinogenicity of vinyl chloride in animal experiments, and some 150 cases are now known to have occurred in Western Europe, North America, and Japan. Men manufacturing vinyl chloride polymer had been exposed to several thousand parts per million (a thousand times more than industrial workers are exposed to now) and it is doubtful whether the amounts to which the general public were exposed, when minute amounts leaked out of plastic containers, caused more than a handful of cases altogether, if indeed they caused any at all.

Cancer of the liver is almost uniformly fatal and it is fortunate that it is so rare in developed countries. That it is so rare must raise doubts about the value of the mouse model as an indicator of carcinogenic risk to humans, as so many chemicals to which humans have been exposed induce liver tumours in mice.

Gall bladder and extrahepatic bile ducts

Cancers of the gall bladder and extrahepatic ducts are commonly classed together and, as with cancers of the colon and rectum, this is unfortunate as the causes are certainly different. Cancer of the gall bladder is more than twice as common in women as in men, is strongly associated with obesity, and is nearly always preceded by cholelithiasis, whereas cancer of the extrahepatic bile ducts is more common in men than in women, is increased in incidence by clonorchiasis, and possibly also by long-standing ulcerative colitis. Both types are uncommon, constituting in combination only about 0.7 per cent of all cancer in Britain; and their incidence is not very different anywhere else. The highest rates (four times that recorded in Britain) are recorded in Jewesses in Israel, particularly in those who have migrated from Europe and America.

The incidence of cancer of the gall bladder has fallen sharply in the United States in the past 20 years, due possibly in part to the decrease in the consumption of animal fat but certainly in part to an increased rate of cholecystectomy for gallstones, with the result that most of the gall bladders at risk of developing the disease are removed prophylactically.

Pancreas

Cancer of the pancreas is generally regarded as a disease of the developed world, but the diagnosis is difficult in the absence of a well-developed medical service and much of the recorded geographical and temporal variation is probably due to differences in the availability of medical care. In Britain the disease now accounts for about 3.0 per cent of all cancers and it is probably becoming slightly less common with the passage of time, as it is also in the USA. Cigarette smoking is the most important known cause, increasing the risk of the disease, on average, two or three times. No chemical in cigarette smoke has, however, been isolated that is capable of causing pancreatic carcinoma experimentally. The incidence of the disease is correlated with a high standard of living and is twice as high in diabetics as in the population as a whole. It is, therefore, not surprising that the highest rate in the world (about double that in Britain) is recorded in New Zealand Maoris, a population that smokes heavily and is prone to obesity, hypertension, myocardial infarction, and diabetes. The association that was reported with the consumption of coffee has not been confirmed and seems likely to have been an artefact.

Peritoneum
See under pleura.

Respiratory tract

Nose and nasal sinuses
Cancers of the paranasal sinuses are rare throughout the world and cancers of the nasal cavity extemely rare. Together they account for 0.2 per cent of all cancers in Britain. High incidence rates have, however, been observed in a few specialized industries, most notably in association with nickel refining and, in the extreme case in South Wales, they at one time accounted for 8 per cent of all deaths in the refinery workers. Smaller hazards have also been observed in refineries in Canada, Norway, and the USSR. The specific agent has not yet been determined, but nickel subsulphide, nickel oxide, and soluble nickel salts are probably all implicated. The disease has also been produced in men working with hardwoods, particularly in the furniture workers of High Wycombe following the introduction of high-speed wood-working machinery early in this century, but also (though probably to a lesser extent) in many other groups of hardwood workers throughout the world. Other industries to have given rise to a risk of nasal sinus cancer are the manufacture of isopropyl alcohol and the manufacture of leather goods.

Most occupational and other cancers of this type are squamous carcinomas, but the hazard from hardwood dust characteristically produced adenocarcinomas. This type of nasal sinus cancer is normally so rare that the 5 per cent incidence that occurred in some groups of workers meant that the normal risk had been increased 1500 times.

Larynx
Cancer of the larynx accounts for 0.9 per cent of all cancers in Britain. Like cancers of the buccal cavity, pharynx, and oesophagus, it is closely associated with tobacco smoking and the consumption of alcohol. The two agents act synergistically and in the absence of either the disease would be rare; in the absence of both the incidence would be reduced by about 90 per cent. Cancers of the glottis are particularly associated with cigarette smoking, but cancers of the extrinsic larynx are caused equally by pipe and cigar smoking. Other factors seem likely to have been more important in the past and it seems probable that some other factor (possibly nutritional) became less prevalent in the first half of the century at the time when cigarette smoking became more common, as there was no corresponding increase in the incidence of the disease. Other factors must also account for the higher incidence rates that are observed in parts of Asia, North Africa, and Brazil.

The only occupational hazard to have been established is the manufacture of mustard gas, but a small hazard may also have been produced by exposure to asbestos.

Lung
Bronchial carcinoma became the most common cause of death from cancer in the world in the early 1980s. Until the First World War, bronchial carcinoma had been rare everywhere, apart from a few places where there were foci of gross occupational hazards. In the next 70 years it increased rapidly in incidence, but at different rates at different ages, in each sex, and in different countries. In Britain, where the increase was most notable, it was much greater in men than in women, and a peak in the male rate was reached in 1973, when the disease accounted for 36 per cent of all deaths from cancer in men and 9 per cent of deaths from all causes. Since then the incidence has decreased, most notably in young men in whom the mortality rate in the mid-1980s was less than half what it had been 30 years earlier. In women the incidence is still increasing at all ages except the youngest, and the disease now challenges breast cancer for the distinction of being the cause of the greatest number of cancer deaths. In total it now accounts for about 20 per cent of all cancers in both sexes combined.

The rapid increase in incidence is due everywhere to the increase in the consumption of tobacco and particularly to the increase in the consumption of cigarettes, which produce a smoke that is less irritating than the smoke from pipes and cigars and is easier to inhale. Nicotine in cigarette smoke consequently reaches the alveoli where it is absorbed rapidly and gives rise to a rapid and (to the addict) a gratifying increase in the level in the blood. Nicotine in pipe and cigar smoke is, in contrast, absorbed principally from the mouth. It may eventually give rise to higher blood levels than the nicotine in cigarette smoke, but absorption is slow and the reaction to the sudden increase in blood level is lacking. In Britain, the smoking of tobacco was estimated to have been responsible for nearly 95 per cent of all bronchial carcinomas in men by the mid-1970s and, 10 years later, to over 80 per cent of all cases in women. The reduction in mortality, which began to occur in the early 1960s in the professional classes and in the youngest age groups in all men, has been due partly to a decrease in the consumption of tobacco, but also, and to an important degree, to the progressive introduction of cigarettes that deliver less tar to the bronchial mucosa.

On stopping smoking the rate of increase in the incidence of the disease with age slows down within two or three years, and may even cease altogether for 10–20 years. Tobacco smoke must, therefore, act as a promoting agent as well as an initiator, which is presumably why it acts synergistically with some other carcinogenic agents, such as asbestos, increasing their effects multiplicatively instead of simply adding to them. It has, therefore, been possible to conclude that 80 per cent of the bronchial carcinomas that occurred in a group of heavily exposed asbestos insulation workers could have been avoided if they had not been exposed to asbestos, and that 90 per cent of the same cancers could have been avoided if they had not smoked.

In the absence of smoking, the disease is rare throughout the world and occurs at much the same age-specific rates in all communities, except for Chinese women and some groups of industrial workers. The nature of the hazard to which Chinese women are exposed and which doubles the normal risk in non-smokers has not yet been established firmly, but it seems to be the fumes from cooking oils produced by the characteristically Chinese method of cooking with a 'wok'; that is, a semi-spherical vessel without a lid that can be used to cook food with a minimum of fuel.

All other known causes have been discovered as a result of localized exposures in industry. A few such exposures have caused risks comparable to or greater than that caused by cigarette smoking, such as the high concentrations of radon that used to occur in the mines of Jachymov and Schneeberg, uncontrolled exposure to asbestos, and the conditions in some nickel refineries before the end of the Second World War. The most widespread causes, apart from radon and asbestos, are some of the polycyclic hydrocarbons in the fumes from coal tar that have caused hazards in the manufacture of coal gas and coke and, to a lesser extent, in aluminium factories and iron foundries, arsenic trioxide encountered in the manufacture of arsenical insecticides and in the refining of copper, hexavalent chromium compounds encountered in the manufacture of chromates from chrome ore, zinc chromate, bischloromethyl ether, and mustard gas. Many others have been suspected and may well have caused relatively small increases in risk which could, however, be substantial in absolute terms because the disease is so common. These include man-made mineral fibres, crystalline silica, beryllium and beryllium compounds, diethyl sulphate, and formaldehyde.

Several of the established agents also pollute the ambient atmosphere and must be presumed to cause some risk to the general population if, as generally believed, most carcinogenic agents produce an effect proportional to the dose received at low levels of exposure. The most important has been the pollution of the atmosphere with coal smoke which used to be characteristic of urban life and continues to be in some developing countries. It is still debatable how great an effect this pollution produced, but it seems unlikely that it was ever responsible for more than about 10 per cent of all bronchial carcinomas, even in the most polluted cities in the past, and the relatively very small amount of pollution that is now produced, mostly by internal combustion and diesel engines, is unlikely, on the basis of extrapolation from proven occupational hazards, to cause more than a small fraction of 1 per cent of all cases of the disease. The most important of the many other general pollutants are asbestos, from its use as a building and insulating material in houses and as a lining for brakes; radon, which escapes from the soil and may accumulate in poorly ventilated houses; and tobacco smoke. The last may account for a quarter of all cases of bronchial carcinoma in non-smokers, while radon may cause 6 per cent of all bronchial carcinomas in conjunction with smoking and a substantially higher proportion in parts of Cornwall and Devon.

Not all the histological types of bronchial carcinoma are produced equally by all the known causes. Smoking specifically increases the risks of squamous carcinoma and, to a less extent, of small cell and undifferentiated carcinomas. Whether it affected the risk of adenocarcinoma has been debatable.

Changes in diagnostic criteria make time trends difficult to assess, but there is evidence to suggest that adenocarcinomas have become relatively more common and it is possible that this is due to the introduction of low-tar cigarettes, the smoke from which tends to be inhaled more deeply and may consequently produce a relatively greater risk of peripheral cancers of adenocarcinomatous type.

Most occupational hazards produce all the main histological types of the disease, but there have been few adequate studies that take into account the source of the material. This is an essential requirement for any reliable comparisons, as adenocarcinomas tend to occur peripherally and consequently contribute a higher proportion of cases in any series that is derived from necropsy or thoracotomy material than in one that consists largely of material obtained by bronchoscopy. Two exceptions are radon and bischloromethyl ether, which characteristically produce small cell carcinomas. It is therefore understandable that the lung tumours in the miners of Schneeburg and Jachymov were originally described as sarcomas of the mediastinum. In contrast, the agent that produces the increased risk in Chinese women characteristically produces adenocarcinomas.

Pleura

Cancers of the pleura are nearly all mesotheliomas. Similar tumours occur in the peritoneum and, as both have the same aetiology, they can be considered together. About 80 per cent are caused by occupational exposure to asbestos or by exposure to asbestos in some unusual domestic or environmental circumstances. Some of the remainder may be due to the small amounts of asbestos that are found ubiquitously in the general environment, while some others are presumably due to natural radioactivity. The straight fibres of amphibole asbestos (notably amosite and crocidolite) persist in the body for many years and are more likely to cause the disease than the less persistent curly fibres of the more commonly used chrysotile. There is, indeed, no good evidence to show that the latter have caused any mesotheliomas of the peritoneum. A few pleural and peritoneal mesotheliomas have been caused by other similar mineral fibres that have not been exploited industrially, such as erionite, and several clusters of cases have occurred in Turkish and Greek villages, where rock containing erionite has been used for domestic purposes.

Mesotheliomas seldom occur less than 15 years after first exposure to unusual amounts of asbestos, commonly occur after 20 or 30 years, and may occur up to 50 years after exposure has ceased. The measures that have been taken to reduce exposure have, therefore, not yet been reflected in a decline in the incidence of the disease. The rate of increase, which was rapid in the 1960s has tailed off in the 1980s, and the incidence appears to have stabilized under 50 years of age. Interpretation of the recorded trends is, however, difficult, as the disease used to be overlooked and now tends to be overdiagnosed if the patient gives a history of any unusual exposure to asbestos. Pleural mesotheliomas are 2–4 times as common as peritoneal mesotheliomas, but both are rare in Britain and together account for about 0.2 per cent of all cancers.

Urinary tract

Kidney

Renal cancer contributes 1.4 per cent of all cancers. There are three main varieties, each of which has different causes.

Nephroblastoma is a rare cancer that occurs with approximately equal frequency in all populations. It occurs only in childhood and is occasionally familial. These characteristics suggest that the development of the disease requires two 'spontaneous' mutations, one of which occurs prenatally and may be inherited, while the other occurs postnatally.

Adenocarcinomas are the most common. They increase in incidence with age in the same way as most epithelial cancers and have become more common, albeit slowly, over the past few decades. About a quarter of all cases are due to cigarette smoking, but the association is weak and the conclusion that it is causal has been accepted only because the urine of cigarette-smokers is mutagenic and there is a strong relationship between cigarette smoking and cancer of the bladder.

The third variety, squamous or transitional carcinoma of the renal pelvis, accounts for some 10 per cent of all cases. Four causes are known: cigarette smoking, which is related to the disease more strongly than to adenocarcinoma of the body; the occupational factors that cause bladder cancer; the consumption of phenacetin in large enough amounts to cause renal nephropathy; and the factor that causes Balkan nephropathy in villages along the banks of several rivers in Yugoslavia, Bulgaria, and Romania. Unlike the other factors, that cause only small risks, the Balkan nephropathy factor increases the risk to the inhabitants of the affected villages more than 100-fold.

Bladder

Cancer of the bladder accounts for 4.4 per cent of all cancers. Occupational studies have led to the discovery that four aromatic amines cause the disease, all of which are carcinogenic in experimental studies in animals: namely, 2-naphthylamine, 4-amino-biphenyl, benzidine, and 3,3′-dichlorobenzene. Others that may cause the disease are auramine, magenta, and 1-naphthylamine. Contact with these chemicals has occurred in many different occupations, particularly those involved in the manufacture and use of dyes and rubber and in biological laboratories. One of these chemicals (2-naphthylamine) is so potent a human carcinogen that all of one group of 19 men who were employed in distilling it developed the disease. Trace amounts occur in coal tar fumes and this may account for the excess incidence of bladder cancer in coal gas retort house workers. Discovery of these occupational hazards has led to the elimination or control of these agents in industry and the proportion of cases attributable to occupational hazards, which used to be of the order of 10 per cent, is now reduced.

By far the greatest number of cases, about half the total, is caused by cigarette smoking. This is not surprising as cigarette smoke contains small amounts of 2-naphthylamine and cigar-ette smoking leads to the excretion of increased amounts of mutagens in the urine.

Three other causes are chlornaphazine (N,N′-bis(2-chloro-ethyl)-2-naphthylamine), cyclophosphamide, and infestation with *Schistosoma haematobium*. The first was used briefly (though not in the UK) for the treatment of myelomatosis. The second is used primarily in the treatment of cancer, but also as an immunosuppressant. The third accounts for the exceptionally high incidence of the disease in Egypt and Tanzania. The schistosomes are presumably not carcinogenic in themselves, and they may cause the disease secondarily by causing persistent bacterial infection with a consequent local production of carcinogenic nitrosamines. All these agents cause transitional cell carcinoma, except for schistomiasis, which characteristically causes squamous cell carcinomas.

Several dietary causes have been postulated, partly on the basis of animal experiments (namely, cyclamates and saccharin) and partly on the basis of epidemiological observations (namely, coffee). The experiments incriminating cyclamates were, however, misleading, as the material used contained carcinogenic impurities and the totality of the epidemiological evidence relating to the use of saccharin could hardly be more negative. Whether the consumption of coffee increases the risk of bladder cancer is uncertain. The observed association is weak and inconsistent and the evidence fails to allow adequately for the effect of confounding with the much stronger association with cigarette smoking.

Reproductive organs

Breast

Cancer of the breast is the most common fatal cancer in women throughout most of the developed world, being resonsible for 20 per cent of all female cancer deaths, but overall it accounts for little more than 10 per cent of all cancers in both sexes (11.8 per cent in the UK). It is less common in Eastern Europe and much less common in Asia and in the black African populations south of the Sahara. Incidence rates are tending to rise slowly in most countries, but rapidly in countries like Japan, where the pattern of cancer incidence is coming to resemble that in the West.

No cause has been clearly established but hormonal factors are indicated by the effect of early menarche, late menopause, and late age at first full-term pregnancy, all of which increase the risk of the disease. Full-term pregnancies after the first and abortions before the first pregnancy have little effect, which suggests that the determining factors is age at first lactation. Duration of lactation is, however, of only slight importance, prolonged lactation slightly reducing the risk of the disease.

Many clues point to an effect of diet, particularly the close positive correlations between the consumption of fat and the incidence of the disease in different countries. Within countries the evidence is conflicting. In sum, it seems likely that saturated fat increases the risk of the disease, but it is difficult to separate the effect of fat from that of total intake of calories. A high calorie diet in childhood will increase risk by bringing forward the age of menarche and possibly also by increasing the size of the breast. After the menopause it will do so by causing obesity and, consequently, an increase in circulating oestrogens which are formed from adrenal hormones in adipose tissue. Before the menopause, however, obesity is associated with a decreased risk, due presumably to its association with irregular menses and ovarian dysfunction.

Studies of hormonal levels in blood and urine have given inconsistent results in the past, but evidence is beginning to accumulate that the risk of the disease increases with the concentration in the blood of oestradiol that is physiologically available: that is, the free and albumin-bound oestradiol, excluding the amount bound to sex-hormone-binding globulin. This is supported by the observation that the long-term use of oestrogens medicinally after the menopause slightly increases the incidence of the disease. Whether the use of steroid contraceptives, including both oestrogens and progestogens, has any effect is unclear. The totality of the evidence suggests that long-term use early in life may increase the risk premenopausally but that it has little or no effect later in life.

Genetic differences between individuals within a population have a substantial effect on susceptibility to the development of the disease; but they do not seem to play an important part in explaining the differences between national groups.

Cervix uteri

Cancers of the cervix uteri constitute 2.1 per cent of all cancers. They were much more common at the beginning of the century than now and they are still one of the most common types of cancer throughout much of Africa, Asia, and Latin America. The disease was long thought to be related to child-bearing as the incidence was much greater in multiparous than in nulliparous women. It is now clear, however, that child-bearing is irrelevant and that the great majority of cases owe their origin to an infection spread by sexual intercourse. This was proved when it was shown that the risk of the disease increased not only with the number of sexual partners that a women had had, but also, in the case of women who had had only one sexual partner, with the number of his sexual partners. The crucial factor seems to be infection with some of the many types of human papilloma virus (HPV). These are not the types that cause the majority of vulval warts (types 6 and 11) but other types that produce less obvious lesions (principally, but not only, types 16 and 18). Infection with these viruses is, however, extremely common and there must be other factors that determine whether the viral genome is integrated into the host's DNA and whether this leads to the progressive development of dysplasia, carcinoma *in situ*, and invasive cancer. Two other factors that probably contribute to the development of the disease are cigarette smoking and the use of oral contraceptives. Both are confounded with sexual activity, but they seem also to have independent, though relatively minor, effects. That cigarette smoking should have an effect became comprehensible when it was discovered that smoking caused the appearance of mutagens in the cervical mucus.

The disease is extremely uncommon in Jewesses and less common in Muslim women than in Hindu or Christian women living in the same country, and this has suggested that male circumcision might reduce the hazard. No such effect is, however, apparent within communities in which some men are circumcised and others are not, as in Christian communities in Britain and the USA.

The great majority of all cancers of the cervix are squamous carcinomas, and the less common adenocarcinomas may have different causes. Adenocarcinomas have not been shown to be related to sexual intercourse, but their incidence may be increased by the use of steroid contraceptives.

Endometrium

Endometrial cancers constitute 1.9 per cent of all cancers and are almost as common as cervical cancers. Their epidemiological features are, however, very different. Histologically the tumours are nearly always adenocarcinomas. They are common in developed countries and rare in poor countries; common in nulliparous women and progressively less common in women with increasing parity; unrelated to sexual intercourse, but like cancer of the breast, positively associated with early menarche and a late menopause. They are common in association with ovarian tumours that secrete oestrogen; increased in incidence by the use of sequential oral contraceptives in which oestrogen and progestogen are given at different periods of the menstrual cycle; and increased in incidence by the use of oestrogens post-menopausally and by adiposity. The last, like most of the other factors that are positively associated with the disease, increases the level of serum oestrogen, since the adrenal hormone, androstenedione, is converted to oestrogen in adipose tissue. Conversely, the risk of the disease is reduced by the use of steroid contraceptives in which oestrogen is always opposed by progestogen, and by cigarette smoking, which tends to bring forward the menopause and decreases the level of serum oestrogens. All these findings point to the same conclusion: that the risk of the disease is proportional to the extent to which the endometrium is exposed to oestrogen unopposed by progestogen.

Choriocarcinoma

Most choriocarcinomas occur as a result of malignant degeneration of the remnants of a hydatidiform mole left behind after a miscarriage, but a few occur after completion of an apparently normal pregnancy. They are extremely rare, occurring in about 1 in 30 000 pregnancies. Nothing is known about their aetiology except that they are somewhat more common in Maoris, Hawaiians, Malays, American Indians, and in some groups of Chinese than in other populations.

Ovary

Cancers of the ovary constitute 2.3 per cent of all cancers. There are many different histological types and each may have different causes. Most are too rare to have been the subject of separate epidemiological investigation, and the epidemiological features that have been recognized may refer only to the adenocarcinomas, which are by far the most common type. These features resemble, in some respects, the features of endometrial cancer, in that the risk of the disease is greater in developed countries than in undeveloped, increases with the length of time between menarche and menopause, decreases with increasing number of pregnancies, and decreases with the duration of use of steroid contraceptives combining both oestrogen and progestogen. The features differ in that ovarian cancer is not produced by medication with oestrogens, and it seems probable that the risk is proportional to the total number of ovulations.

Prostate

Cancers of the prostate constitute 3.8 per cent of all cancers. The disease increases in incidence with age more sharply than any other type of cancer, so that it has come to be increasingly prominent with the shift in the age distribution of the population towards the oldest age groups. Foci of cells indistinguishable from malignant cells are found in a high proportion of normal prostates in elderly men, and the recorded incidence rate can be increased dramatically by increasing the number of prostatic biopsies. Age-specific death rates have changed very little, and the true incidence of the disease has probably also remained steady. Two epidemiological observations stand out: the high incidence in Blacks in the USA and the low incidence in Japanese in Japan. Both may reflect differences in genetic susceptibility, but they are not wholly due to genetic factors as Blacks and Japanese both have higher rates in the USA than in Africa and Japan.

Hormonal factors presumably play an important part in the production of the disease, but none has been identified. Early reports of an occupational hazard of the disease in cadmium workers have not been borne out by later investigations.

Testis

Testis cancers constitute 0.4 per cent of all cancers. Both the main types (teratomas or embryonal carcinomas and seminomas) begin to appear in late adolescence, occur most frequently between 20 and 34 years of age (with teratomas peaking before seminomas), and then became progressively less common with increasing age. After 50 years of age most so-called cancers of the testis are lymphomas. The disease has increased in incidence since before the Second World War in the UK, North America, and several European countries, but it has continued to be rare in Blacks, Japanese, and Chinese, irrespective of the society in which they live. The only known aetiological factors are incomplete descent of the testis at birth and maternal obesity during pregnancy. The former increases the risk of the disease about tenfold, the latter increases it by about 50 per cent.

Penis

Cancers of the penis account for 0.1 per cent of all cancers. Circumcision carried out within a week or two of birth almost completely prevents the disease; carried out later it reduces the risk, but to a much smaller extent. Absence of circumcision is not, however, the only factor, and the incidence of the disease varies greatly between different African tribes which do not practise circumcision. Personal cleanliness seems to be an important factor, as is the frequency of infection with different types of the human papilloma virus (HPV). There is some weak association between the occurrence of penile and cervical cancer in marital pairs, which cannot be accounted for simply by confounding with socio-economic class, and this, combined with discovery of the same type of HPV in penile cancer cells as in cervical cancer cells, suggests that viral infection is likely to be a crucial factor in the development of the disease.

Lymphatic and haemopoietic tissue

Hodgkin disease

Hodgkin disease accounts for 0.7 per cent of all cancers. Despite its name it may not be a pathological entity, but the histological and clinical varieties have not been distinguished with sufficient clarity long enough for their epidemiological features to have been determined separately. Considered as one disease, the incidence rises from childhood to about 25 years of age, declines to about 45 years of age, and then rises into the oldest age groups. The clinical and histological characteristics, however, vary with age, and the unusual age distribution seems likely to result from the combination of a disease with a peak incidence in early adult life and another that increases in incidence progressively with age.

Reports that clusters of cases have occurred in young people in which those affected have all had personal contact with each other have suggested that the disease may be due to a virus. Spread by personal contact has not, however, been confirmed when looked for in controlled studies. Other evidence of an infectious origin derives from the observation that in many tropical and subtropical parts of Sub-Saharan Africa and Central and South America the disease is unusually common in children. As the standard of living rises, the childhood cases become less common and are replaced by a larger number in young adults. This changing pattern is reminiscent of what happened with poliomyelitis in the first half of the century, and suggests that the disease may be due to an infectious agent that becomes less widespread as hygiene improves. One agent to have been implicated is the Epstein–Barr virus, as the incidence of Hodgkin disease is increased slightly 5–20 years after an attack of infectious mononucleosis. The virus is not, however, found in the malignant cells, and any contribution that it may make to the development of the disease is likely to be non-specific, e.g. by stimulating the division of the relevant stem cells.

Non-Hodgkin lymphoma

If Hodgkin disease is a label attached to two or three aetiologically different diseases, other lymphomas classed under the umbrella of non-Hodgkin lymphomas, embrace many more. The recorded incidence of these lymphomas, which now account for 1.4 per cent of all cancers, has increased since the end of the Second World War and has continued to rise in the oldest age groups in the past decade. It is still uncertain, however, whether this reflects a true increase in incidence or a change in diagnostic habits and skills.

One type of non-Hodgkin lymphoma that has been distinguished histologically and epidemiologically is the B-lymphocyte lymphoma named after Burkitt. It affects children throughout the world, but is rare everywhere except in a few places where malarial infection is heavy and widespread. In these areas the incidence is 100 times that in Europe and North America. The localization of high incidence rates to areas where the annual rainfall was at least 20 inches and the daily temperature consistently above 60 °F led Epstein to suspect that the tumour was due to an insect-borne virus and to the isolation of the EB virus from the malignant cells. Laboratory research, combined with the observation that the disease occurs characteristically in children who had previously had exceptionally high levels of antibodies to the capsid antigen of the virus, has established that the virus plays an essential part in the production of the disease, but the localization proved to be because the disease occurred in epidemic form only when infestation with malaria was heavy and widespread. The EB virus plays no part in the few cases of Burkitt's lymphoma in children that occur in other parts of the world, but it is a cause of the few cases of B-cell lymphomas that occur in patients who are immunosupressed to receive organ transplants or for therapeutic reasons, and in patients with acquired immunodeficiency syndrome (AIDS).

Another type of non-Hodgkin lymphoma that occurs at all commonly only in restricted areas is the lymphoma that constitutes part of the syndrome of adult T-cell leukaemia/lymphoma. Occasional cases may occur anywhere, but the disease is common only in Japan, particularly in the southernmost islands of Kyushu and Shikoku, and in the Caribbean. The human T-cell leukaemia/lymphoma virus type I (HTLV-I) is a cause of the disease; but, as with the EB virus and Burkitt lymphoma and the hepatitis B virus and hepatocellular carcinoma, one or more other factors seem to be required to produce clinical disease, as infection is common in the epidemic areas and only a small proportion of affected people develop the disease.

A third type is the primary upper small intestinal lymphoma, known by the acronym of PUSIL, which affects young people in many populations with a low standard of living. Many cases of the disease have been described in Iraq, Iran, Algeria, Syria, Lebanon, Tunisia, and Greece, which led to the alternative name of Mediterranean lymphoma. This, however, is inappropriate as the disease also occurs in Africa south of the Sahara, and in Central and South America. The disease is preceded by malnutrition and repeated attacks of gastroenteritis, which lead eventually to small intestinal villous atrophy with proliferation of lymphocytes and plasma cells in the lamina propria of the small intestine. Malnutrition and gastroenteritis are, however, not sufficient cause, as the disease is rare in other countries where these are common, such as Bangladesh. Intestinal lymphomas in people over 50 years of age are unrelated to PUSIL and have no special geographical localization.

The epidemiological features of the tumours that constitute the vast majority of the non-Hodgkin lymphomas in Europe and North America are unrevealing. There have been isolated reports of an increased incidence in chemists, agricultural workers, and men exposed to phenoxyacetic acid herbicides but no specific occupational hazards have been established.

Myelomatosis

Myelomatosis accounts for 0.9 per cent of all cancers. The recorded incidence has increased greatly in all developed countries; but it is difficult to decide whether this reflects an increase in the risk of developing the disease or is due to improved diagnosis, made easy first by marrow biopsy and then by serum electrophoresis, and further facilitated by the improved treatment of renal failure, which was often the immediate cause of death. The rapid and progressive increase in incidence with age, which is similar to that observed with most epithelial cancers, suggests that it may be due to prolonged exposure to some environmental carcinogen. No such cause is established, apart from ionizing radiation; but there is accumulated evidence to suggest that there may be some special risk associated with farming and agriculture.

Differences in genetic susceptibility may be important as the disease is rare in Japanese, irrespective of where they live, and it is twice as common in American Blacks as in American Whites.

Leukaemia

Leukaemia, which accounts for 2.1 per cent of all cancers, is not properly a disease but a sign that accompanies a variety of different malignant diseases of the lymphatic and haemopoietic tissues, and the term should not normally be used without some qualification to indicate the type of cell that has given rise to the malignant clone.

One of this group of diseases is chronic lymphatic leukaemia (CLL), which increases in incidence with age in the same way as most of the common epithelial cancers. In Europe, North America, and Israel, where it is common, it is a disease of B-lymphocytes. It is extremely rare in Chinese, Japanese, and Indians, which is presumably due to genetic differences in susceptibility, as it continues to be rare in these racial groups even after migration to countries in which it is generally common. In Japan, the few cases that do occur mostly arise from T-lymphocytes. Unlike other types of leukaemia, CLL does not appear to be induced by ionizing radiations at all easily, possibly because the relevant stem cells are so sensitive to damage by ionizing radiations that they are killed before any increase in the incidence of CLL can be detected.

Acute lymphoblastic leukaemia (ALL) accounts for nearly half of all childhood cancers. Its incidence in children is at a maximum at 2–3 years of age and then declines to about age 15 years. Most cases, and all those accounting for the early peak in incidence, arise from the precursors of B-lymphocytes, possess a distinctive antigen, and are described as 'common acute lymphoblastic leukaemias' (or c.ALL). Untreated cases are rapidly fatal, either as a direct result of the malignant process or indirectly by diminishing the response to acute infections, and the apparent rarity of the disease in undeveloped countries (and elsewhere before the 1930s) is probably the result of a high fatality rate in the early stages of the disease before the diagnosis is clinically obvious. The T-cell ALLs, which are relatively uncommon in developed countries and occur at a more-or-less constant rate throughout childhood, are less rapidly fatal, present with enlarged lymph glands, and are diagnosed with relative ease. The high ratio of T-cell ALL to c.ALL in countries with limited medical services may, therefore, be a diagnostic artefact. Alternatively, the geographical differences may be real, c.ALL being produced more commonly in developed countries as a result of delayed stimulation of the immune system associated with better hygiene and reduced social contacts. Clusters of cases of childhood ALL have been reported periodically, particularly in recent years in the vicinity of nuclear installations. They cannot have been produced by the amounts of radioactive waste known to have been released. They may have been due to mutations by irradiation of parental spermatids and sperm or to the sociodemographic features of the local population which have enhanced the factors that normally cause the disease.

ALL in adult life is a different disease. It is induced relatively easily by ionizing radiations, but few other epidemiological features have been defined. One type, which does not normally occur in Britain (ATLL), has been described under non-Hodgkin lymphoma.

Acute myeloid leukaemia (AML) occurs at all ages. Its incidence increases slowly from childhood on, and it is the principal type of leukaemia in young adult life. In this age-group, its incidence is less variable throughout the world than that of any other common type of cancer. Chronic myeloid leukaemia (CML) is, in contrast, very rare in youth, but it increases in incidence with age more rapidly than AML, and becomes more common than AML after about 50 years of age. Both types of myeloid leukaemia are induced more readily by ionizing radiations than are other cancers (except perhaps for thyroid cancer), and an increase in the incidence of myeloid leukaemia raises the possibility of a radiation hazard.

Myeloid leukaemia, and particularly its rare variant erythroleukaemia, is an occupational hazard of workers exposed to benzene. Cases tend to be preceded by a bout of aplastic anaemia and it is uncertain whether doses that are insufficient to cause anaemia are able to cause leukaemia. Myeloid leukaemia may also be produced by two drugs. One, melphalan, is an alkylating agent and is presumably mutagenic. The other, busulphan, is not and has been observed to cause leukaemia only after producing aplastic anaemia. Both risks are too small to weigh heavily against the therapeutic benefits of the drugs.

Several types of leukaemia occur particularly commonly in childhood in association with congenital and hereditary abnormalities. The incidence of ALL is increased many times in children with ataxia telangiectasia and Bloom syndrome, and of AML in children with Fanconi congenital aplastic anaemia, while the rare acute megakaryocytic leukaemia is increased approximately 600-fold in children under 3 years of age with Down syndrome with all childhood leukaemia being increased about 20 times.

Other causes

Bone

Bone tumours, according to national vital statistics, have caused progressively fewer deaths over the past 50 years. This is partly due to improved treatment of bone tumours in childhood leading to a reduced fatality, but mainly to improved diagnosis, with the result that metastases to bone are more often diagnosed correctly and less often erroneously described as primary tumours of bone. The disease now accounts for 0.2 per cent of all cancers and the incidence has probably been more-or-less static.

There are many different histological types, and some have different causes. The rare Ewing tumour occurs only in children and is almost unknown in Black populations, irrespective of the society in which they live. Osteosarcomas are responsible for most of the cases that cause a peak incidence in adolescence, and for the increase in incidence after 45 years of age. This last is entirely due to the rapid increase with age of Paget osteitis deformans, a disease that so predisposes to the development of osteosarcoma that tumours develop in 1 per cent of all affected people.

The only other known cause is ionizing radiations. Iatrogenic cases of osteo-, chrondro-, and fibrosarcoma have been produced by intensive radiotherapy and by the medicinal use of thorium, a bone-seeking radionuclide; and occupational cases have been produced by the ingestion of radium in the course of applying luminous paint.

Connective tissue

Sarcomas of the soft tissue constitute 0.4 per cent of all cancers. They include many different types of tumours, all of which are rare throughout the world, with the single exception of Kaposi sarcoma. One type of Kaposi sarcoma affecting elderly people occurs sporadically everywhere but particularly affects Jews in, or from, Eastern Europe. Another affects principally young men in central Africa, and in some parts is so common that it constitutes 8 per cent of all cancers. A third type is a common complication of AIDS, particularly in male homosexuals in whom it seems to be due to a specific virus spread at the same time and in the same manner as the human immunodeficiency virus. Whether the three types of Kaposi sarcoma are all the same disease with the same cause, modified in their clinical course by the age of infection and the immune status of the subject, is an open question. A few cases of other types of soft-tissue sarcoma are caused by ionizing radiations, but the causes of the great majority are unknown. Some may be due to exposure to phenoxyacetic acid herbicides, but the relationship is not proven.

Skin

Melanomas of the skin have become progressively more common over the past 50 years in all countries with a predominantly White population and they now constitute 0.8 per cent of all cancers. Their incidence varies inversely with the amount of skin pigmentation. In White people melanomas occur most commonly on the legs in women and or the trunk, head, and neck in men, the incidence varying roughly in proportion to the flux of ultraviolet light in the countries in which they live. Melanomas tend to be more common in indoor than in outdoor workers, perhaps due to the lack of protection from a semipermanent suntan, and they tend to be associated with periodic bouts of sunbathing. The disease is extremely rare in Black people in the USA, but is more common in Africa, where it occurs at the junction of the pigmented and unpigmented skin on the foot. Like basal and squamous cell carcinoma of the skin, it is particularly common in people with the defect in DNA repair that characterizes xeroderma pigmentosum. The evidence suggests that ultraviolet light is the principal cause, but there are some discrepant observations and other factors (possibly hormonal) may play a part.

Squamous carcinomas of the skin are produced by many different agents, including ultraviolet light, some polycyclic hydrocarbons in natural oils, coal tar, pitch, and soot, arsenic trioxide, immunosuppressive drugs, and some types of the human papillomas virus. Ultraviolet light causes cancers of the exposed skin of the face, head, and neck. Polycyclic hydrocarbons in the industrial environment cause cancers on different sites, depending on the nature of the industrial processes; in the past they commonly focused on the scrotum; now, on the rare occasions when exposure leads to cancer, it is mostly on the forearms. Arsenic caused cancers anywhere on the skin, but characteristically on the hands and pathognomonically on the palms. Human papilloma viruses cause flat warts, which frequently progress to carcinoma in patients with the inherited defects of cell-mediated immunity that present as epidermodysplasia verruciformis, and they are probably responsible for the increased incidence of carcinomas of the exposed skin in patients given intensive immunosuppression to permit organ transplantation. Many different types of the virus appear to be involved.

Other causes operate in Kashmir, where the habit of carrying a *Kangri* or small stove, inside the clothes for warmth in winter has led to cancers on the skin of the abdomen; in India, where the continual friction of the dhoti cloth localizes cancers to the groin and waist; and in tropical Africa where squamous carcinomas are common complications of chronic ulceration of the legs.

Basal cell carcinomas (or rodent ulcers) are the most common type of skin cancer in Britain, occurring about three times as often as squamous carcinomas. Nearly all cases occur on the face, head, and neck, and are due to exposure to ultraviolet light. They are consequently more common in fair-skinned people and almost unknown in Blacks, unless they suffer from albinism. People with the defect of DNA repair that characterizes xeroderma pigmentosum develop large numbers of both basal cell and squamous carcinomas at an early age unless they are protected from even mild exposure to sunlight. Registered cases of basal or squamous cell carcinoma constitute 10 per cent of all cancers, but the precise proportion is unknown as many cases of basal cell carcinoma, being so easily treated, escape registration. In Queensland it is estimated that three-quarters of the population have developed at least one skin cancer if they survive to 75 years of age.

Brain and nervous tissue

Benign tumours of the brain and spinal cord are commonly classed with malignant tumours for purposes of cancer registration and epidemiological enquiry, as both can cause death by local pressure and the two types are not always distinguished clinically. Classed together, they account for 1.7 per cent of all cancers. The tumours are of many different histological types and have different epidemiological features. Medulloblastomas occur characteristically in childhood, glioblastomas in adult life, and astrocytomas at all ages. Most tend to be more common in males, but meningiomas are more common in females. Several occupational hazards have been suspected, particularly in the chemical industry, but none has been established. No large differences in geographical distribution are known.

Thyroid

Thyroid cancers account for 0.4 per cent of all cancers. Together with myeloid leukaemias they are particularly easily induced by ionizing radiation, in the sense that the background incidence is increased proportionately more than that of other cancers, and many cases have been observed in the survivors of the atomic bomb explosions over Hiroshima and Nagasaki and in young people whose necks were irradiated in infancy for the treatment of what was, at one time, regarded as a dangerously large thymus. The tumours caused by ionizing radiation are characteristically papillary and follicular carcinomas, which respond well to treatment.

The incidence of the disease varies geographically, but has no simple relationship to iodine intake. Moderately increased rates are observed in Switzerland and Colombia, in association with iodine deficiency and endemic goitre, but still higher rates (approximately five times those in Britain and North America) are observed in Iceland and Hawaii, where iodine intake is high. These increased rates are due principally to follicular carcinomas in the iodine-deficient areas and papillary carcinomas in the high-iodine areas. No factors have been associated with the medullary and anaplastic carcinomas, apart from the genetic factors responsible for the multiple endocrine syndrome of which medullary thyroid carcinomas fom a part.

Eye

Cancers of the eye are rare, accounting for only 0.2 per cent of all cancers, and retinoblastomas are exceptionally rare, accounting for only one-tenth of eye cancers. The epidemiology of retinoblastoma is, however, of interest as it has led to the construction of a model for the origin of the disease, which has served, in its turn, as a model for the origin of nephroblastoma and childhood lymphoblastic leukaemia. Twelve per cent of children with a retinoblastoma have a family history of the disease, but another 26 per cent develop tumours in both eyes and, like the obviously familial cases, are believed to be genetic in origin. A third of the genetically determined cases present within the first 6 months of life, while the sporadic cases tend to present about 2 years later. No cases present after 10 years of age and very few after 5 years of age: those that do are clinically advanced, indicating delay in diagnosis. These findings have suggested that the disease is due to two mutations, one of which occurs prezygotically, thus accounting for the familial cases, while in the sporadic cases both mutations occur during the development of the retina.

Nearly all other cancers of the eye are melanomas. No noteworthy epidemiological features have been reported, except that they tend to occur in people with blue eyes and in rural rather than urban areas, suggesting an aetiological role for sunlight.

9.7.5   Further reading

Doll, R. and Peto, R. (1981). The causes of cancer: quantitative estimates of avoidable risks of cancer in the United States today. *Journal of the National Cancer Institute* **66**, 1191–308.

Knudson, A. G. (1985). Hereditary cancer, oncogenes, and anti-oncogenes. *Cancer Research* **45**, 1437–43.

Schottenfeld, D. and Fraumeni, J. F. (1982). *Cancer epidemiology and prevention*. Saunders, Philadelphia.

9.8   Endocrine effects of tumours

J. G. Ratcliffe

9.8.1   Introduction

Tumours produce endocrine effects directly by hormone secretion or, more commonly, by indirect mechanisms. Indirect effects may be due to alterations in normal endocrine control or homone metabolism secondary to intercurrent illness, compromised renal, respiratory, hepatic, or central nervous system function, or destruction of an endocrine gland by tumour infiltration; or they may be associated with concomitant chemotherapy. In general indirect effects are not specific to particular types of tumour, and are insensitive markers of early disease.

Endocrine effects result less frequently from direct secretion of hormones by tumour cells. Primary tumours arising in endocrine glands frequently produce hormones characteristic of the gland. For example, pituitary tumours produce growth hormone, prolactin, or ACTH; parathyroid tumours produce PTH; and adrenal tumours, corticosteroids. Hormones characteristic of the endocrine tissue in which the tumour has arisen are termed 'eutopic'. Typically, all the tumour cells synthesize the hormone and secretion is related to the viable number of tumour cells, although it is relatively unresponsive to normal control mechanisms. For example, hyperglycaemia does not suppress growth hormone (GH) secretion by GH-producing pituitary tumours.

Endocrine effects may also be produced directly by hormone secretion from tumours arising outwith classical endocrine glands. On occasion the resulting endocrine and metabolic disturbances are more life-threatening than the presence of the tumour itself. Tumour hormones that are not characteristic of the tissue in which the primary tumour has arisen are termed 'ectopic'. Ectopic hormones may be produced by benign and malignant tumours. Typically, not all the cells of the tumour produce or secrete the ectopic hormone to the same extent. Hormone secretion is then poorly related to the viable tumour cell mass and usually unresponsive to normal endocrine control mechanisms. This section is concerned with the pathological concepts underlying the endocrine effects of ectopic hormones, and their clinical relevance. Some of these aspects are discussed in greater detail in Ratcliffe (1982), De Bustros and Baylin (1985), and *Recent results in cancer research* (1985).

The classical definition of an ectopic hormone is 'a hormone produced by a neoplasm derived from a tissue not normally engaged in the production of that hormone'. This definition requires that the tumour synthesizes the hormone and, implicitly, that the normal sites of production of hormones are known. While the evidence for production of many hormones by 'non-endocrine' tumours is now firmly established, it has become clear that many peptide hormones are produced in small amounts by normal adult tissues (e.g. brain, lung, gut, gonads) and in non-neoplastic proliferating tissues outside the major endocrine glands.

Thus, the term 'ectopic' as originally defined does not accurately describe the presence of hormones in neoplastic tissues. Nevertheless, until there is a better understanding of the pathogenesis of tumour hormones, it is convenient to retain it to describe increased and inappropriate hormone production by 'non-endocrine' neoplasms, particularly when clinical syndromes result.

Despite these terminological inexactitudes, the biology of hormone production by 'non-endocrine' tumours has become more understandable by the realization that there exists an extensive diffuse endocrine system in which cells with neuroendocrine characteristics occur, albeit sparsely, in many 'non-endocrine' tissues. The existence of a diffuse endocrine system was originally based on the demonstration of 'clear' cells which stain poorly on conventional histology. Many of these endocrine-type cells have been shown to have characteristic amine-handling properties, stain with antisera specific for peptide hormones, and contain membrane-bound dense-core cytoplasmic granules on electron microscopy.

These properties have been encapsulated by the term 'amine precursor uptake and decarboxylation' (APUD). While APUD properties were originally postulated to identify cells with a common embryological origin from neural crest, it is now apparent that APUD cells can be derived from all germ layers. APUD properties are probably related to the presence of the complex intracellular structures and functions involved in post-translational steps required for packaging and secreting intact, active small-peptide hormones. The term is now only a shorthand way of describing neuroendocrine-type cells dispersed in normal tissues, which produce and package peptides for secretion. It does not imply a particular embryological origin of those cells.

Basic concepts
Establishment of the basis of endocrine syndromes
The association between endocrine syndromes and 'non-

endocrine' neoplasms has been described in case reports for over 50 years. The idea that this may be due to tumour hormone production was formulated in the 1940s and 1950s, when it was suggested that hypercalcaemia might result from tumour peptides with PTH-like activity, and hyponatraemia from tumour peptides with antidiuretic hormone activity. However, the hypothesis was only put on a firm basis by Liddle and colleagues in the 1960s in their seminal studies of the ectopic ACTH syndrome (Liddle *et al.* 1969). They demonstrated that in patients with Cushing's syndrome and 'non-endocrine' neoplasms, the tumours contained bioactive ACTH, and plasma ACTH levels were elevated. Furthermore, tumour ACTH resembled authentic ACTH in many biological, immunological, and physicochemical properties.

Subsequently, other endocrine syndromes associated with 'non-endocrine' neoplasms were recognized, as well as increased and inappropriate tumour hormone production without clinically overt syndromes (Table 9.14).

Proof of hormone production

Demonstration of hormone synthesis by a 'non-endocrine' tumour is necessary but not sufficient proof of a cause-and-effect relationship with an endocrine syndrome. Many criteria for hormone production have been used, which have given rise to a literature of uneven and frequently misleading quality. These include:

1. association of a tumour with a clinically apparent endocrine syndrome and elevated circulating hormone levels;

2. regression of clinical manifestations of hormone excess and fall in circulating hormone levels after removal of the tumour;

3. persistent endocrine syndrome after removal of the normal gland of origin of the hormone;

4. significant arteriovenous gradient of hormone levels across the tumour;

5. demonstration of hormone in tumour tissue in amounts greater than in adjacent non-involved tissue;

6. demonstration of hormone synthesis and/or specific mRNA expression in the tumour *in vitro*.

The weakest, but most commonly advanced, evidence is based on the first criterion. Criteria two, three, and four are often not feasible clinically. Criterion five requires application of specific quantitative methods of hormone analysis and rigorous controls, particularly when immunohistochemical methods are used, since tumour hormone levels are often very low. Criterion six is the most convincing but requires more sophisticated isotope, cell culture, and DNA-RNA hybridization techniques. Furthermore, hormone-secreting ability may be lost during culture and demonstration of hormone secretion in cell lines does not prove that the tumour secreted pathologically significant amounts of hormone *in vivo*.

Hormones produced

There is now good evidence for the production of many of the recognized peptide and protein hormones, including hypothalamic hormones (Table 9.14). It is notable, however, that some peptide hormones are produced rarely, if at all. These include parathyroid hormone (PTH), insulin, pituitary glycoproteins (TSH, LH, FSH), prolactin, gastrin, and glucagon. Nonpeptide hormones (catecholamines, steroids, and thyroid hormones) have not been demonstrated to be synthesized *de novo*, although tumours may interconvert steroid precursors. Perhaps this is not surprising, since synthesis would require the concerted expression and structural organization of all the enzymes of specialized biosynthetic pathways.

Table 9.14 Endocrine syndromes associated with non-endocrine tumours

Clinical syndrome	Biochemical clues	Tumour-derived hormone	Tumour associations
Non-metastatic hypercalcaemia (humoral hypercalcaemia of malignancy)	Hypercalcaemia	Parathyroid hormone-related protein	Lung (squamous), renal
Syndrome of inappropriate ADH secretion	Hyponatraemia	Arginine vasopressin	Lung (small cell)
Ectopic ACTH syndrome	Hypokalaemic alkalosis	ACTH (CRH)	Lung (small cell)
Acromegaly	—	GHRH (GH)	Carcinoid
Gynaecomastia/precocious puberty	—	HCG	Lung (non small cell) hepatoblastoma
Diabetes mellitus, steatorrhoea, gallstones	Hyperglycaemia	Somatostatin	Carcinoid
Hypoglycaemia	Hypoglycaemia	Uncertain	Mesenchymal tumours
Watery diarrhoea	—	Vaso-active intestinal peptide	Lung (small cell)
No overt syndrome	—	Calcitonin	Lung (all types)
No overt syndrome	—	Gastrin-releasing peptide	Lung (small cell)

Hormones in parentheses indicate that they are rare causes of the clinical syndrome.

Frequency and tumour associations

When originally described, ectopic hormone syndromes were considered rare and bizarre features of neoplasia. With increasing clinical awareness and the application of sensitive immunological and molecular biological techniques, it has become apparent that ectopic hormone production is associated with certain types of tumour relatively commonly. It has been suggested, but not yet proven, that hormone production is a universal concomitant of neoplasia. Estimates of prevalence vary widely according to the criteria applied.

Clinical endocrine syndromes attributable to hormone production occur in about 10 per cent of unselected patients with lung cancer, the malignancy for which the most complete data are available. There is a clear association of the ectopic ACTH syndrome and ectopic ADH syndrome with small cell lung cancer (SCLC) with prevalences of 2–3 per cent and 5–10 per cent, respectively. Hypercalcaemia in the absence of bone metastases occurs in up to 15 per cent of patients with squamous cell lung cancer, but rarely with other histological types of lung cancer.

While overt clinical endocrine syndromes are unusual, detailed clinical and biochemical investigation suggests that hormone production by 'non-endocrine' tumours is more common. Impaired suppression of corticosteroids is found in about 50 per cent of patients with small cell lung cancer in the absence of clinically apparent syndromes. Positive immuno-activity of ACTH-related peptides in tumour extracts and immunoperoxidase staining is detected in the majority of small cell and carcinoid lung tumours, at levels within the range found in proven cases of ectopic ACTH syndrome. Secretion of ACTH- and calcitonin-related peptides has also been demonstrated in about half the cell lines established so far from small cell lung cancers. Production of bombesin-like immunoactivity is even more common in small cell lung cancer cell cultures. Some cell lines produce multiple hormones, with up to 10 being detected in a single cell line. Although most reported hormone-secreting hormone cell lines originate from SCLC or carcinoid tumours, it is clear that non small cell lung cancers (NSCLC) may secrete a similar spectrum of peptides, although less frequently. Placental hormones, such as human chorionic gonadotrophin (HCG) and its β-subunit, are particularly associated with NSCLC.

While many investigations do not satisfy the most stringent criteria, the evidence overall suggests that hormone production detected biochemically or by immunohistochemistry is much more common than clinically overt endocrine syndromes. This may be due to lack of obvious clinical effect in the short term, or because clinical syndromes associated with ectopic hormone secretion are poorly defined, or because the tumour hormones have significantly reduced biological activity. Production of an ectopic hormone with well-defined feedback control may suppress secretion by the normal gland of origin so that the rate of tumour hormone secretion must exceed eutopic hormone secretion before signs of hormone excess become evident. Furthermore, tumour hormones may be secreted intermittently, and secretion of one hormone may mask the clinical effect of another.

Endocrine syndromes occur rarely with common neoplasms other than lung, such as breast, colon, skin, urogenital tract. There is little rigorous and systematic biochemical data on hormone production by these tumours, although elevated plasma levels of chorionic gonadotrophin and calcitonin are reported in a minority of patients with tumours of the gastrointestinal and urogenital tract.

Chemical nature of hormones

The structure of ectopic hormones is a central issue of biological and clinical importance. The full amino-acid sequences of ectopic hormones have rarely been determined, although recombinant DNA–RNA techniques will make this more feasible in the future. The application of classical techniques of protein analysis is difficult because hormone concentrations in 'non-endocrine' tumours are often several orders of magnitude lower than those in normal endocrine glands.

Present evidence suggests that peptide hormones are synthesized in 'non-endocrine' tumours as larger molecular weight preprohormones, which are subsequently processed to prohormones, biologically active hormones, and hormone fragments which may or may not have biological activity. Processing is by proteolytic enzymes specific for dibasic amino-acid sequences. However, while the primary transcription products of 'non-endocrine' tumours closely resemble their normal counterparts, their post-translational processing may differ both quantitatively and qualitatively, yielding greater heterogeneity. Thus, whereas the authentic hormone is the major stored and secreted form in the normal endocrine gland, precursors and/or subunits and fragments are often the major tissue and circulating forms found in 'non-endocrine' tumours. Furthermore, each tumour is to some extent unique, there being considerable variation in the degree of post-translational processing and modification (e.g. glycosylation, amidation, acetylation) between tumours. Some tumours process the hormone precursor by pathways typical of normal tissues other than the major eutopic site. For example, ectopic ACTH is often cleaved almost completely to N- and C-terminal fragments resembling α-melanocyte stimulating hormone (α-MSH) and ACTH 18–39 (corticotrophin-like intermediate lobe peptide, CLIP), which is characteristic of cells of neurointermediate lobe origin.

The range of peptides produced depends upon the precise complement of tumour enzymes and their organization in intracellular structures such as the Golgi apparatus and secretory granules. Precursor forms may not be incorporated into mature storage granules, and so escape normal processing and release mechanisms.

Such differences can account for reported structural abnormalities in ectopic hormones, such as abnormal ratios of biological to immunological activities, C- to N-terminal immunoactivities, or minor differences in amino-acid composition.

9.8.2 Pathogenesis

Several hypotheses have been proposed over the past 25 years to explain the origin of ectopic hormones, although none is fully convincing (Baylin and Mendelsohn 1980).

1. Abnormal genome. Since the genetic information for synthesis of cell proteins is present in every diploid cell, mutations in nuclear DNA could give rise to synthesis of peptides, some of which may possess amino-acid sequences required for biological activity. Expression of the abnormal genome would then be associated randomly with any type of tumour and the primary structure of hormones so produced would be abnormal. Neither prediction is supported by current evidence.

2. Derepression. Most genes are repressed in differentiated tissues. Derepression of previously inactive genes could give rise to peptide products identical to their normal counterparts. However, in its simple form this fails to explain the observed tumour associations of ectopic hormone syndromes, and there is no general increase in gene transcription in neoplastic cells. Furthermore, there is increasing evidence that gene transcription for peptide hormones is never completely repressed in normal 'non-endocrine' adult tissues.

3. Endocrine cell. This postulates a change in gene function in neoplastic cells derived from differentiated cells of the diffuse endocrine system. An endocrine cell origin seems plausible for small cell lung carcinomas and carcinoids, which are often considered to be tumours distinctive in origin, behaviour, and hormone synthesizing capabilities. However, the distinction between the pathogenesis of tumours from endocrine or non-endocrine cells is becoming difficult to sustain. Thus, lung cancers often contain mixtures of small cell and non small cell histologies, appearing as complex mixtures of all types rather than multiple primary lesions. Lung cancers show a similar gradation of biochemical phenotypes with some non small cell cancers expressing endocrine markers. *In vitro*, small cell lung cancer cell lines show phenotypic transitions to a form of non small cell cancer with surface antigen expression characteristic of both small cell (SCC) and non small cell cancer (non-SCC). Furthermore, in experimental regenerating bronchial mucosa, large undifferentiated cells are related to each of the main differentiated cell types. Large cell undifferentiated cancer of SCC lineage may represent a neoplastic counterpart to such an indifferent cell, which has totipotent differentiation capabilities for each of the major types of normal and neoplastic cells in the bronchial mucosa. It therefore seems unlikely that small cell lung cancer is derived from a terminally differentiated endocrine cell, but rather suggests a unitary stem cell of origin for both endocrine and 'non-endocrine' neoplasms arising in complex epithelial mucosa.

4. Abnormal differentiation. This suggests that neoplastic events affect a proliferative cell occurring in small numbers in normal mature tissues, but larger numbers in a regenerating tissue. In the repair processes in bronchial mucosa occurring during chronic injury (e.g. cigarette smoking) it is postulated that there is an increase in a transient endocrine cell population uncommitted to a particular differentiation pathway, which is the target for transformation events. Depending on the nature of these events, neoplastic cells become committed to more complete endocrine differentiation (e.g. small cell cancer) or towards non-SCC phenotypes, thus mimicking the spectrum of normally differentiated mucosal cells.

A schematic diagram of one of the hypotheses proposed to relate normal differentiation within the bronchial epithelium to the development of the spectrum of human lung cancer, is shown in Fig. 9.100. Endocrine cell differentiation represents an early transient multipotent stage of maturation. Only a small proportion of these cells normally undergo differentiation to mature endocrine cells, the majority maturing via an indifferent cell type to mucous and ciliated cells which constitute the main mucosal cell population. This hypothesis is compatible with the observations that SCC can differentiate towards non-SCC (usually large cell undifferentiated) phenotypes; that early hyperplasia is associated with a large population of cells with

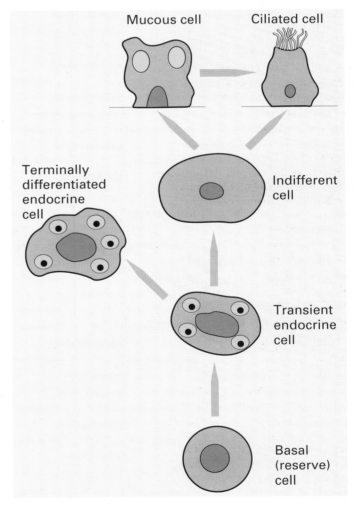

Fig. 9.100 The differentiation pathway of cells within the normal bronchial epithelium: a hypothesis proposed by Baylin (1985).

endocrine features, which are lost as the final neoplasms do not have SCC histology; and that the SCC phenotype is common in lung cancer, yet mature endocrine cells are very sparse in the normal adult bronchial mucosa.

Role of tumour hormones

Hormones produced by endocrine-type cells in tumours may be important in regulating the direction of differentiation and rate of tumour growth, so that hormone-producing cells are selected for the evolution of the tumour. The ability of cancer cells to produce growth factors and to respond to these factors via simultaneously expressed cell-membrane receptors suggests that tumour hormones may have an autocrine function and that transformed cells maintain autonomous growth by autocrine secretion. This possibility has been elegantly explored for bombesin-like activity (BLI) in SCLC (bombesin is homologous to the C-terminal 14–27 sequence of gastrin-releasing peptide). Small cell lung cancer cells injected into athymic nude mice give rise to tumours that can be prevented by early treatment with specific monoclonal antibodies to bombesin, but not non-specific antibodies. Furthermore, exogenous bombesin, but not inactive analogues, stimulates colony formation of SCLC.

Whether similar autocrine or paracrine mechanisms occur with other hormone-related peptides has yet to be determined but, if so, would emphasize the potential importance of ectopic hormones in tumour biology and suggest novel therapeutic approaches.

It is also possible that hormonal growth factors are controlled by the expression of oncogenes. Some oncogenes function by directing the synthesis of a growth factor and/or its receptor or structurally altered receptor, which may allow constitutive activity of the receptor in the absence of the ligand, or free cells from negative regulatory factors. Amplification of several oncogenes occurs in lung cancer, although their relationship, if any, with expression of tumour hormones or their receptors is not known.

9.8.3 Selected examples

Hypercalcaemia of malignancy

Hypercalcaemia is the most common endocrine manifestation of malignancy, with a prevalence similar to that of primary hyperparathyroidism. Three pathological associations are recognized though there may be overlap in their underlying mechanisms.

1. Hypercalcaemia associated with skeletal metastases from solid tumours, such as breast and lung cancer, is the commonest cause. The plasma phosphate and nephrogenous cyclic AMP levels are usually normal. It is probably due mainly to direct resorption of bone by enzymes released by tumour cells and osteolytic factors from tumour cells or active immune cells. A variety of osteolytic factors are identified, of which prostaglandins may be particularly important in metastatic breast cancer. *In vitro*, prostaglandins of the E series are potent stimulators of

bone resorption, and prostaglandins probably act locally but are not the sole paracrine factors involved. Humoral factors with PTH-like activity are also implicated as renal tubular calcium reabsorption is increased and phosphate reabsorption decreased.

2. Hypercalcaemia associated with haematological malignancies, such as multiple myeloma, acute lymphocytic leukaemia, and lymphomas. Most of the associated malignancies arise from B-lymphocytes, which produce a family of bone resorbing peptides, originally termed osteoclast activating factors (OAF), which are distinct from PTH, prostaglandins, and vitamin D. Most of the bone resorbing activity previously attributed to OAF is due to cytokines, such as tumour necrosis factors (TNF) α (cachectin) and β (lymphotoxin), and interleukin--1. These factors are released *in vitro* by myeloma cells and mononuclear leucocytes. It seems likely that cytokine release at the site of tumour deposit is the main cause of hypercalcaemia in these malignancies, but the impaired ability of the kidney to excrete calcium, common in myeloma, may be an important contributory factor.

3. Hypercalcaemia not associated with skeletal metastases (non-metastatic hypercalcaemia, humoral hypercalcaemia of malignancy, HHM). This is typically associated with squamous cell carcinomas, especially of lung, and renal carcinomas. Tumour factors are secreted, which act humorally on the skeleton to increase bone resorption and on the kidney to decrease calcium excretion and increase phosphate excretion. Nephrogenous cyclic AMP excretion is increased and there is often a mild hypokalaemic, hypochloraemic alkalosis.

Important progress has been made recently in elucidating the humoral factor involved (Burtis *et al.* 1988). Patients with HHM resemble those with primary hyperparathyroidism in some respects, e.g. hypercalcaemia, increased phosphate excretion, increased nephrogenous cAMP excretion, increased osteoclastic bone resorption. These features support the idea that PTH itself is involved, but other observations are not explained:

1. hypercalcuria for a given serum calcium level is greater in HHM than in primary hyperparathyroidism;

2. circulating 1 : 25-dihydroxyvitamin D levels are typically reduced in HHM, whereas they are increased in primary hyperparathyroidism due to PTH stimulation of renal 1-hydroxylation;

3. osteoblastic bone formation is decreased in HHM in contrast to primary hyperparathyroidism, while osteoclastic bone resorption is increased in both syndromes;

4. circulating parathyroid hormone levels measured by specific two-site immunometric assays are low in HHM but inappropriately raised in primary hyperparathyroidism;

5. PTH mRNA has not been detected reliably in tumours associated with HHM using DNA–RNA hybridization assays, although there are occasional cases in the older literature reporting arteriovenous gradients of PTH across tumours.

Overall, the evidence suggests that PTH is rarely, if ever, the cause of HHM.

These difficulties appear to have been resolved by the isolation and characterization of the same factor that stimulates the PTH-sensitive adenyl cyclase assay from squamous lung, renal, and breast cancers associated with HHM. Subsequently, the cDNA encoding it was characterized. The factor, PTH-related protein (PTHRP) contains 141 amino acids and is synthesized in an extended precursor form typical of peptide hormone synthesis. There is high sequence homology with PTH in the N-terminal 13 amino acids, which may explain common effects on bone resorption, adenyl cyclase stimulation, and inhibition of phosphate reabsorption. The structural differences may explain the previously variable results with PTH radioimmunoassays in HHM, and differences in renal calcium handling, vitamin D metabolism, and osteoblastic activity. While there are many unanswered questions relating to PTHRP, not least its normal role in keratinocytes and its transforming growth factor activity, it provides a convincing explanation of the clinical, biochemical, and histological manifestations of the syndrome of HHM.

PTHRP has also been identified by immunohistochemical staining of tumours from patients without hypercalcaemia, commonly in squamous cell carcinomas from many sites, renal cell and breast carcinomas, malignant melanoma and, surprisingly, small cell lung cancer, but rarely in adenocarcinomas. This suggests that PTHRP may be a useful histogenetic marker.

However, PTHRP may not be the only humoral mediator of hypercalcaemia. Transforming growth factors α and β (TGF-α, -β) are produced by many tumours (rhabdomyosarcoma, lung cancer, malignant melanoma) and are powerful stimulators of bone resorption *in vitro*, in addition to their effects on transforming normal to malignant cells. Further assessment of the pathogenetic role of TGFs is required, but it is unlikely that they can explain the renal features of HHM.

Cytokines (e.g. interleukin-1 and TNF) are produced by solid tumours as well as haematological malignancies. Tumour secretion of interleukin-1 may cause hypercalcaemia directly by its potent bone resorbing activity and indirectly by stimulating prostaglandin synthesis by adjacent fibroblasts. It is also possible, but not proven, that cytokines may be humoral agents in HHM. They could be produced directly by the action of tumour factors on circulating lymphocytes or indirectly by interaction with monocytes, and hence act synergistically with tumour-derived hypercalcaemic agents.

It thus seems that hypercalcaemia of malignancy is caused by several mechanisms, depending on tumour type and presence of skeletal metastases. In solid tumours without metastases, e.g. squamous cell carcinomas of lung, skin, head and neck, and carcinomas of kidney, pancreas, and ovary, PTHRP seems the likely hypercalcaemic factor, though transforming growth factors and cytokines could play synergistic roles. In haematological malignancies, e.g. multiple myeloma, leukaemia, and lymphomas, local lymphokines are implicated. In metastatic hypercalcaemia due to carcinomas of breast, lung, kidney, and ovary, local osteolytic factors, such as prostaglandins and tumour enzymes, are involved, in addition to an uncertain contribution by humoral factors. Overall, there is evidence of an underlying humoral mechanism in 80–90 per cent of cases with hypercalcaemia associated with unselected solid tumours.

Hypercalcaemia is important clinically whatever the cause, and severe hypercalcaemia (serum calcium > 3.5 mmol/l) requires immediate treatment. Hypercalcaemia causes symptoms related to the gut (nausea, vomiting, abdominal pain, constipation), kidney (polyuria, polydipsia, thirst leading to dehydration and renal failure), and central nervous system (drowsiness and eventually coma). Hypercalcaemia causes renal tubular damage, and resulting potassium loss may induce hypokalaemic alkalosis. Distinguishing features from primary hyperparathyroidism include its acute onset, absence of nephrocalcinosis, and subperiosteal bone erosions, and suppressed immunoactive PTH levels.

Ectopic ACTH syndrome

Most of the basic concepts of ectopic endocrine syndromes were established by investigation of this syndrome. In particular, the presence of increased concentrations of biologically active hormone in tumour and plasma, the chemical nature of tumour hormones, abnormal control of tumour hormone release, and specific tumour associations of the syndrome (Liddle *et al.* 1969).

The ectopic ACTH syndrome is restricted to a limited range of tumours and is not related to the degree of malignancy. It is most commonly associated with small cell or carcinoid tumours arising in lung, thymus, thyroid, gut (especially pancreas), genito-urinary system (especially prostate and ovary), and rarely with chromaffin cell tumours such as phaeochromocytoma, ganglioneuroma, neuroblastoma. A similar pro-opiomelanocortin (POMC) gene appears to be expressed in tumours associated with ectopic ACTH syndrome as in the normal anterior pituitary, but processing of the translated product differs. Characteristically, tumours associated with the syndrome produce greater proportions of ACTH precursors (e.g. POMC, pro-ACTH) and fragments. Some process ACTH extensively to an N-terminal peptide resembling α-MSH and CLIP (ACTH 18–39), a pathway typical of the neurointermediate lobe. β-Lipotrophin (LPH) may be processed to fragments (e.g. β-MSH) not normally found in the anterior pituitary, and β-endorphin to smaller molecular forms with varying degrees of acetylation and to methionine enkephalin.

The major circulating forms of POMC peptides in the syndrome are pro-ACTH, N-proopiocortin (N-POC), ACTH, β- and γ-LPH, and β-endorphin. While plasma ACTH levels do not discriminate ectopic from pituitary sources, ACTH precursor levels are characteristically higher in the ectopic ACTH syndrome and may prove to be useful in the differential diagnosis. It is not yet clear whether the increased fragments (e.g. α-MSH, CLIP, β-MSH) demonstrated in tumour extracts are reflected consistently in the circulation.

Several peptides derived from POMC have biological activities. Thus, although ACTH is the major corticosteroidogenic hormone, pro-ACTH has some intrinsic activity, and both pro-ACTH and N-POC may potentiate ACTH-induced steroidogenesis. It has been suggested that the elevated levels of pro-ACTH commonly found in the ectopic ACTH syndrome may give rise to the characteristic hypokalaemia by enhancing secretion of mineralocorticoids. N-POC may have adrenal mitogenic activity and its C-terminal fragment (γ-MSH), hypertrophic activity. The function of LPH is unknown, apart from serving as a prohormone for β-EP. Methionine enkephalin and β-endorphin have opioid activity but their endocrine roles are uncertain in modulating pain sensation, influencing psychiatric state, or their neurotransmitter effect on regulating other pituitary hormones.

Clinically, overt and occult presentations of the syndrome can be distinguished:

1. Most commonly the syndrome occurs in a middle-aged male with a history of weight loss and heavy cigarette smoking. The underlying malignancy is usually disseminated small cell lung cancer and the prognosis is very poor, with survival less than 6 months. The full stigmata of Cushing syndrome are seldom present, and the clinical features are dominated by the metabolic effects of high corticosteroid levels, such as muscle weakness, carbohydrate intolerance, hypertension, and oedema. The biochemical hallmark is hypokalaemic alkalosis (plasma potassium < 3 mmol/l, bicarbonate > 30 mmol/l), secondary to potassium loss induced by corticosteroids with mineralocorticoid activity. Urine and serum cortisol levels are grossly elevated, and fail to suppress with high-dose dexamethasone or rise in response to corticotrophin-releasing hormone. The circadian rhythm of circulating cortisol is lost. Plasma ACTH levels are uniformly elevated and usually higher than those found in Cushing's disease (Chapter 26).

2. A less aggressive syndrome occurs typically with carcinoid tumours, thymomas, and some pancreatic and adrenal medullary tumours. The patients are often younger, female, and present with features of Cushing syndrome, including psychiatric disturbances, before a tumour is evident. Hypokalaemia and carbohydrate intolerance are less pronounced, plasma corticosteroid and ACTH levels are only modestly elevated, and may suppress partially with high-dose dexamethasone. The clinical and biochemical features can thus be indistinguishable from Cushing disease. Although the occult syndrome is relatively rare, accurate diagnosis is important since, in contrast to the overt syndrome, the underlying tumours are often resectable.

Ectopic corticotrophin-releasing hormone

The demonstration of tumour peptides with corticotrophin-releasing bioactivity in pancreatic and small cell lung cancers suggested that ectopic corticotrophin-releasing factors (CRF) might cause Cushing syndrome. The role of CRF has been more precisely delineated since the structure of the hypothalamic peptide, corticotrophin-releasing hormone (CRH), was characterized. Tumour production of CRH has been implicated as a cause of Cushing syndrome by two mechanisms. In both situations exogenously administered CRH would be expected to increase plasma ACTH and cortisol levels, in contrast to its lack of effect in the ectopic ACTH syndrome.

1. Tumour CRH production in the absence of ACTH. Immunoactive and bioactive CRH was demonstrated in a prostatic carcinoma which had metastasized adjacent to the pituitary. The tumour stained for CRH but not ACTH, there was pituitary corticotroph hyperplasia, elevated plasma CRH and ACTH, and non-suppressible hypercortisolism. A similar situation was described in a patient with medullary thyroid carcinoma. However, the absence of immunostaining for ACTH does not exclude ACTH production.

2. Concomitant tumour CRH and ACTH production. In the majority of tumours containing CRH, ACTH is also produced. These include bronchial carcinoids, small cell lung cancer, paraganglioma, and medullary thyroid cancer. In such cases, CRH may stimulate autocrine or paracrine release of tumour ACTH, or of pituitary ACTH by an endocrine mechanism.

In addition to CRH, other tumour peptides may contribute to Cushing syndrome. Gastrin-releasing peptide (bombesin-like) has weak CRF activity, potentiates CRH action, and occurs commonly in small cell lung cancer, carcinoids, medullary thyroid carcinoma, and phaeochromocytomas associated with Cushing syndrome. Ectopic gastrin-releasing peptide may thus contribute to either pituitary or tumour ACTH production.

Ectopic vasopressin (antidiuretic hormone) syndrome

The ectopic vasopressin syndrome is characterized by marked hyponatraemia, persistent urinary sodium loss, impaired urinary dilution, and elevated plasma and tumour vasopressin concentrations. It is only one cause of the syndrome of inappropriate ADH secretion (SIADH)—this term should not be used indiscriminately to describe patients with serum hyponatraemia and abnormally high ratios of urine to serum osmolality. Many patients with malignant and non-malignant disease have the latter pattern of serum and urine electrolytes, but with low or undetectable plasma vasopressin levels, suggesting that the antidiuresis is mediated by other factors.

Ectopic vasopressin is most commonly due to small cell carcinoma of lung, and rarely to bronchial carcinoids, thymomas, and gastrointestinal tumours. The diagnosis is suspected in such a patient who has hyponatraemia (serum sodium < 130 mmol/l), low serum osmolality (< 275 mosm/kg), hypertonic urine containing inappropriate levels of sodium, and who is unable to excrete a water load. High plasma vasopressin levels strongly suggest the diagnosis since other causes of inappropriate vasopressin (e.g. bronchopneumonia, TB, central nervous system disease, myxoedema) are associated with hormone levels comparable to those in healthy adults, though clearly inappropriate to the serum hypotonicity. In addition to secreting vasopressin, tumours can cause inappropriate release of vasopressin from the posterior pituitary by resetting the osmostat by unknown mechanisms.

Mild hyponatraemia may not cause overt symptoms. Clinical manifestations of water intoxication (e.g. lethargy, weakness, irritability, confusion, fits, and coma) usually occur only when excessive fluid is taken in the presence of high circulating vasopressin levels, and are related to the serum sodium, which may be <110 mmol/l in severe cases.

Tumour vasopressin is chemically, immunologically, and biologically similar to arginine vasopressin (AVP). *In vitro* studies of small cell lung cancer associated with the syndrome indicate that a glycosylated precursor (propressophysin) gives rise to AVP and its carrier protein, neurophysin, by post-translational processing similar to that in the hypothalamus. Circulating propressophysin has been detected in patients with small cell lung cancer, but not in patients with inappropriate antidiuresis due to central nervous system disease. The specific neurophysin associated with vasopressin is elevated in the plasma of a high proportion of patients with small cell lung cancer, particularly those with extensive disease, and its measurement may be useful in monitoring disease status. As with other ectopic hormones, the true frequency of ectopic vasopressin is not reflected in the prevalence of the clinical syndrome, since vasopressin production occurs in the absence of metabolic abnormalities.

Oxytocin (and its associated neurophysin) is also usually found in ectopic vasopressin-producing tumours, but is not associated with obvious clinical manifestations.

Ectopic gonadotrophins

Two endocrine syndromes are associated with ectopic gonadotrophin production:

1. Isosexual precocious puberty in young boys with hepatoblastoma. Secondary sexual characteristics develop prematurely, together with advanced skeletal maturation and hyperplasia of the prostate and interstitial cells of the testis. Serum gonadotrophic activity and testosterone levels are increased.

2. Gynaecomastia without galactorrhoea in middle-aged males, usually with undifferentiated carcinoma of lung and less commonly with tumours of gastrointestinal and urogenital tract. Some patients show hypertrophic pulmonary osteoarthropathy, interstitial cell hyperplasia of testis, and increased oestrogen production. The latter appears to be due to tumour conversion of DHA sulphate to oestradiol, a characteristic of trophoblastic tissue. High oestrogen levels may suppress FSH, leading to atrophy of the seminiferous tubules and small testes.

Histologically these tumours typically contain choriocarcinoma elements or giant cells resembling syncytiotrophoblast, suggesting a possible germ-cell origin. Chemically, the tumour gonadotrophin resembles human chorionic gonadotrophin (HCG) rather than LH or FSH.

These endocrine syndromes are rare but production of HCG-related peptides in the absence of clinical manifestations is more common with elevated serum levels in 10–20 per cent of non-trophoblastic tumours. HCG-related peptides also occur in many normal tissues (e.g. liver, colon, testis), as well as placenta. HCG in non-trophoblastic tumours and normal tissues is less glycosylated than placental HCG. In addition, ectopic α- and β-HCG subunits are frequently produced in a disordant fashion, with β-subunits in the absence of α-HCG and vice versa. It has been suggested that the detectability of HCG-related peptides in serum is related to the degree of their glycosylation and molecular size. Thus carbohydrate-poor HCG and HCG subunits produced by non-trophoblastic tumours are cleared much more rapidly than intact HCG derived from placenta or trophoblastic tumours.

These considerations have renewed interest in measuring HCG-related peptides in urine as potential markers of non-trophoblastic tumours. The major form of immunoreactive HCG in urine from patients with malignancy is β core fragment, a biologically inactive peptide consisting of residues 6–40 disulphide linked to 55–92 of β-HCG. Minor concentrations of intact HCG, free β-HCG, and asialo β-HCG are also present. β core fragment and asialo β-HCG in urine may derive from intracellular processing of β-HCG in malignant cells and/or from renal metabolism of β-HCG. Elevated concentrations of β core fragment occur much more commonly than intact HCG in urine from cancer patients, and levels are more closely related to stage of disease. In gynaecological cancers (e.g. ovary, cervix, endometrium) the urine β core fragment test is sufficiently sensitive and specific to merit its further exploration as a prognostic and monitoring marker. It may extend significantly the clinical usefulness of serum HCG and subunit assays.

Ectopic growth hormone

Ectopic secretion of growth hormone (GH) is very rare and in only one case has it been shown to cause clinical acromegaly. This intramesenteric islet cell tumour fulfilled strict criteria for tumour secretion; with a high arteriovenous gradient across the tumour, rapid decrease in GH after tumour resection, positive immunostaining for GH, and *in vitro* synthesis with expression of GH mRNA. Plasma growth hormone releasing hormone levels were undetectable. The similarities between acromegaly (Chapter 26) and hypertrophic pulmonary osteoarthropathy (HPOA) led to the suggestion that the latter is one manifestation of ectopic GH secretion. However, there is no evidence that HPOA is either caused by tumour GH hypersecretion or is associated with non-suppressible GH or paradoxical increases in GH after glucose loading.

Ectopic growth hormone releasing hormone

The primary structure of hypothalamic GHRH was determined initially from pancreatic GHRH-secreting tumours associated with acromegaly. Although a rare cause of acromegaly overall, ectopic GHRH causes the syndrome more commonly than ectopic GH, and is particularly associated with slow-growing bronchial carcinoid and pancreatic tumours, both malignant and benign. Plasma GHRH and GH levels are markedly elevated, increase in response to TRH but do not suppress with glucose. The pituitary is usually enlarged, with somatotroph hyperplasia and preservation of the reticulin network.

Ectopic somatostatin

Ectopic somatostatin is associated with thymic, bronchial carcinoid tumours, small cell lung cancer, phaeochromocytoma and retinoblastoma. A syndrome of mild diabetes mellitus, steatorrhoea, and cholelithiasis may result from markedly elevated somatostatin levels, but is rarer with ectopic than eutopic somatostatin production.

Ectopic calcitonin

Although calcitonin (CT) production by extrathyroidal tumours is not associated with a characteristic endocrine syndrome, it merits attention because elevated serum levels of CT occur quite commonly in neoplasia and there is good evidence for tumour synthesis *in vivo* and *in vitro*. CT production is particularly common in small cell carcinoma of lung. A wide range of other malignancies, including NSCLC and some forms of leukaemia, are also associated, albeit less frequently, with increased tissue and serum levels.

As with other small bioactive peptides, CT is synthesized as a larger precursor of 136 amino acids. The major immunoactive forms of CT detected in lung tumours are larger than CT monomer (32 amino acids) and presumably precursor forms, in contrast to the small molecular weight forms typical of medullary thyroid carcinoma (MTC). Not all of the high molecular weight species are well recognized by CT antibodies, emphasizing the need to use immunoassays with carefully defined specificities.

The CT gene encodes two alternative mRNA products, one the precursor for CT and the other a precursor for calcitonin gene-related peptide (CGRP), both of which share a common N-terminal sequence. The expression of these genes is relatively tissue-specific, with CT the main product expressed in the thyroid and CGRP mainly in the central nervous system. Both CT and CGRP are expressed in lung cancer cell lines, with a higher ratio of CGRP to CT mRNA than in a MTC cell line, suggesting differential processing in these tissues. The mRNA species are also larger in lung carcinomas than in MTC. Whether selective mRNA splicing (see Chapter 2) of the calcitonin gene, giving differential expression of CT and CGRP, is related to tumour differentiation and progression has yet to be determined. In this context, it is relevant that tumour receptors for CT and a CT-responsive adenylate cyclase were demonstrated in a squamous cell lung cancer line, whereas no receptors for high molecular weight CT were found.

Endocrine syndromes of uncertain cause

There are rare tumour-associated endocrine syndromes whose hormonal basis is poorly understood. These include:

1. Hypoglycaemia associated with non-islet cell neoplasms, particularly large mesenchymal tumours in the abdomen and thorax (e.g. fibrosarcoma), adrenocortical carcinomas, and hepatoma. There is no proof that this syndrome is due to tumour production of insulin. There is some evidence for tumour production of factors with insulin-like biological activity (non-suppressible insulin-like activity) belonging to the family of insulin-like growth factors (somatomedins) but this proposal needs rigorous testing by DNA–RNA hybridization techniques. Excessive glucose utilization by these large tumours and failure of compensatory hyperglycaemic mechanisms are other possible contributing factors.

2. Hyperthyroidism associated with tumours of trophoblastic origin (e.g. choriocarcinoma, testicular teratoma) is almost certainly due to the weak thyrotrophic activity of HCG. There are no proven cases of ectopic production of TSH-related peptides.

3. Galactorrhoea was reported in a case of hypernephroma, with elevated serum prolactin levels which declined after tumour resection and *in vitro* secretion of prolactin. With this exception there is no definite evidence that galactorrhoea is caused by ectopic prolactin. There is *in vitro* evidence that some tumours can synthesize prolactin but are unable to secrete the hormone.

4. Erythrocytosis has been associated with uterine fibromyomata and cerebellar haemangioblastoma and elevated tumour or cyst erythropoietin levels. More rigorous and systematic investigation, using modern techniques of measuring erythropoietin gene products, are required.

9.8.4   Hormones as tumour markers

The demonstration that hormone-related peptides are produced frequently by tumours in the absence of overt endocrine syndromes suggests that their measurement in serum or urine may have clinical utility. An ideal diagnostic marker must fulfil several criteria with respect to tumour specificity, ability to detect disease at a stage which is curable, high prevalence of a positive marker, correlation of blood or urine levels with viable tumour mass, and availability of a simple and cheap assay. While these criteria are met in large part for hormone-related markers applied to classical endocrine neoplasms, they have not yet been satisfied generally for hormone-related markers in 'non-endocrine' tumours. The most systematic information is available for hormone markers in lung cancer, though there are difficulties in comparing results of different studies due to variation in patient selection, staging procedures, cut-off limits, and assay specificity.

Plasma CT has some promise as a tumour marker in SCLC, in which the prevalence of elevated levels is about 50 per cent but with wide differences between studies. Elevated levels are found less frequently in non-SCLC. Assay specificity is clearly important in determining the clinical value of plasma CT. Although plasma CT levels do not detect early disease reliably, high pretreatment levels unresponsive to treatment indicate a poor prognosis. In contrast, decreasing CT levels after initial chemotherapy correlate well with, and give an early indication of, clinical response and are associated with a better prognosis. Plasma CT levels are less reliable in detecting relapse after remission. This may be related to the greater sensitivity of CT-producing tumour cells to chemotherapy.

The possibility that plasma ACTH measurements might be a useful tumour marker was suggested by the high prevalence of ACTH production in lung cancer, particularly SCLC. However, elevated plasma ACTH occurs in only 20–30 per cent of patients with SCLC, and levels are poorly related to the stage of disease and clinical course. Plasma ACTH measurements seem less useful than plasma CT in monitoring response to therapy. ACTH assay may have some value in CSF for early diagnosis of brain metastases in SCLC. As with CT, assay specificity is important since the major tumour-associated POMC species are of high molecular weight. Preliminary evidence suggests that plasma assays for ACTH precursors (e.g. pro-ACTH) may discriminate ectopic from eutopic sources better than plasma ACTH, since the proportion of high molecular weight forms is greater with an ectopic source and usually comprises more than 50 per cent of total ACTH immunoactivity.

Assays for neurophysins derived from proprossophysin (VP–NP) and prooxyphysin (OT–NP) have advantages over those for vasopressin and oxytocin since neurophysins are more stable and can be measured directly in plasma. Elevated plasma VP–NP levels are found in about half the patients with SCLC and indicate a poorer prognosis, independent of the number of metastatic sites.

In summary, current hormone markers do not have an established role in diagnosis in the absence of clinically suspected endocrine syndromes, but they may have some utility in monitoring therapy and prognosis. There is as yet insufficient experience with recent markers of important potential, such as PTHRP and β-HCG core fragment. No tumour-specific hormone marker has been identified, and seems unlikely on theoretical grounds. However, with improved knowledge of the structure and control of genes for tumour hormones and the way in which tumour-derived hormones are processed, it may be possible to identify subtle tumour-related differences that can be exploited in the design of sensitive assays with improved tumour specificity. Because of the cellular heterogeneity, which changes during tumour progression, it seems likely that a panel of markers that reflect different stages of tumour differentiation may have greater utility than a single marker.

9.8.5 Bibliography

Baylin, S. B. (1985). The implications of differentiation relationships between endocrine and non-endocrine cells in human lung cancers. In *Peptide hormones as mediators in immunology and oncology* (ed. R. D. Hesch), Serono Symposium No. 19, pp. 1–12. Raven Press, New York.

Baylin, S. B. and Mendelsohn, G. (1980). Ectopic (inappropriate) hormone production by tumours: mechanisms involved and the biological and clinical implications. *Endocrine Reviews* 1, 45–77.

Burtis, W. J., Wu, T. L., Insogna, K. L., and Stewart, A. F. (1988). Humoral hypercalcaemia of malignancy. *Annals of Internal Medicine* 108, 454–6.

De Bustros, A. and Baylin, S. B. (1985). Hormone production by tumours: biological and clinical aspects. *Clinics in Endocrinology and Metabolism* 14, 221–56.

Liddle, G. W., Nicholson, W. E., Island, D. P., Orth, D. N., Abe, K. and Lowder, S. C. (1969). Clinical and laboratory studies of ectopic

humoral syndromes. *Recent Progress in Hormone Research* 25, 283–314.

Ratcliffe, J. G. (1982). Ectopic production of hormones in malignant disease. In *Recent advances in endocrinology and metabolism* (ed. J. L. H. O'Riordan), No. 2, pp. 187–209. Churchill Livingstone, Edinburgh.

Recent Results in Cancer Research (1985). Volume 99. Springer-Verlag, Heidelberg.

9.9 Paraneoplastic neurological syndromes

M. M. Esiri

Several different forms of neurological dysfunction, unrelated to local tumour growth or metastasis, may develop in patients with carcinoma and other neoplasms (Table 9.15). The incidence of clinically significant neurological paraneoplastic syndromes is generally low. They probably occur in 3 per cent of those with carcinoma of the lung, the form of cancer with which they are most commonly associated. However, the incidence of mild, clinically trivial, or subclinical involvement of the nervous system with similar pathology is almost certainly considerably higher. In some cases the neurological manifestations precede recognition of the existence of a tumour and give rise to considerable diagnostic difficulty, whereas in other cases the presence of a tumour is obvious before any neurological symptoms occur. The neurological conditions tend to run a progressive course and may eventually be fatal. Not infrequently, it may take painstaking care on the part of a pathologist performing an autopsy examination to demonstrate the existence of a tumour which, in some cases, may measure less than a centimetre in diameter and may not have metastasized further than (or even to) the local lymph nodes. The most common tumour to be associated with these neurological syndromes is a small cell (oat cell) carcinoma of the lung. Paraneoplastic syndromes are also occasionally associated with other carcinomas, myeloma, and various lymphomas.

The four main categories of neurological disorders that are discussed here are a subacute encephalitis, cerebellar degeneration, various forms of peripheral neuropathy, and a disorder of neuromuscular transmission, the Lambert–Eaton myasthenic syndrome. Of these, the commonest is peripheral neuropathy. Some patients suffer from more than one of these disorders either simultaneously or consecutively. Tumours may also be associated with cachectic myopathy, dermatomyositis or necrotizing myopathy, neurological complications of hypercalcaemia, paraproteinaemia, and alterations of clotting (Chapter 24), Wernicke's encephalopathy and other vitamin deficiencies, central pontine myelinolysis (Chapter 25), toxic effects of radiotherapy or chemotherapy, and opportunistic

Table 9.15 Paraneoplastic syndromes

Syndrome	Associated with
Subacute encephalitis	Carcinomas: small cell lung cancer (much the commonest), other anaplastic cancers of lung, ovary, breast, stomach, uterus, larynx Thymoma Hodgkin disease
Cerebellar degeneration	Carcinomas: small cell lung cancer (commonest), other anaplastic cancers of lung, ovary, breast, uterus, stomach, large bowel, larynx
Peripheral neuropathy	Carcinomas: small cell lung cancer (much the commonest), other anaplastic cancers of lung, kidney, thyroid, stomach, large bowel, oesophagus, breast, ovary, pancreas, prostate, uterus Synovial sarcoma Thymoma Hodgkin and non-Hodgkin lymphomas Myeloma
Lambert–Eaton myasthenic syndrome	Carcinomas: small cell lung cancer (much the commonest); cancer of breast, prostate, rectum, stomach

infections (Chapter 6). A suggested association between neoplasia and motor neurone disease is generally regarded as controversial.

9.9.1 Subacute encephalitis

This is an inflammatory condition which predominantly affects grey matter of the brain. The spinal cord may also be affected (myelitis), and rarely tracts of white matter (e.g. optic nerves, pyramidal tracts) may be prominently involved. Although occasionally generalized, it is usual for one or a few regions or groups of nuclei to be predominantly affected. This topographic localization is reflected in the clinical features. Thus, in one form the hippocampus, amygdala, and related limbic cortex are affected and the principal clinical features in such cases are behavioural disturbances, memory loss, and confusion. In another form the striatum is the focus of inflammatory change, and in yet another, the brain stem. The brain, examined postmortem, usually shows few naked-eye changes, but in histological sections the affected regions show mononuclear cell perivascular infiltrates, astrocytic and microglial reactions, and neurone loss (Fig. 9.101). The severity of each of these features does not always go hand in hand.

9.9.2 Cerebellar degeneration

In patients presenting with progressive ataxia as the chief manifestation of paraneoplastic neurological disease, one of two different forms of cerebellar pathology is usually found, though exceptionally they may occur together. The first is a form of encephalitis of the type described above, but affecting predominantly the dentate nuclei of the cerebellum. In this form of cerebellar degeneration, the neurones of the dentate nuclei are severely depleted and there are inflammatory infiltrates in the

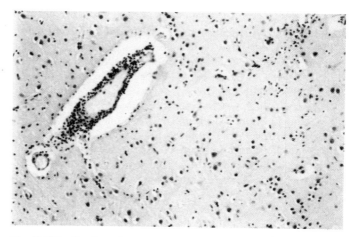

Fig. 9.101 Section of temporal lobe cortex from a case of paraneoplastic encephalitis. There is perivascular and parenchymal lymphocytic infiltration.

nuclei and their efferent tracts in the superior cerebellar peduncles. Some loss of Purkinje cells may be evident in the cerebellar cortex, but this is inconstant. In the other form the pathological changes are confined to the cerebellar cortex, where they affect the Purkinje cell layer. There is severe loss of Purkinje cells throughout the cerebellum, particularly in the superior folia, with variable astrocytosis and no inflammation (Fig. 9.102). The granule cell layer of the cortex may also show some cell loss, but this is much less severe than the Purkinje cell depletion.

9.9.3 Peripheral neuropathy

Clinically, cases of paraneoplastic peripheral neuropathy may be subdivided into those with a purely sensory deficit, those

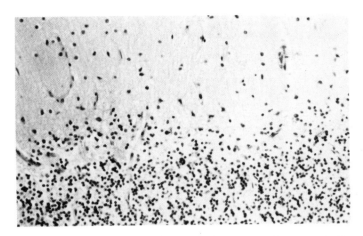

Fig. 9.102 Section of cerebellar cortex from a case of paraneoplastic cerebellar degeneration with loss of Purkinje cells.

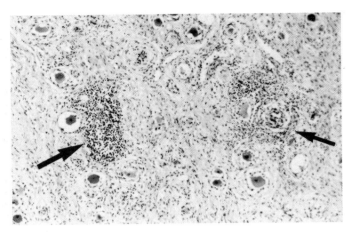

Fig. 9.103 Section of a cervical dorsal root ganglion from a case of paraneoplastic sensory neuropathy. Lymphocytic inflammatory infiltrates (large arrow) and degeneration of ganglion cells with proliferation of satellite cells (small arrow) are present.

with motor weakness, and those with mixed sensory and motor nerve involvement. Occasionally autonomic disturbances are also present. The first of these is generally due to a ganglionitis and radiculitis (nerve roots) affecting the spinal sensory system. Spinal sensory ganglia and roots show perivascular mononuclear inflammatory cell infiltrates, with loss of ganglion cells and axons and focal proliferation of satellite cells (Fig. 9.103). The central axons of the ganglion cells degenerate so that the posterior columns appear pale in myelin-stained sections of the spinal cord. In the sensorimotor and motor forms of neuropathy there may be combined features of segmental demyelination and axonal degeneration (see Chapter 25) in peripheral nerves, and a variable lymphocytic and macrophage infiltrate. Axonal degeneration tends to predominate. Rarely, the deposition of amyloid (see Chapter 4) in nerves may be responsible for neuropathy associated with myeloma.

9.9.4 Lambert–Eaton myasthenic syndrome

This syndrome affects a few patients with carcinoma (usually small cell lung carcinoma) who complain of excessive fatigability of their muscles and varying degrees of persisting muscle weakness. Characteristic electrical responses to motor nerve stimulation serve to distinguish the syndrome from myasthenia gravis (Chapter 25). The underlying defect is an abnormality of acetylcholine release from the pre-synaptic motor nerve endings. There are no constant pathological changes found on conventional muscle histology but freeze-fracture electron microscopy of the motor end plates has demonstrated alterations in the number and distribution of membrane particles on the pre-synaptic membranes.

9.9.5 Pathogenesis of paraneoplastic neurological syndromes

It is thought likely that many of these syndromes are due to immune-mediated damage which is triggered by the presence of

the tumour. Evidence for this view is strongest for the Lambert–Eaton myasthenic syndrome, in which it has been shown that circulating IgG from patients will passively transfer the disease to mice. In cortical cerebellar degeneration, there is evidence of high titre serum antibodies that bind specifically to Purkinje cells. Such antibodies are not present in the serum of patients with Purkinje cell degeneration due to other causes. Circulating IgG in a few patients with paraneoplastic sensory neuropathy has been found to react both with a tumour antigen and a neuronal nuclear protein. The particular association of small cell carcinoma of the lung with many of these neurological syndromes is of interest in view of the neuroendocrine origin of the likely cell lineage of this tumour, and the demonstration of shared antigens between oat cell tumours and dorsal root ganglion cells. Earlier suggestions that paraneoplastic encephalomyelitis might be of viral origin have not been supported by any recent evidence.

9.9.6 Further reading

General

Henson, R. A. and Urich, H. (1982). *Cancer and the nervous system.* Blackwell, Oxford.

Dropcho, E. J. (1989). The remote effects of cancer on the nervous system. *Neurologic Clinics* **7**, 579–603.

Subacute encephalitis

Booss, J. and Esiri, M. M. (1986). *Viral encephalitis.* Blackwell, Oxford.

Dorfman, L. J. and Forno, L. S. (1972). Paraneoplastic encephalomyelitis. *Acta Neurologica Scandinavica* **48**, 556–74.

Cerebellar degeneration

Cunningham, J., Graus, F., Anderson, N., and Posner, J. B. (1986). Partial characterisation of the Purkinje cell antigens in paraneoplastic cerebellar degeneration. *Neurology* **36**, 1163–8.

Greenlee, J. E. and Brashear, H. R. (1983). Antibodies to cerebellar Purkinje cells in patients with paraneoplastic cerebellar degeneration and ovarion carcinoma. *Annals of Neurology* **14**, 609–13.

Peripheral neuropathy

Bell, C. E., Seetharam, S., and McDaniel, R. C. (1976). Endodermally derived and neural crest derived differentiation antigens expressed by a human lung tumour. *Journal of Immunology* **116**, 1236–43.

Graus, F., Elkon, K. B., Cordon-Cardo, C., and Posner, J. B. (1986). Sensory neuropathy and small cell lung cancer. *American Journal of Medicine* **80**, 45–52.

Lambert–Easton myasthenic syndrome

Fukunaga, H., Engel, A. G., Osame, M., and Lambert, E. H. (1982). Paucity and disorganization of presynaptic membrane active zones in the Lambert–Eaton myasthenic syndrome. *Muscle and Nerve* **5**, 686–97.

Lang, B., *et al.* (1981). *Lancet* **2**, 224–6.

9.10 Immunology of cancer

N. A. Mitchison

9.10.1 Immune surveillance and viral cancer

It was at one time hoped that tumour cells might bear antigens able to evoke protective immunity in their host. Thus, some 30 years ago Sir Macfarlane Burnet and Lewis Thomas independently proposed that the immune system might operate an 'immune surveillance of cancer' which would ensure that many early cancers would be destroyed before they reach the level of detection. A natural corollary of this view is that those cancers that escape the surveillance mechanism may nevertheless bear weak antigens, and that it makes sense to try to design treatments able to enhance the response to these antigens up to an effective level.

It is worth recalling that the theory of immune surveillance was proposed at a time when the functions of T-cells were poorly understood, and almost their only known activity was in the rejection of transplants. An attractive feature of the theory was that it provided a plausible purpose for that component of the immune system. That merit has disappeared with the passage of time and a better understanding of the role of T-cells in immunoregulation (Chapter 4) and resistance to infection. The other supports for the theory were: (1) the supposed high incidence of cancer in immunosuppressed individuals, and (2) the presence of tumour-specific transplantation antigens (TSTA) on animal tumour cells. Each of these merits discussion.

Extensive data are available concerning the incidence of cancer in immunosuppressed patients. Table 9.16 is taken from a recent UK/Australian survey, mainly of kidney transplant recipients. This and other similar surveys establishes that for most forms of cancer the relative risk does not significantly increase as a result of immunosuppression and hence, in general,

Table 9.16 Relative risk of developing cancer in immunosuppressed patients (from Kinlen *et al.* 1983)

Non-Hodgkin lymphoma	49
Skin	9
Melanoma	9
All others	1.4

that the immune system does not appear to protect against cancer. There are however, notable exceptions, most of which are for forms of cancer that are likely to be of viral origin. In non-Hodgkin lymphoma, Epstein–Barr virus (EBV) is implicated, and in skin cancer, human papilloma virus (HPV). The number of skin cancers occurring in immunosuppressed individuals from which HPV has actually been isolated is still too small to permit a firm conclusion to be reached, but the pattern of cancer incidence is certainly highly suggestive.

Turning briefly to other forms of immunosuppression, it is surprising how highly selective is the impact on cancer incidence. In X-linked lymphoproliferative disease (XLPD, or Duncan's syndrome; see Chapter 4) for instance, a congenital T-cell defect predisposes strongly for uncontrolled EBV infection, leading to non-Hodgkin lymphoma. HIV infection, on the other hand, predisposes to Kaposi sarcoma, where a viral aetiology has not been definitely established. Thus while the details remain obscure, the rule seems clear: immune surveillance applies to viral but not other forms of cancer, and the immune system protects us essentially only against viral infection.

Much the same conclusion can be drawn from animal experiments. Nude mice lack a thymus and therefore do not develop T-cells. A substantial study of these animals produced the following conclusion (Rygaard and Poulson 1974): 'Approximately 6,300 nudes were observed . . . spontaneous malignant tumours were not observed in any animal.' On the other hand, nude mice are highly susceptible to polyoma virus infection and develop tumours in consequence, but this only confirms the importance of T-cells in resistance to viral infection. Indeed, it is an animal oncogenic virus that provides the only example of successful large-scale immunoprophylaxis against cancer: vaccination with turkey herpes virus protects chickens against subsequent infection with chicken herpes virus, the agent of Marek's lymphoma.

The epidemiological evidence for immune surveillance of viral cancer is likely to be superseded in the fairly near future by the outcome of vaccine trials. Retrospective sero-epidemiology and other evidence implicates the following viruses as agents of cancer in man: hepatitis virus B (HVB) for primary hepatocellular carcinoma; Epstein–Barr virus (EBV) for Burkitt lymphoma and for nasopharyngeal carcinoma; human papilloma virus (HPV) for carcinoma of the cervix, bladder, and skin; and human leukaemic virus (HTLV) types I and II for certain T-cell leukaemias. For the first of these, vaccine trials are already underway in Taiwan; and for the second and third, vaccines are under active development.

9.10.2 Tumour-specific transplantation antigens

Tumour-specific transplantation antigens (TSTA) have a long history in transplantation biology. For many years confused with histocompatibility antigens (see Chapter 4), they were eventually dissected out as distinct entities some 30 years ago by transplantation experiments with tumours in inbred strains of mice. Tumours that arise within an inbred strain can usually be transplanted freely within that strain (syngeneic transplantation), provided that large numbers ($> 10^6$) of cells are given. Transplantation of small numbers of cells, or of cells that have been sterilized by irradiation or appropriate chemical treatment, often induces immunity that makes the host resistant to subsequent larger transplants. This immunity is highly specific to each individual tumour, so that in an extreme case two tumours that arose on either side of a mouse did not cross-react. It is mediated by T-cells, and precisely the same T-cell subsets seem to be involved as are responsible for tissue allograft rejection. Certain tumours, such as skin tumours induced by UV irradiation or strong chemical carcinogens, are much more highly immunogeneic than others. Indeed, the extraordinarily close parallel between the immunology of skin cancer in mouse and man, and the individual-specific TSTA that the mouse tumours display, does raise a doubt about the simple explanation of the surveillance data offered above.

The molecular biology of TSTA has not been resolved, in spite of a great deal of effort. This is mainly because these antigens are defined by T-cell assays, and monoclonal antibodies cannot be used with any confidence to investigate them. Thus while cytolytic T-cell clones specific for certain TSTA are readily available, such powerful techniques as radioimmune precipitation or Western blotting cannot be used. In this connection it is fair to add that minor transplantation antigens, such as the male-specific antigen H-Y, enjoy the same mysterious status, despite substantial molecular efforts. And the problem has become all the more baffling, now that it is known that T-cell-derived epitopes are not necessarily derived from cell-surface macromolecules.

Recent work on TSTA suggests that these structures represent mutations in normal cell proteins, and possibly mainly among the MHC glycoproteins. Thus under extreme chemical mutagenesis tumour cells develop new TSTA at high frequency. Subsequently, transplantation selects strongly for loss of these antigens. Among the highly immunogeneic TSTA present on UV-induced skin tumours, mutant class I MHC molecules have been identified by means of T-cell assays and analysis of such loss variants.

TSTA similar to those of mice have been discovered in other rodents such as rats and guinea-pigs, but not in man. This is disappointing, particularly when one recalls that lung cancer, for instance, is just as clearly a product of chemical carcinogenesis as the mouse tumours that bear strong TSTA. There are those who argue that this is largely a technical problem and that TSTA in mice would have been hard to discover using only the limited range of immunological methods available for examining human T-cells. At best, however, the case for human TSTA remains unproven.

9.10.3 Monoclonal antibodies and cancer

The proteins made by a cancer cell reflect the differentiated state of the normal cell from which it was derived. Of particular interest are the glycoproteins (and glycolipids) of the cell surface that constitute the 'surface phenotype', and also any characteristic proteins that are released into body fluids. Many of these molecules were first identified by means of monoclonal antibodies, and even when they have been fully characterized by gene cloning and in other ways, monoclonal antibodies remain the most convenient tools for recognizing and manipulating them.

These macromolecules are of special value as markers if they can be used to distinguish cancer cells from surrounding normal ones. This is likely to be the case if:

1. the marker forms part of the phenotype of an early developmental stage in a cell lineage [e.g. the common lymphoid leukaemia antigen ('CALLA') present in some leukaemias and a small number of normal thymocytes and bone marrow cells];

2. the marker is induced on cancer cells by the special features of their microenvironment (e.g. the Ca-1 antigen that is believed to develop on cancer cells in response to their acid environment, and otherwise occurs only on cells lining the genito-urinary tract and in some hyperplasias);

3. the marker occurs in the original environment of the cancer cell, but not in a site to which it has metastasized (e.g. α-keratins, that occur in large amounts in epithelium but not in lymph nodes, and so distinguish carcinomas from their surroundings in lymphoid metastases); or

4. the marker occurs at higher density on cancer cells than on most normal cells (e.g. the transferrin receptor).

There are no known examples of markers defined by monoclonal antibodies that are unique to cancer cells, i.e. that do not occur also on normal cells, and the information provided in the foregoing account of immune surveillance makes such a possibility unlikely.

Monoclonal antibodies against cancer cells and their products have a variety of uses: the more immediate lie in diagnosis and monitoring; the more distant in imaging and therapy. Thus monoclonals against cell components are being used to detect micrometastases in histopathology: to stage carcinomas according to the derangement of cytoskeletal elements, and leukaemias according to their surface phenotype; and to detect early leukaemia relapse from bone marrow biopsies. Monoclonals (and also conventional polyclonal antisera) are used to detect proteins produced by tumours, for instance chorionic gonadotrophin produced by choriocarcinoma, placental alkaline phosphatase by ovarian carcinoma, and carcinoembryonic antigen by colon carcinoma. Cancer imaging by means of monoclonal antibodies coupled to γ-emitting isotopes (^{131}I, ^{111}In) is finding a place in nuclear medicine. And, for the more distant future, high hopes are held for immunotoxins (antibodies coupled to toxins) and other conjugates of monoclonal antibodies that could be used to deliver poisonous agents to tumour cells. Meanwhile, panels of monoclonal antibodies directed at cell-surface antigens are being tested in clinical trials for their ability to purge bone marrow of cancer cells prior to auto-transplantation.

9.10.4 Natural killer (NK) and lymphokine-activated killer (LAK) cells

While hunting for lymphocytes that are reactive with cancer antigens in the blood of cancer patients, it was observed that lymphocytes from normal control individuals could kill some, but not all, tumour cells. These cells, termed natural killer cells (NK cells), express the CD16 (Fc$_\gamma$ receptor) antigen, are large granular lymphocytes (LGL), mostly express asialo-GM1 glyco-lipid, and mostly do not express CD3 or the $\alpha\beta$TcR. These properties are shared with killer cells (K-cells), so that NK and K activities presumably represent different functions of the same cell population. The surface phenotype resembles that of immature T-cells, and it is generally believed that this cell population is derived from precursors that branch off the main T-cell lineage prior to $\alpha\beta$TcR gene rearrangement in the thymus (athymic nude mice display high NK activity); thus they lack the normal T-cell receptor repertoire, and if they recognize target cells at all must do so through other unidentified recognition structures (see Chapter 4).

Lymphokine-activated killer (LAK) cells represent an operationally defined lymphocyte population that can lyse NK-resistant fresh tumour cells upon culture with IL-2. These cells are derived from precursors within the NK population but are much enriched for CD3-expressing cells. There is evidence that these CD3$^+$ cells with NK or LAK activity express the $\gamma\delta$TcR; as such they manifest a repertoire that is probably smaller than that of $\alpha\beta$TcR T-cells. Functions such as primitive defence against pathogens or amplifying the activation of $\alpha\beta$TcR cells have been proposed for this population; the matter has not yet been resolved, but meanwhile it is worth noting that NK/LAK cells may have major functions other than tumour recognition.

Attempts to demonstrate a physiological anti-tumour function for the NK/LAK population have yielded inconclusive results. Anti-tumour effects, but minor ones, have been noted in mice depleted of NK cells congenitally (the *beige* mouse) or experimentally (e.g. by treatment with antibodies to asialo-GM1), or by comparing congenitally high- and low-NK strains. In man, clinical trials with LAK cells are currently under way.

A major problem of work with NK/LAK cells is that normal T-cells can acquire non-specific cytolytic activity as a result of being grown *in vitro*. To give one particularly dramatic example, the entire population of lymphocytes from the mouse thymus acquire this non-specific killer phenotype if cultured in the presence of an excess of feeder cells.

9.10.5 Macrophages

By the beginning of the present decade a large body of research had raised a suspicion that macrophages might exercise control of cancer growth. Thus, treatment with the macrophage stimulant BCG, or its derivative MER (methanol-extracted residue), or *Corynebacterium parvum* slightly delayed the effect of chemical and viral carcinogens in rodents, and reduced metastasis of some transplanted rodent tumours. Macrophages activated by these and other agents could kill or inhibit proliferation of certain rodent and human tumour cells *in vitro* (a current estimate is that 60 per cent of tumours are susceptible to this effect). Activation of macrophages depended on factors released by T-cells, and was known to proceed in stages in which the ability to kill or damage tumour cells is acquired progressively, in parallel with the ability to kill bacteria and parasites. The macrophage content of animal tumours showed an erratic correlation with tumour growth: the percentage of macrophages is proportional to the immunogenicity of the tumour and inversely proportional to the frequency of metastasis, but only for certain carcinogen-induced tumours and in certain species of rodents; for others, no such correlation could be found. Similar correlations have been reported from time to time in man, but no systematic trend is evident.

All this inspired attempts to perform cancer immunotherapy in man by administration of BCG or other macrophage stimulants, a wave of activity that peaked in the 1970s and has not yet entirely died out. Extensive clinical trials of treatment with BCG conducted under the auspices of the National Cancer Institute (USA) and the MRC (UK) eventually proved entirely negative (with the possible exception of local treatment of bladder cancer). Related forms of treatment are still employed on a large scale in Japan, but not elsewhere. The view gained ground that the presence of macrophages within tumours might reflect activities other than control of tumour cell growth, and that the effects seen in rodents were either slight or reflected the special features of carcinogenesis in those species.

There the matter might have rested, had not rapid progress been made recently in identifying the factors that mediate macrophage activation and activity. Among these the most significant are tumour necrosis factor (TNF) and γ-interferon (γ-IFN); the functional relationships of these well-defined (and cloned) proteins to one another and to other cytokines is illustrated in Fig. 9.104. TNF is produced by macrophages and is the agent mainly responsible for their cytotoxic and cytostatic effect on tumour cells, mentioned above. Direct killing by cell–cell contact, mediated by reduced oxygen species, can be demonstrated but plays a less important part; antibodies to TNF potently inhibit the cytotoxic activity of macrophages. Macrophages are activated to release TNF and reduced oxygen species principally by γ-IFN, a cytokine that is able to perform this function by itself. Its activity in this respect shows synergy with another cytokine, lymphotoxin (LT), and also with TNF itself

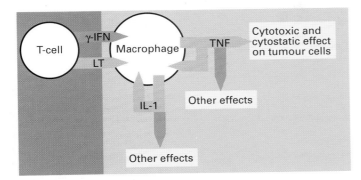

Fig. 9.104 Activation of macrophages by γ-IFN, in synergy with LT, IL-1, and TNF. Activated macrophages produce TNF, which has many effects including acting on tumour cells.

and another macrophage product, interleukin-1 (IL-1). *In vivo*, all these four cytokines presumably act in concert to control the level of macrophage activation. Note that activation occurs in stages (see above and Chapter 4).

TNF acts on tumour cells (and on other cells) via specific receptors on the cell membrane. A simple and appealing hypothesis is that a membrane oncogene such as *c-erb-2* promotes, say, breast cancer cell growth by its activity as a tyrosine phosphokinase; and TNF receptors, activated by binding TNF, neutralize this by acting as phosphatases. However, it must be emphasized that TNF has many important activities unrelated to cancer; it almost ended up with the less beguiling title of cachexin, and might equally well be termed a shock-factor.

Any hypothesis that points to cancer immunotherapy needs to be regarded with the utmost scepticism, on the basis of past experience and the epidemiology of immunosuppression.

9.10.6   Bibliography

Azuma, I. and Yamamura, Y. (1985). Stimulation of host-defence mechanisms with immunoadjuvants. In *Macrophage biology* (ed. S. Reichard and M. Kijuma), pp. 597–611. Alan R. Liss, New York.

Kinlen, L., Doll, R., and Peto, R. (1983). The incidence of tumours in human transplant recipients. *Transplantation Proceedings* **15**, 1039.

Lachmann, P. J. (1982). The immune response to tumours: *in vitro* aspects. In *Clinical aspects of immunology*, Vol. 2 (ed. P. J. Lachmann and D. K. Peters), p. 1263. Blackwell, Oxford.

Mitchison, N. A. (1982). The immune response to tumours: protective immunity *in vivo*. In *Clinical aspects of immunology*, Vol. 2, (ed. P. J. Lachmann and D. K. Peters), p. 1273. Blackwell, Oxford.

Rygaard, J. and Poulson, C. O. (1974). The mutant nude mouse does not develop spontaneous tumours. *Acta Pathologica Microbiologica et Immunologica Scandinavica* **82**, 99.

Stern, K. (1983). Control of tumours by the RES. In *The reticuloendothelial system*, Vol. 5 (ed. R. B. Herberman and H. Friedman), pp. 59–176. Plenum Pess, New York.

Excellent sections on the immunology of cancer are in:

Progress in immunology, Vol. V (1984). (ed. Y. Yamamura and T. Tada). Academic Press, Japan.

Progress in immunology, Vol. VI (1986) (ed. R. G. Miller). Academic Press, London.

9.11   Cytokines in neoplasia

C. E. Lewis

9.11.1   Introduction

Cytokines are a multifunctional group of signalling proteins (ocasionally still referred to as monokines or lymphokines) which mediate, in part, the paracrine communication between cells of the immune system (Table 9.17). As such, they play a crucial role in the regulation of both the development and activation of immune cells, and thus control their relative contributions to immune and inflammatory mechanisms. Many of these soluble mediators were originally identified by their involvement in embryogenesis. differentiation/growth, and tissue repair (Arai *et al.* 1990).

Cytokines interact with specific, high-affinity receptors on the plasma membrane of their target cells. This signal is then amplified and conveyed, by intracellular events, to the nucleus where genetic activity and the resultant protein synthesis is altered (see Section 2.3). Individual cytokines have multiple, overlapping functions which can vary with local concentration, duration of stimulus, and the influence of other cytokines and/or hormones on the responsiveness of the target cell. Thus, cytokines do not work in isolation but rather as a complex network of interdependent signals. Investigation of the factors that regulate the synthesis and action of these compounds has been greatly facilitated by the recent advent and application of DNA technology to generate larger quantities of human cytokines, together with their respective monoclonal antibodies.

Malignant human tumours are markedly heterogeneous, often comprising a variety of cell types other than just the malignant cell population. The latter are to be found in intimate contact with such infiltrates as T-cells, macrophages, natural killer (NK) cells, and granulocytes. Although this array of effector cells exist within tumours, their interaction with tumour cells rarely results in an effective antitumour activity, but rather the suppression of such a response. Investigations into the cellular mechanisms underlying this tumour-specific immuno-regulation have largely focused on the aberrant role of certain cytokines in disrupting the ability of these cells to mount an appropriate response to tumour-associated antigens (TAA) present on malignant cells.

Fig. 9.105 illustrates the range of cytokines which could potentially be generated by the cell types present in human tumours and play a part ultimately in the disregulated growth of malignant cells. Certain individual cytokines are known both to influence directly the proliferation and metastatic potential of the tumour cells themselves, and to perturb the host–tumour relationship in a variety of ways. However, it should also be noted that cytokines can be used as a potent force for good. Recent clinical trials have demonstrated their therapeutic potential in the restoring something of the cytokine imbalance

Table 9.17   The current list of human cytokines

Cytokine (+abbreviations)	Alternative name(s)	Subtypes	Molecular weight (kDa)	Cellular source	Target cells
Interleukin (IL-)					
1	EP, TPF, LAF	α, β	17.5	Monocytes/macrophages, endothelial cells, NK cells, B- and T-cells, fibroblasts, epithelial cells, osteoblasts, keratinocytes	B- and T-cells, thymocytes, fibroblasts, synovial cells, chondrocytes, endothelial cells, hepatocytes, osteoclasts, NK cells
2	TCGF, TSF		15.5	T-cells, NK cells	B- and T-cells, NK cells, macrophages
3	Multi-CSF		28	T-cells, keratinocytes, some tumour cell lines	Haematopoietic progenitor cells, mast cells, macrophages
4	BSF-1		20	T-cells, NK cells	B- and T-cells, fibroblasts, monocytes/ macrophages, granulocytes, mast cells, lymphoma cell lines, megakaryocytes, NK cells
5	EDF, TRF, BCGF-2		45	T-cells	B-cells (?), eosinophils
6	IFN-β2, BSF-2,		26	B- and T-cells, fibroblasts, macrophages, endothelial cells, keratinocytes, NK cells, various tumour types, myeloma cells	B- and T-cells, NK cells, hepatocytes, thymocytes, fibroblasts, myeloma cells
7			25	Thymocytes, splenocytes	T-cells, B-cell progenitor cells, thymocytes
8	MDNCF, NAP, GCP, MIP-2		7	Monocytes/macrophages, T-cells, fibroblasts, endothelial cells	T-cells, granulocytes, and NK cells
Interferon (IFN)					
α		15	18–20	B- and T-cells, macrophages	B- and T-cells, granulocytes, fibroblasts, NK cells, some tumour cells
β			23	Fibroblasts, epithelial cells	B-cells, NK cells
γ			20–25	T-cells, NK cells	B- and T-cells, NK cells, macrophages, some tumour cells
Tumour necrosis factors (TNF-)					
α	Cachetin		17	B- and T-cells, NK cells, macrophages, thymocytes	NK cells, endothelial cells, adipocytes, osteoclasts, fibroblasts, macrophages, chondrocytes, hepatocytes, granulocytes
β	LT		25	T-cells	Granulocytes, osteoclasts
Colony-stimulating factors (CSF-)					
CSF-α	GM-CSF		23	T-cells, macrophages, fibroblasts, endothelial cells	Granulocyte/macrophage progenitor cells
CSF-β	G-CSF		20–30	Fibroblasts, some tumour cells lines, monocytes	Granulocyte progenitor cells
CSF-1	M-CSF		47–76	Monocytes, endothelial cells, fibroblasts, placenta	Macrophage progenitor cells, monocytes/ macrophages
Transforming growth factor (TGF-)					
α			6	Keratinocytes, some tumour cells, e.g. melanoma	Keratinocytes, fibroblasts, some epithelial cells and tumour cell types
β		1–5	25	Platelets, macrophages, T-cells, malignant cells, numerous other cell types	B- and T-cells, fibroblasts, thymocytes, smooth muscle cells, NK cells, monocytes/macrophages, some tumour cell lines

in cancer and augmenting the immune response of the host to the tumour.

This section outlines the most recent developments in our understanding of the role of cytokines in the development, metastatic spread, and immunotherapy of human cancer. For further information on this topic, the reader is referred to the excellent recent monographs by Sinkovics (1988) and Balkwill (1989).

9.11.2   Interleukins

The term 'interleukin' was first coined in 1979 to denote the molecular mediators involved in communication between leucocytes. Hitherto, names for these proteins had been loosely based on their biological activities. In fact, we now know that their cellular sources and target cells are by no means restricted to leucocytes alone. However, for various historical reasons certain cytokines such as the interferons, transforming growth factors, and colony-stimulating factors have retained their original, if a little out-dated, nomenclature.

Interleukin-1 (IL-1)

Many cell types can synthesize IL-1, although the monocytes and macrophages are widely considered the major source of the secreted form of IL-1 (Table 9.17). This cytokine is initially

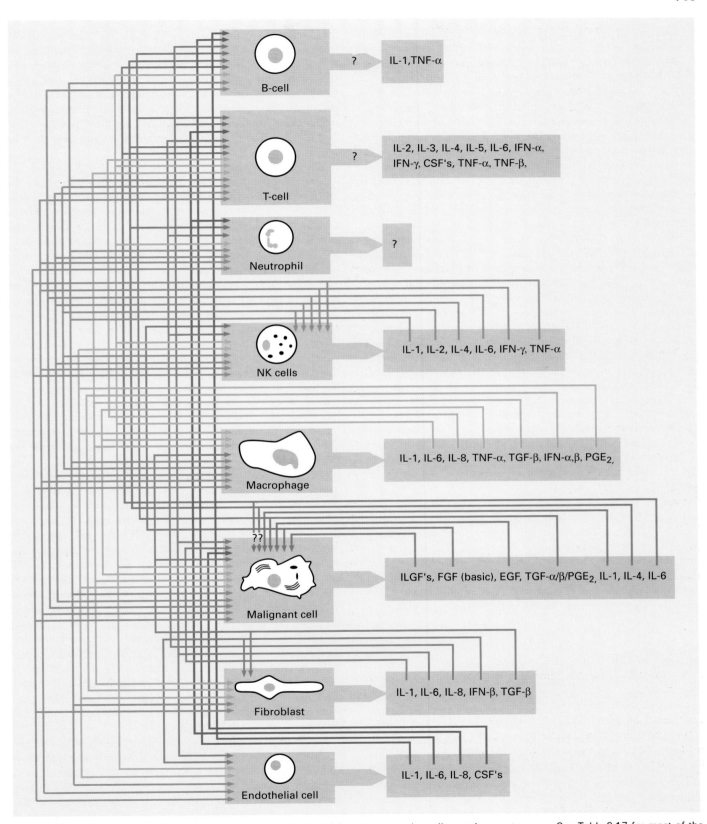

Fig. 9.105 Various aspects of the complex cytokine network which may operate in malignant human tumours. See Table 9.17 for most of the abbreviations cited (except: EGF, epidermal growth factor; FGF, fibroblast growth factor; ILGF, insulin-like growth factor). Very little is known of the regulation of these factors within the microenvironment of the tumour. Hence, the diagram is speculative and represents only the possible cytokine products of these tumour-infiltrating cells. Their release by these cell types has been suggested in studies using either blood leukocytes or stromal cells isolated from other tissues.

synthesized as a 33 kDa precursor and subsequently cleaved into a small, biologically active form (17.5 kDa). The pathway for IL-1 secretion is at present unknown. But since the larger IL-1 precursor lacks a classical hydrophobic signal sequence, IL-1 is thought not to be a conventional secreted product and, indeed, may play its most important immunoregulatory role while lodged in the plasma membrane. There are at least two distinct IL-1 genes encoding the α and β forms, which differ in their amino-acid sequences and isoelectric points, but bind to the same receptor and exert similar biological activities (Mizel 1989). The pleiotrophic actions of IL-1 are reflected in their influence on wound healing, inflammation, immunity, acute phase response to trauma, fever, sleep patterns, and weight loss (Dinarello 1989).

The role of IL-1, if any, in tumour biology is also somewhat unclear. Myelomonocytic leukaemia cells, together with skin and renal carcinoma cells, can secrete elevated levels of IL-1. In addition, IL-1 also stimulates such cells as endothelial cells to secrete colony-stimulating factors (CSFs), which, in turn, stimulate the proliferation of such leukaemic cells (see Sections 1.1–1.5). Furthermore, IL-1β may itself act in an autocrine manner to stimulate proliferation of this malignant cell type, thereby inferring that up-regulated IL-1 may act as one of the signals for overproliferation in such disorders (Balkwill 1989). By contrast, monocytes of patients with colorectal carcinoma or malignant melanoma release only small amounts of this cytokine. This is hardly surprising in light of the finding that human malignant cells can secrete such IL-1 inhibitors as prostaglandin E_2 (PGE$_2$), and that IL-1α and β can both inhibit the growth of various carcinoma cell lines (e.g. breast) and be directly cytotoxic to melanoma cells (reviewed by Sinkovics 1988).

Very few studies have been performed on the therapeutic possibilities of IL-1, either as a single agent or in combination with various other cytokines/drugs. However, using mice bearing Meth A sarcoma, Nakata *et al.* (1988) found that administration of IL-1α resulted in a high (86 per cent) complete response rate. Interestingly, when given together with indomethacin (which would block IL-1α-induced PGE$_2$ production in these animals), the antitumour efficacy of this cytokine was significantly increased.

Interleukin-2 (IL-2)

IL-2 (formerly T-cell growth factor) is a 15 kDa glycoprotein secreted by two cell types; T-cells activated by exposure to mitogens, antigens, contact with antigen-presenting cells, and/or such macrophage-derived signals as IL-1 or IL-6; and NK cells. Activated T-cells also express high- and low-affinity receptors for IL-2 and so become responsive to their own autocrine growth factor, which then stimulates clonal expansion of antigen-specific T-cells. Specific effector cells performing helper, suppressor, and cytotoxic T-cell functions are the usual downstream products of this IL-2-mediated event (Mizel 1989).

Apart from promoting T-cell proliferation and function, IL-2 is also known to augment cytokine production and the non-MHC-restricted cytotoxicity of NK cells (see Section 9.10.4). Such cells, called lymphokine-activated killer (LAK) cells are then capable of destroying autologous and NK cell-resistant malignant cells (Balkwill 1989; Hellmann 1989). However, it is not clear whether the antitumour effects of LAK cells *in vivo* reflect a direct cytotoxicity of LAK cells on tumour cells, or rather their enhanced production of such cytokines as TNF-α, IL-1α, γ-IFN with potential tumoricidal activities (Limb *et al.* 1989).

With these antitumour effects in mind, IL-2 has been used extensively over the past few years in attempts to stimulate the immune system of the host (i.e. to generate such effector cells as LAK cells *in vivo*) in response to the tumour. Despite its marked toxicity at the high levels needed for it to be effective in anti-cancer human therapy, IL-2 infusion alone has been partially effective (5–10 per cent show durable complete responses), albeit mainly restricted largely to cases of renal carcinoma and melanoma. Limited activity has also been seen in preliminary studies in patients with other tumour types, including colon carcinoma, ovarian carcinoma, neuroblastoma, lymphoma, and mesothelioma (Hellmann 1989). This form of immunotherapy has only been applied to patients with advanced cancer which is refractory to standard forms of radio- or chemotherapy. Little is known of the efficacy of such novel forms of treatment at earlier, untreated stages of the malignancy. A second, more effective model has been used recently in which IL-2 is administered together with the patient's own LAK cells (generated *ex vivo*). Substantial regressions were reported, although significant toxicity was again associated with the treatment (reviewed by Hellmann 1989).

Recent clinical trials, involving predominantly melanoma patients, have utilized a different type of activated killer cell; those derived from surgically excised tumours—tumour-infiltrating lymphocytes (TIL). Unlike LAK cells, TIL are cytolytic T-cells (rather than NK cells) which can be expanded in culture by IL-2 *in vitro*, and after re-infusion into the patient will traffic back to tumour sites to mediate greater tumour regression than that elicited by the adoptive transfer of blood-derived LAK cells (Balkwill 1989; Hellmann 1989). Although these IL-2 activated TIL do migrate to metastatic sites, their generation *in vitro* is lengthy, labour intensive, and expensive. A further disadvantage of TIL therapy is that of their cytotoxicity, which is both antigen-dependent and MHC-restricted. Since high levels of TAA and MHC molecules are not ubiquitously found in human tumours, further studies incorporating such cytokines as α-interferon and/or γ-interferon (see Section 9.11.3) into these protocols are planned to maximize the expression of such epitopes.

The abnormal release of IL-2 and expression of its receptor (IL-2R) by T-cells has been demonstrated in various forms of human malignancy. As both regulate the proliferation of T-cells, it is hardly surprising that T-cell leukaemia cell lines express high levels of IL-2R. However, there is no correlation between high levels of IL-2 secretion or IL-2R expression in adult T-cell leukaemia, thereby making autocrine stimulation unlikely as the major mechanism underpinning this proliferative disease. Elevated levels of IL-2R (released by malignant B-cells) have also been found in the plasma of patients with B-cell leukaemia (Balkwill 1989). By contrast, peripheral blood mononuclear cells of patients with breast carcinoma display markedly suppressed levels of IL-2 secretion and IL-2R expression. This phenomenon may play an important part in the immunosuppression seen in such forms of cancer.

Interleukin-4 (IL-4)

This pluripotent cytokine acts on a variety of cell types, including B- and T-cells, NK cells, macrophages, and granulocytes. IL-4 has been shown to greatly enhance the cytotoxicity of T-cells and macrophages (Paul and Ohara 1987; Widmer et al. 1987). This cytokine is also known to augment the activity of LAK cells preactivated by IL-2 (Kawakami et al. 1989). These recent findings have implications for the potential use of IL-4 as an immunotherapeutic agent in cancer, especially as a possible co-stimulant with IL-2 in adoptive therapies using both LAK cells and TIL. Although elevated levels of IL-4 receptors have been localized in tumours of epithelial origin, their function(s) have not been determined (Jabaari et al. 1989).

Interleukin-5 (IL-5)

Little is known of the possible role of IL-5 in the cytokine network of malignant tumours. It is known to be secreted by lung carcinoma and lymphoma cells and to be a potent regulator of eosinophil activation. This led Balkwill (1989) to speculate on a possible link between IL-5 production by the tumour and the eosinophilia present both in IL-2/LAK-treated patients and certain forms of cancer. IL-5 can also induce the expression of high-affinity IL-2 receptors on thymocytes and enhance the generation of cytotoxic T-cells (Mizel 1989).

Interleukin-6 (IL-6)

Far from being merely a B-cell growth and differentiation factor or antiviral agent as originally thought, this 26 kDa protein exhibits a broad spectrum of biological functions. The main immunoregulatory role of IL-6 is on immunoglobulin production by B-cells and IL-2 release by activated T-cells. IL-6 also has limited antigrowth effects on some carcinoma, leukaemia, and lymphoma cell lines (Hirano et al. 1989). By contrast, IL-6 may be an autocrine growth factor in human myeloma, since these cells can both secrete and respond to this cytokine. Thus, antibodies to IL-6, or application of specific antagonists to IL-6, may have therapeutic potential in the treatment of this condition.

Interleukins 7 and 8 (IL-7, IL-8)

These two new cytokines were cloned in 1988. IL-7 is known to stimulate the proliferation of immature forms of B- and T-cells, while also acting as a comitogen for mature T-cells. In the latter case, IL-2 secretion and expression of IL-2R is augmented. This, then, would seem to indicate that IL-7, in combination with or preceding IL-2 administration, may well prove useful in the immunotherapy of cancer. The possible interactions of IL-7 with other cytokines (such as IL-6 and IL-3, already nominated as likely candidates for synergism with IL-7) have yet to be fully researched.

Recently, definitive evidence that IL-8 regulates the chemotaxis and activation of granulocytes has emerged. This cytokine is also chemotactic for T-cells, which express fewer IL-8 receptors, albeit of higher affinity. Studies are currently in progress to examine the relationship between IL-8 and the prevalence of granulocyte infiltrates in human tumours.

9.11.3 Interferons (IFNs)

These were discovered in 1957 and called interferons since they were produced in response to viral infections and could confer resistance on other cells to a wide range of viruses. The IFNs are a multigene family encoding proteins in three main categories; α-IFN, β-IFN, and γ-IFN. While there is only one gene for β-IFN and γ-IFN, there are at least 23 different α-IFN genes, of which 15 correspond to functional genes. Stimuli for α-IFN and β-IFN include viral infection, bacteria, and a variety of pathogens which stimulate only their transient release. γ-IFN, which is thought to be secreted constitutively in some instances, has an extensive role in immunoregulation and is thus augmented by exposure to antigenic/mitogenic stimulation. The IFNs also play a vital part in the regulation of the cytokine network of the body and, as such, are responsive to regulation by a variety of cytokines including IL-1, IL-2, IL-4, IL-6, TNF-α, and the colony-stimulating factors. The major immunomodulatory functions of IFNs include activation of macrophage function, and the cytotoxicity of T-cells, NK cells, and granulocytes. They also induce class I/II histocompatibility antigens on potential target cells for cytotoxic lymphocytes and modulate antibody responses. (see Sinkovics 1988; Balkwill 1989).

α-IFN and β-IFN are known to inhibit the growth of malignant cells in vitro; an antitumour activity that has subsequently been confirmed in clinical studies. α-IFN is particularly effective in the treatment of such haematological malignancies as hairy-cell leukaemia, chronic myeloid leukaemia, multiple myeloma, and lymphoma. α-IFN treatment of patients with breast carcinoma increased oestrogen-receptor expression and sensitized breast carcinoma cells to tamoxifen. Intralesional administration of β-IFN was found to be more effective than α-IFN in patients with metastatic skin melanoma. However, most clinical studies indicate that although β-IFN can be safely administered at higher doses, α-IFN is the more effective tumoricidal interferon of the two. Results of clinical trials indicate poor efficacy of IFNs in the case of the more common solid tumours such as lung, colon, breast, and prostate carcinoma. Despite the fact that γ-IFN is a more powerful immunoregulator than α-IFN or β-IFN, this has yet to be reflected in clinical trials, with only a low rate of partial responses in a range of human malignancies (e.g. renal and colon carcinoma, melanoma). Although γ-IFN does not appear to be any more effective than α-IFN, it is possible that their combined effects may prove more beneficial in cancer studies, and this is the subject of current studies. Recent reports have suggested that the immunostimulatory effects of γ-IFN may be partly counteracted by a direct effect of this cytokine on tumour cells, reducing their sensitivity to lysis by LAK cells. This has fuelled speculation that relatively high levels of γ-IFN may exist within the tumour microenvironment to disrupt the host–tumour relationship. However, γ-IFN pretreatment of autologous tumours enhances susceptibility to lysis by IL-2-stimulated TIL, although this cytokine is more effective in combination with TNF-α than as a single agent.

9.11.4   Tumour necrosis factors (TNFs)

The genes for cachectin/TFN-α and lymphotoxin/TNF-β are closely linked to the MHC genes on chromosome 6 and tightly regulated by such factors as endotoxin, antigens, and various cytokines (γ-IFN, GM-CSF, IL-1, etc.). A wide range of cells possess receptors for TNFs, reflecting far-reaching effects of these two cytokines on immunity, inflammation, angiogenesis, viral infection, and bone resorption (reviewed by Balkwill 1989). Both TNFs can be either cytostatic or cytotoxic for human tumour cells. Indeed, local injection (rather than systemic administration) has been effective in reducing tumour size in patients with hepatoma and subcutaneous tumours. TNF-α is also known to directly inhibit the proliferation of myeloid leukaemia cells and modulate the growth of some carcinoma cell types in a dose-dependent manner. Recent data suggest that TNF-α, especially when acting in synergy with γ-IFN, may be involved in both the induction and effector phase of LAK cell and macrophage-mediated cytotoxicity. Whether the membrane-bound form and/or its secreted counterpart mediate the killing mechanism has not been resolved. The molecular basis for susceptibility or resistance to TNFs has also to be determined. It is noteworthy that TNF-α or -β elicit considerable toxicity but have yet to be shown in clinical trials to induce durable complete or partial remissions in cancer patients.

9.11.5   Colony-stimulating factors (CSFs)

This group of factors regulate the proliferation and differentiation of myeloid progenitor cells in bone marrow. As their names depicts, the effects of CSFs are specific for granulocytes and macrophages (Table 9.17). The CSFs are not only able to stimulate the development of these cell types but also their cellular functions as mature cells (phagocytic activity and tumour cell lysis). Various studies have indicated, although often with contradictory results, that CSF regulation is disrupted in human myeloid leukaemia. CSFs can enhance not only the growth of such leukaemic cells, but also their terminal differentiation, and thus suppression. However, more information is required concerning their role in this disease before therapeutic strategies involving CSF manipulation can be established. Since radiotherapy and chemotherapy are usually accompanied by relatively severe myelosuppression, CSFs may have considerable importance in combination with these more conventional forms of therapy to stimulate the recovery of the immune status of the patient.

9.11.6   Transforming growth factors (TGFs)

The biosynthesis, structure, and receptors for both the α and β forms of TGF have been fully described by Burgess (1989) and Hsuan (1989), respectively, and so will not be discussed here. Initially discovered by virtue of their ability to cause reversible phenotypic transformation, the TGFs are now thought to be centrally involved in the regulation of tumour cell growth. Human tumours have elevated levels of mRNA for TGF-α and TGF-β. Whereas both normal and malignant cells express both mRNA and receptors for TGF-β, only non-neoplastic cells are sufficiently responsive to the growth-inhibiting influence of this factor. Neoplastic cells appear to have lost this ability, thereby contributing to their disregulated growth. TGF-β1 and TGF-β2 also inhibit B- and T-cell function, the cytotoxicity and generation of cytokines by LAK cells, and expression of class II MHC antigens. The secretion of these subtypes of TGF-β by tumour cells may, therefore, mediate some of their immunosuppressive effects. Recent evidence suggests that TGF-β may modulate the metastatic potential of malignant cells by controlling the ability to break down and penetrate basement-membrane barriers (Welch et al. 1990). The biologically active form of TGF-α is structurally related to epidermal growth factor (EGF) and, in many instances, acts through the receptor for this agent. Malignant cells readily produce TGF-α which then acts as an autocrine (or indeed paracrine) growth promoter. Many types of human carcinoma and sarcoma cells express elevated levels of mRNA for TGF-α along with EGF receptors. TGF-α is also involved in angiogenesis within malignant tumours, and stimulates vascularization of the tumour mass.

9.11.7   Concluding remarks

Cytokine biology, though still in its infancy, is an exciting and rapidly expanding area of cancer research. We are far from understanding the complexities of the cytokine network sufficiently to describe the local imbalances generated within the tumour. Thus, its exploitation in the immunotherapy of malignancy has proved somewhat elusive. Until this stage is reached, it is at least hoped to optimize the effects of cytokine therapy by careful attention to such factors as dose levels and schedules, and route of infusion (local to the tumour or systemic). Since many cytokines only exert their full biological effects when working in synergy with others, the immunomodulatory and therapeutic effects of various cytokines combinations are currently being evaluated in clinical trials. It is hoped that these may prove considerably more effective than the use of single agents alone.

9.11.8   Bibliography

Arai, K., et al. (1990). Cytokines: coordinators of immune and inflammatory responses. Annual Review of Biochemistry 59, 783–836.

Balkwill, F. R. (1989). Cytokines in cancer therapy. Oxford University Press, Oxford.

Burgess, A. W. (1989). Epidermal growth factor and transforming growth factor α. British Medical Bulletin 45, 401–24.

Dinarello, C. A. (1989). Interleukin-1 and its biologically related cytokines. *Advances in Immunology* **44**, 153–205.

Hellmann, K. (ed.) (1989). International Symposium on IL-2. *Cancer Treatment Reviews* **16** (Suppl. A).

Hirano, T., *et al.* (1989). A multifunctional cytokine (IL-6/BSF-2) and its receptor. *International Archives of Allergy and Applied Immunology* **88**, 29–35.

Hsuan, J. J. (1989). Transforming growth factor β. *British Medical Bulletin* **45**, 425–37.

Jabaari, B. Al., Ladyman, H. M., Larche, M., Sivolapenko, G. B., Epenetos, A. A., and Ritter, M. A. (1989). Elevated expression of the interleukin-4 receptor in carcinoma: a target for immunotherapy? *British Journal of Cancer* **59**, 910–15.

Kawakami, Y., Custer, M. C., Rosenberg, S. A., and Lotz, M. T. (1989). IL-4 regulates IL-2 induction of lymphocyte-activated killer activity from human lymphocytes. *Journal of Immunology* **142**, 3452–61.

Limb, G. A., *et al.* (1989). Release of cytokines during generation of lymphokine-activated killer (LAK) cells by IL-2. *Immunology* **68**, 514–19.

Mizel, S. B. (1989). The interleukins. *FASEB Journal* **3**, 2379–88.

Nakata, K., Kashimoto, S., Yoshida, H., Oku, T., and Nakamura, S. (1988). Augmented antitumour effect of recombinant human interleukin-1α by indomethacin. *Cancer Research* **48**, 584–8.

Paul, W. E. and Ohara, J. (1987). B cell stimulatory factor 1/interleukin-4. *Annual Review of Immunology* **5**, 429–78.

Sinkovics, J. G. (1988). Oncogenes and growth factors. *CRC Critical Reviews in Immunology* **8**, 217–98.

Welch, D. R., Fabra, A., and Nakejima, M. (1990). Transforming growth factor β stimulates mammary adenocarcinoma cell invasion and metastatic potential. *Proceedings of the National Academy of Sciences (USA)* **87**, 7678–82.

Widmer, M. B., Acres, R. B., Sassenfeld, H. M., and Grabstein, K. H. (1987). Regulation of cytolytic cell populations from human peripheral blood by B cell stimulatory factor 1 (IL-4). *Journal of Experimental Medicine* **166**, 1447–55.

9.12 Cachexia

K. C. Calman

9.12.1 Introduction

Cachexia provides an important example of a tumour–host interaction, having pathological, endocrine, metabolic, and immunological components. Cachexia is often, though not always, associated with anorexia.

The term cachexia is derived from the Greek 'kakos' (bad) and 'hexis' (condition). It is common feature of malignancy; its incidence varies with tumour type and stage, but ranges between 8 and 73 per cent of patients. It is most common in lung cancer and gastrointestinal malignancy. In terms of symptoms, it is commoner than pain in patients with advanced disease.

The syndrome of cachexia is characterized by the features of anorexia and early satiety, weight loss and marked muscle weakness, anaemia of a non-specific type, and altered host metabolism. It is not directly correlated with food intake, size, or site of the primary tumour, or the histological type. It can occur with a very small primary tumour, and cachexia can be the presenting feature of the disease. It is not necessary for the primary tumour to be large for the syndrome to occur.

The weight loss associated with the cachexia, although it is only one part of the syndrome, does have considerable prognostic value. This is particularly true of small tumours. Those patients who have lost weight have both a poorer prognosis and response to chemotherapy. The assessment of weight loss is, therefore, of clinical value as it can be readily measured by non-invasive techniques.

While there are a number of features in common, there are important differences between cachexia and starvation, and the metabolic problems associated with sepsis and trauma. In acute starvation there is rapid breakdown of protein from lean body mass, with mobilization of amino acids. After the initial loss, the body then conserves protein and energy. In sepsis and trauma, the magnitude of this response is greater and it is normally associated with a degree of hypercatabolism. The patient with cancer cachexia shows features of both, but the picture is more like sepsis and trauma. An important feature is that in starvation appropriate nutritional support reverses the problem, whereas in cancer cachexia this is not normally achieved.

9.12.2 Animal models

Numerous animal tumour models have been used in the investigation of cachexia, the most common being in mice or rats. All of them have drawbacks, though they have provided useful data in the pathogenesis of the syndrome. The most commonly used model is the Walker 256 carcinosarcoma. There are many different strains of this tumour line and it can be difficult to compare data from one laboratory with another. Animal models have been used to study aspects of cachexia such as tumour uptake of nutrients, use of experimental diets, production of tumour-specific products, and endocrine factors associated with the syndrome. Parabiotic experiments and the injection of tumour products into normal animals have been part of this. Such models have raised a number of questions, but in the complex pathogenesis of cachexia it is necessary to test these in humans.

9.12.3 Clinical and laboratory features of cachexia

In addition to the weight loss already noted, a number of other findings are commonly present in patients with cachexia. Because of the complexity of the syndrome and its multifactorial origin, some of these features may also be present in other diseases. Anthropometric tests reveal loss of subcutaneous fat and lean body mass. This can be confirmed in a variety of laboratory tests, including whole-body neutron activation analysis, which shows loss of nitrogen, calcium, potassium, and fat. The clinical signs and laboratory data show evidence of multiple vitamin deficiencies. Trace metal deficiencies are common, as is a low serum albumin value. Raised acute phase reactants are a well-recognized feature. Estimation of protein turnover shows that in some patients there is a raised catabolic rate, in others a decreased synthesis rate, and in some a mixture of both. A range of measures to estimate the capacity to respond immunologically have shown that patients with cachexia frequently have abnormal responses to skin testing, and *in vitro* estimations of immunological reactivity and capacity to synthesize antibodies are diminished. In some instances the immunological reactivity is used as a measure of cachexia, though this is not uniformly employed.

A number of other symptoms can exacerbate the cachexia, including pain, breathlessness, and the psychological response of the patient. These aspects are important in management.

The clinical features described above show evidence of the diverse nature of the problem and its possible pathogenesis. It is now generally recognized that a number of factors are involved in its aetiology.

9.12.4   The pathogenesis of cachexia

In the following section the significance of each factor will depend on the individual patient. It is likely, however, that more than one factor operates in each patient.

Deficient food intake

This can be related to a malignant lesion of the head and neck, or to an obstructive lesion further down in the gastrointestinal tract. Pain, in almost any part of the body, can be associated with a decreased food intake. Taste abnormalities are common in patients with cancer. Normally attractive food tastes bitter, and the texture appears altered. The extent of the abnormality can be correlated with the stage of the disease. The mechanism is unknown, though there is a suggestion that it may be related to trace metal abnormalities, notably zinc.

Anorexia

This is a very common feature, and a particularly difficult symptom to manage. Anorexia may be defined as that set of signals which guide the selection and consumption of foods. Anorexia occurs, therefore, when these signals are absent or abnormal. Appetite is thought to be regulated by two systems. The long-term feedback system controls body weight over a long period despite changes in food intake. The short-term system regulates the food consumption from meal to meal. The hypothalamus seems to be the focus for the long-term feedback system, while the short-term system is based on numerous factors, including blood glucose levels, free fatty acids, or amino acid concentrations, altered neuronal activity, distension of the gastrointestinal tract, and the activity of a variety of hormones such as insulin, glucagon, bombesin, and cholecystokinin. Many cancer patients have abnormalities in the above and these may contribute to the anorexia. The metabolism of serotonin in the brain may also be altered in patients with anorexia. This may influence neurotransmitter concentrations in the hypothal-

amus and so alter the appetite centre. As with cachexia, it is likely that several mechanisms are involved.

Excessive loss of body protein

This is unlikely to be the sole cause of cachexia, but may well contribute. Ulceration, haemorrhage, diarrhoea, and repeated vomiting would be examples of this. Large volumes of ascites or pleural fluid may also be relevant.

Malabsorption

This is an interesting finding in patients with advanced malignant disease. It has been well recognized and its incidence appears to vary with tumour type. There is flattening of the villi, and biochemical tests of malabsorption are abnormal (see Chapter 16). The mechanism of these changes is not clear.

Alteration in metabolic rate

An early finding in the study of cachexia was the observation that patients with cachexia had an increased basal metabolic rate. This contrasts with starvation in which the metabolic rate is depressed. More recent work, using calorimetry, suggests that the picture is more complicated than the earlier work would suggest. Some patients do have an increased energy expenditure, but about 30 per cent of patients have a normal rate of expenditure, and 30 per cent are hypometabolic. It will clearly depend on the exact population studied. However, even a 'normal' rate of energy expenditure in a semi-starving patient would be abnormal.

The mechanisms by which the energy expenditure is increased or inappropriate are unknown. It has been suggested, however, that energy-dependent cycles, such as protein metabolism or the glucose lactate cycle (Cori cycle) are increased. As will be discussed later, the tumour may be a source of increased energy requirements which affect the metabolic rate of the host.

Altered host metabolism

A number of the metabolic abnormalities in cachetic patients have already been noted. The metabolism of carbohydrates is particularly interesting as, in contrast to starvation, the rate of gluconeogenesis from alanine, lactate, and glycerol are increased. In addition, the early observation that the rate of glucose metabolism via glycolysis in tumours is increased has been confirmed recently. This high glucose demand may be important in the aetiology of cachexia, in that fat and protein are used to provide substrates for gluconeogenesis. Glycolysis is an inefficient way of metabolizing glucose, and there may be energy loss. However, as cachexia can occur with a very small tumour, this cannot be the whole explanation.

Protein metabolism also differs from that in uncomplicated starvation. There is known to be a decreased rate of protein synthesis and an increased rate of protein degradation in skeletal muscle, resulting in a reduction in lean body mass. The reduced protein synthesis in muscle is consistent with that in starvation. However, in several tumour types liver protein synthesis may increase. This increase in the synthesis of protein in liver and in the tumour, together with a decreased synthesis in muscle protein, results in an overall increase in whole body protein synthesis and turnover. This is in contrast to the effects in starvation.

Fat, a major energy reserve, is mobilized in the cachectic patient to provide substrates for gluconeogenesis. In starved patients this effect is mediated via insulin, but not so in cachexia. Such patients often show insulin resistance.

As described before, there are abnormalities in trace metal and vitamin metabolism in this group of patients. Numerous hormonal changes have been noted.

The nitrogen trap

Based mainly on animal work, it was suggested that a major reason for cachexia was the uptake of proteins and amino acids by the tumour. Limb perfusion studies in patients with sarcoma have confirmed the uptake of such metabolites by the tumour. There is little doubt that this mechanism occurs, but it is unlikely to be the only component of cachexia.

Tumour products

For almost every abnormality noted above it has been postulated that a 'tumour product' is implicated. In animal models such products have been reported to have an effect on almost all metabolic processes. They were originally called toxohormones and, although they were chemically uncharacterized, they were isolated and purified. In humans it was difficult to confirm that such compounds existed.

In recent years, however, the situation has changed considerably. With more sophisticated isolation and measurement techniques, a range of compounds has been identified, best known perhaps as tumour-associated products, which may be important in cachexia. These include bombesin, tumour necrosis factor, cachectin, and interleukin-1. These are host products produced by the tumour or in response to injury or infection. They do seem to enhance fat mobilization, and amino acid release in skeletal muscle. These short-term metabolic mediators may well provide a key to the mechanism of cancer cachexia.

Treatment associated

All forms of cancer treatment, surgery, radiotherapy, chemotherapy, and hormone therapy can have an effect on host metabolism. Iatrogenic malnutrition is perhaps more common than realized, and should be included as a contributory factor in any account of cachexia.

9.12.5 The management of cachexia and anorexia

While the management of these problems are not strictly relevant to this text, three points can be made. The first is that a greater understanding of the pathogenesis is required before a rational method of treatment can be instituted; there are enormous gaps in our knowledge. Secondly, almost all attempts to reverse cachexia by a variety of methods or nutritional support have failed. Cachexia is different from simple starvation. Finally, the most successful way of reversing the cachexia is to remove the tumour. Where this can be done the patient will put on weight and become metabolically normal.

9.12.6 Associated problems

The patient with advanced cancer, in addition to developing cachexia, may also develop a range of other clinical problems, associated with the disease. While these will be covered in detail elsewhere, they are collected here for completeness.

Neurological syndromes are rare, but of considerable interest (Section 9.9). The neuromuscular problems such as dermatomyositis and the progressive muscle weakness of the myasthetic syndrome (Lambert–Eaton syndrome) can be the presenting feature of the illness and can be very troublesome to the patient.

Dermatological syndromes such as acanthosis nigricans and acquired icthyosis (Chapter 28) can indicate the presence of an internal malignancy and can antedate the clinical presentation of the tumour by some years. A variety of erythematous conditions occur, including erythroderma, telangiectasis, and thrombophlebitis. Perioral pigmentation occurs in the Peutz–Jeghers syndrome.

Haematological effects (Chapter 23), particularly anaemia, are common. While this may be due to marrow infiltration, fibrosis, blood loss treatment, or malabsorption, non-specific anaemia of a hypochromic microcytic type is also frequently present. Pure red cell aplasia may be associated with thymic tumours.

9.12.7 Further reading

Balkwill, F., *et al.* (1987). Evidence for tumour necrosis factor/cachectia production in cancer. *Lancet* **ii**, 1229–31.

Brennan, M. F. (1977). Uncomplicated starvation versus cancer cachexia. *Cancer Research* **37**, 2359–64.

Calman, K. C. and Fearon, K. C. H. (1986). Nutritional support for the cancer patient. *Clinics in Oncology* **5**.

Dinarello, C. A. (1985). An update on human interleukin I: from molecular biology to clinical relevance. *Journal of Clinical Immunology* **5**, 287–97.

Jeevanandam, M., Horowitz, G. D., Lowry, S. F., and Brennan, M. F. (1984). Cancer cachexia and protein metabolism. *Lancet* **i**, 1423–6.

Lundholm, K., Edstrom, S., Karlberg, I., Ekman, L., and Schersten, T. (1982). Glucose turnover, gluconeogenesis from glycerol and estimation of net glucose cycling in cancer patients. *Cancer* **50**, 1142–50.

Strain, A. J. (1979). Cancer cachexia in man: a review. *Investigative Cell Pathology* **2**, 181–93.

10

Environmental pathology

10 Environmental pathology

10.1 Dust diseases

A. R. Gibbs and J. C. Wagner

10.1.1 Introduction

The reaction of the lung to the inhalation of particulate materials is referred to as pneumoconiosis. This can be separated into two groups:

1. that caused by the inhalation of minerals, which may take the form of dusts, fumes, or mists; and

2. that caused by the inhalation of vegetable and animal dusts.

The lung's reaction to inhaled particulates ranges from no reaction to severe life-threatening problems and is dependent on several factors (Tables 10.1 and 10.2). In this section we shall discuss the general principles of how the lung reacts to different dusts and give specific examples.

10.1.2 Factors influencing the reaction of the lung to particulate minerals

Physical properties

The size, density, shape, and solubility of the particulates are important. The larger particles, i.e. those that have a diameter greater than 5 μm, are filtered out in the respiratory tract proximal to the terminal bronchiole. Particles with a diameter between 0.5 and 5 μm can reach the respiratory portion of the lung and are referred to as the respirable portion. However, it

Table 10.1 Factors determining reaction to inhaled dust

Physical
Chemical
Concentration
Duration
Other minerals
Host

Table 10.2 Inhaled agents and type of pulmonary reaction

Agent inhaled	Type of reaction
Tin	Accumulation of non-fibrogenic dust
Coal	Mild centrilobular fibrosis
Silica	Severe centrilobular fibrosis
Asbestos, talc, kaolin	Diffuse interstitial fibrosis
Cadmium, beryllium	Diffuse alveolar damage
Isocyanates	Asthma
Mouldy hay	Extrinsic allergic alveolitis
Beryllium	Granulomatous disease
Cadmium	Emphysema
Tuberculosis in silicosis	Infection and fibrosis
Asbestos	Pleural fibrosis
Asbestos, arsenic, nickel	Lung cancer
Asbestos	Mesothelioma

should be realized that not all the respirable particles reach the lung parenchyma; many are deposited in the nose and conducting airways. In the case of fibres, i.e. particles with a length:diameter ratio of greater than 3, it appears that those with a length greater than 8 μm and a diameter less than 0.25 μm have the potential to cause lung fibrosis, while those with a length greater than 8 μm and a diameter less than 0.5 μm have the potential to cause mesothelioma (Stanton *et al.* 1972). It is unclear whether this is because of shape or increased surface area. Solubility is an important determinant: insoluble agents, such as silica, cause a local reaction whereas relatively soluble agents, such as beryllium, can cause systemic as well as local effects.

Chemical properties

According to the site of deposition and the pH of the particle, interference with ciliary function, particle clearance, and cellular metabolism may occur. Some agents are more fibrogenic than others, e.g. tin is inert and almost non-fibrogenic whereas silica is cytotoxic and very fibrogenic. Some agents may in themselves possess, or be contaminated by materials possessing, antigenic properties and cause immunological lung disease. An example of this is farmer's lung, which is caused by fungal spores contaminating mouldy hay (see Section 13.4).

Concentration and duration of exposure

With certain agents the responses of the lung may vary according to the severity and duration of exposure. For example, acute exposures to high concentrations of beryllium produce severe diffuse alveolar damage, which can result in death in the acute phase (see section 13.4) whereas chronic exposure to low concentrations produces a disease similar to sarcoidosis.

Presence of other materials

Pure exposures to one particular agent are rare in the human situation; almost all are complex exposures to more than one material. The majority of animal experiments have been concerned with exposures to pure materials and it is only comparatively recently that research has begun to address the complex interactions of materials. Much knowledge still needs to be acquired in the understanding of these interactions. For example, there is good evidence that the fibrogenic effect of free silica can be modified by the presence of other materials such as carbon, kaolin, and mica.

Host factors

These include genetic, acquired, and environmental factors. In a small number of individuals genetic abnormalities may result in impairment of ciliary or immunological function. Some individuals clear particles relatively rapidly from the conducting airways whereas others do it relatively slowly; this pattern of clearance appears to be genetically determined and may influence the development of disease. Occupational asthma is more likely to develop in persons with an allergic diathesis (see Chapter 4). The pneumoconiosis observed in coal workers may be modified in those with a rheumatoid diathesis (Caplan's syndrome).

In the respiratory portion of the lung, the main defence against foreign materials is the macrophage system. Macrophages endeavour to phagocytose particulate material and digest it but some persists and is transported by the macrophages to the terminal bronchioles where it may be removed either by the mucociliary apparatus or the lymphatic system. Air pollutants, cigarette smoking, drugs, temperature, and humidity may interfere with mucociliary and/or macrophage function.

10.1.3   Silica

Lung fibrosis caused by the inhalation of free silica (silicosis) is known to have occurred for centuries; silicotic nodules having been described in Egyptian mummies. Quartz is the commonest form of free silica and is present in almost all types of igneous, sedimentary, and metamorphic rocks. It can be appreciated that the potential for exposure to quartz exists in a very wide range of industries, including mining and quarrying of a variety of materials, stonecutting, abrasive manufacture, foundry work, and ceramics. Despite strict controls, silicosis is still observed in developed countries, as well as in underdeveloped countries where controls are few or non-existent.

Quartz is intensely fibrogenic. When quartz particles (below 5 μm in diameter) reach the lung parenchyma they become engulfed by macrophages and polymorph neutrophils. They are then incorporated into lysosomes within the cell, which then rupture, with consequent death of the cell. This cytotoxic property is associated with the crystallinity and surface properties of the silica particles. During the process, a variety of chemoattractants and fibrogenic factors are released, with the result that more macrophages and polymorph neutrophils are attracted to the site. The quartz particles are then phagocytosed again and the cycle repeated. After a short time macrophages become the dominant cell and fibrosis occurs, with the collagen becoming arranged into a concentric layer to become the fully developed classical whorled silicotic nodule (Fig. 10.1). These nodules are characteristic of silicosis and are different from any other pneumoconiosis. Usually disease progresses gradually with more and more nodules developing in the lungs; these nodules, which measure a few millimetres on average, may become fused together (conglomerate) to form large lesions, which may measure several centimetres in diameter. Clinical manifestations are not usually observed until 20 years of exposure have occurred and are then associated with large lesions (progressive massive fibrosis, see Chapter 13).

In rare situations exposure to high concentrations of very fine particulate silica may occur, e.g. in sandblasting, when pulmonary disability may become apparent within three or four years. In these cases the pathological reaction is quite different from classical silicosis; nodules are absent or inconspicuous and the picture is that of filling of the alveoli with amorphous, eosinophilic, granular fluid, which is rich in lipid. This is termed acute silicoproteinosis. It is due to direct damage to type 2 pneumocytes, which release phospholipid (surfactant) from the cells into the alveolar spaces.

Another interesting feature of silica exposure is that it increases the patient's susceptibility to mycobacterial infection.

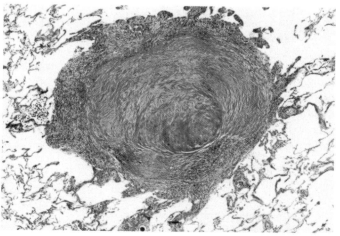

Fig. 10.1   A silicotic nodule, showing circumferentially arranged collagen that is partly hyalinized and encompassed by dust-laden macrophages.

Prior to antibiotic therapy tuberculosis was a common cause of death amongst silicotics. This synergism is unexplained.

10.1.4 Coal

It is comparatively recently that the pulmonary disease that develops in coal workers has been recognized as being pathologically different from silicosis. The majority of coal workers are exposed to dust which contains a low percentage of silica (less than 5 per cent). Coal dust, unlike silica, has relatively low fibrogenic potential. When coal dust particles reach the lung parenchyma they can be digested by macrophages without causing death of the cell. The characteristic lesion of coal workers is therefore a black macule which consists of a dense sleeve of coal-laden macrophages admixed with a small amount of collagen fibres situated around the respiratory bronchiole (Fig. 10.2). The respiratory bronchiole associated with this is usually dilated—so-called focal emphysema (Chapter 13). When the lungs show only these macules, each of which averages 2–4 mm in diameter, the disease is referred to as simple pneumoconiosis, but when lesions above 1 cm in diameter are present it is referred to as complicated pneumoconiosis or progressive massive fibrosis. Pulmonary disability usually occurs in association with complicated pneumoconiosis. Simple pneumoconiosis does not usually cause disability. The precise mechanisms involved in the development of complicated pneumoconiosis are not understood, but factors implicated include heavy dust exposures, the type of coal to which exposure has occurred, mycobacterial infection, and immunological mechanisms (see Chapter 13).

10.1.5 Asbestos

Asbestos is the generic term given to a number of naturally occurring fibrous inorganic silicates. This group is subdivided into serpentine and amphibole groups according to the physical characteristics determined by electron microscopy (Table 10.3). This is not simply of academic interest but important because the shape and dimensions of the fibres are a good predictor of disease potential. Long, thin, straight fibres are the most dangerous, which is why crocidolite produces more neoplasms than amosite. Chrysotile, because of its shape, has a different aerodynamic behaviour and in its pure form causes little or no significant disease (Fig. 10.3). Commercially, chrysotile is the most frequently used type of asbestos but, unfortunately, it is often contaminated by the more dangerous amphibole fibres. The interval between the presentation of disease and the exposure to asbestos can be as long as several decades, which is why it is often overlooked.

Table 10.3 Classification of asbestos minerals

Group	Physical configuration (EM)	Important minerals
Serpentine	Wavy and coiled	Chrysotile (white)
Amphibole	Long and straight	Amosite (brown) and crocidolite (blue)

Asbestos is widely used in industry and large numbers of people have been exposed. Exposure is not always direct, as in the asbestos cement, asbestos textile, asbestos mining, shipyard, and insulation industries, but may occur indirectly when the subject is in the vicinity of other workers directly handling asbestos. Other members of the household may be exposed as a result of handling the clothes of an asbestos worker and some of these have developed asbestos-related diseases. Inhalation of asbestos can result in a variety of pathological reactions (Table 10.4).

Pleural plaques are pearly white areas of scarring located on the parietal pleura. They are not pre-malignant and serve merely as a marker of asbestos exposure. They appear to be related to amphibole exposure but the fibres have broader dimensions than those usually associated with mesothelioma.

Asbestosis is the term given to pulmonary interstitial fibrosis caused by inhalation of asbestos. The pathological clue that the pulmonary fibrosis is due to asbestos is the presence on light microscopy of asbestos bodies in the vicinity of the fibrosis (Fig. 10.4). Asbestos bodies consist of a transparent, thin, fibrous

Table 10.4 Pathological reactions to asbestos exposure

Pleura	Effusion
	Plaques
	Diffuse fibrosis
	Mesothelioma
Lung	Diffuse interstitial fibrosis
	Carcinoma

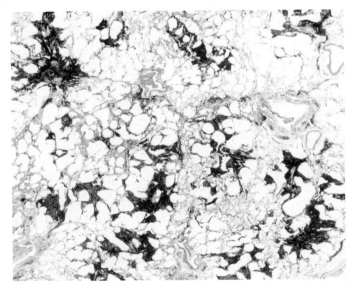

Fig. 10.2 Stellate black coal-dust macules with adjacent dilated respiratory bronchioles and alveoli.

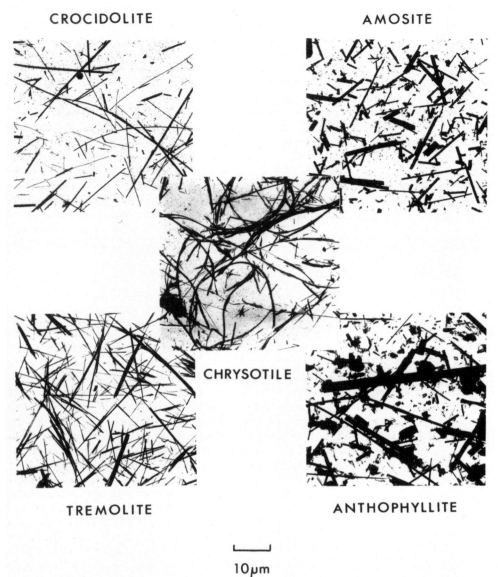

CROCIDOLITE

AMOSITE

CHRYSOTILE

TREMOLITE

ANTHOPHYLLITE

10μm

Fig. 10.3 Electron microscopic appearances of the various types of asbestos minerals. Chrysotile has a curly shape whereas the amphiboles (crocidolite, amosite, tremolite, and anthophyllite) are straight. Crocidolite is the thinnest and anthophyllite the thickest. (Courtesy of Mr Griffiths.)

core partly covered by golden-brown beaded haemosiderin and glycoprotein. In its severe form asbestosis can cause impairment of pulmonary function and finally respiratory failure and death of the patient. Heavy exposures to asbestos are needed to produce severe asbestosis so that it is rarely seen in Britain nowadays.

Lung cancer may occur in association with asbestosis and the risk rises with the severity of exposure. The effects of smoking and asbestos exposure on the incidence of lung cancer are multiplicative, of the order of 20–100 times. There is usually a latent interval of at least 20 years between exposure and pre-

sentation of lung cancer. All major histological types occur but adenocarcinoma is the most frequent (see also Section 9.7).

Mesotheliomas of both pleura and peritoneum may result from asbestos exposure. There is a latent interval of several decades between exposure to asbestos and the development of mesothelioma and the exposure may have been relatively slight. This explains why the incidence of mesotheliomas is still rising despite the public health measures brought in during the past few decades. Again, mesotheliomas appear to be related to amphibole exposure, particularly crocidolite. There is little evidence to support an association with chrysotile exposure (see also Section 9.7).

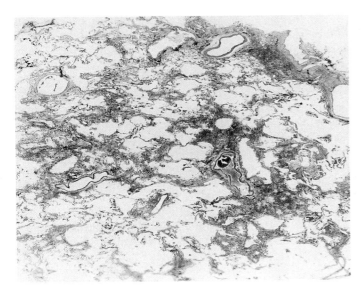

Fig. 10.4 Fibrotic, thickened alveolar septa that are linking up and caused by asbestos.

10.1.6 Further reading

General

Gibbs, A. R. and Seal, R. M. E. (1982). Atlas of pulmonary pathology. *Current histopathology*, Vol. 3, pp. 83–102. MTP Press, Lancaster.

Occupational lung disease

Gibbs, A. R. (1987). Industrial lung disease. In *Recent advances in histopathology*, Vol. 13 (ed. P. P. Anthony and R. N. M. Macsween). Churchill Livingstone, Edinburgh.

Morgan, W. K. C. and Seaton, A. (1984). *Occupational lung diseases* (2nd edn). W. B. Saunders, Philadelphia.

Stanton, M. F. and Wrench, C. J. (1972). Mechanism of mesothelioma induction with asbestos and fibrous glass. *Journal of the National Cancer Institute* **48**, 797.

Wagner, J. C. and Elmes, P. C. (1981). The mineral fibre problem. In *Recent advances in occupational health*, Vol. 1 (ed. J. C. McDonald). Churchill Livingstone, Edinburgh.

10.2 Environmental pollution

A. E. M. McLean and S. P. Wolff

Patterns of disease vary widely between social groups, and between populations living in different environments. We need to know whether the chemical composition of the general environment (e.g. food, air, soil, and water) is a determining factor in disease. We also need to know if particular contaminants will cause harm to some individuals.

There are numerous examples of a clear-cut relation between environmental contamination and disease. Catastrophic release of volcanic gases from deep lakes (mainly hot carbon dioxide) recently caused over 1000 deaths in one event in Africa. Inhalation of asbestos-like fibrous minerals from surface rocks caused lung disease among villagers in Turkey. Escape of industrial chemicals at Bhopal caused the sudden death of more than 2000 persons from asphyxiation due to pulmonary damage from the reactive, volatile methyl isocyanate. In contrast, the slow release of mercury into enclosed waters at Minamata in Japan led to the gradual formation of fat-soluble methyl mercury by sea-bed micro-organisms. This accumulated in fish and so was passed on to the human fish-eating population, and even their domestic cats. Lethal neurotoxic and embryo-toxic effects went on for years, even after the cause of the disease was unearthed, before the plastics factory that was the mercury source was stopped from contaminating the bay (Hunter 1975; Wohl 1983).

10.2.1 Natural and synthetic molecules

These spectacular localized events are noticed because high concentrations of contaminants lead to doses that are toxic to large numbers of the population. This raises several questions: do the lower doses found in the general environment have lesser degrees of adverse effects; or cause major effects in a small proportion of the exposed population; or is there no adverse effect at all because a threshold dose is not reached? At the same time we must consider whether molecules synthesized in the chemical factories are different in principle, and should be regulated differently, from the molecules made by plants or micro-organisms. For instance, there is considerable agitation about food additives such as the antioxidant butylated hydroxytoluene (BHT), which protects fats from rancidity due to oxidative attack, because BHT in large doses causes cell injury and carcinogenic effects in rats. However, BHT may well also be a factor in the decline in gastric carcinoma in Western countries over the past 50 years. In contrast, there is little public concern over the indole-glucosynolates found in brassicas (the mustard and cabbage family) where they probably form part of the evolutionary defence against insect attack and give a sharpness of taste. These compounds have marked physiological effects in that eating cabbage causes major increases in P_{450} drug metabolizing enzyme activity by inducing synthesis in the small and large intestine and liver. In animal experiments enzyme inducers can either enhance or decrease the carcinogenic effects of exposure to mutagenic chemicals. Clearly, we need assurance that new chemicals used as drugs or pesticides do not have unexpected and unacceptable toxic effects at the doses to which patients or spraymen are exposed; this is the major objective of toxicity assessment of new chemicals. However, there are unsettled problems of how to deal with environmental exposure to low levels of molecules that are found to have biological effects when tested at vastly higher dosages. This is particularly true for molecules that have irreversible effects such as teratogenesis or carcinogenesis. For these 'low-level' effects the 'natural' and the 'man-made' molecules pose exactly similar problems. The key questions can be listed as follows: Is there a threshold of effect? Are the risks quantifiable? Can one infer human risk from results of animal experiments? Is the risk worth the proposed benefit? We have definitive answers to none of these questions.

10.2.2   Pollution of the general environment

By the early nineteenth century the industrial activities of man reached a scale which permitted massive pollution of the environment. Smoke from coal fires and the emission of hydrochloric acid from alkali works were able to blight large cities, great tracts of countryside, rivers, and water supplies.

The emission of smoke and hydrochloric acid was gradually controlled by the efforts of government agencies such as the Alkali Inspectorate (the precursor of the Factory Inspectorate and the Health and Safety Executive). The London smog of 1952 in which many old people, and people already suffering from heart and lung disease, were rapidly killed off by high concentrations of sulphur dioxide mixed with particles of soot and oxides of nitrogen was a major event. It helped to push through further Clean Air Acts in Britain that eventually led to a marked reduction in the amount of smoke pollution of the air in cities (Royal Commission on Environmental Pollution 1976).

The major, self-evident contaminations of the air we breathe have been controlled somewhat in most of the developed parts of the world. They remain a major problem as countries undergo a process of industrialization.

Agro-chemicals

At the same time as heavy industry grew up so agriculture developed the new techniques whereby a few workers in the fields could produce food for many in the factories and towns. New varieties of crop plants and new fertilizers (especially phosphate and potassium mined from distant rock formations) and nitrogen from the fixation of atmospheric nitrogen gave heavier yields; new farm machinery enabled one man to cultivate large areas. These allowed massive increases in yields per acre and even more per man hour.

The next great phase of increase in agricultural productivity from the 1940s onwards lay in the prevention of crop and harvest spoilage by use of fungicides and insecticides, and in the great reduction in labour required for cultivation by use of herbicides. In addition, rodenticides and other substances were designed and used extensively to kill particular organisms that prevented the smooth flow of agricultural productivity.

Pesticides

The use of arsenical and copper sulphate mixtures to inhibit the growth of fungi, especially the mildew on grape vines, and the use of poison bait, such as strychnine or arsenic, to kill off rats and mice goes back more than 100 years. Crude chemical means, such as sulphuric acid spray, were used to kill the tops of potato plants.

From the late 1930s onwards a great wave of new chemicals of increasing potency and specificity came into use in agriculture. Dinitro-*ortho*-cresol (DNOC) is a potent uncoupler of oxidative phosphorylation (like dinitrophenol) and was used as an insecticide and selective herbicidal spray in the 1940s. The bright yellow colour of the solution was not enough warning to prevent heavy contamination of the skin, and a number of fatal poisonings from ordinary working practice resulted. Arsenical sprays were known to have a high acute toxicity in overdose, but what became clear after prolonged use was that, even at the lower levels of contamination found during normal use, workers with arsenical sprays developed an excess of skin cancers (there is still no adequate animal model for this effect). In the UK a scheme of testing and control of pesticides was agreed by the Ministry of Agriculture, the agrochemical manufacturers, and wholesalers (Pesticide Safety Precaution Scheme, PSPS). This successfully controlled the use of pesticides for 30 years and was replaced by a statutory government scheme in 1986 (Hunter 1975; Royal Commission on Environmental Pollution 1979; Ministry of Agriculture, Fisheries and Food (MAFF) 1988). The manufacturers have to test new pesticides for efficacy, measure various kinds of toxicity (e.g. acute, carcinogenic, reproductive, etc.), and submit the proposal for use on particular crops at particular concentrations and by defined modes of application. The Advisory Committee on Pesticides then suggests appropriate licensing for sale.

The DDT events

In the 1940s DDT was a tremendous advance in pesticide design. Insects are highly susceptible to the neurotoxic effect and readily absorb DDT from surface contact. In contrast, mammals, including man, are relatively insensitive to the neurotoxic effects, and hardly absorb it at all from the skin. DDT holds open the sodium channels of nerve cell membranes, and as a result a train of multiple action potentials and convulsions are set off by a stimulus that would normally produce a single spike. Because its skin absorption is low, 50 per cent DDT powder could be widely used, even shaken down the trousers, to eliminate lice and fleas. DDT is credited with stopping the epidemic of typhus that was threatening Naples at the end of the Second World War in 1944, and with the enormous decrease in malaria in many parts of the world, following spraying of houses and mosquito-infested ponds. DDT has such low cutaneous toxicity to man that spraymen could mix their DDT/detergent mixture with water by stirring it with their hands and come to no ill effects, even when they contaminated their food with their hands. This was a bad lesson to learn as more advanced and more toxic materials came into use, but it means that we have a generation of spraymen who used DDT and were heavily exposed. At follow up, so far, no adverse effects due to occupational or accidental exposure to DDT have been found in people. Successful suicides took place from drinking kerosene in which DDT had been dissolved, but it was the kerosene not the DDT which proved fatal, producing lung lesions without any signs of the neurotoxic effects of DDT. A couple of instances of suicide with DDT powder are recorded in persons strong-minded enough to eat about 200 g of the material. A famous Chinese family in Taiwan is recorded as having used 50 per cent DDT powder instead of flour in making meatballs. One child had minor convulsions and others noted pre-epileptic symptoms, mainly twitching in the thumbs. There were no continuing adverse effects from an ingestion of several grams of DDT.

The low mammalian toxicity of DDT led to widespread, indiscriminate use on many crops, to kill caterpillars, aphids, and other insects. It was used in dusting livestock, including pigeons, and it was among the hawks who preyed on racing pigeons that the first long-term adverse effect on wildlife was noticed. There was a drastic drop in the hawk population, which coincided with the introduction of DDT. There was failure to breed and the eggs that were laid had thin shells that broke in the nest. Investigation of hawks showed that DDT accumulated in the tissues presumably because each hawk had eaten many pigeons; and, similarly, herons had eaten many fish, which in turn had accumulated DDT from waters contaminated either by anti-mosquito sprays or water runoff from fields. Experimental studies showed similar lesions in laboratory birds treated with DDT. The dilemma posed was that here was an adverse effect not predicted by experimental studies on other species, with a profound effect on reproduction, and a threat to the existence of a whole species of aesthetically valuable wildlife. On the other hand, DDT was a cheap and effective way of pest control. For developed countries there was, in the long run, no question about the choice. It was not acceptable to wipe out the hawks for a very minor reduction in the cost of pest control, especially as DDT was out of patent and other insecticides became available. However, there was a long and bitter battle between those who pointed out that the widespread use of DDT was affecting the environment and becoming less effective as resistant insects were selected and the pesticide industry and those involved in its regulation, who first doubted the reality of the adverse effects and later on suggested that the effects were minor and tolerable. In the course of the bitter arguments, best exemplified by Rachael Carson's book *Silent spring*, it was suggested that DDT would cause cancer in people, would block photosynthesis, would lead to the death of waters and oceans, and was an enormous threat to the health of the people. The other side accused Rachael Carson of being unscientific and inaccurate in her statements (Royal Society 1979; Moriarty 1988).

The real dilemma seemed to be that it was impossible to move the regulatory authorities and the agrochemical companies without a massive shift of public opinion to say that DDT should no longer be used. This massive shift in public opinion could only be achieved by wild exaggerations of the dangers posed to people. A rational and accurate set of statements explaining that it was wrong to wipe out a beautiful and valued set of species of birds of prey for very minor economic gain, and that widespread contaminants pose unpredictable levels of risk seemed insufficient. The arguments which took place over DDT continue in their varied forms over many other substances, such as the polychlorinated biphenyls (PCB) and food colourings, to this day.

10.2.3 Low-level contamination by carcinogens

For DDT and similar organochlorine compounds such as aldrin and dieldrin questions arise over the liver cancers produced in rodents by prolonged treatment at very high dosage (Moriarty 1988). Lifelong feeding of DDT at around 100 mg/kg diet [i.e. 100 parts per million (p.p.m.) in the diet] produces tumours. DDT and other pesticides are normally present in amounts far less than 1 p.p.m. in food (MAFF 1982). Epidemiological studies have never shown any increase in liver cancer or adequate evidence for any carcinogenic effect in workers exposed to these organochlorine insecticides. The mechanisms by which these compounds produce an increase in liver tumours, benign and malignant, in rodents seems to be related to their ability to induce massive synthesis of microsomal P_{450}-linked enzymes and to cause a great increase in liver size. All compounds having these properties, including phenobarbitone, polychlorinated biphenyls, and many others, seem to be able to promote liver tumour development in rats pretreated with initiating doses of genotoxic carcinogens. (We classify as 'genotoxic carcinogen', compounds like the alkyl N-nitrosamines, which are metabolized to reactive molecules that insert alkyl groups covalently into DNA and cause mutations or chromosome abnormalities). We now have a paradox; N-nitrosamines are found at very low levels in many natural foods and are also formed in the gastrointestinal tract (in microgram quantities) from dietary amines and nitrates. Then why does exposure to enzyme inducers not cause liver cancer in man (White *et al.* 1979)? For some of the tumour-promoting enzyme inducers, tumours are produced in mice or even rats without previous deliberate exposure to initiating genotoxic compound. Since tests for genotoxicity in DDT, PCB, aldrin, and dieldrin have always been negative, one assumes that these pesticides act as promotors of liver tumour development. The argument put against all compounds that cause an increase in tumour incidence (i.e. carcinogens, broadly defined) is that there is 'no safe dose for any carcinogen'. As dose decreases the probability of tumours developing decreases, but there is no dose where probability becomes zero. At low dose the risks for the individual may be small yet it might be regarded as unacceptable to have an unnecessary death rate of one in a million persons exposed, per year. It is reasonable to examine this line of argument for genotoxic compounds where a low dose might cause an increase in the load of mutagens from the environment and so increase the overall risk of cancers by a small fraction. However, as the dose of a potential mutagen/carcinogen decreases, so the site and chemical pattern of metabolism may well alter. For instance, many natural flavourings go into a harmless pathway of metabolism at low dosage, and only at high dose are the low-affinity P_{450} enzymes engaged, with a resultant production of reactive mutagenic metabolites. In these circumstances, which often arise when mutagenic components are found in natural foodstuffs, one can only assess the quantity of risk as best one can in the light of prevailing risks. Where the risk is small in comparison with the background mortality from other causes, one might regard it as acceptable, depending on the various costs of removing the potential mutagens. For substances that act as tumour promoters there is no good evidence of any increased risk at the low doses associated with human exposure. There is good epidemiological evidence for DDT, and for phenobarbitone used as an anticonvulsant. For DDT, doses in the region of 100 mg/kg of diet were needed to produce liver tumours in rodents. The human population was exposed to doses of 0.03 mg/kg of diet from the widespread use of DDT in the 1960s (MAFF 1982). This was not enough to produce a measurable increase in drug metabolism in the liver and it seems most unlikely that there was ever any danger to human beings from environmental, accidental, or occupational exposure to DDT (Royal Society 1979; White *et al.* 1979; IARC 1987).

10.2.4 Development of new pesticides

The great drive of increased productivity in agriculture, together with the outcry against the persistent organochlorine insecticides, especially aldrin and dieldrin, led to the rapid development of more potent and more specific insecticides, herbicides, and fungicides.

For insectides, the organochlorine compounds that dominated the 1940–1950s era were gradually replaced, particularly by organophosphate (OP) compounds. The active OP compounds are those organic phosphate ester molecules (e.g. tetra ethyl pyrophosphate) that are cholinesterase substrates and at first reversible, then irreversible, inhibitors of the enzyme in mammals, insects, and other species. Inhibition of cholinesterase leads to accumulation of acetylcholine at motor end-plates with muscle fasciculation and paralysis, which can cause death. At the same time, cholinergic effects, such as excessive production of mucus in the bronchi and dilation of the pupils, lead to respiratory and visual disturbance. These compounds were developed in the late 1930s and their potential as war gases was seized upon so that a series of extraordinarily toxic compounds were made with a view to their use against people (the LD_{50} for Soman is in the region of 2 mg/person, that is one breath of the vapour). After the Second World War other directions of development were taken to produce OP compounds of low mammalian but high insect toxicity, and OP compounds were synthesized which were 'prodrugs', metabolized to the active cholinesterase substrate to a very much greater extent in most insects than in mammals. At the same time it became clear that some of the OP compounds, in addition to their acute neurotoxic effects, which wear off within a few days of exposure, also had chronic irreversible neuropathy as part of their spectrum of adverse effects. After a number of tragic incidents involving some of the research workers engaged in the development of OP compounds, it was found that, in addition to inhibition of esterases in the peripheral tissues, these compounds which caused irreversible neuropathy also caused an inhibition of one of the esterases found in the brain (neurotoxic esterase). The work by Dr M. Johnson of the MRC Toxicology Research Unit at Carshalton has made it possible to screen potential insec-

ticides to ensure that they do not have the irreversible neurotoxic effect (Murphy 1986).

10.2.5 Conditions for safety for insecticide use

A high degree of insect specificity has been achieved, especially through the use of thiocompounds where a sulphur replaces the oxygen of the cholinesterase-inhibiting OP compounds. In insects the sulphur is replaced with oxygen by P_{450}-linked enzymes, while in the mammalian system other routes of metabolism lead to detoxification rather than to lethal synthesis. Compounds such as malathion have exceedingly low mammalian toxicity in contrast to malaoxon, which is the metabolite produced in insects. The use of potent insecticidal compounds in agriculture can be achieved safely given adequate protection of workers against undue exposure; the education of workers in safe use and hygiene; and the provision of adequate protective gear, such as enclosed cabs on spray machinery (which allow application without excess exposure of the operators), and provision of methods of hygiene, such as water for washing (Code of Practice, MAFF 1988).

In addition, it is important that the insecticidal preparation should be of good quality, not contaminated by impurities that arise in faulty manufacture or storage, and properly labelled.

These conditions are notably absent in some countries, where technical, economic, and social conditions result in heavy exposure of workers. For instance, in California migrant labourers are regularly exposed to organophosphorus compounds, leading to episodes of poisoning. In India, highly toxic impurities in the OP compounds used for mosquito control in the antimalaria campaign have led to a number of deaths amongst spraymen. In Brazil, fatal exposure of field workers to older, cheaper, non-specific organophosphorus compounds is widely reported.

Frequently, the official laws of a country do not reflect the reality of safety of use of insecticides, which depends more on social and cultural development than on the laws enacted in a distant capital.

10.2.6 A herbicide controversy—245T and dioxin

Herbicides are probably the economically most important pesticides, and for many years analogues of the plant hormone auxin have been used to kill broad-leaved plants, such as brambles and brushwood, while leaving grasses undisturbed to maintain soil structure. The most widely used of these were 2,4,5-trichlorophenoxyacetic acid (245T) and its dichloro-analogue 24D. These compounds have come under increasing adverse comment, because 245T (but *not* 24D) was contaminated with trace amounts of 2,3,7,8-tetrachlorodibenzodioxin (TCDD). Dioxin levels of 2 mg/kg of 245T were common in the 1960s (up to 45 mg/kg in 'agent orange' in Vietnam) and were brought down to 10 μg/kg by the 1980s (MAFF 1982). TCDD has an unusually high degree of persistence and toxicity, and causes lethal effects in guinea-pigs at a dose of 2 μg/kg body weight. Rats and people seem far more resistant. TCDD may act by blocking cell surface receptors for epidermal growth factor. Certainly, the signs of toxicity are unusual in that the animals fade away, with slow loss of cells from various tissues, especially the liver, over many days. In addition to the lethal effects, TCDD causes a massive increase in liver weight and induction of the cytochrome P_{448} family of mixed function oxidase enzymes, promotes liver tumour growth, and has numerous embryo-toxic effects. In humans the most notable effect of exposure to TCDD is the development of chloracne, a persistant and disfiguring form of acne, especially of the face, arms, and shoulders, found in workers exposed to TCDD in chlorinated naphthalenes or in other processes in which TCDD or similar compounds are produced. In particular there have been a number of cases where trichlorophenol manufacture has run out of control, overheated, and exploded, with the formation of relatively large amounts of TCDD; the most notable example being the explosion at Seveso in Italy. Heavily exposed workers had not only chloracne but other debilitating effects. However, neither carcinogenesis nor embryo toxicity have been shown to increase above background incidence in human populations exposed to trace amounts of TCDD. It appears that dioxins are less toxic to human beings than to some animal species, and in the absence of chloracne none of the other severe adverse effects are found.

There are many other chlorinated compounds, such as the chlorinated biphenyls, which may either have effects like TCDD, perhaps because they block the same receptor site, or are contaminated with active materials. There are rigid structure activity rules and many of the chlorinated dibenzodioxins are notably non-toxic because the chlorines are in the wrong position for toxicity. This makes it hard to measure the effective contamination of an environment with biologically active dioxins (Royal Commission on Environmental Pollution 1979).

245T and related herbicides were used to defoliate forests and destroy food crops by spraying from the air during the war in Vietnam. There was extensive damage to the environment and reports of teratogenic effects in the Vietnamese population, which had been sprayed from the air as well as being bombed and starved. A campaign against the use of 245T in the USA was mounted by organizations claiming to work for protection of the environment, the consumer, and agricultural workers. No evidence of injury was ever produced and chloracne was not observed in exposed populations. However, the appalling circumstances of human exposure to dioxin, in war and in factory explosions, together with its potent and wide-ranging toxic effects, especially in tumour promotion and teratogenesis, have outweighed the low level of contamination found in present-day samples of 245T and have given the herbicide a bad name, which was sufficient to have it banned in many places. Highly chlorinated compounds such as dioxin and the polychlorinated biphenyls (used in electric transformers until banned) have extraordinary persistence in soil and water and may accumulate in fish and fish-eating animals. It looks as if these compounds will be present in the environment at p.p.b. (parts per billion, $\mu g/kg$ of water, food, etc.) levels for very many years.

Fortunately, it looks so far as if there are no adverse effects at these levels and that the introduction of these chemicals and contaminants over the last 40 years will not lead to another disaster of the scale that has followed the introduction of cigarettes about 100 years ago.

10.2.7 The newer pesticides

The acute toxicity of a compound (Table 10.5) gives only one dimension of its potential adverse effects. However, it is notable that new pesticides, such as the herbicide glyphosate, have a remarkable specificity, and low toxicity for mammals in comparison to their efficacy against target pests. Glyphosate interferes with plant growth by preventing the new synthesis of aromatic amino acids, a pathway that is important for plants but does not exist in mammals. Similarly, when one compares modern pyrethroids with the organophosphorus compounds one notices that while the acute toxicity of the pyrethroids is not remarkably low their extreme potency as insecticides means that they can be applied in such dilute solutions and at such low quantities per hectare, that mammalian toxicity from the dilute spray becomes most unlikely.

High specificity for some plant biochemical system does not always guarantee safety to mammals. For instance, paraquat attacks the redox system of the chloroplast, the photosynthetic

Table 10.5 Some acute toxicity measurements (British Crop Protection Council 1979; Merck Index 1983; Vale and Meredith 1981).

Substance	Usage	LD$_{50}$*
Pesticides		
Parathion	Old OP pesticide	10 mg/kg
Decamethrin	Pyrethyroid insecticide used at 11 g/ha†	130 mg/kg
Malathion	New OP insecticide	1.3 g/kg
Paraquat	Herbicide at 1 kg/ha	100 mg/kg
Glyphosate	Newer herbicide at 1 kg/ha	4.3 g/kg
Comparators		
Botulinus A toxin	Food contaminant	15 ng/kg
Soman	OP war gas, volatile, 3 mg/litre air	60 μg/kg
Paracetamol	Analgesic	5 g/kg in rats, 0.7 g/kg in humans
Ethanol	Euphoriant	5 g/kg
Sucrose	Food (osmotic haemoconcentration in overdose)	25 g/kg

* LD$_{50}$: Dose causing 50 per cent mortality in groups of rats in the week following a single dose (usually oral).

LD$_{50}$ may vary between species, strain, and testing laboratory by an order of magnitude or more. Substances with similar LD$_{50}$ values may vary greatly in associated risk. Decamethrin is highly potent and used in very dilute solution, while paraquat is sold as a 50 per cent solution. Dermally absorbed materials (such as parathion) may be more readily absorbed to toxic dose levels than non-penetrating materials.

† 1 hectare (ha) = 100 m × 100 m.

apparatus of green plants, in a light-dependent fashion, causing death of these cells. Mammals contain no chloroplasts, but paraquat attacks a different system. It is actively taken up by the lung and, in the presence of the high oxygen concentration, sets off oxidative damage to lung cells with cell death and fibrosis. However, paraquat is not persistent and environmental contamination does not seem to be a problem, damaging doses being found only in accidental or deliberate overdose, usually from misuse of the concentrate, which contains 25 per cent paraquat. Here poisoning risks are reduced by adding colour and odour to the formulation, so making it more difficult to slip paraquat into cups of tea without causing surprise or suspicion.

Overall, the pesticide industry has been under persistent attack for contaminating the environment, for encouraging overuse of pesticides with destructive effects on wildlife, and for neglecting improved methods of agriculture that will reduce the need for pesticides. As a response, the industry has produced pesticides that are less persistent in the environment, more potent, and therefore used in smaller quantities, and far more selective in their toxicity towards target organisms rather than having sheer biocidal activities. None of these prevents misuse or accidental contamination of the wrong target, whether gardens or people, or widespread use of the wrong materials because of wrongly formulated policies. In particular, developing countries are vulnerable to being sold out of date, impure, wrongly labelled materials, which are then used by populations that have not been warned or educated about pesticides.

In developed countries pesticides and environmental contaminants, such as lead, are often a cause of anxiety, in the absence of any evidence to justify it. This does not absolve the medical profession from the need for vigilance to see whether some new and unsuspected adverse effect will crop up from widespread exposure to new pesticides and environmental contamination.

10.2.8   Bibliography

British Crop Protection Council (1979). *The pesticide manual: a world compendium* (6th edn) (ed. C. R. Worthing). BCPC, Croydon.

Hunter, D. (1975). *The diseases of occupations* (5th edn). Hodder and Stoughton, London.

IARC (1987). *Monographs on the evaluation of carcinogenic risks to humans, Supplement 7. Overall evaluation of carcinogenicity: an updating of IARC monographs, Volumes 1–42.* WHO, Lyon.

Merck Index (1983). *An encyclopaedia of drugs, chemicals, and biologicals,* (10th edn). Merck and Co. Inc., New Jersey.

Ministry of Agriculture, Fisheries, and Food (1982). *Report of the working party on pesticide residues (1977–1981).* Food Surveillance Paper, No. 9. HMSO, London.

Ministry of Agriculture, Fisheries, and Food (1988). *Revised draft code of practice for the agricultural and commercial horticultural use of pesticides.* HMSO, London.

Moriarty, F. (1988). *Ecotoxicology. The study of pollutants in ecosystems.* Academic Press, London.

Murphy, S. D. (1986). Toxic effects of pesticides. In *Casarett and Doull's toxicology. The basic science of poisons* (3rd edn) (ed. C. D. Klaassen, M. O. Amdur, and J. D. Doull), pp. 519–81. Macmillan, London.

Royal Commission on Environmental Pollution (1976). *5th Report. Air pollution control: an integrated approach.* HMSO, London.

Royal Commission on Environmental Pollution (1979). *7th Report. Agriculture and pollution.* HMSO, London.

Royal Society of London (1979). *Long term hazards from environmental chemicals.* The Royal Society, London.

Vale, J. A. and Meredith, T. J. (eds) (1981). *Poisoning: diagnosis and treatment.* Update Books, London.

White, S. J., McLean, A. E. M., and Howland, C. (1979). Anticonvulsant drugs and cancer. A cohort study in patients with severe epilepsy. *Lancet* ii, 458–60.

Wohl, A. S. (1983). *Endangered lives. Public health in Victorian Britain.* J. M. Dent and Sons, London.

10.3   Nutritional disorders

Martin Eastwood

10.3.1   Introduction

Good health requires an adequate intake of nutrients. A deficiency or excess of overall calorie intake, or of individual nutrients, may result in nutritional disorders. Nutritional studies have resulted in the definition of requirements for essential nutrients, amino acids, fatty acids, vitamins, and trace elements. These requirements vary and are dependent upon diverse factors such as growth, pregnancy, and illness. Therefore the so-called recommended daily amounts (RDA) are very much approximations.

It is not possible to live for more than 2–3 minutes without oxygen. However, life can continue without water for between two and seven days, depending upon the ambient temperature and the amount of exercise being taken. Survival without any food at all, but with water, may be for up to 60 days, depending upon the body stores. Thus females and those with considerable subcutaneous fat survive for longer than slightly built males.

There are individual responses to nutritional deficiency and excess. Weight increases in association with overall excessive eating. Weight loss is associated with inadequate dietary intake. The failure to provide the essential amino acids, fats, vitamins, and trace elements leads to specific lesions, which may progress to morbidity and death. The response to a dietary deficiency varies. It may be that some apparently essential vitamins are synthesized by some individuals. When scurvy was a problem in the Royal Navy the fleet would come into land every two months to reduce the prevalence of scurvy. Yet on long voyages some individuals died quite quickly of scurvy and others appeared to be unaffected. Similarly, the different types of beriberi suggest individual metabolic responses to thiamine deficiency. This is, however, an unexplored aspect of nutrition.

Until there is an understanding of such nutritional mechanisms confused advice will continue to be disseminated wherein the pathology which is provoked by the response of even a small proportion is applied to the population as a whole.

10.3.2 Satiety and nutrition selection

Thirst

The sensation of thirst is produced by dehydration in a series of receptors. Osmotic dehydration stimulates osmoreceptors in the forebrain. Intravascular dehydration stimulates stretch receptors in the low pressure side of the circulation. Extensive volume losses result in arterial hypotension which stimulates baroreceptors in the high pressure side of the circulation and also renal renin secretion through angiotensin. The precise sequence of signals which contribute to thirst are not known.

Hunger

It is not clear how the brain controls food intake or how eating and complementary processes form an integrated control of caloric homeostasis. It used to be believed that a dual mechanism was involved in hunger, with a feeding centre and a satiety centre in the hypothalamus controlling the onset and completion of eating, with feedback systems maintaining glucose homeostasis and body fat stores. However, it is now realized that the hyperphagia resulting from damage to the ventromedial hypothalamus not only results in loss of satiety but has effects on the autonomic nervous system, decreasing sympathetic tone and increasing the responsiveness of the parasympathetic system to food consumption. This allows a shift in the direction of energy flux towards fat cells and lipogenesis.

Biological basis of hunger and satiety

The requirements for nutrient intake can be regarded as continuous or intermittent. The basic vegetative activities of the cardiorespiratory system, renal, endocrine, liver, nervous, and brain stem activity ensure the housekeeping of the body. The intermittent activities range from trivial movements to maximal activity where brain and the voluntary muscular systems are utilized to their limit.

Food intake may be continuous, as in the ever-eating sparrow or fieldmouse, or intermittent, as in the eagle or the lion. These creatures appear quiescent between bursts of energy during which the prey is secured prior to the resumption of passivity.

Control of appetite

No centre controlling satiety has been identified in the brain. In man the needs for metabolic fuels are substantial and continuous, yet eating is episodic. It is unlikely that there is a central receptor monitoring caloric flux and therefore moderating food intake. There may be important, non-central controls, e.g. the liver which monitors gastric emptying and the distribution of insulin and energy sources.

The passage of energy-rich food from the stomach to the intestine is regulated. Concentrated solutions empty slowly, whereas dilute solutions empty rapidly, producing the same net delivery of calories to the intestine. Satiety may result from a feeling of gastric distension and rate of gastric emptying. After a meal, metabolism is stimulated by nutrients entering the circulation from the gastrointestinal tract, with excess energy being stored as glycogen or triglyceride. Intestinal absorption provokes insulin secretion and shifts hepatic metabolism from mobilization to storage, thus providing a second signal of satiety. When both satiety signals have disappeared, liver and adipose tissue energy stores are mobilized and hunger begins. Hunger cannot reflect a biological need for food, as thirst does for water.

There may be specific stimuli to appetite, e.g. sodium chloride in salt deficiency, disease states, and heat. Other effects on appetite are social influences, e.g. culture, religion, learned preferences and aversions, and hedonic factors, e.g. taste, texture, and odour.

Perception is an important factor in specific appetites. An animal ensures adequate nutrition by consuming a widely varied range of foods. Experiments in newly weaned infants and in adults show that when more than one food is available there is a natural tendency to switch between foods rather than to consume only the most preferred one. A nutritious but monotonous diet, given to military or even starving refugees may eventually be refused. The aversion may persist for several months. It is possible that the decline in acceptability of a particular food, consumed in excess is due to some innate automatic mechanism directing food selection; a sensory-specific satiety. Proteins are less likely to cause satiation than carbohydrates. Variations in the flavour and shape of food can prevent satiation.

Heavy sedation decreases food intake. Alcohol may decrease food intake because of gastritis, though alcohol itself is a food. Corticosteroids may increase the appetite and food intake.

It has been suggested that diet affects behaviour. In some ancient cultures certain foods were thought to have magical qualities capable of giving special powers of strength, courage, health, happiness, and well-being. It is possible that food constituents may affect the synthesis of brain neurotransmitters and thus modify brain functions. In this way, what we eat could, ultimately, influence what we like.

Endogenous and exogenous determinants of food selection

Society and culture influence the choice of food. The delicacies of peoples of one part of the world are elsewhere regarded with abhorrence. Finance may determine the availability of nutrients. Religious beliefs also influence eating patterns, dictating fasting and forbidden foods, e.g. the vegetarian diet of Hindus and, more specifically, the banning of pork and shellfish, etc. for the Moslem and Jewish faiths.

There are endogenous determinants of energy intake such as gender, wherein a male, growing to a greater height and weight, will eat more than his contemporary female. As people grow older food intake declines, in part because of reduced physical activity.

10.3.3 Nutrients

Cell metabolism may, in part, be regarded as a balance between oxidation and reduction. Vitamins play an essential part in this oxidation and reduction interplay. Table 10.6 gives some

Table 10.6 Approximate daily requirements for a fit adult living in a temperate climate

Nutrient	Requirement	Source
Total energy	130–150 kJ/kg body weight	
Water	2–3 l	
Protein	1 g/kg body weight	Plant and animal
Fat	30–35% of energy intake	Vegetable and animal source
Carbohydrate	50–60% of energy intake	Plant
Vitamins		
Vitamin C	30–60 mg	Fruit, milk, liver
Thiamine (B$_1$)	100 μg/MJ	Fresh vegetables, liver, cereal grain husks
Riboflavin (B$_2$)	130 μg/MJ	Most foods, especially milk and meat
Niacin (B$_3$)	1.6 mg/MJ	Liver, lean meats, cereals, and legumes
Pyridoxine (B$_6$)	2 mg	Meats, cereal, lentils, some fruits and vegetables
Pantothenic acid	3–10 mg	Liver, meat, cereals, milk, egg yolk, and fresh vegetables
Choline (synthesized by man)		Muscle meats, egg yolk, legumes, cereals
Biotin	30 μg	Yeast, meat, grains, vegetables
Folic acid	350 μg	Muscle meats, egg yolk, legumes, cereals
Vitamin B$_{12}$	3 μg	Micro-organisms, liver, meat, fish
Vitamin A	800 μg	Dairy products, eggs, liver, fatty fish, green vegetables
Vitamin D	10 μg	Sunlight, fish oils
Vitamin K	40 μg	Greens, colonic bacteria
Tocopherol, Vitamin E	8 μg	Vegetables, seed oils, corn oil, sunflower seed, wheat germ oil
Minerals and trace elements		
Sodium	70–100 mmol	Salt, meat, processed foods
Potassium	50–150 mmol	Vegetables, fish
Iron	10–20 mg	Meat, vegetables
Magnesium	15 mmol	Cereals and vegetables
Zinc	15 mg	Meat, whole grain, legumes, oysters
Copper	2 mg	Green vegetables, fish, oysters, liver
Selenium	100 μg	Cereals and meat
Cobalt	?	Vitamin B$_{12}$
Molybdenum	0.5 mg	Legumes, cereal, grains, milk
Manganese	8 mg	Cereal, legumes, leafy vegetables, tea
Iodine	2 μg	Water, fish
Calcium	500 mg	Milk, cheese
Phosphorus	500 mg	Meat, poultry, fish
Fluoride	1 p.p.m.	Water

indication of the dietary requirements of the major and essential nutrients, vitamins, and minerals. This is an area of controversy and the recommendations are constantly being changed. The requirements vary from individual to individual, with energy expenditure, the climate and also the stage of growth, pregnancy, lactation, and also the state of health. Trauma and illness can increase nutritional needs. Therefore the requirements of a pregnant young woman suffering from multiple infections, undertaking heavy work in extremes of climate (cold or hot) will be quite different from those of the elderly, retired man living in a temperate climate with all services provided.

Energy

Total energy or total calorific intake is measured in Joules, which have replaced the once familiar calories.

1 kcal = 4.2 kJ; a daily 2500 kcal intake is 10.5 MJ (1 MJ = 10^6 J).

Protein provides 17 kJ per gram of energy (4 kcal per gram), carbohydrate 17 kJ per gram (4 kcal per gram), alcohol (ethyl alcohol) 29 kJ per gram (7 kcal per gram), and fat 38 kJ per gram (9 kcal per gram).

In the United Kingdom energy intake estimates for men vary. The elderly retired require 9–10 MJ per day; university students 12–13 MJ per day; and coal miners 15–16 MJ per day. In contrast, an elderly housewife would expend 8–9 MJ per day; female university students 9–11 MJ per day; and female bakery workers 10–11 MJ per day. Energy expenditure in bed is 2 MJ per 8 hours. The energy intake for children is high because of their activity and growth: 3–4 MJ per day are required for a child under one year; 9–10 MJ per day for a child between 7 and 9 years; 12–13 MJ per day for a male adolescent between 16 and 19 years, and 9–10 MJ per day for a female adolescent between 16 and 19 years. Recommended intakes are reduced in tropical areas by 5–10 per cent per day if the mean annual temperature exceeds 25°C.

Pregnancy requires an overall increase of energy intake of about 325–350 MJ. An increase in daily intake of 1.6 MJ is required over the last 6 months of pregnancy but depends on the difference in energy needs between the pre-pregnancy and pregnancy period. Extra fat laid down during pregnancy provides a reserve of energy. An additional dietary intake of 2.0 MJ per day is recommended during pregnancy. Lactation creates an enhanced caloric demand. A lactating mother requires about 3.0 MJ extra per day for 6 months to maintain weight and to provide milk with a value of 2.5 MJ.

Energy value of food and activity

When sufficient food is available, food intake, storage, and metabolism are balanced. Water, the major constituent of all living cells, is closely regulated. The total body fat in a 70 kg man is approximately 588 MJ, protein 100 MJ, and carbohydrate (as glycogen) 3.3 MJ.

Carbohydrate stores are replenished each day, whereas the daily fat and protein intake contribute only 1 per cent of the total store. Body fat stores are many times larger than fat intake, implying a much greater storage capacity for fat and a much longer time to achieve balance.

Muscle and skin metabolism uses 18 per cent of total energy expenditure at rest, increasing to more than 50 per cent during physical activity. Brain and visceral metabolism contribute a more significant and constant usage of energy. The brain requires 20 per cent of the total basal energy expenditure, utilizing only glucose and so has a respiratory quotient of 1. Visceral tissues use fatty acids or ketones and only small amounts of carbohydrate, depending on diet or exercise. Skeletal muscle uses carbohydrate and fat according to training and the intensity and duration of exercise. During short bouts of intense exercise the major fuel is glycogen stores within muscles. After prolonged exercise (45–70 min) muscle fatty acid oxidation increases and the respiratory quotient falls. A major difference between the muscles of a physically trained person and those of an untrained person is the ability to store glycogen and oxidize fatty acids during exercise and rest.

Water

Water is the largest single component of the human body, about 40 litres in a 65 kg man; 25 litres being intracellular and 15 litres extracellular. The essential water intake includes free fluid and water in ingested food. Additional metabolic water is formed by nutrient oxidation. A gram of starch may yield 0.6 g of water, protein 0.41 g, and fat 1.07 g. The fluid intake with an 8.8 MJ per day diet would be 2500 ml; 1100 ml from the solid food, 1200 ml from fluid, and the remainder from metabolic water. Water is inevitably lost in the urine, faeces, and by evaporation from the skin and lungs. Water intake must compensate for these continuous, inevitable losses.

Carbohydrates

Carbohydrates are an important contributor to energy in all human diets, providing some 85 per cent for poor people on marginal diets and 40 per cent of the diet of the prosperous.

The primary units of carbohydrates are fructose, glucose, mannose, deoxyribose, arabinose, and xylose. Important dietary sugars are disaccharides, e.g. sucrose, lactose, and maltose. Sucrose is domestic sugar, processed from sugar cane or sugar beet. Lactose is present in milk; maltose is a breakdown product of the malting of starch. Trialose is present in mushrooms, other fungi, and insects.

Starch is a complex polysaccharide stored in root granules and plant seeds. There are two types, amylose is a long unbranched chain with α-1,4 linkages and amylopectin, a highly branched molecule, with α-1,6 linkages, with glucose units in each branch, the branches joined by α-1,4 linkages. Amylopectin is the major component of most starch grains. Dextrins are hydrolysis products of starch, and are important as sources of carbohydrates in oral supplemented feeds. Glycogen is the animal equivalent of starch and is present in liver and muscle. An oyster contains about 6 per cent of its wet weight as glycogen.

Protein

Proteins contribute some 10–15 per cent of the energy in all natural diets and renew proteins in cell walls, plasma proteins, muscles, enzymes, and collagen. The amino acids of protein can be deaminated and provide an energy source in their own right.

The recommended human dietary intake of protein is approximately 1 g per kg of body weight of protein. Protein is needed for growth, and the protein intake of an infant should be 2–3 g per kg body weight during the first 6 years of life. At 5 years, growth is sustained on an adult diet whereby 10 per cent of the energy intake comes from protein.

Proteins are large molecules, polymers of amino acids which vary in size from 1000 to >1 000 000. The amino acids are classified by the number of amino and carboxylic groups and the presence of sulphur or an aromatic group (Fig. 10.5). Uncombined free ornithine, citrulline, taurine, and β-alanine are found in cells. Man can synthesize most non-essential amino acids from glucose and ammonia. The synthesis of tyrosine requires the availability of phenylalanine, and cysteine synthesis requires methionine. Both phenylalanine and methionine are essential amino acids and, if they are present in the diet at or below minimum requirement levels, tyrosine and cysteine may then become essential amino acids. The aromatic amino acids are important in hormone synthesis—tyrosine for thyroxine and catecholamines, adrenaline and noradrenaline, and tryptophan for serotonin.

Proteins differ in biological quality, due to different proportions of essential amino acids. A relative lack of an amino acid in one dietary protein can be compensated for by another protein with a more adequate complement of essential amino acids. The amino-acid composition differs between dietary plant and animal proteins with nutritional consequences.

To measure the biological value of a protein, individual proteins are fed to animals and the capacity to maintain the nitrogen balance or promote growth is measured. In any protein the amino acid present in the smallest amount relative to the recommended daily allowance (RDA) is the limiting amino acid. Tryptophan is a limiting amino acid in maize protein, lysine in

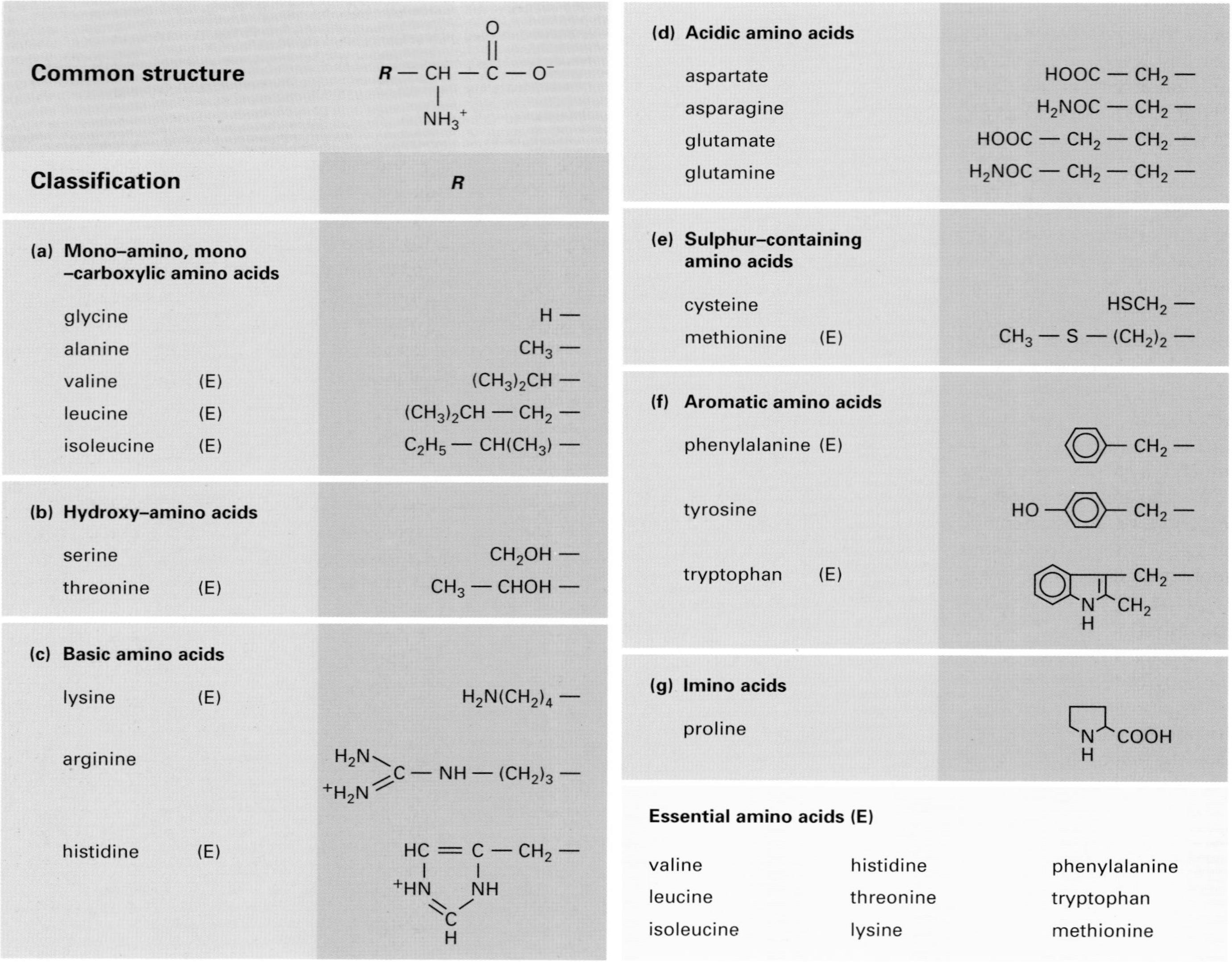

Common structure	$R - \overset{\displaystyle \underset{NH_3^+}{|}}{CH} - \overset{\displaystyle \overset{O}{\|}}{C} - O^-$

Classification	**R**

(a) Mono–amino, mono –carboxylic amino acids

glycine		H —
alanine		CH_3 —
valine	(E)	$(CH_3)_2CH$ —
leucine	(E)	$(CH_3)_2CH - CH_2$ —
isoleucine	(E)	$C_2H_5 - CH(CH_3)$ —

(b) Hydroxy–amino acids

| serine | | CH_2OH — |
| threonine | (E) | $CH_3 - CHOH$ — |

(c) Basic amino acids

lysine	(E)	$H_2N(CH_2)_4$ —
arginine		$\overset{\displaystyle H_2N}{\underset{\displaystyle ^+H_2N}{\diagdown}}C - NH - (CH_2)_3$ —
histidine	(E)	$HC = C - CH_2$ — with ^+HN, NH, $\overset{C}{H}$ ring

(d) Acidic amino acids

aspartate	$HOOC - CH_2$ —
asparagine	$H_2NOC - CH_2$ —
glutamate	$HOOC - CH_2 - CH_2$ —
glutamine	$H_2NOC - CH_2 - CH_2$ —

(e) Sulphur–containing amino acids

| cysteine | | $HSCH_2$ — |
| methionine | (E) | $CH_3 - S - (CH_2)_2$ — |

(f) Aromatic amino acids

phenylalanine	(E)	benzene — CH_2 —
tyrosine		HO — benzene — CH_2 —
tryptophan	(E)	indole $- CH_2$ / CH_2

(g) Imino acids

| proline | pyrrolidine N $COOH$ |

Essential amino acids (E)

valine	histidine	phenylalanine
leucine	threonine	tryptophan
isoleucine	lysine	methionine

Fig. 10.5 Amino acids.

wheat protein, and the sulphur-containing amino acids methionine and cysteine in beef protein.

$$\text{The biological value of a protein} = \frac{\text{retained N}}{\text{absorbed N}} \times 100$$

The protein efficiency ratio (PER) is the weight gain per weight of protein eaten by young rats.

Fat

Dietary fat is a heterogeneous mixture of lipids, predominantly triglycerides but includes phospholipids and sterols. Triglycerides are the principle lipids in foodstuffs and fat stores in man. They consist of esters of glycerol and fatty acids, both saturated or unsaturated.

Fatty acids

Fatty acids have the basic formula $CH_3(CH_2)_nCOOH$ where n can be any even number, the three major classes of fatty acids being distinguished by the number of double bonds (Fig. 10.6).

Unsaturated fatty acids can undergo further desaturation and chain lengthening or extension. Desaturation enzymes only act on the bond between the two carbon atoms, two places away from a double bond and towards the carboxyl end (Fig. 10.7).

The prefix ω or n indicates that numbering is from the terminal methyl end. A numbering nomenclature from the COOH end is chemical and called the Geneva system. The main families of dietary polyunsaturated fatty acids are ω-3, ω-6, according to the position of the first double bond relative to the methyl

Saturated acids	C	
Butyric acid	4:0	Short
Caproic acid	6:0	chain
Caprylic acid	8:0	
Capric acid	10:0	Medium
Lauric acid	12:0	chain
Myristic acid	14:0	
Palmitic acid	16:0	Long
Stearic acid	18:0	chain
Arichidic acid	20:0	
Behenic acid	22:0	
Monounsaturated acids		
Palmitoleic acid	16:1	ω-9
Oleic acid	18:1	ω-9
Erucic acid	22:1	ω-9
Polyunsaturated acids (PUFA)		
Linoleic acid	18:2	ω-6
γ-Linolenic acid	18:3	ω-6
Eicosatrienoic acid	20:3	ω-6
Arachidonic acid	20:4	ω-6
Eicosapentaeonic acid	20:5	ω-3

Fig. 10.6 Important natural fatty acids. C = ratio of number of carbon atoms to number of double bonds.

carbon atom. This double bond determines the number of double bonds that can be inserted. The essential fatty acids all belong to the ω-6 and possibly ω-3 groups but not ω-7 and ω-9. If ω-7 or ω-9 fatty acids are extended these extended fatty acids cannot substitute for the essential fatty acids.

α-Linolenic acid (C18:3 ω-6) can extend to eicosapentaenoic acid (C20:5 ω-3). Linoleic acid, γ-linolenic, and oleic acid can extend to eicosatrienoic acid (C20:3 ω-6).

Unsaturated fatty acids exist in two isomeric forms. *cis*-Isomers are present in both plants and animals. The *cis* form is required for the essential fatty acid activity. *cis*-Isomeric fatty acids may be converted into the *trans* forms during heating and as such are not incorporated into structural lipids and can no longer function as essential fatty acids. The *trans* fatty acids are oxidized and serve only as tissue fuels.

In all freshwater plant or animal life the unsaturated C_{16}, C_{18}, C_{20}, and C_{22} fatty acids predominate. The important saturated fatty acid is palmitic acid, which is usually present as 10–18 per

cent of total fatty acids. In the marine world polyunsaturated C_{20} and C_{22} fatty acids containing up to six double bonds predominate. In land animals the unsaturated oleic acid and saturated palmitic acid (hard fats with a low melting point) predominate. Dietary fats contain small amounts of short-chain C_4 and C_8 fatty acids. In plant seeds oleic acid and palmitic acid are predominant, with linoleic acid an important minor component. A diet rich in linoleic and linolenic acid can be obtained by eating vegetable seed oils, e.g. olive oil. Arachidonic acid is not present in vegetable oils but is synthesized from linoleic acid. Erucic acid (C22:1) is the principle fatty acid in rape-seed oil and is toxic to the myocardium. A developed variety of rape seed, cambra, contains only 2 per cent of erucic acid.

Polyunsaturated fats are susceptible to oxidation but are protected by coincident natural antioxidants (vitamin E).

Cholesterol

Cholesterol is found in all animal tissues. Most Western diets provide about 500 mg per day. Cholesterol is a structural component of cell membranes, a precursor of bile acids, adrenal and gonadal hormones, and vitamin D. It also can accumulate in atheromatous lesions of arterial walls.

Dietary fibre

This complex consists of the polymers of the plant cell wall—cellulose, hemicellulose, pectin, and lignin. It is an important but not essential constituent of the diet. Fibre contributes to the British diet to a varying extent (15–40 g per day). A recommended intake of dietary fibre is 30 g per day, half taken from non-fermentable sources, such as wheat bran, and half from fermentable sources, such as fruit and vegetables. Fibre passes along the gastrointestinal tract acting as a sponge, and modulates function by delaying gastric emptying, slowing the absorption of nutrients from the jejunum, possibly modifying bile acid absorption from the ileum, providing nutrition to caecal bacteria, and increasing faecal weight.

The variation in the relative amounts of pectin, cellulose, hemicellulose, and lignin in different plant sources accounts for the varying effects in the modulation of events along the gastrointestinal tract. The viscous guar gum slows gastric emptying and nutrient absorption. Pectin reduces the serum cholesterol and increases faecal bile acid excretion.

Fibres which contain pectin and hemicellulose, and to a lesser extent cellulose, are degraded by bacteria in the caecum. Faeces are 75 per cent water, and of the dry weight 40 per cent is

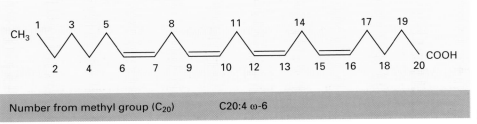

Number from methyl group (C_{20})   C20:4 ω-6

Fig. 10.7 The structure of arachidonic acid.

residual fibre and 40 per cent bacteria. The range of faecal wet weight in Britain is 50–300 g per day. The residual fibre and the bacteria which have proliferated on the fibre dictate the amount of stool passed.

Wheat bran, a complex compressed fibre, which is hardly fermented, increases stool weight by virtue of its water-holding capacity. The fibre in fruit and vegetables can be fermented and so increase the faecal bacterial mass and weight.

The solubility of cholesterol in bile is influenced by the amount of bile acids in the enterohepatic circulation. The ratio of cholesterol to bile acids can be influenced by ingested wheat bran. An increased concentration of biliary bile acids results in a reduction of the lithogenic properties of bile and hence an inhibition of the development of cholesterol gallstones.

Vitamins

Vitamins are essential organic, water- and fat-soluble, dietary nutrients required in relatively small amounts for metabolism. In general they cannot be synthesized by the body. The water-soluble vitamins are: vitamins B_1 (thiamine), B_2 (riboflavin), B_3 (nicotinic acid, niacin), and B_6 (pyridoxin), pantothenic acid, folic acid, vitamin B_{12}, cobalamin, biotin, choline, and vitamin C (ascorbic acid). The fat-soluble vitamins are vitamin A, vitamin D, vitamin E, and vitamin K.

Mineral

The minerals and trace elements that are necessary for regulating cell metabolism, cell and body structure, and growth are readily available in the Earth's crust.

Elements are absorbed at different points along the gastro-intestinal tract. There is some absorption of copper and selenium in the stomach. There is absorption of iron, zinc, calcium, selenium, and copper in the upper small intestine; chromium, manganese, fluoride, and molybdenum in the lower upper small intestine; and magnesium in the ileum. Sodium, potassium, and chloride are absorbed in the jejunum, ileum, and colon. It has been suggested that there is absorption of magnesium in the colon. Disease in the stomach, jejunum, ileum, and colon may affect the status of each of these elements, depending upon the part of the gut affected.

The role of vitamins and trace metals in metabolic reactions

Thiamine (B_1) is utilized as thiamine pyrophosphate, a cofactor in a variety of reactions, especially oxidative decarboxylations requiring ATP generation, e.g. oxoglutarate dehydrogenase and pyruvate dehydrogenase. Riboflavin (B_2) is incorporated into flavin mononucleotide and flavin adenine dinucleotide, which are necessary for oxido-reduction reactions. Nicotinic acid (niacin) is incorporated into NAD and NADP.

Pyridoxine (B_6) is metabolically important in its coenzyme form, pyridoxal 5-phosphate; ATP is catalysed by pyridoxal kinase. A number of enzymes require pyridoxal phosphate, especially those involved in amino acid metabolism, transamination, and decarboxylation. Biotin is a coenzyme for enzymes where ATP hydrolysis is coupled to the carboxylation

of biotin to form N-1 carboxybiotin, e.g. acetyl-CoA carboxylase. Pantothenic acid forms part of the coenzyme-A molecules and is involved in major metabolic pathways, including fatty acid synthesis.

All folates are derived from pteroylmonoglutamic acid. Pteridine is linked by a methylene bridge to p-amino benzoic acid, which in turn is linked by an amide link to glutamic acid. The commonly found folates in food may be modified in a number of ways. The folates are reduced to give 5,6,7,8,-tetrahydrofolate (H_4PteGlu). Up to eight glutamate residues may be linked by a γ-carboxyl group to pteroylmonoglutamic acid, and this glutamate chain attaches to enzymes (H_4PteGlu). Various carbon groups, e.g. $-CH_3$, $-CHO$, $-CH=NH$, and $-CH_2$, may be attached to nitrogen atoms at positions 5 or 10, or may form a bridge between them. These structures are fundamental to the activity of folate, e.g. 5,10-CH_2-H_4PteGlu$_5$.

Folates form prosthetic groups for enzymes involved in one-carbon unit transfer, e.g. from the β-carbon of serine, the α-carbon of glycine and the carbon 2 of the imidazole ring of histidine. This transfer of one-carbon units is important in purine nucleotide synthesis, pyrimidine nucleotide synthesis, and the conversion of homocysteine to methionine, which also requires vitamin B_{12} and the methylation of transfer RNA.

The structure of vitamin B_{12} is complex, with four linked pyrrole rings co-ordinating with a cobalt atom at the centre. The fifth ligand is the ribonucleotide of 5,6-dimethyl benzimidazole. In the stomach secreted intrinsic factor binds to vitamin B_{12}. Following ileal absorption as the intrinsic factor complex, vitamin B_{12} provides prosthetic groups to two classes of enzymes. The first group includes methylmalonyl-CoA mutase, which is involved in intramolecular group transfers (isomerizations), while the second group consists of methyltransferase reactions. The functional relationship between folate and vitamin B_{12} in the tetrahydropteroylglutamate methyl transferase reaction can cause a deficiency of intracellular folate resulting in megaloblastic anaemia. In vitamin B_{12} deficiency, homocysteine cannot be converted to methionine so that 5-CH_3-H_4PtGlu cannot be converted to H_4PteGlu in which form it is retained within the cell by conversion to the polyglutamate form (pentaglutamate). Only H_4PteGlu can be converted to polyglutamate forms. Hence a deficiency of intracellular folate occurs in bone marrow cells, the so called 'methylfolate trap'.

Iron is present in all cells of the body and plays a key role in many biochemical reactions. It is central to oxygen metabolism in that 2.5 g circulates chelated into haemaglobin and 150 mg is present in myoglobin. Dietary iron absorption roughly depends on iron stores, the lower the stores the more is absorbed. Although 10–15 mg of iron is ingested each day in a steady state, only 1 mg is absorbed. Absorbed iron is either taken up by bone marrow and incorporated into haemaglobin, or into the reticuloendothelial tissue stores. Increased dietary iron is absorbed during growth, blood loss, or pregnancy.

Zinc is essential for a number of enzyme functions, e.g. alkaline phosphatase, alcohol dehydrogenase, connective tissue and foetal thymidine kinase, pancreatic carboxypeptidase A, and liver nuclear DNA-dependent RNA polymerase. Copper is present in many enzyme systems, e.g. cytochrome oxidase, dopamine hydroxylase, superoxide dismutase, and lysyl oxidase. Iron metabolism is dependent on copper. Magnesium plays a key role in enzymatic reactions in intermediate metabolism, e.g. phosphokinases, oxidative decarboxylation, and amino acid acyl synthetases, also in protein synthesis through ribosmal aggregation, messenger RNA binding to ribosomes, the synthesis and degradation of DNA, and the formation of cyclic AMP. Manganese is a cofactor in phosphorohydrylases, phosphotransferases, and metal–enzyme complexes. The role of cobalt is solely as part of vitamin B_{12}. Molybdenum is involved in the early stage of fetal development. The enzyme sulphite oxidase requires molybdenum. Phosphorus is important in calcium homeostasis, and it is a major constituent of important organic phosphoric esters, including ATP.

Vitamins and trace elements in reduction reactions

Vitamin C (ascorbic acid) is a powerful reducing agent present in all tissues and is important in synthetic processes and energy exchanges. Ascorbic acid is a cosubstrate in a number of oxidoreduction reactions. Vitamin E consists of a group of eight naturally occurring tocopherols found in vegetable-seed oils, corn oil, sunflower-seed or wheatgerm oil. Vitamin E is an antioxidant, a scavenger for oxygen free radicals. It is found in all cell membranes and may prevent the non-enzymatic oxidation of polyunsaturated fatty acids by molecular oxygen.

Selenium is a constituent of human red cell glutathione peroxidase. Selenium and vitamin E are important in the synthesis of glutathione peroxidase which protects against oxidative damage to lipid membranes.

Vitamins, trace elements, and endocrine hormones

Cholecalciferol is the natural form of vitamin D (D_3), produced by the ultraviolet irradiation of 7-dehydrocholesterol sterol in the skin. Fish oils are the sole dietary source. Ergocalciferol (D_2) is derived from a fungal sterol converted by ultraviolet irradiation. The active form of vitamin D is 1,25-$(OH)_2$-vitamin D. The active form is formed only in the kidneys by 1-hydroxylation of the 25-OH-vitamin D (25-hydroxylation occurs in the liver). Vitamin D is a hormone rather than a vitamin, functioning with parathyroid hormone and calcitonin, and regulating calcium and phosphate metabolism and hence bone formation. 1,25-OH-vitamin D promotes intestinal calcium and phosphate absorption and mobilizes bone calcium.

Iodine is essential for the biosynthesis of the thyroid hormone, thyroxin. Arachidonic acid and linoleic acid are the precursors of prostaglandins which are present in all tissues. In this way essential fatty acids are involved in hormone metabolism.

Vitamin involvement in specific activities

Vitamin A consists of a group of biologically active compounds closely related to the plant pigment carotene. Vitamin A is stored as retinyl esters with long-chain fatty acids in animal tissue, especially the liver. Vitamin A is essential for photoreception by the eye retinal cells, and for normal function and development of epithelial surfaces. Retinol is present in butter, cheese, egg yolk, liver and fatty fish. Another important source of vitamin A is pro-vitamin A, found in green vegetables and split by a 15,15^1-oxygenase in the intestinal mucosa to two retinol molecules during absorption.

Dietary vitamin K is provided in two forms. Vitamin K_1 (phylloquinone), of plant origin, and Vitamin K_2 (menaquinone), the daily requirements. Vitamin K_1 is a cofactor for the hepatic synthesis of proteins active in coagulation (prothrombin and factors VII, IX, and X), through the post-translational carboxylation of glutamate residues in proteins to γ-carboxyglutamate.

Essential nutrient involvement in body structure

Protein and a sufficiency of essential amino acids are a requirement for the synthesis of cell membranes, collagen, and skeletal structure. Ascorbic acid is important in collagen formation for the post-translational hydroxylation of proline. This is important in wound and bone healing.

Vitamin D, in the form of its 1,25-hydroxy-vitamin D, promotes intestinal absorption of calcium and phosphate and is involved in the calcification of the matrix of bone. The bony skeleton is a protein matrix upon which insoluble calcium salts are deposited. Dietary calcium is important during growth and is needed in small amounts in adults. The bones of a young adult male contain 30 mol of calcium and those of a new-born baby 750 mmol. The total weight of the skeleton in the young adult is 9 kg; this is composed of 1.8 kg protein, 2.25 kg water, 0.45 kg fat, and 4.5 kg minerals. In bones the ratio of calcium to phosphorous is constant and greater than 2:1.

Fluoride is a normal component of calcified tissues, the concentration depends on dietary intake, usually from drinking water at 1 p.p.m. Copper deficiency of nutritional or genetic origin results in a failure of collagen and elastin cross-linkage in arteries and lungs.

The body sodium and potassium pools are similar (3900 mmol and 4300 mmol, respectively, in the 65 kg man) but the distribution is quite different. Sodium is predominantly an extracellular cation (2000 mmol), and a smaller amount occurs in cell water (400 mmol) and in a distinct non-exchangeable bone compartment (1500 mmol). Potassium is predominantly an intracellular-fluid cation (4000 mmol) with only 80 mmol in the extracellular fluids.

Calcium has a major role in muscle and cell excitation as well as in the endocrine and nervous systems.

10.3.4 Assessment of nutrition

A man weighing 65 kg consists of 40 kg of water, approximately 11 kg of protein, 1 kg of carbohydrate, 4 kg of minerals, and 9 kg of fat. Most of the protein forms essential cell components. All but 1 kg of fat is present in fat stores.

Energy

Cell repair and growth continuously use energy, whereas work uses energy intermittently. Nutrient ingestion is intermittent.

Much of the nutrient energy available in food is dissipated as heat during conversion to mechanical energy. Some 25 per cent of nutrient energy is used for mechanical work. Less than 10 per cent is used for tissue maintenance, e.g. cardiac and respiratory contractions. Rates of work or energy expenditure are calculated in watts (W = kJ/second). Twelve people sitting talking in a room produce heat at 60 kJ per minute, equivalent to a 1 kW electric fire.

Measurements of energy expenditure

Direct calorimetry measures the heat produced by the metabolism of foods and the excretion of by-products, e.g. water and carbon dioxide as in the Atwater and Rosa respiratory chamber.

Indirect calorimetry measures oxygen consumption, which is proportional to the energy and heat production. The ratio of excreted carbon dioxide to oxygen is peculiar to a particular nutrient, i.e. the respiratory quotient, glucose oxidation = 1, animal fat = 0.7, and protein = 0.8. Measuring the urinary nitrogen allows an estimate of the protein being metabolized. Oxygen consumption can be measured over long periods in respiration chambers or in closed circuit systems, e.g. the Benedict Roth spirometer, Douglas bag, or the Max Planck respirometer.

The energy expenditure for light work is less than 170 W (2.5 kcal per minute); examples are golf, assembly work, gymnastic exercises, bricklaying, painting. Moderate work 350–500 W (5–7.4 kcal per minute), includes general labouring with a pick and shovel, agricultural work, ballroom dancing, and tennis. Very hard work 650–800 W (10–12.5 kcal per minute), includes lumber work, work done by furnace men, cross-country running, and hill climbing.

Energy expenditure at rest—basal metabolic rate (BMR)

At complete rest and without physical work some energy is required for the activity of the internal organs and to maintain body temperature (basal metabolic rate, W/m^2). Surface area (m^2) is used to standardize measurements of BMR in individuals of varying size. The surface area is calculated from height and weight by normograms. BMR is more closely related to lean body mass than to surface area. During sleep the overall metabolic rate approaches the BMR.

Energy requirements of man, methods of assessment—dietary survey

Dietary surveys are one of the most precise and demanding exercises in nutrition, requiring full co-operation between dietitian and subject. At their most precise such surveys entail the weighing of all food coming into the house, on the plate, and the residue after eating. An inventory of the food in the house is made at the beginning and at the end of the survey period. Simpler and less accurate methods include diet diaries and dietitian interviews.

Assessment of nutritional status

Four methods are used:

1. clinical examination;
2. physical measurements;
3. biochemical and other tests;
4. the dietary survey.

Signs of malnutrition are shown in Fig. 10.8. Height and weight are important indices of growth in children and adults. Life Assurance Company tables give acceptable weights for a range of heights. Approximate measurements of muscle mass and body mass are made by the mid-arm circumference and triceps skinfold thickness. The lower 10 per cent of the range indicates significant underdevelopment. In the upper 10 per cent of the range individuals can be regarded as obese. Possibly the most effective diagnostic examination is to look at the patient and to decide whether the patient is underweight, normal, or overweight.

There are precise and important laboratory methods for measuring nutritional status for vitamins, electrolytes, and trace elements. These are summarized in each of the sections devoted to these substances.

More general biochemical measurements are the plasma albumin and protein concentrations. Albumin has a half-life of 20 days and is therefore a slow indicator of nutritional abnormality. A plasma albumin of under 25 g/l suggests severe malnutrition (or liver disease etc.). Plasma proteins include transferrin and retinol binding protein, complement component (C3), and fibronectin, which have shorter half-lives and therefore more rapidly reflect nutritional status. There is as yet no consensus as to which of these plasma proteins are the best to use for routine assessment.

The nitrogen loss in urine is measured by measuring the total urea in a 24-hour urine collection. Total nitrogen loss = 24 h urinary urea × 0.035 + 2 g.

10.3.5 Food availability along the gastrointestinal tract

Water is essential to life. The mineral content of certain fluids in the body are similar to those of sea-water. An important function of the intestine is to regulate the intake of minerals that are essential though poisonous in excess. Most organic compounds are readily absorbed from the jejunum. An excess of protein, carbohydrate, or fat is usually stored as fat. Many water-soluble vitamins, if eaten in excess, are excreted in the urine.

The uptake of food is dependent upon the total intake and bioavailability. Bioavailability can be defined as

$$\frac{\text{absorbed and utilized}}{\text{ingested}} \times 100$$

No food is of value to the individual until it has been absorbed through the intestinal mucosa.

The availability of foods for absorption is dependent upon a number of factors:

1. mucosal absorption function;
2. pathological factors altering intestinal absorption function;
3. alterations in lumenal availability, e.g. interaction between accompanying nutrients within a meal.

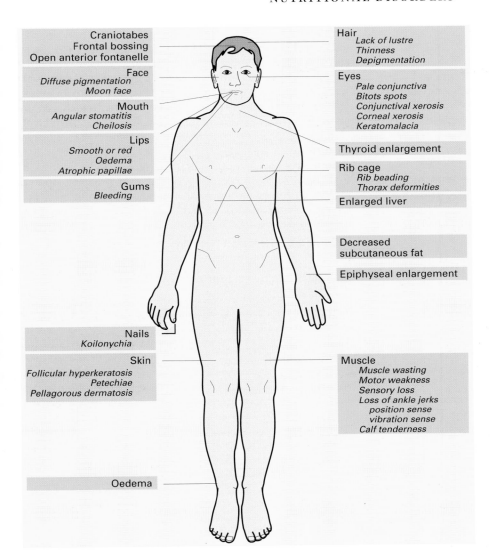

Fig. 10.8 Clinical features associated with abnormal nutritional status.

Other factors that may affect absorption include deficiency of necessary intestinal secretions and competing enteric bacteria, medicinal drugs, and surgical procedures; for example, partial gastrectomies or gastroenterostomies will alter gastric emptying time and accelerate absorption, endocrine response, and cause hypoglycaemia, i.e. dumping syndrome.

The uptake by the mucosa of various nutrients may depend on the individual's needs. Intestinal absorption may be inhibited either partially or totally. There follows a sequence of consequences. When nutrient absorption is slowed there is a resulting modulation of rate of nutrient passage to the plasma which results in a less marked increase of plasma nutrient concentrations but the increase extends over a prolonged period. This results in a modified endocrine response. A further consequence is that the renal excretion of nutrients may be reduced.

Gastric emptying time modifies the rate of intestinal absorption. A dilute glucose solution will empty from the stomach rapidly and hence be absorbed from the jejunum more rapidly than a more concentrated glucose solution. Fat has a slower gastric emptying time than carbohydrate.

Gastric mucosa

Alcohol can cause gastritis which reduces gastric mucosal alcohol metabolism. Gastritis can suppress appetite and hence can modify food intake.

The mucoprotein intrinsic factor complexes with and is essential for vitamin B_{12} absorption. This factor is deficient in pernicious anaemia. Thus, although the vitamin is dietarily adequate, pernicious anaemia develops.

Small intestinal effects on nutrient availability

Lactose is absorbed by the intestinal mucosa and readily hydrolysed into glucose and galactose by the mucosal enzyme, lactase. Intestinal lactase is present in all infants, except in a rare congenital deficiency. However, in Black races and some Asian races the adult becomes lactase deficient, whereas 90–97 per cent of North European communities have persistent mucosal lactase activity.

Protein absorption includes breakdown to dipeptides, tripeptides, and amino acids. Dietary protein intake is approximately 100 g per day and, in addition, 170 g of protein are secreted into the intestine as enzymes and shredded cells. The faecal excretion of protein-derived nitrogen is about 10 g per day or less, indicating an effective absorption of protein.

Specific defects of intestinal amino-acid transport systems can occur. Cystinuria is a failure of the small intestinal and renal tubule transport systems for the basic amino acids, lysine, ornithine, arginine, and cystine. In Hartnup's disease several neutral amino acids, e.g. tryptophan, are not absorbed from the intestine at normal rates. Yet if these amino acids are introduced to the small intestine as peptides they are efficiently absorbed. In less specific malabsorption states, e.g. coeliac disease, amino-acid absorption is markedly reduced while peptide transport is less severely affected.

In some instances only a proportion of a nutrient, e.g. trace elements, is absorbed. The absorption of calcium is dependent upon the 1-α,25-dihydroxy-cholecalciferol status of the individual. Where there is reduced exposure to solar ultraviolet light then vitamin D status can be compromised and calcium absorption is reduced.

The intestinal muscosal permeability to small molecules may be increased in children with food allergy, suggesting that permeability may be an integral part of the atopic constitution.

Triglycerides and fat-soluble vitamins A, D, and K require high lumenal concentrations of bile acid for absorption. Triglycerides containing predominantly short-chain and medium-chain fatty acids (to 12 carbon length) are hydrolysed independently of bile acids and micelles, and are readily absorbed and enter the circulation through the portal blood bound to albumin.

Folic acid is present in food predominantly as a polyglutamate which is hydrolysed by a conjugase at the γ-glutamyl bond before absorption. Folic acid is very labile but is protected from oxidation by ascorbic acid. Vitamin C and folic acid are heat labile and readily destroyed by cooking.

Cooking may modify absorption of other nutrients. Raw starch is poorly digested by amylase but during cooking starch granules are disrupted and become readily digested. When the starch in bread, potatoes, and puddings is stored in the cold after cooking then the starch hardens by a process of retrogradation. Retrograde starch is not readily hydrolysed by pancreatic amylase though this retrogradation is partially reversed by heating.

The colon

The colon is a conserving organ, containing a large bacterial mass. The bacteria modify the enterohepatic circulation of chemicals secreted in bile, e.g. bile acids, hormones, and drugs. The caecal bacterial breakdown of proteins is followed by the absorption of amino-acid derivatives. Dietary fibre is not hydrolysed in the small bowel and passes through to the colon. Wheat bran is minimally fermented in the caecum. Pectin, hemicellulose, gums, and retrograde starch yield volatile fatty acids, acetate, butyrate, and propionate. Hydrogen, methane, and other gases are produced. Absorption from the colon is somewhat specific. Colonic bacteria are able to synthesize vitamin K_2 (multiprenylmenaquinones) and vitamin B_{12}, which are not absorbed. The faeces from subjects with pernicious anaemia contain unabsorbable vitamin B_{12} which is more than sufficient for their needs. The relatively modest large bowel absorption of polar molecules, e.g. hormones, toxic agents, and drugs, results from small colonic pores. Such pore size probably protects against toxins being absorbed. Changes in colonic pore permeability can be induced by drugs and disease, e.g. colitis. Fatty acids and dihydroxy bile acids increase permeability and pore size, allowing oxalic acid to be absorbed.

Interactions between nutrients and the effect on bioavailability

Nutrients may interact chemically and physically to increase or decrease bioavailability. The complexing of vitamin B_{12} with intrinsic factor allows absorption of vitamin B_{12} from the ileum.

Alcohol may reduce thiamine absorption, particularly if there is coincidental folate deficiency. Niacin is held in cereals in a bound form which is not enterically absorbed unless released by dilute alkali or roasting. Failure to release niacin is a factor in the development of pellagra, i.e. vitamin B_6 deficiency. Biotin is bound to avidin, a protein in raw eggs, which renders biotin unavailable for absorption. The binding of calcium to oxalate and phytate reduces calcium absorption. The human intestinal tract mucosa contains no phytase. Yeast cells contain phytase, which hydrolyses phytic acid during the leavening of dough. Calcium absorption is reduced in populations who habitually eat unleavened bread. Dietary fibre, a cation exchange binder, may reduce mineral absorption.

Intestinal zinc absorption is reduced by the coincidental presence of cadmium, copper, calcium, ferrous iron, phytate, and proteins which have undergone Maillard reactions. Zinc absorption is, however, increased by methionine, histidine, cysteine, citrate, and picolinic acid.

Nutrient interactions may enhance nutrient absorption. Intestinal calcium absorption is enhanced by lactose, unsaturated fatty acids, lysine, arginine, and glucose polymers. Iron in the form of haem is readily absorbed by mucosal cells. Haem itself is poorly soluble in water but when haemaglobin is digested the resultant peptides render the haem more soluble. Non-haem iron is absorbed by a separate transport system in an ionic form. Absorption is increased by a coincidental presence of meat, fish, and vitamin C, and is inhibited by phytate and tannin. Selenium is better absorbed as the selenomethionine form than as sodium selenite.

The underlying mechanism, between these seemingly unrelated enhancements and inhibitions of absorption, is water solubility. Insoluble calcium salts, e.g. calcium phytate and fatty acids, are not absorbed. If a trace mineral, e.g. zinc or magnesium, is bound to phytic acid then calcium can displace the trace element, which can then be absorbed, particularly if the trace element is in the form of a soluble, readily absorbable amino-acid salt.

Competition for nutrients

Small intestinal bacterial colonization can develop in jejunal diverticulosis or in a surgically formed stagnant loop. There is nutrient competition between host and bacteria for vitamins, iron, proteins, fats, and carbohydrates. The most dangerous inhibitor of absorption is the cholera vibrio; its enterotoxin stimulates a cyclic-AMP-mediated secretory process with profound water loss.

Drugs can cause malabsorption and diarrhoea, e.g. neomycin precipitates bile acids. Specific amylase blockers in beans slow the hydrolysis of amylose and retard the absorption of starch breakdown products.

Systemic adverse effects of nutrients

Iodine is essential to the synthesis of thyroid hormones. There are natural dietary inhibitors of thyroid synthesis called goitrogens. Linamarin produced in the processing of cassava releases the goitrogens hydrocyanic acid and thiocyanate. Cabbage, rape and mustard contain isothiocyanates which are natural goitrogens.

10.3.6 Nutritional disorders

Excess of nutrients and obesity

An excess of carbohydrate, fat, and protein can lead to obesity. Obesity does not appear to have a single cause, but represents a variety of conditions with differing aetiologies. Obesity can be classified by adipose tissue morphology and the age of onset. Obesity can be identified as hypertrophic, with enlarged fat-cell size; or as hyperplastic–hypertrophic, characterized by both excess fat-cell number and enlarged fat-cell size. Though there are many exceptions, hypertrophic obesity is usually associated with the adult onset of obesity, while hyperplastic–hypertrophic obesity is associated with juvenile or childhood onset. It has been shown that increased fat-cell number is better related to increased body size than with age of onset of obesity. The hypertrophic and hyperplastic–hypertrophic obese types differ in their response to treatment. Obesity may also be associated with endocrine disorders, such as Cushing's disease.

The term generalized or diffuse obesity indicates that the fat is uniformly distributed throughout the body, including the extremities. There are also gynoid female-like and android male-like states, dependent on whether the fat is distributed on the hips and thighs, or chest, abdomen, and arms.

In humans a weight/height² (w/h²) index (Quetelet Index) of more than 30 or a weight that is 120 per cent greater than recommended, results in a rapid increase in mortality and morbidity, e.g. cardiovascular disease, type II diabetes mellitus, and osteoarthritis. The decreased respiratory excursion in obesity results in an increased likelihood of chest infections. The obese are statuesque but severely at risk of a shortened life. It is

important, however, that a distinction is drawn between those plump individuals whose Quetelet Index is between 25 and 30 (Grade I) and the obese (Grade II, III). The mortality risk in Grade I (plump) is minimal. Grade II represents a transition range from clinically trivial to clinically crippling obesity with a mortality double that of people in the desirable weight range. Grade III is virtually incompatible with normal employment.

Many individuals who are lean, even underweight, owe their leanness to cigarette smoking. Cigarette smoking is a high-risk factor in itself and therefore the risk factors for mortality describe a J-shaped distribution.

There are socio-economic differences in the acceptability of obesity. Poorer, leaner, pre-adolescent girls become poorer, fatter, adult women; while richer, fatter girls mature into richer, leaner women. The reversal takes place at adolescence around the age of 15. Wallis Warfield Simpson is quoted as saying 'No woman can be too rich or too thin'. A trim figure is easiest achieved by eating a high unrefined carbohydrate and fibre, low fat diet, and exercising to maintain muscles at moderate degrees of training.

An excess intake of vitamin C can lead to excess excretion of oxalic acid in the urine and oxylate stones. The fat-soluble vitamins can be poisonous in excess. An excessive intake of vitamin A may result in lethargy, abdominal pain, headaches, and increased intracranial pressure. Polar bear and seal livers are very rich in retinol and eating liver from these animals can be poisonous, as polar explorers found to their cost. An excess dietary intake of vitamin D can result in abnormal absorption of calcium and hence hypercalcaemia, anorexia, loss of weight, nausea, depression, and irritability. The irritability may influence the myocardium and hence cardiac abnormal rhythms can occur, which are sometimes lethal.

Excessive dietary intake of all minerals can be poisonous. The role of the intestinal mucosa is to modulate the intake of these very important but potentially lethal constituents, whether sodium, potassium, or trace elements.

Alcohol

Prolonged and excessive alcohol intake can result in pathological changes in the liver, pancreas, and neurological systems (see Chapters 16, 17, 18, 25).

Alcohol can cause an enlarged liver due to fatty accumulation. During alcoholic liver decompensation an acute 'hepatitis' change can be found in central areas. Chronic alcohol ingestion results in an increased consumption of oxygen, due largely to increased mitochondrial reoxidation of NADH. In the liver this is associated with a steeper oxygen gradient along the sinusoid length so that necrosis develops in zone 3 (centrilobular). Thus the necrosis may be hypoxic in origin. The cells show lytic necrosis and clumps of refractile, dense, eosinophilic materials, the so-called alcoholic hyaline of Mallory, are to be found in the cytoplasm. These materials are complex glycoproteins with antigenic properties. Polymorphs surround the necrosing liver cells. Cholestasis and jaundice develop. The portal zones show stellate fibrosis, and pericellular fibrosis may develop around hepatic veins. In the final stages the liver collagen forms a network dividing the residual liver into small regular nodules. This can lead to re-routeing of the portal vasculature, the formation of varices at the lower end of the oesophagus, and an increase in the portal vein pressure. A transudate type of ascites can develop which contain a low albumin concentration (less than 250 g/l).

A heavy alcohol intake is also associated with an extremely painful chronic relapsing pancreatitis, though in some individuals progressive loss of pancreatic function can occur without pain. A possible mechanism for pancreatitis is oedema or spasm of the ampulla of Vater.

Behavioural changes of a violent nature can occur in bout-drinking. Peripheral neuropathies and brain atrophy occurs in prolonged drinking, in part due to nutritional deficiencies.

Alcoholic patients often have a red cell macrocytosis (MCV greater than 95 fl) due to a direct effect on bone marrow, although vitamin B_{12} and folate deficiency may be contributory factors.

Starvation and anorexia nervosa

There are many causes of starvation (Table 10.7). When food is unavailable the body has to rely on its own stores of food. The crucial provision of glucose for the brain and elsewhere depends on total liver glycogen and subsequently on the synthesis of glucose by both the liver and kidneys, initially from muscle protein amino acids. Collagen proteins, which represent 25 per cent of muscle, are preserved (4 kg protein). The liver, intestine, skin, brain, and adipose tissue can contribute 1 kg of protein amino acid. Fat is a high-density energy source, which makes fat a highly economic storage fuel. Muscle glycogen falls progressively during the first five days of starvation and may contribute 140 g of glucose to the brain after hepatic glycogen reserves are exhausted and circulating blood ketones are insufficiently concentrated to supply the brain. Muscle protein catabolism releases mainly alanine and glutamine. Alanine is the preferred substrate for gluconeogenesis in the liver and glutamine contributes to gluconeogenesis in the kidneys. In prolonged starvation, the flow of alanine from muscle falls and this is reflected in a steady decline in urea synthesis and excretion. Glutamine release tends to persist, since after 10 days of fasting ammonia becomes the main urinary nitrogen product.

During fasting there is an increase of ketone bodies from fatty acids in the liver, to be used by most tissues including the brain.

Table 10.7 Causes of starvation

Insufficient food available

Digestive tract malfunction and malabsorption, specific or total nutrient

Impaired appetite: disease, e.g. cancer
                               psychological, e.g. anorexia nervosa

Abnormal tissue metabolism: renal disease
                                               hepatic disease
                                               hyperthyroidism

Severe long-standing infection

Voluntary political hunger strike

Initially ketone production is small; as fasting continues it increases progressively so ketones become the dominant substrates. Two main ketones, acetoacetate and 3-hydroxy butyrate, are formed by acetyl-CoA in the liver (and are found in urine).

Atrophy of all tissues except the brain is the most characteristic feature of starvation. The wasting and loss of weight is initially rapid, but gradually slows down. The actively metabolizing cell mass is reduced and requires less energy to maintain activity. Unnecessary voluntary movements are curtailed. A healthy, non-obese subject can lose 25 per cent of weight without endangering life. During starvation 70 per cent of fat is lost, intracellular water is reduced from 25 kg to 19 kg; and 3 kg of protein, 6.5 kg of fat, and 200 g of carbohydrate can be lost in a 65 kg man. These represent 300 MJ reserves of nutrition, and are lost over approximately 50 days. The major weight loss in the first week is 1.5 kg of body water, when water-bound glycogen is released and excreted. A gram of glycogen binds 3–5 g of water. Protein deficiency in starvation causes a fall in concentration in plasma albumin, which also contributes to oedema.

Most people, with primary undernutrition, recover rapidly with access to food. Over 20 MJ per day may be consumed when free food is available.

Protein energy malnutrition

The term protein energy malnutrition (PEM) is applied to a spectrum of clinical conditions of both adults and children, kwashiorkor, famine oedema, marasmus, and cachexia. Young children with kwashiorkor weigh between 60–80 per cent of the international standard for age, have oedema, and slight reduction in weight for their height. Marasmic children weigh less than 60 per cent of the international standard, and exhibit a marked weight defect relative to height, but do not have oedema. Infants with marasmic kwashiorkor are 60 per cent of the ideal weight for their height and exhibit oedema. Severe undernutrition in adults is found in famine or is secondary to a specific illness, such as anorexia nervosa.

Protein energy malnutrition is the most important social health problem in underdeveloped countries and is an important factor in the high mortality in children under five years of age. Marasmus is caused by a lack of dietary energy, protein, and other nutrients in the growing infant. Kwashiorkor is due to quantitative and qualitative deficiencies of proteins, with an otherwise adequate energy intake. These two conditions may be discrete conditions. It is also possible that they represent success (marasmus) or inability (kwashiorkor) to adapt to a poor diet by preserving body function at the expense of growth.

Marasmus occurs in infants under one year in urban populations eating insufficient food. All elements of the diet are restricted. The mother has frequent pregnancies, early and abrupt weaning, followed by dirty and dilute artificial feeding of the infant. Repeated infections develop and the child may be treated with water, rice water, and other non-nutritious foods. This condition is found in the young baby who is cachectic, alert, and ravenous. Marasmus also occurs in total starvation.

Not all organs of the body are uniformly affected by malnutrition. The organs most affected are those least essential to life, with a reduction in the gastrointestinal tract mucosa, reduced salivary glands, fat stores, muscle mass, heart, liver, pancreas, reproductive organs, and thymus. The baby may have a mildly normochromic anaemia, which is due to reduced haemopoietic activity. The brain size is unaffected, though it is difficult to know whether the change in size of an organ *per se* is conclusive evidence of altered function. The marasmic child is more sensitive to bacterial, viral, and fungal infection, due in part to a reduced thymus size and circulating T-cell population. The spleen and adrenals may be increased in size. The patients readily succumb to infective diarrhoea and hence malabsorption occurs. As a result, kwashiorkor may develop in addition to marasmus. There is a range of clinical signs in the child which, in the one extreme, can be called marasmus and, in the other, kwashiorkor. All gradations between these two are seen clinically and can occur at all ages. Each of the clinical signs has a singular metabolic basis and the changing signs characteristic of protein energy malnutrition must reflect different metabolic abnormalities.

The term 'kwashiorkor' was introduced into modern medicine by Cecily Williams in 1931, and the Ghanaian word means 'the sickness which the second child gets when the next baby is born'.

Kwashiorkor occurs in the second year of life after a prolonged period of breast feeding. The child is weaned to a traditional diet which, because of poverty, is deficient in protein. The condition is, in part, due to an inadequacy of protein in a diet which is otherwise adequate. There is a failure of growth. Pitting oedema is always found in kwashiorkor. The oedema is both dependent and periorbital. The reason for the oedema is the low serum albumin and the consequent reduced hydrostatic pressure created by the plasma proteins. Because of this there is a failure to bind water by hydrophilic proteins. In addition to this there is a leakage of fluid from the vascular compartment into the extracellular tissues, which may be due to increased permeability. Sodium and water retention in the extracellular fluid may reach 50 per cent in severe cases. There may be accumulations of fluid in the peritoneum, pleural cavity, or pericardium. In severe cases the entire body and internal organs may be oedematous. There is inappropriate distribution of sodium and water throughout the compartments of the extracellular fluids. The intravascular volume may be depleted. The combination of loss of soluble proteins, and the excess of sodium and water, is responsible in part for the oedema. There are frequent deficiencies of other intracellular ions, e.g. magnesium, zinc, phosphorus, iron, and copper, with consequent effects on metabolism.

Children with protein energy malnutrition are apathetic while resting but cry when they are nursed. Adults become introspective and apathetic. The higher cerebral functions are most affected. Feeding the infant usually results in a restoration of function and growth. However, cerebral function may make only a partial recovery.

Water and electrolyte loss

The clinical features of water and electrolyte losses usually co-exist. Clinical evidence of dehydration includes sunken features (especially the eyes), dry, inelastic skin and tongue. Severe and rapid dehydration results in oligaemic shock with peripheral vasoconstriction, high pulse rate, and low systolic blood pressure (see Chapter 12). Pure sodium deficiency may present with behavioural abnormalities; this is diagnosed by a low serum sodium concentration (less than 135 mmol/l) and a low daily sodium excretion in the urine. The differential diagnosis is with water concentration conditions where there is inappropriate antidiuretic hormone secretion (ADH), e.g. associated with carcinoma of the lung. Sodium deficiency is treated by oral and intravenous saline replacement. Sodium and potassium are usually excreted in the urine but may be lost in faeces during profound diarrhoea. Sodium is also lost in sweat in hot humid conditions and where excess exercise is undertaken in such conditions. Water deficiency can also be a problem with marathon runners who fail to drink at the feeding stations. In humid hot conditions, sodium and potassium sweat loss results in a rapid onset of cardiovascular decompensation. In all these conditions failure to effectively replace the water and electrolytes results in patients becoming seriously depleted and very ill. Tissue wasting, diabetes mellitus, malnutrition, and trauma are important causes of potassium deficiency because of muscle wasting. A reduction in muscle mass of 1 kg results in the loss of 105 mmol of intracellular potassium and 200 g of protein. Potassium depletion is characterized by lethargy and mental confusion. The measurement of serum potassium (under 2.5 mmol/l) is an important diagnostic step. The ECG can also be abnormal.

Deficiency of vitamins and micronutrients

Thiamine Deficiency results in beriberi which presents in three forms.

Dry beriberi is a neurological condition affecting the motor and sensory nerves, spinal cord, and brain stem. The result is a polyneuropathy with a symmetrical distribution. The brain stem changes involve the medulla, pons, cerebellum, and dorsal root ganglion. The overall change is of fatty degeneration of the myelin sheath. Clinically there are two syndromes: Korsakoff's syndrome, which is a psychosis with memory loss and intellectual impairment, and Wernicke's syndrome, wherein there is focal degeneration with mental confusion, nystagmus, extraocular palsies, and prostration. Both may occur together. Which syndrome predominates depends on the area of brain stem most affected (see Chapter 25). It is ironic that in the Western world the commonest cause of the condition is excessive alcohol intake, so that an apparent drunken state is retained in perpetuity.

Wet beriberi is clinically associated with neuromuscular change and oedema. In cardiac beriberi the right side of the heart particularly becomes dilated. There is dilatation of the peripheral vasculature with increased blood flow and consequent high-output cardiac failure.

Riboflavin Deficiency causes minimal morbidity but is associated with cheilosis, angular stomatitis, and superficial interstitial keratosis of the cornea. Nasolabial seborrhoea can occur.

Nicotinic acid (niacin) Deficiency results in pellagra which is characterized by diarrhoea, dermatitis, and dementia. The diarrhoea is a result of mucosal atrophy in the oesophagus, stomach, and colon. The dermatitis is symmetrical and is most pronounced on the face, the dorsum of the hands, wrists, and elbows, and the lesion is sharply demarcated from normal skin. The skin is hyperkeratotic, and at a later stage becomes thickened and fibrosed. The tongue is swollen, red, and beefy. Dementia is associated with degeneration of the brain and spinal cord ganglia.

Pyridoxin This vitamin has a major role in the intermediatory metabolism of amino acids. Nevertheless a deficiency is only seen in alcoholics and with certain drugs, e.g. *para*-aminosalicylic acid. This deficiency condition may result in hyperoxaluria with a tendency to urinary stone formation. In infants there may be hyperirritability, convulsions, and anaemia.

Pantothenic acid This is found in most foods so a deficiency state is rare.

Folic acid Deficiency is an important cause of megaloblastic anaemia. The functional relationship between folic acid and vitamin B_{12} is in the tetrahydropteroylglutamate methyl transferase reaction determining intracellular folate. In B_{12} deficiency homocysteine cannot be converted to methionine, and $5\text{-}CH_3\text{-}H_4PteGlu$ cannot be converted to $H_4PteGlu$; the latter is retained in the cell. A cellular deficiency develops and the synthesis of purines and pyrimidines is reduced. In the bone marrow cells red cell formation also is reduced and a megaloblastic anaemia results. This is called the 'methylfolate trap'.

Vitamin B_{12} This is important in methyl transferase reactions. A deficiency of vitamin B_{12} results in megaloblastic anaemia and neurological disorders, especially in the posterolateral columns of the spinal cord (subacute combined degeneration of the cord, see Chapter 25).

Vitamin A This is important in the detection of light by the retinal cells of the eye. The aldehyde (retinol) in the retina is associated with the proteins opsin, in rods, and iodopsin, in cones. These form part of the structural light-sensitive pigment of the rod cells, rhodopsin. When light impinges on the retina there is a stereoisomerism of 11-*cis*-retinol to the 11-*trans* form, which alters the configuration of the protein and triggers transmission of a nerve impulse along the optic nerve. A deficiency of vitamin A leads initially to poor night vision, though there may be impairment of overall vision. Vitamin A is also involved in the maintenance of epithelial surfaces and a deficiency leads to epithelial metaplasia in the respiratory tract, mucous membranes, especially the eyes, gastrointestinal tract, and genito-urinary tract. The mucosa is replaced by inappropriately keratinized stratified squamous epithelium.

Vitamin K This vitamin is a cofactor for the hepatic synthesis of proteins active in coagulation, e.g. prothrombin and factors VII, IX, and X, through the post-translational carboxylation of glutamyl residues in proteins to γ-carboxyglutamate. Deficiency of vitamin K, therefore, leads to problems with coagulation.

Vitamin C Deficiency (scurvy) results in a failure of support structures, viz. collagen, osteoid, dentine, and intercellular cement formation, which leads to a loose cellular connective tissue. Hydroxyproline is important in collagen synthesis and is formed from proline. This requires prolyl hydroxylase, which in turn is ascorbic acid dependent. In the absence of ascorbic acid hydroxyproline production is negligible. The result is poor wound healing, perifollicular haemorrhage and other evidence of bleeding, gingivitis, coiled hair, arthralgia, neuropathies, anaemia, and Sjögren's syndrome. Capillary haemorrhage is due to a defect in the basement membrane joining the epithelial cells together. Wounds fail to heal through defective scar tissue. Bone cartilage and dentine fail to develop because of a defect in the extracellular matrix in which chondroblasts, osteoblasts, and ondotoblasts lay down minerals. The collagen molecule is important in all of these matrices.

Vitamin D Deficiency is associated with a failure of mineralization of the bone matrix. An important cause of vitamin D deficiency is lack of sunlight and to a lesser extent dietary deficiency. Deficiency of the active forms of vitamin D, which might also be regarded as hormones, can occur in diseases such as chronic renal failure and congenital conditions such as Fanconi's syndrome, where activation of cholecalciferol by 1:25 hydroxylation is impaired (Chapter 27), or in malabsorption of vitamin D, e.g. in coeliac disease, liver disease, and during anticonvulsant therapy. The failure of mineralization of the osteoid matrix results in a soft bone. The bony abnormalities which accrue depend on the age of onset and the way in which gravity stresses the bone. The infant in the cot lying all day develops craniotabes, frontal bossing, and abnormalities in the sternum giving rise to pigeon chest, and enlarged costochondral junctions (called the rachitic rosary). The toddler develops abnormalities in the pelvis, long bones, and vertebral column. The adult with a mature bone structure suffers from osteomalacia (see Chapter 27) with fractures characterized by radiological abnormalities called 'Loosers zones'.

Iron Deficiency is associated with a low serum iron and usually associated with excess loss of blood either in menstruation or pregnancy, or loss from lesions in the gastrointestinal tract.

Iodine Deficiency leads to goitre. This is a hypertrophy of the thyroid gland compensatory to inadequate supplies of iodine for thyroid hormone synthesis.

Magnesium Deficiency is caused by excess faecal loss in diarrhoea; and the result is apathy, muscular weakness, and occasionally tetany and convulsions. This condition is diagnosed by the measurement of a low serum magnesium concentration.

Zinc Deficiency in man results in characteristic skin lesions, starting on the face as erythematous crusted lesions, papulopustular eruptions or vesico-bullous lesions, which spread to the perineum, fingers, and toes. The patients may also show growth retardation, anorexia, hypogonadism in males, mental lethargy, and skin changes. Zinc deficiency exacerbates vitamin A deficiency and the associated night blindness.

Copper Deficiency in humans has never been recorded. Copper deficiency in experimental animals can result in failure of collagen and elastin cross-linkage in arteries and lungs.

Fluoride This element is a natural component of calcified tissues and at optimal levels of intake is beneficial in reducing the rate of dental caries. Epidemiological studies with human populations have not shown any evidence that fluoridated water (1 p.p.m.) causes or exacerbates disease.

Special nutritional states

Pregnancy

An expectant mother needs an adequate mixed diet both before and during pregnancy, adequate in total number of calories, protein, vitamins, and minerals. Her weight and diet should be monitored. Iron, calcium, and folic acid supplements (as milk) are important. A woman should gain weight during the first two trimesters and thereafter gain 0.5 kg per week until term, with a total gain of 12.5 kg: this is made up of 4.8 kg fetus, placenta and liquor, 1.3 kg uterus and breasts, 1.25 kg blood, 1.2 kg extracellular water, and 4 kg fat. When the expectant mother is obese, hypertension is a dangerous complication.

Formerly, undernutrition during childhood and adolescence stunted growth with a resulting small pelvis. This contracted pelvis led to a difficult and prolonged labour. It is now a rarity in Western obstetric practice, due to improved nutrition.

The birth weight of infants of well-fed mothers are on average higher than those of less well-fed women. The lower weight may be due to the baby being born prematurely or to retarded intrauterine growth. When a baby's weight is less than 2500 g the chances of survival are reduced. Other causes of low birth-weight babies are smoking and excess alcohol consumption. Premature babies may require specialized tube or intravenous feeding in order that growth and development are normal. Critical cerebral developments occur at this stage and appropriate nutrition is mandatory.

Lactation

Human breast milk (containing 29 kJ per 100 g) is the best food for babies. For the first 5 days after delivery the milk is rich in colostrum and immunoglobulins. The nitrogen content of human milk falls rapidly during the early weeks of lactation and slowly thereafter. The nutrient content of human milk is very adequate at parturition, except for iron (0.6 mg/l at 2 weeks, declining thereafter to 0.3 mg/l at 20 weeks); the infant is born with substantial iron stores. After 10 days the milk composition remains unchanged. Healthy infants at 2, 4, and 6 months need about 800, 900, and 1000 ml of milk daily. Most mothers can meet the needs of their baby at 4 months but only a minority at 6 months. Supplementary feeding starts when the baby is between 3 and 4 months. In general, the mother is able to maintain milk production even in poor communities, though an alternative feed is modified cow's milk. Cow's milk has a high sodium content of between 20 and 25 mmol/l (human milk is 7 mmol/l). If modified milk is incorrectly made up, it can lead to contamination of the milk or a high sodium intake.

Childhood and youth

Food is essential for growth and high activity. The progress of growth can be followed by regular weight and height measurements which are compared with tables for that population. During adolescence there are increased nutritional requirements for calorie intake, protein, vitamins, and minerals; this is especially so at the pubertal growth spurt when boys grow 20 cm in height and gain 20 kg in weight. Girls grow rather less during this phase.

Middle and old age

During middle age fat stores usually increase and there is a decline especially of pulmonary and renal capacity, which reduce by half between the ages of 30 and 90. The decline in function is gradual except for the abrupt cessation of ovarian function at the menopause. The two most important factors in longevity are heredity and luck. It is, however, not possible to choose one's parents, culture, or exposure to war or fatal accidents.

As age advances physical activity declines and so less dietary energy is required. Once old age has been attained alteration of the diet, e.g. to reduce obesity, has no effect on longevity. Osteomalacia and other results of long-standing malnutrition should be corrected. Osteoporosis, a loss of bone trabeculae and skeletal shrinkage is common in old age (see Chapter 27). There is no clear association with diet in this condition.

Trauma and surgery

Following all forms of trauma there is a loss of body nitrogen. The trauma may range from a fracture to surgery to skin burns. Following even uncomplicated surgery there is increased urinary nitrogen loss. The degree depends very much on the severity of the surgery. Even immobilization of a normal healthy individual in a leg plaster results in increased nitrogen loss. There is a gradation of increasing urinary nitrogen loss following the operations of appendicectomy, partial gastrectomy, colectomy, infection and fever superimposed on the operation, and fractured neck of femur. However, in diarrhoea the loss may be by the faecal route, and in burns through the damaged skin surface. The body requirements of protein therefore increase. The requirements for individual amino acids may also increase, e.g. for glutamine. If this protein loss is not recognized, then there may be a slowing down of convalescence or prolonged reduction in muscle mass.

Nutrition and disease therapy

For most of the history of medicine, diet has been the major recommendation available to a physician, particularly when working with poor insights into disease processes. In the Western world luxious amounts of clean nutritious food have resulted in a life expectation in excess of three-score years and ten. In 1911, the average citizen in the USA died at 52 years. By 1950 this had risen to 73 years, and by 1980 to 79 years.

There is an important fundamental distinction between the

two extremes of nutritional status. Overall malnourishment takes no account of the genetic background of the individual; starvation is indiscriminate in its destruction of the individual, though pre-existing body stores such as fat may favour women with an inherent advantage for the continuation of the species.

Overfeeding exposes an individual's inherent susceptibility to disease processes with a familial predisposition, e.g. cardiovascular disease, diabetes mellitus, gout, and possibly hypertension and colon cancer. Many population studies suggest that dietary fat, and particularly saturated fat, is an important contributor to coronary artery disease, increasing weight, compromising lipoprotein metabolism, and depositing cholesterol on arterial intima. A combination of genetic susceptibility, high fat and salt intake, cigarette smoking, and weight excess causes large numbers of men to suffer from cardiovascular, particularly coronary artery, disease (see also Chapters 2 and 12). Factors which reduce the risk of premature death from coronary artery disease include not smoking, exercising, being of normal weight for height, and eating a diet containing reasonable levels of fat (with significant polyunsaturated fat). This advice is particularly pertinent in men with a family history of this disease.

The modification of metabolic strains on a failing organ is of particular interest in clinical medicine and nutrition. In diabetes there are two major clinical groups, the young insulin-dependent diabetic and the older obese diabetic. In the first instance, a balance has to be achieved between maintaining energy input and weight, and modulating the needs for insulin. In the older group the important requirement is to lose weight.

In gout, the increased plasma uric acid can be modified by restricting purine intake. In renal failure there are the contrasting problems of accumulating protein-degradation products and urinary loss of protein. The dietary protein intake has to be restricted and a high-energy intake encouraged. In liver disease a compensatory mechanism is required for the failure of the liver to synthesize protein. Where there is portal hypertension and hepatic encephalopathy, the requirement is a reduction in the dietary protein intake. In ascites a low salt intake with adequate protein is important. In symptomatic diverticular disease wheat bran can reduce pressure and symptoms in the sigmoid colon.

10.3.7 Further reading

Anderson, G. H., Lovernberg, W. M., Lubin, H., and Morris, D. (1986). Diet and Behaviour. A multidisciplinary evaluation. *Nutrition Reviews* **44** (Supplement).

Bray, G. A. (1987). Obesity, a disease of energy imbalance. *Nutrition Reviews* **45**, 33–43.

Cannon, G. (1987). *The politics of food*. Century, London.

Crisp, A. H. (1980). *Anorexia nervosa*. Academic Press, London.

Davidson and Passmore (1986). In *Human nutrition and dietetics* (ed. R. Passmore and M. A. Eastwood) (8th edn). Churchill Livingstone, Edinburgh.

Garrow, J. W. (1981). *Treating obesity seriously. A clinical manual*. Edinburgh.

Hoyem, T. and Kvale, O. (eds) (1977). *Physical, chemical and biological changes in food caused by thermal processing*. Applied Science Publishers, London.

Le Fanu, J. (1987). *Eat your heart out. The fallacy of the health diet*. Macmillan, London.

Present knowledge in nutrition (1984). The Nutrition Foundation, Washington, DC.

Stricker, E. M. (1984). Biological basis of hunger and satiety: therapeutic implications. *Nutrition Reviews* **42**, 333–40.

10.4 Adverse reactions to drugs

J. K. Aronson and D. G. Grahame-Smith

10.4.1 Introduction

From the earliest times drugs have been recognized as being potentially dangerous. Indeed, it is a maxim that unless a drug is capable of doing some harm it is unlikely to do much good. For the most part adverse drug reactions are the province of clinicians, but pathologists can contribute in several ways:

1. By making a definitive tissue diagnosis, e.g. by bone marrow examination in aplastic anaemia, by renal biopsy in interstitial nephritis, or by the immunopathological investigation of the drug-induced lupus-like syndrome.

2. By developing strict pathological criteria for the diagnosis of drug-induced disease, on which formal studies of adverse drug reactions may be based.

3. By applying their techniques to the elucidation of the mechanisms of adverse drug reactions.

In this section we shall discuss the classification of adverse drug reactions, and give examples of the different ways in which such reactions may occur. A discussion of the precise types of specific organ pathology that occur as a result of drug action will be found in the appropriate chapters of Volume 2.

10.4.2 History

Public and professional concern about adverse drug reactions first arose between 1870 and 1890, when it became necessary to investigate sudden deaths occurring during chloroform anaesthesia, now known probably to be due to increased myocardial sensitivity to the arrhythmogenic effects of catecholamines in the presence of chloroform. Since then there have been many adverse drug effects that have caused public concern, or that have resulted either in the complete withdrawal of a drug from the market (e.g. benoxaprofen) or in a restriction of its indications (e.g. practolol); for other examples see Table 10.8.

However, the major incident that revolutionized attitudes to adverse drug reactions occurred in 1961, when there was an outbreak of congenital defects, particularly phocomelia (virtual absence of limbs), in new-born babies. It was shown subsequently that thalidomide, a non-barbiturate hypnotic, was to blame. This incident led to a public outcry, to the institution all

Table 10.8 Drugs of note in the history of adverse reactions

Drug	Date	Adverse reaction	Outcome
Sulphanilamide	1937	Liver damage	Solvent changed→FDA established
Diododiethyl tin	1954	Cerebral oedema	Withdrawn
Thalidomide	1961	Congenital malformations	Withdrawn→Dunlop Committee→The CSM established
Chloramphenicol	1966	Blood dyscrasias	Uses restricted
Clioquinol	1975	Subacute myelo-optic neuropathy	Withdrawn
Practolol	1977	Oculomucocutaneous syndrome	Uses restricted
Benoxaprofen	1982	Liver damage	Withdrawn
Zimeldine	1983	Hypersensitivity	Withdrawn
Zomepirac	1983	Anaphylaxis	Withdrawn
Indoprofen	1984	GI bleeding and perforation	Withdrawn
Osmosin®	1984	GI ulceration and perforation	Withdrawn
Phenylbutazone	1984	Blood dyscrasias	Uses restricted
Aspirin	1986	Reye's syndrome (children)	Uses restricted
Bupropion	1986	Seizures	Not marketed
Nomifensine	1986	Haemolytic anaemia	Withdrawn
Tocainide	1986	Neutropenia	Uses restricted
Suprofen	1987	Renal impairment	Withdrawn

® = Trade name.

around the world of drug regulatory authorities, to the development of a much more sophisticated approach to the preclinical testing and clinical evaluation of drugs before marketing, and to a greatly increased awareness of adverse effects of drugs and methods of detecting them.

From time to time events occur which result in further modifications of drug regulatory habits. For example, within a year or two of the introduction in 1982 of a novel anti-inflammatory drug, benoxaprofen, there were reports that it could cause severe liver damage, particularly in elderly patients. This led to an increased awareness of the need for pre-marketing testing in subjects (especially the elderly) representative of those who are going to receive the drug in regular therapy, and emphasized the need for post-marketing surveillance.

10.4.3 Incidence of adverse drug reactions

It is very difficult both to be certain how commonly adverse reactions occur overall, and to know what proportion of those that do occur are trivial or serious. However, the following are representative figures, gleaned from the results of major studies:

1. *hospital in-patients*, 10–12 per cent suffer an adverse drug reaction;
2. *deaths in hospital in-patients*, 0.24–2.9 per cent are due to adverse drug reactions;
3. *hospital admissions*, 3.0–6.0 per cent of hospital admissions are due to adverse reactions;
4. *general practice*, one in 40 consultations is due to an adverse reaction and up to 40 per cent of all patients have an adverse reaction of some kind at some time.

10.4.4 Classification of adverse drug reactions

No classification of adverse drug reactions is entirely satisfactory. However, we have proposed the following classification into four types:

1. dose-related effects;
2. non-dose-related effects;
3. long-term effects (related to both dose and duration of exposure);
4. delayed effects.

The various subdivisions of these four categories are shown in Table 10.9.

10.4.5 Dose-related adverse effects

Dose-related adverse effects occur when there is an excess of a known pharmacological effect of the drug. The pharmacological effect which proves adverse may be that through which one hopes to achieve the therapeutic effect (e.g. pseudomembranous colitis due to superinfection with *Clostridium difficile* following the eradication of other bowel flora by clindamycin); or it may be due to some other effect occurring in parallel with the therapeutic effect (e.g. asthma in patients taking β-adrenoceptor antagonists).

Dose-related adverse reactions have led to the concept of the therapeutic index, or the toxic:therapeutic ratio. This indicates the margin between the therapeutic dose and the toxic dose. The bigger the ratio the better. For example, if a patient is not hypersensitive to penicillins, then for that patient penicillins will have a high therapeutic index, or a high toxic:therapeutic

Table 10.9 Classification of adverse drug reactions

(1) Dose-related effects
    (a) Pharmaceutical variation
    (b) Pharmacokinetic variation
        (i) Pharmacogenetic variation
        (ii) Hepatic disease
        (iii) Renal disease
        (iv) Cardiac disease
        (v) Thyroid disease
        (vi) Drug interactions
    (c) Pharmacodynamic variation
        (i) Hepatic disease
        (ii) Altered fluid and electrolyte balance
        (iii) Drug interactions

(2) Non-dose-related effects
    (a) Immunological reactions
    (b) Pseudo-allergic reactions
    (c) Pharmacogenetic variation

(3) Long-term effects
    (a) Adaptive changes
    (b) Rebound phenomena
    (c) Long-term tissue damage

(4) Delayed effects
    (a) Carcinogenesis
    (b) Effects concerned with reproduction
        (i) Impaired fertility
        (ii) Teratogenesis—adverse effects on the fetus during the early stages of pregnancy
        (iii) Adverse effects on the fetus during the later stages of pregnancy
        (iv) Drugs in breast milk

ratio, since one can safely use much higher doses than one needs to treat the patient effectively. Some examples of commonly used drugs with a low toxic: therapeutic ratio (i.e. for which a small increase in dose beyond the therapeutic dose may result in toxicity) are:

- anticoagulants (e.g. warfarin, heparin);

- hypoglycaemic drugs (e.g. insulin, sulphonylureas);

- anti-arrhythmic drugs (e.g. lignocaine, amiodarone);

- cardiac glycosides (e.g. digoxin, digitoxin);

- aminoglycosides (e.g. gentamicin, netilmicin);

- oral contraceptives;

- cytotoxic and immunosuppressive drugs (e.g. methotrexate, azathioprine);

- antihypertensive drugs (e.g. hydralazine).

Dose-related adverse reactions may occur because of variations in the pharmaceutical, pharmacokinetic, or pharmacodynamic properties of a drug, often due to some disease or pharmacogenetic characteristic of the patient. The following are examples of such mechanisms.

Pharmaceutical variation

Although adverse drug reactions can occur because of some peculiarity of the pharmaceutical formulation, such reactions are uncommon. A striking example was the outbreak of pheny-

toin intoxication among epileptic patients in Australia in the late 1960s, which was found to be due to a change in one of the excipients in the phenytoin capsules from calcium sulphate to lactose, causing increased phenytoin absorption. Adverse reactions may also occur because of the presence of a contaminant, e.g. pyrogens or even bacteria in i.v. formulations, if quality control breaks down. Out-of-date formulations may sometimes cause adverse reactions, because of degradation products. For example, outdated tetracycline may cause Fanconi syndrome, because it is degraded to anhydrotetracycline and epiandrotetracycline. The omission of the preservative citric acid from tetracycline formulations has reduced the risk of this effect, but has not removed it completely. Paraldehyde that has been sitting on the shelf for 6 months degrades to acetaldehyde, which is then oxidized to the toxic product acetic acid.

Pharmacokinetic variation

There is a great deal of variation among normal individuals in the rate of elimination of drugs. This variation is most marked for drugs that are cleared by hepatic metabolism, and is determined by several factors which may be genetic, environmental (e.g. diet, smoking, alcohol), or hepatic (blood flow and intrinsic drug metabolizing capacity). On top of this normal variation there may occur specific pharmacogenetic or hepatic abnormalities that may be associated with adverse reactions. In addition, renal and cardiac disease can cause alterations in drug pharmacokinetics.

Pharmacogenetic variation

Pharmacogenetics is the study of the influence of heredity on both the pharmacokinetics of drugs and the pharmacodynamic responses to them. A list of pharmacogenetic defects is given in Table 10.10.

We shall discuss here polymorphic drug acetylation as a pharmacogenetic variable of pharmacokinetic type which can lead to adverse drug reactions. Several drugs are acetylated by the hepatic enzyme N-acetyl transferase, and the distribution of rates of acetylation in the population is bimodal (Fig. 10.9). The difference between fast and slow acetylators depends on the amount of hepatic N-acetyl transferase, rather than a change in its properties. It is known that fast acetylation is inherited as an autosomal dominant character, while slow acetylation is thought to be recessive. The ratio of fast: slow acetylators differs with race; for example, 40:60 in Europe, 85:15 in Japan, and 95:5 in the Inuit.

Drugs whose acetylation is genetically determined in this way are isoniazid, hydralazine, procainamide, phenelzine, dapsone, and some sulphonamides (e.g. sulphamethoxypyridazine and sulphapyridine). However, not all drugs which are acetylated are affected, since some are acetylated by a different enzyme outside the liver. The exceptions include sulphanilamide, *para*-aminobenzoic acid, and *para*-aminosalicylic acid.

The clinical consequences of these differences are that in slow acetylators there may be an enhanced response to treatment, but also an increased risk of drug toxicity. Thus, slow acetyl-

Table 10.10 Some genetic defects that can cause adverse drug reactions

Drug(s)	Basis of reaction	Inheritance
Pharmacokinetic defects		
Debrisoquine, phenformin, perhexilene	Poor/extensive metabolism (hydroxylation)	AR
Ethanol	Reduced metabolism	Racial (Inuit and Oriental)
Isoniazid, hydralazine, procainamide, some sulphonamides, phenelzine, dapsone	Slow/fast metabolism (acetylation)	AR/AD
Suxamethonium	Impaired metabolism (pseudocholinesterase)	AR (three types)
Pharmacodynamic defects		
Corticosteroids	Glaucoma	AR
Drugs listed in Table 10.11	Haemolysis (G6PD deficiency)	XICD
	Haemolysis (methaemoglobin reductase deficiency)	AR
	Haemolysis (glutathione reductase deficiency)	AD
Numerous	Porphyria	AD
Suxamethonium, halothane	Malignant hyperthermia	AD
Warfarin	Resistant Vitamin K epoxide reductase	AD

AD, autosomal dominant; AR, autosomal recessive; XICD, X-linked incomplete codominant.

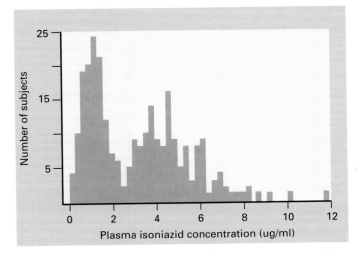

Fig. 10.9 Polymorphic acetylation, illustrated by the bimodal frequency distribution of plasma concentrations of isoniazid 6 hours after the oral administration of 9.7 mg/kg to 267 individuals of 53 families. Those with lower plasma isoniazid concentrations are fast acetylators, those with higher plasma isoniazid concentrations are slow acetylators [Adapted from Evans, Manley, and McKusick (1960). *British Medical Journal* ii, 485, with permission.]

ators have been reported to require lower doses of isoniazid and hydralazine than fast acetylators in the treatment of tuberculosis and hypertension, respectively. They are also more likely to develop the lupus erythematosus-like syndrome (see Chapter 4) caused by isoniazid, hydralazine, and procainamide, and the peripheral neuropathy (see Chapter 19) caused by isoniazid (which can be prevented or treated with pyridoxine). The interaction between isoniazid and phenytoin, in which phenytoin metabolism is inhibited by isoniazid, resulting in phenytoin toxicity, occurs more frequently among slow acetylators.

In contrast, if a metabolite were toxic, fast acetylators would be theoretically more at risk. Isoniazid is acetylated to N-acetyl-isoniazid, which in turn is hydrolysed to acetylhydrazine, and this is thought to be the precursor of a hepatotoxic metabolite. However, acetylhydrazine is itself acetylated polymorphically to diacetylhydrazine, and acetylhydrazine would therefore be expected to be removed more quickly in fast acetylators. Furthermore, although it was at one time thought that the hepatic damage associated with isoniazid was more common among fast acetylators, more recent studies suggest that the incidence of liver damage is not greater among fast acetylators, and the question is clearly more complicated than was originally thought.

The acetylator status of an individual may be easily assessed by giving a sulphonamide, such as sulphadimidine or sulphapyridine, orally and measuring the relative proportions of acetylated and total sulphonamide in a sample of urine passed 5–6 h later.

Hepatic disease

In view of the central role of hepatic metabolism in the pharmacokinetics of many drugs, it might be expected that hepatic disease would frequently be associated with impaired drug elimination. However, such is the reserve of the liver parenchyma that in practice adverse reactions due to impaired hepatic metabolism are not all that common (see Chapter 17). Nevertheless, in the presence of severe liver disease care must be taken, particularly with drugs with a low toxic:therapeutic ratio and those which are subject to extensive first-pass elimination.

Theoretically, liver dysfunction can affect drug disposition and elimination in several ways, and the outcome in an individual case may be complex and difficult to predict.

1. *Hepatocellular dysfunction*, as in severe hepatitis or advanced

cirrhosis, may reduce the clearance of drugs for which the capacity of the liver is limited, for example phenytoin, theophylline, and warfarin.

2. *Portosystemic shunting* in portal hypertension, associated with cirrhosis, reduces the clearance of drugs normally cleared by the liver, for example morphine and other narcotic analgesics, propranolol, labetalol, and chlorpromazine.

3. *A reduction in hepatic blood flow*, as in heart failure, can reduce the hepatic clearance of drugs which have a high extraction ratio. Such drugs include lignocaine, propranolol, morphine, and pethidine.

4. *Decreased plasma protein (albumin) production* by the liver in cirrhosis may lead to reduced protein binding of drugs.

5. *Drugs which are hepatotoxic* may cause reduced clearance of other drugs, even in patients with previously normal liver function.

Renal disease

If a drug or active metabolite is excreted by the kidney it will accumulate in renal failure and toxicity will occur. Important examples include digoxin, the aminoglycoside antibiotics, lithium, allopurinol, methotrexate, and procainamide. There are some drugs which are nephrotoxic and which should be avoided or used in reduced doses in patients with renal impairment. Important examples of these include nitrofurantoin, amphotericin B, the aminoglycoside antibiotics, and vancomycin.

Cardiac disease

Cardiac failure, particularly congestive cardiac failure, can alter the pharmacokinetic properties of drugs by several mechanisms:

1. *Impaired absorption*, due to intestinal mucosal oedema and a poor splanchnic circulation, can alter the efficacy of frusemide.

2. *Hepatic congestion and reduced liver blood flow* may impair the metabolism of some drugs (e.g. lignocaine).

3. *Poor renal perfusion* may result in decreased renal elimination (e.g. procainamide).

4. *Reductions in the apparent volumes of distribution* of some cardioactive drugs, by mechanisms which are not understood, cause reduced loading dose requirements (e.g. procainamide, lignocaine, and quinidine).

Thyroid disease

The hepatic metabolism of some drugs is increased in hyperthyroidism and decreased in hypothyroidism, but it is not possible to make general statements about all drugs that are metabolized. Drugs reportedly affected are methimazole (the active metabolite of carbimazole), propranolol, practolol, tolbutamide, and hydrocortisone. Plasma digoxin concentrations are increased in hypothyroidism and decreased in hyper-

thyroidism, partly because of changes in the apparent volume of distribution, and partly because of changes in renal clearance.

Drug interactions

There are many drug interactions in which the pharmacokinetics of one drug is altered by another. The most important mechanisms involved are inhibition or induction of drug metabolism and inhibition of renal excretion. Important examples include the inhibition of warfarin metabolism by antifungal imidazoles (e.g. metronidazole), chloramphenicol, and cimetidine, which can result in bleeding; the induction of oestrogen metabolism by rifampicin, carbamazepine, and phenytoin, which can result in pregnancy in a woman taking an oral contraceptive formulation; and the inhibition of lithium excretion by some diuretics, which can result in lithium toxicity.

Pharmacodynamic variation

As with pharmacokinetic variability, there is a great deal of pharmacodynamic variability within the general population, and that variability may be compounded by the effects of disease.

Hepatic disease

There are several mechanisms whereby hepatic disease may influence the pharmacodynamic responses to certain drugs:

1. *Reduced blood clotting.* In cirrhosis and acute hepatitis production of clotting factors may be impaired and patients may bleed more readily.

2. *Hepatic encephalopathy.* In patients with, or on the verge of, hepatic encephalopathy (hepatic coma or pre-coma), the brain appears to be more sensitive to the effects of drugs with sedative actions, and if such drugs are used coma may result (see Chapter 17). Diuretics used for the treatment of ascites and peripheral oedema may precipitate hepatic encephalopathy, particularly if there is too rapid a diuresis. This seems to be associated with the production of a hypokalaemic alkalosis, which in turn causes renal ammonia synthesis, resulting in ammonia retention, one of the factors which contributes to hepatic encephalopathy.

3. *Sodium and water retention.* In hepatic cirrhosis sodium and water retention may be exacerbated by certain drugs, including indomethacin and phenylbutazone, corticosteroids, carbamazepine, carbenoxolone, and preparations containing large amounts of sodium, e.g. some antacid mixtures and sodium salts of penicillins.

All of these problems may also be exacerbated by drug-induced liver damage.

Altered fluid and electrolyte balance

The pharmacodynamic effects of some drugs may be altered by changes in fluid and electrolyte balance. For example, the effects of cardiac glycosides are potentiated by both hypokalaemia and hypercalcaemia, while the effects of some anti-arrhythmic drugs, such as lignocaine, quinidine, procainamide, and disopyramide, are reduced by hypokalaemia. Hypocalcaemia prolongs the action of skeletal muscle relaxants such as tubocurarine, and fluid depletion enhances the hypotensive effects of antihypertensive drugs.

Drug interactions

There are many drug interactions in which the pharmacodynamic action of one drug is altered by another. Important examples include the potentiation of the actions of drugs acting on the brain (e.g. antihistamines, benzodiazepines, phenothiazines, lithium) by alcohol; the potentiation of the actions of cardiac glycosides due to potassium depletion secondary to diuretic therapy; and the increased risk of severe bleeding in patients taking warfarin because of impaired platelet function secondary to aspirin or sulphinpyrazone or because of gastric ulceration secondary to non-steroidal anti-inflammatory drugs.

10.4.6 Non-dose-related adverse reactions

The mechanisms of adverse reactions which are not related to dose are immunological and pharmacogenetic.

Immunological reactions (drug allergy or hypersensitivity reactions—see also Chapter 4)

The following are the features of allergic drug reactions:

1. There is no relation to the usual pharmacological effects of the drug.

2. There is often a delay between the first exposure to the drug and the occurrence of the subsequent adverse reaction.

3. There is no formal dose–response curve, and very small doses of the drug may elicit the reaction once allergy is established.

4. The reaction disappears on discontinuation of the drug.

5. The illness is often recognizable as an immunological reaction, e.g. rash, serum sickness, anaphylaxis, asthma, urticaria, angio-oedema, etc.

The factors involved in drug allergy concern the drug and the patient.

The drug

Macromolecules such as proteins (e.g. vaccines), polypeptides (e.g. insulin), and dextrans can themselves be immunogenic. Smaller molecules may act as haptens and combine with body proteins to form antigens. Little is known about the exact nature of many of the haptens (drugs or their metabolites) involved in immunological reactions to drugs. One exception is penicillin, for which the major antigenic determinant is known to be the penicilloyl group which is formed after the splitting of the β-lactam ring.

The patient

Some patients are more likely to develop allergic drug reactions than others. These include patients with a history of atopic disease (eczema, asthma, or hay fever), those with hereditary angio-oedema, and those with a history of previous allergic drug reactions.

There is evidence that the syndrome mimicking systemic lupus erythematosus produced by hydralazine occurs with increased frequency in patients with the HLA DR4 tissue type.

Drug allergy—a mechanistic approach

Drug allergy and its manifestations are classifiable according to the classification of hypersensitivity reactions, i.e. into four types, Types I–IV. However, in practice it is not so easy to classify allergic drug reactions in this fashion because they present as clinical syndromes.

Type I reactions (anaphylaxis; immediate hypersensitivity)

In this type of reaction the drug or metabolite interacts with IgE molecules fixed to cells, particularly tissue mast cells and basophil leucocytes. This triggers a process which leads to the release of pharmacological mediators (histamine, 5-hydroxytryptamine, kinins, and arachidonic acid derivatives) which cause the allergic response.

Clinically, Type I reactions manifest as urticaria, rhinitis, bronchial asthma, angio-oedema, and anaphylactic shock. Drugs likely to cause anaphylactic shock include penicillins, streptomycin, local anaesthetics, and radio-opaque iodide-containing X-ray contrast media.

Type II reactions (cytotoxic reactions)

In Type II reactions a circulating antibody of the IgG, IgM, or IgA class interacts with a hapten (drug) combined with a cell membrane constituent (protein), to form an antigen–antibody complex. Complement is then activated and cell lysis occurs. Most examples are haematological: thrombocytopenia associated with quinidine or quinine ('gin and tonic purpura'), digitoxin, and occasionally rifampicin; neutropenia due to phenylbutazone, carbimazole, tolbutamide, anticonvulsants, chlorpropamide, or metronidazole; haemolytic anaemia due to penicillins, cephalosporins, rifampicin, quinine, and quinidine.

Type III reactions (immune-complex reactions)

In Type III reactions antibody (IgG) combines with antigen (drug hapten–protein) in the circulation. The complex thus formed is deposited in the tissues, complement is activated, and damage to capillary endothelium results.

Serum sickness is the typical drug reaction of this type and is manifested most commonly by fever, arthritis, enlarged lymph nodes, urticaria, and maculopapular rashes. Penicillins, streptomycin, sulphonamides, and antithyroid drugs may be responsible. Another example of a Type III reaction is the acute interstitial nephritis which may be caused by penicillins and some non-steroidal anti-inflammatory drugs.

Type IV reactions (cell-mediated or delayed hypersensitivity reactions)

In Type IV reactions T lymphocytes are 'sensitized' by a drug hapten–protein antigenic complex. When the lymphocytes come into contact with the antigen an inflammatory response ensues. Type IV reactions are exemplified by the contact dermatitis caused by local anaesthetic creams, antihistamine creams, and topical antibiotics and antifungal drugs.

Pseudo-allergic reactions

We include these reactions here for convenience. 'Pseudo-allergy' is a term applied to reactions which resemble allergic reactions clinically but for which no immunological basis can be found. An example is the asthma and skin rashes caused by aspirin. In a proportion of asthmatics aspirin may trigger an attack of asthma. This may be associated with nasal polyposis in cases of extrinsic asthma and with sinusitis in intrinsic asthma (see Chapter 13). Aspirin-sensitive asthmatics are often sensitive to other salicylates and to other non-steroidal anti-inflammatory drugs, such as indomethacin and ibuprofen. In addition, about 50 per cent of aspirin-sensitive asthmatics are also sensitive to tartrazine, a yellow dye used as a colouring agent in some drug formulations and foodstuffs. In about a third of patients with chronic urticaria, aspirin may make the rash worse.

In some patients the administration of ampicillin or amoxycillin causes a maculopapular erythematous skin rash which resembles the toxic erythema which can occur in penicillin hypersensitivity. However, there is no evidence that the ampicillin rash, as it is called, is immunological in origin. It can be distinguished from true penicillin hypersensitivity on the basis of two features. First, it has a later onset after the first time of administration (typically 10–14 days compared with 7–10 days in penicillin hypersensitivity, although there is some overlap). Secondly, the ampicillin rash does not necessarily recur following re-exposure to ampicillin or amoxycillin, and it is not associated with an increased risk of a serious allergic response to other penicillins. This contrasts with penicillin hypersensitivity, in which further exposure to any member of the penicillin group is contraindicated because of the high risk of a fatal allergic reaction. The ampicillin rash occurs in about 1 per cent of the normal population, but its incidence is greatly increased in some groups of patients, and it occurs almost invariably in patients with some viral infections (e.g. infectious mononucleosis, cytomegalovirus infection, measles), lymphomas, and leukaemias. It is also more common in patients who are also taking allopurinol; the reason for this is not known.

Drug allergy—a clinical approach

As mentioned above, the mechanistic approach does not always fit the clinical presentation. The following are the syndromes with which one is usually faced in clinical practice.

Fever
- For example, this can occur with penicillin, phenytoin, hydralazine, and quinidine therapy.

Rashes (see also Chapter 28)
- Toxic erythema, commonly due to antibiotics (e.g. penicillins), sulphonamides, thiazide diuretics, frusemide, sulphonylureas, and phenylbutazone.
- Urticaria, e.g. penicillins, codeine, dextrans, and X-ray contrast media.
- Erythema multiforme and Stevens–Johnson syndrome, e.g. penicillins, sulphonamides, barbiturates, and phenylbutazone.
- Erythema nodosum, e.g. sulphonamides and occasionally oral contraceptives.
- Cutaneous vasculitis, e.g. sulphonamides, phenylbutazone, thiazide diuretics, allopurinol, indomethacin, phenytoin, and alclofenac.
- Non-thrombocytopenic purpura, e.g. corticosteroids, thiazide diuretics, and meprobamate.
- Exfoliative dermatitis and erythroderma, e.g. gold salts, phenylbutazone, isoniazid, and carbamazepine.
- Photosensitivity, e.g. sulphonamides, thiazide diuretics, sulphonylureas, tetracyclines, phenothiazines, and nalidixic acid.
- Fixed eruptions, e.g. phenolphthalein, barbiturates, sulphonamides, and tetracyclines.
- Toxic epidermal necrolysis (Lyell's syndrome), e.g. phenytoin, sulphonamides, gold salts, tetracyclines, allopurinol, and phenylbutazone.

Connective tissue disease
- Lupus-like syndrome, e.g. hydralazine, procainamide, phenytoin, and ethosuximide.
Polyarteritis nodosa, e.g. sulphonamides.

Blood disorders
- Thrombocytopenia, neutropenia, haemolytic anaemia, and aplastic anaemia may all occur as adverse drug reactions to a large number of drugs.

Pharmacogenetic variation causing non-dose-related reactions

Some pharmacogenetic abnormalities that can result in altered pharmacodynamic responses to drugs are listed in Table 10.10. Here we shall discuss glucose-6-phosphate dehydrogenase (G6PD) deficiency and porphyria.

Glucose-6-phosphate dehydrogenase (G6PD) deficiency

There are three different but functionally related enzymes in erythrocytes responsible for the maintenance of the oxidative status of the cell. They are glucose-6-phosphate dehydrogenase (G6PD), glutathione reductase, and methaemoglobin reductase, and the metabolic interrelationships of the reactions which they catalyse are shown in Fig. 10.10. G6PD catalyses the oxidation of glucose-6-phosphate to phosphogluconate, from which pentose-5-monophosphate is eventually generated. Although this phosphogluconate pathway is relatively unimportant as a route of glycolysis, it is important as a source of reduced NADP (i.e. NADPH). NADPH in turn is an important

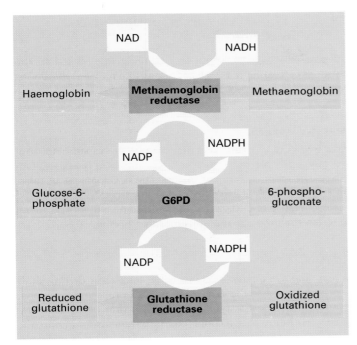

Fig. 10.10 The reactions catalysed by glucose-6-phosphate dehydrogenase (G6PD), methaemoglobin reductase, and glutathione reductase in red cells, and their metabolic interrelationships. Deficiency of G6PD or of glutathione reductase may result in haemolysis on exposure to certain drugs (see Table 10.11). Deficiency of methaemoglobin reductase may result in methaemoglobinaemia on exposure to these drugs. (Drawn after Grahame-Smith and Aronson 1984, with permission.)

electron donor in the reaction, catalysed by glutathione reductase, in which oxidized glutathione is converted to reduced glutathione, which in turn is necessary for the prevention of the oxidation of various cell proteins. Although NADPH also acts as an electron donor for the reduction of methaemoglobin by one

of the enzymes in the methaemoglobin reductase complex, this is a relatively unimportant pathway for methaemoglobin reduction, and the enzyme for which NADH acts as an electron donor is more important (see below).

Lack of G6PD in erythrocytes results in diminished production of NADPH. Consequently, oxidized glutathione (and to a lesser and insignificant extent methaemoglobin) accumulates. If the erythrocyte is then exposed to oxidizing agents, haemolysis occurs, probably because of unopposed oxidation of sulphydryl groups in the cell membrane, which are normally kept in reduced form by the continuous availability of reduced glutathione. The prevalence of this defect varies with race. It is rare among Caucasians, and occurs most frequently among Sephardic Jews of Asiatic origin, of whom 50 per cent or more are affected. It also occurs in about 10–20 per cent of Blacks.

Inheritance of the defect is complex, the enzyme being heterogeneous. There are, broadly speaking, two enzyme varieties, the Negro and the Mediterranean. In the Negro variety G6PD production is probably normal, but its degradation is accelerated, so that only old red cells (those older than about 55 days) are affected. In this form acute haemolysis occurs on first administration of the drug and lasts for only a few days. Thereafter continued administration causes chronic mild haemolysis (Fig. 10.11). In the Mediterranean variety the enzyme is abnormal, and both young and old cells are affected. In this form severe haemolysis occurs on first administration and is maintained with continued administration.

The commonly used drugs which may cause haemolysis in susceptible individuals are listed in Table 10.11. The reaction is sometimes called 'favism' because it may result from eating broad beans (*Vicia faba*), which contain an oxidant alkaloid.

Deficiencies of both glutathione reductase and methaemoglobin reductase also occur and are associated with haemolysis on exposure to oxidant drugs such as those listed in Table 10.11.

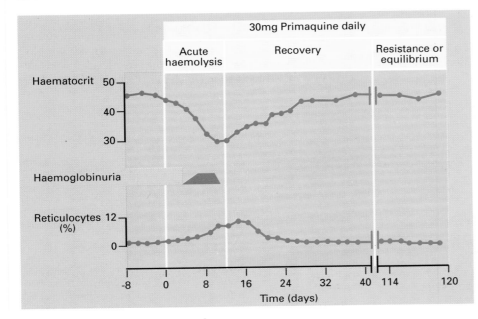

Fig. 10.11 The time-course of haemolysis on exposure to primaquine in a subject with the Negro variety of G6PD deficiency. The abnormality in this variety is accelerated degradation of G6PD. (Drawn after Alving, Johnson, Tarlov, Brewer, Kellermeyer, and Carson (1960). *Bulletin of the World Health Organization* **22**, 621, with the permission of the WHO.)

Table 10.11 Drugs which may precipitate haemolysis in subjects with G6PD, methaemoglobin reductase, and glutathione reductase enzyme deficiencies

(a) **Drugs with the most marked effect**	(b) **Drugs with possible risk in some individuals**
Dapsone and other sulphones	Analgesics
Methylene blue	antipyrine, salicylates
Nalidixic acid	Antimalarials
Niridazole	chloroquine, mepacrine,
Nitrofurantoin	quinidine, quinine
Pamaquine	Sulphonamides other than
Primaquine	those listed in group (a)
Sulphonamides	Others
sulphafurazole	chloramphenicol,
sulphamethoxazole	dimercaprol,
sulphanilamide	probenecid,
sulphapyridine	vitamin K
sulphasalazine	

Note: Warfarin and phenylbutazone have been implicated in glutathione reductase deficiency, and nitrates in methaemoglobin reductase deficiency.

Porphyria

The hepatic porphyrias, which include acute intermittent porphyria and porphyria cutanea tarda, are characterized by abnormalities of haem biosynthesis. The main biochemical pathways are shown in Fig. 10.12.

The activity of δ-aminolaevulinic acid (ALA) synthase, the rate-limiting enzyme, is increased in porphyria, resulting in excess production of ALA and porphobilinogen (PBG), and of the porphyrins down the pathway alternative to haem biosynthesis. Haem normally acts as a repressor of ALA synthase activity, and this action is reduced because of reduced haem synthesis. The mechanisms by which some drugs may precipitate an attack of porphyria are not fully understood, but involve an increase in ALA synthase activity. Drugs which are enzyme inducers (e.g. carbamazepine, phenobarbitone, phenytoin, rifampicin) may act by diverting haem to the synthesis of cytochrome P_{450}, thereby derepressing ALA synthase activity.

Many drugs have been incriminated as being likely to precipitate acute attacks of porphyria in susceptible subjects, and extensive lists can be found elsewhere (Moore and Disler 1983).

10.4.7 Long-term effects causing adverse reactions

Adverse effects listed under this heading are related to the duration of treatment as well as to dose, and may be regarded as being related to some function of the two.

Adaptive changes

Adaptive changes can sometimes occur in response to drug therapy, and sometimes such changes can form the basis of an adverse reaction. Examples include the development of tolerance to and physical dependence on the narcotic analgesics and the occurrence of tardive dyskinesia in some patients receiving long-term neuroleptic therapy for schizophrenia.

Rebound phenomena

When adaptive changes occur during long-term therapy sudden withdrawal of the drug may result in rebound reactions. Examples include the typical syndromes that occur after the sudden withdrawal of alcohol (delirium tremens) or of narcotic analgesics. Sudden withdrawal of barbiturates may result in restlessness, mental confusion, and convulsions. A similar syndrome, in which anxiety features prominently, may occur after the sudden withdrawal of benzodiazepines. Sleeplessness may also be a feature of the sudden withdrawal of these and a variety of other hypnotic drugs. Sudden withdrawal of some antihypertensive drugs may result in rebound hypertension and is particularly common with clonidine. Sudden withdrawal of β-adrenoceptor antagonists may also cause rebound effects, especially worsening of pre-existing cardiac ischaemia.

In a separate category is the effect of the sudden withdrawal of corticosteroids. During long-term treatment with corticosteroids there is interference with the normal feedback system involving the hypothalamus, pituitary gland, and adrenal glands. As a result, the hypothalamus and pituitary become unable to react normally to the stimulus of low circulating concentrations of corticosteroids and the adrenal glands atrophy. After sudden withdrawal the syndrome of acute adrenal insufficiency occurs. The extent to which this effect occurs depends on

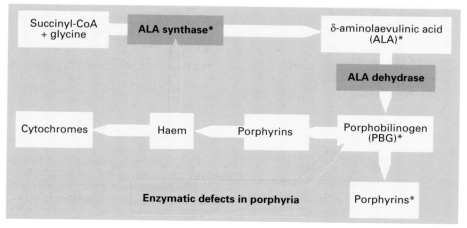

Fig. 10.12 Some abnormalities of haem biosynthesis in patients with porphyria. *Increased in hepatic porphyria. (Drawn after Grahame-Smith and Aronson 1984, with permission.)

both the daily dose and the duration of treatment, and it can to some extent be minimized by giving twice the usual dose but on alternate days. If corticosteroids have to be given every day, in cases where the therapeutic response is poor with alternate-day therapy, hypothalamic–pituitary–adrenal axis suppression can be reduced by giving the dose in the morning.

Reversal of the effects of heparin with protamine sulphate may be associated with rebound hypercoagulability and an increased risk of thromboembolism.

Long-term tissue damage

Chloroquine, used in malaria prophylaxis, has a particular affinity for melanin. It may accumulate in the corneal epithelium, causing a keratopathy, and in the retina, causing a pigmentary retinopathy. The former occurs in about 30–70 per cent of patients after 1–2 months of therapy, but although the latter is less common it is more serious. The risk increases with daily doses of over 500 mg and in patients also taking probenecid.

Chronic ingestion of analgesic mixtures, particularly those containing phenacetin, causes papillary and medullary necrosis in the kidneys, accompanied by renal tubular atrophy (see Chapter 18). Later the degenerative and fibrotic changes may extend into the cortex and produce glomerular damage and an interstitial nephritis. There is still some confusion about the precise type of analgesic responsible for analgesic nephropathy. Undoubtedly phenacetin was the main culprit in the past. However, some have suggested that the nephropathy associated with phenacetin was due to the combination of phenacetin with aspirin, and it is possible that phenacetin metabolites are concentrated in the renal medulla, and that the normal tissue response there to oxidative damage is impaired by aspirin.

Some of the long-term adverse effects of amiodarone are caused by the deposition in the tissues of lipofucsin, and may mimic the appearances of systemic lipoidoses. These effects include a neuropathy, pulmonary alveolitis, liver damage, microdeposits in the cornea, and an increased sensitivity of the skin to sunlight.

10.4.8 Delayed effects causing adverse reactions

A simple example of a delayed adverse drug effect is that of hypothyroidism occurring years after the treatment of hyperthyroidism with radioactive iodine, ^{131}I. However, this is a recognized and acceptable risk of this form of treatment, whereas our other examples are adverse effects which are highly unacceptable.

Carcinogenesis

The subject of the production of tumours in man through the actions of drugs is a confused and difficult one. Because it is seldom possible, on clinical and pathological grounds, to distinguish in an individual a 'naturally occurring' tumour from one produced by an identifiable chemical carcinogen, one has to rely on statistical associations, and these are not easy to observe

in a condition whose pathogenesis involves an indefinite period of exposure to a carcinogen (and possibly other chemical substances) and a latent period for development (see Section 9.6). There are three major mechanisms that are currently considered to be important in carcinogenesis.

Hormonal

There is a clear increase in the occurrence of vaginal adenocarcinoma in the daughters of women who have received stilboestrol during pregnancy for the treatment of threatened abortion. The extent to which there are changes in the incidences of various tumours in women taking oestrogens, and in particular oral contraceptive formulations, is not settled. However, there is probably an increase in the incidence of uterine endometrial carcinoma in women receiving oestrogen replacement therapy for menopausal symptoms, and oral contraceptives increase the incidence of benign liver tumours.

Gene toxicity

This term is used to cloak the mystery of what happens when certain molecules bind to nuclear DNA and produce changes in gene expression, leading to abnormalities of cell growth and the production of tumours. In man it is sometimes difficult to divorce this mechanism from suppression of the immune response (see below). There are some examples of drug-induced tumours which might fall into this class:

1. the increased risk of bladder cancer in patients taking long-term cyclophosphamide;

2. carcinomas of the renal pelvis associated with phenacetin abuse;

3. the occurrence of non-lymphocytic leukaemias in patients receiving alkylating agents, such as melphalan, cyclophosphamide, and chlorambucil.

Suppression of immune responses

Patients receiving immunosuppressive drug regimens, such as azathioprine with corticosteroids, have a greatly increased risk of developing lymphomas. This has been noted mainly after renal transplantation, but has been seen in other patients also. In immunosuppressed patients there also seems to be an increased risk of cancers of the liver, biliary tree, and bladder, of soft tissue sarcomas, bronchial adenocarcinoma, squamous carcinoma of the skin, and malignant melanoma.

There is probably an association between the occurrence of lymphoma and the long-term use of phenytoin, although at present this does not influence the prescribing of phenytoin for the treatment of epilepsy.

Adverse effects associated with reproduction

Impaired fertility

While impaired fertility due to drugs in women is a desired effect in the case of oral contraceptives, it may be an unwanted effect of other drugs. For example, cytotoxic drugs may cause female infertility through ovarian failure. Impairment of male fertility can be caused by impairment of spermatozoal production or function and may be either reversible or irreversible:

1. Reversible impairment may be caused by sulphasalazine, nitrofurantoin, monoamine oxidase (MAO) inhibitors, and antimalarials.

2. Reversible impairment leading to irreversible impairment, due to azospermia, can be caused by cytotoxic drugs, such as the alkylating agents cyclophosphamide and chlorambucil.

Teratogenesis—adverse effects on the fetus during the early stages of pregnancy

Teratogenesis occurs when a drug taken during the early stages of pregnancy causes a developmental abnormality in a fetus. The potential for doing harm to the fetus by prescribing drugs for the mother during pregnancy is considerable, as was emphasized by the thalidomide disaster. It is thought that about 35 per cent of women take drug therapy at least once during pregnancy and 6 per cent during the first trimester (this excludes iron, folic acid, and vitamins). The most commonly used drugs are simple analgesics, antibacterial drugs, and antacids.

For a drug to affect the development of a fetus it must first pass across the placental barrier. Most drugs pass across the placenta by simple diffusion, which depends in part upon molecular size, degree of ionization, and lipid solubility. Thus, drugs that are of low molecular weight, poorly ionized at physiological pH, and very fat soluble will pass across the placenta readily. The drugs that do not pass across the placenta illustrate these principles. For example, heparin is ionized and of high molecular weight; tubocurarine is ionized and relatively lipid insoluble; neither of these drugs crosses the placenta. However, most drugs in the maternal circulation do reach the fetus to some extent, and since the thalidomide incident great care has been taken about prescribing drugs during pregnancy, particularly during the early stages (i.e. the first trimester). Furthermore, during the development of a drug its potential for teratogenesis has to be explored if there is any likelihood of its being promoted for use in women of child-bearing age. The first trimester of pregnancy, and particularly the period from the second to the eighth weeks of gestation, the period of organogenesis, is the most critical. During this time drugs may cause structural abnormalities. Later in fetal life drugs may affect the subsequent growth, development, and integrity of body structures, particularly the brain.

Table 10.12 lists the drugs that should be avoided during early pregnancy because of the effects on the fetus, or because of a slightly increased risk of fetal abnormality.

Adverse effects on the fetus during the later stages of pregnancy

There are some drugs that are not teratogenic, but which may cause adverse effects in the fetus if given later in pregnancy. These include drugs that may be given immediately before and during labour, and which can cause problems in the neonate. Some of these drugs should also be avoided during early pregnancy. Table 10.13 lists drugs which should be avoided or used with care during later pregnancy. Note that some of these drugs also appear in Table 10.12.

Adverse reactions to drugs in breast milk

Certain drugs are excreted in breast milk to an extent that is

Table 10.12 Drugs to avoid during early pregnancy

Drug	Effect
Drugs with a high risk of producing abnormalities (known teratogens)	
Androgens	Virilization and multiple congenital defects
Antineoplastic agents	Multiple congenital defects
Corticosteroids in high dosages	Cleft palate
Diethylstilboestrol	Vaginal adenosis and adenocarcinoma in daughters
Tetracyclines	Yellow discoloration of teeth, inhibition of bone growth
Warfarin	Multiple congenital defects
Drugs under strong suspicion of producing abnormalities (slightly increased risk)	
Chloroquine (do not withhold in acute malaria)	Deafness
Lithium	Cardiovascular defects
Phenytoin (do not withhold if absolutely necessary for control of epilepsy)	Multiple congenital defects
Other drugs to avoid (theoretical risk from animal and other studies)	
Co-trimoxazole, rifampicin, sulphonylureas, trimethoprim	
There is a possible teratogenic risk from general anaesthesia during early pregnancy	

Table 10.13 Drugs to be avoided or used with care during later pregnancy

Drug(s)	Risk to fetus or neonate
Aspirin	Kernicterus, haemorrhage (also maternal)
Aminoglycoside antibiotics	Eighth nerve damage
Antithyroid drugs	Goitre and hypothyroidism
Benzodiazepines	Floppy infant syndrome
Chloramphenicol	Peripheral vascular collapse ('grey syndrome')
Oral anticoagulants	Fetal or retroplacental haemorrhage, microcephaly
Sulphonylureas	Hypoglycaemia
Pethidine	Respiratory depression
Reserpine	Bradycardia, hypothermia, nasal congestion with respiratory distress
Sulphonamides and novobiocin	Kernicterus
Tetracyclines	Abnormalities of bones and teeth
Thiazide diuretics	Thrombocytopenia

likely to affect the infant, while others are known to be safe. The problem of adverse drug effects in infants because of ingestion via the breast milk is determined by the following factors:

1. the passage of the drug from the maternal blood into the milk;
2. the concentration of the drug in the milk;
3. the volume of milk sucked;
4. the pharmacokinetics of the drug in the infant, particularly his/her ability to eliminate the drug;
5. the inherent toxicity of the drug.

A list of drugs that may cause adverse effects in a breast-fed infant is given in Table 10.14.

This list includes drugs that are excreted in breast milk to an extent likely to cause dose-related adverse effects in the infant, and drugs that do not necessarily enter the milk in large amounts, but whose adverse effects are not dose-related. The latter include drugs that may cause hypersensitivity reactions even in the small quantities excreted in breast milk (e.g. penicillins and sulphonamides), and drugs that are hazardous to babies with G6PD deficiency (e.g. nitrofurantoin; see Table 10.11). Some drugs are hazardous for more than one reason (e.g. sulphonamides, which can cause kernicterus in any baby and haemolysis in G6PD-deficient babies).

10.4.9 Surveillance methods used in detecting adverse drug reactions

During the period of clinical trial which a drug undergoes before its general release none but the most frequent of adverse reactions will be picked up, despite meticulous monitoring, because so few patients are studied. Table 10.15 shows the numbers of patients usually studied during the various stages of the de-

Table 10.14 Drugs and breast feeding

Some drugs to be avoided in breast-feeding mothers
Antineoplastic drugs
Antithyroid drugs
Benzodiazepines
Chloral derivatives
Chloramphenicol
Corticosteroids (high dosages)
Ergot alkaloids
Erythromycin
Immunosuppressive drugs
Indanedione anticoagulants
Isoniazid
Lithium
Methysergide
Metronidazole
Nalidixic acid
Nitrofurantoin
Oral contraceptives
Oral hypoglycaemics
Penicillins
Phenytoin
Radioactive iodine
Streptomycin
Sulphonamides
Tetracyclines
Vitamin D
Xanthines

Some drugs that appear to be safe
ACTH (corticotropin)
Adrenaline
β-adrenoceptor antagonists (but monitor neonate for bradycardia and hypoglycaemia)
Amitriptyline
Anti-asthmatic drugs (inhalations)
Antihistamines (H$_1$ antagonists)
Carbamazepine
Heparin
Hydralazine
Imipramine
Insulin
Methyldopa
Neuroleptics (moderate dosages, e.g. chlorpromazine, haloperidol)
Nortriptyline
Thyroxine
Valproate
Warfarin

velopment of a drug before it is marketed for sale or prescription. The total is usually less than 2500.

In contrast, Table 10.16 shows the numbers of patients one would have to study in order to detect only one, two, or three adverse events for a given incidence of adverse reactions in the treated population. On this basis only adverse reactions with a relatively high incidence will be picked up before marketing. Note, however, that the numbers in Table 10.16 refer to an adverse event which has no background incidence, i.e. which does not occur as a 'natural disease' or as one that is induced by something other than a drug. However, not many adverse drug reactions are like that—they tend to mimic the signs and symptoms of non-drug-induced diseases. In these circumstances it becomes even more difficult to detect an adverse drug reaction.

If only the most common of adverse reactions are going to be

Table 10.15   Numbers of patients usually recruited in pre-marketing studies

Phase I	Volunteer or very early patient studies	25–50
Phase II	Clinical pharmacology in patients	50–100
Phase III	Dose-finding and early efficacy studies	100–250
Phase IV	Extended clinical studies leading to marketing	250–1000 (rarely >2000)
Total		Usually fewer than 2500

Table 10.16   Numbers of patients one would need to observe to have a 95 per cent of detecting 1, 2, or 3 cases of an adverse reaction at a given incidence of the reaction (with no background incidence of the reaction)

Expected incidence of adverse reaction	Numbers of patients to be observed to detect one, two, or three events		
	1	2	3
1 in 100	300	480	650
1 in 200	600	960	1300
1 in 1000	3000	4800	6500
1 in 2000	6000	9600	13 000
1 in 10 000	30 000	48 000	65 000

detected during the pre-marketing stage, it is important to devise methods for detecting adverse reactions as quickly as possible after marketing, for confirming that the events detected are truly adverse reactions, and for assessing their overall incidence, in order to be able to make some evaluation of the balance of benefit and risk.

Methods of surveillance

Anecdotal reporting

We are still largely dependent upon anecdotal reports from individual doctors that a patient has suffered some peculiar effect for the majority of 'first reports' of adverse drug reactions. An example of the value of astute observation by individuals was the detection in 1974 of the oculomucocutaneous syndrome (dry eyes, corneal damage, a skin rash which was likened to psoriasis, and sclerosing peritonitis) due to practolol. The propensity of halothane to cause jaundice on repeated administration was first brought to light by anecdotal reports, as was the effect of chloramphenicol in causing neutropenia. Of course, such anecdotal reports need to be verified by further studies, and these sometimes fail to confirm a problem. Nevertheless, the skill of individual observant clinicians is still a valuable force in the detection of adverse drug reactions. Pathologists also have a role to play, since they may be able to detect pathological events that occur in association with drug use, e.g. small bowel ulceration and perforation due to potassium in some types of delayed- or slow-release formulations (see also Chapter 16).

Voluntary but organized reporting

In the UK the Committee on Safety of Medicines (CSM) has established a scheme for the voluntary reporting of suspected adverse drug reactions. Doctors are encouraged to report suspected adverse drug reactions as soon as possible after detection on a yellow form (the 'yellow card') and may at a later date receive a follow-up request for more information. Every doctor is urged to report a suspected adverse reaction to the CSM on a yellow card. At that stage it does not matter if the reported reaction is a true reaction, since the system is designed to detect patterns of reporting that may implicate a particular drug from the conjunction of a handful of similar reports.

This system suffers from various problems. For example, it is difficult to be ingenious enough to spot an adverse effect which you do not know exists. Furthermore, there is a natural desire to report an adverse reaction that one has just heard about, and not to report those about which everybody already knows; this introduces an element of bias into the system. Finally, there is a tendency to under-report, mainly because of indolence. Despite these difficulties, this organized voluntary system of reporting in the UK has provided extremely useful information on the occurrence of adverse drug reactions in the national community. Coupling these occurrence figures with the figures on the numbers of prescriptions issued (information which is available from the Prescription Pricing Authority, UK) the frequency of a given adverse drug reaction can be very roughly calculated. Although the system has not often been responsible for the initial detection of an adverse reaction, it has been helpful in monitoring adverse drug reactions in the national community, in validating adverse reactions, and in assessing in a large population the risk of an adverse reaction relative to the potential benefit of treatment. This in turn has led to the formulation of specific advice to doctors about prescribing, or warnings not to prescribe a drug in particular cicumstances. In serious cases a drug may be taken off the market or have its uses restricted because of this kind of monitoring, as happened with benoxaprofen and practolol. In those cases the risk of adverse reactions was thought to be greater than the potential benefits.

Other systems of post-marketing surveillance

Because of the imperfections of voluntary reporting systems other surveillance methods have been tried or considered, but for various reasons none has yet proved completely satisfactory. What one needs is: speed of detection; an estimate of the incidence or prevalence of the reaction in the population receiving the drug; and clues to the factors involved (e.g. age, sex, concurrent diseases, concurrent drug therapy). From information of this kind one may be able to estimate the benefit:risk ratio and even be able to give advice that will allow the prescriber to prevent the adverse reaction.

The types of systems that have been developed include inten-

Table 10.17 Advantages and disadvantages of various post-marketing surveillance schemes

Scheme	Advantages	Disadvantages
Anecdotal reports	Simple; cheap	Rely on individual vigilance and astuteness; detect only common effects
Voluntary organized reporting	Simple	Under-reporting; bias by 'bandwagon' effect
Intensive event monitoring	Easily organized	Selected population studied; monitoring for only a short time
Cohort studies	Can be prospective; good at detecting effects	Very large numbers required; very expensive
Case-control studies	Excellent for validation and assessment	Will not detect new effects; expensive
Population statistics	Large numbers can be studied	Difficult to co-ordinate; quality of information may be poor; too coarse
Record linkage	Excellent if comprehensive	Time-consuming; relies on accurate records; retrospective; expensive

sive event recording, cohort studies (prospective studies), case-control studies (retrospective studies), the use of population statistics, and record linkage. The various advantages and disadvantages of the different schemes are outlined in Table 10.17.

10.4.10 Further reading

Benet, L. Z. (ed.) (1976). *The effect of disease states on drug pharmacokinetics*. American Pharmaceutical Association, Academy of Pharmaceutical Sciences, Washington, DC.

D'Arcy, P. F. and Griffin, J. P. (1986). *Iatrogenic diseases* (3rd edn). Oxford University Press, Oxford.

Davies, D. M. (ed.) (1986). *Textbook of adverse drug reactions* (3rd edn). Oxford University Press, Oxford.

Dukes, M. N. G. (ed.) (1989). *Meyler's side effects of drugs*, Vol. 11. Elsevier, Amsterdam. (With yearly update volumes.)

Eskes, T. K. A. B. and Finster, M. (1985). *Drug therapy during pregnancy*. Butterworths, London.

Grahame-Smith, D. G. and Aronson, J. K. (1984). *The Oxford textbook of clinical pharmacology and drug therapy*. Oxford University Press, Oxford.

Mann, R. D. (ed.) (1987). *Adverse drug reactions*. Parthenon, Lancashire.

Moore, M. R. and Disler, P. B. (1983). Drug-induction of the acute porphyrias. *Advances in Drug Reactions and Acute Poisons Review* **2**, 149.

Rubin, P. C. (ed.) (1987). *Prescribing in pregnancy*. British Medical Journal, London.

Stockley, I. (1981). *Drug interactions*. Blackwell Scientific Publications, Oxford.

Walker, S. R. and Goldberg, A. (eds) (1983). *Monitoring for adverse drug reactions*. MTP Press, Lancaster.

10.5 Photopathology

I. A. Magnus

10.5.1 Historical introduction

Medical photobiology of the modern era started at the end of the nineteenth century with the discoveries of Niels Finsen, a medical and scientific investigator of exceptional talent. He studied the therapy of lupus vulgaris, a skin disease, now rare but then very common, due to the tubercule bacillus. Finsen found that ultraviolet radiation (UVR) in the narrow wavelength region of what is now known as UV-B was the most effective therapeutically. The radiation was focused with hollow quartz lenses filled with water to reduce heat transmission. Glass lenses were ineffective because they absorbed too much UVR, but quartz lenses were satisfactory because they allowed UVR transmission. These simple observations are basic in the understanding of radiative and photobiological processes and illustrate well simple scientific methods and logical assessment of medical therapy.

Finsen died young at the turn of the century and in the immediate subsequent decades medical photobiology underwent a decline. The use of light for therapy (phototherapy) for the most part became debased and a part of quack medicine. Since then, and until more recently, it had become widely accepted that UVR was generally noxious and that visible light was interesting only because of its part in vision. Sunlight exposure of the skin became a leisure cult and tanning associated with the idea of good health. Only slowly has it been accepted that solar exposure has an important role in provoking skin ageing and cancer.

Photobiology has now even entered media sensationalism and popular controversy through the issues of 'environmental' chemical pollution. Thus an increase in atmospheric CO_2 is thought possibly to raise the Earth's temperature through the 'greenhouse' effect. But depletion of the atmospheric ozone layer is thought possibly to lead to an increase in the UVR reaching the Earth's surface. Present evidence confirms this. Increased solar UVR could be very likely to have widespread harmful effects, both biological and physical. For instances UVR reduces cell-mediated immune responses by inactivating epidermal Langerhans cells with subsequent elicitation of T-suppressor lymphocytes (see Chapter 4).

The only definitely beneficial action of UVR on humans turned out to be its role in vitamin D synthesis. Vitamin D is synthesized from precursors in the skin, mostly in the malpighian and basal layer, after absorbing radiation in the UV-B spectrum in sunlight. The main precursor is 7-dehydro-cholestrol and is photoconverted to pre-vitamin D_3. The latter undergoes thermal isomerization and is carried in the bloodstream to the liver where it is hydroxylated to 25-hydroxy-vitamin D_3 and then in the kidney to 1,25-dihydroxyvitamin D_3. The last is the active anti-rachitic vitamin.

The importance of sunlight treatment (heliotherapy) and UVR from artificial light sources (phototherapy) in providing vitamin D soon disappeared, as in many instances the vitamin is more easily supplied in the diet or an oil or tablet by mouth. Also, heliotherapy for tuberculosis was superseded by efficient antibiotic drugs such as streptomycin.

More recently, phototherapy and photomedicine have made a comeback. It is noteworthy that modern phototherapy, unlike that in an earlier era (1910–40), is supported by a seemingly sound theoretical background, as in the photochemical processes underlying so-called photodynamic action. But, with two exceptions, dependable clinical success still evades many kinds of phototherapy. The exceptions are PUVA photochemotherapy for psoriasis and blue-light therapy for neonatal jaundice. Lasers exploit mostly the thermal effects of very intense radiation; as a 'light knife' they are beginning to show promise in some branches of surgery.

10.5.2 Photobiology: theoretical background

An understanding of the physiological and pathological effects of non-ionizing radiation requires a grasp of the properties of the electromagnetic spectrum. From this, one can understand basic photochemistry and photobiology. These photobiological and photochemical effects, it must be noted, should be clearly separated from radiobiological and radiochemical effects, dealt with in another section (see Section 10.6.2).

Electromagnetic spectrum

This is depicted in Fig. 10.13 in terms of wavelength, which is convenient for characterizing the ultraviolet and visible parts of the spectrum. However, photochemical reactions are more easily described in terms of the quantum theory, viz. with photons instead of wavelengths.

The diagram shows on the right the longest wavelength regions in which lie radio wavelengths. As we move towards shorter wavelengths, we pass through the microwave and infra-red regions, both of which have heating rather than chemical effects. Next appears the relatively narrow visible light region, that part to which the human retina responds, and the UVR spectrum. These two regions, the visible (c.800–400 nm) and the UVR (400–10 nm), are those that are responsible for photochemical effects and thus are of main concern in photobiology/pathology. Further to the left of the scale, in even shorter wavelengths, lie the X-ray and gamma-ray regions. These cause ionization and radiobiological effects. It should be noted that the borders of the various spectral regions overlap and that the titles are arbitrary, mostly arising out of the historical circumstances of their discovery.

Laws of photochemistry

The first law This states that for radiation to produce a photochemical effect, photons must first be absorbed by a molecule or atom. Not all molecules or atoms readily absorb UVR and visible radiation, and where they do the wavelengths absorbed are quite specific and characteristic for the molecule or atom.

The second law This refers to the reciprocity of the dose of radiation for a given effect and the power and length of time of exposure. Thus, the same effect can, according to this law, be produced by a low power or slow rate of delivery of photons given over a long time as where the power is high and exposure time is short, as long as the total number of photons is the same.

The third law This is concerned with the efficiency of the photochemical reaction, the so-called quantum yield or efficiency. Essentially, this is that the absorption of one photon of radiation will cause one molecule or atom to undergo photochemical change. Where this appertains, the quantum efficiency is said to be 1.0 or 100 per cent. In practice, the efficiency is nearly always far less, viz. 0.001 or 0.1 per cent.

The first law of photochemistry (specific absorption) is an essential of the idea that absorption of photons leads to a photochemical increase in reactivity of an atom or molecule and thus to chemical change. The first law also leads to the idea of an absorption spectrum. This is a very useful practical characteristic, much used for identification and quantification. Fig. 10.14, which illustrates an action spectrum, also conveys the

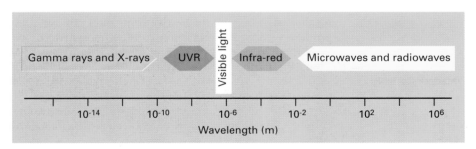

Fig. 10.13 Simplified diagram of the electromagnetic spectrum. The borders between each region overlap and are arbitrary. Ultraviolet radiation (UVR) is subdivided into UV-A (315–400 nm), UV-B (280–315 nm), and UV-C (10–280 nm). Visible light may be subdivided according to colour, viz. violet (400–420 nm), green (500–560 nm), red (650–760 nm), etc.

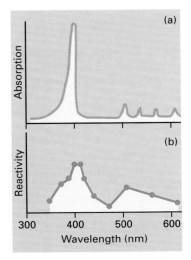

Fig. 10.14 (a) Absorption spectrum. This example is of protoporphyrin in solution; note peak at about 400 nm (violet light), lesser points of absorption at 500–620 nm (green and yellow light). (b) Action spectrum. This shows spectral reactivity of protoporphyrin in the skin as indicated by abnormal responses (erythema, urticaria, etc.) produced with an irradiation monochromator. Compare with absorption spectrum.

idea of spectral effectiveness, an important notion in photobiology.

The second law of photochemistry (reciprocity of dose) is of practical importance in the laboratory, for instance for the investigation of dose–response effects.

The third photochemical law (quantum efficiency) is essential for basic characterization of photochemical and photobiological reactions. Other laws of photochemistry will be quoted as necessary.

Basic photochemical reactions

Photochemical reactions, as compared with ordinary chemical reactions, are exemplified by the formation of 'excited species', i.e. molecules or atoms that are raised to a reactive chemical condition by absorption of photons. These 'excited species' are unstable and tend to return to the 'unexcited' or so-called 'ground state'. When they do this they will re-emit some of the absorbed energy, either as heat or as photons of light.

Relatively little is known about the photochemical reactions that occur in the physiological processes of human photobiology. In theory, a large variety of possibilities exist, but in practice, probably only a few classes of photochemical reactions seem to be important. The main types are; (1) photodynamic action, (2) photodimerization, (3) photo-adduct formation, and (4) photoisomerization. These are described briefly in a later section, but first the initial stages of a photochemical reaction must be examined. They are believed to be as follows:

$$A + h\nu \rightarrow A^1$$

Here, A represents an atom or molecule which is susceptible to a photochemical change after absorption of a photon. The latter is depicted by the term $h\nu$. On absorbing a photon A enters a reactive state shown as A^1. The symbol for photon, $h\nu$, consists of h, which is Planck's constant, and ν which represents the frequency of the radiation associated with the photon; the term A^1 refers to the atom or molecule in a short-lived reactive state known as 'excited singlet'. The peculiar terms 'singlet' and 'triplet' (see below) arise from historical circumstances in early spectroscopy.

Very frequently, the excited singlet returns rapidly to its initial state, namely:

$$A^1 \rightarrow h\nu^f + A$$

The term $h\nu^f$ is meant to show that the photon emitted is different, i.e. of lower energy and longer wavelength, to the photon that was originally absorbed, and in this instance is fluorescent light.

Sometimes, however, the first reaction will proceed to a second stage,

$$A^1 \rightarrow A^3$$

where the symbol A^3 refers to the original atom or molecule in a new long-lived 'excited state'. Superscript 3 refers to the name of the excited state, viz. 'triplet state'. The crucial point is that as the atom or molecule is reactive for a relatively long time, so a photochemical reaction is more likely to occur. Thus:

$$A^3 + B \rightarrow AB$$

which, in this example, represents a photo-adduct process between A^3, the triplet, and B, some other reactant. However, the triplet frequently undergoes return to ground state or decay without a photochemical reaction and the atom or molecule will revert to its original state:

$$A^3 \rightarrow h\nu^p + A$$

Here, A is the original unexcited species, the term $h\nu^p$ refers to a photon of phosphorescent light and differs from fluorescent light by having a relatively long lifetime.

All these photochemical reactions may also undergo decay by the absorbed energy being merely emitted as non-quantized heat:

$$A^1 \rightarrow \text{heat} + A,$$

or

$$A^3 \rightarrow \text{heat} + A$$

These thermal processes degrading the 'excited singlet' or 'triplet' molecule are very common and are how initial photochemical processes mostly end up unless in favourable circumstances, e.g. immobilized in a solid or frozen, or fixed on to some biological structure or membrane.

Sunlight

The solar spectrum, as it reaches the Earth's surface, is comparatively wide, making the possibility of photochemical reaction most diverse. Apart from parts of the visible and near infra-red spectrum utilized in photosynthesis, UVR is the spectral region most responsible for photochemical reactions arising from sunlight. Fading of paintwork by the sun is an everyday example.

Although the sun in outer space emits more or less the whole electromagnetic spectrum, the Earth's atmosphere considerably reduces the extent and power of its spectrum. The shorter wavelength limit of sunlight in midsummer at midday is at about 300 nm in the UVR, the longer wavelength limit in the infra-red region is very variable and may end, for practical purposes, at about 1000 nm. Likewise, the power of UVR at 300 nm is variable and mostly very weak, depending on the height of the sun in the sky. The latter depends on the time of day, season of the year, geographical location, altitude above sea-level. Thus, the sunlight spectrum at its shortest wavelength limit at the Dead Sea, 397 m below sea-level, is at longer wavelengths than at the peak of Mount Everest, 8848 m above sea-level. These differences result from attenuation of UVR by different thickness of atmosphere, chiefly due to oxygen and ozone (Fig. 10.15).

The difference of attenuation of UVR and visible light in the atmosphere is highly complex and wavelength-related. Sunlight undergoing attenuation in the atmosphere does not necessarily follow the simple straight line paths of geometrical optics, but is scattered in all directions. The scattering processes are complicated and not completely understood. For shorter wavelengths, the scattering and attenuation is mostly by very small particles, namely gas molecules, and is related thus:

$$\text{Scattering} \propto \frac{1}{\lambda^4}$$

In other words, attenuation is inversely proportional to the fourth power of the wavelength. The Greek letter λ refers to wavelength. This process, associated with the name of Lord Rayleigh, helps to explain various atmospheric effects, such as blue skies and red sunsets. The attenuation of UVR and invisible light by larger particles such as dust or water droplets is less wavelength-dependent than in Rayleigh scattering:

$$\text{Scattering} \propto \frac{1}{\lambda}$$

This is associated with the name of the German physicist, Mie. So-called Mie scattering differs from Rayleigh scattering in that the former is more forward directed, whereas in the Rayleigh process scattering occurs more or less in all directions. Mie scattering also helps to explain certain meteorological or atmospheric effects, such as the colour of clouds or fogs.

Environmental pollution by chemicals of the soil, water, food, and air around factories and cities, has been reviewed in Section 10.2. Pollution of the upper atmosphere, in particular the ozone layer, however, comes under the purview of photobiology. One of the earliest hazards to the ozone layer was thought to lie in the effects of the exhausts of the engines of supersonic aircraft. The contamination of the ozone layer leading to its depletion by chlorofluorocarbons (CFCs) was another. Recent evidence of an actual reduction of O_3 and its allowing of increased UVR from the sun to reach the Earth's surface by CFCs is now becoming more convincing. The clear demonstration of the so-called Antarctic ozone 'hole' has resulted in efforts to ban the use of CFCs, especially in their application as refrigerants. Increased power of UV-B at the Earth's surface and shift of the lower spectral limit to shorter wavelengths are likely to lead to manifold changes, particularly if, as seems very probable, they are global. To humans these would include increased prevalence of skin neoplasia, certain eye diseases (cataract, keratoconjunctivitis, snow blindness) and suppression of the immune system. Extensive damage to plant and marine life would also be expected. (See the UNEP report of 1989.)

Ultraviolet radiation

UVR is a relatively wide region of the electromagnetic spectrum and is generally divided for convenience into three regions, referred to as UV-A, UV-B, and UV-C. (The infra-red spectrum is also similarly subdivided into three regions.)

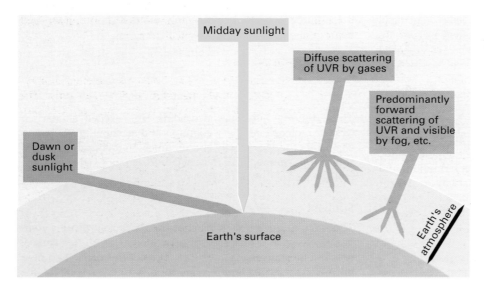

Fig. 10.15 Diagram to illustrate some effects of the Earth's atmosphere on sunlight. The height of the sun in the sky governs the thickness of atmosphere the direct ray has to pass through. Midday sunlight has the shortest path and delivers all of the visible spectrum and UVR down to c.300 nm. With the sun lower in the sky UVR is attenuated more than visible radiation and the shortest wavelength is 350 nm or longer. Diffuse-type scattering by gas molecules strongly attenuates UVR; forward-type scattering by larger particles (fog) is less wavelength-dependent.

UV-A, by a convention proposed at an international congress in 1935, extends from 400 nm, which is at the border of the violet part of the visible spectrum, to 315 nm. This spectral region is of relatively high power in sunlight and, although relatively lower in photon energy than other parts of the UVR, is effective in promoting many photochemical and photo-biological reactions.

The UV-B region extends from 315 nm to 280 nm. This region is highly noxious to many biological systems and in the case of the human is responsible for the phenomena of sunburn, suntan, snow blindness, and probably of skin ageing and cancer (see below).

The UV-C region extends from 280 nm to shorter wave-lengths; generally 10 nm is taken to be the lower limit. UV-C is the most highly toxic to biological processes and is therefore sometimes known as 'germicidal radiation'. However, its pen-etration through the terrestrial atmosphere is extremely poor and none of it reaches us from the sun. To obtain UV-C, one has to use an artificial source, such as a mercury vapour lamp.

The wavelength region around 260 nm in UV-C is specially important for its ease of production by mercury vapour lamps and its specific absorption by DNA. Hence, it is widely used in experimental work, especially in microbiology.

Artificial sources of UVR and visible light

The radiant power and wavelength emission of artificial sources are important factors in considering their possible uses, e.g. in therapy and experimental work, or their potential adverse side-effects in industrial applications. Gross errors can arise from using an inappropriate source, e.g. where mimicry of sunlight is required, the most useful is the xenon arc, *not* the low pressure mercury vapour arc (Fig. 10.16 and Table 10.18).

There are two main types of lamp. The most familiar is the

Table 10.18 Lamp and light characteristics

Type of lamp	Approximate radiant emission*
Tungsten	Visible light, but mostly infra-red
Tungsten–halide	Visible light (mostly infra-red) with a small amount of UV-A
Discharge lamps	
Mercury vapour	
low pressure	Mostly 260 nm region (UV-C)
medium pressure	Many emission lines, mostly UV-B
high pressure	Strong continuum mostly UV-B, UV-A, and some visible
Fluorescent lamps 'phosphor' powder on envelope	Depending on phosphor and transmission of envelope, selected parts of UV-A, UV-B, or visible
'Doped' discharge lamps	Mostly UV-A and visible
Xenon arc	Similar to terrestrial sunlight

* Nature of envelope of lamp may filter emissions.

filament lamp, where the tungsten filament becomes incandes-cent by heating it electrically. The other class of lamp is where an electrical discharge is formed in a gas, the latter being enclosed usually in an envelope of glass or sometimes quartz. The now largely obsolete carbon arc, however, burns un-enclosed in the air. So-called 'doped lamps', usually mercury vapour arcs, a modern development especially for street light-ing, have considerable promise in photobiological experiments. The doping refers to traces of metals, e.g. germanium, added to the mercury vapour, their nature being an industrial secret. The compositions of the phosphor powders applied to the tubes in fluorescent mercury vapour lamps are also commercial secrets, but are mostly alkaline oxides and salts.

Photochemical reactions

A large variety of photochemical reactions are possible. But the photochemical reactions important in photobiology, photo-therapy, and photopathology are relatively few. Lasers in sur-gical use operate mostly, though not entirely, by causing heat rather than specific photo-chemical processes.

Photodynamic action

This term was coined in 1904 and refers, somewhat inappro-priately, to processes involving molecular oxygen only. The name is strongly implanted into the literature and probably im-possible to change.

Photodynamic action is particularly associated with a number of natural pigments, e.g. porphyrins and flavins, and certain artificial dyes, such as eosin. It is also associated with a number of diseases connected with porphyrin photo-sensitization. This is seen in sheep and cattle, and in humans, in the group of diseases known such as the porphyrias. In all these disorders, the skin is rendered abnormally sensitive to sunlight. The porphyrins are intermediates of the normal biosynthesis of haem, which occurs principally in the liver and bone marrow. Flavins are more widespread, e.g. in muscle, liver, and kidney,

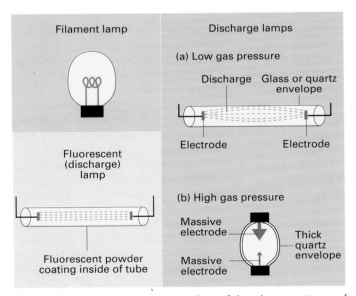

Fig. 10.16 Diagrammatic representations of three important types of artificial light sources.

but in low concentration generally; it will be recalled that they play important parts in physiological mechanisms associated with energy production and electron transfer. Eosin is an example of a large number of heterocyclic compounds that are highly photoreactive. Many of them are used in the dye industry, others as food colours, e.g. erythrosine. A typical photodynamic compound has a ring chemical structure that is planar and has alternating single and double bonds.

In photodynamic action it is supposed that the photosensitive molecule (porphyrin, flavin, etc.) absorbs a photon of light and is then raised to an 'excited singlet state' and next to a 'triplet state'. In the latter condition, a photo-oxidative reaction occurs. This may be either via an energy transfer process with molecular oxygen directly, which is converted into 'excited singlet oxygen', or via various free radicals in an electron transfer process. The former, energy transfer, is illustrated below.

$$(1) \qquad P + h\nu \rightarrow P^1 \rightarrow P^3;$$

$$(2) \qquad P^3 + O_2 \rightarrow O_2^* + P;$$

$$(3) \qquad O_2^* + S \rightarrow O_2 + SO_2.$$

In process (1), triplet formation of a porphyrin molecule is illustrated and the absorbed photon, $h\nu$, would be in the visible or nearby UV-A spectrum, typically about 380–410 nm, i.e. violet visible light. For flavin, the absorbed wavelength would be 340–360 nm, i.e. UV-A. In (2), an oxygen molecule is shown to go into a reactive state, O_2^*. (Oxygen is peculiar in that the excited singlet is most reactive for photochemical reactions.) According to (2), the photosensitizer, porphyrin, is reformed so that it can react once more. Process (3) shows excited singlet oxygen reacting with a substrate molecule, S, which might be a biomolecule in a cell or micelle membrane, such as lipoprotein. The oxide form of this, SO_2, would initiate a cellular lesion.

Alternatively, photodynamic reaction may occur via free radical formation and electron transfer types of processes:

$$P^3 + RH \rightarrow PH^{\cdot} + R^{\cdot}$$

Here, triplet state photosensitizer, P^3, reacts with a receptor substrate, RH, to form free radicals $PH^{\cdot}$ and $R^{\cdot}$. These can react with molecular oxygen to form various superoxides:

$$PH^{\cdot} + O_2 \rightarrow P + HO_2^{\cdot}$$

Superoxides, e.g. $HO_2^{\cdot}$, are highly reactive and react with biological target molecules in a similar way to excited singlet oxygen.

In passing, note that these photochemical processes have uses in clinical diagnosis. Animals or humans with the porphyrias often excrete excess porphyrin; this can be detected with UV-A light, which makes the porphyrin fluoresce a red colour. This is a very sensitive diagnostic test.

Photodimerization

This process is exceedingly common in photochemical reactions. In photobiology it is also important with respect to DNA lesions. Photochemical reactions with DNA, especially by photodimerization, are suspected to cause cell death,

mutations, and carcinogenesis. Dimerization is conveniently studied quantitatively in bacteria, particularly in *E. coli*, and has resulted in a large corpus of important data. Photodimerization affects DNA by linking adjacent pyrimidines in the same chain of the DNA duplex. The best-known dimer is between two thymines, although similar links can occur with other pyrimidines, viz. between two cytosines or between cytosine and thymine (see Fig. 10.17).

Other photochemical changes in DNA, due to UVR, are less well characterized, namely DNA–protein interactions and various types of methylation and hydroxylation of pyrimidines. Thymine dimers are best understood because they are readily detected and measured by simple extraction and chromatographic separation in bacterial or human cell culture. Although large numbers of pyrimidine dimers are lethal to a cell, a relatively small number of them can often be repaired and the cell survives.

DNA repair Three main repair processes are known, namely excision repair, post-replication repair, and lastly, photo-reactivation repair. Of these, the role of the last process is of most significance in lower taxonomic groups, of less importance in higher forms, and virtually absent in mammalians including humans. Excision repair and post-replication repair are well established thoroughly studied processes in cell cultures of human material and have been exhaustively investigated in bacteria, in particular *E. coli*. Failure of repair processes is thought to underlie some of the rarer genetic disorders in humans such as in xeroderma pigmentosum, a condition with a very strong tendency to the early development of skin cancer (see Section 9.61).

Photo-adducts

This type of photochemical reaction is again important with DNA. The other molecule concerned, a photosensitizer, may be various, viz. an acridine dye, but of particular importance in human photobiology are the furocoumarins, also known under the trivial chemical name of botanical derivation, as psoralens. These plant substances seem to play a defensive role against fungal and bacterial invaders. Photo-adducts are formed by the furocoumarin molecule intercalating into the DNA duplex and forming a mono-adduct with a pyrimidine, either thymine or cytosine (see Fig. 10.17). Where furocoumarin forms a di-adduct, this will bridge the DNA duplex; this is thought to be a more serious lesion than the mono-adduct. These photo-adducts cause cell death when present in large quantity. In lesser quantity, they appear to be capable of being repaired, though the mechanism is not well known. As with the thymine dimer, probably the furocoumarin–pyrimidine photo-adduct interferes with cell duplication and DNA synthesis. This property, it is supposed, may cause mutation and cancer. However, in low doses, plus UV-A radiation, furocoumarins are probably safe if properly supervised in so-called PUVA photochemotherapy for psoriasis and certain malignant reticuloses (see below).

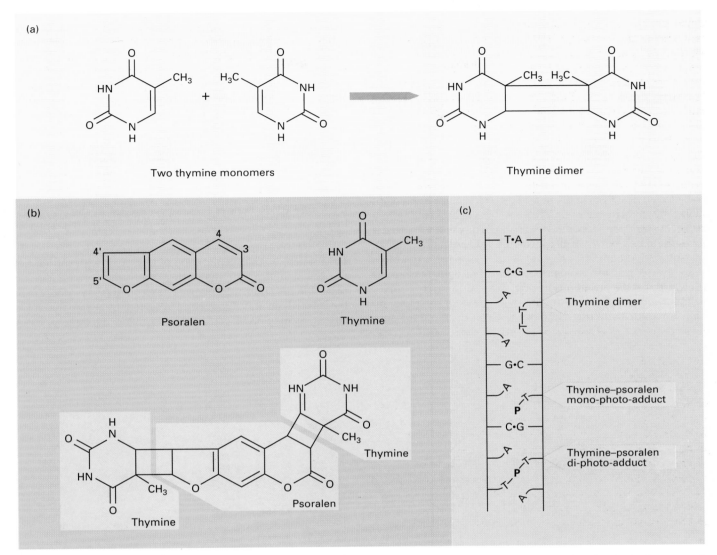

Fig. 10.17   (a) Chemical structure of thymine dimers. (b) Furocoumarin photo-adducts. Note two different reactive sites in the furocoumarin molecules, viz. the 4,3 and 4′,5′; these allow, therefore, mono-photo-adducts or di-photo-adducts. (c) Diagrammatical representation of thymine dimer, furocoumarin mono- and di-photo-adducts in the DNA duplex; the latter a cross-link. P = psoralen (i.e. furocoumarin).

Other photochemical reactions

Certain therapeutic drugs cause skin photosensitivity as an adverse side-effect when a patient is exposed to the sun. These include tetracyclines, sulphonamides, non-steroidal anti-inflammatory drugs and phenothiazines. In the last case, this is evidently due to actual photo-products formed from pheno-thiazine in the patient's skin. However, the nature of these photo-products and the mechanism are unclear, though photo-dynamic action may play a part.

Reflection, transmission, and absorption of UVR and visible light by biological tissues

Skin

For human skin, only qualitative information is available. It is relatively simple to separate the skin into several layers and to measure their optical properties with an instrument such as an absorption spectrophotometer. But almost certainly the very removal of the epidermis from the dermis and from the sub-cutaneous layers alters their optical properties. In addition, skin is most inhomogeneous and its thickness and surface irregular. These properties also differ markedly from one body location to another, e.g. palmer and plantar epidermis is considerably thicker than that of volar forearm, thus the former will transmit far less UVR and visible light. The relatively much thicker horny layer of the epidermis seems to be the important attenuating optical filter.

Reflection of UVR from the skin surface is small. Most UVR is scattered and absorbed on passing into the skin. The absorption occurs at various depths, largely depending on wavelength, but details are lacking. However, the mode of passage of visible light is different. Much is diffusely reflected out of the skin, again chiefly by a complex forward scattering, perhaps similar to the Mie process. (One should separate *diffuse* reflection from *specular* reflection, as from a mirror; together the two are known as *remission*, the reflecting process in non-homogeneous tissues such as skin.) The visible light that is transmitted, partly absorbed and 'remitted' is responsible for the phenomenon of skin colour. This is complex and controversial. The chief factors, apart from wavelength, are the concentration of the pigments melanin, oxyhaemoglobin, and haemoglobin, and, probably, the depth at which these lie in the skin. Thus, due to so-called subtractive colour mixing, haemoglobin, in blood in dilated dermal blood vessels, absorbs green light resulting in a red colour, whereas melanin lying superficially in the epidermis gives the skin a brown or black colour. This probably is due to melanin attenuating the blue end of the visible spectrum more than the red; to the human eye weak red light appears as brown. But if the melanin is in high concentration in a superficial location of the skin, attentuation could be complete, no light is remitted and the skin looks to be black. But if melanin

lies deep in the dermis, as occurs in certain birthmarks or in tattoos, the colour appears blue (see Fig. 10.18). Probably what happens here is that blue light is strongly remitted in the more superficial layers of the skin above the dermis, whereas the green-yellow-red part of the visible spectrum is attenuated in the deeper-lying melanin or tattoo pigments.

Eye

The main transmission characteristics in the human eye can be summarized as follows for the different types of UVR. Visible light, of course, is transmitted very well through the cornea and vitreous to reach the retina.

UV-C and UV-B Both of these are absorbed in the superficial layers of the cornea and sclera; none reach the anterior chamber or lens.

UV-A There is some penetration of the sclera with substantial transmission through the cornea and anterior chamber to reach the iris and lens. Complete absorption of UV-A occurs in the lens, which may fluoresce a bluish colour. Where the lens is absent, as may occur congenitally or following surgery, UV-A

(a)

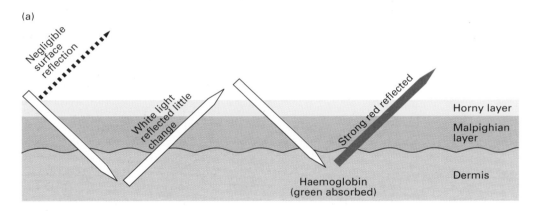

(b)

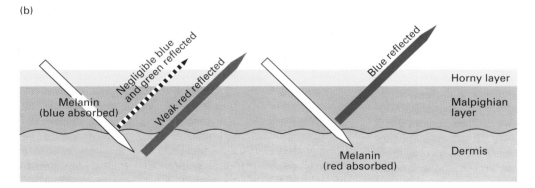

Fig. 10.18 Suggested scheme for 'skin optics'. Transmission depends on wavelength; shorter wavelengths are absorbed and/or remitted superficially, longer wavelengths more deeply. (a) Skin without much haemoglobin or melanin transmits and remits white light little changed. With increased haemoglobin, strong green absorption leads to light remission giving pink or red colour. (b) With increased melanin lying superficially, weak red light is remitted giving a brown colour. Where no light is remitted, the colour is black. With increased melanin lying deeper, blue is remitted.

will reach the retina and appear to the patient as a blue-violet colour.

Visible and near infra-red Substantial transmission through the cornea, anterior chamber, and lens occurs. On reaching the retina, further transmission is blocked by the melanin pigment layer behind the retina. There is partial transmission of visible and infra-red through the sclera.

Far infra-red Essentially there is complete absorption by the sclera and cornea.

Visible light and near infra-red (400–1400 nm) are potentially hazardous, causing severe retinal damage, because this part of the spectrum is focused optically to form an image on the retina. This may result in a small area of very high irradiance and a severe burn.

10.5.3 Normal photobiochemical responses in the skin

Sunburn and suntan

Sunburn and suntan are familiar normal acute responses. The erythema of sunburn is due to dilatation of dermal arterioles, capillaries, and venules of the subpapillary vascular plexus. The time course of the erythema development depends on the power and emission spectrum of the UVR source causing the reaction. Terrestial sunlight in moderate dose, say in an exposure lasting 30 minutes at midday in midsummer, may cause erythema to appear in 30 minutes, reach a maximum after about 24–36 hours, and then gradually fade away over about a week. The response to irradiation with narrow wave-band UV-B, say from a medium-pressure mercury vapour arc, is different to that caused by the very broad wave-band of sunlight, and this suggests that the two sources cause different photochemical, cellular, and other processes. With narrow wave-band UVR at about 300 nm, the spread of erythema and its time course has been described in terms of classical diffusion theory (Fick's law) by van der Leun (1966) with some success.

Mechanism of UVR-induced erythema For erythema in normal white skin, a threshold dose of monochromatic 300 nm is 10–20 mJ cm^2 and the response has a latent period of 8 hours. But with monochromatic 360 nm, this dose is about 1000 times higher and there is often no latent period, or the response is biphasic. These variations in time response and dose with wavelength point to different processes being responsible for the sunburn reaction. The role of inflammatory chemical mediators in sunburn erythema is highly complex (see Chapter 5). The action spectrum for UVR erythema is shown in Fig. 10.19. The splitting of the curve (I,II) in the shorter wavelength region arises from variations in time-course and dose–response. As the longer wavelength region is not affected, this again suggests that several complex mechanisms are responsible at different parts of the spectrum.

Suntan This is the browning effect, delayed for a day or so after solar exposure, due to new melanin pigment formation. This

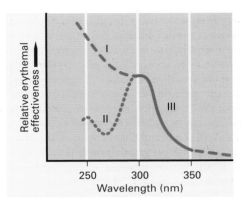

Fig. 10.19 The action spectrum for erythema induced by monochromatic UVR in normal white skin. Effectiveness is plotted against UVR wavelength. The upper dashed line (I) (from 250 to *c*.300 nm) shows the approximate spectral effectiveness if the responses are measured at an early stage of the time course, with UVR doses near threshold. Maximum effectiveness is at 250 nm. The lower dotted curve (II) shows effectiveness measured later in the time course, with UVR dose higher than threshold. The effectiveness is biphasic with maximum effectiveness at *c*.300 nm. The continuous line curve (III) on the right is less affected by time-course and dose–response. That part of the effectiveness curve, which is shown in a dashed line, from 350 to 400 nm, is partly conjectural and based on sparse data. These complex spectral results indicate that several mechanisms underlie the normal sunburn erythema response.

occurs in melanocytes in the basal layer of the epidermis. (Immediate tanning is different, due to photo-oxidative darkening of existing melanin.) The biochemical process of melanogenesis is thought to depend on the enzymatic conversion of tyrosine to deoxyphenylalanine (DOPA), followed by the formation of a series of quinone, indole, and hydroxy-indole-like structures, which join together to form the large lattice-like molecule known as melanin. The latter occurs as two types, probably mixed together to varying degree: eumelanin (black and brown) and the cysteine-containing phaeomelanin (yellow and red).

The photobiological mechanisms responsible for melanogenesis are not known, and it is often assumed that suntan is merely a non-specific result of the inflammation accompanying the erythema of sunburn. This remains conjecture. The threshold dose for delayed suntan and its action spectrum and time course are not dissimilar to those of sunburn erythema. (Immediate tanning, however, is mostly due to UV-A and is often a transient response.)

Melanin supposedly acts mainly as an optical filter of UVR and, to a lesser extent, of visible light; but it also appears to 'trap' electrons and free radicals arising from photochemical and other reactions. Melanin probably has a similar trapping action (unrelated to light) in deeper tissues, viz. the cochlea, substantia nigra, and other parts of the central nervous system.

Cellular turnover and other effects

These changes occur in both epidermis and dermis and are relatively delayed responses to solar and UV irradiation. Most studies have been done using UV-B and measuring epidermal nuclear division and cellular differentiation by determining autoradiographically the incorporation of tritiated thymidine into skin or skin cells. It can thus be shown that UVR interferes with normal DNA synthesis; there is a reduction for 1–6 hours followed by an increase of DNA synthesis over a day or so. Similar changes occur with RNA and protein synthesis and with epidermal mitotic rates. Thickening of the epidermis and, to a lesser extent the dermis, accompanies the above changes and its extent depends on whether multiple or single exposures are given. With regular multiple intermittent exposures, as occurs normally in outdoor workers such as farmers, thickening occurs especially of the stratum corneum of the epidermis. There is evidence that this is the change responsible for induction of tolerance to UVR-induced erythema in people who are habitually exposed to solar radiation, though increased melanin pigment also plays a role. Possibly immunological factors play a part. Better established as UVR induced is a reduction in immune functions, as manifest in hyposensitivity to contact-dermatitis-inducing chemical agents and failure to reject the grafting of neoplasms into the skin in mice.

Histological changes

In sunburn, a sparse mononuclear, or round-cell, infiltrate in the dermis is a feature. It is evident about 8–72 hours after adequate UV-B exposure. Neutrophils also occur but are less obvious. Increased capillary and venular permeability also can be demonstrated up to about 72 hours. A more striking change in the epidermis after solar or UV-B exposure is the appearance of so-called 'sunburn cells', present from 1–7 days after exposure. These are dyskeratotic cells with an eosinophylic homogeneous cytoplasm and pyknotic nucleus. The title 'apoptosis', borrowed from botany, has been applied and sunburn cells are sometimes called 'apoptotic cells'. They occur dispersed, singly, throughout the epidermis and lend themselves readily to quantitative study. Sunburn cells also occur after UV-C, but not after UV-A, unless the skin has been photosensitized with furocoumarin. Apoptosis also occurs in locations where UV-B or solar irradiation plays no part, such as in deep organs, especially the gut, and in tissues in which a high cellular turnover is normal. But apoptosis is also produced by certain drugs and infections and has also been observed in neoplastic tissue. Its significance is a matter for conjecture (see Chapter 4).

Skin neoplasia

In white-skinned persons basal cell and squamous cell carcinoma are amongst the commonest neoplasms. Squamous cell carcinoma is unmistakably associated with solar exposure, and epidemiological studies over several decades, mostly in Australia and southern USA, have demonstrated convincing evidence for clear dose–response effects. But for basal cell carcinoma the evidence is less sure. More recently, a role for solar exposure has been claimed for malignant melanoma of the skin, but the mechanistic relationship to solar exposure is obscure. It has been suggested that there is a link between solar induced immunological suppression and precipitation of malignant mel-

anoma. If this were important and solar UV-B were increased because of atmospheric ozone depletion, higher prevalence of the neoplasm would be expected. This would be most serious because of the poor response to therapy and the high mortality of malignant melanoma.

Animal models for linking skin cancer to UVR exposure confirm many of the ideas arising from clinical and epidemiological work in humans. But with malignant melanoma, no animal model is available as yet.

PUVA therapy with high-dose UV-A, or with certain previous treatments, e.g. radiotherapy, has been shown clearly to lead to an increased prevalence of skin cancer as an adverse side-effect. This increased prevalence is especially evident in patients with previous radiotherapy and suggests possible initiation and promotion as in two-stage oncogenesis (see Section 9.6.1). This and other considerations have led to the view that DNA lesions induced by UVR play an important role in the mechanism underlying neoplastic formation. The deficient repair of UVR-induced lesions in DNA which occur in xeroderma pigmentosum, the rare genodermatosis associated with greatly increased prevalence of skin cancer, is another example supporting this concept.

Diseases due to sunlight

These are well established, mostly on clinical grounds, in the field of dermatology. Except for a role in the provocation of cataract and the cause of photokeratitis, photoconjunctivitis, and retinal burns, sunlight seems to play a small part in eye diseases. Table 10.19 shows a classification of some of the so-called photodermatoses. The first group, of unknown aetiology other than its connection with solar exposure, is generally believed to have some kind of immunological basis. The second group has some obvious underlying cause, endogenous or exogenous. Here, photobiological lesions can be explained as due to photodynamic action, as in the porphyrias; to DNA lesions arising from pyrimidine photodimers, as in xeroderma pigmentosum; or exposure to plants containing furocoumarins which form photoadducts with DNA pyrimidines. See Frain-Bell (1985) for further details of the photodermatoses.

Again, if the wavelength range of UV-B in sunlight were widened and its power increased by ozone depletion, both the prevalence and severity of the photodermatoses would be expected to rise. New therapies would have to be developed, for

---

Table 10.19 Pathogenesis of photodermatoses

Primary (unknown aetiology)
Polymorphic light eruption
Actinic or summer prurigo (Hutchinson)
Actinic reticuloid or chronic actinic dermatitis

Secondary
Metabolic porphyrias, xeroderma pigmentosum, other rare genodermatoses
Exogenous therapeutic drugs, industrial chemicals, botanical materials (furocoumarins)

instance sun-barrier creams with formulations suited to the new solar spectrum.

10.5.4 Phototherapy

Two types of phototherapy have been well established in the past 15 years. These are (1) PUVA for skin diseases, especially psoriasis; and (2) blue-light therapy for neonatal jaundice. A third therapeutic use is that of light as a surgical instrument—using a laser for cutting, destruction, and coagulation.

Skin diseases

As mentioned above, since Niels Finsen in the late 1890s started modern photobiology with the first successful treatment of the skin disease lupus vulgaris, the chief uses of phototherapy have remained in the field of dermatology. This has continued using mostly traditional styles of irradiation apparatus with medium-pressure mercury vapour arcs or fluorescent tubes emitting UV-B. UV-B therapy has been chiefly successful in psoariasis and acne vulgaris. UV-A irradiation therapy has only achieved special popularity when combined with the taking of oral furocoumarin, usually 8-methoxy psoralen. Thus the treatment is more correctly termed photochemotherapy. An hour or so before irradiation, the patient is temporarily (c.2 hours) photosensitized to UV-A by ingesting furocoumarin; which is why it is called PUVA, an acronym where P stands for psoralen, the trivial botanical name for furocoumarin. Special lamp arrays, 4–6 feet long fluorescent tubes of relatively high output UV-A, have been developed to cater for this therapy. It is supposed that the mechanism for the beneficial effect in psoriasis, mycosis fungoides, and other proliferative diseases is by interrupting DNA synthesis. But PUVA is also known to suppress certain immune processes. How much this contributes to therapeutic effects is not clear.

Neonatal jaundice

The bile pigment, bilirubin, has been long known to be susceptible to fading from light exposure. It is this photochemical property that is used to treat jaundice in the new-born. In most instances, the susceptible infant is unable to conjugate bilirubin because of deficient activity in its hepatic uridine diphosphate glucuronyl transferase enzyme system. Bilirubin-glucuronide, being relatively water-soluble, is excreted in the urine, but with deficient enzyme activity the free, water-insoluble bilirubin accumulates in the body. This enzyme deficiency, often a manifestation of prematurity, resolves after a few weeks. But the icterus is potentially serious in leading to the risk of irreversible brain damage (see Chapter 17).

Less common and more severe is so-called haemolytic disease of the new-born, a serious condition formerly with high morbidity and mortality. This is usually due to maternal Rh blood-group incompatibility. Less often there are other genetic disorders, e.g. deficient glucose-6-phosphate dehydrogenase activity.

For phototherapy, irradiation of the jaundiced infant was originally with fluorescent tubes emitting white light, but now blue light is preferred, as the maximum absorption of bilirubin is near 420–480 nm. The mechanism of the bleaching effect is complex. It involves the solubilization of bilirubin by photo-isomerization from a relatively insoluble to a relatively water-soluble form. The latter is then rapidly removed from the blood lying in the skin and fatty subcutaneous tissue and is excreted in the urine. Bilirubin is also photo-oxidized to a complicated variety of products.

When as a result of phototherapy the plasma bilirubin falls towards normal again, insoluble bilirubin diffuses from deeper tissues, especially fat, and hyperbilirubinaemia recurs. The phototherapy exposures then have to be repeated as necessary.

Other phototherapies

These remain largely experimental and include in particular the use of photodynamic dyes to treat advanced neoplasia and recurrent virus infections, especially herpes simplex. Unfortunately, in the treatment of herpetic keratitis in this way, photo-induced keratitis and uveitis occur as serious side-effects. In other forms of recurrent herpes (lip and genital organs), this treatment seems to be of no avail. But some success is claimed in eczema herpeticum. As there is evidence for potential neoplastic change from photodynamic transformation of certain viruses, including herpes simplex, there may similarly be a clinical risk of neoplasia. In fact animal experiments lend some support to this and in certain circumstances photodynamic therapy appears to unmask neoplasia.

Notwithstanding these discouraging results, a very large effort has been made in investigating the potential of photodynamic action in the treatment of advanced neoplasia, especially of the urinary bladder. It has been claimed that neoplastic tissue will take up porphyrin compounds (in particular haematoporphyrin or so-called 'haematoporphyrin derivative') preferentially to normal tissue and that this has helped in identification and localization of neoplastic lesions. In the case of bladder neoplasia (usually papillomas), haematoporphyrin has been given intravenously and the tumours examined cytoscopically and treated by light, usually laser, delivered by fibre optics. (Here the laser light is acting photochemically not thermally.) Unfortunately, the preferential uptake of porphyrin, as shown by fluorescence, is disappointing in practice, and the overall therapeutic results are unimpressive.

Apart from bladder cancer, many other types of neoplasia have been treated with photodynamic dye and irradiation, usually laser. Other photodynamic dyes have also been suggested, in particular phthalocyanines, merocyanines, and benzophenoxazines. A large collection of review articles on these and other relevant matters was published by Gomer (1987). At present it is difficult to predict whether any good will come out of these endeavours.

10.5.5 Further reading

Cronly-Dillon, J., Rosen, E. S., and Marshall, J. (eds) (1988). *Hazards of light*. Pergamon Press, Oxford.

Environmental Effects Panel Report, *Environmental Effects of Ozone Depletion*; November 1989, United Nations Environmental Programme (UNEP). Copies obtained from US Environmental Protection Agency, Washington, DC, USA, *or* J. C. v.d. Leun, Institute of Dermatology, Heidelberglaan 100, Utrecht, The Netherlands.

Frain-Bell, W. (1985). *Cutaneous photobiology*. Oxford University Press.

Gomer, C. J. (1987). Photodynamic therapy. *Photochemistry and Photobiology* **46**, 561–952.

Regan, J. D. and Parrish, J. A. (eds) (1982). *The science of photomedicine*. Plenum Press, London.

10.6   Ionizing radiation

J. Denekamp

Since his appearance on Earth, man has been exposed to ionizing radiation, emanating from natural radionuclides in the environment, or as cosmic rays from space. This background radiation may even have had a major impact on the evolutionary development of the Earth's flora and fauna; it can cause breaks and translocations in DNA, leading to the genetic variation that is necessary for evolutionary trends. Ionizing radiation cannot be detected by any of the common senses. Its existence has therefore been recognized relatively recently. In 1895, Röntgen discovered a 'new' kind of ray from a gas discharge tube that would blacken a photographic film although it was not visible. Shortly thereafter, in 1898, Becquerel noticed the damaging effect of radium when he developed a skin ulcer caused by radium which he had left in his pocket. He also identified that the rays from this natural radioisotope blackened a film when both were stored in a drawer. Thus X- and γ-rays (man-made and natural forms of the same sort of radiation) were recognized almost simultaneously. Their remarkable property in allowing radiographs to be made of bony structure was quickly recognized and made them of great interest to the medical community (and to science fiction writers!). Within a year or two they were also being used to treat malignant tumours, which sometimes 'melted away'.

10.6.1   Basic physics

X- and γ-rays are part of the electromagnetic spectrum, with wavelengths below those of UV (approximately 10^{-8} cm), and with a photon energy that is high enough to excite or eject electrons from their normal atomic orbits. This latter process leads to disruption of atomic bonds by ionizing the molecules. Damage in critical molecules may occur by direct ionization or by the attack of radicals produced in adjacent water molecules by the ionizing radiation. The energy dissipated in such an event is typically about 33 eV, much higher than the bond strength of a $C≡C$ bond (4.9 eV).

The total thermal energy dissipated in a man from a lethal radiation dose is very small. It is less than that imparted from a warm cup of coffee. However, the energy is imparted as discrete packages, with the special property of disrupting molecular bonds. Most of these disruptions will be irrelevant because the cell may be capable of chemically rejoining the bond, of biochemically repairing the molecule, or simply generating another copy of the molecule. Lesions in the genetic codes carried by DNA may, however, be irreparable and the cell may then lose the capacity to produce the gene product encoded in that region. This is why genetic damage is much more sensitive to radiation than most cellular functions.

Radiation lethality

Although radiation is widely used in Western medicine, in radiodiagnostic procedures and radiotherapy of malignant disease, it is perceived by the general public as a mainly hazardous rather than helpful agent. The short-term deaths after the atom bombs dropped on Hiroshima and Nagasaki, and the long-term genetic abnormalities in offspring and in the form of induced cancers have gained widespread news coverage over the past 40 years. Arguments rage about the dose needed to kill half the population, with estimates ranging from 1.5 Gy to 12 Gy (UNSCEAR Report 1988). This wide range of values results from the paucity of data and from the confounding factors associated with each accidental exposure of human populations. Calculations of the lethal dose after the atom bombs in Japan yield figures of 3–4 Gy, but most of the population near the epicentre suffered also from blast injury, thermal burns, and the problems of infection resulting from the disruption of the water and sewage system and of all hospital facilities. Recent evidence from the Chernobyl nuclear power plant disaster indicates a value of about 9 Gy. Once again, however, the workers were exposed to thermal burns and to radiation burns resulting from skin contamination with β-emitting radionuclides. These skin doses were 10–20 times higher than the dose to bone marrow and other deep-seated organs. Ninety per cent of the casualties who died had extensive skin burns, which were the main cause of death (UNSCEAR Report 1988).

Whole body irradiation is nowadays used quite widely prior to bone marrow transplantation in patients with disseminated leukaemia or lymphoma. It is also used in the pretreatment of patients before organ transplant in order to minimize the immune rejection of the graft. These and other medical uses of whole body irradiation suggest that the LD_{50} in man can be as high as 10–12 Gy if the dose is given at a low dose rate (e.g. 5 cGy/minute) or as a series of acute fractions of 2–3 Gy at daily intervals, and if the patients receive intensive medical support. Sensitivity to radiation depends upon the type of ionizing radiation, its rate of energy deposition (dose rate), its energy and hence depth of penetration, and several other physical and biological factors, as outlined below. Thus it is impossible to quote a single value for the LD_{50} for man.

Measurement of radiation

Since ionizing radiation is invisible, inaudible, tasteless, and odourless, how can it be measured? As mentioned earlier, it can produce latent images which can be developed and fixed on photographic film. Densitometry can then be used to estimate the amount of radiation to which the film was exposed. This is the principle of the original 'film badges' used as a personal radiation monitoring system for many hospital and laboratory staff. The quality of the radiation is also important and this can be judged from its ability to penetrate through appropriate shielding. Film-badge holders have thin layers of lead and aluminium over a section of the film so that a comparison can be made of the dose in the shielded and unshielded portions of the film.

More accurate dosimetry is usually performed with ionization chambers, with chemical dosimeters (e.g. ferrous sulphate) or thermoluminescent crystals. These techniques all depend on measuring the ionizations produced by the passage of the 'rays' through the monitor. An ionization chamber is usually a hollow device containing air or a 'tissue equivalent' gas. It has a fixed electrical charge across the cavity which is altered if the contained air is ionized so that electrons and positive ions can leak to the electrodes. The well-known clucking Geiger counter is a crude version of such an ionization chamber, in which the number of clucks per minute indicates the dose rate.

Thermoluminescent dosimetry, mainly using lithium fluoride came into use in the 1960s. It depends upon charge being trapped in impurities in the crystal structure when the material is irradiated. This charge or energy is stable at room temperature, but can be released if the crystals are heated to about 300 °C, and can be measured in the form of emitted light or luminescence. The availability of a convenient material that can be formed into rods or enclosed in capsules has allowed much more accurate dosimetry inside tissues, and inside body cavities.

The amount of radiation that is absorbed is measured in grays, where 1 Gy is 1 joule per kilogram. The original unit was 1 rad, i.e. 100 ergs per gram. 1 Gy = 100 rads. Medical exposures to the organ of interest during diagnostic procedures, usually give a dose of a few micrograys, rising to a centigray or two for a prolonged fluoroscopy examination, e.g. cardiac angiography or computerized axial tomography (CAT scan). By contrast, the exposures given to a malignant tumour in curative radiotherapy may be as high as 60–75 Gy, conventionally given as a series of daily 2 Gy fractions over 6–7.5 weeks.

Types of ionizing radiation

Many different forms of ionizing radiation now exist. The forms first recognized were photons, electrons, and α-particles. Photons are called X-rays when they are generated in a machine, usually by firing electrons at a target. Photons are electromagnetic radiation which can be regarded as having characteristics of both wave and particles. If such photons are emitted from a naturally unstable isotope, e.g. from ^{60}cobalt or ^{137}caesium, they are termed γ-rays and would then have a characteristic energy, depending upon the isotope source. The ability of X- or γ-rays to penetrate tissue depends upon their energy, with highly energetic radiation being capable of pene-

trating to greater depths. Their energy may be expressed either as the voltage of the machine (e.g. 30 kV, 3 MV) or, more exactly, as the energy of the photons expressed in 'electron volts' (e.g. 50 keV, 18 MeV). Diagnostic X-ray sets are usually run from electrons at a few tens of thousand volts, e.g. 30–50 kV, whereas the machines used for therapy range from superficial X-rays (∼ 30 kV) to penetrating supervoltage X-rays from linear accelerators of 20 MV. ^{60}Co γ-rays are also considered as supervoltage, having an energy of about 1.25 MeV.

Electrons themselves are a form of ionizing radiation, and are termed β-rays if emanating from a natural radioisotope. For example, tritium emits a β-particle, energy 18 keV, with a range in tissue of only a few microns, whereas ^{14}carbon has a much more penetrating β-ray of 155 keV.

When some radionuclides decay, they do not simply lose energy as photons (or electrons), but they may undergo an explosion of their nuclear core emitting protons, neutrons, or helium ions (2 protons + 2 neutrons). The latter are described as α-particles. These products of nuclear disintegration were first discovered in the 1940s and it is the massive energy from such nuclear fission that is harnessed in the atomic bomb and in nuclear power plants.

10.6.2 Basic biology

Linear energy transfer

As ionizing radiation travels through tissue, it encounters the clouds of electrons orbiting around each nucleus. The number of orbiting electrons and the size of the nucleus increase with increasing atomic number, and therefore the likelihood of encountering either an electron, or even the central nucleus increases in heavier materials. For this reason, heavy metals, e.g. lead, are very efficient as shielding materials. It is this atomic number dependency that gives X-rays their ability to distinguish bony tissue from soft tissue and from air space. The absorption (and hence the residual transmission on to the film) depends both on the tissue density and on its atomic content.

Very high-energy machines have been devised since the 1940s that can accelerate stripped ions, e.g. protons, deuterons, or α-particles, to very high levels of kinetic energy. These are used to bombard various targets so that the constituent atoms are 'smashed', and the components of the nuclei can be identified. In this way mesons and muons can be produced. Also even heavier charged particles such as carbon$^+$ or silicon$^+$ nuclei can be accelerated. Beams of these particles have been produced in various centres (e.g. the American National Laboratories in Berkeley and Los Alamos) and their potential for radiotherapy as an alternative to X-rays has been investigated (Fowler 1981).

The rate at which beams of radiation give energy to the material they are traversing is called the linear energy transfer (LET) and is measured in keV per micron. High LET radiations, e.g. neutrons or α-particles, give up more energy per micron and are more damaging biologically than conventional X-rays. This is measured by comparing the dose of each radiation required to give the same damage as a dose of 250 kV X-rays:

the Relative Biological Effectiveness (RBE). Because the response of cells to each radiation follows a different pattern at low and high doses, the RBE is not a fixed value for one type of radiation. It depends also on the type of organism irradiated, the level of effect being observed, and the dose rate. In general, the RBE is highest at low dose levels and falls towards unity at very high dose levels.

Cell kill in tissues

Ionizing radiation seldom causes instant cell death. Cells may continue to function, e.g. in respiration and protein synthesis, for hours, days, or even many months after single doses of 10–20 Gy. The radiosensitive aspect of a cell's life is its ability to divide and produce viable offspring. This may be influenced by a dose of a few gray, and after 10 Gy less than 1 per cent of cells are likely to retain their reproductive potential. For this reason, it is the rapidly proliferating tissues in the body that most quickly express their radiation damage. For example, the cells in the crypts of the small intestine normally divide every 12 hours, providing a supply of cells which move up to cover the villi, and are worn off at the tip of each villus after about 4 days. After irradiation, cell production is halted when the cells die in abortive mitoses. The cells on the villus surface continue to be worn off, the villi become eroded and if the dose is high enough, the animal will die of epithelial denudation within 4–7 days (Fig. 10.20). Death is due to water loss into the intestine and bacterial invasion from the intestine into the bloodstream.

Other tissues, with a slower turnover of their cells will show damage at a later time, when the differentiated cells have been worn out and there has been a failure to replace them from the proliferating subset. Fig. 10.20 shows that death from bone marrow failure occurs after lower doses, but not until 30 days. If only the thorax is irradiated, the oesophageal damage gives rise to early deaths whereas lung damage leads to deaths after 3–6 months.

The clonogenic assay

The effect of radiation can be studied *in vitro* by growing cells in dishes and scoring the survival of those capable of making a colony after irradiation. This is the clonogenic assay. If a cell is capable of producing a colony of at least 50 cells within 7–10 days, it is regarded as having retained its reproductive integrity and is scored as a survivor. Non-surviving cells may divide two, three, or even four times before petering out. They may therefore form small or slow-growing colonies which contain 10, 20, or even more cells, which are biochemically active, but these are regarded as reproductively dead in the clonogenic assay. If they were still inside an intact tissue, they would be unable to maintain the integrity of that tissue indefinitely because they fail to continue to produce viable offspring.

Studies of cells *in vitro* have shown that this 'killing' effect is not linear with dose. The first few gray are quite ineffective, giving the appearance of a shoulder before cell killing becomes evident (Fig. 10.21). In this shoulder region, there is some evidence of damage, so it is not a true threshold, but rather a curve that becomes steeper with increasing dose. The exact shape of the curve can be modified by the type of radiation, the cell's stage in the cell cycle, its nutritional status, and the amount of radical scavengers (e.g. glutathione) and electron acceptors (e.g. oxygen) that are present (Fig. 10.21). High LET radiations give a steeper response in the shoulder region. Thiols and other radical scavengers, including ascorbate, have a radioprotective effect. Oxygen and other electron acceptors have a radiosensitizing effect. Cells in mitosis are very sensitive, with no evidence of a shoulder. Cells in DNA synthesis, when all the enzymes for DNA repair are likely to be available, are least sensitive and have a very broad shoulder.

The subcellular target

The critical target for reproductive killing is the DNA of the cells. Using very shallow-penetrating α-particles, it has been shown that huge doses can be given to the cytoplasm without causing cell death, but if the radiation reaches inside the nuclear membrane the cells appear sensitive. Various biochemical techniques have been developed to look at the sorts of lesion produced in DNA. Many types of injury occur, the most common being single-strand breaks due to damage to a single base. There are also intra-strand cross-links, inter-strand cross-links, or

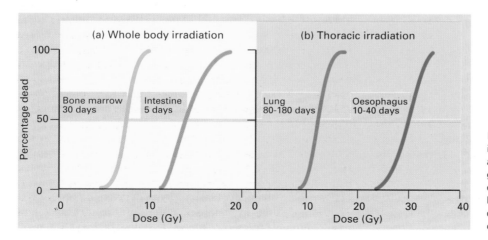

Fig. 10.20 Schematic illustration of lethality in mice after whole body or partial body irradiation. (a) The most rapidly proliferating tissue gives rise to early morbidity if the dose is high enough. (b) Slowly proliferating tissues can lead to later deaths even after much higher doses. Time of death ascribed to failure of each organ is indicated.

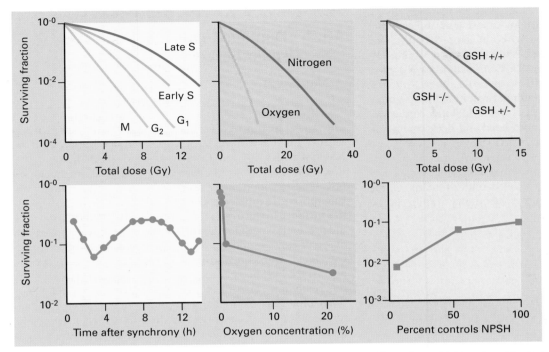

Fig. 10.21 Survival curves measured with clonogenic assays of cells *in vitro*. The radiosensitivity varies with stage in the cell cycle (left panels), with oxygen content (middle panels), and with glutathione content (right panels).

alteration of individual bases. One of the least common lesions, but the only one that correlates well with cell death is the double-strand break. This consists of damage on both strands of the double helix, either directly opposite or within a few base pairs of each other.

Cells are capable of removing most lesions in DNA, using the opposite strand as a template to replace the appropriate bases. Presumably, if the opposite strand is also damaged, this becomes much more difficult. Rejoining of double-strand breaks does occur in cells, and it is the residual unrepaired lesions that correlate best with cell killing. However, it seems likely that the repaired DNA may often be inaccurate (or misrepaired). This may be fatal; or may simply give rise to a mutation, which may even be a carcinogenic event. It is because the genetic material is the target that the anomaly exists that ionizing radiation may be both beneficial (by killing clonogenic tumour cells) and hazardous (in producing potentially carcinogenic or teratogenic mutations).

Sparing effect of fractionation

It is well recognized, both *in vitro* and *in vivo* that radiation is much less damaging if it is divided into a series of smaller doses, or fractions, instead of being given as a large single dose. Repair of the first set of lesions can occur before the next set is inflicted. In this way, interaction of lesions is minimized and/or the enzymes responsible for the repair process are less likely to be overwhelmed or depleted.

Radiotherapy for malignant tumours is used in both a palliative mode and in a curative mode. For palliation of a local tumour in a patient with known disseminated disease, it is relatively easy to kill 99 per cent of the local tumour cells, with single doses or a few large fractions. When the aim is curative, however, e.g. in patients without metastases, it becomes much more important to give the treatment in a way that will maximize its effect on tumour cells while minimizing its effect on surrounding normal tissues. To do this requires an extensive understanding of the radiobiology of tumours, of acutely responding tissues, and of late-responding tissues (Thames and Hendry 1987). Tumours and acutely responding tissues both contain rapidly proliferating cells. They are sensitive to alterations in the fractionation schedule that involve lengthening or shortening it (because they proliferate between fractions) but are not much influenced by the size of the individual fractions. Late-responding tissues are slowly proliferating. They are insensitive to changes in overall time, but are very much influenced by the size of the individual fractions. They are particularly harmed by large doses of radiation. Deviations from the convention of 2 Gy per day, five times a week, must therefore be approached with caution.

The possibility of shortening treatment duration and cutting down the workload of a busy radiotherapy department by giving a few large fractions has been shown to give equal acute side-effects but disastrous late morbidity. The current trend is towards reducing the fraction size below 2 Gy (which spares late-reacting tissues) and shortening treatment times (which damages tumours, but also increases acute reactions) by giving several fractions on each day. Animal experiments indicate that the interfraction interval needs to be at least 6 hours. One extreme example of this approach is under study at Mount Vernon Hospital (UK) using three fractions a day for 12 days (including the weekend) with a 6–6–12 hours interval (Saunders *et al.* 1988). The preliminary results show a significant increase in local control at 2 years of lung carcinoma (12→35 per cent) and of advanced head and neck carcinoma (35→63 per cent). The acute reactions, as predicted, are increased but there is no sign of increased late morbidity. This emphasizes the need to understand that all normal tissues will not behave alike, and that a detailed understanding of the underlying biology is needed before laboratory results can be translated into clinical practice.

10.6.3 Summary

Ionizing radiation damages cells by causing ionizations in DNA, either directly, or indirectly by producing toxic radicals in the immediate vicinity. The effect of radiation is mainly on the reproductive capacity of the cell. The cell can continue to function biochemically after very high doses if it is not called upon to divide. The clonogenic assay is the best measure of the loss of proliferative potential. Survival curves after X- or γ-rays are shouldered, but these can be altered by oxygen, thiols, the cell cycle state of the cell, by dose rate, LET, or fractionation. Cells are capable of repairing most of the lesions inflicted by radiation but misrepair may lead to mutations. The time at which damage appears in normal tissues in the body depends upon the cell kinetic features of that tissue. Radiation will halt division in the proliferative subpopulation, but this will only be reflected in tissue malfunction when the differentiated cells have been lost by normal wear and tear. It may be manifest within days (in intestine) or may be latent for many months (e.g. lung, liver, heart, spinal cord).

10.6.4 Bibliography

Alper, T. (1979). *Cellular radiobiology*. Cambridge University Press, Cambridge.

Denekamp, J. (1982). *Cell kinetics and cancer therapy* (ed. W. C. Dewey). C. C. Thomas, Springfield, Illinois.

Fowler, J. F. (1981). *Nuclear particles in cancer treatment*, Medical Physics Handbook 8. Adam Hilger, Bristol.

Hall, E. J. (1988). *Radiobiology for the radiologist* (3rd edn). Lippincott, Philadelphia.

Johns, H. E. and Cunningham, J. R. (eds) (1969). *The physics of radiology*. C. C. Thomas, Springfield, Illinois.

Saunders, M. I. *et al.* (1988). Radiotherapy employing 3 fractions on each of 12 consecutive days. *Acta Oncologica* **27**, 163–8.

Thames, H. D. and Hendry, J. H. (eds) (1987). *Fractionation in radiotherapy*. Taylor & Francis, London.

UNSCEAR Report (1988). *Sources, effects and risks of ionizing radiation*. United Nations Publications, New York.

10.7 Damage to normal tissues due to radiotherapy

A. Michalowski

The radical treatment of cancer by means of ionizing radiations aims at, and often appears to achieve, the sterilization of all the neoplastic cells. The pre-eminent efficacy of radiotherapy does not, however, rely on highly selective sensitivity of malignant cells, and radiation interferes similarly with cell production in tumours and in proliferating normal tissues, which are of necessity included in the irradiated volume. Consequently, the standard procedures of radiation treatment, which have been arrived at empirically, amount to balancing the gravity of prognosis associated with uncontrolled tumour growth and spread, against the likelihood and severity of complications incurred by the treatment. The perception of price worth paying in the currency of normal tissues for the prospect of cure from cancer is widely shared by the patients and physicians alike; it defines the limits to the intensity of treatment and is loosely referred to as the 'therapeutic ratio'.

10.7.1 Mechanisms of tissue damage

Various side-effects of radiotherapy differ in their temporal relation to the treatment and are therefore divided into two broad categories. The early reactions occur within hours to weeks after exposure to radiation and are usually short-lived, whereas the late complications take months to decades to become noticeable and are often persistent or even progressive. Reactions of both types may sequentially affect the same organ or structure; when early lesions are more severe and prolonged than usual, they merge with, and are likely to contribute to, the late damage.

Most of the early untoward reactions to irradiation are due to depletion of rapidly turning-over cell lineages, such as those which provide the diverse epithelial lining to various segments of the alimentary canal. Irradiation interferes with the otherwise continual process of new cell production necessary to replace the short-lived functional cells. After exposure the loss of these cells proceeds at the normal speed, resulting in rapid depopulation and a corresponding reduction in the overall lineage-specific functions (Michalowski 1990). The depletion is made good by vigorous regeneration from the remaining homologous precursor cells unaffected by the randomly sterilizing action of radiation.

The pathogenetic mechanisms involved in late side-effects of radiotherapy are controversial and less well understood. Although these effects have some common features uncharacteristic of early responses (Michalowski 1986), they are often presented as strict analogues of the latter, dominated by depopulation of slowly turning-over parenchymal cell lineages, with a correspondingly longer time-scale of development

(Michalowski 1989). In the opposite view, the crucial primary damage somehow takes the form of a protracted increase in endothelial permeability to plasma constituents. The leakage results in arterio- and arteriolosclerosis with progressive ischaemia, parenchymal cell degeneration and atrophy, and widespread deposition of collagen.

These issues have recently gained in practical importance with the realization that the late effects depend to a greater degree than the early ones on the size of each fractional dose administered in the course of radiation treatment, and less on the overall duration of treatment (Thames and Hendry 1987). The difference is possibly exploitable in the clinic and calls for departure from standard treatment schedules. The questions addressed at present (Hendry *et al.* 1986) include the important distinction between direct radiation damage and various reactions to it; the latter, when noxious, may prove amenable to judicious drug treatment (Michalowski 1989, 1990) only seldom attempted at present.

The problem of individual sensitivity to ionizing radiations (Sabovljev *et al.* 1985) has received insufficient attention, except for patients with ataxia telangiectasia who are both prone to develop tumours and are abnormally radioresponsive (Waldmann *et al.* 1983). Nevertheless, the trait does not eliminate its bearers from radiotherapy for cancer provided that the doses are appropriately reduced (Hart *et al.* 1987).

The following outline of systematic human radiopathology (cf. Fajardo 1982; Lett and Altman 1987) is naturally biased towards the rare instances of severe damage caused by the treatment. In the majority of patients (around 90–95 per cent) curative radiotherapy is administered without exceeding the tolerance of any normal tissue, i.e. no permanently debilitating or life-threatening lesions are produced. The total absorbed dose of radiation is obviously important in determining the incidence and severity of complications; however, the quality of radiation, fraction size, dose rate, overall treatment time, and the irradiated proportion of the structure in question are all contributory (see Section 10.6). Administration of cytotoxic drugs tends to lower the radiotolerance. No single common criterion could possibly be devised to compare radiosensitivity of all the different anatomical entities which carry out their diverse functions, yet the lens, gonads, haemo- and lymphopoietic tissues, and lungs are considered to be among the most vulnerable, whereas the locomotor system in adults is one of the least responsive.

10.7.2 Nervous system

Therapeutic irradiation of the brain may lead to acute cerebral oedema with an associated increase in intracranial pressure. The so-called 'early delayed' reactions that develop within a few months after exposure consist of multifocal demyelination of the white matter, possibly reflecting the damage suffered by oligodendroglia. Severe late reactions affect predominantly the hemispheres, and present as foci of coagulative or, less often, colliquative necrosis (see Chapter 3). The unresorbed dead tissue may undergo granular calcification. In the immediately adjacent white matter the number of glial cells is moderately increased (gliosis), and the necrotic foci are usually surrounded by areas of demyelination. These late lesions are associated with vascular pathology. The intracerebral arteries and arterioles may have their lumina narrowed by endothelial proliferation or subendothelial deposits of collagen. The entire vascular wall may undergo hyalinization or 'fibrinoid necrosis'. Some arteries lose their patency as a result of thrombosis. The capillaries become tortuous and dilated (telangiectasiae).

Radiation lesions of the spinal cord are similar in nature to those of the brain.

10.7.3 Cardiovascular system

Acute or protracted pericarditis develops after a lag period of variable duration, with the accumulation of fibrinous and/or serous exudate sometimes leading to heart tamponade. The extravasated fibrin later becomes organized by dense connective tissue infiltrated with scanty inflammatory cells. Constrictive pericarditis is only seldom encountered. The capillary network of the heart muscle gradually decreases in density, with the concomitant development of diffuse myocardial fibrosis.

The major blood vessels do not ordinarily show signs of therapeutic radiation damage. Lesions affecting the visceral vasculature are described under individual organs.

10.7.4 Respiratory system

Upper respiratory tract

The most notable early complication is laryngeal oedema, coinciding with or closely following the course of fractionated radiotherapy. Late lesions consist of stromal fibrosis with glandular atrophy. Aseptic chondronecrosis may develop and lead to purulent chondritis and perichondritis.

Lung

Early lesions termed 'acute radiation pneumonitis' are dominated by exudation of plasma constituents into the alveolar walls and lumen, on occasion leading to hyaline (fibrin) membrane formation resembling the adult respiratory distress syndrome (see Chapter 13). The various cells lining the alveoli are reduced in number, hypertrophied, and distorted. The scanty cellular inflammatory infiltrates may include foamy macrophages invading the air spaces. The late damage consists of deposition of collagen and elastic fibres in the walls of collapsed alveoli, sometimes progressing to solid scar formation. The involvement of large fractional volumes of the lungs leads to respiratory insufficiency with an increase in pulmonary arterial blood pressure.

Total body irradiation with bone marrow transplantation, as used for treatment of haematological disorders and early disseminating tumours of childhood, is quite often associated with pulmonary morbidity. The condition is caused not by radiotherapy alone but also by cytostatic drugs, prolonged immunodeficiency leading to respiratory infections, and graft-versus-host reactions.

10.7.5   Digestive system

Oropharynx

Early epithelial depopulation may progress to erosive mucositis whereas late damage shows as submucosal fibrosis. Mandibular osteonecrosis (which is fortunately infrequent) can be accompanied by chronic oral ulcers.

Salivary glands

The serous glandular cells are prone to rapid degeneration and necrosis with only mild cellular inflammatory reaction. Later, the glands undergo patchy though severe interstitial fibrosis with parenchymal atrophy and arteriolosclerosis.

Oesophagus

Early damage shows as transient erosive oesophagitis, whereas the most frequent delayed lesion is a fibrotic stricture of the oesophagus.

Stomach

Relatively mild fractionated irradiation of the stomach was formerly used to treat peptic ulcer, since it rapidly resulted in a protracted reduction in gastric acid secretion which at present is achieved with drugs, particularly those blocking the H2 histamine receptors. More attention is now given to rare instances of gastric or duodenal ulcer allegedly induced by upper abdominal irradiation for cancer treatment.

Intestines

Acute radiation enteritis is due to continuing loss of short-lived enterocytes with impaired production of replacement cells in the crypts of Lieberkühn. The absorptive surface of the gut is thus reduced; when denuded of its epithelial cover, the mucous membrane oozes the interstitial fluid and may be invaded by the luminal micro-organisms. These diffuse lesions are responsible for acute diarrhoea with water and electrolyte losses. Resumption of successful cell divisions in the crypts leads to their hyperplasia followed by replenishment of the villous epithelium.

Late consequences of intestinal irradiation are reflected in malabsorption of nutrients and persistent diarrhoea. Stenosis with ileus, ulceration, haemorrhage, perforation, fistula, or adhesions sometimes develop against the background of a widespread chronic radiation damage to the intestine. The latter is characterized by mucosal atrophy and fibrosis of the enteric wall associated with vascular lesions (arterial intimal fibrosis and thickening of the media; capillary thrombosis).

Liver

Early stages of radiation damage are characterized by intravascular coagulation, with deposits of fibrin selectively obstructing the centrilobular outflow venules and larger hepatic (but not portal) veins. The vascular lesions lead to congestion and secondary degeneration and atrophy of hepatocytes. The condition is termed 'hepatic veno-occlusive disease' and is similar to that caused by ingestion of pyrrolizidine alkaloids. With time, the fibrin is substituted by collagen and reticulin fibres, which also replace the missing parenchymal cells. Severe injury of a large fractional volume of the organ is associated with ascites and jaundice.

Pancreas

In man, only late effects have been characterized morphologically as interstitial fibrosis, sometimes associated with atrophy of the exocrine parenchymal cells and arteriolosclerosis.

10.7.6   Urinary system

Kidney

An insidious development of radiation nephropathy takes months to decades before the condition becomes clinically manifest as progressive renal failure or a stable functional deficit. Even then, it only occurs if a large fractional volume of the kidneys has been irradiated; otherwise the circumscribed damage is compensated for by hypertrophy of the intact nephrons. Within the irradiated renal tissue, tubular lesions are invariably present in the form of atrophy or denudation, affecting predominantly the proximal convoluted tubules. The lesions are associated with interstitial fibrosis and sparse lymphocytic infiltration. Arteriolar and microvascular damage, including that of the glomerular tufts, is variable both in its severity and character. A gradual loss of the glomerular endothelial cells may lead to capillary thrombosis. Arteriolosclerosis and segmental or diffuse glomerular sclerosis and hyalinization are seen most often. In some cases both the afferent arterioles and glomeruli undergo 'fibrinoid necrosis'. It is far from clear whether these vascular lesions represent direct radiation damage or are secondary to either benign or malignant hypertension, which affects a large proportion of patients suffering from radiation nephropathy, presumably due to malfunction of the myoepithelial cells of the afferent arterioles which normally participate in regulation of blood pressure by secreting renin.

Another systemic effect of radiation nephropathy is normocytic normochromic anaemia, compatible with morphologically undefined damage suffered by cells involved in renal production of erythropoietin.

Urinary bladder

Early reactions consist of transient depopulation of the urothelium and mucosal oedema. Late damage is dominated by fibrosis which may affect all layers of the wall and lead to rigid contraction of the organ, while telangiectatic mucosal vessels tend to bleed. The overdosed areas are prone to develop chronic ulcers or even fistulae.

10.7.7   Endocrine system and gonads

Hypothalamus and pituitary

Inclusion of the hypothalamus in a therapeutically irradiated volume of tissues may result years later in subnormal secretion of one or more of the following hypophysiotrophic hormones: growth hormone releasing factor and thyrotrophin, corticotrophin and luteinizing hormone releasing hormones; this leads to a corresponding secondary hypopituitarism. Radiation-induced failure of an inhibitory function of the hypothalamus is reflected in hyperprolactinaemia.

The adenohypophysis may also suffer from direct radiation damage with impaired synthesis and secretion of growth hormone (which in children results in retarded growth), as well as the thyroid stimulating hormone, adrenocorticotrophic, luteinizing and follicle stimulating hormones. In the extreme cases, the endocrine anterior pituitary cells undergo atrophy associated with interstitial fibrosis.

Thyroid

Apart from following radiation damage to the hypothalamic–pituitary axis, hypothyroidism may develop after external beam irradiation of the thyroid gland itself. Moreover, thyroid insufficiency requiring replacement therapy (thyroxine) frequently succeeds an euthyroid phase in patients treated with oral $Na^{131}I$ for thyrotoxicosis. Direct radiation damage to the gland is strikingly dose-dependent in its timing and severity. The follicles decrease in size and colloid content, and are lined with either atrophic or irregularly enlarged cells possessing expanded, sometimes hyperchromatic nuclei. The amount of the intervening connective tissue is increased, with individually variable density of lymphocytic infiltration.

Ovary

Direct radiation insult results in disappearance of both primary and growing follicles, as well as stromal cells of the ovarian cortex, leaving behind dense collagen deposits. Such severe lesions are associated with infertility, amenorrhoea, and high gonadotrophin levels.

Testis

The spermatogenic cells, and particularly spermatogonia, are much more radiosensitive than mature spermatozoa or Sertoli and Leydig cells. Irradiation results within hours in cell death and depopulation of the rapidly proliferating seminiferous epithelium, followed weeks later by oligo- or azoospermia whose duration (measured in years) is directly dose-dependent. Severe damage leads to permanent collapse of the tubules with marked thickening and hyalinization of the basal lamina and a reduction in Leydig cell numbers. Such lesions are associated with rises in follicle stimulating and luteinizing hormones, and low testosterone levels.

10.7.8 Other organs

Lymphoid tissues

Quiescent (non-proliferating) lymphocytes are exceptional in that, when even mildly irradiated, they die and disintegrate within hours of exposure; most other cells are lost only during or after post-irradiation mitotic division. This makes lymphocytes vulnerable to radiation not only if resident in the exposed volume of tissues but also while circulating in blood. Consequently, repeated large-field irradiation tends to result in early and selective lymphopenia.

Irradiation of the solid lymphoid tissue in any location (the thymus, lymph nodes, white pulp of the spleen, tonsils, Peyer's patches) leads rapidly to local massive nuclear damage; this is evident morphologically as pyknosis and karyorrhexis of small lymphocytes followed by their disappearance. Replenishment takes months and may never be complete. Such reactions are taken advantage of in total body irradiation which, in addition to eradicating widely disseminated malignant cells, serves to induce immunological tolerance required for subsequent successful allogeneic bone marrow transplantation. Total nodal or lymphoid irradiation has also been used in attempts to control some autoimmune conditions.

Bone marrow

Irradiation is followed by a steady local reduction in the number of nucleated cells, reaching a nadir approximately at the time of completion of the fractionated treatment. Repopulation takes months and may be incomplete, with hypocellular bone marrow partially replaced by adipose or loose connective tissue. These lesions only infrequently reach clinical significance since the exposed fractional volume of the erythro-, leuko-, and thrombopoietic tissue is ordinarily small.

Eye

The most frequent sequel of irradiation is opacity of the lens (cataract). It begins locally at the posterior pole and spreads both in the plane parallel to that of the capsule and anteriorly. The opacity is due to degeneration and liquefaction of lens fibres which normally contain transparent crystalline proteins, and is accompanied by posterior migration of the superficial epithelial cells.

Skin

Early reactions include erythema, inflammatory oedema with variable white blood cell extravasation, alopecia, scaling, and increased pigmentation. More severe exposure leads to transient multifocal or confluent loss of the irradiated epidermis. Late damage is reflected in epidermal thinning, non-uniform pigmentation, sparsity of hair follicles, as well as sebaceous and sweat glands, and telangiectasiae. The dermal connective tissue is less cellular and denser than normal.

10.7.9 Bibliography

Casarett, G. W. (1980). *Radiation histopathology*, Vols 1 and 2. CRC Press, Boca Raton, Florida.

Fajardo, L. F. (1982). *Pathology of radiation injury*. Masson Publishing, New York.

Hart, R. M., Kimler, B. F., Evans, R. G., and Park, C. H. (1987). Radiotherapeutic management of medulloblastoma in a pediatric patient with ataxia telangiectasia. *International Journal of Radiation Oncology* **13**, 1237–40.

Hendry, J. H., Potten, C. S., Moore, J. V., and Hume, W. J. (eds) (1986). Assays of normal tissue injury, and their cellular interpretation. *British Journal of Cancer* **53**, suppl. VII.

Lett, J. T. and Altman, K. I. (eds) (1987). Relative radiation sensitivities of human organ systems. *Advances in Radiation Biology* **12**. Academic Press, Orlando.

Michalowski, A. (1986). The pathogenesis of the late side-effects of radiotherapy. *Clinical Radiology* **37**, 202–7.

Michalowski, A. (1989). Radiopathology of normal tissues: are clonogenic survival and cell kinetics all that matter? In *XVth Berzelius Symposium: Somatic and genetic effects of ionizing radiation*, T. Stigbrand (ed.). Nyheterna Tryckeri, Umeå, pp. 67–73.

Michalowski, A. (1990). On radiation damage to normal tissues and its treatment. I. Growth factors. *Acta Oncologica* **29**, 1017–23.

Patt, H. M. and Quastler, H. (1963). Radiation effects on cell renewal and related systems. *Physiological Reviews* **43**, 357–96.

Sabovljev, S. A., Cramp, W. A., Lewis, P. D., Harris, G., Halnan, K. E., and Lambert, J. (1985). Use of rapid tests of cellular radiosensitivity in radio-therapeutic practice. *Lancet* **ii**, 787.

Thames, H. D. and Hendry, J. H. (1987). *Fractionation in radiotherapy.* Taylor & Francis, London.

Waldmann, T. A., Misiti, J., Nelson, D. L., and Kraemer, K. H. (1983). Ataxia telangiectasia: a multisystem hereditary disease with immunodeficiency, impaired organ maturation, X-ray hypersensitivity, and a high incidence of neoplasia. *Annals of Internal Medicine* **99**, 367–79.

Withers, H. R., Peters, L. J., and Kogelnik, H. D. (1980). The pathobiology of late effects of irradiation. In *Radiation biology in cancer research*, (ed. R. E. Meyn and H. R. Withers), pp. 439–48. Raven Press, New York.

11

Principles of developmental pathology

J. S. Wigglesworth

11

Principles of developmental pathology

J. S. Wigglesworth

11.1 Nature and importance of developmental pathology

Developmental pathology encompasses pathological processes related to placentation, embryogenesis, fetal growth, the process of birth, and adaptation to extra-uterine life and neonatal development. During the period covered there are immeasurably greater changes occurring in form and function than over the whole of the rest of life. The subject differs fundamentally from the pathology of adult life in that many of the abnormal processes seen are the result of deviations of normal development. The drive of growth can translate a minor developmental programming error into a lethal malformation. The sequential processes of growth are associated with varying susceptibilities to damage, so that a particular disease process may have widely differing effects according to the stage of development at which the embryo or fetus may be exposed to it. Conversely, a single gross end-result, such as distorted limbs and undersized lungs, may result from a genetic abnormality of the CNS or muscle fibres or one of several problems arising during pregnancy, including a severe anoxic–ischaemic episode which injures the fetal CNS or chronic loss of amniotic fluid following rupture of the placental membranes. The prognosis for future pregnancies is critically dependent on recognizing which form of process is involved. In the case of an autosomal recessive genetic disease there will be a 25 per cent recurrence risk, but an accurate diagnosis may allow the possibility of antenatal diagnosis or exclusion at an early stage of any succeeding pregnancy. Recognition of a condition that has arisen during pregnancy

may lead to a far better prognosis for future pregnancies and a strategy to limit the risk of recurrence, e.g. of premature rupture of membranes. Study of developmental pathology thus demands an understanding of the dynamic background of normal structural and functional development which may become pathologically disturbed or upon which pathological processes may be superimposed.

Despite the increasing attention of specialists in fetal medicine including, in some departments, the performance of needle biopsies of fetal organs *in utero*, the practice of fetal and perinatal pathology remains, on the whole, an autopsy specialty. Unlike the adult autopsy, which may be regarded as an end-point of largely academic interest, that of the fetus or infant is often of major importance to the family as a prognostic indicator for future children. It would be realistic to think of the dead fetus and placenta, or the infant, as a particularly complex form of surgical sample from which the pathologist may be asked to assess the future reproductive potential of the parents. Much effort in recent years has been expended on improving techniques of prenatal diagnosis, particularly in the case of genetic disease. Improved ultrasound techniques, amniocentesis, and chorion villous sampling have resulted in the ability to detect abnormalities at an ever earlier stage of pregnancy, often within the first trimester. This has allowed the pathologist to study fetal disease processes close to the time of inception and to gain new insights into their mode of development. It does, however, impose the demand that the pathologist be able to dissect and recognize the abnormalities within these small fetuses. In future one can imagine the developmental pathologist undertaking much of his/her work with the aid of the dissecting microscope or even the scanning electron microscope.

The ability to diagnose fetal abnormalities *in utero* means that the pathologist is often asked merely to confirm a diagnosis already made, and to check that there are no additional lesions. Prenatal diagnoses are sometimes incorrect, and in about 35 per cent of cases where a correct diagnosis has been made there are additional abnormalities unrecognized by prenatal procedures such as ultrasound. In the case of unexpected still births no such studies may have been undertaken and it is equally important to exclude the presence of some unrecognized abnormality as to attempt to establish a diagnosis. In deaths during or soon after labour the problems of avoidable asphyxia and trauma require consideration.

Patients, in general, now have a more critical view of medical practitioners than in the past. The relatively low frequency of death in the perinatal period leads parents to expect a live, healthy baby from each pregnancy. Unexpected death of a fetus or infant, or birth of a handicapped infant, may prompt searching questions as to the cause of the disaster. The pathologist has the responsibility of ensuring that, in the case of the dead infant, a full explanation can be given wherever possible. Fatal pathology in the perinatal period is often an end-point of a range of disease which includes a significant group of surviving handicapped individuals. Thus the various patterns of haemorrhagic and ischaemic brain damage seen in the dead fetus or infant have their counterparts in surviving neonates. Since the lesions have often been recognized in life by obstetricians or neonatologists, they may be the focus of informed concern by the clinician when a fetus or neonate is referred for post-mortem examination. Clinicians may reasonably expect the pathologist to have a similarly informed approach.

Deaths in the neonatal period, particularly those of preterm infants from neonatal intensive care units, may be associated with some unforeseen complication of therapy. Close cooperation between pathologist, obstetrician, paediatrician, and clinical geneticist is essential for a proper approach to investigation of these various types of case, since the critical diagnostic investigations are often non-histological (radiology, cytogenetics, microbiology, biochemistry, or haematology may be involved) and it may be important to investigate the mother as well as her dead infant (e.g. in cases of possible congenital infection or inherited metabolic disease).

The pathology of development provides a wide field for research. Currently, the rapid advances in location of the molecular basis of genetic disorders using DNA technology hold centre stage. Conditions that are fatal in the perinatal period are a fruitful area for this type of investigation. The effects of pathological processes on development of organs or body systems may provide important insights into the physiology of normal development. Studies prompted by the observation of hyaline membrane disease and lung hypoplasia represent examples. Conversely, the need to explain developmental pathological processes may prompt more detailed studies on areas of normal development which have been neglected by embryologists, anatomists, or developmental physiologists. Thus many studies on human fetal brain development in the past few years have been performed by pathologists requiring more detail of the basis for perinatal brain damage.

11.2   Pathology of early fetal development

11.2.1   Early fetal loss

It is not possible to assess accurately total embryonic loss rates as many embryos fail to implant or are lost before the mother recognizes that she is pregnant. Some 15 per cent of clinically recognized pregnancies result in spontaneous abortion during the first trimester, with the highest loss rates in the earlier weeks. Chromosomal abnormalities are present in some 60 per cent of the conceptuses aborted in the earlier weeks of development. The major defects are ones seen rarely in surviving fetuses, including trisomy 16, monosomy X, and triploidy. Often no embryo can be detected in early spontaneous aborted conceptuses and the placental villi show absence of blood vessels, suggesting failure of circulatory development as a primary defect. Deaths at a later stage, from 20 weeks on, include an increasing proportion due to problems that have arisen during pregnancy, such as infections, premature rupture of the membranes, and a range of problems resulting in impairment of uteroplacental transfer.

Much of this loss can be regarded as a necessary deletion of reproductive failures, neither preventable nor treatable. Within this unavoidable loss it might, however, be extremely difficult to recognize the influence of any environmental factor that prevented implantation or caused early embryonic disruption or lethal malformation.

11.2.2   Congenital malformations

A malformation can be defined as a primary structural defect that results from a localized error of morphogenesis. Such defects arise during the period of organogenesis within the first 8 weeks following conception. More subtle defects within organs can arise at a later stage of development, e.g. abnormalities of migration of neurones within the cerebrum in the second trimester. In addition, the remodelling during later growth of tissues which have been damaged after normal organogenesis can result in an abnormal structure by the time of birth. These disruptions or deformations should be recognized as distinct from true malformations, being of different causation and prognosis. Deformations in one organ may result from a malformation in another. Thus, lack of formation of the kidneys results in failure of urine production, with consequent lack of amniotic fluid leading to limb distortion and impaired lung growth. Malformations may involve any system or organ and often present in the form of groups of associated abnormalities, or syndromes.

Causes of malformations

Malformations may be due to either genetic or environmental causes or may be of multifactorial causation. Genetic causes are subdivided into chromosomal and single gene abnormalities.

Chromosomal causes of malformation

Gross chromosomal abnormalities arise in a number of ways. An extra full set of chromosomes (triploidy) may be the result of double fertilization of the ovum or failure of the ovum to exclude a polar body during meiosis. An additional full chromosome (trisomy) or absence of a chromosome (monosomy) arises by errors in assortment of chromosomes during meiotic divisions of the gamete or the first mitotic division of the zygote. Chromosome breakage during cell division may result in partial monosomy or a duplication deficiency translocation chromosome, according to whether loss or rearrangement follows the initial breakage of chromosomal material. Details of the various patterns of chromosomal breakage and rearrangement are to be found elsewhere.

Single gene defects

Single gene mutations account for most disorders that are commonly recognized to be of genetic origin. The inheritance pattern may be autosomal dominant, autosomal recessive, or X-linked (either recessive or dominant). Most of the genetic abnormalities that are lethal at, or soon after, birth are autosomal recessive. Examples include the form of short-limbed dwarfism known as achondrogenesis and infantile polycystic kidney disease. Autosomal dominant conditions tend to show wider variation in expression among affected individuals than autosomal recessive disorders, although lethal dominant disorders may present as new mutations (thanatophoric dwarfism and the lethal form of osteogenesis imperfecta).

Polygenic or multifactorial causation

In most common malformations it is believed that polygenic inheritance accounts for a major part of the tendency to recurrence within families, although environmental factors play some part.

Environmental causes of malformation

These include drugs, industrial and agricultural chemicals, radiation, and infections. The potential teratogenic effect of drugs administered to pregnant women was widely investigated following the thalidomide disaster. Many drugs have been suspected of causing fetal malformations but teratogenic activity has been confirmed in relatively few of them. Drugs used for cancer therapy, including folate antagonists (aminopterin and methotrexate) and alkylating agents (6-mercaptopurine, busulphan, chlorambucil, and cyclophosphamide) may cause microcephaly, growth deficiency, and limb abnormalities. Other teratogenic drugs include: androgenic steroids (female virilization), anticonvulsants (cardiac, skeletal, brain, and facial anomalies with mental retardation), warfarin (nasal hypoplasia, optic atrophy, skeletal abnormalities, and mental retardation), and alcohol (microcephaly, facial and joint abnormalities, and growth deficiency). Other drugs suspected, but not proven, to cause malformations include: oral hypoglycaemic agents used in the treatment of diabetes, sex hormones, amphetamine, tranquillizers, salicylates, and antibiotics. Establishing a causal

relationship between a drug and a malformation in human pregnancy may present considerable problems. The malformation could be due to the disease for which the drug is given rather than the drug itself; the defect could be due to synergistic action of several drugs; the timing of fetal exposure or the drug dosage may be critical; and information on drug dosage and timing may be unreliable.

Of industrial chemicals, methyl mercury poisoning (Minamata disease) in pregnancy causes impaired fetal growth, microcephaly, and limb deformities. Evidence for teratogenic effects of other chemicals remains controversial.

Exposure to large doses of radiation *in utero* causes microcephaly associated with mental retardation. The effect is mediated in the second trimester when formation of cortical neurones is most active.

Of infections, the rubella virus is known to be teratogenic in the first 4 months after conception, with the highest risk to the fetus at 8–10 weeks. Effects on the fetus include growth retardation, microcephaly, microphthalmia, and cardiac septal defects or patent ductus arteriosus. Other effects of the rubella virus, as well as most of the effects of other infectious agents in pregnancy, are those of a continued infection or destruction of fetal tissues by the infectious process.

Major patterns of malformation

A detailed description of the enormous range of human malformations is beyond the scope of this chapter. The patterns of malformation that are of major importance are those that allow survival until late pregnancy or birth. The individual organ systems most frequently involved by serious malformations are the CNS and the cardiovascular system. Important CNS abnormalities are those related to failure of neural tube closure, anencephaly, and spina bifida. Serious cardiac anomalies are those that involve the great arteries and arterial outflow from the ventricles. These include aortic hypoplasia (hypoplastic left heart syndrome), pulmonary atresia, and transposition of the great arteries. In a condition such as transposition of the great arteries, in which the aorta arises from the right ventricle and the pulmonary trunk from the left ventricle, the baby may appear normal at birth but becomes severely cyanosed when the ductus closes in the first few days of life. Other important internal abnormalities include: oesophageal atresia with tracheo-oesophageal fistula and congenital diaphragmatic hernia. The former condition is due to abnormal separation of the tracheal groove from the primitive foregut during the fourth week of development. If occurring as the sole malformation, the prognosis following corrective surgery is good, but the condition is often associated with malformations of other systems, including the cardiovascular system and renal tract.

Congenital diaphragmatic hernia is due to a persistent pleuroperitoneal canal, most often the left, with consequent herniation of liver, stomach, and spleen into the thoracic cavity. This malformation has a poor prognosis despite early diagnosis and surgery as there is usually severe hypoplasia of the lung on the affected side and, to some extent, also on the opposite side. Intra-uterine operative repair has been attempted as an experimental procedure to allow catch-up growth of the lungs before birth.

A very large number of malformation syndromes have been recognized and are listed in several major texts. Some important syndromes are associated with chromosomal defects, including trisomies of chromosome 13, chromosome 18, and chromosome 21 (Down syndrome).

Trisomy 13 is characterized by moderate microcephaly, eye defects including microphthalmos or coloboma, and cleft lip and/or palate. There is often polydactyly of the hands, and internal abnormalities of the brain, heart, and kidneys.

Infants having trisomy 18 are often severely growth retarded with a small placenta, single umbilical artery, and polyhydramnios. The head shows a prominent occiput and narrow bifrontal diameter; there are low-set malformed ears, short palpebral fissures, a small mouth, and micrognathia (Fig. 11.1). The hands tend to be clenched with the index finger overlapping the fourth finger. The most frequent internal malformations are ventricular septal defects, although many other defects may be present

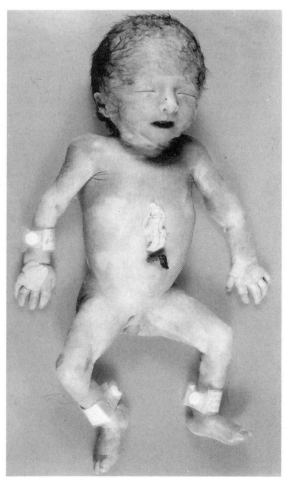

Fig. 11.1 Preterm infant with trisomy 18. The small low set ear, small mouth, and small lower jaw can be seen.

involving the brain, kidneys, lung, diaphragm, gastrointestinal tract, skeletal tissues, endocrine organs, and genitalia.

Infants with either of these syndromes tend to die in the first few weeks after birth, although the conditions are often recognized prenatally with consequent termination of pregnancy.

Trisomy 21 is usually not fatal in the perinatal period but some cases present as spontaneous abortions or still births, and some of the associated malformations may prove fatal in early life. These infants show brachycephaly with a relatively flat occiput and mild microcephaly. The face is flat with a small nose with a low bridge and inner epicanthic folds. The palpebral fissures slope upward from inner to outer canthus. The ears are small with a folded angulated upper helix. There tends to be excess skin on the back of a short neck and there are short metacarpals with hypoplasia of the midphalanx of the fifth finger. There are characteristic dermatoglyphic patterns. Cardiac anomalies, present in 40 per cent of cases, include atrioventricular canal, ventricular and atrial septal defects, persistent patent ductus arteriosus, and tetralogy of Fallot. Common gastrointestinal defects include duodenal atresia and tracheo-oesophageal fistula.

Among the non-chromosomal malformation syndromes one of the more frequent and important is Potter syndrome, now more often described as 'oligohydramnios sequence'. These infants have growth impairment. The face shows prominent epicanthic folds, low-set cartilage-deficient ears, a beak-like nose, and a small lower jaw (Fig. 11.2). The upper limbs have large spade-like hands and the legs show talipes and often distortion and congenital dislocation of the hips. These features are all due to lack of amniotic fluid, and identical features are seen in cases in which the oligohydramnios is caused by failure of renal output (renal agenesis or severe cystic renal dysplasia), lower urinary tract obstruction, or chronic amniotic fluid leakage dating from early in the second trimester. Internally, the syndrome is characterized by hypoplastic lungs.

11.3   Problems of placentation

Fetal growth and nutrition is dependent on development and maintenance of an adequate materno-fetal exchange mechanism through the placenta. Details of placental structure and development are beyond the scope of this chapter and it is possible only to outline the types of problem that may interfere with materno-fetal exchange across the placenta. The human placenta varies considerably in shape as placental villi are formed initially over the entire surface of the chorion as the conceptus implants within the decidua but later become restricted to the basal decidua, where the villi can establish and maintain a close relationship with the maternal circulation as the conceptus enlarges. Placentas of different shape, thickness, or number of lobes may function equally well. In addition, various lesions of no significance can be seen within the normal mature placenta.

with passive transfer of the maternally acquired antibodies. IgA and IgM can be produced in the fetal organs in response to antigenic stimulation from about 20 weeks. Thus, at term, the fetus has a degree of immunity to those organisms to which efficient IgG antibodies are present. The placenta gives some protection against certain maternal infections, including most bacteria, but does not hinder passage of a number of viruses or of *Treponema pallidum*, *Listeria monocytogenes*, or *Toxoplasma gondii*.

Congenital syphilis is rare in Europe, although still very common throughout much of the African continent, and will not be discussed here.

Listeriosis has received considerable publicity recently, with the recognition of the high concentration of the organism achieved in many popular products in the supermarket chill cabinet, including soft cheeses and pâtés. This particular organism can multiply at a temperature marginally above freezing. The current increase in perinatal fatalities from this infection is likely to persist unless the onus is placed on supermarkets to supply relatively clean food, rather than on pregnant women to guess which supermarket products are lethally contaminated. The diphtheroid-like organism produces abscesses in the placenta and readily crosses the placental barrier to cause a fetal septicaemia. Equally, it may infect the maternal vagina and reach the fetal respiratory tract by way of the placental membranes and amniotic fluid (Fig. 11.4). The fetus infected *in utero* may be growth retarded and may have multiple small abscesses, resembling miliary tuberculosis, in almost any organ but particularly the gastrointestinal tract and central nervous system. Stillbirth, or early neonatal death from septicaemia or meningitis, are common outcomes.

Toxoplasmosis is acquired from cats or from uncooked meat, particularly in some continental countries. It is currently relatively uncommon as a perinatal infection in the UK. The fetal central nervous system is most at risk and may show focal necrosis, calcification, and hydrocephalus, with the presence of encysted organisms round the margins of affected areas.

Rubella infection has been mentioned as a cause of anomalies. With the widespread immunization of young girls against rubella, cytomegalovirus and parvovirus infections may be more important. Cytomegalovirus infection involves the CNS in a high proportion of cases, but causes lesions in many organs, including liver, kidneys, pancreas, and lungs. Non-specific foci of inflammation may be associated with the presence of the characteristic owl-eyed cells. Parvovirus B19 infection has only recently become recognized as an important fetal problem. In children and adults the infection causes a minor illness known as slapped-cheek syndrome. In the fetus it causes a haemolytic anaemia and sometimes hepatosplenomegaly with oedema and ascites (one form of non-immunological hydrops). Intranuclear viral inclusions are seen in the plentiful normoblasts within the liver, spleen, and capillaries.

11.5 Problems of the birth process

During the process of birth the infant is at particular risk to asphyxial and traumatic processes. Concern over death in such circumstances centres on the potentially avoidable nature of the lesions. Few of the asphyxial and traumatic lesions seen at autopsy are necessarily fatal and similar ones can be recognized in life or are assumed to have occurred in a large number of surviving infants. Although most concern attaches to such lesions in infants delivered at term, it should be remembered that similar problems can develop in preterm infants.

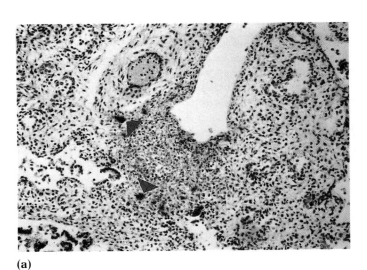

(a)

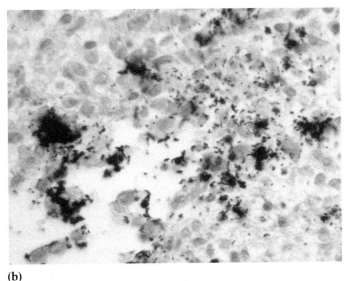

(b)

Fig. 11.4 (a) Lung of a stillborn fetus showing a small abscess due to *Listeria monocytogenes* in a bronchiolar wall with masses of organisms (arrowheads). (b) Gram stain on same lung shows masses of short rod-shaped Gram-positive organisms.

11.5.1 Birth asphyxia

The uterine contractions of labour inevitably cause some decrease in uteroplacental blood flow, which may be enhanced by factors such as the pressure of the pregnant uterus on the inferior vena cava when the mother is supine. Maternal disorders such as pre-eclampsia, or placental factors such as obstruction or entanglement of the umbilical cord, or placental infarction, will also lead to a risk of fetal asphyxia during labour. Growth-retarded fetuses are liable to be at increased risk of birth asphyxia, as mentioned above. Usually it is not clear why a particular infant should show signs of acute asphyxia, such as prolonged bradycardia after uterine contractions (Type 2 dips) on the fetal heart monitor.

The post-mortem findings in infants who die as a result of birth asphyxia include external features such as evidence of growth retardation and, often, meconium staining. There may be evidence of excessive moulding of the head if labour was prolonged.

Internally there may be relatively few signs other than petechial haemorrhages over heart and lungs, and intense congestion of some internal organs, such as the liver. On histology the lungs may show evidence of inhalation of meconium or amniotic debris, as deep gasps are a feature of the terminal stage of acute fetal asphyxia.

If the asphyxia was due to retroplacental haemorrhage, there may be acute congestion of all internal organs, with large echymoses or streaky haemorrhages over lungs and heart, due to overloading of the fetal circulation by blood forced back from the compressed placental villi. Acute renal tubular necrosis and anoxic–ischaemic damage to adrenals, liver, and/or brain are histological features of infants who survive acute perinatal asphyxia for some hours or days.

Infants who appear to be acutely asphyxiated during birth may sometimes be suffering from other disorders. Infection can be acquired from the birth canal during labour so that the infant is born with a developing pneumonia. The Group B β-haemolytic streptococcus is an organism that often causes an intrapartum infection of this type.

In addition, an infant who is difficult to resuscitate at birth may be suffering from cerebral anoxic–ischaemic damage that has been induced by episodes of prenatal asphyxia, induced many hours or days before the mother was admitted to hospital in labour. Disasters occurring during delivery, such as an acute fetal haemorrhage (e.g. from a torn fetal placental vessel) or direct fetal trauma, may also result in birth of a collapsed, apparently 'asphyxiated' infant.

11.5.2 Birth trauma

The process of birth is necessarily traumatic, involving the forcing of the baby through the birth canal. Significant traumatic injury to the infant during birth is now uncommon in developed countries, due largely to a ready recourse to Caesarean section as an alternative to complicated instrumental deliveries. Trauma does still occur and requires some mention.

The three major situations where trauma develops are:

1. forceps deliveries in cephalic presentations, particularly rotational forceps deliveries;
2. vaginal breech deliveries; and
3. deliveries of abnormal babies (very large infants, infants with tumours, infants with neuromuscular abnormalities, etc.).

Minor forms of trauma include haemorrhages beneath the pericranium (cephalhaematoma) and fractures of long bones. Serious forms of intracranial trauma include subdural haemorrhage from veins bridging between the brain and cranial sinuses, tears of tentorium and falx, and separation of the squamous and lateral parts of the occipital bone. These injuries result from excessive antero-posterior and oblique pressures applied to the skull during birth.

Trauma is often associated with asphyxia and the relative contributions of each to handicap or death of an infant can be difficult to determine.

11.6 Problems of adaptation to extra-uterine existence

At birth the infant has to undergo a series of major physiological changes in order to survive in the extra-uterine environment. One of the most obvious and major changes which must be accomplished within minutes of birth is the onset of gaseous respiration. This involves commencement of regular deep respiratory movements of thorax and diaphragm, replacement of the liquid which has filled the lungs *in utero* by air, and the increase of pulmonary circulation by closure of the ductus and foramen ovale and reduction in pulmonary arterial pressure. There is an overall redistribution of circulation as the placenta is no longer in the circuit. The infant has to commence enteral nutrition and rely on his or her own enzymes for metabolizing nutrients, including carbohydrates, amino acids, fatty acids, and bilirubin, and producing waste products such as urea. Any deficiencies in these functions can no longer be compensated for by clearance through the maternal blood traversing the placenta and will rapidly become apparent as overt disease.

The most frequent problem that interferes with the establishment of extra-uterine existence is preterm birth. Perinatal mortality rate is inversely related to birth weight and maturity. Some 70 per cent of infants who die in the perinatal period are preterm, that is less than 37 weeks' gestational age. The lowest gestation at which babies have a realistic chance of survival is about 24 weeks and, of liveborn infants at that gestation, some 80 per cent currently die in the first week after birth.

11.6.1 Pathological problems of prematurity

Respiratory system

Development of the respiratory system is the most important determinant of survival following birth. At the critical 24 week gestational age period the fetal lung transforms from a duct-like canalicular structure to a saccular structure.

The essential features of the saccular lung are the approximation of the capillaries of the pulmonary circulation to the airspace walls and differentiation of the airspace-lining epithelium from a simple cuboidal form into type 1 and type 2 pneumocytes. The flattened type 1 pneumocytes stretch over the capillaries, bulging into the airspaces to form the future blood–air barriers, and the type 2 cells are responsible for secretion of surfactant.

Pulmonary surfactant is a complex, water-insoluble, particulate material with surface-tension-lowering properties, consisting principally of phospholipid, neutral lipids, and proteins. This material spreads to form a monomolecular epithelial lining layer and prevents collapse of airspaces over a wide pressure range. In the immature infant, particularly below 30 weeks' gestation, the quantity of surfactant produced is low and readily displaced or denatured to disrupt the integrity of the epithelial lining layer. Consequently, the saccules tend to collapse at the end of each respiration. Spontaneous respiratory efforts or mechanical ventilatory pressures expand the respiratory bronchioles, disrupt the bronchiolar epithelium, and lead to exudation of plasma and red cells. The mixture of plasma exudate and cell remnants becomes plastered round the respiratory bronchioles to form eosinophilic 'hyaline' membranes, the hyaline membrane disease of prematurity. Clinically, the affected infants become cyanosed with rapid respirations, in-drawing of the chest wall, and a typical X-ray appearance.

The condition is frequent in infants below 33 weeks' gestation but is predisposed to by conditions that enhance surfactant destruction, such as asphyxial deliveries. Surfactant secretion can be enhanced by glucocorticoid administration to women in threatened preterm labour, and the stimulation of natural glucocorticoid secretion by stress may explain the decreased frequency of hyaline membrane disease in infants born to women with pre-eclampsia.

The secretion of surfactant is stimulated by birth and the condition naturally resolves within 3–4 days. The high oxygen tensions and high mechanical ventilatory pressures, needed to maintain an immature infant alive until resolution occurs, often result in a series of secondary complications which may prolong illness or lead to death. The high ventilatory pressures may lead to rupture of respiratory epithelium, resulting in interstitial emphysema or pneumothorax.

The combination of high pressures and high oxygen tension may cause bronchopulmonary dysplasia, a form of diffuse alveolar damage. To some extent this is an exaggeration of the normal repair process, since the phagocytic removal of hyaline membranes is normally accompanied by a temporary focal oedema and a fibroblastic reaction around the respiratory bronchioles (Fig. 11.5). In bronchopulmonary dysplasia the oedema

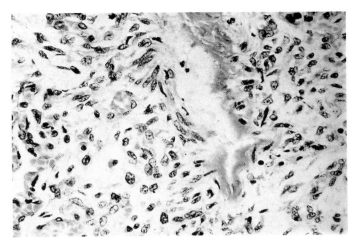

Fig. 11.5 Resolving/organizing hyaline membrane disease in lung of a 3-day-old preterm infant. Persistent hyaline membrane lines a small bronchiole with early fibroblast proliferation in adjacent tissue. With prolonged survival the condition might have resolved or progressed to bronchopulmonary dysplasia.

and fibroplasia persist as prominent reactions and lead to continued impairment in oxygenation and a distortion of subsequent airspace development.

Preterm infants with chronic hypoxia, due to conditions such as hyaline membrane disease and bronchopulmonary dysplasia, may have a persistently high pulmonary artery pressure with failure to close the ductus arteriosus. A long-term result may be development of pulmonary hypertension and right-sided heart failure.

Cardiovascular system

The preterm infant may not be able to maintain an appropriate circulation to various internal organs. The brain is mentioned specifically below. Ischaemic damage to kidneys, intestine, or the myocardium itself may be additional results of the attempts to maintain very small preterm infants alive in intensive care units.

Central nervous system

The two main problems of preterm birth are the development of subependymal/intraventricular haemorrhage and periventricular leukomalacia. Currently, both of these conditions are considered to be due to alterations in blood flow to the preterm infant brain. Periventricular leukomalacia is a purely ischaemic lesion, whereas intraventricular haemorrhage represents hyperfusion or reperfusion following ischaemia. The essential problem in both is the difficulty in maintaining an appropriate circulation to an organ that represents some 12 per cent of body mass (as compared with 2 per cent in the adult).

The conditions are described in Chapter 25 and will not be discussed further here.

Alimentary system

Immaturity of gastrointestinal enzyme systems may make it difficult to maintain nutrition and growth in small preterm infants. Hepatic immaturity is associated with a lack of glucuronyl transferase and the inability to conjugate bilirubin. Jaundice due to a raised circulating level of unconjugated bilirubin is a frequent complication of immaturity but, in the face of modern management, seldom leads to bilirubin toxicity with kernicterus (staining of brain nuclei with bilirubin and consequent neuronal damage). More frequent is the problem of cholestasis due to conjugated bilirubin in the livers of infants maintained on intravenous feeding for a prolonged period.

Ischaemic necrosis and non-specific inflammation of the bowel wall, necrotizing enterocolitis, is a relatively frequent problem in very small preterm infants. The process is considered to be due to the combination of the osmotic effects of enteral feeds on the intestinal epithelium, regional bowel ischaemia, and invasion by gut organisms.

Other systems

All other systems of the preterm infant are susceptible to damage or disease in various forms. Thus the immaturity of the reticuloendothelial system renders the preterm infant at particular risk of infection. At the same time, the thin skin with lack of a cornified layer is easily breached by infections. Internal organs such as the kidneys, adrenals, and liver, in addition to those already mentioned, are readily damaged by hypoxic episodes in the neonatal period.

11.6.2   Inborn metabolic errors

Inborn metabolic errors are individually uncommon but represent an important group of infants who fail to adapt to the extra-uterine environment. Some types of defect influence development adversely before birth. Thus infants suffering from abnormalities of lysosomal enzymes involving storage of lipids or mucopolysaccharides may be born with enlarged livers and spleens, and abnormal skeletal development, in association with the presence of specific types of storage cell in many tissues, including bone marrow, spleen, liver, and the placenta. Examples include Niemann–Pick disease type A, Gaucher's disease, and mucopolysaccharidosis type VII. Although these conditions are often compatible with prolonged neonatal or infant survival, severely affected infants may be stillborn or die in the neonatal period.

Other forms of inborn metabolic error may be entirely compensated for prenatally by transfer across the placenta. Following birth there is a build-up of toxic metabolic products or failure to metabolize an essential nutrient, with consequent rapid onset of acute illness. Examples of this type of inborn metabolic error include: disorders of carbohydrate metabolism, such as galactosaemia (the inability to metabolize the disaccharide lactose with consequent liver damage and hypoglycaemia); deficiency of various enzymes of the urea cycle, resulting in acute respiratory failure associated with hyperammonaemia; and a variety of disorders of amino-acid metabolism. Infants with one of these defects may appear quite well at birth but become acutely ill within the first few days. Correct diagnosis in some cases, such as galactosaemia, can lead to appropriate treatment, but in others, such as the urea cycle defects, respiratory failure and death are inevitable. There may be distinctive pathological findings in those conditions that affect the fetus adversely *in utero* but in most cases definitive diagnosis depends on biochemical studies in life or on fresh tissues or cell cultures set up after death.

11.7   Developmental tumours

Developmental tumours are rare as a cause of death in the fetal or neonatal period. Malignant neoplasms do, however, account for significant morbidity and mortality in childhood, being second only to accidents as a cause of death in the first 14 years of life. The difference between what one might call a perinatal view of malignant tumours, as rare, and a paediatric view of such tumours, as common, relates to the time of appearance of most of the important developmental tumours after the neonatal period. Congenital acute leukaemia is the most frequent cause of death attributable to cancer in the first month of life and has been recorded in stillborn infants.

The two most frequent forms of tumour recognized in the neonatal period (as compared with the most frequently fatal tumour) are teratomas and neuroblastomas.

11.7.1   Types of developmental tumour

The three major groups are hamartomas, teratomas, and embryomas.

Hamartomas are tumour-like masses comprising an excess of tissues which are normal to the site of occurrence. Their capacity for growth normally parallels that of the host and they usually behave in benign fashion. There may sometimes be difficulty in distinguishing between a hamartoma and a congenital malformation, or between a hamartoma and a neoplasm. Terminology such as 'congenital fibrosarcoma-like fibromatosis' expresses the latter difficulty. The group of hamartomas include a number of extremely common benign lesions, such as congenital haemangiomas and melanotic naevi, as well as more serious autosomal dominant conditions, including tuberous sclerosis, neurofibromatosis (von Recklinghausen), and syndromes of multiple angioma.

Teratomas are neoplasms derived from more than one cell layer. They commonly contain tissues of ectodermal, mesodermal, and endodermal origin, many of them foreign to the site of origin of the tumour. The tumours are usually partly cystic and contain a disorganized mass of tissues such as brain tissue, epidermis with hair and dermal glands, fat, cartilage, bones, and muscle. Other tissues that may be found include intestinal epithelium, thyroid, pancreas, salivary gland, adrenal, and kidney. Organoid structures such as tooth buds may be present. The most frequent site of congenital teratomas is the sacrococcygeal region where they may be attached to the sacrum or coccyx, or arise from the soft tissues of the pelvis. Other sites include the neck, the pharyngeal region, the mediastinum, and retroperitoneal region. The tumours are often large and may obstruct delivery. Increase in size of a teratoma in the neonatal period may be due to distension of cystic spaces with products of the lining cells or proliferative activities of the cellular constituents.

Teratomas seldom contain malignant constituents at birth, but not infrequently undergo malignant transformation beyond 4 months of age if not removed earlier. The most frequent malignancy is a large-cell adenocarcinoma.

Embryomas are tumours arising in organs and tissues which are at a primitive stage of development but are already committed to differentiate into a particular histogenetic type. The tumours are thus restricted either to specific organs or to specific tissues and consist of cells that display features of an early stage of development of the organ or tissue concerned.

A number of types of embryoma may present at birth. These include the neuroblastoma, arising from primitive neuroblasts (Fig. 11.6), the hepatoblastoma, arising from primitive hepatic parenchyma, and the retinoblastoma, arising from the primitive retinal epithelium.

11.7.2 Associations between tumours and malformations

A number of malformations are known to be associated with the development of tumours after birth. Wilms' tumour is reported to develop with undue frequency in a variety of conditions, including hemihypertrophy and the Beckwith–Wiedemann syndrome (enlargement of body organs including tongue and kidneys, cystic dysplasia of the renal medulla, and enlarged abnormal cells of the adrenal fetal cortex). Sacrococcygeal teratomas are one form of congenital tumour associated with malformations. The associated anomalies usually involve the hindgut region, including imperforate anus and rectovaginal fistula. Down syndrome is associated with an increased incidence of leukaemia, including both acute lymphoblastic and congenital acute myelogenous forms.

11.7.3 Causation of congenital tumours

The development of neoplasia during fetal life is of interest in relation to the problems of the aetiology of cancer in general. There is little time for environmental agents to act, so that one might expect genetic factors to play a major role. In fact, some childhood tumours (e.g. some cases of retinoblastoma) may show a direct autosomal dominant inheritance pattern or may be associated with a recognizable chromosomal abnormality (partial deletion of the long arm of chromosome 13 in cases of retinoblastoma). Knudsen and Strong proposed that two successive mutations are necessary within a somatic cell for neo-

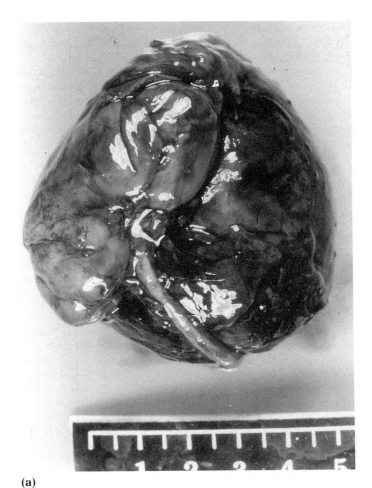

(a)

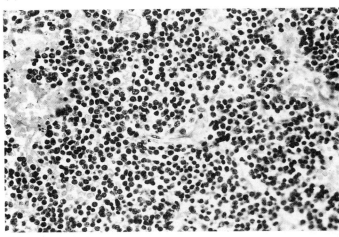

(b)

Fig. 11.6 (a) Kidney and adrenal of a new-born infant with a large mass arising from the adrenal. (b) Histological appearance of mass showing a tumour of uniform round cells typical of neuroblastoma.

plastic change to occur. If the first mutation occurs within a germ cell, only one subsequent mutation during development can lead to tumour formation. In such instances the tendency for neoplasia will be hereditary, as in bilateral retinoblastoma. If the first mutation was teratogenic, this would explain the association between teratogenesis and tumour formation.

At the experimental level it can be shown that embryonic tissues may be highly susceptible to induction of tumours by some chemical agents, such as urethane and alkylnitrosamines, which are also teratogenic. Such agents may cause malformations if administered during organogenesis, and tumours if given at a later stage of development. Although the tumours resulting from such experiments are not present at birth, the findings do confirm the close relationship between malformations and tumours.

The equivalent situation in humans is represented by the development of clear-cell vaginal adenocarcinoma at adolescence in girls whose mothers were given diethylstilboestrol to prevent threatened abortion. The development of the tumours is related to the presence of primitive sex duct vestiges, known as vaginal adenosis, which may represent a teratogenic effect of the drug. The observations provide further evidence of the association between teratogenic and oncogenic effects which may be relevant to the development of congenital tumours.

11.7.4 Further reading

Keeling, J. W. (1987). *Fetal and neonatal pathology*. Springer-Verlag, London.

Reed, G. B., Claireaux, A. E., and Bain, A. D. (1989). *Diseases of the fetus and newborn*. Chapman and Hall, London.

Wigglesworth, J. A. (1984). *Perinatal pathology*. Major Problems in Pathology No. 15. W. B. Saunders, Philadelphia.

Wigglesworth, J. S. and Singer, D. B. (1991). *Textbook of fetal and perinatal pathology*. Blackwell Scientific Publications, Oxford.

Index

Pages 1–792 appear in Volume 1, pages 793–1682 in Volume 2a, and pages 1683–2344 in Volume 2b

antigens (*cont.*)
  antibody interactions 219
  classes **207–8**
  denaturation, immunocytochemistry and 2282
  failure of presentation 295
  immunologically privileged sites 295
  lymph nodes 1750
  mechanisms of tolerance to 295
  nature 198–200
  presentation to B-cells 211–12, 267–8
  role of HLA antigens in presentation 201–2
  routes of immunization 199–200
  T-cell-dependent 207–8, 211–16
  T-cell-independent type 1 (TI-1) 208, 216
  T-cell-independent type 2 (TI-2) 208, 216
  tolerogens 293, **296**
  transformed cells 576
antiglobulin test 1701
anti-glycophorin C, lymphoma typing *581*
antihypertensive drugs, sudden withdrawal 754
anti-i 1708
anti-idiotypic antibodies 199, 272
  immunological tolerance and 295–6
  self-non-responsiveness and 293
anti-lymphocytic serum 296–7
antimicrobial drugs
  acute interstitial nephritis 1482
  altered cellular permeability to 433–4
  broad-spectrum therapy 436, 468, 476
  enzymic inactivation 430–3
  hospital-acquired infections and 492
  hypersensitivity reactions 1766–7
  immunoproliferative small intestinal disease 1789
  mode of action *431*
  nephrotoxic 1509
  neutropenic patients 1707
  normal gut flora and 436, 468, 1209
  prophylaxis of hospital-acquired infections 493
  pseudomembranous colitis and 1225
  teratogenicity 783
  see also specific drugs
antimicrobial resistance **428–34**, 479
  biochemical mechanisms 430–4
  intrinsic 429
  mode of origin 429–30
  multiple 429
  mutational 429
  transferable 429–30
antimitochondrial antibodies 1319, 1322
antimycin A 184

antioestrogens, breast carcinoma 1667
anti-oncogenes (tumour suppressor genes) 636, 638, 678, 1661
antioxidants 150–1
  in food 725
  natural 150–1, 737
anti-perspirant, granulomatous reactions 401
anti-phospholipid antibody syndrome 1862
antiretroviral therapy **292**
antistreptolysin O (ASO) titres 868
antithrombin III 508
  deficiency *110, 111, 123*, 508
  heparan sulphate proteoglycan binding 796
antithyroid drugs 1706, 1948
α-1-antitrypsin (AAT, α₁ proteinase inhibitor) **107**, 1894
  accumulation in hepatocytes 1318, 1357, 1358
  function 508–9, 1356–7
  serum levels 1290–1
α-1-antitrypsin (AAT) deficiency 1318, *1350*, **1356–8**, *1378*, 2163
  liver disease in adults 1357–8, 1392
  liver disease in infancy/childhood 1293, 1295, 1357
  molecular pathology **107**, *110*
  neutrophil function and **329**
  paucity of intrahepatic bile ducts 1294
  phenotypes 1357
  pulmonary disease 976, 978–9
anti-tumour necrosis factor (TNF) monoclonal antibodies 471
Antoni A and B areas, schwannomas 1110, 1892, 2122, 2123
antrochoanal polyp 1114
anus **1275–80**
  Crohn disease 1244, 1277
  haemorrhoids 1275–6
  infections 1277–8
  inflammation 1276–7
aorta
  coarctation 866, 1994
  congenital malformations 866
  extracellular matrix 64
  normal anatomy 795–6, 856
aortic aneurysms 847, 848
  dissecting 848–9
  formation 815
  'inflammatory' **817–18**, 819, 822
  syphilitic 846
aortic arch 856
aortic atherosclerosis **812–22**, 1523
  aneurysm formation 815
  chronic periaortitis 815–22
  terminology 822
aortic body tumour 1996
aortic hypoplasia 783
aortico-pulmonary bodies 1993
aortico-sympathetic glomera 1993
aortic regurgitation **870–2**
  cusp abnormalities 870

aortic regurgitation (*cont.*)
  pathophysiology 904–5
  root disease 870–2
  syphilis 846, 871, 872
aortic root 852, 854
  dilatation 871, 905
  disease 870–2
  inflammatory disease 871–2
aortic valve
  bicuspid 869, 903
    calcific stenosis 870
  calcification 868, 904
  disease, pulmonary oedema 1002
  normal appearances 854, 855–6, 857
  pathology **869–72**
  Takaysu disease 845
aortic valve stenosis **869–70**
  congenital 869–70, 903, 1015
  pathophysiology 903–4
  rheumatic 870, 871, 903
  senile tricuspid 870, 871
aortitis
  idiopathic retroperitoneal fibrosis 1523
  rheumatoid arthritis/related conditions 843–4, 871–2
  syphilitic 846
  Takayasu disease 845
aortocoronary bypass grafts **899–903**
  collateral blood supply 903
  failure 900–1
    early 900
    late 900–1
  graft sources 899–900
  healing 852, 901–3
aortopulmonary septal defects (windows) 865, 1022
aphthoid ulcers, Crohn disease 1242, 1246
aphthovirus (foot-and-mouth disease virus) 446
aplasia, pure red cell 1702, 1817
aplastic anaemia **1702**
  bone marrow changes 1702, 1703
  causes 752, 1702, 1817
  see also Fanconi anaemia
apnoea, sleep 1007, 1122
apocrine adenocarcinoma 1580
apocrine carcinoma 2179
apocrine sweat glands 2142, 2179
apocrine sweat gland tumours **2179–80**
apolipoprotein(s) 126–7, 802
  embryonic synthesis 601
apolipoprotein A (apo A) 126–7, 802
apolipoprotein AI (apo AI) 127
  serum levels, apo AI–CIII–AIV RFLPs and 132–3
  Tangier disease 129
apolipoprotein AI–CIII–AIV (apo AI–CIII–AIV) gene cluster *128*, 132, 136
  RFLPs and apo AI/HDL levels 132–3
  RFLPs and atherosclerosis 130, *131*

apolipoprotein AII (apo AII) 127, *128*
apolipoprotein B (apo B) 126–7, 802
  abetalipoproteinaemia 129
  gene *128*
    expression 94
    identification of 'mutations' 135
    RFLPs and atherosclerosis 130–2
    RFLPs and cholesterol levels 133–4
    RFLPs and hypertriglyceridaemia 132
  hypobetalipoproteinaemia and 135
apolipoprotein B-100 (apo B-100) *802*
  familial defective (FDB) **128**
apolipoprotein C (apo C) 126–7, 802
apolipoprotein CII (apo CII) 127
  deficiency 129, 802
apolipoprotein E (apo E) 126–7, 802
  polymorphism and hyperlipidaemia 132
apolipoprotein E–CI–CII (apo E–CI–CII) *128*
apophyseal joints 2075
apoptosis **142–7**, 168, 563
  calcium-activated endonucleases and 146, 147, **190–1**
  definition 141
  germinal centre 213
  graft versus host disease 319, 1255
  immunologically mediated 155–6
  incidence 142
  initiating stimuli 146–7
  kinetics 145
  mechanisms 144–7
  morphology 142–4
  priming 146, 147
  recognition mechanism 146
  solar/UV-B irradiation-induced 768
  thymocytes 1810
  triggers 146–7
  tumour 154–5
apoptotic bodies 142, 144, 145, 169
apo-SAA 412
appendices epiploicae 1180
appendicitis **1218–22**
  actinomycosis 1221
  acute **1218–19**
    aetiology and pathogenesis 476, 1218
    complications 1219
    pathology 1218–19
  Campylobacter 1223
  chronic (grumbling appendix) 1219–20
  granulomatous 1220, 1221
  schistosomiasis 1221–2
  tuberculous 1220

CD45 (leucocyte common antigen)
    236, *2278*
  isoforms 233, 271
    lymphoma diagnosis *581, 1748*
CD45RA *2278*
  CD4 T-cells 233–4
  CD8 T-cells 234
  lymphoma typing *581*
CD45RO (UCHL1) *2278*
  CD4 T-cells 233, 234, 271
  CD8 T-cells 234
  lymphoma diagnosis *581*
CD61 *581, 2278*
CD68 (KP1) *581, 2278*
cdc2⁺ gene 90
cell(s)
  adaptation and injury **158**
  atrophy 162, **562–3**
  bacterial multiplication in 420
  bacterial penetration/invasion
    420–1
  bacterial sequestration 480
  diversity 33–8
  hypertrophy **563–5**
  potential lethal damage (PLD)
    repair 662, 669
  redox activity, reactive oxygen
    intermediates and 151
  structure and function **3–52**
  'very dark' 142
  virus entry mechanisms **444–7**
  virus spread between 448
cell adhesion **37–8**
  fibronectin and 26, 61, 62
  inflammatory response 356–7
  proteoglycans and 60
cell adhesion molecules (CAMs) **26,**
  38
  Ca⁺⁺-dependent 26
  Ca⁺⁺-independent 26
  endothelial cells 357
  phagocytic cells 357
  primary 26
cell coat (glycocalyx) 8–9, 162
cell cultures
  environmental modulation of
    differentiated phenotype 40
  nomenclature 575
  saturation density 576
  teratoma stem cells 603–4
  transdifferentiation and
    dedifferentiation 40–1
  tumour cells 573–4
  types 574
cell cycle 43, 44
  analysis by flow cytometry 2335,
    2337
  control 555–6
  critical control point 555
  kinetics, breast carcinoma 1667
  nucleolar organizer regions and
    588
cell death **141–57**
  bacterial exotoxins 423–4
  bacteria-mediated· 420
  definition 157–81
  identification and measurement
    141–2
  immunologically mediated
    155–6
  neutrophil-mediated 353–4

cell death (*cont.*)
  radiation-induced 669, 772
  tumours 141, 154–5
  see also apoptosis; necrosis
cell divisions, amplifying 46
cell fusion, activation of metastatic
    behaviour 620–1
cell injury
  abnormal inclusions 172–5
  adaptation and 158
  artefacts 159–60
  biochemical changes following
    182–3
  biochemical mechanisms 183–91
    calcium homeostasis and
      189–91
    interference with endogenous
      substrates/effectors 183–4
    lipid peroxidation 188–9
    reactive intermediates 184–7
  classification of causes 181
  cytoplasmic changes 160–71
  limitations of morphology 159
  mechanical damage 181
  mechanisms **181–93**
  menadione-induced 185, 186,
    187, **192–3**
  nuclear changes 175–80
  organelle pathology **157–81**
  outcomes of non-lethal 181
  paracetamol-induced 152, *183*,
    185–7, **191–2**
  protective mechanisms 181
cell interactions **25–31**
  early mammalian development
    598–601
  extracellular matrix 26, 60
  injured cells, changes in **162–3**
  morphological expressions 30–1
  morphologically specialized
    junctions 26–30
cell lineages **43–52**
  definitions 46
  epidermal 47–9
  haematopoietic 46, 47
  hierarchical organization 46,
    51–2
  small intestine 49–51
  spermatogenic 46–7, 48
  tumours 640–1
cell lines
  established 575
  immortalized 575
  nomenclature 575
  senescent 575
  side 576
  stem 576
  transformed 575–6
cell loss factor, tumours 141
cell-mediated immunity 198,
    228–36
  disorders 279, *280*
  leprosy 398–9, 403, 482–3
  non-specific **439**
  pulmonary 947
  specific **439–40**
  syphilis 403
  tuberculosis 400–1
  viral reactivation and 485
cell membrane, *see* plasma
    membrane

cell migration
  inflammatory reaction 357–8
  skin wounds 367–8, 373
cell morphology, tissue-specific
    variation **34**
celloidin (cellulose tetranitrate)
    2272
cell populations
  cell types in proliferating 44, 45
  conditionally renewing 43, 44,
    46, 366
  hierarchical organization 46,
    51–2
  renewing 43, 44, 46–52, 366
  static (non-renewing) 43, 366
cell proliferation
  analysis by flow cytometry 2335,
    2337
  control **555–60**
  in disease 556
  early mammalian development
    598, 600–1
  growth factors and 556–60
  healing tissues 366
  measures in tumours 588–9
  nucleolar organizer regions and
    587–8
  partial hepatectomy 382–3
  pulmonary cells 385
  skin wounds 367–8
cell rests of Malassez 1081, 1082,
    1083
cell shape, apoptotic cells 145
cell size
  apoptotic cells 142, 145
  changes in **161–2**
  decreased 162
  tissue-specific variation 34
cell sorting, flow cytometry 2334
cell strains 575
cell surface **8–11**
  apoptotic cells 142
  expression of viral proteins 486
  injured cells 162, 183
  metastatic tumour cells 618
  proteoglycans 59, 60
  specializations 9–10
  staphylococci 464
  streptococci 462
  transformed cells 576
cell-surface glycoproteins/proteins
  endothelial cells 499
  lymphocytes 228, 229
  metastatic tumour cells 618
  phagocytic cells 357
  platelet 510
  thymocytes 1810–11
  transformed cells 576
  tumour cells 707
  see also CD antigens
cell-surface receptors
  endocytosis and 10–11
  macrophage, *see* macrophages,
    plasma membrane receptors
  neutrophils 322
  virus entry via 443–4
cell suspensions, lymph nodes 1750
cell swelling 161–2, 182, 183
  necrosis 148
cellular differentiation, *see*
    differentiation

cellular organization 3
cellular transformation, *see*
    transformation, cellular
cellulitis 463, 478, 926
cellulose 735
cell wall
  fungi 489
  Gram-negative bacteria 468–9
  pneumococcus 464
  staphylococci 464, 544
  streptococci 462
cementifying fibroma 1090, 1119
cement lines, bone 2019
  hyperparathyroidism 2043
  Paget disease 2045
cementoma *1087*
centimorgan (cM) 70, 124
central-core disease 2100, 2101
central nervous system (CNS)
  adrenal medulla connections
    1987
  axonal regeneration 385
  congenital malformations 783,
    1923
  demyelinating diseases **1867–73**
  enterovirus-induced disease
    280–1
  healing after injury 366
  hypertension and 839
  infections **1835–50**, 1924
  ischaemia **527–8**
  microglia 253–4
  monocyte recruitment 254
  preterm infants 789
  schistosomiasis 1849, 2259
  staining methods 2273
  vascular anomalies 917,
    1855–6, 1894
  virus-associated diseases 449,
    1839–47, 2288
central pontine myelinolysis 1857,
    1861, 1872
centrioles 16
centroacinar cell metaplasia,
    pancreatic 1441
centroblastic/centrocytic lymphoma
    1779–80, 1807
centroblastic lymphoma 1781
centroblasts
  centroblastic/centrocytic
    lymphoma 1779
  centroblastic lymphoma 1781
  lymph nodes 1746, 1747
  Peyer's patches 1752
  phenotype *215*
  response to immunization
    212–13, 215
  tonsillitis 1123
centrocyte-like cells
  gastric lymphoma 1789, 1790
  immunoproliferative small
    intestinal disease 1789,
    1791
  pulmonary lymphoma 1792
  salivary gland lymphoma 1791,
    1792
  thyroid gland lymphoma 1791
centrocytes 213, *215*, 217
  centroblastic/centrocytic
    lymphoma 1779
  centrocytic lymphoma 1780

factor XI 504, 505, 506, 508
  deficiency **1739**
factor XII (Hageman factor) 504–5, 508
  deficiency **1739**
  inactivator 334
factor XIII (fibrin stabilizing factor) 505, 506
  deficiency **1740**
Factor B 200, 259, 260
Factor D 259, 260
Factor H 259, 260, 262
Factor I 259, 260, 264
  cofactors 262
  deficiency 265
faecal continence 1181–2
faecal–oral route of infection 454
faeces, fibre content 735–6
faggot cells 1721
Fallopian tube **1609–14**
  ampulla 1609
  cysts 1612–13
  development 1565
  ectopic pregnancy 1635–6
  endometriosis and 1634
  histology 1609–10
  inflammation 1610–12
    ascending infection 1610–12
    blood-borne infection 1612
    lymphatic infection 1612
  infundibulum 1609
  interstitial segment 1609
  isthmus 1609
  macrophages 253
  plicae 1609
  rupture complicating ectopic pregnancy 1636
  tumours 1613–14
Fallopian tube adenocarcinoma 1613–14
Fallot's tetralogy, *see* tetralogy of Fallot
family linkage studies 85
Fanconi anaemia 692, 1341–2, 1702, 1717
Fanconis syndrome 748, 1499
F-antigens 418
farmer's lung 278, 721, 983, *984*
fascia adhaerens 27, 28
fasciitis
  cranial 2108
  intravascular 2108
  necrotizing 463
  nodular 2107–8
  parosteal 2108
  proliferative 2108
Fasciola (fascioliasis) 1311, 1411, 2254, **2262–3**
  clinical features and pathology 2263
  diagnosis and treatment 2263
  ectopic 2263
  life cycle and morphology 2255, 2262–3
Fasciolopsis 2254
fat
  brown 2105
  dietary **734–5**
    breast carcinoma and 688–9, 1660

fat (*cont.*)
  dietary (*cont.*)
    colorectal carcinoma and 684, 1264
    daily requirements 732
    disease susceptibility and 746
    hypertension and 838
    subcutaneous 2141
      panniculitis **2162–3**
    total body 733
    see also lipid(s)
fat embolism **524**
  cerebral 524, 1853, 1927
  pulmonary 1009
fat embolization syndrome 524
fat necrosis
  acute pancreatitis 1437
  breast 1652, 1675
fat tumours **2103–6**
fatty acids **734–5**
  adrenoleukodystrophy 1986
  essential 735
  hepatic oxidation 1325, 1337
  polyunsaturated 735
  saturated 735
  unsaturated 734–5
fatty change 173–4
  heart 885
  liver, *see* fatty liver
fatty cysts, liver 1326
fatty liver (hepatocyte steatosis) 173–4
  alcoholic liver disease **1325–7**, 1336, 1337
    clinical presentation 1325
    pathogenesis and prognosis 1327
    pathology 1325–6
  diabetes mellitus 1367
  intestinal bypass operations 1367
  kwashiorkor 1367
  macrovesicular (large droplet) 1325, 1336–7
  microvesicular (small droplet) 1325, 1336, 1337–8
  of pregnancy, acute 1337
  Wilson disease 1363
fatty streaks **798**, 799, 801
  experimental studies 804–7
  regression 812
favism 753, 1701
Fc receptors (FcR) 222, 223, 358
  IgG binding 223
  macrophages 241, 337–8, 339, 340, 344
  mast cells/basophils 227–8, 332–3
  neutrophils 322
febrile neurophilic dermatosis, acute (Sweet syndrome) 2165
feline leukaemia virus 658
feline sarcoma virus 658
Felty syndrome 1706
female genital tract **1565–639**
  barriers to infection 197
  development 1565–6
  diffuse neuroendocrine system 2013, *2014*
  malformations 1566–8
    aetiology and pathogenesis 1568

female genital tract (*cont.*)
  malformations (*cont.*)
    classification 1566–8
    incidence and clinical features 1568
    metaplasias 567
    pregnancy-related abnormalities 1635–9
female pseudohermaphroditism 1569, 1978
feminization, testicular 1547
feminizing adrenocortical tumours 1981
femoral capital epiphysis
  necrosis (Perthes disease) 2031, 2076
  slipped 2076
femoral head
  avascular necrosis 2030, 2080
  congenital dislocation 2028, 2076
femoral nerve palsy, haemophilia 1736
ferritin 19–20, 1370, 1693–4
  idiopathic haemochromatosis 1372
  serum levels 1374, 1375, 1702
fertility, impaired, *see* infertility
c-*fes* oncogene 672
v-*fes* oncogene 658
fetal alcohol syndrome 783, **1858**
fetal cells, polymerase chain reaction 2298
fetal granular layer of Obersteiner 1891
fetal growth **786–7**
fetal growth retardation 785, **786**
  birth asphyxia and 788
  malnutrition form 786
  symmetrical 786
fetal infection 450, **786–7**
fetal loss, early 73, 782, 1635
feto-maternal transfusion, placental effects 785
α-fetoprotein (AFP)
  congenital nephrotic syndrome 1455
  embryonic synthesis 600, 601
  hepatic synthesis 1291
  hepatoblastoma 1397
  hepatocellular carcinoma 584, 1392
  hepatocyte proliferation and 1383, 1384
  large intestinal adenomatous polyps 595
  testicular germ cell tumours 584, 1556, 1557, 1558, *1560*
  yolk sac tumours 1629
fetor, hepatic coma 1422, 1423
fetus
  adverse drug effects 756
  chronic anaemia 785
  immune function 211, 222, 225
fever
  acute phase response 438
  drug allergy 752
Feyrter, Kulschitsky cells, *see* endocrine cells
F fusion protein 445
fibre, dietary **735–6**, 740

fibre, dietary (*cont.*)
  colorectal carcinoma and 1264
  diverticular disease and 1256
  gallstones and 1406
fibre-type disproportion, congenital 2100
fibrillary centres, nuclear 5, 6, 587–8
fibrillar zone, epidermis 2139
fibrillation, osteoarthritic cartilage 2084
fibrillin 58
fibrin 504, 505, 2273
  clot formation 507–8
  monomer 519
  synovial membrane 2081
  thrombi, *see* microthrombi
fibrin(ogen) degradation products (FDPs) 519
fibrinogen 503, 504, 505, *506*, 507–8
  defective (dysfibrinogenaemia) **1740**
  deficiency **1739**
  hepatic failure 1418–19
  ischaemic heart disease and 823
fibrinoid necrosis 1475–6
  erythema multiforme 2156
  haemolytic-uraemic syndrome 1476
  malignant hypertension 836, 1475–6
  polyarteritis nodosa 842
fibrinolytic activity, metastatic cells 619
fibrinopeptide A 519
fibroadenoma, breast, *see* breast fibroadenoma
fibroblast growth factor (FGF) 499
  acidic (aFGF) 675, *676*
  atherogenesis and 808, 810
  basic (bFGF) 675, *676*
  hepatocyte proliferation and 1384
  induction of mesoderm 40
  oncogenes and 675
  wound healing and 376
fibroblast growth regulator (FGR) *678*
fibroblastoma, giant-cell 2130–1
fibroblasts
  connective tissue metaplasias and 567
  desmoplastic fibroma 2062, 2063
  endoneurial 1892
  granulomatous diseases 397
  growth pattern in culture 576
  nodular fasciitis 2107, 2108
  portal tract, collagen synthesis in cirrhosis 1381
  silicosis 405–6
  of specialized stromal origin 1624
  wound healing 369–70
fibrocartilage, proliferation in osteoarthritis 2085
fibrocystic breast change 1644, **1650–1**, 1671, 1672, 1673
fibrodysplasia ossificans progressiva 2129

G-cells 1150, *1184*, 2005
G-CSF, *see* granulocyte colony-
    stimulating factor
gelatinous lesions, arteries 798,
    799
gender, *see* sex
gene(s)
    cancer 124–5
    candidate, *see* candidate genes
    fusion *110*, 111–12
    housekeeping 34, 95
    structure in eukaryotes 91–3
    structure and function in
        eukaryotes **88–99**
    tandem arrays 90, 92
    'unique' 89, 90
gene amplification
    nucleolar organizer regions and
        587
    tumour cells 1661, 1885
gene deletions **110–11**
    breast carcinoma 1661
    clinical phenotypes 115–16
    neural tumours 1885, 1903
    see also tumour suppressor genes
gene disorders, single
    congenital malformations 783
    historical background 100–1
    levels of abnormal gene expression
        101–2
    molecular pathology **100–17**
    patterns of inheritance 69, 83–4
    phenotype–genotype relationships
        115–16
    reduced amount of protein product
        causing 109–15
    synthesis of abnormal proteins
        causing 102–9
gene dosage methods 85–6
gene expression
    abnormalities in single gene
        disorders 101–2
    alterations in cancer cells
        639–40
    differentiated cells 38–9
    mechanisms **91**
    regulation 93
gene inversions *110*, 112
gene locus 69
gene mapping 70, 84–7, 2287
gene mutations, *see* mutations
general paralysis of the insane 1837
gene therapy 126, 630–1
genetic disorders **121–6**
    congenital malformations 783
    DNA methods for diagnosis and
        carrier detection 87–8
    identification of mutant locus
        122–4
    'new' 124
    patterns of inheritance 69, 83–4,
        121–2
    polygenic 100, 116, 783
    prenatal diagnosis 125–6
    see also gene disorders, single
genetic distance 70, **123–4**
genetic exchange, antimicrobial
    resistance 429–30
genetic linkage 70, **124**
genetic predisposition
    adverse drug reactions 748–9

genetic predisposition (*cont.*)
    auto-immune diseases 298–301
    breast carcinoma 1660
    cancer 124–5, 644–7
    cataract 1918
    congenital tumours 791
    Graves disease 1950
    hypertension 838
    infection susceptibility 415, 441,
        481
    ischaemic heart disease 126
    malignant melanoma 2174
    nervous system tumours 1885
    plexogenic pulmonary
        arteriopathy 1003
genetics
    basics 69–71
    inherited disorders **121–6**
metastatic drive 620–2
    population 121–2
    reverse 84–7, 116
gene transfection, *see* DNA
    transfection
genital prolapse **1586**
genital ridges 1547
    tumour development from 1555
genital tract
    diffuse neuroendocrine system
        2013, *2014* female, *see*
        female genital tract
    lower
        normal microbial flora *436*
        virus transmission via 447,
            448
    macrophages 252–3
    male **1535–62**
    schistosomiasis 2261
genome
    human, DNA sequencing 86–7
    organization in eukaryotes 88–9,
        90
gentamicin, structure 433
geographic stomatitis **1058**
germ cell neoplasia, intratubular
    (ITGCN) 1555
germ cell tumours
    immunocytochemistry *581*
    lineage relationships 602, *603*
    nervous system **1894–51** ovary
        1628–31
    sex chromosome disorders 1572
    testicular, *see* testicular germ cell
        tumours
    thymic 1814, **1818**
germinal centres, B-cell follicles
    209, 217
    lymph nodes 1746–7
    persistent generalized
        lymphadenopathy 1766
    Peyer's patches 1752, 1753
    progressive transformation 1757,
        1758, 1772
    reaction to immunization
        212–14, 215
    T-cells 234, 235
germinal epithelium, testes 1544
germinal inclusion cysts, ovarian
    1616
germinoma 1939
    cerebral (pineal) 1894–5
    thymic 1818

Gerstmann–Straüssler syndrome
    411, 1882
GH, *see* growth hormone
Ghon focus 398, 969
giant axonal neuropathy, familial
    1902
giant-cell (temporal, cranial) arteritis
    514, **844–5**, 1862
giant-cell carcinoma, lung 1039
giant-cell epulis 1058–9, 1090
giant-cell fibroblastoma 2130–1
giant-cell granuloma
    central 1090
    jaws 1090
giant-cell myocarditis 883
giant-cell pneumonia 962
giant cells
    alveolar rhabdomyosarcoma
        2121
    de Quervains thyroiditis 1953
    epithelioid cell-derived 1760
    Langhans-type, *see* Langhans'
        giant cells
    malignant melanoma of soft
        tissues 2127
    measles pneumonia 962
    osteoclast-like
        aneurysmal bone cyst 2070
        chondroblastoma 2056
        giant-cell granuloma 1090
        giant-cell tumours 2060,
            2114–15
        hyperparathyroidism 2043
        malignant fibrous histiocytoma
            2117
    pleomorphic lipoma 2104
    proliferative fasciitis 2108
    reticulohistiocytoma 2115
    sarcoidosis 990, 1760
    silicosis 405
    Warthin–Finkeldey 962, 1766
    Wegener disease 1029
giant-cell tumours
    bone (osteoclastoma) **2059–60**
    giant-cell granuloma vs. 1090
    malignant 2060
    pancreatic, osteoclast-type 1447
    tendon sheath 2114–15
    tendon sheath and synovium
        (pigmented villonodular
        synovitis) **2090–1**, 2114–15
giant condyloma of
    Buschke–Loewenstein 1279,
    2170
giant stereociliary degeneration
    1109–10
giardiasis (*Giardia*) 1217, **2198–9**
    genetic susceptibility 441
    immunodeficiency and 1202
    malabsorption 1199, 2198
Giemsa stain 2320
gigantism 1931, 2023
Gilbert syndrome *1351*, **1364**,
    1424
gingiva
    inflammatory lesions 1058–9
    mucosa 1053, 1054
gingival crevicular fluid 1093
gingival cyst of adults *1085*
gingival hyperplasia, cyclosporin-
    associated 899

gingivitis **1091–6**
    acute (necrotizing) ulcerative
        (Vincent infection) 472,
        476, **1056**, 1092
    animal studies 476
    chronic marginal 1091
    clinical manifestations 1091–2
    histopathology 1093–4
    hyperplastic 1058
    microbiology 1092–3
    pathogenic mechanisms 1094–6
    ulcerative, HIV infection 1092
gingivostomatitis, primary herpetic
    1056
glanders 971
glandular fever, *see* infectious
    mononucleosis
glandular metaplasia **566–7**
    bladder epithelium 566, 1517,
        1520
    see also gastric metaplasia;
        intestinal metaplasia
Glanzmann disease (thrombasthenia)
    1733, 1734
glaucoma **1905–7**, 1916
    angle-closure 1905, 1906–7
        primary 1906
        secondary 1906–7
    congenital 1907
    corticosteroid-induced *749*, 1906
    open-angle 1905, 1906
        primary 1906
        secondary 1906
    phacolytic 1906, 1918
    pigmentary 1906
    post-thrombotic (thrombotic)
        1913, 1914
    pupillary block 1905–6
glial cells **1832**
    immunological markers 1832
    progenitor 40, 1832
    transdifferentiation 41
    see also astrocytes;
        oligodendrocytes
glial fibres, cerebral infarction
    1851, 1852
glial fibrillary acidic protein (GFAP)
    19, *36*, 581, 584, 1832
    astrocytic tumours 1886, 1888,
        1889
    ependymomas 1890
    pituicytoma 1939
    pituitary cells containing 1931
    reactive astrocytes 385, 386
glial nodule encephalitis 1846
glioblastoma 693, **1887–8**
    giant-celled 1888
    multiforme 1885, 1887, 1888
glioma **1886–92**
    aetiology and pathogenesis
        1884–5
    epidemiology 1883
    hypothalamic 1939
    immunocytochemistry 580,
        581 nasal **1117**, 1895,
        2122
    optic 1889
    progressive multifocal
        leukoencephalopathy and
        1845
gliomatosis cerebri 1892

Kaposi sarcoma (*cont.*)
  oral mucosa 1066
  patch-stage 937
  plaque-stage 937
  skin 2181
  stomach 1172
  Western 937
Kaposi sarcoma growth factor (ks)
    675, *676*
Kartagener syndrome (immotile cilia
    syndrome) 17, 167, 168,
    948
karyolysis 148, 177
karyorrhexis 177, 1925
karyotype analysis 71–3
Kasabach–Merritt syndrome 931
Kasai procedure, extrahepatic biliary
    atresia 1294
Kashin–Beck disease 2086
katacalcin 2023
Katayama syndrome (acute
    schistosomiasis) 2255–6
Kawasaki disease (mucocutaneous
    lymph node syndrome) 843,
    1764
Kayser–Fleischer rings 1363
K-cells 155, 310
  antimicrobial activity 440
  endometrium 1596
  gut *1184*
  tumour cell killing 708
Kell null (McLeod) phenotype 1709
keloids 375, 2107
keratan sulphate 37, 59, 60, 2073
keratinization 19
keratin layer (stratum corneum)
    2140–1
keratinocytes
  growth pattern in culture 576
  keratin expression in culture 40
keratin (epithelial) pearls
  lung carcinoma 1037, 1038
  oral carcinoma 1059, 1060
  squamous cell carcinoma 601
keratins, *see* cytokeratins
keratitis
  Acanthamoeba 1910, 2204
  onchocerciasis 2246
  stromal, herpes simplex 1909
keratoacanthoma **2171**
  perianal skin 1280
  vulva 1577
keratoconjunctivitis
  Encephalitozoon cuniculi 2224
  primary herpetic 1909
  sicca 1073
keratoconus 1917
keratohyalin 2140–1
keratopathy, band 1916, 1917
keratopoiesis **47–9**
keratosis pilaris 2164
Kerley B lines 1001, 1015
kernicterus (bilirubin
    encephalopathy) 790, 1364,
    1425, 1925
Keshan disease 885
2-keto-3-deoxyoctonate (KDO) 478
ketones, fasting 742
17-ketosteroid
    dehydrogenase/reductase
    deficiency 1553

17-ketosteroid excretion, Klinefelter
    syndrome 1548
kidney **1451–531**
  bilateral absence 1452
  congenital diseases 1452–5
  crossed ectopia 1452
  duplex 1517
  dysplastic 1453
  extracellular fluid volume control
    531–2
  extracellular matrix 64–5
  granular contracted 836, 1474,
    1475
  growth response to unilateral
    nephrectomy 383–4
  heart failure and 909
  horseshoe 1452–3
  interstitial space 1452
  macrophages 253
  medullary sponge **1454**, 1455
  multicystic disease, acquired
    1454, 1503
  polycystic disease, *see* polycystic
    kidney disease
  in pregnancy 1496–7
  radiation-induced damage 776,
    1482
  schistosomiasis 2259
  shock-induced lesions **548**, 549
  simple ectopia 1452
  structure 1451–2
  unilateral atresia 1452
  uraemic medullary sponge **1455**
  Wegener granulomatosis 1115
Kienbock disease 2031
Kikuchi disease 1764
Kimura disease 934
Kingella kingae 467, 468
kininogen, high molecular weight
    (HMWK) 504, 505–6
  deficiency 1739
kininogenase *334*
kininogens 363
kinins 363, 839–40
c-Ki-*ras* gene *672*
  colorectal carcinoma 595,
    1260, 1266
v-Ki-*ras* oncogene 658
Klatskin tumours 1415
Klebsiella 436, 467, 472
  hospital-acquired infections *493*
  urinary-tract infections 1477,
    1518
Klebsiella pneumoniae
  nitrogenase protein 204
  pneumonia **959–60**, 968
Klebsiella rhinoscleromatis 1113
Klinefelter's syndrome 75, **1547–8**,
    1572
  isochromosomes 80
  mosaicism 1548
  46,XX (XX males) 84
Klippel–Trenaunay(–Weber)
    syndrome 918, 932, 1209
Klüver–Barrera myelin stain 1870
knee joint, haemophilia 1735,
    1736
Koch's postulates 471
Koebner phenomena 2146, 2148
Kogoj, spongiform pustule of 2147
Kohler disease 2031

Köhlmeier–Degos syndrome 1206
Kohn, pores of 946
koilocytes 2166
  cervical smears 2310
  cervical warts 1588
  HPV integration and 2290
koilocytosis
  perianal warts 1278
  squamous cell papilloma of larynx
    1128
koilonychia 1694–5
Kopf, acrokeratosis of 2167
Korsakoff syndrome 743
Kostmann disease 1707
Krabbe disease (globoid cell
    leukodystrophy) *1351*,
    1361, 1873
Krukenberg tumours 1171,
    1631–2
Kugelberg–Welander disease *2096*
Kupffer cells 240, 243, 248, **251**,
    341
  drug-induced changes 1341
  falciparum malaria 1310, 2192,
    2193
  haemosiderin deposition 1372,
    1373
  hepatic sinusoids 1288
  Niemann–Pick disease 1362
  tropical splenomegaly syndrome
    2195
kuru 411, 1881, 1882
Küttner tumour 1071
Kveim (Kveim–Siltzbach) test
    401–2, 990, 1761, 1839
kwashiorkor 742–3
  heart involvement 885
  intestinal mucosal changes 1202
  liver disease 1367
  marasmic 742
  oedema 540, 743
  pancreatic features 1435
  pneumonias 966
kyphoscoliosis, hypoxic pulmonary
    arteriopathy 1007
kyphosis, tuberculous osteomyelitis
    2036

labia majora 1572
labia minora 1572
labyrinth
  bony 1105
  membranous 1105–6
lacis cells, juxtaglomerular
    apparatus 1452
lacrimal glands, chronic graft versus
    host disease 321
β-lactamases 428, 429, **430–2**
lactase deficiency 739–40, 1202
lactate dehydrogenase (LDH) serum
    levels 1417, 1723, 1727
lactation 745
  energy requirements 733
lacteal 1177, 1178
lactic acidosis, alcohol-induced
    1325
lactobacilli
  oral 1097
  vaginal (Doderlein bacilli) *436*,
    437, 2306, 2307

Lactobacillus acidophilus 1581
lactoferrin 324, 354, 437, 438
lactose intolerance 739–40, 1202
lacunae, cerebral 1852
Laemli loops 70
Lafora bodies 1366
Lafora disease (myoclonus epilepsy)
    1352, 1366
Lambert–Eaton syndrome, *see*
    Eaton–Lambert syndrome
Lambl's excrescences 867, 892
lamellar bodies 945
lamina cribrosa 1903, 1904
lamina densa, *see* basal lamina
lamina lucida 2139
lamina propria 1515, 1516
  large intestine 1179
  lymphoid tissue 1752, **1753**
  oesophagus 1133
  small intestine 1177
    Whipple disease 1201
  stomach 1149–50
lamina rara interna/externa,
    glomerular basement
    membrane 1451, 1452
laminin 26, 37, **62–3**, 925
  function 63
  growth factor interactions 557
  molecular structure 62–3
  properties 62
  receptors 26, 322, 1661
lamins 36
lamps 763
Langer–Giedion syndrome 81
Langerhans islets of, *see* islets,
    pancreatic
Langerhans cell granules, *see* Birbeck
    granules
Langerhans cell histiocytosis, *see*
    histiocytosis X
Langerhans cells 237, 240, **251–2**,
    2141
  histiocytosis X 1767, 1768,
    2068
  oral mucosa 1053
Langhans giant cells 255, 256, 397
  beryllium/zirconium-induced
    granulomas 401
  sarcoidosis 990
  tuberculosis 969, 2077–8
laparotomy, staging, Hodgkin
    disease 1769–70
large-cell anaplastic lymphoma, B-
    cell 1783
large-cell carcinoma, lung 697,
    1036, **1039**, 2319
large intestinal adenomas 595–6,
    684–5, 1259–61
large intestinal carcinoma, *see*
    colorectal carcinoma
large intestinal glands (crypts)
    1178–9
large intestinal infections **1222–33**
  bacterial 1223–7
  fungal 1229–30
  helminthic 1232–3
  pathogens causing *1210*
  protozoal 1230–2
  sexually transmitted 1227–9
  viral 1230
large intestinal mucosa 1178–9

lipomatous hypertrophy, atrial
　　septum 892
lipopolysaccharide, bacterial (LPS),
　　see endotoxins
lipoprotein lipase (LPL) 127, 801
　　binding by endothelial cells 497
　　deficiency **129**, 802
　　gene *128*
lipoproteins 126–7
　　atherosclerosis and 801–3
　　macrophage metabolism
　　　813–14, 815
　　oxidization by endothelial cells
　　　499
　　see also high-density lipoprotein;
　　　low-density lipoprotein; very-
　　　low-density lipoproteins
liposarcoma **2105–6**
　　clinical features 2105–6
　　histopathology 2106
　　myxoid 2106
　　nasopharyngeal 1122
　　pleomorphic 2106, 2107
　　round cell 2106
　　well-differentiated 2106
liposclerosis 928
liposome-encapsulated
　　immunomodulators,
　　macrophage activation 629
lipoteichoic acid 462
β-lipotrophin (LPH) 699, 700,
　　1932
lipoxygenase pathway 361–2
lissencephaly, Miller–Dieker
　　syndrome of 81
Listeria monocytogenes 459–60,
　　480, 494
　　entry into macrophages 344
　　HIV infection and 288, 460
α-listeriolysin 460
β-listeriolysin 460
listeriosis **459–61**
　　congenital 460, 787
　　epidemiology 461
　　granuloma formation 255
　　meningitis/meningo-encephalitis
　　　460, *1835*
　　neonatal 460, 952, 1924
　　pathogenesis 460–1
lithium, goitrogenic effects 1948
littoral cells, lymph node sinuses
　　1758, 1795, 1796
liver **1287–426**
　　amyloidosis 411
　　anatomical anomalies 1292
　　atrophy of left lobe 1292
　　bacterial infections 1309
　　biliary system 1288–9
　　blood supply 1287–8
　　chemoreceptors 539
　　compensatory hypertrophy of
　　　caudate lobe 1344, 1385
　　congenital disorders 1291–5
　　fatty change, see fatty liver
　　function 1290–1
　　graft versus host disease 318,
　　　319, 320, 321, 1345
　　gross structure 1287
　　hydatid disease 1311, 2252,
　　　2253

liver (*cont.*)
　　iron overload, *see* iron overload,
　　　hepatic
　　macrophages, *see* Kupffer cells
　　malaria 1310, 2192, 2193
　　microanatomy 1289–90
　　parasitic diseases 1310–11
　　radiation-induced damage 776,
　　　1345
　　regeneration **381–3**, 560, 561,
　　　1382
　　shock-induced lesions **549**,
　　　1343–4
　　supernumerary lobes 1292
　　tropical splenomegaly syndrome
　　　1310, 2195, 2197
　　vascular disorders 917–18,
　　　920–1, **1343–8**
liver acinus 1289–90
liver biopsy 1348
　　Hodgkin disease 1774
　　quantification of iron stores 1374
liver cell-adhesion molecule (LCAM)
　　26, 27, 28
liver disease
　　alcoholic, *see* alcoholic liver
　　　disease
　　bleeding disorders 750,
　　　1418–19, 1740
　　circulatory failure and 1343–4
　　Crohn disease 1246
　　diet in 746
　　drug clearance and 749–50
　　drug- and toxin-induced
　　　1330–43
　　end-stage, *see* cirrhosis
　　gastritis 1154
　　hepatocyte hyperplasia 1385–7
　　metabolic disorders **1348–68**
　　neurological disorders 1860–1
　　pathobiology **1417–26**
　　pulmonary vascular disease
　　　1003
　　schistosomiasis 1310, 1311,
　　　1345, **2256–8**, 2262
　　ulcerative colitis 1241
liver function tests 1290–1
liver lobule 1289–90
liver membrane antibodies (LMA)
　　1300
liver transplantation 1347,
　　1398–400
　　acute rejection 313, 314, 1398
　　chronic rejection **315–16**,
　　　1398–9
　　differential diagnosis 1400
　　hyperacute rejection 312, 1398
　　mechanism of rejection
　　　1399–400
'lizard skin' 2245
Loa loa (loiasis) 1849, **2242–3**
　　cryptic 2242
lobules
　　breast 1644, 1645
　　liver 1289–90
　　pulmonary 943
locomotor system **2019–135**
locus
　　gene 69
　　identification of mutant 122–4,
　　　125

locus coeruleus 1826, 1827
　　multiple system atrophy 1877
　　Parkinson disease 1875, 1876
locus coeruleus noradrenergic
　　complex 1826, **1827–8**
　　ascending fibres 1827–8
　　coeruleocerebellar fibres 1827
　　descending fibres 1827
locus control regions (LCRs) 92
locus homogeneity 122, 125
Löeffler fibroplastic endocarditis
　　873, 881
Löeffler syndrome, *see* eosinophilic
　　pneumonia, acute
long bones
　　adamantinoma **2065**
　　bowing 2040, 2041
　　gross organization 2019
loop diuretics, ototoxicity 1108
loose bodies in joints 2086–7
Looser's zones 744, 2041
low-density lipoprotein (LDL) 127,
　　802
　　clearance rate, apo B gene
　　　polymorphisms and 134
　　endothelial metabolism 499, 807
　　macrophage metabolism
　　　813–14, 815
　　metabolism 802–3
　　oxidation 499, 813, 820
low-density lipoprotein (LDL)
　　receptor 116, 127
　　defective, molecular pathology
　　　107, 111
　　endothelial cells 499
　　familial hypercholesterolaemia
　　　801, 803, 815
　　gene 128
　　modified (scavenger receptors)
　　　802–3, 815
　　smooth muscle cells 501
lower limbs
　　chronic ischaemia 526
　　oedema 535
　　varicose veins 918–19
　　venous 'stasis' 2161
　　venous thrombosis 512, 513–14,
　　　521, 919
low-resistance pathways through
　　interstitium 923–4
LT (heat-labile) toxin, *Escherichia coli*
　　423, *424*, *425*, 470
Lucke renal adenocarcinoma of
　　Leopard frog 619, 620,
　　1501
lung(s)
　　adenomatoid malformation
　　　948–9
　　conducting zone 946
　　congenital anomalies **948–9**
　　defence mechanisms 947
　　development 789, 943
　　fissures 943, 944
　　functional zones **946–7**
　　gangrene 967
　　gas-exchanging (respiratory) zone
　　　946–7
　　Gough–Wentworth sections 979
　　graft versus host disease 321,
　　　955
　　honeycomb 985, 986, 994–5

lung(s) (*cont.*)
　　innervation 946
　　lobes 943, 944
　　lobules 943
　　lymphatics 930
　　macrophages, *see* alveolar
　　　macrophages
　　radiation-induced damage 775,
　　　1002
　　regeneration and growth
　　　capabilities 385
　　shock, *see* respiratory distress
　　　syndrome, adult
　　structure 943, 944
　　transitional zone 946
　　uraemic **991–2**
　　vascular anomalies 916–17
lung abscess **967–8**, 1042
　　bacterial pneumonia 958, 960,
　　　965, 968
　　blood-borne infections 968
　　bronchial neoplasms 968, 1033
　　causes 968
　　cryptogenic 968
　　inhalation 967–8
　　multiple 971
　　Nocardia 971
　　Pseudomonas aeruginosa
　　　pneumonia 960
　　septic thromboemboli 1014
　　trans-diaphragmatic spread 968
　　traumatic 968
lung adenocarcinoma 566, 1036,
　　1037–8
　　aetiology 687
　　malignant mesothelioma vs.
　　　1047
　　respiratory tract cytology 2319
lung biopsy, surgical 1035
lung carcinoid (neuroendocrine)
　　tumours 696, **1041**, 1273,
　　2320
　　atypical 1041
lung carcinoma **1032–41**
　　asbestos-induced 686, 687, 724
　　central necrosis 1033
　　classification 1036
　　criteria for diagnosis and
　　　classification 1037–40
　　cytology 1034–5, 2315,
　　　2318–20
　　diagnosis 1034–5
　　ectopic hormone production 695,
　　　696, 697–8
　　epidemiology 679, 680, **686–7**,
　　　1034
　　genetic susceptibility 646
　　heterogeneity in relation to
　　　histogenesis 1039–40
　　hormone markers 702–3
　　hypertrophic pulmonary
　　　osteoarthropathy 2032
　　latent period 681
　　local complications 968, 1033
　　macroscopic features 1033
　　mixed tumours 1039, 1040
　　paraneoplastic neurological
　　　syndromes 703, 1040–1
　　precursor lesions 1035–6
　　radiation exposure and 669,
　　　689, 1034

malaria (*Plasmodium* infections) (*cont.*)
cerebral (CM) 525, 544, 1847, **2193–5**
clinical features and pathology 2192–7
congenital 2193
diagnosis and treatment 2197
epidemiology 2191
falciparum, *see Plasmodium falciparum*
glucose-6-phosphate dehydrogenase deficiency and 1701, 2193
life cycle and morphology 2191–2
liver 1310, 2192, 2193
quartan, *see Plasmodium malariae*
sickle-cell disease and 122
splenectomy/hyposplenism and 1801
splenic involvement 1805, 2192
tropical splenomegaly syndrome 1805, 2195
malarial nodules (granulomas) of Dürck 1847, 2194
Malassez, cell rests of 1081, 1082, 1083
malathion 728, *729*
male
pseudohermaphroditism 1547, 1569
XX 84, 1547
male generative system **1535–62**
diffuse neuroendocrine system 2013, *2014*
malignant cells
ascites fluid 1421
seeding after fine-needle aspiration biopsy 2327
serous effusions 2321–4
urine cytology 2324–5
malignant disease, *see* cancer
Mallory bodies (MBs, alcoholic hyaline) *149*, *175*, *176*
alcoholic liver disease 741, 1327–8, 1330
drug- and toxin-induced liver disease 1338
hepatocellular carcinoma 1393
primary biliary cirrhosis 1321
Mallory–Weiss syndrome 1137
malnutrition
cancer risk and **682–3**
heart involvement 885
hepatocyte steatosis 1336
infection susceptibility 286, 441
intestinal mucosal changes 1202
pancreatic features 1435
protein energy, *see* protein energy malnutrition
signs 738, 739
thymic effects 1814
malondialdehyde 151, 189
MALT, *see* mucosa-associated lymphoid tissue
mammary epithelial cells, casein expression 40
mammary tumours
animals, radiation-induced 669

mammary tumours (*cont.*)
murine
chemically-induced 644
colonization potential 617
metastatic capability 618, 619
organ-conditioning of tumour cells 627–8
organ-specific metastasis 624
virus-induced 657
see also breast carcinoma
mammillary body (Rokitansky tubercle) 1630
mammography 1644, 1660, **1671–80**
ANDI (aberrations of normal development and involution) 1672
benign breast disease 1671–5
breast cancer screening 1677–9
differentiation of benign/malignant lesions 1671, *1672*
malignant breast disease 1675–7
Wolfe classification 1677, 1679
mandibular cysts, median 1084
mandibular torus 1091
manganese
absorption 736
dietary requirements *732*
metabolic function 737
poisoning 1876
mannose-6-phosphate 99
receptors 118, 119
mannosyl, fucosyl receptors (MFR), macrophages 251, 337, 339, 340, 341
mantle zone
lymph nodes 1746
Peyer's patches 1752, 1753
mantle-zone lymphoma, *see* centrocytic lymphoma
Mantoux reaction 278
maple syrup urine disease 1499
marasmic kwashiorkor 742
marasmus 742–3
marble bone disease (osteopetrosis) **2027**
Marburg virus infection 544
Marek disease virus 651, 706
Marfan disease 124
arterial disease 846–7
bleeding disorders *1732, 1733*
cardiac valve disease 869, 871
marginal zone
B-cells 206, 209–10, 212, *213*, 214
Peyer's patches 1752, 1753
splenic white pulp 209–10, 1796, 1797
Maroteaux–Lamy syndrome *1349*, 1356
masculinization, incomplete 1979
mast cell-restricted colony-forming cells (Mast-CFC) 1686
mast cells **332–6**
activation secretion coupling 333, 335
activation signals 226–7, 332–3
anaphylaxis and 276, 544
connective tissue 332, *333*
granules 20, 21

mast cells (*cont.*)
inflammatory reaction 352, 355
mediators 332, *334*
biological activities 334–5
pharmacological modulation of release 335
mucosal 332, *333*
type I allergic responses 275, 276
mastectomy, lymphoedema 929
mastitis
acute 1675
granulomatous 1652
obliterative 1649
mastoid air cells 1105
mastopathy, fibrous 1652
matrix attachment sites, DNA 90
maturation, definition 45–6
maturing cells, post-mitotic 46
maxillary antrum infections 474
maxillary sinuses 1112
maxillitis, neonatal 1083
May–Grunwald Giemsa stain 2302
Mazotti skin reaction 2245, 2246
M-cells (microfold cells) 1752
M-CSF, *see* macrophage colony-stimulating factor
mean corpuscular volume (MCV) 1693, 1694, 1700
measles 94
achalasia and 1136
acute post-infectious encephalomyelitis 1872
bronchial involvement 954
corneal involvement 1909–10
epidemics 455
immunosuppressive encephalitis 1845
impairment of host defences 441
lymph node reactions 1766
pneumonia 961, 962
subacute sclerosing panencephalitis 1844–5
mechanoreceptors, extracellular fluid volume control *531*
Meckel's diverticulum 1159, **1188**, *1189*
Meckel syndrome 1923
meconium aspiration 788, **950**
meconium ileus 1193, 1194, 1365
media 497
aneurysm development and 847, 848–9
arteries 795, 796, 851
chronic periaortitis 819
inflammation in giant cell arteritis 844
pulmonary arteries 946, 999, 1024–5
vascular grafts 901–2
veins 497, 500, 914–15
medial atrophy, pulmonary arteries 1020
medial fibrosis, congestive pulmonary vasculopathy 1015, 1016
medial forebrain bundle 1827
medial necrosis, cystic 847, 848, 871
medial sclerosis, Monkberg 846
medial septal nucleus, cholinergic cells 1825, 1826

medial thickening
benign hypertension 834–5
congestive pulmonary vasculopathy 1015, 1016
lung fibrosis 1019, 1020
pulmonary arteries 1003, 1004, 1008, 1024
pulmonary veins 1008
medial thinning
coronary arteries 826
pulmonary arteries 1020, 1021, 1025
mediastinal fibrosis, idiopathic (IMF) 816
mediastinal tumours 1002, **1814–20**
mediastinitis
fibrosing 1002
sclerosing 972
Mediterranean fever, familial 410, 411, 2084
Mediterranean lymphoma (primary upper small intestinal lymphoma) 691, 1200, 1789
medulla oblongata, compression 1853
medullary carcinoma
breast 1656, 1664, 1676, 1677
thyroid, *see* thyroid medullary carcinoma
medullary cords, lymph nodes 1746, 1747
medullary sponge kidney **1454**, 1455
uraemic 1455
medulloblastoma 693, 1884–5, **1891**
age-related incidence 680
desmoplastic 1891
medulloepithelioma 1887
mefenamic acid, intestinal toxicity 1196, 1200
megacolon
Chagas disease 1232, 2210
toxic
amoebic dysentery 1231
Crohn disease 1246
ulcerative colitis 1235–6, 1237
megakaryoblast progenitors (CFU-Mk), primary thrombocythaemia 1730
megakaryocyte colony-stimulating factor (Meg-CSF) *1687*
megakaryocyte-restricted colony-forming cells (Meg-CFC) 1686, 1687
megakaryocytes
chronic myeloid leukaemia 1727
large mononuclear 1724
myelodysplastic syndromes 1724
polynuclear 1724
megakaryocytic leukaemia, acute 692, 1721
megaloblastic anaemia **1695–8**
blood and marrow changes 1695
causes 744, 1216, 1695–7
development 1697
diagnosis 1698
megamitochondria 164, 1328

pemphigus foliaceus **2151–2**, 2153
  Fogo Selvagem variant 2151
pemphigus vegetans 2152, 2153
pemphigus vulgaris 2151, **2152–3**
  clinical features 2152
  differential diagnosis 2152–3
  histopathology 2140, 2152
  HLA associations 300
  pathogenesis 2153
Pendred syndrome 1948
penetrance 83
penetration
  bacterial 420–1
  peptic ulcers 1162
penicillamine, adverse reactions
    989, *1459*
penicillin-binding proteins (PBPs)
    431, 432, 434
penicillins
  haemolysis induction 1701
  hypersensitivity 752
  resistance 428–9, 430–2, 434
penile cancer, epidemiology **690**
penile fibromatosis (Peyronie disease)
    375, 2111
pentagastrin, medullary carcinoma
    of thyroid 1958
pentraxin 409
pepsin, hypersecretion 1174
pepsinogen *34*
peptic ulcer **1159–64**
acute 1159
  aetiology 1163–4, 2005
  chronic 393, 1159–60
    cicatrization zone 1160
    exudative zone 1160, 1161
    granulation tissue zone 1160,
      1161
    healing 379–80, 1161
    necrotic zone 1160, 1161
  complications 1161–3
  haemorrhage 1161–2
  Meckel's diverticulum 1159,
    1188
  morphological features 1160–1
  oesophagus 1140, 1141
  pathogenesis 1174–5
  penetration 1162
  perforation 1162
  see also duodenal ulcers; gastric
    ulcers
peptide histidine isoleucine
    (methionine) (PHI(M))
  genitourinary system *2014*
  gut *1184*
  respiratory tract *2010*, 2011–12
  skin *2015*
peptide histidine methionine-
    secreting tumour (PHMoma)
    2007
peptides, regulatory
  diffuse neuro-endocrine system
    2010–16
  region-specific antibodies 1272
  see also neuropeptides
peptide yy (PYY) *1184*
peptidoglycan
  gingivitis/periodontal disease and
    1095, 1096
  Gram-negative bacteria 469
  staphylococcal 464, *465*

peptidoglycan (*cont.*)
  streptococcal 462
peptidoleukotrienes, *see*
    leukotriene(s)
Peptococcus 960
peptostreptococci *472*, 960
perchlorate 1948
Perenyi's fluid 2271
perforation
  appendix 1219
  bile duct 1404
  colonic diverticular disease 1258
  gall bladder 1410
  intestinal
    Crohn disease 1246
    typhoid 1212
    ulcerative colitis 1236
  oesophagus 1137
  peptic ulcers 1162
  peritonitis and 1281
perforins 153, 155, 156, 439
perhexiline maleate, hepatotoxicity
    1332, 1336, 1338
periadenitis, syphilitic 1764
perianal pruritus, *Enterobius
    vermicularis* 2225, 2226
perianal skin
  amoebiasis 2199, 2201, 2202
  basal cell carcinoma 1280
  Bowenoid papulosis 1280
  Bowen disease 1279
  condylomata acuminata 1278–9
  infections 1277–8
  keratoacanthoma 1280
  Paget disease 1280
peri-aortic fibrosis 820
periaortitis, chronic **815–22**
  idiopathic retroperitoneal fibrosis
    and 816–17
  inflammatory aneurysms and
    817–18
  pathogenesis 818–22
periapical dental abscess 1083
periapical granuloma 1083, 1101
periapical periodontitis 1083
peri-arteriolar lymphoid sheath
    (PALS) 1796, 1797
periarteritis, chronic 818–22
pericardial adhesions 890
pericardial cysts 890, 893
pericardial disease **886–91**
  chronic 890
pericardial effusion **887**
  cholesterol-containing 887
  malignant disease 893
  myocardial infarction 889
  serous 887
pericardial tumours **890**, 893
  benign 890
  malignant 890
  secondary 893–4
pericarditis **887–90**
  caseous 888
  constrictive 887, 890, 911,
    1420, 1421
  drug reactions 890
  fibrinous 387, 887
  haemorrhagic 888
  in immune-mediated disease 889
  infectious 888–9
  myocardial infarction 889

pericarditis (*cont.*)
  pathogenesis 888–90
  primary 888
  purulent 887–8
  radiation-induced 775
  renal failure 890, 991
  rheumatic fever 867, 889
  serofibrinous 887
pericardium 852
  heterotopic tissue 893
  milk spots 890
  oblique sinus 852, 853
  response to injury 387
pericholangitis, ulcerative colitis
    1241
perichromatin granules 5
pericoronitis 1084
pericrypt fibroblastic sheath 1177,
    1179
pericytes, capillary
    haemangioblastoma 1894
perifollicular zone, splenic white pulp
    1796
peri-intestinal abscesses 1247,
    1257–8
perinephric abscess 1523
perineurial cell 1892
perineurium 1897
perinuclear cisterna 6
peri-ocular tumours **1918–19**
periodate, lysine and
    paraformaldehyde (PLP)
    fixative 2275
periodic acid-Schiff method 1231,
    1232, 2273
periodic paralyses 2101
periodontal abscess, acute 1092
periodontal cyst
  inflammatory lateral *1085*
  lateral *1085*
periodontal disease **1091–6**
  clinical manifestations 1091–2
  histopathology 1093, 1094
  microbiology 1092–3
  pathogenic mechanisms 1094–5,
    1096
  therapy 1096
periodontal ligament 1081
periodontitis
  chronic adult 1092
  juvenile 1092, 1093
  periapical 1083
  rapidly progressive 1092
perioophoritis, chronic 1616
periosteum 2019
periostitis 2032
peri-ovarian adhesions 1616
peripartal heart disease 880
peripheral nerves **1897–903**
  axonal regeneration 385–6,
    1898, 1899
  general pathology 1899–900
  normal 1897–9
  pathology of diseases 1900–2
  schwannomas 1892, 1902
  tumours *1901*, 1902–3
peripheral nerve sheath tumour,
    malignant (MPNST) **2125–6**
  epithelioid 2126
  rhabdomyoblastic differentiation
    2126

peripheral nervous system
  demyelinating diseases 1867
  monocytes/macrophages 254
peripheral neuropathies 1897,
    1900–2
  demyelinating *1901*, 1902
  diabetes mellitus 1861–2, 1902
  diphtheria 954
  drug-induced 1863, 1864
  glue-sniffers 1864
  multiple myeloma 1715
  muscle changes **2097**
  paraneoplastic 703, 704–5,
    1863
  pernicious anaemia 1859
peripheral vascular resistance
    541–2, 909
perisinusoidal cells, *see* Ito cells
peritoneal cysts 1282
  Fallopian tube 1613
  vulva 1576
peritoneal dialysis, pleural effusion
    1049
peritoneal fluid, cytology 2320–4
peritoneal macrophages 240, 242,
    1634
peritoneal mesothelioma 687–8,
    1282–3
peritoneal tumours **1282–3**
  benign 1282
  malignant 1282–3, 1634
  secondary carcinoma 613, 1171,
    1283, 1604, 1613, 1623
peritoneo-venous shunting,
    neoplastic ascites 624–7
peritoneum **1281–3**
  endocervicosis 1634
  endometrial metaplasia 1633
  endosalpingiosis 1634, 1635
  response to injury 387
  tuberculosis 1282, 1421
peritonitis **1281–2**
  acute 1281
  amoebic 2199
  ascariasis 2230
  biliary 1404, 1410
  chronic 1281–2
  Fitz–Hugh–Curtis syndrome
    1309
  perforated peptic ulcers 1162
  salpingitis 1610, 1612
  spontaneous bacterial 1420,
    1423
peritonsillar abscess 473
perivascular cuffing
  glomus tumour 2181
  nervous system lymphomas
    1893–4
  viral encephalitis 1840, 1841
perivascular pseudorosettes,
    ependymomas 1889, 1890
periventricular leukomalacia 789,
    1925
permeabilization, mRNA *in situ*
    hybridization 2292–3
pernicious anaemia 277, **1698–9**
  atrophic gastritis 1155, 1173–4,
    1696, 1698
  diagnosis 1698
  experimental development
    1698–9

Proteus (cont.)
  otitis media 1108
  pneumonia 960, 966
  urinary-tract infections 1477,
    1518
Proteus mirabilis 1477
prothrombin (factor II) 505, *506*,
  507
  deficiency **1738**
  index 1290, 1417–18, 1425
prothymocytes 229, 1810
proton balance, renal failure 1513
proto-oncogenes, *see* oncogenes,
  cellular
protoplasts, recurrent urinary-tract
  infections 1477
protoporphyria, erythropoietic
  1349, 1352, 1353
protozoa, intracellular 166, 167
protozoal infections **2191–224**
  blood and tissue flagellates
    2205–15
  cervix 1587–8
  coccidian 2218–24
  eye 1910
  free-living amoebae 2203–5
  granulomatous 404–5
  intestinal 2198–203
  intra-erythrocytic 2191–8
  large intestine 1230–2
  liver 1310
  lymphadenitis 1764–5
  microsporidian 2224
  myocarditis 883
  nervous system **1847–8**
  pneumonias **964**
  small intestine 1217–18
  splenic involvement 1805
  see also specific infections
prune belly syndrome 1193
pruritus
  aquagenic 1729
  gravidarum 1365
  onchocerciasis 2244, 2245
  polycythaemia rubra vera 1729
pruritus ani, *Enterobius vermicularis*
  2225, 2226
psammoma bodies
  meningioma 1117, 1893
  papillary carcinoma of thyroid
    1957
psammoma-bodies endosalpingiosis
  1634
PSC, *see* primary sclerozing
  cholangitis
pseudoacanthosis 560
pseudo-allergic drug reactions 752
Pseudoallescheria 1835
pseudocholinesterase *749*
pseudodiploidy 575, 591
pseudoepitheliomatous hyperplasia,
  granular cell tumour 2124,
  2125
pseudoexfoliation (exfoliation)
  syndrome, open-angle
  glaucoma 1906
pseudogenes 89, 90
pseudogout 2088
pseudohermaphroditism
  female 1569, 1978
  male 1547, 1569

pseudohypoparathyroidism 1966,
  1967
  principles of treatment 1968
  type I 1967
  type II 1967
pseudoinclusions, intranuclear 7,
  177, 178
pseudointima 901
pseudomembranes, ischaemic
  intestinal 1204, 1205
pseudomembranous colitis 476,
  1204, **1224–6**
  pathology 1225
  role of *Clostridium difficile* 1226
Pseudomonas 467
  antimicrobial resistance *431*,
    432
  chronic granulomatous disease
    1709
  endocarditis 876
  exotoxin A *425*, 544
  hospital-acquired infections *493*
  otitis media 1108
  urinary-tract infections 1477
Pseudomonas aeruginosa 467, 468,
  494
  antimicrobial resistance *431*,
    434
  corneal ulceration 1908
  exotoxin A 544
  penicillin resistance 429
  pneumonia 953, **960**, 965, 966,
    968
Pseudomonas cepacia 467
Pseudomonas mallei 971
Pseudomonas pseudomallei 971
pseudo-mosaic appearance,
  hyperparathyroidism 2043
pseudomyxoma ovarii 1621
pseudomyxoma peritonei **1282**
  mucinous cystadenocarcinoma of
    appendix 1268
  mucinous ovarian tumours
    1282, 1621–2
  mucocele of appendix 1220,
    1282, 1622
  mucocele of gall bladder 1408
pseudo-palisading, glioblastoma
  1888
pseudopelade of Brocq 2164
pseudo-pseudohypoparathyroidism
  1967
pseudopuberty, isosexual precocious
  1625, 1628, 1629, 1980
pseudo-pyloric metaplasia 1155
pseudorosettes, olfactory
  neuroblastoma 1117
pseudosarcoma (spindle-cell
  carcinoma), larynx 1130
pseudosinuses, splenic 1804
pseudotabes, diabetes mellitus 1862
Pseudoterranova 2234
pseudo-tubercles, schistosomiasis
  398
pseudoxanthoma elasticum
  1732–3
psittacosis 963
psoralens, *see* furocoumarins
psoriasiform drug reactions 2147
psoriasiform skin lesions **2146–7**
psoriasis 556, 560, 1759, **2146–7**

psoriasis (*cont.*)
  clinical features and aetiology
    2146
  differential diagnosis 2147
  drug-induced 2147
  histopathology 2146–7
  phototherapy 769
  pustular 2147
psoriatic arthritis 2083, 2146
pteroylmonoglutamic acid 736
pterygium 1916
ptyalism (sialorrhoea) 1069
puberty, precocious, non-endocrine
  tumour-associated 695, 701
puerperium, pituitary infarction
  1939–40
pulmonary agenesis 948
pulmonary alveolar proteinosis
  986–7
pulmonary arterioles 946, 1000
  muscularization 1003–4, 1007,
    1008–9, 1015
  vasoconstriction 913
pulmonary arteriopathy
  congestive 1015–16
  hypoxic **1007–9**
    causes 1007
    mechanisms 1007
    morphology and pathogenesis
      1007–9
  lung fibrosis **1018–19**
  plexogenic **1003–7**
    aetiology 1003
    morphology and pathogenesis
      1003–7
    primary 1003, 1020
    reversibility 1007
  thrombotic **1013–15**
pulmonary arteriovenous fistulae
  1022–3
pulmonary arteriovenous
  malformations 916–17,
  1732
pulmonary arteritis
  septic thromboemboli causing
    1014
  Wegener granulomatosis 1029
pulmonary artery(ies) 915, 946,
  999
  age-related changes 1025
  aneurysms 1025, 1026
  congenital malformations 866
  developmental anomalies
    1020–4
  dilatation lesions 1004, 1005,
    1025
  diminished pulse pressure and flow
    1020, 1021
  elastic 946, 999
  fetus and newborn infant 1000,
    1001
  fibrinoid necrosis 1004, 1006
  intra-acinar 999, 1000
  lobar 999
  major, lesions **1024–6**
  medial thickness and structure
    1024–5
  muscular 946, 999, 1000
  pulmonary veno-occlusive disease
    1018, 1019

pulmonary artery(ies) (*cont.*)
  segmental 999
  stenosis 1022
  supernumerary 999
  thrombosis 1020, 1021
  unilateral absence 1022
  vein-like branches 1004, 1005
pulmonary artery sling 948
pulmonary atresia 783, 866
pulmonary capillary
  haemangiomatosis 1020
pulmonary collapse, *see* atelectasis
pulmonary disease, *see* lung disease
pulmonary embolism 516, **521–3**,
  1009–12
  air and gas 1010, 1011
  amniotic fluid 1010
  fat 1009
  foreign body 1009, 1010
  massive 521–2, 542, 1011–12
  moderate-sized emboli 523
  pulmonary infarction 523, 529,
    1012
  recurrent 1012, 1026
  risk factors 521
  small emboli 522–3
  tissue 1009
  tumour 1009
  see also pulmonary
    thromboembolism
pulmonary endothelium 946
pulmonary fibrosis, *see* lung fibrosis
pulmonary haemorrhage
  drug-induced **989**
  massive, perinatal **951**
  Pseudomonas aeruginosa
    pneumonia 960
  shock-induced 547
  tuberculosis 969
pulmonary hypertension **911–14**,
  999, **1002–20**
  causes *913*, 1002
  cor pulmonale 913–14
  cryptogenic fibrosing alveolitis
    985
  developmental anomalies of
    pulmonary vessels 1022
  medial changes in pulmonary
    trunk 1024
  mitral regurgitation 907
  plexogenic pulmonary
    arteriopathy 1003–7, 1020
  preterm infants 789
  pulmonary embolism 523
  schistosomiasis 2259
  silent embolic 1012, 1020
  unexplained/primary *913*,
    1002–3, 1018, **1020**
pulmonary hypoplasia 949
pulmonary infarction 529,
  1012–13
  dirofilariasis 2247
  haemorrhagic 1012–13
  pathology 526–7, 1012–13
  pulmonary embolism 523, 529,
    1012
pulmonary infections
  anaerobic and mixed 473–4,
    960, 967
  chronic **968–74**
  fungal **971–4**